A
CENTURY
OF
SURGERY

VOLUME TWO

A
CENTURY
OF
SURGERY

THE HISTORY OF THE
AMERICAN SURGICAL ASSOCIATION

MARK M. RAVITCH, M.D.

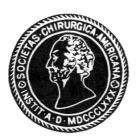

J.B. LIPPINCOTT COMPANY PHILADELPHIA, TORONTO

Library of Congress Cataloging in Publication Data

Ravitch, Mark M
  A century of surgery.

  Includes index.
  1. American Surgical Association—History.
2. Surgery—United States—History.   I.   Title.   [DNLM: 1.   Societies, Medical—History—United States. 2.
  Surgery—History—United States.   WO1   A518R]   RD1.A43R38   617′.006′073   80-21381
ISBN 0-397-50479-9

C O N T E N T S

THE 1900'S

The 1910's

The 1920's

The 1930's

The 1940's

The 1950's

The 1960's

The 1970's

A
CENTURY
OF
SURGERY

1940s

THE NEW YORK TIMES—WEDNESDAY, MAY 1, 1940—THE FIRST DAY OF THE MEETING OF THE AMERICAN SURGICAL ASSOCIATION IN ST. LOUIS, MISSOURI

Norway had been invaded. Britain was concerned for the safety of its ships in the Mediterranean, "Hungary was fully convinced of German friendship and relied upon it." The Italians were "shocked" that Britain was diverting traffic from the Mediterranean. Pittsburghers offered $1,000,000 for Hitler captured "Alive and Unhurt". [The Presidential Address of Allen O. Whipple, "The Critical Latent or Lag Period in the Healing of Wounds", never so much as mentioned the war in Europe. At the second Executive Session, the motion by W. J. Mixter and Harvey B. Stone, dealing with the war, was accepted,- "The President shall appoint a Committee to inquire into the professional needs of the country in the event of war, in the broadest way, with power to organize subcommittees and to call upon the individual members as they see fit. The purpose of this Committee shall be to assist the surgeon-general in every way possible, and it shall place its findings and recommendations in his hands."]

"All the News That's Fit to Print."

The New York Times.

LATE CITY EDITION
Scattered showers, continued mild today, showers and thunderstorms tonight. Tomorrow rain, cooler.
Temperatures Yesterday—Max., 67; Min., 46

Copyright, 1940, by The New York Times Company.

VOL. LXXXIX...No. 30,048. Entered as Second-Class Matter, Postoffice, New York, N. Y. NEW YORK, WEDNESDAY, MAY 1, 1940. PP THREE CENTS NEW YORK CITY and Vicinity | FOUR CENTS Elsewhere Except in 7th and 8th Postal Zones.

NAZIS REPORT DOMBAAS, STOEREN TAKEN; ALLIED LANDING BASE POUNDED BY PLANES; BRITISH SHIPPING TO QUIT MEDITERRANEAN

WAGE BILL BEATEN; REPUBLICANS JOIN WITH NEW DEALERS

Barden Fights Own Measure to Amend Wage-Hour Act After Drastic Changes

STANDING VOTE 156 TO 66

Ramspeck Proposals Shunned, Leaving Norton Amendments, Mildest of All, Up Next

By HENRY N. DORRIS
Special to THE NEW YORK TIMES.

WASHINGTON, April 30—A coalition of New Dealers and Republicans in the House today defeated, by a standing vote of 156 to 66, the Barden bill to change the Wages and Hours Act. This was after the Barden bill itself had been loaded with drastic amendments by the combined forces.

The House also refused to consider the so-called Ramspeck amendments to the Wages and Hours Act, and instead voted to reopen the whole question by taking up the Norton amendments, which are considered the mildest of all.

Representative Barden of North Carolina, author of the amendments which had been under consideration for two days, refused to vote for his own bill. He asserted the House had made a hodge-podge of it. Instead, he said, he would fight to have the Norton bill amended in virtually the same form as he first proposed.

The Republicans privately explained their votes by saying the Democratic leadership, as the result of Senate hints that the legislation would receive "a proper burial for this session, had put them "on the spot." The Republicans said they willingly accepted the challenge and their votes on several amendments went further toward courting the friendship of labor than perhaps any proposals ever offered by the New Deal.

Farm Funds Play a Part

Another consideration was the situation affecting farm benefit payments, to be voted upon as soon as the House completes action on the Wages and Hours admendments. The New Dealers have openly sought farm votes to defeat the Barden bill, offering their votes in turn for $212,000,000 in farm parity payments, $85,000,000 for surplus-crop disposal and $50,000,000 in farm-tenant loans.

President Roosevelt this afternoon strengthened the hand of New Dealers in the House by sending to Speaker Bankhead a letter saying he has no objections to the Senate provision for $50,000,000 in farm tenant loans. The letter said the disagreement in the conference committee of the two branches had been called to his attention, and that he was "anxious" that provision be made for the farm tenant program. The Bureau of the Budget had recommended $25,000,000.

Few now believe there will be any wages and hours legislation this session, in view of the log-rolling over farm appropriations, and the apparent Republican determination to make its bid for the labor vote on the record to be written tomorrow and probably next day on the Norton bill.

Representative Mary T. Norton of New Jersey, chairman of the House Labor Committee and author of the amendments now up for consideration, conceded that, in view of the turn of events, her measure probably would be "loaded" with amendments and become much the same "hodge podge" as the Barden bill. If this happened, she said, there was little chance of the Senate "sticking out its neck" in a campaign year by attempting to salvage the legislation.

Allows No Exceptions

The amendment which made the Barden measure too repugnant to the majority was sponsored by Representative Brown, Republican of Ohio. It put an absolute floor under wages, and allowed no exemptions. It negated part of the Barden amendment to "repeal" the area of production ruling as to agriculture.

Mr. Brown's amendment was adopted by a voice vote, with a thunder of "ayes" from the Republican side and a smattering "aye" vote on the Democratic side. A few murmured "no."

The Ohio Republican started consideration of his amendment by taunting the Democratic side.

"My proposal is a simple one," he said. "We all have heard a lot of talk here that no member of Congress wants to reduce wages below 30 cents an hour. This is an excellent chance for all members to prove that they are sincere."

Another amendment, by Representative Bland of Virginia, proposing to exempt from the law canners of fruits and vegetables who also process other products as a sideline, was adopted. This was opposed also by Mr. Barden, who protested that the amendment went too far.

Mr. Barden took the floor to en-

Continued on Page Thirteen

21 U. S. Seamen Arrested By British at Port Said

By The United Press.

SAN FRANCISCO, April 30—Twenty-one American seamen of the Matson Navigation Company steamer Ewa were arrested by British authorities at Port Said, Egypt, when they refused to obey their captain, the company stated tonight.

The seamen were paid off and seventeen of them were ordered deported to the United States, said Hugh Gallagher, Matson operations manager. Four seamen were held in the port detention home, where they have begun a hunger strike, Mr. Gallagher added.

The United States Consul was arranging transportation for the returning men. It was reported that British authorities intervened because of labor trouble arising from wage demands. The Ewa, under Captain W. G. Leithead, is under charter to the Isthmian Steamship Company.

SEC ORDER BRINGS WILLKIE CHALLENGE

He Says 'Death Sentence' for His Utility Would Violate Law, Public Interest

The $1,000,000,000 Commonwealth and Southern Corporation, which operates utility properties in ten States, yesterday challenged the right of the Securities and Exchange Commission to enforce against its system the "death sentence" provisions of Section 11 of the Public Utility Holding Act, and declared, in a formal answer filed in Washington to the commission's show-cause integration proceedings, that any attempt by the SEC to force the corporation to dispose of its subsidiaries would be "detrimental to the public interest."

The corporation's brief was signed by its president, Wendell L. Willkie, frequent critic of the Administration and of the SEC's policies. He declared that any order which might be issued by the commission "purporting to be in pursuance" to the provisions of Section 11—the "death sentence"—requiring Commonwealth and Southern to divest itself of any securities or properties now owned would be contrary to the intent and provisions of the act, would be unlawful and would be in violation of the Constitution of the United States.

Obtained Delay in Answer

The Commonwealth and Southern Corporation, along with eight other major utility holding companies, were cited on March 6 by the SEC with orders to show cause why they should not be required to meet certain standards of geographic integration and corporate simplification as laid down in the provisions of the Holding Company Act. Commonwealth and Southern originally was scheduled to file its answer with the commission April 16, but obtained a two-week delay.

While the position taken by the corporation in its answer was necessitated by the desire to preserve completely its legal rights, Mr. Willkie asserted, it was not to be construed as an indication that it intended to fight the constitutionality of the act to the highest court in the land.

If it is at all possible, Mr. Willkie said in a statement here last night, "I am willing to make a sincere effort to work out the entire integration problem of our system at a round table conference with members of the Securities and Exchange Commission."

The Commonwealth and Southern system, which comprises ten operating properties serving a population in excess of 5,600,000, is providing electric service to residential consumers at an average cost of 2.93 cents a kilowatt hour, while the average use for each customer is 1,226 kilowatt hours annually, according to Mr. Willkie's answer to the commission.

Offers General Comparison

Commonwealth and Southern's residential rates are, therefore, Mr. Willkie added, 27 per cent lower than the national average for the country and the use 37 per cent higher, saying that in 1939 the national average rate was 4 cents a kilowatt hour and the national use 897 kilowatts.

Citing the low rates and high use throughout the Commonwealth and Southern system as a clear-cut indication that it was serving the "public interest," Mr. Willkie declared that the "facts that the Commonwealth companies bettered the national average to such an extent and at the present time have such a high average residential consumption" are attributable primarily to two outstanding achievements:

1. The Commonwealth and Southern Objective Rate Plan, whereby sharply reduced rates are made available for additional consumption.

(2) The service rendered by the Commonwealth and Southern Service Corporation in rendering assistance to the operating properties in their aggressive sales appliance

Continued on Page Forty-two

$1,000,000 for Capture of Hitler 'Alive and Unhurt' Is Offered Here

Pittsburgh Group Headed by S. H. Church Would Try Nazi Fuehrer Before a World Court for 'Crimes Against Peace'

A reward of $1,000,000 in cash to the person or group who will deliver Adolf Hitler "alive, unwounded and unhurt" into the custody of the League of Nations was offered yesterday in behalf of a group of Pittsburgh residents by Samuel Harden Church, president of the Carnegie Institute.

Mr. Church made public his offer through a letter to the editor of THE NEW YORK TIMES which appears on the editorial page of this newspaper today.

In the letter he said the German Fuehrer should be delivered "for trial before a high court of justice for his crimes against the peace and dignity of the world."

After the letter had been received, Mr. Church added, in a telephone interview with THE TIMES, that he believed the United States should be represented on the tribunal that would try the Fuehrer if the offer were successfully taken up. It was learned that the plan had been put forward without the knowledge of the State Department.

The proposal is made in good faith, Mr. Church emphasized, and the money will be paid without cavil to any qualified claimant.

The group that is backing the project is not over-optimistic about its chances of achieving its end, but, Mr. Church explained, they do think that even a slim possibility is worth encouraging, on the ground that the capture of Hitler would avert untold suffering.

The offer is for the month of May only. The purpose of that limitation, Mr. Church said, is to make sure that seekers after the reward will act quickly. The decision to post the $1,000,000 was reached by the Pittsburgh group after certain of them had received private advices from Europe that Hitler was determined to strike soon on the Western Front and that he had said he would break through even though it cost the lives of 500,000 Germans.

"The question of offering the reward has been under discussion by a group of members of the Duquesne Club here for two or three months," Mr. Church said. "Finally the project has taken shape, and I was selected to make the offer public. There are, in the group of present sponsors, about fifty persons, some of them women.

"I have held back quite a while,

Continued on Page Six

THREAT TO SLOVAKS ISSUED BY HUNGARY

Csaky Warns on Treatment of Magyar Minority, Stressing Close Ties With Reich

By Telephone to THE NEW YORK TIMES.

BUDAPEST, Hungary, April 30—Count Stephen Csaky, the Hungarian Foreign Minister, issued a sharp warning today to German-protected Slovakia that the treatment of the Magyar minority in Slovakia must be improved.

Replying in the upper house to charges of the abuse of Hungarians in Slovakia, brought by Dr. Geza Szuelke, former champion of Hungarian interests in Czecho-Slovakia, the Foreign Minister declared that Hungary was nearing the end of her patience on this issue.

Hungary did her best, he asserted, to come to friendly terms with Slovakia. She was the first to acknowledge the independence of the small neighboring State and the first to conclude a commercial agreement with the Slovaks.

Moreover, he declared, the Hungarian Government had exercised its patience to the utmost limit and had often "shut its eyes to dangerous symptoms." That patience, however, he concluded, would come to an end unless the rights and property of Hungarians in Slovakia were respected.

Faith Pinned on Reich

Count Csaky stated that the Slovaks, confident of German protection, had attempted to play off Germany against Hungary. This, he asserted, was a mistaken effort, since Hungary was fully convinced of German friendship and relied upon it.

"It might prove to be an error," he remarked, "to suppose that Hungary is weak. Hungary may have to take risks for the protection of her national honor.

"The Hungarian Government will pay no attention to provocations, but it will act at the appropriate moment."

The House had received with some consternation the bitter attack of Dr. Szuelke on the treatment of the Magyars. He had suggested that the German Government should rebuke the attitude of the Slovaks and had warned that the Hungarian Government would hit back if its rights were violated.

"In Neutra, last Saturday," he reported, "Rodolf Tucek, commander of the Hlinka Guard, declared amid the applause of a vast crowd that the tongue must be torn out of the mouth of any one who dared to speak Hungarian."

Legation Is Attacked

"On the same day university students and tradesmen smashed the windows of the Hungarian Legation in Bratislava with the connivance of the police. Leaflets are being distributed claiming the return of the territories ceded to

Continued on Page Five

GOLF DRIVING RANGE OPEN Day-Night. Pel. Pk'w'y, Eastch'ster Rd.—Advt.

ITALIANS SHOCKED BY BRITAIN'S MOVE

See No Reason for So Grave a Step as Rerouting Ships—Holy See Paper Assailed

By CAMILLE M. CIANFARRA
By Telephone to THE NEW YORK TIMES.

ROME, April 30—Great Britain's decision to divert Mediterranean traffic to the Cape route was learned by the Italians with surprise and apprehension. They thought that it was out of all proportion to the present state of Anglo-Italian relations, which, though tense, have not shown signs of aggravation recently.

They could see no new factor that could have induced the British Government to take such a grave step, which, they thought, would have repercussions on all Mediterranean trade. The press campaign, it was pointed out, was no stronger today than it was a week ago and, indeed, it seemed, if anything, to have become less violent.

Moreover, it was said that no unusual military or naval preparations were under way in Italy that would justify Britain's alarm. There was a strong resentment in some quarters, because it was thought that the British step would tend to make Italy appear as an aggressor before world public opinion.

If Italy were preparing for a sudden attack against the Allies, it was argued, she would have seen to

Continued on Page Four

DETOUR IS ORDERED

'Precaution' Is Taken in View of Attitude of Italian Leaders

NORWAY RETREAT HINTED

'Withdrawal' Trial Balloon Stirs Liberal Chief to Urge Parliament to 'Act'

By RAYMOND DANIELL
Special Cable to THE NEW YORK TIMES.

LONDON, April 30—British merchant ships have been ordered to keep out of the Mediterranean, as they were in the opening days of the war, when it was half expected that Premier Mussolini would cast Italy's fate in with that of his Axis partner.

Tonight, that uncertainty exists again. The British and French are reinforcing their naval forces and freeing them from the task of protecting merchant shipping purely as a precautionary rather than as an offensive gesture.

Hostile utterances from Italy in recent days, coupled with the blows the Allies' expeditionary forces in Norway have suffered, have caused considerable anxiety here about possible repercussions in other parts of the world, notably that part where the Italian dictator exercises powerful influence.

Navy Freed for Action

The effect of the order sending British ships around the Cape of Good Hope instead of through the Mediterranean and Suez short cut is to help the navy clear its decks for action if the war spreads to that sector. That eventuality, while unexpected, is not excluded as a possibility.

British merchantmen already in Mediterranean waters are ordered to get out as quickly as possible. Those outside are directed to stay out. The purpose is to relieve the navy of duties that would devolve upon it if it became necessary under war conditions to escort these vessels to safe waters.

While it may be taken for granted that the Admiralty's decision to send ships in trade with parts of the Empire East of Suez around the Cape was not made lightly, it should not be taken as an indication that the British expect Italy to enter the war on Germany's side. They do not know which way the cat is going to jump. Recognizing the strategy of fence-sitting, they are taking no chances in view of what has been happening in Norway, where Chancellor Hitler has lost a third of his fleet to gain a foothold from which it is growing increasingly apparent it will be a long, difficult and costly job to dislodge him.

Things have not gone well with the expeditionary force the British sent to Norway as much for political as for strategic and military reasons. Its job was to demonstrate to the world, especially to Italy and the Balkans, that Allied help could be given quickly and effectively to a threatened country.

Members of the House of Com-

Continued on Page Four

Taft Wins Adherence of a Chamber Group At Unofficial Meeting During Convention

By TURNER CATLEDGE
Special to THE NEW YORK TIMES.

WASHINGTON, April 30—The annual convention of the Chamber of Commerce of the United States took a sudden and wholly unofficial practical political turn today when 75 to 100 delegates slipped quietly away for an off-the-record conference with Senator Robert A. Taft, one of the contenders for the Republican nomination for President.

As a result of the meeting at the Metropolitan Club, while the rest of the 1,500-odd convention participants gathered at the Mayflower Hotel for a luncheon forum on business problems, a sizable Taft boom was taking shape among the delegates tonight.

Spokesmen from thirty to thirty-five States were invited to the Taft luncheon, arranged by Morris Edwards, executive vice president of the Chamber of Commerce of Cincinnati. The Senator made no set speech. He talked informally about the situation in Congress, predicting that little legislation, aside from the appropriation bills, would be passed in the rest of the session.

Chamber officials said that the conference was the personal affair of Senator Taft and the business men who attended; that the organization still adhered to its unbroken policy of strict "nonpartisanship" in politics.

The formal program was featured tonight by the submission by Brig. Gen. Charles G. Dawes, first director of the Federal budget, of a four-point program whereby he reasoned that "the next President" might balance the budget. He spoke at "the Organization Night Dinner," sponsored by the National Association of Commercial Organization Secretaries.

"The Federal budget can be balanced," said the general. "If the next President is a fighter and will, without qualification, pledge himself in his conscience before his people—and before Congress—to fight for a balanced budget, he should not fail. But he must be made of stern stuff."

General Dawes proposed that the "next President" return as soon as possible to the system of executive control and governmental coordination established in 1921, under which, he said, "national deficits were converted into na-

Continued on Page Eighteen

The International Situation

Officers who had led a German motorized column across the perilous mountains of Central Norway shook hands yesterday with the leaders of another column that had smashed its way down from Trondheim to a point southwest of Stoeren. The meeting marked the junction of the Reich's forces in the Oslo and Trondheim zones and dashed Allied hopes of quickly dislodging the invaders.

Germany's High Command announced that simultaneously Nazi troops advancing up the Gudbrandsdal had "reached" the important railway junction at Dombaas, but the German news agency, D. N. B., which is usually a step ahead of the communiqués, proclaimed the capture of that place and Stoeren, too. Regardless of whether the points were actually taken—and London simply said it lacked information on the subject—it seemed evident that the junction of German forces would make the Allies' position in that region untenable and throw them back upon the immediate vicinities of their landing bases at Aandalsnes and Namsos.

At the far northern port of Narvik the situation apparently was the reverse. There the Allies were reported carrying on a drive that threatened to dislodge the Germans after they had been attacked from the air. [All the foregoing, Page 1.]

Following up their success in the central region, the Germans smashed at the Allied beachheads. In addition to attacking toward Aandalsnes, they pounded Namsos from the air in six separate raids covering ten hours, during which a British destroyer was set afire and wrecked. [Page 1.]

This was not the only British naval setback recorded during the day. The Admiralty announced the loss of two submarines and two naval trawlers, presumably in the Norwegian operations. Berlin asserted that since the campaign began thirteen British submarines had been destroyed in the Skagerrak. In that body of water another sea battle was reported by Swedish sources. [Page 3.]

The day's developments drew from Chancellor Hitler a glowing proclamation to his troops, in which he declared that their "inexorable advance" had "conclusively nullified" Allied efforts to force the Reich to its knees. He also announced the rewarding of the Nazi commander in Norway, General von Falkenhorst, with one of Germany's highest decorations. [Page 1.] The Chancellor himself, incidentally, was the object of a reward of $1,000,-

Continued on Page Four

NAZI BOMBERS RAID NAMSOS TEN HOURS

Destroyer Wrecked in One of Six Attacking Waves—Two Planes Reported Downed

By The United Press.

ALLIED HEADQUARTERS, Namsos, Norway, April 30—Six waves of German planes bombed this British landing base for ten hours today with a heavy toll of life and the destruction of a British destroyer, which was left a blazing shell.

The German planes, before flying away from the bombing attack, were alleged to have machine-gunned civilians in the streets.

The big, swastika-marked bombers swept upon the city and port in six separate attacks between 7 A. M. and 5 P. M.

The British destroyer was struck squarely aft and within a few minutes was blazing as depth bombs stored in her holds went off with detonations that shook the entire area. Despite the fact that the destroyer was in flames, the British succeeded in beaching it.

Many houses were shattered by the high explosive bombs of the raiders, who, in the last thirty-six hours have raided Namsos ten times, laying waste whole areas of the town and taking a high toll of dead and wounded.

German Plane Hit

British anti-aircraft guns, newly arrived aboard transports, hit one of the German planes, which disappeared, leaving a trail of black smoke.

The guns also kept the raiders at high altitude.

During the last forty-eight hours persistent German reconnaissance flights had been staged over Namsos, indicating a big-scale aerial attack intended to cripple Allied operations here.

Among the casualties thus far in the aerial attacks have been twenty-seven French officers and soldiers killed by German bombs.

Many incendiary bombs have been dropped by the Nazis.

A French soldier, coming out of an air raid shelter after yesterday's raids, said:

"We wish our people would send us some planes to beat off the Germans."

A British soldier added:

"Blimey! They fly over us here as if they were over their own air field. They gave us hell during the recent fighting."

Most of the French soldiers here are of the Alpine Chasseurs of "Blue Devils" of World War fame, but all branches of the French Army are represented. The British troops are from all parts of the British Isles, and among the ac-

Continued on Page Two

Dispatches from Europe and the Far East are subject to censorship at the source.

TROOPS IN NORWAY THANKED BY HITLER

Nazi Victories Block Allied Effort to Beat Germany to Her Knees, He Asserts

By The United Press.

BERLIN, April 30—Chancellor Hitler, in a jubilant proclamation to his soldiers in Norway tonight, boasted that German victories there have "conclusively nullified" the Allies' efforts to beat Germany to her knees on the Scandinavian battle front.

Herr Hitler, self-described "first soldier of the Reich," said in his order of the day that Oslo and Trondheim had been linked during the day by an "inexorable advance of German troops."

As a reward, he announced that he was conferring upon General Nikolaus von Falkenhorst, Nazi commander in Norway, the Chevalier's Cross of the Iron Cross, one of Germany's highest honors.

TEXT OF ORDER OF DAY

The text of Herr Hitler's order of the day follows:

Soldiers of the Norwegian scene of war!

The inexorable advance of German troops today established land connections between Oslo and Trondheim. Thereby the Western powers' intention still to force Germany to her knees by the subsequent occupation of Norway has been conclusively nullified.

Units of the army, navy and air force in exemplary cooperation brought about an achievement reflecting the highest honor on the daring of the young German armed forces.

Officers, non-commissioned officers and men! You have fought on the Norwegian war scene against all inclemencies of sea and land and in the air and against the resistance of the enemy.

You have fulfilled the tremendous task which I, in faith in you and your powers, was forced to set for you.

The nation through me expresses thanks. As an external sign of recognition and of this gratitude I decorate the Commander in Chief in Norway, General von Falkenhorst, with the Chevalier's Cross of the Iron Cross.

On the recommendation of your Commander in Chief, I will also decorate the bravest among you. The highest award for you all can already be the conviction that you have made a decisive contribution in the most severe and fateful battle of our people for existence or non-existence.

I know you will further fulfill the tasks set for you.

Long live the Great Germany!

Symbolic of the unanimous jubilation in German quarters over the reported successes, the newspaper Nachtausgabe said editorially that the importance of the German establishment of a continuous line

Continued on Page Six

GERMAN UNITS JOIN

Mountains Scaled to Link Oslo and Trondheim in a Furious Advance

ALLIES ARE IN DIFFICULTY

Large Forces May Be Trapped —Defenders Keep Hold at Namsos, Press at Narvik

By OTTO D. TOLISCHUS
By Telephone to THE NEW YORK TIMES.

STOCKHOLM, Sweden April 30—The battle for the Dombaas-Stoeren railroad line, the Allied key position in the heart of Norway, ended today with a German victory, the full extent of which must still be determined but of whose decisiveness there can be no doubt.

According to German claims, the German forces that have been battering against that line for many days have captured both Dombaas and Stoeren and have therewith established overland connection between their main force around Oslo and the hitherto isolated German troops in Trondheim.

What is perhaps even more important, they have therewith also ended any immediate Allied chance of an offensive not only against Oslo but also against Trondheim, and have thrown the Allied forces back to the immediate vicinity of their landing bases, against which German offensives may be expected immediately.

Germans Press Advantage

In fact, these offensives appear to be already under way. For the Germans are keeping on the heels of the Allied forces retreating from Dombaas in the direction of Aandalsnes and Molde, and they have likewise launched attacks against the Allied lines north of Steinkjer, in the direction of Namsos, where French and Norwegian troops are in the first lines and the British in reserve.

Simultaneously, it appears that both landing bases are being subjected to new, intensive air bombardment, partly, no doubt, to paralyze the debarkation of reinforcements and supplies, but mostly to keep the Allied Navy at a distance. And whether the Allies can hold their landing bases without the support of the heavy naval guns is now the question that may decide the whole Norwegian campaign.

So far in that campaign German air supremacy has proved superior to Allied sea supremacy, in which connection it must be remembered that the principal German objective in Norway is to obtain closer air bases for a crushing air attack on Britain itself.

The battle for the Dombaas-Stoeren railroad—the Norwegian Battle of the Marne—was decided in favor of the attacking Germans when to the four columns trying to reach that railroad along the mountain passes in a northwestward direction was added a fifth column, detached from the reinforced German troops in Trondheim, which attacked the Allies at Stoeren from the north at the same time that the Germans were battering against Dombaas itself, as well as Hjerkinn and Ulsberg.

Whether the Germans also attacked Stoeren from north of Roeros is still unknown, but inasmuch as light troops were reported to have passed the damaged bridges that had stopped the previous advance from that direction, it may be assumed that they participated in the battle.

German Claims Accepted

The report of the German victory comes so far only from German sources, but they meet no denials and in neutral quarters are accepted as true. According to these reports, Stoeren was taken during the night and Dombaas at midday today. This left the question open as to whether the Allied forces that had occupied Stoeren and the railroad line to Dombaas have been able to escape.

According to the German reports, the German troops advancing through Stoeren from the north reached Opdal today, but from Opdal leads a mountain road to Sunndals, where Allied forces were reported to have landed with tanks, artillery and other material. It may be assumed, therefore, that the Allied forces from Stoeren are falling back along that road.

But considerable Allied troops were also concentrated at Hjerkinn, from where heavy fighting was reported during the night. The fate

Continued on Page Two

LVIII

1940

The 1940 meeting was held May 1, 2, and 3, in St. Louis, at George Warren Brown Hall, Washington University, President Allen O. Whipple, of New York, Professor of Surgery, Columbia University; Director of Surgical Service, Presbyterian Hospital, in the Chair. That year had seen the deaths of, among others, George E. Brewer, Harvey Cushing, and of Charles H. Mayo, and William J. Mayo, and of the interestingly named Dr. Gatewood.

* * *

The meeting opened with a series of physiologic papers about blood,- not remarkably, since the Program Committee consisted of Frederick A. Coller, Alfred Blalock, and Thomas G. Orr.

John P. Peters, of New Haven, Connecticut, Professor of Medicine at Yale, by invitation, *The Structure of the Blood in Relation to Surgical Problems,* opened the symposium, illustrating the effects on the serum electrolytes of pyloric obstruction and ileal obstruction. For the first time the Association heard the statement that "The best way to rest the alimentary canal is to give it nothing to do . . . if no water or food is given to dogs after ligation of the pylorus, vomiting ceases after a short interval." Complete withdrawal of fluids and food by mouth was required and "The term 'complete' permits no compromises nor exceptions, not even water in sips or cracked ice . . . The introduction of water into

the obstructed bowel or stomach seems to provoke the excretion of further fluid as well as salt." Nevertheless, he felt it necessary to add that if, "The courage of the physician fails, care should be taken that as little fluid as possible is introduced and that all food or fluid given by mouth or through the tube contains enough salt to make it isotonic with blood serum." As for the volume of fluid which was to be administered "Only enough is required to establish an adequate volume of urine. The patient who is excreting 1,000 to 1,500 cc. of urine daily is seldom a subject for anxiety."

* * *

Also by invitation, David C. Bull and Charles R. Drew, of New York, from the Department of Surgery, College of Physicians and Surgeons, Columbia University, *The Preservation of Blood,* informed the members about the changes in the blood caused by storage, in the then relatively new blood banks. The cell count did not change in stored heparinized blood for 30 days, but slowly dropped in the second fortnight in citrated blood, at the same time that the hemoglobin content of the plasma rose. Whereas fresh transfused cells survived 95 days in the recipient, the survival of transfused cells of stored blood dropped from 60 days in ten-day old blood to 20 days in 14-day old blood. The white blood cell count of stored blood dropped 50% in the first 24 hours and white cells disappeared, for the most part after the second week. The platelet count fell rapidly, prothrombin fell rapidly, plasma potassium rose with the length of storage. The cells of placental blood fared no better than the cells of adult blood. There was some concern that the amount of potassium in the serum of bank blood could be lethal if several liters of blood were administered. The plasma potassium was higher in cadaver blood than in donor blood. Blood stored nine days or more was much more likely to produce transient jaundice than was fresh citrated blood.

* * *

John Scudder, of New York, by invitation, from the laboratories of the Rockefeller Institute for Medical Research, *Studies in Blood Preservation.* The Stability of Plasma Proteins, had just written a book on shock and was heavily involved in the active field of blood storage and blood transfusion. Whereas whole blood deteriorated with storage, plasma could be preserved indefinitely. Plasma was not antigenic, red cells were. Experimental studies suggested it was much safer to use plasma than serum, which seemed to produce a variety of reactions in man and in animals. There might be some danger in the use of untyped plasma, so type AB plasma should be kept on hand for emergency use. Refrigerated plasma could be kept for months, and lyophilized plasma had been kept for years and found safe to use. "Plasma approaches the ideal physiologic perfusion fluid, and is superior to acacia, glucose, salt, and serum." Scudder's electrophoretic studies of serum and blood plasma were the first such studies to be presented before the Association. Minor changes in the electrophoretic pattern were observed with storage, whereas unrefrigerated plasma, reconstituted lyophilized serum, and autopsy plasma were grossly abnormal. [Scudder did not specifically refer to the Russian use of cadaver blood, which was exciting great interest, stating only that "Postmortem blood appears abnormal; this may not apply to blood collected from those who have met sudden death."]

* * *

Walter G. Maddock, Associate Professor of Surgery, University of Michigan Medical School and Hospital, and Frederick A. Coller, Professor of Surgery, University of Michigan; Director of Department of Surgery, University Hospital, *Sodium Chloride Metabolism of Surgical Patients,* presented another in their series of papers elucidating the subject. Their paper was a physiologic review of the effects of the reduction of salt intake, of abnormal losses of fluid containing salt, and of retention of salt and water in certain disease states. As to the patient on total parenteral support ". . . if no abnormal losses of sodium chloride have occurred, each patient should be given half a liter of Ringer's solution daily, and the remainder of the fluid needs should be supplied by 5 or 10 percent dextrose in distilled water." The conservation of electrolytes by the kidneys was pointed out. In reference to abnormal salt losses they referred to the recommendations of O'Shaughnessy, and the experience of Latta in the treatment of cholera patients with intravenous saline solution in 1831, and Rogers' success in treating cholera patients in 1916 with hypertonic solutions of sodium bicarbonate and salt. They reminded the Fellows of the cardinal demonstration by Hartwell and Hoguet in 1912, and the subsequent contributions of Haden and Orr, that dogs with intestinal obstruction could be kept alive by infusion of sodium chloride. They brought forth again their formula that 0.5 of a gram of sodium chloride per kilogram of body weight was required for each 100 milligrams that plasma chloride level needed to be raised to reach the normal 560 milligrams per cent. Since "modern surgical practice requires intubation of the gastro-intestinal tract", the loss of the withdrawn fluid demanded volume-for-volume replacement with physiologic saline or Ringer's solution, as was true for bile drainage. With ileostomy drainage and diarrhea, they said only that " the base loss is greater than the chloride loss . . . the surgeon is dealing chiefly with upper alimentary tract losses which generally have an excess of chloride ions and the pediatrician is at the other end of the canal and deals with excess base loss . . . Gamble has repeatedly emphasized that the same two solutions [sodium chloride and 5% glucose,- Gamble was on the eve of recognizing the need for potassium] will, in the vast majority of cases, correct the electrolyte imbalance associated with losses from either end of the canal. Edema in surgical patients . . . is nearly always the surgeon's error" and the result of hypoproteinemia and excessive administration of salt. They pointed out that while "it would be extremely handy if the plasma chloride or sodium level would increase proportionately to the salt retained and be an index of excessive administration" that did not happen, admitted it was a paradox and offered no explanation.

Discussion

Waltman Walters, of Rochester, Minnesota, opening the Discussion, spoke about "the clinical aspects of dehydration toxemia", an indication of which was decrease in urinary output, reminding the Fellows that if "the cooperation of men skilled in biochemical tests is not available . . . " they might remember that "one sees the red cheeks of such patients due to the alkalosis, the dry skin and tongue, and in addition the blood pressure usually is found to be below normal." In his practice, he avoided the production of edema by giving no more than 1000 cc of normal saline solution above that required to replace the gastrointestinal secretions lost. Owen H. Wangensteen, of Minneapolis, repeated Dr. Peters' "emphasis on the matter of distention as related to the absorption of fluid and to the prophylaxis of distention after abdominal operations." He was interested in Peters' comments about taking saline by mouth if any fluid at all, but found it "difficult to get patients after operation to ingest more than half a liter of saline solution unless the salt is given in capsules. Patients do enjoy the refreshment of cool water." With respect to obstruction, he reminded the Fellows of his paper of the previous year showing that a dog with complete ileal obstruction survived remarkably well if his esophagus was transected so that he could not swallow air. In postoperative patients, Wangensteen emphasized the loss of fluid from perspiration during and after operation, and obviously gave much larger volumes of fluids than the others, "For a patient who has had a protracted operation under anesthesia, and who has not lost large quantities of fluid from the gastrointestinal canal, 5 Gm. of sodium chloride and 3,000 to 4,000 cc. of fluid will usually suffice, and insure a satisfactory urine output, during the first 24-hour period." In older patients, they had returned to the subcutaneous route for administration of fluids, "Patients with malignancies in the upper age-brackets not uncommonly have coronary sclerosis with diminished cardiac reserve. Intravenous administration of fluid to such patients not uncommonly elicits cardiac pain and may provoke pulmonary edema. I have come to insist on the subcutaneous administration of fluid to such patients and find it eminently satisfactory." Wangensteen brought up the matter of nitrogen balance, "Up until now, surgeons have concerned themselves solely with the item of proper water and electrolyte balance and the administration of enough glucose to prevent ketosis. Why not also, maintenance of patients in proper caloric and nitrogen balance?" In patients with gastric outlet obstruction, "Five hundred cubic centimeters of human plasma daily usually suffices to maintain nitrogen equilibrium" and an equal amount of whole blood did as well. "Recent experience with the intravenous administration of amino-acids (F. Stearns & Co., Detroit) suggests that this is a simple and practical manner in which to supply patients with a source of nitrogen when the gastrointestinal canal is not available for feeding." They had been experimenting with the "feasibility of administering bovine plasma to man intravenously." They had been able to give rather large quantities, found it was retained and not excreted in the urine, had given from 100 cc. to 1,500 cc. in over 50 patients. "There have, of course, been some reactions. We have had only one anaphylactoid reaction, in an asthmatic. There have been no deaths." He was "hopeful that the method may become useful in the treatment of shock and contracted protein stores in man, both in civil and war surgery. It is not unlikely that separation of the albumin and globulin fractions may pyramid the usefulness of the method, for the globulin fraction appears to be the more toxic." [Edgar Cohn, at Harvard, was engaged in this fractionation at the time and the bovine plasma albumin was shortly available in large quantities but proved to be too foreign a protein for human use.] John P. Peters, closing, addressed "this business of excessive chloride." He thought excessive chloride intravenously might be dangerous, "My own practice is to administer saline chiefly under the skin, as Doctor Wangensteen has suggested, and to reserve the vein for hypertonic glucose, if it was necessary." Walter G. Maddock, closing, commented upon the edema in the face of low or normal plasma electrolytes, feeling that it was "because more than usual of the saline solution goes to the interstitial spaces."

* * *

W. Osler Abbott, of Philadelphia, by invitation, from the Gastro-Intestinal Section, Hospital of the University of Pennsylvania, *Fluid and Nutritional Maintenance by the Use of an Intestinal Tube,* described his double lumen tube, the end of one channel could be used for jejunal feeding, while the more proximal openings in the second channel permitted constant gastric suction. The fluid could be given by drip, by pump, or by intermittent syringe injection. He discussed the use of his long tube in intestinal obstruction, "When a patient with a low obstruction is treated by the passage of a small intestinal tube, strained fluids should be started at once provided that salt is given as described. While the tube is in the stomach this constitutes gastric lavage. As soon as it traverses the duodenum the fluid begins to contribute to his maintenance. When the tube is progressing down the jejunum, strained soup, tea, coffee, melba toast, puffed rice and clear jellies are cautiously tried. To this may be added zwieback, Holland rusks, boiled rice, cream cheese, well cooked eggs and finally strained cereal, chicken and lean beef and lamb . . . On such a regimen the patient should be able to take 1,500 to 1,800 calories daily for two to three weeks in spite of complete obstruction if the nasal and throat irritation from the tube can be combatted for that long a period." He cited such a case in detail, in which a patient was obstructed after an appendectomy, for 24 days, but was maintained because "A long intestinal tube was passed into the stomach by Dr. Richard Warren" on the third day. The patient recovered without an operation.

* * *

Robert Elman, of St. Louis, Associate Professor of Clinical Surgery, Washington University School of Medicine, *Parenteral Replacement of Protein with the Amino-Acids of Hydrolyzed Casein,* had obtained his material from Mead Johnson and Co. His amino acid solution with glucose and electrolytes had been given to 35 adult patients "as the *sole* source of alimentation, with the particular purpose of parenteral protein replacement." Positive nitrogen balance was achieved, the serum protein concentration rose, and the patients responded well clinically. In many of the patients, there was a large urinary nitrogen excretion. During the discussion, on the virtues of plasma, the use of lyophilized plasma in "the present military emergency" was mentioned.

* * *

Henry W. Cave, of New York, Attending Surgeon to the Roosevelt Hospital, Assistant Clinical Professor of Surgery, Columbia University, College of Physicians and Surgeons, and by invitation, William F. Nickel, Jr., *Ileostomy,* discussed their experience with ulcerative colitis at the Roosevelt Hospital. For ileostomy the bowel was to be divided six or eight inches from the ileocecal valve, the distal end brought through a left-sided stab wound and the proximal end brought through a right McBurney incision. Two inches of ileum should protrude from the abdominal wall and a large tube be tied in place in it. A transfusion was given immediately following ileostomy. They sutured the ileal mesentery to the fascia and since doing that had had no instances of prolapse, and no instances of retraction. The emergency indication for ileostomy was perforation. Massive bleeding, formerly an indication for ileostomy, was found always to result fatally if an ileostomy was performed. The bleeding could be controlled by administration of vitamins K and C. The mortality

of ileostomy was still high. From a questionnaire to the members of the American Surgical, Southern Surgical, and Western Surgical Associations, they found a mortality of 33% for patients who had had an ileostomy and retained it. "Cattell's mortality of 22 per cent; Kunath's 83 per cent mortality following ileostomy in 12 patients, and our total mortality of 23 per cent, all emphasized the necessity of earlier surgical intervention and better preparation for operation." Twenty-two patients in the questionnaire response, or 59% of those whose ileostomy had subsequently been closed, had been restored to health with an average follow-up of nine years, nine or 25% had had a recurrence and there had been six deaths or 16.7% after closure, early or late. Cave and Nickel agreed that "It is impossible to say that after any given period of freedom from activity the disease will not recur." On their own service, they had done 11 emergency ileostomies with a 45% mortality and 19 elective ileostomies with an 11% mortality. They had abandoned the practice of closing and dropping the distal end back into the peritoneal cavity for fear of an ultimate blow out resulting from obstruction of the diseased colon. In the Roosevelt Hospital series, the ileostomy was always performed "as a preliminary step to the radical removal of the diseased colon and rectum."

Discussion

Harvey B. Stone, of Baltimore, discussed the paper at length, stating that after ileostomy, some patients continued to deteriorate, some improved systemically but the bowel remained diseased,- the most numerous group,- and in a very small group, the patient improved and the disease healed. He urged earlier operation based on progressive radiologic signs showing stiffening and shortening of the bowel. In three cases, Stone had created a pouch of bowel proximal to the ileostomy by a technique similar to that of a Finney pyloroplasty and had found the secretions to be thickened and discharge slowed. Frederic W. Bancroft, of New York, had closed the ileostomy in four patients, in one of whom there was a rapid recurrence resulting in death, the other three being well for one, four and eight years, despite the fact that in the last patient the X-rays of the colon were still grossly abnormal. Frank H. Lahey, of Boston, was "sure that a great many patients die needlessly every year due to the fact that we do not get the gastroenterologists and the medical men to cooperate well enough with us about early ileostomies . . . this late delivery of patients with ulcerative colitis, who are candidates for ileostomy . . . results in most of the mortality of this disease." Nevertheless, an ileostomy was an unpleasant arrangement and he did not agree with Dr. Stone that beginning rigidity of the colon was an indication for the operation, "I wonder if I, myself might not possibly accept a fairly rigid colon with some hazard rather than ileostomy." They had done 70 ileostomies, representing 59% of the cases they had seen. The divided ileostomy was indeed the best, but requires considerable technical manipulation" which ill patients might not tolerate, and in profoundly ill patients a loop ileostomy was performed first. He agreed with the use of a tube on suction, in the ileostomy. He indicated that subsequent colectomy was the expected outcome. Vernon C. David, of Chicago, endorsed early ileostomy. He brought up the question of carcinoma occurring in the retained colon, ". . . these long-standing ulcerations with polyposis have really serious significance." Edwin M. Miller, of Chicago, with his interest in pediatric surgery, presented a slide of a child of six with an ileostomy ". . . the skin has always been in excellent condition. She has spent most of her nights and a part of the time during the day face down upon a frame in which there is an opening, so that the contents of the proximal ileum drains directly into a receptacle, and during the day, at intervals, the nurse irrigates this area with a little sterile water." He hoped some day to close the ileostomy. Henry W. Cave, closing, did not argue with Dr. Stone's preference for early ileostomy nor did he care for the pouch ileostomy. He thought he would prefer the Devine technique although he had not used it. Cave thought the incidence of carcinoma superimposed upon chronic ulcerative colitis was "3 per cent of the patients who have reached an irreversible stage of pseudopolypoid degeneration . . ."

* * *

William Crawford White, of New York, Assistant Clinical Professor of Surgery, Columbia University; Associate Attending Surgeon, The Roosevelt Hospital, *Irradiation Burn of the Intestine*, spoke of injuries to the bowel after irradiation for carcinoma of the cervix,- rectovaginal fistula, rectal stricture, cicatricial contracture of the small bowel, ulceration of both large and small bowel, and symptoms, in these various conditions, of pain and diarrhea. Lesions above the peritoneal floor might be resected and the bowel reconstructed, but "it is very important to go sufficiently wide of the lesion to assure good blood supply."

* * *

The paper of Rudolph Matas, of New Orleans, now 80 years of age, *Personal Experiences in Vascu-*

lar Surgery, discussed the political and governmental history of Louisiana, as well as the history of medicine in that area and the history of vascular surgery, listed all the 622 operations upon the blood vessels which he had done from 1888 to 1940 with their results, and then gave his own complete bibliography of 108 papers on vascular surgery.

* * *

Emile Holman, of San Francisco, Professor of Surgery and Executive Head, Department of Surgery, Stanford University Medical School; Chief Surgeon, Lane-Stanford Hospitals, *Clinical and Experimental Observations on Arteriovenous Fistulae*, had been working on this problem since 1923. Holman challenged some of the 1923 observations of Thomas Lewis and A. N. Drury. In his remarkably clear delineation of the problem, he stated that a secondary or fistulous circuit was created and that "the lowered peripheral resistance in this secondary circuit results in a diversion of blood from the primary circuit with its high capillary resistance, the extent of such diversion depending upon the size of the fistula and its location in the arterial tree . . . That the diversion of blood from the normal arterial bed through the fistula into the capacious venous system proximal and distal to the fistula results in the lowering of blood pressure in the primary circuit . . . the general blood pressure is lowered, the diastolic pressure permanently . . . the systolic pressure is gradually restored . . . by . . . an increased cardiac output . . . and an increased total blood volume." The increased venous return to the heart could be accommodated by increased cardiac work, but gradual dilatation of the heart and of the artery proximal to the fistula resulted, "the final result being a dilatation of the entire circulatory bed through which the short-circuited blood flows." Closure of the fistula reversed all of these changes and in evidence he provided abundant clinical illustrations. His experimental work in animals showed that following the creation of a large arteriovenous fistula, there was an immediate decrease in cardiac size followed by return to normal and progressive enlargement "which may be apparent within four or five days." The increase in blood volume which occurred was commensurate with the size of the fistula. "The physiologic effect of a fistula . . . depends upon the volume of blood diverted through the fistula and, therefore, upon its size."

Discussion

Mont R. Reid, of Cincinnati, said Holman's data were "most convincing. We have not been able

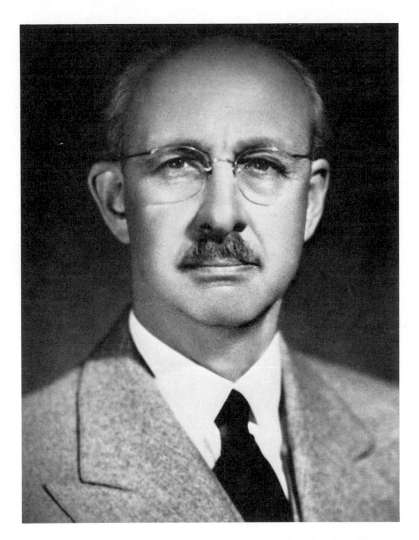

Emile Holman 1890-1977, M.D. Johns Hopkins, 1918, Vice-President 1949. After the long Halsted residency training—he was the last resident to finish under Halsted—went briefly with Cushing to Harvard and the Peter Bent Brigham and in 1926 accepted the call to Stanford, from which he had gone as a Rhodes Scholar in 1914. Established a productive, scientific Department of Surgery at Stanford, the first academic Department of Surgery in the West. A thoughtful, precise, cultured and unprejudiced man, his surgical interests were broad, but increasingly in matters of cardiothoracic surgery. At Hopkins, he began his clinical and laboratory investigations of arterio-venous fistulae and unequivocally demonstrated in a series of classical papers, the physiological changes produced early and late by production of and closing of the fistulae—changes in pulse contour, rate, blood pressure, blood volume, vessel size, heart size and in 1930, for this work, received the prize named for the founder of the Association. He continued, even after retirement, to work on and elucidate these problems. Although of "the older group of surgeons", he introduced cardiac surgery to the West, performing the first operations there for patent ductus, for coarctation of the aorta, for Tetralogy of Fallot, for mitral stenosis and provided the impetus for the important program in open heart surgery which followed at Stanford.

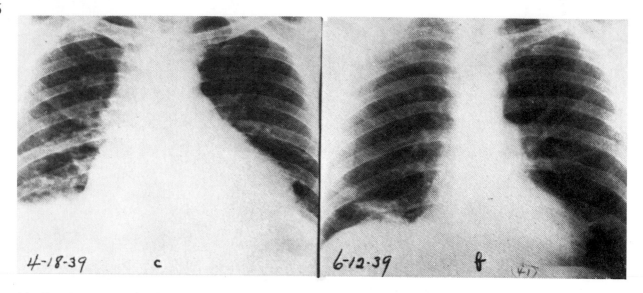

4-18-39   c   6-12-39   f   (4.7)

(c) Roentgenogram showing a massive cardiac enlargement and some pulmonary infiltrate in a patient six-and-a-half years after a right subclavian-jugular fistula resulting from a knife wound.
(f) X-ray 33 days after operation. Holman resected the clavicle, tied and divided the internal jugular vein and ligated the subclavian artery.
     Holman showed that production of an arteriovenous fistula was associated with a lowered diastolic blood pressure, increased blood volume, increased cardiac output, dilatation of the heart and dilatation of the artery proximal to the fistula and that all these changes were reversible.
     Emile Holman, *Clinical and Experimental Observations on Arterio-Venous Fistulae,* Volume LVIII, 1940.

to completely confirm his blood volume studies and I do not know why . . . I grant that we see very few, in which the heart is badly damaged, in which there is not an increase in the total blood volume." He asked whether Holman had undertaken any studies of cardiac output immediately upon opening the fistula. Reid had found an immediate very large increase in output. Reid ended by saying plaintively "Of course, Doctor Holman and I have argued this question many, many times. He is probably right. I have never been able to agree with him that simply because there is an increased vascular bed there must of necessity be an increase of blood volume." In reply, Holman said, to his old Hopkins associate, "I should like to ask Doctor Reid what fills this increased vascular bed—air? Humor? There must be something to fill this enlarged vascular bed and it is blood. Doctors [William] Dock and [Tinsley] Harrison, at the Peter Bent Brigham Hospital, in 1923, showed a doubling of cardiac output the moment we introduced a fistula into the circulatory system, and that was shown not only the day after the introduction of the fistula, but it was shown months later, with an increase in cardiac output during that time. There is no question about the increase in cardiac output the moment a fistula is introduced into the

circulatory system." Fistulae in Reid's patients, who had no increase in blood volume, were small fistulae Holman said, and there was no change in pulse rate or blood pressure when the fistulae were closed, so that an increase in blood volume should not have been expected.

* * *

Isaac A. Bigger, of Richmond, Virginia, Professor of Surgery, Medical College of Virginia; Surgeon-in-Chief, Medical College of Virginia Hospital; *The Surgical Treatment of Aneurysm of the Abdominal Aorta.* Review of the Literature and Report of Two Cases, One Apparently Successful, commented that "Clinically, recognizable aneurysms of the abdominal aorta occur infrequently . . ." but 65 had recently been collected from the Charity Hospital and perhaps it was not so rare. In those cases, the symptoms were of brief duration, less than a year in 87% and death occurred within a month of admission in 38. He cited the history of aortic ligature beginning with Astley Cooper. Out of the total of 30 operated cases, Barney Brooks' patient had died of intestinal obstruction three months after an apparently successful ligation of the aorta, LaRoque's patient with an iliac aneurysm was well 14 months af-

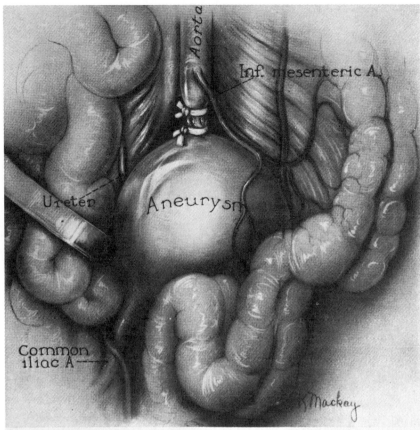

FIG. 1.—The appearance of the aneurysm at operation. Double ligation, with cotton tape, between the inferior mesenteric artery and the bifurcation.

Elkin placed two cotton tapes to occlude the aorta completely in a 61-year-old man with a steadily increasing pulsation of six-months' known duration. Eleven months later, the patient was well with a small mass, slightly pulsating, and with good extremity pulsations.

Daniel C. Elkin, *Aneurysm of the Abdominal Aorta,* Volume LVIII, 1940.

ter partial ligation of the abdominal aorta, and Bigger and Dan Elkin had surviving patients. Bigger's successful case [he had failed in an earlier attempt at ligating the aorta for an arteriosclerotic aneurysm in a man of 54] was of a man of 25 who had been shot with buckshot just a year earlier and came in now with what was diagnosed as a bleeding abdominal aneurysm. The aneurysm, 8 to 10 cm. in diameter, "arose from the anterior wall of the abdominal aorta at the level of the inferior mesenteric artery." The hole in its anterior surface was filled with firm clot and not bleeding at the moment. The aorta was ligated with fascia lata. There had been a thrill felt before ligation which had disappeared afterwards and was assumed to be due to an arteriovenous fistula. Paraplegia, which appeared after operation, gradually improved, but the pulsation returned. The patient was reexplored and from within the aneurysm the opening of a large vessel was successfully sutured. The patient recovered, his neurologic defect cleared, but he subsequently had a continuous abdominal bruit which suggested an arteriovenous fistula. The peripheral pulses of his extremity had re-

turned. They presumed that the lumen of the aorta had been restored.

* * *

Daniel C. Elkin, of Atlanta, Professor of Surgery, Emory University; Surgeon-in-Chief, Emory University Hospital, *Aneurysm of the Abdominal Aorta.* Treatment by Ligation, provided almost exactly the same historical list of previous cases as had Bigger, discussing them in somewhat more graphic language. His own patient was a 61-year-old male with a pulsating abdominal mass known to have been present for six months. The dilatation of the aorta began just below the inferior mesenteric artery. The aorta was ligated below this artery with two pieces of heavy cotton tape, "until the pulsation in the aneurysm was almost completely obliterated and until the pulsation of the femoral vessels could scarcely be felt . . . Six months later the mass could be felt but was much smaller than originally. There was a slight pulsation in it and a definite systolic bruit could be heard over it." The patient was still well 11 months after operation, free from pain and fully restored, "It would appear that the partial ligation has so slowed the current of blood through the aneurysm as to bring about partial clotting but complete occlusion has not been accomplished."

Discussion

I. A. Bigger said that ligation could not be attempted if a vital vessel, such as the superior mesenteric arose from the aneurysm and in any case he doubted whether proximal ligation could ever be more than palliative in most cases. Rudolph Matas, of New Orleans, initiating his remarks by introducing himself "As a pioneer in this field", congratulated Elkin and Bigger, mentioned "Doctor Owings' experimental success in the segmental obliteration of the lower thoracic and abdominal aortic tract by his method of gradual occlusion" [James Owings, of Baltimore, suggested rubber band occlusion]. He said that "surgery is gradually approaching some mastery over one of its most rebellious provinces." The old gentleman discussed in detail the cases of Bigger and Elkin, went into the literature, and discussed endoaneurysmorrhaphy throughout the world.

* * *

[In the *Transactions,* there then follows a long paper by Matas on *Aneurysm of the Abdominal Aorta at Its Bifurcation into the Common Iliac Arteries.* The evidence suggests that the papers of Bigger and of Matas were submitted after the meeting, to complement Elkin's paper.]

* * *

Herman E. Pearse, of Rochester, New York, Assistant Professor of Surgery, University of Rochester School of Medicine and Dentistry, *Experimental Studies on the Gradual Occlusion of Large Arteries,* in that day before arterial replacement was a reality, presented a lucid and beautifully illustrated review of the methods of gradual occlusion of large arteries [including even the method of Milton, 1891, passing a rubber tube around the aorta and vertebral column and out the back where it could be progressively tightened]. As Pearse pointed out, the various types of ligature and compression clamps, all resulted in erosion and those which led to some tightening devices on the outside resulted in infection as well. By injecting irritant materials into the dog aortic wall, he was unable to produce sufficient inflammation to produce a complete occlusion. He had

previously reported the insertion of ". . . a coiled tubular spring . . . introduced through a puncture wound and screwed into the lumen" to avoid the hazard of opening the artery. This caused a gradual closure by thrombosis which gradually recanalized in the dog aorta but with a very small lumen. He had his greatest success from wrapping "Ordinary DuPont cellophane No. 300 P.T." around the aorta snugly, but without compression. "Cellophane was found to be an extreme tissue irritant, for, with but two exceptions, an extensive change occurred around it. This consisted of an intense reaction with either purulent or gelatinous fluid in the center about which the tissue contained many phagocytic, mononuclear cells interspersed among fibrous tissue. This fibrocollagenous layer became partly hyalinized. This process causes a steady progressive constriction of the vessel and an eventual obliteration of the lumen in some instances." He had been led to try cellophane because of I. H. Page's 1939 report of hypertension produced by wrapping cellophane about the kidney.

Discussion

Emile Holman opened the Discussion, commenting in passing that Van Allen, some years earlier, had suggested wrapping the lung in cellophane to produce a fibrous constriction before lobectomy was undertaken, Holman mentioned a recently incomplete operative closure of a patent ductus and wondered whether the cellophane technique might not provide added assurance. Of the basic principle, he said, [without suggesting that it be applied to the very problem of the patent ductus which he had just mentioned] "With reference to the ligation of large arteries in continuity . . . all [methods] have the inherent danger of the fact that this ligature is applied at a fixed point and that the distending force of pulsation is directed at this point with each beat of the heart, with gradual rupture of the tissue and rupture of the vessel . . . Following division of the artery, there is no fixed point. The force of each pulsation is used up in the lateral expansion and in the lengthening of this proximal segment, so that there is no tendency for rupture of the tissues at the point of ligation. I think we should endeavor, in every instance, to divide a large artery between ligatures rather than to ligate it in continuity." Rudolph Matas, of New Orleans, who had already spoken at length of aortic surgery, now provided another two-and-a-half pages of discussion, recapitulating some of the history of experimental large artery occlusion, reminding the Association of his own attempts at repeated longitu-

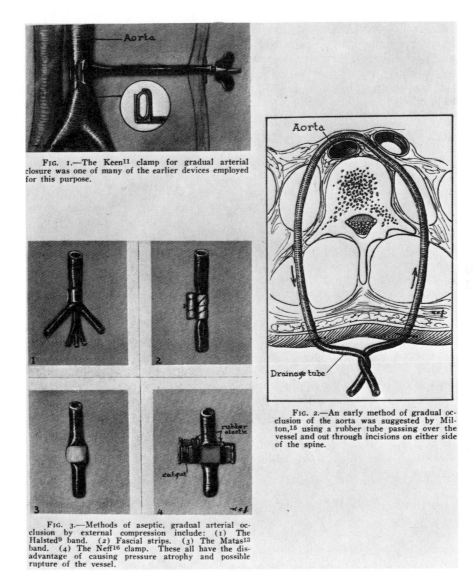

FIG. 1.—The Keen[11] clamp for gradual arterial closure was one of many of the earlier devices employed for this purpose.

FIG. 2.—An early method of gradual occlusion of the aorta was suggested by Milton,[15] using a rubber tube passing over the vessel and out through incisions on either side of the spine.

FIG. 3.—Methods of aseptic, gradual arterial occlusion by external compression include: (1) The Halsted[9] band. (2) Fascial strips. (3) The Matas[13] band. (4) The Neff[16] clamp. These all have the disadvantage of causing pressure atrophy and possible rupture of the vessel.

TECHNIQUES OF GRADUAL ARTERIAL OCCLUSION

Pearse had great success with an internally placed coiled tubular spring "introduced through a puncture wound and screwed into the lumen" and even more with wrapping of cellophane about the artery which produced "a terrific reaction long-continued and persistent but not associated with ordinary inflammation." In some instances, the dog aorta became completely occluded. He reviewed the problems inherent in all the methods previously employed.

Herman E. Pearse, *Experimental Studies on the Gradual Occlusion of Large Arteries,* Volume LVIII, 1940.

dinal plication of the aorta [see page 469, Volume XXXI, 1913] and went on for the second time at the meeting to mention "Dr. James C. Owings, a young and capable experimenter—assistant to Dr. Harvey B. Stone in the Surgical Hunterian Laboratory at Baltimore—" and described Owings' use of a broad rubber band sutured around the aorta and progressively resutured more tightly at three-week intervals until complete occlusion has occurred. [The author of this history may have been the only surgeon to apply this clinically. The patient succumbed within a few days of the first-stage operation, almost certainly from too tight an application of the rubber band, producing insupportable distal ischemia.] The indefatigable Matas corresponded with Owings again after the meeting and includes in his discussion a May 21, 1940 letter from Owings, "Since my last letter I have cut across the aorta below the point of constriction, ligating the two ends with ordinary black silk and allowing them to retract. All three animals have done very well." Frank Lahey, of Boston, asked the obvious question "How does cellophane cause this reaction?" Pearse responded, "I do not know". [It was several years before Yeager, of the University of Maryland (see page 919, Volume LXVI, 1948) demonstrated that the irritating substance was di-cetyl phosphate.] "It is a terrific reaction, long-continued and persistent but not associated with ordinary inflammation. There are very few polymorphonuclear leukocytes in the tissue. There are many large phagocytic cells often containing fragments of cellophane, which would lead one to believe that it is a foreign body reaction."

* * *

Mims Gage, by invitation, and Alton Ochsner, of New Orleans, Professor of Surgery and Head of the Department, School of Medicine, Tulane University, *The Prevention of Ischemic Gangrene following Surgical Operations upon the Major Peripheral Arteries by Chemical Section of the Cervicodorsal and Lumbar Sympathetics,* recommended the use of novocaine blocks of the sympathetics in a variety of situations, with or without operation, in which there was threatened ischemia.

Discussion

Once more, the redoubtable Matas discussed the paper at great length [and very possibly discouraged any other discussion]. The lovely introductory paragraph to his remarks provides a sidelight on the development of the presentation of papers, "*Rudolph Matas* (New Orleans, La.): The excellence of Doctor Gage's presentation suggests a contrast between the past and present methods of introducing papers at these meetings which are no doubt best appreciated by the older members, who, like the speaker, have lived to enjoy the modern outlook so strikingly exhibited by Doctor Gage. With the marvelous aid of contemporary cinematography and short, crisp, tabloid, lantern-slide condensations, a long dissertion is abridged with enormous economy of words without sacrifice of lucidity or precision. Formerly, we spoke of a bird's-eye view of a scene or subject. Now, we survey an encyclopedic panorama with all the speed, sweep and effectiveness of an airplane view. In this way, our surgical programs are being made increas-

ingly attractive and instructive by their pictorial and epitomized visualizations."

* * *

J. Albert Key, of St. Louis, Clinical Professor of Orthopedic Surgery, Washington University, and by invitation, Charles J. Frankel, *The Local Use of Sulfanilamide, Sulfapyridine and Sulfamethylthiazol,* had been stimulated by recent reports " . . . that the local implantation of sulfanilamide powder in the wound before suturing the debrided compound fracture reduced the incidence of infection . . . from 27 to 5 per cent." Very high concentrations of the sulfanilamides occurred in the wound and slowly diffused into the surrounding tissues and the drugs were only bacteriostatic and not bactericidal, except in very high concentrations. Their experiment consisted in producing compound fractures of the ribs or ulna in rabbits, swabbing the wounds with a broth culture of staphylococci, placing the various drug powders in the wound before it was closed. They studied also the reaction to instilled powders of the drugs in clean wounds of bone, joints, soft tissues, serous cavities. They concluded that "Sulfanilamide, sulfapyridine and sulfamethylthiazol, in the form of powder, are well tolerated by the joints, muscles and connective tissues . . . In solution, they are well tolerated by the joints, pleura and peritoneum . . . are bacteriostatic, but not bactericidal . . . and should be sterilized before they are placed in a clean wound . . . slightly inhibit the early healing of the wound, but do not unduly prolong the period of healing." The experiments did not "permit us to evaluate the efficacy of the drugs in preventing infection in contaminated wounds." But this did not prevent them from recommending, from their own clinical experience and that of others, "the local implantation of sulfanilamide powder not only in contaminated wounds, but also in clinically clean operative wounds where infection is especially to be feared or would be especially undesirable." [One remembers packing sulfanilamide powder and subsequently sulfathiazol powder, not only into appendectomy wounds but into clean, incised wounds of the extremities including those in which multiple divided nerves and tendons had been resutured. At the time, one had enthusiasm for the beneficial effect of this insult and clinically one could not see that any harm was done to the healing of the tissues or the recovery of function.]

Discussion

Kellogg Speed, of Chicago, had used sulfanilamide locally, particularly in secondary amputations,

"We take a small handful of the drug, without measuring its quantity, and place it directly in the closed stump." Apart from prolonged serous drainage, he had seen no harm and thought it was beneficial. Frank L. Meleney, of New York, said he had used the drugs essentially only by mouth or intravenously and was somewhat critical of Dr. Key's experimental protocols, saying that in clinical compound fractures there was a variety of organisms, not the staphylococcus alone, and there was more trauma to the tissues than in Key's clean operative insult. Meleney spoke about possible local toxicity and injury, but did not specifically argue for systemic as against local treatment. Owen H. Wangensteen, of Minneapolis, said that in the laboratory, Richard L. Varco had done 40 or 50 very complicated intestinal transposition operations of a variety of kinds placing "4 to 5 Gm. of sulfanilamide about the suture", and had had only three deaths in the entire group, not a single one from peritonitis. "It is Doctor Varco's impression that the local implantation of sulfanilamide about the anastomosis exerts a bacteriostatic effect upon the bacteria which escaped through needle punctures of the intestinal wall. The presence of pathogenic bacteria on the peritoneal surfaces of the anastomosed segments, Doctor Varco feels, interferes with fibrin formation and stops the healing process. Local implantation of sulfanilamide holds the bacteria in check, preventing the lysis and destruction of fibrin, thus permitting the healing process to continue normally. Doctor Varco failed to observe a similar protective influence when the sulfanilamide was administered subcutaneously." J. Dewey Bisgard, of Omaha, commented that, in experiments, he had studied "the healing of fractures in the presence of large quantities of sulfanilamide . . . and there was as prompt healing in those in which there was sulfanilamide present and as thorough healing as those of the controls." Henry F. Graham, of Brooklyn, New York, directly questioned the preference for local instillation of sulfonamides reminding them that "Doctor Garlock . . . demonstrated in his large colon surgery, that he could perform 25 operations in succession with a little skin infection in one only by the use of sulfanilamide by the mouth or subcutaneously" and recalling " . . . the article of Ravdin's . . . on the use of sulfanilamide subcutaneously . . . local use may be valuable, but it remains doubtful, as yet, whether the introduction of a foreign body directly into the wound is better than its subcutaneous or oral administration." [It is interesting that Graham, Senior Surgeon to the Methodist Hospital; Consulting Surgeon to the Victory Memorial Hospital and the Huntington Hospital, Huntington, Long Island, New York, who had been a Fellow since 1933, had no university position, and seldom spoke before the Association, should have been closer to the mark than the pundits.] J. Albert Key, closing, said that while sulfonamides were effective when given systemically, the wound concentration was greater when they were instilled locally. He said that Trueta's work in Spain had been much to the fore, but that, instead of packing their compound fractures with gauze, "if they had used sulfanilamide most of those same wounds could have been closed." He preferred sulfanilamide because he thought there was less foreign body reaction and "We take care that we do not put in lumps of the drug. You can crush it in your fingers . . . and scatter it thinly over the surface. Then I usually rub it over with my fingers . . . I have used it routinely in bone grafts for the past year or more and have not had any trouble."

* * *

No Discussion is recorded of the paper by Elliott C. Cutler, of Boston, Moseley Professor of Surgery, Harvard University, Surgeon-in-Chief, Peter Bent Brigham, and by invitation, Stanley O. Hoerr, *Total Thyroidectomy for Heart Disease. A Five-Year Follow-Up Study,* in which they summed up their experience with 57 of the cases in the series which had been initially discussed at such great length at the 1934 meeting. There had been 32 operations for angina pectoris and 12 patients were living in November, 1939, 25 for congestive failure and four of those patients were living in 1939. There had been five postoperative deaths in the 57 consecutive patients, four attributable to the heart disease, as had been all but three of the later deaths. Twenty-seven of the angina patients survived more than six months and 26 of these "were relieved of pain in some degree for six months or longer . . . and eight of the 12 five-year survivors had sustained relief." The five-year results in the patients with congestive failure "were disappointing". Twelve of the 15 patients who lived six months or more did have relief. Three of the four five-year survivors showed sustained relief, but two of these died of congestive failure in the sixth year. They felt the results were somewhat better in those with failure from valvular disease than from arteriosclerotic or hypertensive heart disease and concluded " . . . that in a selected group of patients with intractable angina pectoris, total thyroidectomy is a worth while therapeutic measure, and is without unwarranted risk." [Nevertheless the procedure was already being abandoned.]

INTRA SPINAL ROOT SECTION

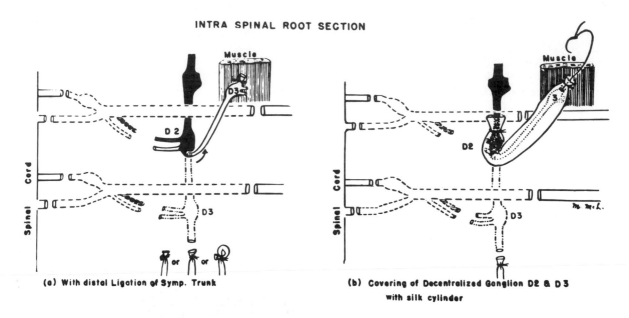

(a) With distal Ligation of Symp. Trunk

(b) Covering of Decentralized Ganglion D2 & D3 with silk cylinder

FIG. 13.—Our present technic combines intraspinal anterior root section with ligation of the distal end of the divided sympathetic trunk. More recently, the decentralized second and third ganglia and intervening trunk have been covered with a fine silk cylinder to further guard against regeneration.

The drawing illustrates the technique at which Smithwick had finally arrived to produce a complete and lasting sympathectomy in the upper extremity. He had first divided the rami to the second and third ganglia, dividing intercostal nerves on both sides of the ganglion, and the trunk below the third ganglion. He had then moved to extraspinal section of the dorsal roots, finally to intraspinal section and now, in addition, ligated the distal stump and covered the proximal stump with a silk cylinder.

Reginald H. Smithwick, *The Problem of Producing Complete and Lasting Sympathetic Denervation of the Upper Extremity by Preganglionic Section,* Volume LVIII, 1940.

* * *

It had long been noted that the results of sympathetic denervation of the upper extremity were less predictable and less lasting than those of the lower extremity, and now Reginald H. Smithwick, of Boston, Instructor in Surgery, Harvard Medical School; Assistant Visiting Surgeon, Massachusetts General Hospital, *The Problem of Producing Complete and Lasting Sympathetic Denervation of the Upper Extremity by Preganglionic Section,* addressed himself to that problem. In the previous five years, he had operated to produce sympathectomy in "151 upper extremities by preganglionic section for the relief of vascular spasm." Cervicodorsal sympathectomy, with postganglionic section had proved unsatisfactory. In his first operation, he had divided the communicating rami of D_2D_3 with associated section of intercostal nerve, divided the sympathetic trunk below D_3 and sutured the divided cephalic end of the trunk up into the wound to prevent regeneration. In his next modification, he not only divided the rami

but divided anterior roots D_2 and D_3, again dividing the intercostal nerve peripherally as well and transplanting the cephalic stump into the wound. In the next modification, the anterior roots were divided "within the arachnoid so that the proximal cut end lies within the spinal canal rather than in the paravertebral space. It is termed intraspinal root section." In his final operation, to this he added ligation of the distal sympathetic, fitting the cephalic end into a cylinder of fine silk "to further guard against regeneration." He concluded that, "The upper extremity can be thoroughly sympathectomized by interrupting the outflow from the second and third dorsal segments and dividing the sympathetic trunk below its third ganglion. The outflow from D_1 is not important in man . . . The immediate results are uniformly satisfactory. The late-results are variable . . . due to cooling of the extremity . . . caused by regeneration of sympathetic motor nerves . . . A number of variations in surgical technic . . . have been made primarily to guard against regeneration. Even in the presence of a considerable degree of regeneration, the blood flow to the extremity is improved, and the result worth while from the patient's point of view. Regeneration is rarely complete". He thought further precautions "which have or can be taken against regeneration will make the late-results even more satisfactory."

Discussion

James C. White, of Boston, and Max M. Peet, of Ann Arbor, both paid tribute to Smithwick's application of modern physiologic principles to arrive at preganglionic section and his technical ingenuity in overcoming the problem of regeneration, but whereas White from the Massachusetts General thought the problem of regeneration had been solved, "it is really fair to say that at the end of a year, or even two years, after preganglionic denervation of the upper, as well as the lower extremities, many of the hands of his [Smithwick's] patients are just as warm as the feet", Peet would only go so far as to say, "Doctor Smithwick's procedure has been very efficient except for the tendency to regeneration. I think perhaps he has overcome that."

The Business Meetings

The 1940 meeting was held May 1, 2, and 3, in St. Louis, at George Warren Brown Hall, Washington University, President Allen O. Whipple in the Chair.

The Suture Committee reported that adequate standards had been set up for the suture materials and that "all sterile surgical products have been included as *drugs* under the new Food and Drugs Act" and placed in the hands of the Food and Drug Administration.

At the Executive Session on the third day, the Association voted to remove the limit on the number of new Fellows elected in any given year, the total to be kept at 175. The meeting at The Homestead, in 1939, the first at a resort, must have been pleasant for it was agreed to hold the meeting the following year at The Greenbrier, in White Sulphur Springs, West Virginia.

The officers elected were David Cheever, of Boston, President; Howard C. Naffziger, of San Francisco, First Vice-President, and Roscoe R. Graham, of Toronto, Second Vice-President and Charles G. Mixter, of Boston, Secretary.

Seventeen men were, this year, elected to Fellowship. Among them were Frank B. Berry, of New York; Richard B. Cattell, of Boston; Grantley W. Taylor, of Boston; Jerome P. Webster, of New York; James Barrett Brown, of St. Louis; Alexander Brunschwig, of Chicago; John H. Gibbon, Jr., of Philadelphia.

The war in Europe had begun and a motion presented by W. J. Mixter and Harvey Stone and passed by vote of the Association reads, "The President shall appoint a Committee to inquire into the professional needs of the country in the event of war, in the broadest way, with power to organize subcommittees and to call upon individual members as they see fit. The purpose of this Committee shall be to assist the surgeon-general in every way possible, and it shall place its findings and recommendations in his hands."

LIX

1941

War was raging in Europe as the Association met,- the last meeting before the entrance of the United States into World War II,- on April 28, 29, and 30, 1941, at The Greenbrier, White Sulphur Springs, West Virginia, President David Cheever, of Boston, Associate Professor of Surgery, Harvard Medical School; Surgeon to the Peter Bent Brigham Hospital, in the Chair. In the previous year d'Arcy Power, a distinguished Honorary Member, had died and there were left only 11 Honorary Members.

Cheever, in his Presidential Address, *War and Aesculapius,* made a passionate statement of the evil let loose on the world by a sinister enemy, ". . . his mailed fist supported by allied ghouls whose nostrils tell them—falsely to be sure—of the expected kill." He ranged over the developments of military surgery through the centuries, the tragedy of disease in the armies, the names and contributions of the great surgeons, singling out among the most immediate advances Orr's treatment of compound fractures, " . . . the method now widely known by his name, foreshadowed by Ollier of Lyon, by Lister himself, and by others, but perfected and brought to the somewhat incredulous attention of the medical world by an American surgeon." There may have been some restraint in the Presidential Addresses on the eve of our entrance into World War I, but no ambiguity for Cheever. The final paragraph of his address reads, "Again Britain and her daughter nations, bleeding but with heads unbowed, stand against this monstrous thing. Again America is moving to their side; again the weight of her power will press down the scale-pan wherein lie liberty and justice. When the victory shall be won, let our care be that mankind shall also win the peace by lavishing on its nurture something of the same energy, treasure, and self-sacrifice which is poured into the lap of Mars."

* * *

The first of 15 papers constituted a symposium on war and surgery entitled *Surgical Preparedness.* L. R. Broster, M.D., F.R.C.S., Senior Surgeon, Charing Cross Hospital, of London, *Surgical Problems of the War,* spoke feelingly of the reaction of the British population to the war and remarked wonderingly, of the evacuation of children from London that ". . . strangely, the town children have shown less strain than those evacuated." In the treatment of war wounds the greatest advance had been ". . . the adoption of the Winnett Orr method based on the experience gained in Spain (Trueta), and the use of sulfonamides for combating infection." The closed method of wound treatment simplified transport and increased comfort, and avoided the constant irrigation and repeated dressings of the open method employed in the first war, although he was compelled to add that "On account of its objectionable smell, it is hoped that it does not remain the final solution to the problem of war wounds in general . . ." Of the special injuries which were seen, he mentioned that "Depth charges are apt to cause rupture of the colon and retroperitoneal hematoma, in men swimming on the surface, and, in ships which have been mined, such curiosities as complete dislocation of the knee, butterfly fractures of the upper end of the femur, and compressed fracture of the spine have been noted." The use of tetanus toxoid had made tetanus uncommon. Sulfanilamide was used by mouth and in the wounds. Shock was treated ". . . by means of rest, warmth, and morphia and transfusion, if necessary." Devitalized muscle and fascia were widely excised, the skin minimally. There was some argument as to how long after wounding it was still worthwhile to debride. Head injuries were treated much as in the first war. Thus far, they had seen relatively few abdominal injuries, "It is manifestly impossible to maintain forward hospitals for an Army falling back. All patients operated before the break-through must be evacuated to the rear, and for the more recently wounded, little more than first aid treatment is possible before evacuation." Nevertheless there had been many successful operations for abdominal wounds in Flanders and at Dunkirk. There was no uniformity among the British as to the treatment of burns. Tannic acid was not satisfactory for the face and hands. The triple-dye,- gentian violet, brilliant green, and acriflavine,- was being used by some, immersion of the burned limb in a water-tight envelope of hypochlorite solution by others, and "The Edinburgh school recommend the application of sulfonamide and glycerin." They had been impressed by the effect of the sulfonamides. He discussed blast injuries and the new entity of crush injury, ". . . characterized by acute renal failure occurring in people who have been trapped under fallen masonry." The renal lesion "resembles that found in cases of incompatible blood transfusion, but occurs without any transfusion . . . It is not clear how much lowered blood volume and diminished renal blood flow or katabolic products, produced by dead or dying tissues, have to do with it."

* * *

Philip D. Wilson, of New York, by invitation, *The Treatment of Compound Fractures Resulting from Enemy Action,* spoke of his experience at the American Hospital in Britain from October 1, 1940 to January 1, 1941 with some 50 air raid casualties. The cases had all been previously treated, generally by the "Orr-Trueta method of closed treatment . . ." If the fracture was well aligned and the patient

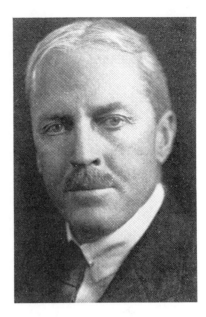

David Cheever, 1876-1955. M.D. Harvard, 1897. Vice-President, 1935; President, 1941. Son of David Williams Cheever (1831-1915) who had been President in 1889, the only other father and son presidencies being those of the Gibbons of Philadelphia. Ultimately Professor of Surgery at Harvard and with John Homans associated from the first with Harvey Cushing and the Peter Bent Brigham, all full time, the first such full-time hospital staff at Harvard.

Portrait courtesy of the Francis A. Countway Library of Medicine, Boston, Massachusetts.

did well nothing more was done. If malalignment, or occasionally fever, required reoperation, ". . . the plaster was removed . . . The cavities were explored, pockets not draining satisfactorily were incised . . . remaining foreign bodies or entirely loose fragments of bone were removed. Cultures from the wound were routinely taken . . . Powdered sulfathiazole was generally introduced locally in doses varying from 3 to 7 Gm., the wound was then packed with vaselined gauze and covered with dry gauze, and a plaster casing reapplied." For maintenance of alignment of the fracture, many of the patients already had pins in the os calcis or tibia, and in others the Americans employed ". . . the Anderson or Haynes systems of machine reduction with the aid of pins inserted in the upper and lower fragment as far away from the wound as possible . . . Under the Orr-Trueta method of treatment, the course of the patients under our care was extraordinarily good. Fever generally subsided in from seven to ten days; thereafter the temperature remained at a normal level, toxic symptoms disappeared, and the appetite improved . . . pain was quite exceptional and when present was always regarded as a sign that something was wrong . . ." The plaster casts were changed at four to six week intervals, usually for softening or loosening of the plaster. There had been ". . . no instance of serious infection about the pins in 28 cases in which the Anderson and Haines methods were employed. The Orr-Trueta method of treatment has taken a firm hold in England and is being widely used. In my opinion, as well as that of many British surgeons of much greater experience, it represents a great advance in the treatment of compound fractures resulting from enemy projectiles over the methods used in the last war. Having had experience with the treatment of similar cases, at that time by the Carrel-Dakin method, I can recall the vast labor required by doctors and nurses to carry out the meticulous technic of those daily dressings and also the pain and horror they caused the patients in spite of the greatest efforts at gentleness . . . What is the secret of the success of the Orr-Trueta treatment? It can only lie in the thoroughness of applying that great surgical principle of rest, which is so frequently disregarded in other methods of wound treatment. Rest favors the walling-off of infection, and the local defensive and reparative forces. The smooth and uniform compression of the extremity by the plaster is also important in preventing the development of edema in the region of the wound and maintains a better circulation in the extremity."

Discussion

Calvin M. Smyth, of Philadelphia, rose to discuss Wilson's paper, pointing out that when he and Doctor [Damon] Pfeiffer ". . . presented this subject before the Association, in 1935, the reception which it was accorded was something less than enthusiastic." However, they had been using the closed method of treatment of compound fracture since 1926 and now had 252 cases of major compound fractures of the long bones, and had been consistently satisfied with it.

* * *

W. E. Gallie, of Toronto, Professor of Surgery, University of Toronto; Surgeon-in-Chief, Toronto General Hospital, who had been Vice-President in 1936, *The Experience of the Canadian Army and Pensions Board with Amputations of the Lower Extremity,* pointed out there was no uniformity amongst the Canadians, the British, and the Americans as to the preference for types of amputations and prostheses. He was speaking only of ". . . the

four principal amputations, namely, the Syme, the midcalf, the Gritti-Stokes, and the midthigh. Our experience with all other amputations has been unhappy." He was well aware of all the arguments, but their experience made them think that ". . . a good Syme is the best of all amputations and if I had the misfortune to have to lose a foot, I would prefer a Syme's operation to all others." He described in detail a technique of maintenance of the position of the Syme's flap and admitted that, "This type of amputation has no place on battlefields or anywhere where there is the slightest risk of infection, or in limbs in which the circulation in the flaps is for any reason impaired." The below-knee amputations were rarely satisfactory, because the side-bearing stump could not bear the constant weight of an active amputee. He mentioned parenthetically that "The old warning against a conical stump does not hold for modern artificial limbs, for a conical shape in these below-knee amputations gives the best chance of a good fitting." It was their practice, if below-knee amputations gave trouble, to convert them to a "Gritti-Stokes type of end-bearing above knee limb." On the other hand, the British ". . . rarely fit a man with an end-bearing limb because, in their experience, such stumps have been painful. I am quite unable to offer any explanation for this . . . on the contrary . . . we are altogether of the opinion that if a workingman must have an amputation anywhere above the level of the Syme, the Gritti-Stokes is the operation of choice." Patients were much more comfortable with the Gritti-Stokes amputation than with amputations in the mid-thigh. Their conclusions were based on 2,448 amputations of the lower extremity.

Discussion

A. B. LeMesurier, of Toronto, strongly supported Gallie's thesis, although he pointed out that whereas the Syme was much better than a mid-thigh amputation, the Gritti-Stokes was only somewhat better than a mid-thigh amputation. "With us the Syme amputation has been excellent and is still excellent, and I think it is about time that something was said in its favor." Colonel N. T. Kirk, of the U.S. Army, said that he had condemned the Syme's amputation until he had seen how well the Canadians performed it, but the American prosthetic makers did not make as good a prosthesis for the Syme as did the Canadians. He could not agree at all to converting a proper below-the-knee amputation to a Gritti-Stokes. This was again a matter of performing the amputation properly, reamputating if necessary, and providing a proper prosthesis. He preferred a supracondylar amputation, as an end-bearing stump, to a Gritti-Stokes. Leo Eloesser, of San Francisco, who supported Kirk, said that "The main trouble with below-the-knee amputations, I think, is the wrangle with the leg maker." The artificial limb had to be made so that the leg did not slip up and down. He pointed out, quite amusingly, that Gritti had proposed his operation because he thought the patella was normally an end-bearing surface, but "We do not kneel on our patellas. We cannot kneel on our patellas unless in kneeling we incline far forward and thrust our thighs far back. Ordinarily, when we kneel, we kneel on our femoral condyles." Nevertheless the operation worked, and he agreed also that "The Syme's or end-bearing stump, I think, is superior to all the other stumps."

* * *

Robert H. Kennedy, of New York, Associate Clinical Professor of Surgery, New York Post-Graduate Medical School, Columbia University; Surgical Director, Beekman Street Hospital, *Present-Day Treatment of Compound Fractures,* emphasized the importance of the immediate application of traction for compound fractures, and debridement as early as possible, rarely after six hours and never after 12. Tetanus antitoxin was given to all cases, always leaving the wound open, using sulfa drugs, and filling the wound with vaseline. The prime requisite was complete immobilization. Skin traction or one-pin skeletal traction did not produce complete immobilization, "A non-padded plaster encasement, with or without internal fixation or two-pin traction, comes nearest to furnishing complete immobilization of the soft parts in order to prevent or allay infection." A window in the plaster interfered with complete immobilization and was to be avoided. Rigid internal fixation or two-pin traction incorporated in plaster permitted mobility of the joints.

Discussion

William Darrach, of New York, agreed in toto, particularly on the importance of rigid immobilization, "Personally, we prefer rigid internal fixation. It is doubtful if that can be carried out in war casualties under many conditions, but it might be done. The nearest approach to that rigid internal fixation is the ideal method, whichever method the individual can best use." J. Albert Key, of St. Louis, said that there was a place for primary closure ". . . if the surgeon who sutures the wound is on the alert

and watches the wound, he can open it up in time to save it. You can shake your heads all you please, but that is true." He was placing both sulfanilamide and sulfathiazole in the same wound, since they were independently soluble.

* * *

Jonathan E. Rhoads, by invitation, William A. Wolff, Ph.D., by invitation, and Walter Estell Lee, of Philadelphia, Professor of Surgery, Graduate School of Medicine, University of Pennsylvania, *The Use of Adrenal Cortical Extract in the Treatment of Traumatic Shock of Burns,* proceeding from the knowledge that ". . . a majority of the fatalities occurred early, within the first three days, and apparently were the result of secondary shock", and because, "Previous studies by other authors have shown that the fundamental cause of this secondary shock is a change in capillary permeability, resulting in the extravasation of a large part of the circulating blood plasma", attempted to "control" the fluid shift by plasma transfusion, which proved not to be as effective as they had calculated it should be. They added to their regimen the administration of ". . . adrenal cortical extract known as Eschatin." Swingle and others had suggested the use of adrenal cortical hormone for shock, and a number of investigators had suggested its use in burns. The Philadelphia group had studied 26 patients with extensive burns. In patients who received plasma only, there was never seen the substantial rise in plasma volume which was seen in those who received adrenal extract as well. They did note "A marked chloride retention . . . in patients receiving adrenal cortical extract."

Discussion

Roy D. McClure, of Detroit, opened the Discussion with a lantern slide of an adrenal gland destroyed by hemorrhage in a burned patient, suggesting ". . . a definite anatomic basis for the treatment advised by Doctor Lee . . ." Alfred Blalock, of Nashville, thought ". . . this is the most convincing evidence as to the effectiveness of adrenal cortical extract that has been offered since the original publication of Heuer and Andrus." [Adrenal extract was widely used in the treatment of burns, for a year or two after this.] He went on to discuss shock, the superiority of plasma or serum over crystalloids in treatment, and the inappropriateness of warming shocked patients, ". . . the blood volume is reduced, in many instances of traumatic shock, very markedly

. . . throughout the body, but more so in the periphery, for the reason that the vital structures, the brain, the heart, the adrenals, need blood very badly, and the proposition that I submit is that it is possible to do harm by trying too vigorously to warm the extremities, unless one at the same time supplements the blood volume by giving plasma and serum or whole blood." Robert Elman, of St. Louis, thought ". . . the evidence presented is most convincing that adrenocortical extract has a therapeutically beneficial effect in the treatment of severe burns by decreasing the amount of plasma necessary to effectively restore the circulation to a safe level . . ." He and McClure both commented that the adrenal extracts contained multiple hormones and varied in effectiveness as received from different manufacturers, "The isolation of the various sterones in the adrenal cortex moreover is handicapped by the fact that all of the adrenals removed from all of the cattle in this country in one year would, it is said, yield only 1000 grams of cortical extract. We must rely therefore upon the synthetic chemist who thus far has produced but few, e.g., desoxycorticosterone."

* * *

Earle B. Mahoney, by invitation, Harry D. Kingsley, by invitation, and Joe W. Howland, by invitation, from the Departments of Surgery and Medicine, University of Rochester, School of Medicine and Dentistry, Rochester, New York, *The Therapeutic Value of Preserved Blood Plasma,* A Summary of One Hundred and Ten Cases, prepared their own plasma, either liquid or lyophilized [plasma had been extensively used for only a relatively short time and the Association obviously felt the Fellows would benefit from the presentation]. They concluded that "Pooled blood plasma may be injected intravenously without regard to blood types . . . The incidence of reactions . . . is 3.5 percent. None . . . severe . . . Plasma is an effective substitute for whole blood in treating peripheral circulatory failure due to trauma, operations, burns, and hemorrhage . . . Plasma is effective in treating temporary hypoproteinemia . . ." And they presented the new data that "Dried plasma retains properties which are effective in treating hemophilia . . . plasma, dried within a few hours after removal from the donor, is effective in treating hemorrhagic disease of the newborn."

* * *

There were papers on *The Medical Department in Naval Warfare,* by Commander Frederick R.

Hook, on *Organization for Evacuation and Treatment of War Casualties,* by Colonel Norman T. Kirk.

Discussion

Commander W. D. Wilcuts, of the U.S. Navy, commented [a remarkable statement, seven months before Pearl Harbor] "We like to think of the Navy as the first line of defense, as being ready. Off the record, may I say that we are ready. We are ready for anything in the western hemisphere; yes, against Japan, against anybody who plays orthodox war. But when we face total war, when we face Europe, it is a different situation." Elliott Cutler's discussion put things in perspective and recounted a little history, "Although I may be one of those who believe that America is about as sound asleep regarding her peril as France was a year and a half before hell broke loose over her, I still think we can take some consolation and feel better after the discussions by the servants of the Federal government this morning. I look back to a trip to visit General Gorgas [the then Surgeon General] in April, 1917, with Doctor Cushing, when the dear old gentleman had to get up ten times in 25 minutes and answer the telephone himself because he did not have a secretary, I look back to the fact that when we arrived in London, in May of 1917, they insisted we go to the American Embassy and get a passport before we could go to France and fight for our country . . . I hope Colonel Kirk will take back with him the idea that we are thoroughly behind him in his work . . . that we realize that the General Staff sometimes does not give to the Medical Department what it wants. We know the months of hard work it took to persuade the General Staff to allow tetanus toxin inoculation of our troops . . . I was a little disappointed in his discussion about front-line work, that he still stuck to the old adage that the Evacuation Hospital had to be a railhead, because I supposed the mobility of modern warfare would leave Evacuation Hospitals anywhere. I recollect being left 25 miles behind a line when we advanced in the last war, and demanding at headquarters that I be moved up with the troops because the sick were dying in the ambulances before they got 25 miles down the line to the hospital, and being told that the big black book of the Medical Department insisted that the Evacuation Hospital had to be on the railhead. I said, 'But the troops are going to Berlin, General. Can't I go with them?' He answered: 'No, you will stay on the railhead.' " Cutler gave Colonel Kirk a little advice, "We should have a new stream-lined sterilizer made out of the best modern, light materials, not the heavy apparatus we had in the last war . . . The next important thing up the line is power. We ought to have a better thing than the old Delco motor, which will run the roentgenologic department and will amply light the field units. Third, and perhaps almost more important, is a laundry. You cannot run an hospital up the line if you need 12,000 sterile towels a day, unless you can wash them. That was forgotten in the last war . . . If the medical profession of America is given the tools, they will see this show through very well."

* * *

The taking of Thiersch grafts had been revolutionized two years before by the description of a new instrument, and Earl C. Padgett, of Kansas City, Missouri, Associate Professor of Clinical Surgery, University of Kansas School of Medicine, *Skin Grafting and the "Three-Quarter"-Thickness Skin Graft for Prevention and Correction of Cicatricial Formation,* presented the results of his experience with his dermatome since January 1938. He thought that the thicker grafts which could be uniformly obtained with a dermatome,- he called them "three-quarter"-thickness grafts,- were better than the usually thinner grafts that were obtained when cut free-hand. He cut his grafts 0.008 to 0.012 of an inch in thickness. The grafts were sutured to the skin with running silk sutures, and if more than one graft was applied in a large granulating area, the grafts were sutured to themselves "in quilt-fashion". Grafts were punctured in "pie-crust fashion" to allow the escape of serum, "A thick roller gauze dressing saturated in boric acid solution is then snugly applied. Above this, cotton pads are laid to hold the moisture . . . This gauze dressing is kept saturated for four days." Afterwards the dressing was changed daily until the graft had healed.

Discussion

Robert H. Ivy, of Philadelphia, and Jerome P. Webster, of New York, were unstinting in their praise of the dermatome. Ivy,- "Doctor Padgett has undoubtedly made one of the lasting contributions to plastic surgery, and his report clearly demonstrates that he is able to obtain results with it that are superior to free-hand methods of skin grafting." Webster,- "Doctor Padgett has definitely added a new principle to the procedure of removing large areas of skin from the body." The grafts could be of uniform thickness and taken from portions of the

body not readily used for free-hand graft cutting. Vilray P. Blair, of St. Louis, concurred,- "I think the dermatome is one of the very, very few really new and useful things that have recently been added to the armamentarium for operative surgery. That combination of a rocking plane and the glue is, as far as I know, something new."

* * *

Peter Heinbecker, of St. Louis, Associate Professor of Surgery, Washington University, and Wesley A. Barton, by invitation, *An Effective Method for the Development of Collateral Circulation to the Myocardium,* reported their technique for producing collateral circulation to the myocardium by the instillation into the pericardium with a grease gun of a mixture of gelatin, aleuronat, starch, glycerin, and water, which was "semi-liquid" at room temperature. Preliminary preparation of this kind permitted six of 14 animals to survive when the anterior descending and left circumflex arteries were ligated four to 12 weeks later. All control animals died. If the heart was surrounded with cellophane after the injection of the irritating material, all animals died after subsequent ligation of the anterior descending and left circumflex branches of the left artery. They pointed out that the vascular bed in the pericardium was not sufficient to provide a really effective collateral circulation. That required ". . . an extrinsic source, and this should contain extrinsic blood vessels in which a high arterial pressure exists." They suggested that this experimental pericarditis might produce sufficient collateral to relieve the degree of myocardial ischemia which caused angina. They discussed the application to man but had not undertaken it. They did indicate that "Experiments are now in progress to determine whether or not an island of retrosternal tissue, with the internal mammary arteries running to it, can be successfully displaced and grafted to the pericardium."

* * *

Cameron Haight, by invitation, and Henry K. Ransom, of Ann Arbor, Associate Professor of Surgery, University of Michigan Medical School, *Observations on the Prevention and Treatment of Postoperative Atelectasis and Bronchopneumonia,* stressed the fact that "The presence of bronchial secretions, and the decreased pulmonary ventilation and cough efficiency subsequent to operation are vitally important factors in the genesis of postoperative atelectasis and bronchopneumonia." They stressed voluntary coughing as the "most important single measure in

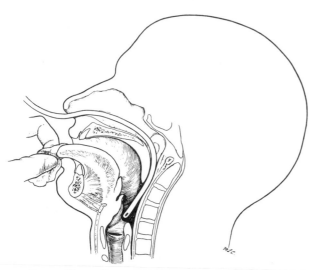

Fig. 7.—Diagram illustrating method for introduction of catheter into trachea. Tongue pulled forward to raise epiglottis, thereby opening passageway for catheter.

Haight and Ransom emphasized the importance of aspirating bronchial secretions retained because of the patient's inadequate cough. The catheter could be passed into the large bronchi and catheter aspiration was ". . . particularly applicable when repeated aspirations are required, perhaps at hourly or two-hourly intervals . . . The patient is placed in the semi-Fowler position, the neck is flexed slightly and the tongue is pulled forward by the operator in order to elevate the epiglottis. The catheter is then introduced through the nose . . . directed posteriorly until the operator feels it touching the larynx. The catheter is then withdrawn 1 or 2 cm . . . and the patient is asked to take a quick deep breath. The catheter is then quickly advanced into the trachea during deep inspiration."

Cameron Haight and Henry K. Ransom, *Observations in the Prevention and Treatment of Postoperative Atelectasis and Bronchopneumonia.* Volume LIX, 1941.

the prevention and treatment of postoperative atelectasis and bronchopneumonia", helping the patient to support the incision while he coughed, employing moderate doses of opiates to release the pain which discouraged coughing, the use of a moist atmosphere, and emphasized the importance of tracheal suction either by bronchoscopy or nasotracheal catheter. As for the cause, "The available evidence suggests that the incidence of atelectasis and bronchopneumonia is not importantly influenced by the anesthetic agent." They agreed with D. F. Jones and W. L. McClure as to ". . . the influence of the transverse upper abdominal incision in reducing the incidence of postoperative complications. As the transverse incision is in the plane of the muscular and aponeurotic fibers of the external and internal

oblique and transversus abdominis muscles, the pull of these respiratory muscles during costal excursion tends to approximate and relax the wound rather than to exert tension upon it, as with the vertical incision."

Discussion

Elliott C. Cutler, of Boston, had had several thousand consecutive operative patients studied by daily vital capacities from the time of admission to the time of discharge. "The reduction [in vital capacity] varies from a median decrease around 59 to 60 per cent for the epigastrium to practically nothing for the extremities; this correlates, almost exactly, with the incidence of pulmonary complications as a whole." He attributed this to painful respiration. Seeking a long-lasting local anesthestic to eliminate wound pain he used ". . . eucupin with oil . . . In a limited number of patients having upper abdominal incisions . . . the reduction in vital capacity is about one-half of that in similar patients, similarly operated upon by the same surgeon, when eucupin is not employed to block the field." They had not yet found an ideal local anesthetic agent for the purpose, but Cutler went on to say that "The chief gift of this paper today . . . seems to me to be this ingenious idea of using such a simple method in the wet, blue patient, as the instillation of a catheter into the trachea; and adequate instructions on how to do this have been given. Most of us, I am sure, suck out the mouth, but the addition of tracheal suction will do much." Walter Estell Lee, of Philadelphia, marveling ". . . of six and one-half- and seven-hour operations, such as Doctor Lahey reported recently . . ." made the appeal "that we should not postpone Doctor Haight's suggestion of tracheal drainage until the signs of bronchial obstruction appear postoperatively, but that routine measures in the form of hyperventilation, with oxygen under pressure, during the operation, and that aspiration of excessive amounts of tracheal secretion at the close of the operation and before the patient leaves the operating table should be practiced routinely." By these measures, they had strikingly reduced the frequency of the necessity for bronchoscopic aspiration.

* * *

Arthur W. Allen, of Boston, Lecturer in Surgery, Harvard Medical School; Chief of the East Surgical Service, Massachusetts General Hospital, and by invitation, Claude E. Welch, *Gastric Ulcer, The Significance of This Diagnosis and Its Relationship to Cancer,* rightly said that *"Gastric and Duode-*

nal Ulcer have been discussed so frequently under the general heading of 'Peptic Ulcer' that a serious confusion has resulted regarding the proper management of these two distinct entities." In the preceding decade they had seen 277 patients with the original diagnosis of gastric ulcer. Of them 14% turned out to have cancer. One hundred-seventy five had been treated medically, and 7.4% of those had cancer. Twenty-three patients had gastro-enterostomy, and 17% of those proved to have cancer. Sixty-nine had resections, under the impression that it was for ulcer, and 43% of them proved to have cancer. They concluded that "Gastric ulcer is, fundamentally, a surgical lesion. This is the direct antithesis of our present concept regarding duodenal ulcer. Gastric ulcer cannot be distinguished from cancer in a high percentage of cases. The gastric cancers that simulate gastric ulcer comprise an especially favorable group for cure. On this basis alone, surgery should be the treatment of choice." They had a five-year 20% cure rate in all cases of gastric cancer, but if they selected out those with a preoperative diagnosis of ulcer, the five-year cure rate was 40%. The mortality from resection for ulcer which proved to be benign had been 6% in 53 cases on the ward service; zero in 36 of their own cases, and in the 51 survivors they had had only two patients with recurrent symptoms. "This is worthy of note when we consider the morbidity frequently associated with prolonged conservative treatment . . . we feel that the results of proper surgery for gastric ulcer justify that form of therapy."

Discussion

Ralph Colp, of New York, was in full agreement based on the Mount Sinai experience. Waltman Walters, of Rochester, Minnesota, indicated that their diagnostic error was only 10%, but did mention the possibility that a malignant ulcer followed radiologically might appear to heal for a time. Their mortality for partial gastrectomy for gastric ulcer in 89 cases was 2.2% in 1939. They had one death in 88 cases in 1940. Allen had performed his Billroth II anastomosis with a posterior gastroenterostomy and Walters agreed and thought this was the commoner practice ". . . abroad, where many more resections have been performed for duodenal ulcer and the posterior method has proved the method of choice." Fordyce B. St. John, of New York, likewise supported Allen, as did Roscoe R. Graham, of Toronto.

* * *

The paper of John H. Gibbon, Jr., of Philadelphia, Surgeon to the Pennsylvania Hospital [the first before the Association of this future President], and by invitation, Clare C. Hodge, *Aseptic, Immediate Anastomosis following Resection of the Colon for Carcinoma,* is of interest chiefly because of the careful description of the development of colon surgery, the discussion of the mortalities in 1941 and the practice of major clinics and hospitals at the time. They reported 24 resections with an aseptic anastomosis ". . . by the Kerr basting-stitch method . . .", three hospital deaths, 13%; and nine patients, 38%, living and well; 14 exteriorization operations, four deaths, 29%, and four living and well, 29%; and 21 open anastomoses with eight hospital deaths, 38%; four living without metastasis, 19%; and strongly preferred ". . . aseptic, immediate anastomosis", from this experience, supported by the recent reports of MacFee [Volume LV, 1937], of Wilkie [1934 and 1939 *Lancet*], and of Stone and McLanahan [*JAMA,* 1939].

Discussion

William B. Parsons, of New York, commented that at the Presbyterian Hospital when resection of the right colon was performed, the mortality without the use of the Miller-Abbott tube was 22%, and with its use was 6.7%. Richard B. Cattell, of Boston, rose to defend the Lahey Clinic's practice of exteriorization resection, "Since 1929, but one case has had a primary resection, with aseptic anastomosis. The rest have all been operated upon in two stages, and 90 percent of all resections by a modified Mikulicz plan." There had been 275 such operations with a 13% mortality and a 53.6% survival without recurrence, of those followed over five years. They thought that the exteriorization principle permitted a great extension of operability. Harry H. Kerr, of Washington, D.C., compared 68 resections by the open method with 39 by his basting-stitch technique. For the open method, the immediate mortality was 35%, for the basting-stitch technique it was 15%. "I do not think there is any question that the profession has accepted the idea that direct end-to-end anastomosis is the most physiologic and the preferred operation for resection, and I do not doubt that the Miller-Abbot tube, and possibly the sulfanilamide groups, will further reduce our mortality." Warfield M. Firor, of Baltimore, [who the year before had reported the use of Sulfanilylguanidine for preoperative bowel preparation] said that in six cases after the Mikulicz procedure as the result of Sulfanilylguanidine ". . . the bacterial count has fallen to an insignificant number. We have felt justified, therefore, in performing an end-to-end anastomosis and replacing the intestine in the peritoneal cavity, thereby shortening the period that is required for closing the bowel in the ordinary Mikulicz operation." Leo Eloesser, of San Francisco, with his usual good sense, suggested that "It may be best to treat carcinomata with obstruction by resection, and exteriorization of the afferent loop, and those without obstruction by resection and immediate anastomosis." He had recently been using the invagination anastomosis [but failed to mention that the first successful entero-anastomosis ever made in a human, by Ramdohr early in the eighteenth century, had been by this technique].

* * *

Warfield M. Firor, of Baltimore, Associate Professor of Surgery, Johns Hopkins Medical School [he was acting Chairman of the Department at the time], and by invitation, Edgar J. Poth, *Intestinal Antisepsis, with Special Reference to Sulfanilylguanidine,* had a few months earlier presented their work on intestinal antisepsis with this poorly absorbed sulfonamide, before the Southern Surgical Association, and now presented a report of their further experience. It took a dose of 0.5 Gm. per kilogram body weight per day, divided into four-hourly doses to produce a uniform and dramatic reduction in the count of coliform drugs in the stool. The drug was much less effective when there was an ulcerative lesion. E. K. Marshall had found that the drug was in fact absorbed from the intestinal tract but almost immediately excreted in the urine. Their paper was devoted entirely to their experimental evaluations and said almost nothing of their clinical results. They had seen only mild toxic reactions in their patients but warned against administering the drug to patients with serious renal disease.

Discussion

Harvey B. Stone, discussing, expressed uncertainty. He had used the drug in preparing some "25-odd cases" for operation upon the large bowel. There were no deaths in the series, but ". . . it is not at all unusual to run a series of 25 cases with the ordinary preoperative preparation, lacking sulfanilylguanidine, without a fatality . . ." He had seen one severe febrile reaction with tachycardia, coma and cyanosis in a patient who recovered within 24 hours. Firor went no farther, in reply, than to say ". . . we do not think sulfanilylguanidine has great merit of its own, and . . . its chief value is that it points the way to a new approach for making surgery of the large bowel safer."

* * *

In many ways, one of the most remarkable reports to appear in the *Transactions* was that by I. S. Ravdin, of Philadelphia, Harrison Professor of Surgery, University of Pennsylvania, School of Medicine; Director, Harrison Department of Surgical Research, and by invitation, Francis C. Wood, *The Successful Removal of a Saddle Embolus of the Aorta, Eleven Days after Acute Coronary Occlusion.* The patient was a 32-year-old physician who had suffered a myocardial infarct and on the eleventh day had an obvious saddle embolus of the aorta. The operation was performed under local anesthesia by Ravdin, "Dr. J. H. Gibbon, Jr. measured the blood which was lost during the operation and controlled the rate of flow and amount of blood which the patient received . . . In order to expedite matters, assistants were arranged for each side—Drs. J. E. Rhoads and W. D. Frazier for the right side, and Drs. N. E. Freeman and K. A. Zimmerman for the left." The femoral arteries were secured in the groin, incised, and cleared with "A modified Babcock veinstripper . . ." and then suction exerted by "A specially prepared catheter, the tip of which had been removed and the end carefully smoothed . . ." The emphasis of the report was on heparin, "Just as the suture line in the right femoral artery was nearing completion, 5,000 units of heparin (Connaught Laboratories) were introduced intravenously . . . After the last arterial suture was placed, an additional 5,000 units of heparin were given . . . Shortly following the operation, Dr. Norman E. Freeman did a left paravertebral injection with 1 per cent novocain." Intravenous heparin was continued for 11 days, the Lee-White coagulation time varying from 14 minutes to one hour and 13 minutes. There was some coldness of the dorsum of the left foot, "Evidently a small embolus had escaped below the site of exposure of the artery. Suction and pressure therapy employed at intervals on this extremity under the direction of Dr. Hugh Montgomery." In spite of the brilliant success of the operation, Ravdin seemed very nearly to be apologizing for it, "Because of the extent and intensity of the ischemia in the lower half of the body of the patient we have just reported, it is our belief that adequate circulation would not have been reestablished without embolectomy. However, three subsequent experiences with major arterial obstruction of the lower extremities have shown us that embolectomy is not always necessary. The use of three conservative measures: (1) Heparin to prevent distal propagation of a thrombus; (2) paravertebral sympathetic block to relieve vascular spasm distal to the arterial obstruction; and (3) suction and pressure therapy to promote circulation in the affected extremity [the Pavaex boot], will bring about a satisfactory result in a certain proportion of these patients." [A particular interest in this case is the fact that the patient was Dr. John Lockwood, whose subsequent and distinguished career in investigative surgery, at Columbia Presbyterian and Memorial Hospitals in New York, was cut short by his death from heart disease ten years after the embolectomy.]

The Business Meetings

The last meeting before U.S. entrance into the war was held April 28, 29, and 30, 1941, at The Greenbrier, White Sulphur Springs, West Virginia, President David Cheever, of Boston, in the Chair.

The Recorder reported an increasing demand for the *Transactions* including that from the Latin American countries.

William J. Mixter reported for The Committee on National Preparedness of the Association that they had offered their services "to the Surgeon-General of the Army who acknowledged our interest and stated that he would use the Committee when the occasion arose." [The same "don't call me, I'll call you" which Dr. Finney had received when he offered similar services to the Surgeons-General for World War I.]

At the Executive Session on the third day, the dues were raised to $25 "due to the loss of dues from the operation of the rule that active fellows are placed automatically on the senior list at the age of 60 years . . ." The Council still required that manuscripts be submitted to the Recorder a month before the meeting to permit early publication in the Annals. The Council recommended "that the American Surgical Association approve in principle the plan proposed by the Health and Medical Committee of the Federal Security Agency to insure continuing and free flow of graduates from our medical schools during the present crisis, to the end that the need of the community and of the armed forces for trained personnel shall not suffer by operation of the Selective Service requirements."

Dr. Irvin Abell, of Louisville, a member of The Committee on National Preparedness, reported that between 4,500 and 9,000 medical officers would be needed annually to replace those completing their one year of military service, that the Medical Reserve Corps would be exhausted as the source of such replacements by 1942, leaving graduates of medical schools as the only source for the continu-

ing supply of medical officers. Of the 5,000 graduates a year, 3,500 might be expected to qualify for military service in the Medical Reserve Officers National Training and Service Program. Drafting medical students as enlisted men would disrupt their medical training and after one year's such service would render them ineligible for draft as physicians after graduation. The Navy had granted commissions as Provisional Ensigns to juniors and seniors in medical school. The Medical Department of the Army had been denied corresponding authority, and in any case, this would not have satisfied the need. ". . . though it may be possible to secure deferment through Selective Service for some medical students, the provision of a continuing supply of essential professional personnel for the armed forces should not be dependent upon the understanding of these needs by 6,000 local Selective Service boards." The Selective Service Act of 1940 did not "provide for deferment or exemption of special groups (other than divinity students and ministers of the gospel) except as individuals", in special cases.

The Health and Medical Committee of the F.S.A. was recommending to the "Co-ordinator of Health, Welfare and other Activities", the presentation to the Secretary of War and Secretary of the Navy of an "offer of appointment, to all physically qualified male students of the first two years in approved medical schools, as Medical Cadets in the Army or as Medical Midshipmen in the Navy . . . to continue only during the period of good standing in the school . . . The commissioning of these Medical Cadets and Medical Midshipmen, on successful completion of the first two years of medicine, as Second Lieutenants in the Medical Administrative Corps . . ." and their commissioning as First Lieutenants or Lieutenants, (j.g.) at the successful completion of the medical school course and ordering them to duty thereafter, only as interns in an Army or Navy Hospital after a year's civilian internship. The medical student could apply for such a commission or could continue under the Selective Service Act risking the draft and a term in the Army or Navy as an enlisted man.

Officers elected were Harvey B. Stone, of Baltimore, President; Loyal Davis, of Chicago, First Vice-President; Daniel C. Elkin, of Atlanta, Second Vice-President; and Charles G. Mixter, of Boston, Secretary.

Among the 16 men elected to Fellowship were Amos R. Koontz, of Baltimore; Charles B. Puestow, of Chicago; Jacob Fine, of Boston; Idys Mims Gage, of New Orleans; and Harold W. Wookey, of Toronto.

LX

1942

In this wartime issue, (as in 1943, 1944, 1945, 1946 and 1947) the *Transactions* were obviously not separately printed, and appear to be simply a rebinding of the Association's papers as published in the June 1942 and October 1942 numbers of the *Annals of Surgery,* and bound with the list of officers, members, etc., of the Association. The pagination is that of the *Annals.* At least one paper by a non-member, and certainly not given at the meeting of the Association, a report of a rectosigmoidal biopsy forceps, appears in this volume of the *Transactions.*

* * *

The 1942 meeting of the Association was held in Cleveland, April 6, 7 and 8.

President Harvey B. Stone, of Baltimore, Associate Professor of Surgery, Johns Hopkins Medical School, *The Defense of the Human Body against Living Mammalian Cells,* found his most cogent arguments in the 1924 paper of Emile Holman on isografting of skin, "Holman doubts that crossgrafts of human skin are ever successful, finds that taking grafts from donors of the same blood group as the host makes little difference in the generally poor results, and attributes these results to the chemical differences between the tissues of host and graft. He thinks the grafts serve as sources of foreign protein intoxication, and lead to the development of a reaction like anaphylaxis. He further cites observations that suggest that this reaction is highly specific against the donor tissue causing it, and does not affect grafts from another donor, which, however, soon develop their own specific destructive chemical reaction." Stone suggested that the clue to the body's tolerance of its own abnormal cells,- cancer cells,- might be found in "an understanding of the defense of the body against alien mammalian cells." He asked whether the rejection of isografts was "mediated through the circulating body fluids or is it a property of the host cells, or do both cells and fluids take part in it? . . . Is it specific against the type of grafted tissue alone, or is it equally effective against all tissues of the donor animal?" He returned to the subject of his 1934 (Volume LII) paper on the use of cultured donor cells grown in the future recipient's serum, stating only that they had now had some clinical success and that others had had mixed results. Aside from the statements that "We hear much these days of military matters. There is a certain analogy between the methods of scientific attack and military offensive", he made no mention of the World War that was going on.

* * *

The Presidential Address is followed in the *Transactions* by the report of Colonel Frederick Rankin, M.C., of Lexington, Kentucky, on *Activities of the Division of Professional Service,* Under the Supervision of the Surgeon-General of the U.S. Army. The Surgeon-General's office had recognized the im-

844

portance of special training and had "adopted a policy of commissioning . . . men in grades commensurate with their age, training, and professional capacity." Whereas previously all first appointments in the Medical Corps were made in the grade of First Lieutenant, men below the age of 37 might now be considered for the grade of Captain or Major by virtue of special evidence such as "Certification by an American Specialty Board . . . fellowship in the American Colleges of Surgery or Medicine . . . membership in other recognized specialty societies or associations . . . training equivalent to that required for examination by an American Specialty Board . . .other recognized training . . ." [At least one future Fellow completing nine years of residency training, having completed Part I of the Boards and with a completed application to the College was commissioned a First Lieutenant.] Rankin assured the Fellows that "there is every indication of a real desire to utilize professional men in professional capacities to a maximum extent, and of avoiding, insofar as possible, pitfalls which developed in a similar rapid expansion during World War I." He mentioned "A striking example of modern medical efficiency in war . . . as demonstrated in the Pearl Harbor engagement, an account of which most of you have had from Doctor Ravdin and Doctor Perrin Long." Rankin spoke in generalities and said nothing about the organization of surgical services in the Army, of the numbers of men that might be required, of the effects upon the medical schools, hospitals and civilian practice, except to urge "upon medical men everywhere the fact that tolerance and patience be a part of their credo, which must recognize certain inevitable dislocations of life and methods in such times of emergency."

* * *

The war, and particularly the large number of burn casualties at Pearl Harbor, had stimulated interest in burns and a symposium took place at the 1942 meeting. It was opened by Vinton E. Siler (by invitation) and Mont R. Reid, of Cincinnati, Professor of Surgery, College of Medicine, University of Cincinnati; Director of Surgical Services, Cincinnati General and Children's Hospitals, *Clinical and Experimental Studies with the Koch Method of Treatment of Heat Burns.* In their application of the treatment of Sumner L. Koch, of Chicago, under general anesthesia, the burned area was washed with soap and water, necrotic skin and blisters removed, and a vaseline gauze pressure dressing applied. They stressed the importance of immediate administration of intravenous fluids through an ankle cut-down and

if no peripheral vein could be found, "one is certainly justified in giving intrasternal plasma transfusion, a route sometimes forgotten." [L. M. Tocantins and J. F. O'Neill, of Philadelphia, had for the previous two years been vigorously espousing intramedullary infusions.] Using the capillary hematocrit,- ". . . very rapid, required much less blood, and is, we believe, more accurate than other methods generally employed . . . for determining the hemoconcentration . . .",- they concluded that "primary pressure dressings may reduce the loss of plasma at the site of, and into the surrounding tissues of, burned areas . . . hemoconcentration may be delayed and perhaps is less severe." In dogs, "The drop of plasma proteins was definitely less". Their patients suffered much less than patients treated by any other method they had employed. They were just beginning to study the use of sulfonamides. They had 37 patients with burns of more than 30% and five deaths, all with burns of 40% or more. Four of the deaths occurred three to 12 hours after admission and one two weeks after admission from pneumonia, empyema, and pericarditis.

Discussion

Wilder G. Penfield, of Montreal, had been in Great Britain looking at the Canadian and British wounded and agreed that "burns are the outstandingly important problem." He reminded the Association that for civilian and military burn injuries in large numbers "what is needed is not a council of perfection in the treatment of burns. What is needed is standardized, simple methods which could be used by a man in a dressing station who has 5 or 50 burns to treat at once, methods that can be used in hospitals that might have to treat hundreds of them." Sumner L. Koch, of Chicago, said that, at the Children's Surgical Service of the Cook County Hospital, they had treated 485 hospitalized patients with severe burns, 19 deaths, 3.9% mortality, but did not state the extent of the "severe" burns. He thought their closed pressure dressing technique was applicable to the care of large numbers of burn patients under emergency conditions and recommended that they "apply over the open wounds an oily dressing containing a sulphonamide, such as was used by Dr. Dragstedt, and his associates, at the University of Chicago, a compression dressing and splint could be quickly added, and the patient evacuated." Leo Eloesser, of San Francisco, California, asked of obvious third degree burns, "Could they not be treated like other wounds . . . by early debridement and an attempt to convert what is certain to become a more or less septic wound into a surgi-

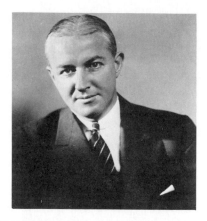

Reginald H. Smithwick (c. 1940), 1899-, M.D., Harvard, 1925. Trained East Service, Massachusetts General Hospital. His contributions to surgery of the sympathetic nervous system, for Raynaud's disease, hypertension, etc., led to his move from Instructor in Surgery at Harvard, to private practice, to Professor and Chairman of the Department at Boston University.

(Portrait courtesy of Charles W. Robertson, M.D., Boston, Massachusetts)

cally aseptic wound. I think perhaps if we could debride third degree burns, especially of the hands and face, early, and immediately skin graft these surfaces we know are doomed to destruction, perhaps the complications which we have been discussing this morning might be avoided."

* * *

W. A. Altemeier (by invitation) and B. N. Carter, Associate Professor of Surgery, University of Cincinnati; Assistant Director of Surgical Service, Cincinnati General Hospital, *Infected Burns with Hemorrhage,* were speaking of the constant loss of blood from infected burn surfaces. They found the application of zinc peroxide to the wounds was effective in controlling the infection and stopping the bleeding, in association with debridement and cleansing.

Discussion

Frank L. Meleney, of New York, rose to discuss the use of the activated zinc peroxide which he had proposed for mixed anerobic infections. He had had similar and somewhat less dramatic experiences in controlling chronically infected wounds.

* * *

Reginald H. Smithwick, of Boston, Instructor in Surgery, Harvard Medical School; Assistant Visiting Surgeon, Massachusetts General Hospital, *Experiences with the Surgical Management of Diverticulitis*

of the Sigmoid, found in the literature, a mortality from diverticulitis of 23.7% for acute perforation, 9.3% for abscesses, and 18.9% for vesical fistulae. The mortality for resection by all techniques was 17%, varying from 11.5% for Mikulicz resection, to 26.3% for one-stage resections with primary anastomosis. In 42 cases from the Massachusetts General Hospital, treated in any way except by resection, there was an immediate mortality of 4.8% and a subsequent death from disease of 12.5%, almost half the patients being considered not well. In 33 resections of the sigmoid at the Massachusetts General Hospital, there was an immediate mortality of 6%, no late mortality, and only 12% of the patients were considered not well. At the Massachusetts General Hospital, the mortality from exteriorizing operations was 13.3%, all the deaths being in the Mikulicz operations, none in Hartmann operations. In 18 primary anastomoses, there were no deaths and there had usually been a prior transverse colostomy or a cecostomy. Smithwick was convinced that cecostomy was ineffective in protecting anastomoses, and transverse colostomy exceedingly effective. He made the valid comment that "There appears to be no contraindication to removing more than the involved segment of bowel. This should place the point of anastomosis in more favorable territory. It would tend to reduce the number of residual diverticula and perhaps the statistical chance of recurrence." He recommended against resection during the acute stage of the disease, and warned of the occasional difficulty in differentiating between carcinoma and diverticulitis. Finally, "Resection of the involved segment of the bowel appears to offer patients suffering from the more severe and complicated forms of diverticulitis the greatest hope for improvement. If carefully planned, the mortality should be low, serious complications few, and unsatisfactory late results infrequent."

Discussion

The Discussion of Henry W. Cave, of New York, indicates the state of colon surgery at the time, "Doctor Smithwick has resected the sigmoid in 33 individuals, with a relatively low mortality rate of 17.1 per cent, considering the nature of the disease. And, in a group of 12 of 33 resections, he had a surprisingly low mortality of 6.1 percent . . . this group of 12, resected because of recurrent attacks of diverticulitis, is one of the principal features of his splendid presentation." [Cave misquoted Smithwick whose mortality in the 33 resections was 6.1%. Presumably since, in any case, Cave had praised the results, Smithwick did not correct him.] Richard B. Cattell, of Boston, without citing any numbers, stated that in diverticular disease they operated only for "complications of inflammation, and . . . most important, the indication of obstruction." For suspected abscess, they delayed until the abscess pointed and usually ignored the abscess and performed a transverse colostomy. They never performed a primary resection if they knew they were dealing with diverticulitis.

* * *

A symposium on thoracic surgery was opened by André Cournand, by invitation, and Frank B. Berry, of New York, Assistant Clinical Professor of Surgery, Columbia University; Director of Chest Surgical Division, Bellevue Hospital, *The Effect of Pneumonectomy upon Cardiopulmonary Function in Adult Patients*. They had studied 11 pneumonectomy patients, eight of them before and after operation and some with additional studies with respect to thoracoplasty. Their conclusions were that "The chief difference between patients after pneumonectomy and normal subjects was the reduction in their breathing reserve in various states of activity. This reduction caused by a decrease in maximum breathing capacity was greater in the older patients because of the cumulative effect of abnormal hyperventilation . . . The decrease in maximum breathing capacity was not proportional to the loss of lung volume, and was greatly influenced by the state of distention of the remaining lung . . . The late effects of pneumonectomy upon gas exchange in the lungs, the state of respiratory gases in the arterial blood, and the cardiocirculatory function were insignificant . . . A supplemental thoracoplasty in four patients did not impair, further, the ventilatory function; and in some patients was of distinct benefit . . . Overdistention of the remaining lung following pneumonectomy, insofar as it impairs the mechanics of the chest bellows, and reduces the efficiency of gas exchange, is physiologically undesirable."

Discussion

Berry had presented the paper and Dr. Cournand opened the Discussion by saying that they had found results remarkably similar in five children after pneumonectomy. The blood gases returned to normal within a few days, and "Persistent arterial oxygen unsaturation after pneumonectomy recognizes three possible causes: . . . a large bronchopleural fistula . . . distention or compression of the remaining lung . . . The additional risk of anoxia

during a period so fraught with other hazards requires that the variation of oxygen saturation in the arterial blood should be carefully followed [a practice which was not generally adopted for years thereafter]." How regularly contralateral emphysema would develop, they did not yet know, but considered it undesirable, and he remarked "The teleologic concept, that the increase in size of the remaining lung to make up for the loss of the other lung, will bring about functional compensation, is not borne out by physiologic studies." Evarts A. Graham commented that "In my first case . . . when I completed the operation I was alarmed at the huge empty space which remained, and I thought that the only thing to do was a thoracoplasty to obliterate it. Consequently, I at the same time removed seven ribs. The patient made an uneventful recovery, although I removed the remaining three ribs at a subseqent date, about three weeks after the operation . . . when Dr. Rienhoff announced that apparently it was not necessary to obliterate this space by thoracoplasty, my own ideas wavered considerably, and after doing several total pneumonectomies without the performance of thoracoplasty, I decided that probably Dr. Rienhoff was right. Since that time, however, my own mind has wavered a good deal back and forth." He indicated that he thought that, presumably because of the prevention of emphysema, "the patient who has had a pneumonectomy would fare better if he had the space completely obliterated by thoracoplasty", and that perhaps it was best not done at the time of the pneumonectomy because of the anticipated increase in the mortality, and that the decision could be postponed to some time after the pneumonectomy.

* * *

Cournand and Berry's paper was followed by William F. Rienhoff, Jr., of Baltimore, Associate in Surgery, Johns Hopkins University; Instructor in Anatomy, Johns Hopkins Medical School; Visiting Surgeon, Johns Hopkins Hospital, and, by invitation, James Gannon, Jr. and Irving Sherman, *Closure of the Bronchus following Total Pneumonectomy*. This was Rienhoff's complete, scholarly and masterful study, beautifully illustrated largely by Leon Schlossberg, which led to the conclusion that "From this study it seems likely that the main point of healing of the bronchus is at the cut end. Every effort must be made to preserve the viability of this portion, not only by gentle handling, which avoids any form of trauma, such as crushing, cauterization, or suturing, but also by preserving the circulation in the bronchial artery. The greatest attention should

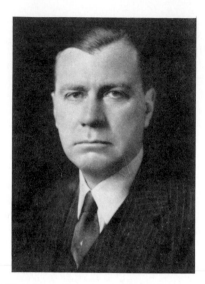

William F. Rienhoff, Jr. (c. 1943), 1894-, M.D. Johns Hopkins 1919, completed surgical residency 1925, always in private practice, ultimately Professor of Surgery. A colorful character and skillful surgeon, Rienhoff first attracted attention with his careful work on the nature of the histologic changes in goiter, particularly nodular. His extensive review with Dean Lewis, of the results at Hopkins with radical mastectomy, may well have been one of the first to recognize the limitations of the radical operation. His first successful pneumonectomy very shortly followed that of Graham. He demonstrated that a complementary thoracoplasty was not required and his histologic studies of the healing of the bronchial stump at once and correctly established the nature of the reparative process and that healing and closure took place at the cut end.

be given to the placing of the occlusion sutures, particularly the number, so that interference with the circulation of the stump will be as little as possible. If the circulation is cut off, the entire end of the cuff distal to the suture line, or at least part of it may slough. Primary agglutination of this open end is thus prevented, so that when any of the occluding sutures give way a bronchial fistula develops at once . . . The use of occluding nonabsorbable sutures is advocated as a means of closing the bronchial tube for a sufficient length of time to permit healing of the cut ends . . . placed as far proximal to the end of the stump as possible and the minimal number of sutures employed to effect an air-tight closure . . . healing of the suture line occurred in only 18 per cent of the experimental animals, a percentage so low that the possibility of such type of healing cannot be regarded as likely in the great majority of instances. The granulation and later fibrous tissue which brings about closure of the cuff-like open end of the bronchial stump is derived mainly from the bronchial walls . . . in the majority of cases the cy-

lindrical open end of the bronchus was filled with a mass or plug of granulation tissue that successfully occluded the stump. The bronchial epithelium grew across the closed end as a modified or somewhat flattened cell-type." In the dog merely sewing the delicate mediastinal pleura over the wide-open end of the main bronchus was sufficient to produce healing in most cases, as secure as that when the bronchus had been closed by sutures and without the infection produced by sutures, so that "the tissue which brought about the final closure of the open end of the bronchus must be considered as being derived mainly from the bronchial walls." Clinically he advocated a sutured bronchial stump closure, tacking the pleura to it. In a series of 48 dogs, there were no operative deaths and no bronchial leaks. [Rienhoff failed to cite Halsted's experimental demonstration (Vol. XXVII, 1909, page 404) that even a ligated bronchus would not heal under the ligature unless the mucosa were crushed or excised.]

Discussion

Appropriately enough, Evarts A. Graham, of St. Louis, opened the Discussion, and agreed that pneumonectomy for carcinoma of the bronchus was going to be more and more utilized and that "securing permanent closure of the bronchus is one of the major problems confronting us . . ." As Rienhoff had said, the clinical problem with the bronchus was greater on the right side than on the left. He had used the same silk mattress sutures that Rienhoff had, but had not realized that they cut through so frequently. He had had difficulty utilizing the gossamer-thin pleura as a flap, but had been persuaded by Dr. Churchill to employ a free pleural graft as well as pedicle flaps from the chest wall pleura with success. The human was different from the dog in the presence of virulent bacteria in the bronchus. He was still championing the thoracoplasty which he had performed in his first and brilliantly successful case. "One way to prevent a serious infection from an open bronchial stump is to do a thoracoplasty at the time of the total pneumonectomy, which will eliminate any pleural cavity to be infected. The dangers of the simultaneous thoracoplasty . . . I have already alluded to . . . if we could do safely a thoracoplasty at the same time as a total pneumonectomy, I do not think the question of closure of the bronchial stump would continue to be anything of major importance." He then set out "to do a little propaganda" on the utility of pneumonectomy for carcinoma, which was being disputed in many quarters. ". . . I have one patient perfectly well and liv-

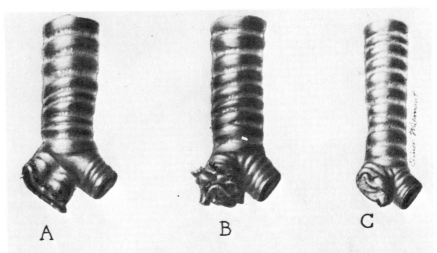

FIG. 9.—Illustration of gross specimens dissected at autopsy, showing three distinct types of healing encountered after suture of the bronchus, as described in the first series of 36 dogs.
A. The conical-shaped bronchus that has healed as it was sutured at operation.
B. The sutures have cut through the wall and the open end is healed with a fibrous tissue mass. Sutures may be seen to lie in the peribronchial tissue.
C. Sutures have cut through, evidently discharged into the lumen of the bronchus. No evidence of them in the peribronchial tissue. Walls of bronchus completely separated and cut end of stump healed over by membranous sheet of tissue.

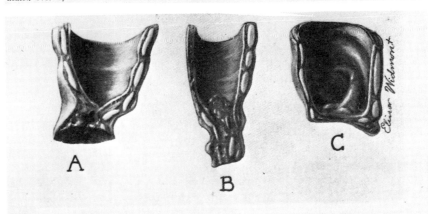

FIG. 10.—Cross-section of gross specimens, shown in Fig. 9, A, B and C.
A. Bronchus healed as sewn at operation.
B. Walls of bronchus, separated as a result of cutting of silk sutures and open end healed by the formation of a fibrous tissue plug or mass occluding the lumen. The internal portion of the mass is covered with bronchial epithelium.
C. Sutures have cut through in the lumen, two may be seen. Bronchial walls have separated and the open end has been occluded by a thin membrane stretching between the cut cartilaginous rings. Internal surface of cylindrical end irregular with elevated ridges flanked by depressed areas on either side of ridge.

Rienhoff, with Gannon and Sherman, who were Fellows in the Hunterian Laboratory, at Hopkins, conclusively demonstrated that the mucosa-to-mucosa closure of the bronchus infrequently healed at the level of the sutures [A in both figures], which either cut through one wall [B] or cut through both walls and were discharged into the lumen [C], sufficient healing having taken place by the organization of the fibrin plug at the cut end, that closure remained secure after the sutures had come loose. They provided overwhelming laboratory and clinical evidence to support the thesis.

William F. Rienhoff, Jr., James Gannon, Jr. and Irwin Sherman, *Closure of the Bronchus Following Total Pneumonectomy*, Volume LX, 1942.

ing nine years afterward; another patient six years and five months afterward; another patient five years; five patients, three years; and a very considerable number less than that, who are living and apparently free from any evidence of recurrence of carcinoma . . . good evidence of the fact that the operation is worth while, and that it is essential . . .that we go on and develop to as good a point as possible technical perfection, so that the mortality will be less." He and Dr. [Brian] Blades had performed 76 total pneumonectomies, 59 of them for bronchogenic carcinoma. Since January 1, 1939,

they had done 48 pneumonectomies for bronchogenic carcinoma with 18 hospital deaths—37%, and in 17 non-cancer cases, they had had four deaths, a mortality of 23%. Norman S. Shenstone, of Toronto, showed a slide of his technique of bronchial closure, applying "light Kocher-style . . . forceps . . . as close as possible to the trachea and the cut margins are approximated anteroposteriorly by three interrupted sutures of fine silk supplemented by a running suture of catgut. Following this procedure the stump is powdered with sulphathiazole, displaced into the mediastinum, and finally covered by pleura." They had done 23 consecutive cases, seven of them for carcinoma, and had only one bronchial fistula, in a patient with active tuberculosis. Alton Ochsner, of New Orleans, had had three failures of bronchial closure in 32 pneumonectomies, two of them in patients who had had extensive preoperative irradiation, which he thought a contributing factor. Like Rienhoff, he stressed covering the bronchial stump with pleura. Alfred Blalock, now of Baltimore, apparently rising to be sure Rienhoff had not been misunderstood, stressed the large number of animal experiments which had been performed and added, "I should not have thought previously that one would be able to produce an air-tight closure of the bronchus simply by approximating with several sutures the thin pleura which lies near the end of the divided bronchus. It is obvious that in the case of patients Dr. Rienhoff does not recommend an omission of sutures in the bronchus . . .The importance of this paper to me is that it is a fundamental study in wound healing in which the particular tissue happens to be the bronchus." Frank H. Lahey, of Boston, arose principally to recall the recent paper in the *JAMA* of Dr. Herbert Adams from the Lahey Clinic, reporting cardiac arrest during a lobectomy in which the heart was massaged for 20 minutes, the patient ultimately recovering well, ". . . this accident will happen in thoracic surgery . . . will happen in war surgery, and it is extremely important for us all to remember that it is possible by cooperation between an anesthetist and a surgeon, either with the patient's chest open or through the diaphragm, to manually maintain circulation while efforts are being made to restore cardiac action." Rienhoff, in closing, reemphasized the cardinal points of his technique. He agreed with Dr. Graham that mediastinal pleura might not always be available in patients, but a flap could be dissected from the parietal pleura, "In our recent cases, the last 30 to be exact, of total pneumonectomy in the human, due to a more deliberate and painstaking mobilization of the pleura, we have not experienced any difficulty in being able to close over the raw area of the hilus of the lung with this membrane." As for thoracoplasties, ". . . we have not found it necessary to perform thoracoplasties at the same time or previous to the total pneumonectomy . . . in three cases, when postoperative bronchial fistulae developed resulting in a rather large infected dead space occupying part of the former pleural cavity, it was necessary to perform a posterior thoracoplasty in three stages." He accepted the fact that thoracoplasty was valuable in certain cases of total pneumonectomy, but ventured the prediction that "Ulti-

mately the conclusion will probably be that the majority of human beings who have a total pneumonectomy will not need a thoracoplasty . . ."

* * *

Edward D. Churchill, of Boston, Chief of West Surgical Service, Massachusetts General Hospital; John Homans Professor of Surgery, Harvard University, and, by invitation, Richard H. Sweet, *Transthoracic Resection of Tumors of the Stomach and Esophagus,* divided the esophagus into fourths, the upper and lower fourths and the two middle fourths taken together as one section, from the clinical, pathologic and operative standpoint. In the first phase of the operation, the abdomen was explored and if there were no malignant lymph nodes, a Beck-Jianu gastrostomy was performed, bringing the stoma up above the costal margin. For the second stage, they recommended a long left thoracotomy through the bed of the seventh or eighth rib, transection and inversion of the distal end of the esophagus, often at the cardia, dropping the stomach back into the abdomen. The esophagus was passed behind the aortic arch after being freed "By working now from above, now from below the aortic arch . . ." and brought out in the neck through an incision on the anterior border of the sternomastoid. The esophagus was then divided an ample distance above the tumor and the upper portion brought subcutaneously and sutured to the skin, as low as it would reach on the chest. In the third stage, the two stomata were connected by a skin tube. They had performed nine such esophagectomies; in two patients, the esophageal reconstruction had been completed, one of these was alive with metastases at four years, and one was alive and well at two years. In a third patient, the reconstruction was still incomplete and the patient was well at two years, and the fourth surviving patient was well a year after operation without reconstruction. For carcinoma in the distal fourth, they advocated a ninth-rib resection and thoracotomy, incising the diaphragm from the costal margin to the hiatus, if resection was to be undertaken. They recommended crushing the phrenic nerve. The stomach was transected below the growth and closed, the esophagus amputated at least two or three inches above the cardia, "because the interruption of the left gastric, the vasa brevia, and the inferior phrenic arteries . . . may deprive the segment just above the cardia of an adequate circulation." The end-to-side esophagogastrostomy was done with "the care and nicety accorded the placement of a vermilion border suture in the lip in the most meticulous plastic operation. Interrupted sutures of fine silk are used throughout." The illustrations show a two-layer interrupted suture repair. They performed resection in 13 cases of carcinoma of the distal esophagus or gastric cardia. Two patients with a total gastrectomy died, one of leakage and the other of soiling at the time of operation. A third patient died of auricular flutter after operation. Two of the ten survivors had died of recurrent disease, the remainder being well and symptom-free three months to two-and-a-half months after operation.

Discussion

Dallas Phemister, of Chicago, called these results "perhaps the best that have been reported, and the series is large enough, in itself, to establish transthoracic resection as the best treatment for tumors in these locations." Phemister had resected carcinoma of the esophagus in 12 patients, four out of five patients survived resection of the midportion of the esophagus, three of seven patients succumbed to an operation for carcinoma of the distal esophagus or gastric cardia, and three patients were alive and well nine months, 14 months, and four years and three months, after operation, "The last . . . is the longest survival that I can find." All patients had a one-stage operation. The stomach was brought up as high as was necessary into the apex of the chest or into the neck to reach the esophageal stump. Alton Ochsner, of New Orleans, said that he was "one of the advocates of the right-sided approach, primarily, because I think it is easier to do, and also because . . . one can remove all of the distal portion of the esophagus." Churchill closed the Discussion of the paper, which Sweet had presented. He stressed once more the absolute precision required for the approximation of the mucous membrane in esophagogastric anastomoses. He challenged Dr. Ochsner, "While Doctor Ochsner points out that the entire esophagus can be removed from the right thorax, I wonder if he would also say that the left gastric artery can be ligated at its point of origin and resected with the lymph nodes that run between that point and the cardiac end of the stomach". Churchill and Sweet had not found it necessary to perform a separate laparotomy to mobilize the stomach, " . . . because we find that the exposure through the diaphragm is adequate to carry out a complete total gastrectomy, should the occasion necessitate."

* * *

Undoubtedly, the most important paper given at this meeting, which appears last in the *Transac-*

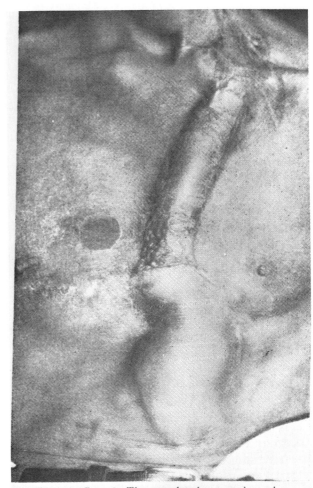

FIG. 4.—Case 6: The completed external esophagus. The prominence opposite the lower portion is caused by the fundus of the stomach.

For tumors of the middle two-fourths of the esophagus, Churchill and Sweet recommended laparotomy, biopsy of the lymph nodes and a Beck-Jianu gastrostomy brought up over the costal margin, and at the second stage, esophagectomy through the left thorax and suture of the proximal healthy cervical esophagus to the chest wall, preferably below the clavicle. In the third stage, the new esophagus was completed with a skin tube. Three out of nine patients were alive and well after esophagectomy; one of them at two years with a completed reconstruction. Another patient with a completed reconstruction was alive, but with metastases, at four years.

Edward D. Churchill and Richard H. Sweet, *Transthoracic Resection of Tumors of the Stomach and Esophagus*, Volume LX, 1942.

tions, was by Charles Huggins, of Chicago, Associate Professor of Surgery, University of Chicago; Attending Surgeon, Billings Memorial Hospital, *Effect of Orchiectomy and Irradiation on Cancer of the Prostate.* Huggins and Hodges had previously shown that prostatic carcinoma "is frequently inhibited by eliminating the testicular androgens by bilateral orchiectomy or by neutralization of androgenic activity by estrogen administration." In the previous 30 months they had treated 45 men with advanced prostatic carcinoma and local infiltration or metastases. All had had bilateral orchiectomy and eight had died, all with extensive metastases to bone. Thirty-one men had a sustained improvement, lasting as long as 30 months, nine had a temporary improvement and five had no improvement following castration. Sometimes the primary tumor decreased strikingly while metastases advanced. In nine men with failure of castration, subsequent estrogen administration by mouth was ineffective. Two patients treated with roentgen radiation of the testis were not benefitted and the Leydig cells were found to be uninjured.

Discussion

Evarts A. Graham, of St. Louis, said he knew nothing about the prostate, but "it would be a pity for such a beautiful presentation as this to go without any discussion". He returned to his thesis of several years ago that the Association had gotten too special, had few but general surgeons in it. It delighted him to point out that Dr. Huggins was one of the specialists who had been elected into the Association as a result of that feeling several years earlier. Graham referred to the fact that "castration for cancer of the prostate is a very old idea". Alfred Blalock rose to give further praise "As a member of the Program Committee." While indeed castration had occasionally been done before, Huggins "demonstrates in this work, I think, the value of a prepared mind" and of his previous scientific training. Of the clinical results, Blalock said, "Having visited in Doctor Phemister's clinic and having seen Doctor Huggins' cases, I can tell those of you who have not seen them that I am sure you will be perfectly amazed. As Doctor Graham has said, if a real contribution is made in cancer in any one field, such as Doctor Huggins has made, at least, it raises our hopes of being able to find out something about cancer in other parts of the body." Huggins, in closing, said "I believe the only person who, knowingly, operated to remove the testes for carcinoma of the prostate was Dr. Hugh Young, who did this in two patients, with negative results. It is unfortunate that his cases apparently were not of that type which responds well. The wave of operations that has been

mentioned for removal of the testes for prostatic conditions, I believe, has been confined otherwise to benign prostatic hypertrophy." [See page 145, Volume XI, 1893, and page 166, Volume XIII, 1895, for the papers of J. William White, of Philadelphia, on castration for hypertrophy of the prostate and the specific reference of Carmalt, of Yale, to carcinoma of the prostate.]

* * *

Herman E. Pearse, of Rochester, New York, Associate Professor of Surgery, University of Rochester, *Vitallium Tubes in Biliary Surgery,* with this presentation stimulated some optimism and considerable activity in the field of biliary reconstruction. In the year since Pearse had presented the technique to the Society of University Surgeons, he had inserted his tubes in a variety of situations in strictures of the biliary and pancreatic ducts. He said nothing about results, complications or recurrences, and indicated that he was planning to use the tubes for malignant strictures.

Discussion

The reaction of Howard M. Clute, of Boston [who had used the tubes], in opening the Discussion, was typical of some of the enthusiastic opinions of the time, "Dr. Pearse's work marks a new era in the management of strictures of the bile duct. He has shown that Vitallium metal tubes can be kept in the common duct for years without harmful results." His own patient with a Vitallium tube in a bile duct stricture had been well two years. Eugene W. Rockey, of Portland, Oregon, had been using metallic magnesium tubes, but thought the Vitallium tube was probably better. Walter G. Maddock, of Ann Arbor, had used the tube in two patients, both of whom had continued to have chills, fever and jaundice.

* * *

Samuel C. Harvey, of New Haven, Connecticut, Professor of Surgery on the William H. Carmalt Foundation, Yale University; Surgeon-in-Chief, New Haven Hospital, and Ashley W. Oughterson, Associate Professor of Surgery, Yale University, *The Surgery of Carcinoma of the Pancreas and Ampullary Region,* had six cases to report, now seven years since Whipple's operation, but the first was a 1932 case with a difficult partial pancreatectomy, and the second, a 1939 case, of a successful transduodenal resection of a carcinoma of the ampulla of Vater by Halsted's technique. The other four were pan-

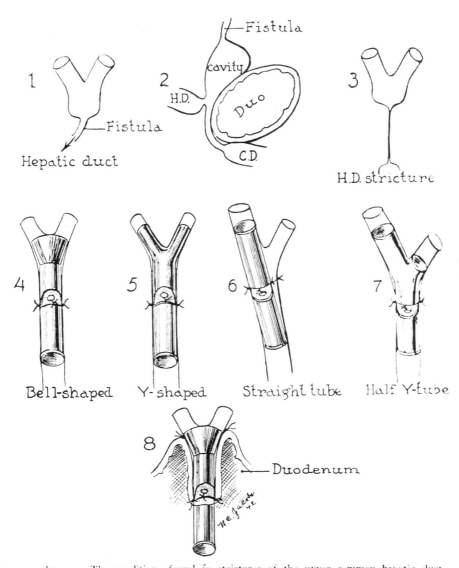

Fistula

Hepatic duct

Fistula

cavity

H.D.

Duo

C.D.

H.D. stricture

4 Bell-shaped

5 Y-shaped

6 Straight tube

7 Half Y-tube

8

Duodenum

FIG. 4.—The conditions found in strictures of the upper common hepatic duct may include an external fistula (1) associated with a functionless common bile duct, a communication with a bile-filled cavity (2) which drains into a fistula and the common duct or, as in (3) a long thread-like channel joining the ends of the ducts.

In 4, 5, 6, and 7, are illustrated the tubes that have been used in high strictures of the common hepatic duct. Here, the inaccessible bifurcation of the hepatic ducts close to the stricture in a short stump of the common hepatic duct creates mechanical problems of management. Zinninger used the bell- or trumpet-shaped tube for hepaticoduodenostomy (8) when the end of the common duct could not be found.

Pearse had presented his Vitallium tubes the year before at the Society of University Surgeons and now had experience with them, for strictures in a variety of locations in the biliary tract and one in the pancreatic duct after a Whipple procedure. While stating that "Injury to the bile ducts which was irreparable by other methods has been successfully treated by the permanent implantation of a Vitallium tube", he gave no figures. The technique was widely and enthusiastically accepted for a few years.

Herman E. Pearse, *Vitallium Tubes in Biliary Surgery,* Volume LX, 1942.

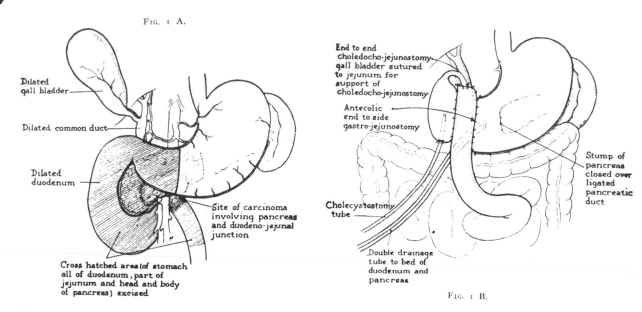

Fig. i A.

Dilated gall bladder

Dilated common duct

Dilated duodenum

Site of carcinoma involving pancreas and duodeno-jejunal junction

Cross hatched area (of stomach all of duodenum, part of jejunum and head and body of pancreas) excised

End to end choledocho-jejunostomy-gall bladder sutured to jejunum for support of choledocho-jejunostomy

Antecolic end to side gastro-jejunostomy

Cholecystostomy tube

Double drainage tube to bed of duodenum and pancreas

Stump of pancreas closed over ligated pancreatic duct

Fig. i B.

Whipple was now persuaded, seven years after his original report, that a one-stage operation was preferable. He had done four two-stage operations with two deaths, and six one-stage operations with one death, had sometimes implanted the stump of the pancreas in the bowel and sometimes simply closed it over as shown in the illustration.

Allen O. Whipple in discussion of Samuel C. Harvey and Ashley W. Oughterson, *The Surgery of Carcinoma of the Pancreas and Ampullary Region,* Volume LX, 1942.

creaticoduodenectomies, with a single operative death from "acute yellow atrophy". The last patient was the only one to have a one-stage operation. The divided surface of the pancreas was closed over in all of them without any attempt at anastomosis. They had two biliary fistulae and two pancreatic fistulae. Three of the four patients with pancreaticoduodenectomy were still alive.

Discussion

Allen O. Whipple, of New York, opened the Discussion. He had been accumulating the figures on the experience around the country, including that of Doctors Harvey and Oughterson, and had records of 64 pancreaticoduodenectomies for a variety of lesions, 41 two-stage operations, 23 one-stage operations, with 20 postoperative deaths overall, 29% mortality for the two-stage operation and 35% for the one-stage operation. There had been 12 biliary fistulae and 18 pancreatic fistulae and two duodenal fistulae. Whipple was able to say, "I am convinced that the one-stage operation, aside from saving the patient two anesthesias, two operations, and very often a very unfortunate delay between the first and second stage . . . avoids the risk, or largely decreases the risk, of the biliary fistula from ligation of the cut end of the common duct by the immediate

anastomosis of the common duct to the loop of jejunum used in the end to side gastrojejunostomy. This is a real advance in the technic and result of the operation." As for the pancreatic stump, he had twice implanted it into the distal opening of the duodenum, once successfully, but the second time resulting in a duodenal fistula, and fatal erosion of a large vessel. Thomas G. Orr, of Kansas City, had previously reported two patients alive 23 and 12 months after operation, and now reported two more, both alive and well. Verne C. Hunt, of Los Angeles, who had reported before the Association the year before four cases of ampullary carcinoma, had since "had occasion to operate upon another similar case, in which I performed a modification of the so-called Whipple radical operation, which makes a total of five cases of ampullary carcinoma that we have successfully operated upon without surgical mortality." Whipple had indicated that Herman E. Pearse, of Rochester, New York, had suggested that it might be safer to use the jejunum rather than the distal duodenum for the reconstruction, and Pearse now said that he had suggested the use of the jejunum "because I excised all the duodenum", and in another case, he had employed the distal duodenum, the circulation of which had been insufficient to support the anastomosis, resulting in a fatal outcome. Oughterson, in closing, said that it was his feeling that the two-stage operation allowed decompression of the liver and improved biliary function, but "I must say Dr. Harvey is rather on the other side."

* * *

Robert Elman, in 1939, had shown the possibility of maintaining nitrogen balance by intravenous administration of casein digest and now Alexander Brunschwig, of Chicago, Professor of Surgery, University of Chicago, and by invitation, Dwight E. Clark, M.D. and Nancy Corbin, M.S., *Postoperative Nitrogen Loss and Studies on Parenteral Nitrogen Nutrition by Means of Casein Digest* [Mead-Johnson], reported their studies on 41 patients with a wide variety of operations from herniotomy to gastric resection and partial colectomy. Clark, Brunschwig, and Corbin had already demonstrated in hypoproteinemic dogs that plasma proteins could be regenerated by the daily intravenous injection of the amino-acid digest. In their control patients, there was always a negative nitrogen balance after operation, depending to a considerable extent upon the patient's normal intake. Casein digest administered intravenously together with proper proportions of glucose was "effective in reducing or even preventing postoperative net loss of nitrogen. Casein digest and glucose intravenously may be employed as the sole source of nutrition, affording at least minimal caloric requirements . . . and . . . an adequate supply of amino-acids to maintain nitrogen equilibrium, or even afford a positive nitrogen balance in patients with depleted protein stores." The reactions to the amigen which they saw were mild, occasionally severe nausea, vomiting, "a generalized disagreeable flushing sensation", decrease in appetite, several patients had severe chills.

Discussion

Owen H. Wangensteen reminded the Association of the contributions of "Doctor Ravdin of this Association" and of George H. Whipple, of Rochester, New York, and of Doctor Robert Elman, of St. Louis. Wangensteen and his associates had shown that nitrogen balance could be maintained by the intravenous injection of human plasma. Brunschwig, in closing, said that jaundice was an absolute contraindication to the use of casein digest in their hands, since each of their three jaundiced patients had severe chills and fever after administration, as had a severe alcoholic, "Apparently the liver, when it is abnormal, cannot cope with a flooding of the circulation by amino-acids, and this reaction results." Brunschwig closed by saying, "It seems sort

of presumptuous to bring up this point again, which has been emphasized by Doctor Wangensteen, namely, that food is important for life, and yet we see patients on surgical wards being given all sorts of vitamins because of the emphasis and the publicity they have received, and yet many of them are starving to death."

* * *

Robert Elman, of St. Louis, Associate Professor of Clinical Surgery, Washington University School of Medicine, and by invitation D. O. Weiner, M.D. and E. Bradley, R.N., *Intravenous Injections of Amino-Acids (Hydrolyzed Casein) in Postoperative Patients*, had studied the use of Mead-Johnson's casein digest Amigen in 312 patients at the St. Louis City Hospital. The only complications were two instances of urticaria, and in 15 patients chills and fever from "pyrogens in some of the distilled water used in its preparation". They had shown in a previous paper that "excellent utilization of the injected material was achieved first because nitrogen retention was marked and persisted even during two weeks of therapy and second, because significant increases of the plasma protein concentration took place." In this study, they were examining patient tolerance and looking for adverse effects in a large series of administrations and did not repeat the studies on the serum proteins. Nevertheless, "from the purely clinical point of view, there was ample evidence of the beneficial, even dramatic, effects of Amigen. In many cases it seemed clear that the addition of the amino-acids to the parenteral glucose, after serious operations, tipped the balance in favor of recovery, although such impressions are, of course, difficult to prove . . . there is no substitute for protein . . . if there is any secret of life it is bound up with protein which is the basis of all living protoplasm . . . we have been lulled into a false sense of security about protein needs because of the presumed 'stores' of protein in the body . . . it is now known that depletion of plasma albumin begins immediately after protein intake is stopped . . . though hypoproteinemia is the only protein deficiency which can be recognized and measured clinically . . . Undoubtedly, other tissues suffer when their protein is depleted. The liver comes to mind . . . "

* * *

Grover C. Penberthy, of Detroit, Professor of Clinical Surgery, Wayne University College of Medicine; Director of General Surgery, Children's Hospital of Michigan, and, by invitation, Clifford D. Benson and Charles N. Weller, *Appendicitis in Infants and Children: A Fifteen-Year Study,* had had 742 acute unruptured appendices, with three deaths, or a mortality of 0.44%; 183 ruptured with local peritonitis, with one death, 0.55% mortality; 94 ruptured with diffuse peritonitis, with 61 deaths, 64.9% mortality, although they indicated that 35 of these patients had not been operated upon; 292 patients with appendiceal abscess, with 11 deaths, a 3.6% mortality. They were encouraged by the results of the recent use of sulfonamides. In the previous three years, 47 patients with abscess or peritonitis had received sulfonamides with one death, a 2.1% mortality, and 67 patients had not, with eight deaths, an 11.9% mortality. It was now their rule to give sodium sulfathiazole intravenously after operation "to all patients with peritonitis of any considerable extent. In addition, during recent months a majority of these patients have received sulfathiazole powder intraperitoneally at the time of operation. In many instances the drug was also placed in the wound layers during closure." Many patients received the drug before operation and the unoperated patients received the drug as well. The condition of the 35 unoperated patients on admission was "critical and attempts to prepare them for surgical intervention were unsuccessful."

Discussion

William E. Ladd, from the Boston Children's Hospital, commented that three years before they had reviewed 466 cases of acute appendicitis with two deaths 0.42%—one due to hemophilia—the same mortality Penberthy had achieved for uncomplicated acute appendicitis. He agreed with Penberthy that delay in children was inappropriate, and reminded the Fellows that "Doctor Ochsner, of Chicago, who was the original advocate of the delayed operation in cases of spreading peritonitis, pointed out over 40 years ago that this practice should not be used in children", although some delay was frequently required to "put the patient in the best possible condition for operation." Penberthy had not been enthusiastic about the McBurney incision, nor was Ladd, "In recent years the McBurney incision has been resurrected, and in my humble opinion rather undue importance has been attached to this incision as a factor in lowering the mortality." He, too, thought that chemotherapy had been helpful. David E. Robertson, of Toronto, Canada, speaking for the Hospital for Sick Children, reported no mortality in 465 cases of acute appendicitis without perforation, and two deaths in 115 with perforation,- 19 of the patients not having been operated upon,- one

of the patients who died never having left the medical service. Robert Elman, of St. Louis, spoke for the use of 10 to 20 cc. of plasma per kilo to offset the loss into the peritoneal cavity and the bowel, and the use of oxygen inhalation to control "anoxia . . . even before it develops."

* * *

Richard B. Cattell, of Boston, Surgeon to the Lahey Clinic, *Closure of Ileostomy in Ulcerative Colitis,* had previously held the position that "once an ileostomy is accepted it must always be maintained." His earlier experience had all been with ileostomy done late for long-established disease. Now performing ileostomy in more hopeful cases, they had undertaken closure of the ileostomy in nine patients, in all of whom there was a "clinical remission of symptoms . . . ", the inflammatory process had been "shown to have healed and be inactive . . . by sigmoidoscopic examinations", though the mucosa might be "granular or scarred and may even bleed somewhat on manipulation with a swab . . . ", and in all of them the colon had been "shown to be distensible by means of a barium enema . . . " Only two of the patients had had the disease for more than five months before ileostomy and these were both failures of operative closure. Of the remaining seven, five were thought to be doing well, although three of them had had recurrences and one had "several stools daily", and none had been followed for more than nine months. There had been no deaths. Cattell still urged early ileostomy to protect the colon from "irreversible structural changes . . . "

Discussion

Henry W. Cave, in opening the Discussion, attributed the 20% mortality of ileostomy to the reluctance of physicians to impose an ileostomy on a patient until the stage of desperation. He complained that he had not been as fortunate as Cattell in having patients turned over to him early, so that he had never seen a patient in whom closure of the ileostomy was justified. Cave seemed to question the ability to tell by sigmoidoscopy whether the disease was truly "inactive". He pointed out that the two failures in patients with disease of three- and six-years' duration, "should have been expected". He mentioned the very brief period of medical management before operation, but said he thought Cattell's results justified the procedure. William E. Ladd, of Boston, said that at Children's they had been somewhat reluctant to undertake early ileostomy. They had closed seven ileostomies which had been present for a considerable period of time, none of them less than two years, and all the children had remained well, one of them for 12 years. Cave had asked about the effect of sulfanylylguanidine and other sulfonamides by mouth and Cattell, in closing, said that their results had not been as satisfactory as some that had been reported.

* * *

The Business Meetings

The 1942 meeting was held at the Cleveland Hotel, Cleveland, Ohio, April 6, 7 and 8, President Harvey B. Stone in the Chair.

Stewart Rodman, Secretary of the American Board of Surgery, reporting to the Association said the percentage of failures in Part I was running 12 to 15% and Part II, 18%. The Board was still "concerned about the percentage of failures in Anatomy and Pathology", 17 and 18% respectively. The American Board of Surgery had "agreed to accept time spent on the surgical service of a regularly constituted Army or Naval Hospital in lieu of an equal amount of time in a civil hospital, but will not curtail the requirement for eligibility nor the examination itself in order to speed up the certification of candidates."

Allen O. Whipple, Chairman of the American Board of Surgery, stated that "The emergency has increased the number of young surgeons desiring to be certified by the Board because there has been a general feeling that those certified by the Board would obtain a higher rank and a better assignment to surgical duties than the general practitioner or uncertified surgeon. This impression, we are very glad to say, is based on fact . . . "

At the Executive Committee Meeting on the third day, dues were reduced to $20 and Fellows on active duty were excused from payment of dues. Separate binding of the *Transactions* for 1942 was to be modified and, "The publishers are directed for 1942 to print and bind in paper 400 extra of the two issues of the Annals, June and October numbers, containing all the published papers . . . " [The 1942 papers had appeared in the June and October numbers of the *Annals of Surgery*, the reason for the gap not stated. The *Transactions* for 1942 have a consecutive pagination, but the tops of the pages carry the dates and numbers of the issues of the *Annals of Surgery* in which the papers were ultimately published, and papers from the October issue frequently appear in this volume before the papers from the June issue.]

Vernon C. David, of Chicago, was elected President; Damon B. Pfeiffer, of Philadelphia, First Vice-President; Edward C. Moore, of Los Angeles, Second Vice-President; Warfield M. Firor, of Baltimore, Secretary. Among the new Fellows elected were Frank Glenn, of New York; Cameron Haight, of Ann Arbor; Robert M. Janes, of Toronto; John S. Lockwood, of Philadelphia; and Harold Neuhof, of New York. Among those proposed as Fellows for the first time were Oliver Cope, of Boston; Howard Gray, of Rochester, Minnesota; Henry N. Harkins, of Detroit; and Richard H. Sweet, of Boston.

LXI

1943

The 1943 meeting was held May 13 and 14 at the Netherland Plaza Hotel, Cincinnati, President Vernon C. David, of Chicago, Chairman, Department of Surgery, Rush Medical College, and Presbyterian Hospital; Secretary in 1932–1936, and Vice-President in 1938, in the Chair. With the war in full force 139 Fellows signed the Register and the meeting was held for two days.

The Presidential Address was titled, *The Importance of Fundamentals in Surgical Education.* Not only had ". . . 47,000 doctors . . . accepted commissions in this war. From our own society fifty are commissioned officers; and many others are serving in an advisory capacity." [Those who were left behind manned departments depleted of staff, had numerous governmental and committee assignments, and it is perhaps more surprising that a meeting was held than that it was in most respects a lackluster meeting.]

* * *

The meeting opened with a symposium on burns, the first paper of which, *The Study of the Prevention of Infection in Contaminated Accidental Wounds, Compound Fractures and Burns,* was presented by Frank L. Meleney, of New York, Associate Professor of Clinical Surgery, Columbia University. A footnote states that he was, "Representing the Subcommittee on Surgical Infections of the National Research Council, and the responsible investigators of the Contaminated Wound and Burn Project, under the Committee on Medical Research of the Office of Scientific Research and Development, Doctors Guy Caldwell, Warfield Firor, Charles Johnston, Sumner Koch, John Lockwood, Perrin Long, Champ Lyons, Roy McClure, Alton Ochsner, Mont Reid, and Frank Meleney, Chairman." [Perrin Long was the only non-surgeon. The rest were all members of the American Surgical Association except Caldwell and Lyons, who became members in 1944 and 1947.] The original plan of the committee had "called for observation on control cases without drugs, and other controls receiving treatment with local bacteriostatic agents other than the sulfonamides. But, said the Pearl Harbor observers: 'You cannot withhold from these patients the benefit of the sulfonamide drugs.' " While they had been planning their study and revising its structure ". . . sulfadiazine had come into use. It was found to be less toxic than sulfanilamide, less nauseating than sulfapyridine, and less likely to block the kidneys than sulfathiazole." The studies were conducted on civilian wounds in hospitals in eight cities, and the seven alternatives were local sulfanilamide and sulfadiazine, local sulfanilamide, "Total local Sulfonamide", no local drug, general sulfadiazine, no general sulfadiazine, general sulfadiazine without local sulfonamide. They had studied 682 soft-part wounds, otherwise analyzed as comparable, 471 compound fractures and 347 burns. The burns had been treated with tannic acid without sulfonamide, Quebracho-tannin, tannic acid with sulfonamide, compression dressings, zinc peroxide with pressure, saline compresses with pressure, total sulfadiazine ointment, total sulfadiazine spray, total sulfonamide film, total sulfonamide powders, total local sulfonamides, general sulfadiazine, no general sulfadiazine. They concluded that ". . . the sulfonamides minimize the general spread of infections and cut down the incidence of septicemia and death . . . We have no evidence that they lessen the incidence of local infection when used as we have employed them . . . If we are going to lessen the incidence of local infection in war wounds and burns, some other forms of the sulfonamides or some other bacteriostatic agents must be found which will be effective against the contaminating organisms in the presence of damaged tissue."

Discussion

Evarts Graham, of St. Louis, said that Meleney's report was satisfactory in terms of the information which it provided but ". . . disappointing, especially after the enthusiastic reports of the success of sulfonamides applied locally, particularly sulfanilamide, in the wounds at Pearl Harbor. I think almost everyone was led to believe that, after all, now we have a panacea which might even perhaps minimize the necessity of surgical asepsis. That is certainly not the case. The day of Listerism is not yet gone. The sulfonamides will not replace surgical asepsis." John S. Lockwood, of Philadelphia, Assistant Professor of Surgical Research and Acting Director, Harrison Department of Surgical Research, Schools of Medicine, University of Pennsylvania, who had been the subject of I. S. Ravdin's remarkable report of aortic embolectomy the year before, and speaking now in his first year as a Fellow of the Association and a member of Meleney's committee said that ". . . as time has gone on, we have become increasingly aware of the fact that no measure designed simply to deal with bacteria in wounds is likely completely to achieve . . . complete prevention of infection in traumatic wounds . . . unless, of course, an agent could be found which would destroy all of the contaminating bacteria." The infections which had occurred in the study had been for the most part local infections and not systemic or invasive or fulminating, and appeared ". . . five, seven, or eight days after wound closure . . . The factors which encouraged bacterial activity were retention of products of tissue injury, tension, and incomplete obliteration of dead space . . . the very same factors which will tend to delay healing and complicate the wound repair, are also factors which tend to inhibit sulfonamide action . . . the outcome of this study certainly justifies a continuing recogni-

tion of the predominant importance of surgical management and of physiologic factors in relation to wound healing and wound infection. At the same time, it points out the fact that the problem of deaths from infection in traumatic wounds should be very significantly minimized with sulfonamides." He added a very strong admonition that "Nothing that has been said about the lack of effectiveness of sulfonamides under the conditions used in this clinical experiment, should contradict the wisdom of the practice of employing sulfonamides routinely in battle casualties, during the period between injury and the time the casualty reaches the hospital for definitive treatment. The problem there is different from the problem which we studied in these wound study projects, and if the multiplication of bacteria in the wound fluids can be delayed for even a few hours during the transport of the wounded . . . from the field of injury to the hospital, that should significantly reduce the likelihood of postoperative infection. This is entirely beside the point of whether or not sulfonamides should be used in the wound if, and when, the wound is closed." Surgeons had been permitted to perform the kind of operative wound treatment they preferred in the study and Lockwood said, "We have plenty of evidence to support the wisdom of the directive, both in the Army and in the Navy, against routine closure of traumatic wounds. If any of us needed to learn the wisdom of that decision, I think we have the evidence." Lockwood added the exciting news that ". . . we now have in penicillin what appears to be an even more powerful weapon in dealing with staphylococcic and *Clostridium welchii* infections." J. Albert Key, of St. Louis, [who commonly at national meetings chose the role of gadfly, devil's disciple or common sense cynic, in this case chose to be a true believer] "I do not know where it is—it may be the unwieldiness of the series, or it may be in the punch-card system—but there is something wrong somewhere. I am perfectly convinced, and this is not emotion, that any report of a series of cases which concludes that the rational implantation of sulfonamides in contaminated wounds after they have been properly debrided does not lower the incidence of infection in these wounds, is wrong, provided the debridements and the after treatment are equivalent. This is a monumental piece of work, backed by a lot of able observers, but I think that a few years from now they will be ashamed of their conclusions." Meleney responded to Key that ". . . I can only say that in our group, at the beginning of the study, we had those who sincerely believed (and I might say that we all hoped), that these drugs would materially cut down the incidence of infection. There was no one in the group who was prejudiced against them. We were simply seeking to find out the facts, and we were not trying to prove anything. I believe that our whole group has come to this consensus of opinion. We all believe that these figures do represent facts and tell the truth." Meleney concluded with a graceful tribute to Graham's Committee on Surgery of the National Research Council and the statement that ". . . it is only fair to report at this time that we all feel that the most efficient unit in this study has been the one carried on here in Cincinnati by our good friends Mont Reid and William Altemeier."

* * *

Allen O. Whipple, of New York, Professor of Surgery, Columbia University; Director of Surgical Service, Presbyterian Hospital, who had been President in 1940, *Basic Principles in the Treatment of Thermal Burns,* gave a very brief and general talk.

Discussion

Sumner L. Koch, of Chicago, responded, saying that "Some years ago Evarts Graham wrote (with Maurice Berck) an admirable paper entitled 'Principles *versus* Details in the Treatment of Empyema.' [See page 726, Volume LI, 1933]. One could well apply his identical words to this discussion of burns . . . The persistent search for some magic substance to apply to the burned area has served chiefly to befog our outlook in the problem of burn treatment and to divert our attention from the principles that Dr. Whipple has stressed so clearly and emphatically . . . Three simple principles cannot be overemphasized . . . concerned particularly with *prevention* of complications . . . prevent infection, the most important *local* complication . . . prevent loss of plasma, the most important *general* complication . . . prevent contractures and long delay in healing . . ." Infection was to be prevented by immediately covering burns with sterile towels until they could be cared for ". . . by masked, gowned and gloved personnel." Local sulfonamides might prove useful. Fluid loss was to be prevented by ". . . an absorbent compression dressing over the cleansed burn surface at the earliest possible moment." As for ". . . early replacement of areas of whole-thickness loss . . . no chemicals, no ointments, and no witchcraft, that have yet been devised, can produce a covering of epithelium when the whole-thickness has been destroyed." Whipple, in closing, returned to the skin coverage problem, mentioning the fact that "I have seen some cases recently, in Harlem Hospi-

tal, where the granulating surface has been frosted with this sulfadiazine, and grafts put on that area adhere very firmly and take amazingly well."

* * *

The National Research Council through its subcommittee on blood substitutes was vigorously stimulating research in this field, and John S. Lockwood, of Philadelphia, Assistant Professor of Surgical Research and Acting Director, Harrison Department of Surgical Research, Schools of Medicine, University of Pennsylvania, reported for his group at the Harrison Department of Surgical Research at the University of Pennsylvania, *Gelatin as a Plasma Substitute: With Particular Reference to Experimental Hemorrhage and Burn Shock.* Dogs tolerated infusion of large volumes of gelatin-saline solution without deleterious effects, and about 50% of the gelatin infused was excreted in the urine. For the treatment of repeated massive hemorrhage, gelatin was superior to saline. Gelatin was as effective as plasma for treatment of ". . . slow, three-stage hemorrhage, with blood pressure maintained at 30 to 40 mm. Hg. for 30 to 40 minutes . . ." Although gelatin was as effective as plasma in the treatment of burn shock, the plasma-treated dogs showed better survival than did the gelatin-treated dogs. [An observation which led to the rather surprising statement that "If a factor can be identified in plasma which accounts for its ability to maintain blood pressure in the severely burned animal during the secondary phase of so-called 'acute toxemia,' the addition of this factor to gelatin would probably result in a more adequate plasma substitute for burns."]

* * *

The symposium on burns concluded with a study by Charles C. Lund, of Boston, Assistant Professor of Surgery, Harvard Medical School, and others "From the Thorndike Memorial Laboratory, Second and Fourth Medical Services (Harvard), and the Burn Assignment of the Surgical Services, of the Boston City Hospital . . .", *Problems of Protein Nutrition in Burned Patients.* They had studied ten patients in detail,- "Increased nitrogen excretion in the urine of some severely burned patients has been established . . . Calculable nitrogen deficits, based upon intake and output studies alone, of some duration and great magnitude have been observed . . . Correction of such a deficit by high protein feeding failed to bring a patient into true nitrogen balance because of incalculable losses which were probably from the burned and granulating surface . . . Heroic intravenous and tube feeding apparently restored . . . true protein balance . . . a level of intake of the equivalent of 2000 Gm. of protein per week . . ." Even so, there was a massive loss in body weight.

Discussion

The Discussion was initiated by Leland S. McKittrick, of Boston, with some comments on the Cocoanut Grove disaster [a night club fire in Boston, the victims from which were treated and extensively studied in the Massachusetts General Hospital with Oliver Cope as the principal figure]. The Massachusetts General Hospital had received 114 people in an hour-and-a-half, 55 were dead on arrival, and 20 died 15 minutes later, leaving 39 patients admitted for treatment. The burns were not cleaned "A simple boric ointment dressing and pressure were applied to wherever the burns might have been." Seven of the 39 died, none within the first 12 hours, and all of pulmonary complications. They concluded that their simple and easily applied local treatment was effective and appropriate. Robert Flman, of St. Louis, agreed with Lund's emphasis on a high protein intake begun early. Evarts A. Graham reminded Lockwood of Hogan's 1912 work with gelatin. Alexander Brunschwig, of the University of Chicago, said they had also been interested in gelatin ". . . from the standpoint of parenteral nitrogenous nutrition." In dogs it maintained positive nitrogen balance when given intravenously for as long as 12 days. They had given it to some patients for four or five days at a time, and he mentioned the various sources ". . . hog or calfskin gelatin, bone gelatin, and fish swim-bladder gelatin." Charles C. Lund, in closing, emphasized the importance of a high caloric diet as well as a high protein diet, as much as 6,000 calories a day and had used intravenous amino-acids for about a third of the nitrogen intake of his severely burned patients. He disagreed with Sumner L. Koch, because, ". . . with deep, extensive, third-degree loss, you are going to get colon bacilli and staphylococci in the area, no matter what treatment. Complete prevention of infection is beyond human capabilities at present." The patient had to be supported so that he could withstand the infection.

* * *

Jacob Fine, of Boston, Assistant Professor of Surgery, Harvard Medical School; Visiting Surgeon, Beth Israel Hospital, and by invitation, Arnold M. Seligman, and Howard A. Frank, *Traumatic Shock,*

An Experimental Study Including Evidence against the Capillary Leakage Hypothesis, presented the first paper on work employing radioisotopes which the Association had heard. "Plasma proteins tagged with radioactive isotopes (S^{35}, Br^{82}, I^{131}) were used to study the capillary leakage hypothesis in hemorrhagic, tourniquet and burn shock. No evidence of leakage due to a change in the permeability of the general capillary bed was found. Tagged plasma proteins escaped into areas of injury in considerable amounts, but not into untraumatized areas . . . There is no evidence to show that the general capillary bed becomes more permeable to plasma proteins or plasma in the late or irreversible phase of shock . . . Data obtained by the use of radioactively-tagged red cells injected intravenously combined with tissue analyses for hemoglobin and tagged red cell content indicate that about one-fifth of the capillary blood becomes stagnant or trapped out of active circulation as the shock phase deepens . . . The progressive decline in shock is not due to a progressive fall in plasma volume but to a progressive fall in the volume of actively circulating plasma . . . The therapeutic problem in shock after adequate replacement of lost blood or plasma has failed is one of restoring volume and velocity flow through capillaries before the integrity of vital tissue processes is inevitably lost."

* * *

In the final paper in the Symposium on Shock, Dallas B. Phemister, of Chicago, *Role of the Nervous System in Shock,* began by repeating the message which Fine had just delivered, "It has been gradually established in comparatively recent years that the outstanding cause of surgical shock is the local loss of blood and/or plasma." Nevertheless he returned to his long interest in neurogenic shock produced in these experiments "by prolonged electrical stimulation of the cardio-aortic (aortic depressor) nerves of the rabbit . . ." Marked and prolonged lowering of blood pressure resulted, with death in five to eight hours. He did say, of course, "The possibility that shock is ever produced by accidental injury of the cardio aortic nerves is so small that it scarcely merits consideration." Transection of the cervical cord of the dog similarly resulted in ". . .prolonged lowering of the blood pressure . . . failure of the circulation and death." Direct stimulation of the somatic nerves never produced impressively severe shock. He thought that "Vasomotor and cardiac afferent depressor impulses from the brain to the medullary center may lower blood pressure and produce syncopy . . .", but the effect was brief, as was the ". . . occasional reflex lowering of pressure in abdominal operations." Combined with the effect of hemorrhage these might, however, be significant. Phemister now essentially discounted neurogenic shock, "A fuller realization on the part of the surgeon of the relatively small importance of hyperactivity of afferent depressor nerve impulses and of the relatively great importance of blood and plasma loss and toxicity of anesthetics in the causation of surgical shock, will lead to greater attention to the latter factors and to further improvement in surgical therapy. The primary cause of shock is probably never a purely reflex vasodepressor reaction."

Discussion

Alfred Blalock, of Baltimore, initiated the Discussion with even-handed comments, "Dr. Phemister and I, and others, have maintained for a good many years that the most important agency in the initiation of traumatic shock is the regional loss of fluid from the blood stream. Most of the pathologists and the physiologists have maintained that there is a general increase in capillary permeability even in the early stages of shock. Now Doctor Fine and his group, Gregersen and Root, at Columbia, Gibson and Aub, in Boston, Evans of Richmond and others, have come to the conclusion that there is not a general increase in capillary permeability in traumatic shock even in the terminal stages. Even though I can find no flaw in their experiments, it is difficult for me to accept this whole-heartedly. It would appear that in the terminal stages there should be a general increase in capillary permeability, but . . . the evidence points in the other direction . . . it makes for a more hopeful outlook in therapy. Certainly, the inability to establish any definite beneficial effect from the use of adrenal cortical extract would indicate that they are correct." The importance of the regional loss of fluid he said had been established. Of the nervous system in shock he said, "It would appear that studies along this line would not be extremely hopeful as making for better therapy . . . attempts to block nerves have not resulted in much benefit in the treatment of traumatic shock . . . the use of spinal anesthesia is not advised in the treatment of traumatic shock . . . as regards the so-called toxemia theory, or what perhaps today had better be spoken of in terms of metabolic disturbance, perhaps the future outlook is somewhat better, for it does appear very likely that there are

chemical hormonal disturbances that might be treated successfully."

* * *

D. E. Robertson, of Toronto, Surgeon-in-Chief to Hospital for Sick Children, *The Medical Treatment of Hematogenous Osteomyelitis,* [in that day when the disease was still prevalent and 90% of the cases were due to staphylococcus, the rest mainly due to the streptococcus] demonstrated from 51 autopsies that this was a general infection,- pericarditis, empyema, lung abscesses, renal abscesses, pyogenic arthritis, and multiple subcutaneous and intermuscular abscesses among the commoner "metastatic" foci. Osteomyelitis was not a local surgical condition ". . . it is, therfore, rational to look for an agent that will assist in preventing this appalling chain of full-blown septicemia." Before sulfonamides, the mortality was 22% in their series. He intimated that the operative therapy of the obvious bony focus might have played a part in the mortality, ". . . we have all seen the late case, one that has survived the early acute phase and has come to hospital with a single lesion, either undrained or opened spontaneously . . . Such cases amply demonstrate nature's ability to deal with the acute phase of osteomyelitis in such a way as to prevent a fatal issue . . . I strongly suspect that so-called undiagnosed and untreated cases would show no such mortality as 20 per cent." Leveuf, of France, withheld operation or operated late and had improved his results. Since the sulfonamide drugs were " . . . capable of effecting a condition in the blood that will inhibit the growth of organisms . . . It would seem rational to attempt to introduce into the blood, at the earliest possible moment, a sufficient quantity of drug to render innocuous, or impotent, organisms that are in the blood stream or in reach of body fluids." They administered 8 to 10 Gm daily to children eight years of age, achieving levels of 6 to 12 mg. percent in the blood. Hoyt two years earlier had published a report of 12 cases of staphylococcal osteomyelitis treated with sulfonamides without any deaths. "This series constitutes a unique record, and must give thoughtful surgeons reason to reassess the whole problem of the treatment of acute osteomyelitis . . . If cases will survive spontaneously on the one hand, and if 12 consecutive cases will survive the acute phase with medication by sulfonamides, the part played by surgical incision of the local lesion is certainly not a factor in saving life . . . Our records of 89 cases, three moribund on admission, show, since sulphonamide administration, 25 not operated upon, and none dead, the others operated upon, and one dead; in all a mortality rate of 1.2 per cent, excluding the cases moribund on admission. These results are not such that, from the mortality standpoint, incision can be altogether condemned when added to sulphonamide medication." He described the effect of sulfonamides,- "In the subsidence in the acute phase a dramatic change takes place. It occurs over a period of 10-12 hours. The general reaction of the patient subsides; the intense swelling of the soft tissues at the local lesion diminishes; the underlying abscess becomes more obvious in its outline; and the patient is comparatively comfortable." The abscess might diminish and disappear or become large and perforate through the skin. Without operative injury, the sequestra tended to be small and fragile, "In drained lesions there is generally a wide destruction of bone together with a large involucrum; sequestration is present in over half of the cases." They did not see " . . . obvious death of a large mass of bone . . . except in rare cases" and sequestration occurred in only 10% to 15% of the cases. They had used sulfathiazole but thought sulfadiazine might be "more readily borne . . . and a higher blood level can be maintained." They used no splinting unless the joint was involved, when traction was sometimes employed.

Discussion

Kellogg Speed, of Chicago, in general agreement, pointed out that it was already apparent that, "The percentage of occurrence of acute infectious osteomyelitis is falling off in some districts because the sulfonamides are widely employed in treatment of nasal and skin infections, acting bacteriostatically before osseous lesions may develop. After early medical treatment by massive doses we can believe that the results in a consecutive series of patients would be even better than the use of the drug plus early local and extensive operation which would interfere with the local blood supply of the bone, lower the resistance locally, and block the bacteriostatic action of the drug." A number of surgeons still used large doses of " . . . potent antistaphylococcic serum until toxemia subsides." He was optimistic, "Additional reports will probably verify Dr. Robertson's results. We await, also, reports on the use of penicillin, which is nontoxic and especially adapted to bacteriostatic action against the staphylococcus and all gram-positive forms of bacteria. While it has not yet proven of value in subacute bacterial endocarditis, in dosages of 30,000 to 40,000 [!], Oxford units in 24 hours according to Herrell, it does clear the blood stream of bacteria and may act favorably in acute

infectious osteomyelitis." Albert Key, of St. Louis, agreed that " . . . the time to treat osteomyelitis with sulfonamides is before it starts . . . the efficiency of the sulfonamide varies inversely with the number of organisms present in a given focus, and inversely with the amount of necrotic tissue present in a given focus . . . for that reason . . . sulfonamides will clear the blood stream and not sterilize the focus in the bone." The question he raised was "Does an incision for drainage—and by that I do not mean an extensive operation but an incision for drainage—lower the resistance locally to infection in the bone or anywhere else?" Failing evidence of this, he believed that " . . . if, you can diagnose the presence of an abscess in bone and your patient is in good condition, that should be drained." How long was sulfathiazole to be continued? He had seen flare-ups after the drug was stopped or after limb use had been resumed, nor was he ready to give up operation, "I still feel that there is a very definite place for surgery in the treatment of acute osteomyelitis, and that that place is the drainage of the abscess as soon as the patient is in condition to stand the operation." Robertson, in closing, responded gently, " . . . when the child is recovering, and is well of the acute phase, and can stand an operation for the drainage of abscess, just consider whether or not it is necessary to drain the abscess. The child has gotten well with an abscess. The secondary soft tissue swelling around the abscess has subsided, leaving the abscess so you can examine it and delineate it easily. It is slightly tender. I think we make a great mistake draining these abscesses just because they are easily accessible . . . when we do attack them, we probably do something that is not in the best interests of the patient . . . when they are left without incision the results are excellent, much better in my opinion than those incised."

* * *

Over the previous several years, there had been increasing interest in surgery of the pancreas, and now Lester R. Dragstedt, of Chicago, Professor of Surgery, University of Chicago, *Some Physiologic Problems in Surgery of the Pancreas,* discussed the results of his experiments in dogs with total resection of the duodenum, total pancreatectomy, and also with ligation of the pancreatic ducts. "Removal of from 80 to 90 per cent of the pancreas causes no defect in carbohydrate or fat metabolism or in the digestion and absorption of foodstuffs, provided the pancreas remnant remains in connection with the duct and its secretion has free access to the upper intestine. Removal of from 90 to 95 per cent of the pancreas, leaving the remnant attached to the duct, produces a diabetes, characterized by marked hyperglycemia and glycosuria, excessive insulin requirement, and hyperlipemia. Digestion and absorption are unimpaired. Lipocaic is usually required. Complete pancreatectomy produces, paradoxically, a less severe diabetes, but which is more difficult to control. Hyperglycemia and glycosuria are not so marked and less insulin is required. Hypolipemia develops and lipocaic is almost always needed. Moderate to severe impairment in the digestion and absorption of fat and protein may be expected. The absorption of carbohydrate is little affected. Permanent occlusion of the pancreatic ducts produces a similar impairment in digestion and absorption. Atrophy of the pancreas results . . . Present information does not indicate that any specific defect will result from removal of the duodenum, but patients who survive for long periods after this operation has been performed should be observed carefully for the possible development of pernicious anemia. The much better nutritive state displayed by animals in which a remnant of pancreas, however small, is left in connection with its duct, as compared with those in which the ducts are occluded or the entire pancreas removed, suggests that this should be attempted whenever possible. In the treatment of carcinoma of the ampulla or head of the pancreas this will, of course, necessitate an implantation of the duct from the pancreas remnant into the stomach or intestines. Methods for accomplishing this have been devised, of which the recent one reported by [Cooper] Person and [Frank] Glenn seems especially promising . . . Substitution therapy is at present only partially effective."

Discussion

Allen O. Whipple, of New York, happily characterized Dragstedt's contribution, "Doctor Dragstedt always presents work of physiologic significance and his inquiring mind has contributed works of fundamental importance to surgery." In their own experiments with duct atrophy, half of the animals had shown no abnormal fat in the liver, and in only two was there more than 25% excess. In three patients with "pancreatic exclusion", they found the patients could digest 85% of their fat intake without supplement, but another patient digested only 40% without supplement. He had just reoperated, three years and eight months after radical pancreaticoduodenectomy upon a patient whose gastroenterostomy had stenosed, and found the liver normal to appearance and by biopsy, but "His pancreas showed a fibrosis, with cystic degeneration." He agreed " . . . that the technic of radical pancreaticoduodenectomy should be changed so as to reestablish the flow of pancreatic juice into the jejunum, in order to improve the existing impaired fat digestion of these patients in whom the flow of pancreatic juice had been blocked for varying intervals, and . . . to avoid the very annoying complication of a pancreatic fistula which so frequently follows the exclusion operation." He had now done seven such operations, in two of them implanting the pancreatic stump into the stomach, in two " . . .implanting the pancreatic fistula into the jejunum at a later operation . . . ", and in three implanting the pancreatic stump into the jejunal loop at the time of the resection. Richard B. Cattell said that in the previous nine months he had done seven radical pancreatoduodenectomies, transplanting the pancreatic duct into the jejunum " . . . by a relatively simple technical procedure that not only implants the cut end of the pancreatic body but also accomplishes actual anastomosis of the main pancreatic duct." The technique of "actual anastomosis" involved pulling the duct through the mucosa of the jejunum, a transfixion suture in the duct being " . . . passed through the jejunal mucosa and tied down tighty as a necrosing suture . . . The necrosing suture will cut through within 48 to 72 hours." In the past nine months he had done radical pancreatoduodenectomy in one stage twice, and in two stages in five patients, without operative mortality. One patient died nine weeks after resection.

* * *

The first mention of the serum amylase test before the Association was by Howard C. Naffziger, of San Francisco, Surgeon-in-Chief, University of California Hospital, who had been Vice-President in 1941, and by invitation, H. J. McCorkle, *The Recognition and Management of Acute Trauma to the Pancreas: With Particular Reference to the Use of the Serum Amylase Test,* by the technique which Somogyi had reported some years earlier. In eight patients who proved to have injury to the pancreas, they found an elevation of the serum amylase so that "In a patient who has received an injury to the abdominal region, an elevation in the serum amylase may be considered to be good evidence that the pancreas has been damaged . . . The significance of elevations in the serum amylase occurring after operations on the pancreas, stomach, duodenum, or lower end of the common duct is probably the same as that of any other trauma to the pancreas."

* * *

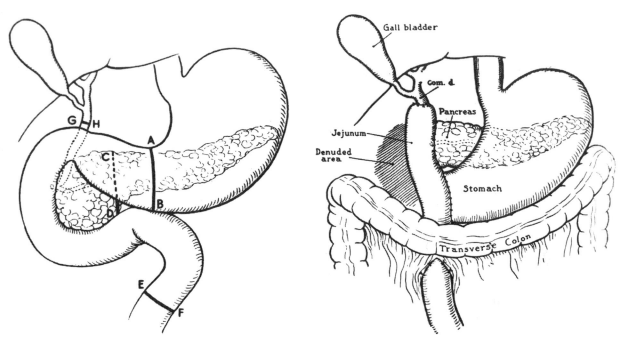

FIG. 2.—Lines of excision. A-B. Stomach. C-D. Pancreas. G-H. Common duct. E-F. Jejunum distal to duodenojejunal angle.
FIG. 3.—The one stage operation, using the distal limb of the jejunum through the rent in the mesocolon for the anastomosis with common duct, pancreatic duct and stomach.

Whipple had already come to the conclusion, now presented by Dragstedt, that the pancreatic secretion should be preserved, and not only to preserve the digestive function but ". . . also to avoid the very annoying complication of pancreatic fistula which so frequently follows the exclusion operation." The illustration shows the pancreas inserted into the side of the jejunal limb, an operation he had done three times, but he had also inserted the pancreatic stump into the stomach twice, and twice, in a secondary operation, implanted a pancreatic fistula into the jejunum.

Allen O. Whipple in Discussion of Lester R. Dragstedt, *Some Physiologic Problems in Surgery of the Pancreas.* Volume LXI, 1943.

A good deal of interest was aroused by the paper of Major Frank C. Shute, Major Thomas E. Smith, Lt. Col. Max Levine, all by invitation, and Col. John C. Burch, Associate Professor of Obstetrics and Gynecology, Vanderbilt University Hospital, who was now Chief of Surgical Service, Brooke General Hospital, Fort Sam Houston, Texas, *Pilonidal Cysts and Sinuses.* This had become a vexing problem in the training camps. The etiology was ascribed to a variety of embryonic malformations. The treatments recommended had varied from injection or painting with escharotics, including fuming nitric acid, roentgenotherapy, and, for the most part, excision and open packing. A variety of techniques of direct closure had been employed and Burch cited the contributions of Dunphy and Matson, Lahey, Cattell, MacFee, Colp, and others. At the Brooke General Hospital, they had treated 77 cases in nine months and found a shorter healing time with the closed method—47 days—than with the open method—77 days. Since October 1942, they had been using the closed method in all cases and had come to applying a technique in which an ellipse of involved tissue was resected down to the sacrococcygeal fascia, flaps of gluteal fascia were dissected to the midline and sutured, and the lateral flaps of gluteus muscle then brought together in the midline. Fifty-nine patients were so operated upon, ten of them recurrent cases, all cases infected. "The block of tissue removed usually measured about 12 × 8 cm. The largest block was 15 × 10 cm." They made the important observation that "In the specimens from recurrent cases, no epithelial tissue was found. Only sinus formation as a result of infection in a dead space was noted . . . we believe the majority of so-called recurrences are the result of incomplete obliteration of dead space." The patients were ambulatory within 12 to 24 hours and pressure dressings were not employed. In 48 of the 59 patients the wounds healed per primam, three wounds separated but were pulled together with adhesive and healed, there were three minor stitch abscesses and five " . . . infections of the lower perianal angle of the wound", and these healed in an average of 22 days. "When healed, the enlisted men returned to duty after an average convalescent period of three weeks, while officers returned in 16 to 20 days following operation . . . "

Discussion

Harvey B. Stone, of Baltimore, whose analogy of the pilonidal sinus to the preen gland in birds they had mentioned, agreed with the principle of primary closure, "I believe that closure should be undertaken, and that it is an unnecessary surrender to pack it open and wait for it to granulate . . . even where closure fails, and where the wound then has to be treated as an open wound and allowed to fill up by granulation, the period of deferred healing is probably less than if no attempt at closure has been made in the first instance." He thought Dr. Burch's method ingenious. Frank H. Lahey, of Boston, said he had just been inspecting Naval hospitals and found the problem of pilonidal sinuses prominent in them, and that duty-days were "saved by primary suture." In civilian practice, Dr. Cattell had told him that out-patient excision and packing with alternate-day redressing was entirely feasible.

The Business Meetings

The 1943 meeting was held May 13, and 14, at the Netherland Plaza, Cincinnati, Dr. Vernon C. David in the Chair. The meeting had been scheduled to take place at Hot Springs, but because of the war had been moved to Cincinnati.

Thirty-four active Fellows were on duty with the Armed Forces, among them, James B. Brown, B. N. Carter, Elliott C. Cutler, John H. Gibbon, Jr., Emile Holman, Walter G. Maddock, Fred W. Rankin, and I. S. Ravdin.

The Recorder explained that in order to maintain the continuity of the *Transactions,* the publishers had been asked to bind the June and October numbers of the *Annals of Surgery* which contained the Association's papers [thus explaining the appearance in that volume of the *Transactions* of papers having nothing to do with the Association or the meeting].

Among those who had died that year were George W. Crile, John M. T. Finney, and Mont Reid, before the Association's meeting in his own city. Louis Herrmann had taken over the arrangements of the Local Committee. There were to be special services for Dr. Reid on the following day at the Medical School, "The ODT [Office of Defense Transportation] has made it impossible for us to get buses to transport the members of this organization to the Medical Building, but we have provided street cars . . . They will take you within a block and a half of the Medical College."

The President said that, "The Council, in discussion of the banquet, has felt that during wartime informal dress at dinner would be in order. Anybody who really has a yen to dress may, but I think this is a time when informal dress, and particularly a uniform, is acceptable."

At the Second Business Meeting on the second and final day, the decision of whether a meeting was to be held in 1944 or not was left to future action of the Council. A letter was read which Mont Reid had sent to the Secretary, W. M. Firor, that February 15, enclosing a copy of the letter which Reid had sent " . . . to the three Surgeons General and to General Hines of the Veterans Administration." There had been news reports that the Army was planning to build a Military hospital in Cincinnati or nearby, and Reid said, "It has seemed to me for some time that such institutions, wherever they are built, should, if possible, be put in close physical contact with good teaching medical centers." This would permit the staff to associate " . . . with the teachers in the medical center . . . It would be far easier for the teachers and specialists in different fields to render their services . . . It seems to me that the time may necessarily come when Government and civic supported hospitals and medical centers will have to supplement each other in the development of a well-rounded program for national health, medical education and investigation . . . In such Government hospitals there is often a great wealth of material dealing with problems which ought to be intensively studied and investigated . . . It might permit studies to be completed in a short time which otherwise might take years simply because of the lack of adequate clinical material. At the same time the patients would be receiving better care." He questioned the wisdom of having placed Government hospitals "in areas like White Sulphur Springs, West Virginia [The Greenbrier had been turned into an Army hospital] . . . it would have been wiser to hospitalize the patients who are now at White Sulphur in Charlottesville, Virginia, where there could have been intimate intercourse between some of the leaders in the field of medicine and the doctors who will have to take care of these patients when the war is over." He pointed out, too, that after the war it would not be easy to staff hospitals in such areas. The Council of the Association endorsed the suggestion and instructed the Secretary to inform the Secretary of War, the Secretary of the Navy, and the Surgeons-General of the Army, Navy, and the Public Health Service of its position. [This may well have been one of the first recorded explicit recommendations which led ultimately to the founding of the Dean's Committee Veterans' Hospitals.]

Frederick A. Coller, of Michigan, was elected President; Urban Maes, of New Orleans, First Vice-President; Arthur M. Shipley, of Baltimore, Second Vice-President; and Warfield M. Firor, Secretary. Fred Coller was not in the room and could not, therefore, be escorted to the platform to accept the applause of his colleagues, but the omission was rectified at the afternoon session when Coller expressed himself as " . . . chagrined and embarrassed at having decided to take early lunch today. That is really what I was doing, in spite of various comments by the members that other things might have caused me to run out."

Among those elected to membership were William Adams, Oliver Cope, Howard K. Gray, Jonathan E. Rhoads, and Richard H. Sweet. Among the new members proposed for action the following year were Michael E. DeBakey, of New Orleans; Donald Walter Gordon Murray, of Toronto; Louis M. Rousselot, of New York; and Captain Harris B. Shumacker, of Baltimore.

LXII

1944

The 1944 meeting was held at Thorne Hall, Northwestern University, Chicago, May 3 and 4, a two-day meeting in deference to the war. President Frederick A. Coller, of Ann Arbor, Professor of Surgery, University of Michigan; Director, Department of Surgery, University Hospital, in the Chair. There were now 56 Active Fellows on active duty with the Armed Forces. Among those who had died that year were Arthur D. Bevan, of Chicago; John Bapst Blake, of New York; Alexander Primrose, of Toronto; Edward P. Richardson, of Boston; and D. E. Robertson, of Toronto.

President Coller spoke on *The State of the Association*. The problems created by the war had required enormous efforts by the Fellows in and out of the Armed Forces, at the same time that it was obvious that the social changes brought about by the war would have a major effect upon surgical practice and education after the war. "Whether the free competitive type of practice under which we have grown up shall in part or wholly be replaced by a controlled and subsidized method of caring for the sick is a possibility that confronts us . . . At present there are forces working to remould Medicine through the more or less violent actions and reactions of pressure groups. The future health of the nation is worthy of greater consideration and if ever it be managed with an appreciation of its worth, it would demand a Minister of Health in the Cabinet with competent advisors from the laity and the profession who together could work out in an orderly fashion a plan that would be for the betterment of all." [With huge numbers of physicians in the Armed Forces, some for five and six years, many of us overseas took it for granted that the opportunity would be seized to "governmentalize" the practice of medicine before our return, so that one form of governmental employment would be replaced by another. We were surprised when that did not happen.] As for medical education, "Under the stern necessity of war there have come almost unbelievable changes in medical education . . . The selection of students for entrance to Medicine is now in part in the hands of the representatives of the Army and the Navy. Premedical training is shortened and its content changed, while the medical course itself is accelerated to a continuous performance. We are all heartily agreed with these or with any courses that will win the war and safeguard the health of our fighting men but . . . these changes are those of expediency and . . . will give birth to vexing problems in the future. A study on medical education at this time discloses a self-confessed deterioration of instruction in many schools with the possibility of a serious breakdown in most . . . Graduate Training worthy of the name has ceased. The present 9-9-9 program [the 9-9-9 plan referred to the *total* duration of house officer training, 9 months internship, 9 months assistant residency, 9 months as Resident] is a distinct aid in caring for sick and injured civilians, but contributes little to what we have come to consider true Graduate Education . . . many men are forced to accept internships in hospitals where training is virtually absent . . . after the war there will be from

20,000 to 30,000 young men who will have had educational opportunities of a character inferior to those offered in the prewar period." The military experience in surgery and in decision making might make up for this in part. In anticipation of this postwar training and retraining problem "There has been set up from our profession a committee for Post-War Planning for Medical Services with representatives from the American Medical Association, The American College of Surgeons, and the American College of Physicians and the Army, Navy, Public Health Service and the Veterans Facility . . . to prepare to fill the needs and wishes of the demobilized medical officers." The Council of the American Surgical Association had appointed a committee to "explore the field and to seek advice and help from every member of the Association. This committee will work with the main committee for Post-War Planning and carry your thoughts and aid to it." He saw the need for refresher courses for well-trained men and the need for further training for men who wanted to prepare themselves for the Specialty Board Examination. The Boards intended "By and large . . . to give credit for one year spent in military service with credit beyond that time given only after careful evaluation of work actually done." Training had to be provided for those returning from the war and for those coming out of medical school so that "we will have to increase the number of available residencies, by increasing the number of hospitals where such training is available and by temporarily at least enlarging the number of residencies in those hospitals where acceptable training is now offered." It was going to be difficult to select men from this large new pool, " . . . many of the men who now will want advanced training would not have qualified for it in the ordinary course of events. It is natural that one will be influenced in choosing a resident by a man's Service record, but this alone is not enough . . . he must be competent and intellectually worthy of this training . . . we should not be satisfied with short measure since, after all, our responsibility is to the American people of the future as well as to aspirants of today." He turned to the question of financing residencies and fellowships, "We should not only seek for funds with which to carry additional residents but we should increase their stipend to a level of financial decency [a consideration almost startling in its radicality] . . . Residents are essential to the proper functioning of a hospital, yet, in the past hospitals have been willing to pay everyone on the staff except the physicians in training." He made the interesting suggestion that, "If every member of this Association, who is not in the Armed Forces sup-

ported a Fellowship for three years, it would be a minor financial burden to us and would give training to 200 men. If we put our minds to it, the financial difficulties could largely be settled within the resources of our own communities." Equally important was it to provide opportunities for research for those "returning men qualified to do and desirous of carrying on research. We should have laboratories and financial support ready for them on their return . . . after this war the torch of science will still be burning in only a few spots on the earth." Coller discussed "specialism" at length and once more made a plea for "a basic examination and surgical fundamentals that would be taken by all those wishing to become candidates for the Boards and for Fellowship in the American College of Surgeons . . . Passing such an examination would be a preliminary to later taking the Final Examination of the Specialty Boards and would admit the successful candidate to Junior Membership in the American College of Surgeons". The matter was under consideration by the American Board of Surgery, American College of Surgeons, and the Board of Orthopedic Surgery. The large number of excellent men produced by the Graduate Training Programs since 1920 had increased the number of surgeons in the country and this with the increase in size of the population suggested that "we could well consider some enlargement of our membership . . . I suggest that, in addition to filling the vacancies that occur each year we add for the next five years five men each year. This would increase our active membership to 200 in that time, certainly not a number larger than would contain the outstanding contributors to surgery in this country and Canada." He joined those who in the past had suggested that the number of papers at a meeting could be increased by limiting the presentation to ten minutes and mentioned, without recommending, "having sections running simultaneously on papers of like interest".

* * *

This volume of the *Transactions* begins with *The Surgical Management of the Wounded in the Mediterranean Theater at the Time of the Fall of Rome*, Colonel Edward D. Churchill, M.C., A.U.S. Churchill had not presented this paper at the meeting and it is preceded by the following note, *"Described by Brigadier General Rankin as 'one of the finest dissertations on management of wounds which has been submitted through the Office of the Surgeon General of the U.S. Army,' this paper by Colonel Churchill, arrived just as we were closing the first issue of the Annals of Surgery devoted to the Transac-*

tions of the American Surgical Association. It was immediately accepted to appear in the Annals with the Transactions as a contribution by Col. Churchill, in absentia. The Editors join the Association in welcoming this fine report from an important battle area, and in congratulating Col. Churchill for his high accomplishment in the field and in reporting such excellent work." Churchill always wrote well and the paper, though relatively brief, is packed with details of the principles and techniques of wound management and care of the wounded. "Plasma is a substitute for whole blood only in the sense that it can be packaged and stored in adequate quantity in areas where blood cannot be obtained. Plasma is not a substitute for whole blood in the physiologic sense. For these reasons a Blood Transfusion Unit procures and processes whole blood in the base and distributes it to the Army installations." Blood was shipped to the Anzio beachhead first by L.S.T. and subsequently by plane. "In approximately four months, over 16,000 pints of whole blood have been drawn and processed for delivery to the Fifth Army." Type "O" blood was used, but "only those with an agglutinin titer less than 1 to 64 are issued as 'universal donor' blood . . . evacuation hospitals maintain their own unit blood banks. Responsibility for the supply of type specific blood other than "O" rests upon the individual hospital." In the field, sulfonamides were given locally and orally, "The value of this procedure is questioned by many surgeons of experience." For all but light wounds, preoperative penicillin therapy was employed, and "At operation, topical application of penicillin is carried out only in wounds penetrating the meninges, serous cavities and joints." There were "two quite different approaches to the application of chemotherapeutic agents to military surgery. The first would utilize these agents to permit delay in wound surgery, and minimize the completeness of the excision of dead tissue. The second employs chemotherapy to extend the scope of surgery and achieve a perfection in results previously considered impossible. The latter policy has guided the surgery of the Mediterranean Theater." It was important to give definitive surgery to the most seriously wounded as far forward as possible and "Initial surgery cannot be carried on as a hasty, slap-dash and bloody spectacle . . . The average operating times for certain types of cases recorded at an evacuation hospital were: one hour 49 minutes for penetrating wounds of the head; two hours for wounds of the abdomen; two hours and a half for wounds of the thorax . . . the small group of first priority cases diverted to the Field Hospital Platoon constitutes approximately one-thirteenth of

the total number . . . Evacuation hospitals handle the great bulk of the wounded in the forward area . . . " He emphasized "the development of what may be called *reparative surgery.* Wounds left unsutured at the initial operation are routinely closed by suture, usually at the time of the first dressing . . . on or after the fourth day . . . Decision to close a wound by suture is based solely on an appraisal of the gross appearance at the time of removal of the dressing . . . smear or culture does not provide information pertinent to this decision or allow the prediction of the result. 'Clean' wounds that heal by first intention after delayed closure may show a profuse and varied flora, both anaerobic and aerobic . . . during the Italian Campaign alone, at least 25,000 soft-part wounds have been closed on the basis of gross appearance only. Healing has resulted in approximately 95 per cent, and no loss of life or limb or serious complications have been reported . . . The topical use of sulfonamides appears to contribute nothing to the favorable results of reparative wound surgery. Parallel series of closures show as satisfactory or better results without the topical application of sulfonamides at the time of suture, as with it." Penicillin therapy was necessary only for established infection. [The most radical advance in wound therapy to come out of the Mediterranean Theater was the experience of the Auxilliary Surgical Groups with the treatment of organizing hemothorax or empyema.] "Radical management of massive organizing hemothorax by thoracotomy, evacuation of the clot and decortication of the lung has proved its effectiveness in returning soldiers to duty and appears to have diminished the incidence of empyema. The same procedure applied to established posttraumatic empyema with penicillin therapy as an adjunct, is followed by immediate healing with a fully expanded lung. It is no longer acceptable to hold that a patient with a penetrating chest wound is making satisfactory progress as long as empyema has not made itself manifest. The focus has been changed from the management of posttraumatic pleural infection to the preservation of lung function. In the history of military surgery this will stand as one of the significant advances of World War II." Churchill's concluding paragraph indicates the difference in wound treatment which was achieved by the efforts and observation of the surgeons in the Mediterranean Theater of Operations, principally the Auxilliary Surgical Groups, under Churchill's enlightened leadership, "It is a satisfaction to note the contrast between the present concept of wound management and the doctrines in vogue scarcely a year ago. The closed-plaster man-

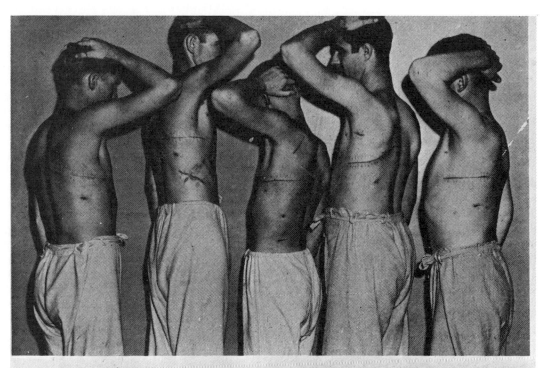

FIG. 9.—Reparative surgery of thoracic wounds.

Five patients, all with severe mixed infection empyema of residual hemothorax following débridement of wounds of the chest in the forward area. Varying degrees of pulmonary collapse and fibropurulent loculation of pleural space. Without preliminary drainage, thoracotomy with decortication of the lung performed on 9th, 16th, 21st, 21st and 21st days after wounding. Penicillin therapy, parental and topical. Complete primary healing, with fully expanded lungs—ready for rehabilitation to duty status.

The formal thoracotomy for the evacuation of clotted hemothorax with decortication, and the postoperative suction drainage of the chest with two or three large tubes, was a radical departure from previous practice and proved to be remarkably successful in saving life and function and shortening the period of disability, particularly in hemothoraces already infected. Churchill correctly said, "In the history of military surgery this will stand as one of the significant advances of World War II."

Col. Edward W. Churchill, *The Surgical Management of the Wounded in the Mediterranean Theater at the Time of the Fall of Rome,* Volume LXII, 1944.

agement of wounds and fractures was designed to conserve life but exacted a high price in skeletal and soft-part deformity. Its use is now limited to certain cases with established infection of bone or with massive defects of soft parts compounding a fracture site. Recommendations that minimized the necessity for a complete initial wound operation or sought to delay it (wound trimming, 'salting down with sulfa drugs,' *etc.*) accepted suppuration as inevitable in a considerable proportion of cases and relied on chemotherapy to hold sepsis within bounds. Resuscitation measures that relied on plasma alone to compensate for loss of whole blood prolonged life but tied the hands of the surgeon in the performance of life-saving surgery. These and other earlier concepts were but faltering steps toward what will emerge as

the ultimate scope of surgery as developed in the present war."

* * *

Vascular Injuries of Warfare, Lt. Col. Daniel C. Elkin, M.C., A.U.S., Professor of Surgery, Emory University; Surgeon-in-Chief, Emory University Hospitals, who had been Vice-President in 1942, discussed the experience at the Ashford General Hospital which had been established at The Greenbrier, White Sulphur Springs, as a vascular surgical center. The paper consisted of a series of detailed case reports, the most interesting of which dealt with arterial aneurysms and arteriovenous fistulae. He pointed out the frequency with which accompanying nerve injuries were missed in the forward installations [one of the nerve repairs at Ashford General Hospital which he reported was performed by Major Barnes Woodhall]. He made no comment about the timing of operation for aneurysm, but for arteriovenous fistulae, said that "While time should be allowed for the development of collateral circulation, operation should not be delayed until cardiac failure has supervened . . . Time should be allowed for the development of collateral circulation about an arteriovenous fistula, usually a matter of three or four months . . . In an arterial aneurysm the use of artificial means to develop collaterals, usually proximal compression of vessels either manually or with the compressor devised by Matas, should be employed . . . Where *large* arterial aneurysms exist without accompanying nerve damage the obliterative endoaneurysmorrhaphy of Matas is the operation of choice. This type, however, is usually the result of arterio-sclerosis or syphilis, and is, therefore, less often encountered in young soldiers." As for the operative treatment of arteriovenous fistula, "On theoretic grounds it would seem best to repair the opening in both artery and vein, but this is technically difficult and may result in secondary hemorrhage, thrombosis, or recurrence. Since collateral circulation is usually abundant, complete excision with ligation of all communicating vessels is the method of choice. Ligation without excision usually results in the recurrence since the fistula will be established rapidly through collaterals . . . "

Discussion

The most interesting comment in the Discussion was that of Allen O. Whipple, of New York, "I had not expected to discuss this paper, but a reference to the work that Doctors Blakemore and Lord have done in this field has not been mentioned, and it seems to me that it is only fair to speak of the original work they have done. Blakemore and Lord have devised a nonsuture method of bridging gaps in main arterial defects, which in a large series of animal experimentations has proven remarkably effective, and has been used in a sufficiently large number of clinical cases to show that it is not only feasible but readily carried out . . . the essential parts of it are that a vein graft is threaded through a vitallium tube on two ends, and the endothelial-covered vein ends are introduced into the ends of artery that have been excised or damaged. This endothelial-to-endothelial lining permits of a reestablishment of circulation through the artery; thrombosis does not result, and the restoration of circulation to the limb is promptly reestablished . . . I have used it myself

in anastomosing the splenic vein to the renal vein in the case of portal obstruction and the patient who had been having repeated gastric or esophageal hemorrhages, and had been tapped a number of times before the operation, has had no recurrence of bleeding or of ascites for nine months . . . it seems to me it is only fair to say that this is a method of reestablishing circulation in a main arterial trunk which must be considered and must be given due study and tried. In a series of eight cases that I saw in Bizerte last summer, seven of them had come to amputation (these were injuries to the popliteal artery) and they had all been previously treated with paravertebral block." Lt. Col. Elkin, in closing,- [and seeing the utility of this method only in the treatment of the original wound and not in reconstruction at the time of excision of aneurysms and arteriovenous fistulae],- "Doctors Blakemore and Lord's work . . . of course is of extreme importance. Doctor Whipple will realize, however, that the patients which I reported here were seen anywhere from six weeks to six months after the origin of the injury, and the application of the principle at that time was hardly applicable."

* * *

Penicillin had been alluded to the previous year by John Lockwood, and Churchill's report from the Mediterranean Theater mentioned its use. Now, from the Harrison Department of Surgical Research [of which he had been director], Schools of Medicine, University of Pennsylvania, John S. Lockwood [carried in the roster as Associate Professor of Surgery, Yale University School of Medicine, where he went in 1944, to return to Columbia in 1946 as Professor and Director of Research], and, by invitation, William L. White and Franklin D. Murphy, *The Use of Penicillin in Surgical Infections,* provided the first in-depth discussion of the new drug before the Association. While sulfonamide therapy had proven its effectiveness in certain areas " . . . contrasting the 38 per cent case fatality rate from meningitis during World War I with a current Army rate of 4 per cent", and similar results "with respect to pneumonia and streptococcic sepsis"; the sulfonamides had been found to "possess certain very definite shortcomings which are of especial significance to the surgeon." Sulfonamide therapy had "modified the invasive aspects of many . . . surgical infections, particularly those due to hemolytic streptococci . . . ", however, they were ineffective once tissue necrosis had developed and were inactivated by-products of tissue breakdown. Their use had been hampered by " . . . the incidence of toxic reactions particularly those resulting from acquisition of drug hypersensitivity, and those affecting the hemopoietic system and the kidneys." Penicillin was shown by Fleming to be particularly effective against staphylococci and other gram-positive organisms, "its activity was not seriously impaired in the presence of proteolytic products of infection . . . it is not inhibited by para aminobenzoic-acid and peptones, as the sulfonamides are . . . " Lockwood said that the production problems involved in making available large amounts of the drug had been solved " . . . as a result of the cooperative efforts of the British Medical Research Council, the Committee on Medical Research, the War Production Board, and several pharmaceutical houses both in Britain and the United States, and the laboratories of the U.S. Department of Agriculture in Peoria, Illinois . . . " The Fellows undoubtedly already knew that "the Committee on Chemotherapeutics and Other Agents of the National Research Council, acting for the Committee on Medical Research, has been responsible for the planning and execution of clinical research on penicillin, using supplies of the drug purchased from the manufacturers by the Office of Scientific Research and Development and allocated for civilian use by the War Production Board. As Chairman of this Committee, Doctor Chester S. Keefer has met urgent requests from civilian physicians for penicillin in treatment of severe sulfonamide-resistant infections in which penicillin therapy might be indicated." The drug was received from the manufacturer as a powder, "varying in color from light yellow to deep reddish-brown . . . highly soluble in water", and stable in the anhydrous state. It had to be given systemically, preferably intravenously. [In the early appreciation of the abuse of antibiotics which has plagued us ever since] he said, " . . . it is perhaps fortunate that the drug must be given parenterally, and therefore, usually in hospitals because, apart from existing legal restrictions, this provides the only effective brake on the indiscriminate use of penicillin for all sorts of minor conditions". The dosage of penicillin had not yet been standardized, but "Most cases of gonorrhea will, for example, respond to 10,000 units every three hours for five doses, a total of 50,000 units . . . in cases of severe staphylococcic bacteremia, the average dose of 120,000 units per day for ten days may at times be increased to 300,000 or 400,000 units per day for a similar period." In areas not readily penetrated by penicillin coming from the bloodstream, it might be used locally,- intrathecally for meningitis, "injected into empyema cavities and infected joints into which the passage of penicillin from the blood is usually quite limited." [Lockwood pointed out quite accu-

rately a fact still perhaps not fully appreciated by physicians treating empyema] "the high local concentrations produced by this method probably aid in causing disappearance of the infecting organisms, but will not necessarily render surgical drainage unnecessary in chronic cases if the cavity is thick-walled and contains large masses of heavily infected fibrin." In the previous 18 months, the group at the University of Pennsylvania had treated 440 patients in various hospitals, usually after failure of intensive sulfonamide treatment. Two-thirds of 57 patients with staphylococcus bacteremia survived, sometimes requiring drainage of suppurative foci. Periorbital cellulitis proved to respond extraordinarily well to penicillin. "Penicillin cannot be expected to have a lasting curative effect in chronic bronchiectasis", but seemed effective in controlling active infection in preparation for operation. Patients with osteomyelitis responded dramatically but "usually developed bone sequestra and have required surgical treatment to complete their recovery." In chronic osteomyelitis, treatment with penicillin improved the local situation to a point at which sequestrectomy and saucerization were substantially safer and freer from complications. In sum, penicillin achieved "Dramatic curative responses in disseminated sepsis, particularly where circulation in localized distributing foci is adequate to effect contact between drug and bacteria. In such cases surgical treatment which would have seemed unavoidable in the past may, with penicillin, be postponed or avoided altogether." In infection within pleural cavity or joints, penicillin produced "Favorable responses characterized by subsidence of toxemia, correction of anemia, rapid healing of infected or seriously contaminated wounds, and elimination of infection . . . " Failures resulted when the organisms were insensitive, when there were other factors besides bacterial infection or when "because of poor circulation or limited transport of the drug" the penicillin did not reach the infected area. "Local penicillin therapy needs further study, but is yielding encouraging results in special cases."

Discussion

Frank L. Meleney, of New York, commented that the data was not yet in on "the prevention of infection in civilian contaminated wounds and burns . . . ." Like Lockwood, he referred to Dr. Champ Lyons' "fine paper reporting the results of his treatment of returned soldiers, mostly with infected compound fractures, all of whom, I would like to point out to Doctor Key, had had sulfonamides." [Albert

Key, of St. Louis, was a vigorous proponent of local sulfanilamide therapy.] At the Presbyterian Hospital, they had treated 150 infections, one-third of them locally. Meleney was inclined to feel that local use of penicillin was effective.

* * *

Harold Neuhof, Professor of Surgery, Columbia University; Attending Surgeon, Mt. Sinai Hospital, now Major, M.C., A.U.S., *The Problem of Embolism of the Pulmonary Artery*. Report of a Transcardiac Operation, had incised the right ventricle in an 18-year-old male with a massive pulmonary embolism and impending exitus. Bleeding from the ventriculotomy was easily controlled by crossed sutures while the catheter was passed into the pulmonary artery, but no thrombus was obtained. The patient died, "Thrombi filled the right and left branches beginning in each instance 2 to 3 cm. from the main trunk. They extended into the smaller branches on both sides."

Discussion

Claude S. Beck, of Cleveland, said Dr. Neuhof's procedure had "much to commend it. I used this same method years ago in the experimental laboratory", but he thought a glass or a metal tube would be better than a catheter. The Trendelenburg operation, he agreed, was much more difficult, "It is difficult to get adequate exposure. It is difficult to place the rubber tube under the pulmonary artery so that it can be elevated and controlled. Orientation is difficult, and the aorta has been opened instead of the pulmonary artery." He thought the important thing was to undertake the operation much earlier, not waiting till death was imminent. Alton Ochsner, of New Orleans, rose in vigorous disagreement, "we, as members of the surgical profession, should try to prevent these complications and not perform an operation that has to be undertaken immediately before death. There is no reason why anyone should ever develop a pulmonary embolism now, I believe." He made the distinction between "thrombophlebitis . . . associated with inflammation of the vein wall . . . and . . . bland thrombus with no associated inflammation of the vein. The latter we have designated as phlebothrombosis,- difficult to diagnose, but "By looking for vein tenderness the condition can be suspected and the diagnosis can be made by phlebography . . . . Ligation of the involved vein above the site of the thrombus will prevent detachment of the clot and pulmonary embolism, obviating the necessity of waiting until the patient becomes moribund, with a massive embolism, in order to perform the acrobatic surgery in order to remove the occluding thrombus in a dying individual." To prevent thromboses, "Every patient past 40 years of age, who is put to bed at all, should have his extremities wrapped from his toes to his groin with ACE bandages . . . when he comes back from the operating room, he should be placed in the Trendelenburg position . . . until he is able to move forcefully his extremities." [He was scornful of the Swedes] who "sat at the patient's bedside after he got his first pulmonary embolism, and waited until he was just about dead, and operated then. They saved a few, it is true, but there is no reason why we should allow this to occur. I hope we will not have any more papers on the removal of pulmonary emboli before this organization, an operation which should be of historical interest only . . . the way to prevent death from pulmonary embolism is to prevent the clot from being detached . . . " Claude S. Beck rose, again, to "take issue with the wishful thinking of Doctor Ochsner concerning pulmonary embolectomy . . . we all go along with him in his attempts to prevent pulmonary emboli but I cannot simply assume that this complication will be wiped out . . . and we need not concern ourselves with removal of pulmonary emboli." Nor were the methods for prevention of emboli established or generally accepted, "An embolus may arise in the vein proximal to the site of ligation and a fair percentage of emboli arises from sources other than the veins of the legs . . . . Until it can be shown that this complication can be prevented, we shall be interested in treating pulmonary emboli."

* * *

The first radical change in the treatment of hyperthyroidism since Plummer's introduction of iodine therapy made thyroidectomy safe, was presented by Howard M. Clute, of Boston, Professor of Surgery, Boston University School of Medicine; Surgeon-in-Chief, Massachusetts Memorial Hospitals, and by invitation, Robert H. Williams, *Thiouracil in the Preparation of Thyrotoxic Patients for Surgery*. The papers of the MacKenzies, of C. P. Richter and Clisby, and of Astwood, all in 1943, had demonstrated the depressive influence of the thiourea drugs "on the functional activity of the thyroid and hence on the basal metabolism." Several clinical reports had followed and Williams and Clute [in a paper in press at the time of the meeting] reported "on the treatment with thiouracil of 72 patients with thyrotoxicosis, the majority of whom obtained a normal metabolic rate and a remission of the disease. They were now reporting 115 patients of whom ". . . 81 were treated with thiouracil without surgery and 34 were treated with thiouracil and surgery." When patients were treated by thiouracil alone, "In the great majority of cases the basal metabolism became normal and the toxic manifestations of the disease disappeared . . . all patients who have continued to take thiouracil have remained in a normal state." In answer to the obvious question "In what cases of hyperthyroidism should we perform a thyroidectomy . . .?", they had adopted the plan "to perform a thyroidectomy . . . . In patients having a very large goiter . . . in patients who live far away and cannot readily have frequent check-up examinations . . . in patients who . . . cannot be depended upon to carefully follow medical treatment; and . . . in the small number of cases who have undesirable reactions to thiouracil." All patients with single discrete adenoma had been operated upon. Patients were usually admitted for the initiation of thiouracil therapy and allowed to go home within a day or two. Operation was generally undertaken after about five weeks of therapy, and patients who had been on Lugol's solution had it withdrawn when therapy with thiouracil was undertaken. Clinical improvement was obvious within a few days of the initiation of therapy and ophthalmic signs usually improved, although in five patients, the edema of the lids increased. The surgeons reported that "There was more bleeding encountered in some of the thiouracil-treated cases than in the iodine-treated cases . . . ." The operations and postoperative courses were remarkably smooth and uneventful, "The striking thing . . . was the absence of anything striking." They had a single death, in a patient with thyroid toxicosis for ten years, under constant iodine treatment, and auricular fibrillation for one year, and thiouracil therapy for eight weeks. " . . . her fibrillation ceased a few days before operation. She died about three hours after an uneventful thyroidectomy, probably from an embolus. Her pulse was 84 and her blood pressure 120/80, 15 minutes before death." They had an additional group of 15 patients with hyperthyroidism "recurrent or persistent after operation" and all had been completely controlled with thiouracil and none had required operation.

Discussion

John deJ. Pemberton, of the Mayo Clinic, said that they too had been impressed by Astwood's work and had used thiouracil. Apparently few or no patients at the Mayo Clinic had been treated with thiouracil alone. He implied that they were treating patients with thiouracil and then performed thyroidectomy, but cited no numbers. Roscoe R. Graham, of Toronto, said that they had had a small experience and shared Dr. Clute's hope that some patients might avoid operation permanently.

* * *

Cameron Haight, of Ann Arbor, Associate Professor of Surgery, University of Michigan Medical School, *Congenital Atresia of the Esophagus with Tracheoesophageal Fistula.* Reconstruction of Esophageal Continuity by Primary Anastomosis, had only the year before reported the first successful case of operation for esophageal atresia with tracheoesophageal fistula by division of the fistula and anastomosis of the esophageal ends. He now reported a series of 16 patients in whom a primary anastomosis had been attempted, two in 1939, both fatal, three in 1941 with one success, three in 1942 with one success, eight in 1943 with four successes, so that six patients out of 16 in whom an operation had been attempted were alive, seven months to three years and one month after operation. In Michigan, the three attempts to perform the "indirect method",- ligation of the fistula, cervical esophagostomy and subsequent antethoracic esophagoplasty,- had all ended in death "before the upper segment was exteriorized" [the method with which Leven, Ladd, and Humphreys had reported successes]. Shaw, Samson, and Lanman had attempted primary anastomosis without success, and since the landmark paper of Haight and Towsley, Shaw, Ladd, Humphreys, and Daniel had had successes. Haight had operated upon 24 patients, had found anastomosis possible only in 17. One might be justified in expending from six to 24 hours to treat any pulmonary aspiration pneumonitis which was present. Their operation had been carried out through a left extrapleural approach in 12 of the 24, and right extrapleural approach in 11. The simpler transpleural approach "was used before it was realized that the respiratory embarrassment would be considerably greater with an intrapleural than with an extrapleural approach." Although their first successful case was with the left extrapleural approach, they now preferred the right extrapleural approach. Through a posterolateral approach he resected the third, fourth and fifth ribs "from the plane of the transverse processes to a point above 1.0-1.5 cm. lateral to the angles of the ribs." The intercostal bundles and periosteum were divided and the pleura stripped away. The azygos vein was divided. A fine clamp on the tracheal attachment of the fistula, the lower end having been cut away, was oversewn with "several figure-of-eight plastic silk

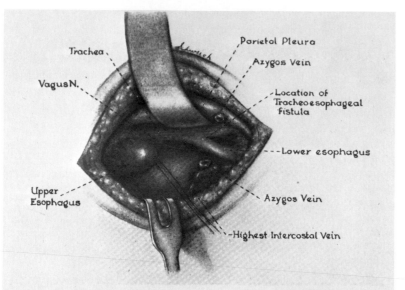

FIG. 6.—The right extrapleural exposure of the anomaly is illustrated. The posterior portions of the third, fourth and fifth ribs have been resected and the parietal pleura has been freed from the thoracic wall. The azygos vein has been divided in order to expose the lower esophagus. The dilated blind upper segment has been partially freed from the posterior wall of the trachea. The relative size of the upper and lower esophagus, and the usual position of the tracheoesophageal fistula are shown. The right vagus nerve serves as a useful guide for locating the lower segment.

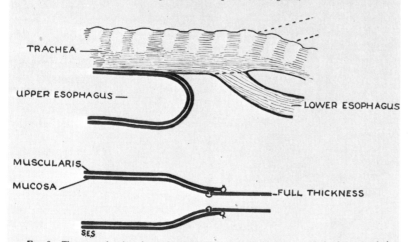

FIG. 8.—The upper drawing shows the blind upper esophageal segment and the lower esophagus arising from the trachea. The relative size of the two segments and the relative thickness of their walls are illustrated.

The lower drawing shows the completed "telescopic" anastomosis. This type of anastomosis is used because of the discrepancy in the size of the two segments and the discrepancy in the thickness of their walls. The relatively thick wall of the dilated upper segment and the extremely thin wall of the smaller lower segment are illustrated. The thickness of the entire wall of the lower segment is usually no greater than the thickness of the mucosa of the upper segment. The inner row of sutures approximates the full thickness of the wall of the lower segment to the mucosa and submucosa of the upper segment. The outer layer of sutures draws the muscularis of the upper segment downward and anchors it to the outer wall of the lower segment at a level several millimeters below the inner layer of sutures. Interrupted sutures of plastic silk are used in the construction of the anastomosis.

Haight's first successful one-stage operation for esophageal atresia and tracheoesophageal fistula had been reported the year before and he now had six living patients. His initial success had been with the left extrapleural approach but he now preferred the right extrapleural approach, as shown. The technique of anastomosis was by the telescoping method shown in his Figure 8.

Cameron Haight, *Congenital Atresia of the Esophagus with Tracheoesophageal Fistula,* Volume LXII, 1944.

sutures." He employed a telescoping anastomosis over a catheter with "the smallest available silk sutures (Deknatel A)". Eight interrupted sutures anastomosed the mucosa of the upper segment to the full thickness of the lower segment, the muscularis of the upper segment was then pulled down over the anastomosis and sutured to the outer surface of the lower segment with a similar number of fine sutures,

and the catheter withdrawn. A minimal amount of subcutaneous fluid was given after operation ". . . a 3 or 5 per cent solution of dextrose, supplemented with the desired amount of a 0.5 per cent solution of sulfadiazine. Physiologic saline solution is not used, except for the minimal amount required in conjunction with blood transfusions. The onset of edema of the extremities is an indication for a transfusion of whole blood . . . . One of the early cases in this series died from pulmonary edema resulting from the administration of an excessive amount of physiologic saline solution, and a more recent patient died from pulmonary edema following a plasma transfusion." X-rays of iodized oil swallows were begun on the second day, and the baby fed if there was no leakage after the examination on the fourth day. They tried to avoid gastrostomy because of the "increased risks . . . . One infant died ten hours after the gastrostomy, and no cause of death could be determined other than the fact that the infant had been subjected to an additional operation and had not had a transfusion in conjunction with the gastrostomy. Three infants died of hemorrhage from the region of the gastrostomy." Three patients developed an external esophageal fistula and all survived but with development of partial stricture. Four of their six successful patients had gastrostomies.

Discussion

William E. Ladd, of Boston, agreed that "extrapleural ligation of the fistula with primary anastomosis is the operation of choice when feasible." At the Children's Hospital, they had seen 72 children with esophageal atresia, "Up until 1939 the experience was valuable largely for furnishing pathologic material, and for teaching us what not to do . . . there has been a rift in the clouds, and we now have 11 living patients. During the past year we have operated upon 13 patients, of whom eight are living. In five of these patients a primary anastomosis was attempted, and two are living. In the other eight patients the fistula was tied off, and esophagostomy and gastrostomy performed, and six of these eight patients are living." Primary anastomosis required great skill and in addition was not feasible if there was a large gap between the segments, so that "multiple-stage operation is a considerably safer procedure, though in some ways less desirable." He used an extrapleural approach on the right, resecting a long segment of the fourth rib and merely dividing the third and fifth. He used a two-layer inverting anastomosis over a catheter leaving the catheter in place. Logan Leven, of St. Paul [whose first successful multistage operation preceded Dr. Ladd's by 24 hours], had since 1939 five surviving children with extrapleural ligation and multistage procedures. He had only attempted two primary anastomoses and lost both children. Rollin A. Daniel, of Nashville, Tennessee, said that at Vanderbilt, they had operated upon seven patients in the previous two-and-a-half years, performing fistula ligation and multi-staged operations in four, and attempting end-to-end anastomosis in the last three, with success in two of them. Cameron Haight, in closing, said that George Humphreys, at Babies Hospital, in New York, had three patients who had survived the multistage procedure, and two after a one-stage procedure, one eight months and one seven days before.

The Business Meetings

The 1944 meeting was held May 3, and 4 at Thorne Hall, Northwestern University, Chicago, Frederick A. Coller in the Chair.

Frank L. Meleney's report of the Program Committee was perhaps the shortest ever made, "Mr. President and gentlemen: The program for the meeting is in your hands. We hope it will meet with your approval."

Arthur W. Elting, reporting concerning the American Board of Surgery, said that the Board felt "very strongly that there should be no relaxation of the standards of surgical training hitherto established by the Board, especially in view of the fact that essentially all medical standards except those of the specialty Boards are under the control of the government. In view of the lowering of medical standards of education and training [he was undoubtedly referring to the lowering of requirements for admission to medical schools and the truncated programs of the medical schools], which will probably be still further lowered, it would seem especially incumbent upon the American Board of Surgery to maintain all its standards for qualification for the postwar era." Since the Army and Navy had officially accepted nine months of internship instead of a full year, the Board had agreed to accept that those entering military service and those going on into residency training would have the first three months of residency training deducted to complete the 12 months of the first year requirement. "The Board also decided to allow one year credit in the five years of graduate work in surgery required, for all who served in the armed forces." Individual allowances might be made after the war for special work and experience of individual candidates. As in President David's address the year before, the suggestion was made that it might be useful to have a uniform examination in basic surgical principles common to all of the Surgical Specialty Boards.

The Committee on Postwar Surgical Training, Chairman, Edward P. Lehman, of Charlottesville, with Lt. Col. D. C. Elkin, Jason Mixter, Nathan Womack, Owen Wangensteen, Fred Coller, ex officio, reviewed the general principles of surgical training, "It is believed that training in the use of English as a tool has been inadequate in recent years and that medical teachers should emphasize and re-emphasize the lack of success of the primary and secondary schools in this regard . . . a liberal education is still . . . essential . . . medical schools, should return to prewar requirements for admission . . . an accelerated medical school program is not desirable for most students . . . the quota system of distributing internships is an important handicap to the development of surgeons . . . It is strongly urged that free choice on the part of both the student and the institution be immediately established in hospitals accepted for graduate surgical training. It is the ultimate hope of the boards of certification that hospitals will not open their operating rooms to uncertified surgeons." There was a fear that incompletely trained men who had acted as surgeons during the war might be tempted ". . . to assume civilian surgical responsibility without adequate fundamental training . . ." The Committee in general approved of the training programs required by the boards and urged consideration ". . . of a period of basic training fundamental to all surgery, and that an examination on this basic training be a prerequisite to specialty certification." The Committee anticipated a substantial postwar deficit of surgeons and the need for increased training facilities, but warned against encouraging ". . . the establishment of surgical training programs in hospitals not well adapted to this purpose . . . ", pointing out with great clarity the problem [which in fact then ensued] that ". . . it would tend to produce surgeons without the fundamental training that those hospitals can give that have adequate material, personnel and medical school contacts. In the second place it would accustom many hospitals to the resident system, which in later years in the absence of a need for increased training facilities could not profitably be employed in the surgical training program." They advised increasing the numbers of residencies and assistant residencies in existing training programs rather than opening many new ones. They advised that the Veterans Administration be ". . . approached with the proposal that these [Veterans] hospitals be organized so as to fulfill the requirements for adequate graduate surgical training." They had not yet been able to complete their statistical study of the need for surgeons or of the number of training programs and their output. They specifically urged the establishment of surgical training programs in the Veterans hospitals and the construction of Veterans hospitals near established medical centers.

Evarts Graham opened the discussion of the report, stating that it was directed to the postwar situation, and "Nobody knows how far off that will be. I am concerned very much indeed with the emergency which exists right now . . . about this whole business of the training of a surgeon." The burden of Evarts Graham's remarks was that the Armed Forces were enthusiastic about the quality of the medical care because of the superbly trained men who had been inducted, but that the Armed Forces had "killed the goose that lays the golden egg. The training which has made these surgeons possible, who are now giving such a splendid account of themselves, that system of training is gone." Eighty-five percent of the medical officers being inducted into the Army had ". . . only nine months of experience in a hospital, and that, for the most part, a rotating service. My God, think of what that means to the wounded men who will fall into their hands!" If the war proved to be short, it would not make much difference; if it lasted three or four years, it would be serious, "There won't be an adequate number of well trained surgeons to take care even of the wounded men in our armed forces, to say nothing of the civilian population . . . I would say, Mr. President, that our concern is not now with a postwar program, but our concern right now is for a program to be revived right now—during the war—and not wait for postwar conditions." Graham proposed a representation by the Association directly to the President of the United States ". . . because I believe that is the only effective way in which anything can be accomplished", pointing out the disastrous effects of disruption of the surgical training programs. General Fred W. Rankin vigorously supported Graham's notion ". . . not only do we need to train more surgeons, but I would go further than that: We need to keep out of Selective Service some pre-medical students."

A motion was passed, the effect of which was to make possible a ". . . protest, in the name of the Society, to the President and to other appropriate people in power . . . ."

Dr. Whipple, for the Committee of the American Board of Surgery on Standardization of Examinations for Specialty Boards of Surgery, once more recommended a basic examination in surgery for all specialties, and hoped that the American Surgical Association would encourage and support such a program, but President Coller said that no action needed to be taken and no recommendations were made.

Since the measures taken by the Army ". . . entering enlisted men as medical students . . . will reduce the number of students entering the medical school by 28 per cent", the Association was empowered to make representations to the President of the United States, Secretary of War, and the Chief of Staff of the United States Army and the Chairmen of the Military Committees in the Senate and House of Representatives, pointing out that "As a result it is to be expected that the output of physicians, when these classes graduate, will be materially diminished, at a time when there will be a great need for such positions", and even that some of the medical schools might have to close.

Once more Council recommended increase of the active membership by five each year, not to exceed 200, and a limitation of Honorary Fellows to 25. Evarts Graham [whose Presidential Address had indicated the need for a significant expansion of the membership] asked ". . . what the line of reasoning was that suggested to the Council that an addition of five members per year would be advisable or would accomplish anything, or be of any use whatever to this organization?" To raise the membership to 200 in five years for a population of 145,000,000, ". . . seems to me to be analogous to the mountain going into labor and producing a mouse." However, President Coller reminded the Association that one of the recommendations of Council's report had been to "appoint a committee to study and to pro-pose ways and means of broadening the influence of this Association", and Secretary Firor said, "The Council thought it might be very likely that this committee might recommend increasing the membership, say, to 300, as one method of increasing the influence of this Association. The Council did not feel that they cared to recommend such a sudden jump in the membership." President Coller, in fact, said that the Committee might perhaps recommend a membership of 500. The motion was put to a vote and carried unanimously.

For the following year, officers elected were William Darrach, of New York, President; Albert O. Singleton, of Galveston, and John deJ. Pemberton, of Rochester, Minnesota, Vice-Presidents; and Warfield M. Firor, of Baltimore, Secretary.

Frederick L. Reichert, when the list of members proposed was read out, asked "Is it possible, next year, to have a list of these new members and their publications, or at least a few of their publications, so if we do not know the men before we come, at least we can have some opinion of their ability?"

Secretary Firor pointed out that some of the candidates had ". . . a bibliography as long as 130-odd articles. I have no intention of copying such a list." There was discussion back and forth and in the end no formal action was taken.

LXIII

1945

No meeting was held in 1945. The *Transactions* for that year represent papers submitted to the Association and published in the October issue of the *Annals of Surgery*. The papers within the volume were printed from the plates of the *Annals of Surgery*, as was to be true for 1946 and 1947. The papers are preceded by a note signed, William Darrach, President, "*A request to Director* [James F., of the Economic Stabilization Board] *Byrnes that the American Surgical Association be allowed to hold its meeting in May was politely but firmly refused. The Council has decided that the papers prepared for this meeting be published as a unit, without discussion, as proceedings of the Association.*" There were of course no discussions.

* * *

Allen O. Whipple, Professor of Surgery, Columbia University, Director of Surgical Services, Presbyterian Hospital, who had been President in 1940, *The Problem of Portal Hypertension in Relation to the Hepatosplenopathies,* agreed with Klemperer and others that the term Banti's disease could be abandoned and accepted Larrabee's term, congestive splenomegaly. Measurements at the time of splenectomy had always shown "an increase of two to five times splenic vein pressure over peripheral venous pressure in cases presenting Banti's syndrome . . . It is our present concept that Banti's syndrome is the result of mechanical obstruction to the flow of blood within the portal bed . . . In the cirrhoses there is a variable amount of portal hypertension, determined by the amount of scar tissue in Glisson's capsule, the relation of the pressure in the hepatic artery to that in the portal vein and the extent of the hepato-fugal collateral circulation. For these reasons splenomegaly, gastrointestinal hemorrhage, leukopenia and thrombocytopenia are not always found in the cirrhoses . . . On the other hand, in our experience, if the extrahepatic portal block, from whatever cause, is sufficient to produce a splenomegaly, Banti's syndrome is nearly always present, and a normal liver is usually found even in the cases of long standing . . . " The diagnosis was entirely clinical aided by the bromsulphalein retention test and the hippuric acid test and other evidences of impaired hepatic function. "The final determination of the site of the extrahepatic block in many patients can be made only at the autopsy table, for the dissection necessary to demonstrate such a block is neither safe nor feasible in the great majority of patients on the operating table. We have been unable to determine the site of the extrahepatic block at the time of splenectomy in more than half of our patients, although in our more recent operations we have demonstrated the block by diodrast venograms taken at the time of determining portal vein pressures with roentgenograms at the operating table." Previous treatment of portal hypertension had been by splenectomy, by extraperitoneal omentopexy and by ligation of the tributaries to the esophageal varices. If the portal block was in the splenic vein, splenectomy would result in permanent cure, but this was uncommon. "We have had only five such cases, but they were all cured, with no recurrence of hematemesis." Even with the block in the main portal vein, the splenec-

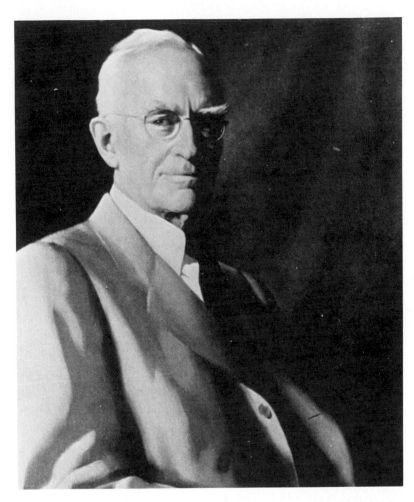

Allen O. Whipple, 1881-1963, President 1940, M.D., College of Physicians and Surgeons, New York, 1908, Valentine Mott Professor and Director of Surgical Services at Presbyterian Hospital, 1921. Eponymously known for his triad of criteria of hyperinsulinism with islet tumors and for the operation of pancreatoduodenectomy (*Whipple's disease* is named after his brother George, the Nobel Laureate pathologist). His more significant contribution was the creation of the Spleen Clinic in his Department of Surgery, the result of which was the Blakemore-Lord technique for porto-systemic shunting, the ultimate development by Blakemore and Voorhees of artificial prosthetic replacement of blood vessels, the continued work with Rousselot and Blakemore on portal hypertension.

Portrait courtesy of Keith Reemtsma, College of Physicians and Surgeons, Columbia University, New York.

tomy, because of the removal of a large area of portal bed" provided relief for a variable period of time. He was dubious about omentopexy of any kind, "In our experience, if the operation is done in the presence of a well-established collateral venous circulation in the abdominal wall, as evidenced by dilated superficial veins, or as shown by infra-red photographs, the results in a few cases are encouraging, but probably due to Nature's efforts rather than to the surgeon's . . . Attempts to ligate the tributaries feeding into the veins of the cardia and the esopha-

geal varices have been very disappointing. Nor have the injection and coagulation methods to obliterate the esophageal varices been any better." Their efforts and those of Gunn, Villard and Tavernier, of Meursing and Bogorts "to anastomose branches of the mesenteric veins to the spermatic, the ovarian and the inferior cava by suture technic" failed usually due to thrombosis of the anastomosis, he thought. They had "discussed the more extensive procedures for portacaval shunt based on the principle of the Eck fistula" but had not attempted it "un-

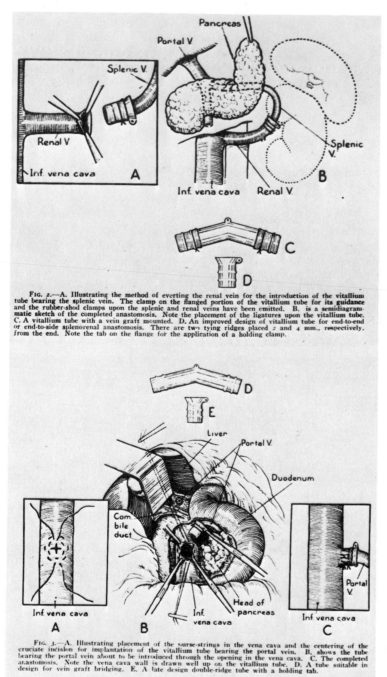

FIG. 2.—A. Illustrating the method of everting the renal vein for the introduction of the vitallium tube bearing the splenic vein. The clamp on the flanged portion of the vitallium tube for its guidance and the rubber-shod clamps upon the splenic and renal veins have been omitted. B. is a semidiagrammatic sketch of the completed anastomosis. Note the placement of the ligatures upon the vitallium tube. C. A vitallium tube with a vein graft mounted. D. An improved design of vitallium tube for end-to-end or end-to-side splenorenal anastomosis. There are two tying ridges placed 2 and 4 mm., respectively, from the end. Note the tab on the flange for the application of a holding clamp.

FIG. 3.—A. Illustrating placement of the purse-strings in the vena cava and the centering of the cruciate incision for implantation of the vitallium tube bearing the portal vein. B. shows the tube bearing the portal vein about to be introduced through the opening in the vena cava. C. The completed anastomosis. Note the vena cava wall is drawn well up on the vitallium tube. D. A tube suitable in design for vein graft bridging. E. A late design double-ridge tube with a holding tab.

For splenorenal anastomosis by the Blakemore-Lord technique (in essence an adaptation of Crile's direct blood transfusion technique), the spleen and left kidney were removed, the Vitallium tube was slipped over the central end of the mobilized splenic vein, a cuff of which was turned back over the Vitallium tube, and the vein-covered Vitallium tube was slipped into the central end of the renal vein and held there by circumferential ligature. For the end-to-side portacaval shunt, the portal vein was divided close to the liver, the hepatic end ligated and the visceral end passed through and everted over a Vitallium tube, which was then inserted into the side of the vena cava through a purse-string suture, which was rapidly tied and the rubber-shod occluding clamps on the vena cava quickly released.

Arthur H. Blakemore and Jere W. Lord, Jr., *The Technic of Using Vitallium Tubes in Establishing Portacaval Shunts for Portal Hypertension,* Volume LXIII, 1945.

til Blakemore, of our Surgical Staff, developed his endothelial-lined Vitallium tube nonsuture technic for bridging large vessel defects. Blakemore and Lord have recently described this technic, and have made a major contribution to vascular surgery." Eck's original publication of the construction of the fistula in animals with a suggestion that it might be used clinically was published in 1877. Vidal, of

France, claimed to have done it in 1903; De Martel, in 1910; Lenoir, in 1914; and Rosenstein, in 1912; Rosenstein's being the only patient that survived. Allen O. Whipple referred also to the work of George H. Whipple [without indicating that he was his brother], who had an extensive experience with Eck fistulae in animals, some of which he had been able to keep in good health for as long as eight years. Of the experience at Presbyterian Hospital, using the Blakemore tube, Allen Whipple said " . . . Dr. Blakemore and I have carried out ten of these major procedures, five consisting of uniting the splenic vein and left renal veins, after removing the spleen and left kidney. In our last five patients we have anastomosed the portal vein to the inferior cava, end-to-side. All these patients have survived their operations. These procedures are as yet purely experimental. They have been carried out in patients that had had repeated severe hemorrhages, and for whom conservative measures offered no hope." Five of the patients had had improvement in liver function with disappearance of ascites and cessation of hemorrhage. He mentioned the fact also that "Four other splenorenal vein anastomoses [these were done by direct vein suture] for portal hypertension have recently been performed by Dr. Alfred Blalock, who writes me that two of these patients have had a disappearance of ascites and are remarkably improved. On the other hand, he says his enthusiasm is somewhat curbed because the other two patients have died since operation from recurrent bleeding from esophageal varices. He thinks this may be due to oc-clusion of the anastomosis as a result of the attendant trauma at time of the operation." Whipple made the prediction that "the large number of men in the armed forces invalided by damaged livers, the result of infectious hepatitis, will become an increasing problem with the development of portal cirrhosis."

* * *

Whipple's paper was followed by that of Arthur H. Blakemore, by invitation, and Jere W. Lord, Jr., also by invitation, *The Technic of Using Vitallium Tubes in Establishing Portacaval Shunts for Portal Hypertension,* which was devoted to the precise technique of the operation. [This was merely a permanent insertion of Crile's transfusion tube (see page 401, Vol. XXVII, 1909).]

[None of the other papers in this slender volume were of the importance of those of Whipple, and Blakemore and Lord, and in the absence of Discussions, which so often make worthwhile an otherwise forgettable paper, none of them have been selected for presentation here.]

LXIV

1946

The 1946 meeting, the first since 1944, the 1945 meeting having been cancelled because the Office of Defense Transportation would not authorize the meeting, was held at Hot Springs, Virginia, April 2, 3, and 4, 1946, President William Darrach, Consultant to Fracture Service, The Presbyterian Hospital; Dean Emeritus and Professor of Clinical Surgery, College of Physicians and Surgeons, Columbia University, in the Chair. The preceding year had seen the deaths of two former Presidents, Edward William Archibald, of Montreal, who had produced hemorrhagic pancreatitis by the intraductal injection of infected bile, proposed sphincterotomy, and issued the Presidential Call that produced the move to form the American Board of Surgery, and Ellsworth Eliot, Jr., of New York, as well as of the Nobel Laureate Fellow, Alexis Carrel, massive contributor to science, but to the Association of greatest interest were his astounding and imaginative feats of vascular anastomosis and replacement, and his brilliant insight into the ultimate potentialities of cardiac and vascular surgery.

Darrach was the first avowed specialist, since the many-sided Harvey Cushing, to be elected President. [His dreary, elementary, and anecdotal account, *Treatment of Fractures,* could have not done much toward persuading the Fellows to elect another orthopedic surgeon as President, assuming that any thought at all is given to the quality of a potential President's Address. In fact, since 1946, only two more specialists have been elected President, Drs. Howard C. Naffziger and Loyal Davis, both representing the specialties of neurosurgery but both Department of Surgery Chairmen.]

* * *

The surgery of Zenker's pharyngeal diverticulum had been discussed at the 1910 meeting, by C. H. Mayo. Now, Frank H. Lahey, of Boston, Surgeon-in-Chief, New England Baptist Hospital; Surgeon-in-Chief, New England Deaconess Hospital, *Pharyngo-Esophageal Diverticulum: Its Management and Complications,* returned to the subject. He now emphasized the incoordination of the action of the constrictor muscles and the cricopharyngeus, in the production of the bulge into the posterior "triangular space bounded above by the lowest fibers of the inferior constrictor and on each side by the oblique fibers of the cricopharyngei. This is known as the pharyngeal dimple and is the weak place in the posterior wall at the pharyngo-esophageal junction." Lahey had finally settled on a two-stage operation. In the first stage, through a longitudinal incision along the anterior border of the left sternocleidomastoid muscle, the sac was dissected out. If it was a small sac, it was fastened to the tissues high in the neck so that it drained downward; if it was a large sac, it was actually exteriorized on the surface of the skin. In the second stage, the neck of the sac

884

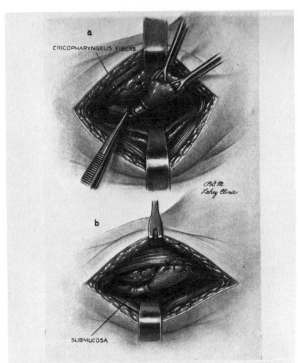

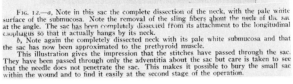

Fig. 12.—*a*, Note in this sac the complete dissection of the neck, with the pale white surface of the submucosa. Note the removal of the sling fibers about the neck of the sac at the angle. The sac has been completely dissected from its attachment to the longitudinal esophagus so that it actually hangs by its neck.

b, Note again the completely dissected neck with its pale white submucosa and that the sac has now been approximated to the prethyroid muscle.

This illustration gives the impression that the stitches have passed through the sac. They have been passed through only the adventitia about the sac but care is taken to see that the needle does not penetrate the sac. This makes it possible to bury the small sac within the wound and to find it easily at the second stage of the operation.

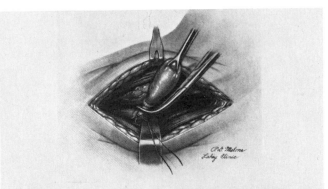

Fig. 14.—This illustration represents the method of ligating the sac at the second-stage procedure when all the fascial planes have been walled-off. One ligature is shown about the sac already tied, the second ligature is about the sac but not yet tied. Note the clamp applied distally to avoid spilling of the infected contents of the sac. Note again that the pale white submucosa, demonstrating how completely the neck of the sac has been dissected, is shown.

Lahey favored an approach along the border of the sternocleidomastoid muscle, under general anesthesia. The inferior thyroid artery was always divided. The operation was a two-stage procedure. Small diverticula were attached to the muscle high up in the neck at the end of the first stage, as in Lahey's 12B. Very large diverticula were brought out into the wound or actually onto the surface of the skin as in Lahey's Figure 10. Lahey's Figure 14 indicates simple ligation of a small diverticulum. Of the opening left by removal of a very large diverticulum, he said, "I would like to say, for the benefit of anyone doing this suture that such are the difficulties of doing it that it is often a far from accurate suture line but, with an indwelling tube, rarely leaks."

Frank H. Lahey, *Pharyngo-Esophageal Diverticulum: Its Management and Complications*. Volume LXIV, 1946.

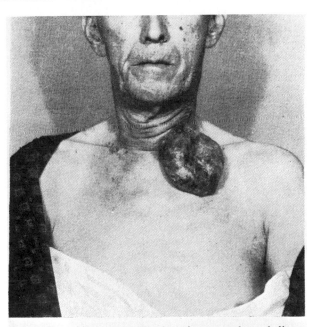

Fig. 10.—This illustrates how in an esophageal diverticulum with a very large sac it is necessary to implant the sac on the neck. One can realize in a sac that has reached this proportion how large the opening into the true esophagus will be and how undesirable it would be to attempt to ligate such a mass of esophageal tissue.

was ligated or sutured. He was reporting 209 cases done by the two-stage method with two deaths, one of uremia four days after an uncomplicated first stage, and one of mediastinitis from unrecognized leakage from the "blind right side of the sac". The principal advantage of the two-stage operation was that if leakage occurred from the closure of the neck of the diverticulum, the mediastinum having been sealed there would be no danger of mediastinitis.

Although he always did the two-stage operation, and if he were to be operated upon himself would have the two-stage operation, he said that he spoke "With no purpose of disparagement of the one-stage operation, with no attempt to persuade those who employ it away from its use, with perhaps an unnecessary sense of caution concerning the possibility of the occurrence of mediastinitis when leakage with the one-stage operation occasionally occurs . . ."

Discussion

Stuart W. Harrington, of the Mayo Clinic, agreed "with Doctor Lahey's statement that pharyngo-esophageal diverticula may be treated surgically by a one-stage or two-stage operation." At the Mayo Clinic, they had 348 operations, the first 25 in two stages and the remaining 146 in one stage. They had one operative death in the 25 two-stage cases, and a temporary fistula in six cases, paralysis of the left vocal cord in one and stricture requiring dilatation in five. The diverticulum recurred in three. In the 146 one-stage operations, they had no mediastinitis and 90% of the wounds had healed by primary intention. There was no operative mortality, five temporary fistulae, one instance of vocal cord paralysis, and two diverticula recurred. Five patients required dilatation. Robert S. Dinsmore, of the Cleveland Clinic, said that mediastinitis was rare with either kind of operation and that if there was much

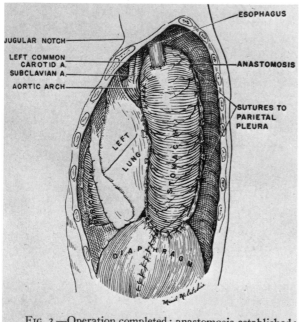

FIG. 3.—Operation completed; anastomosis established; stomach fastened in the chest by sutures to the parietal pleura; diaphragm closed.

Sweet's operation was performed through the bed of the eighth rib on the left, dividing other ribs superiorly as needed. The anastomosis of esophagus to stomach was with three layers of interrupted fine silk sutures. In 32 completed operations, he had eight deaths.

Richard H. Sweet, *Carcinoma of the Midthoracic Esophagus. Its Treatment by Radical Resection and High Intrathoracic Esophagogastric Anastomosis.* Volume LXIV, 1946.

soiling at the primary operation, one could pack the neck and do a secondary closure in 48 hours.

* * *

Richard H. Sweet, of Boston, Visiting Surgeon, Massachusetts General Hospital; Associate in Surgery, Harvard Medical School, *Carcinoma of the Midthoracic Esophagus.* Its Treatment by Radical Resection and High Intrathoracic Esophagogastric Anastomosis. At the Massachusetts General Hospital, they had employed the Torek procedure 14 times, with two initial operative deaths. Only four patients survived to have the external esophagus completed and at the time of reporting, only one was alive and well out of the 14. Of the 66 patients seen in 1944 and 1945 with carcinoma of the midthoracic esophagus, 25 had been inoperable, nine had been only explored, and 32, just under 50%, had had resection with esophagogastrectomy. The chest was entered through a left eighth rib resection and several other ribs divided posteriorly as needed "to provide access to a high growth and for the performance of a very high anastomosis." The esophagus was dissected free below the aortic arch, and from behind the aortic arch, if necessary, the diaphragm was split radially, and the stomach mobilized by division of the short gastric and left gastric vessels. In some cases, the anastomosis had been performed below the aortic arch. The esophagogastrostomy was performed with three layers of fine silk interrupted sutures. He performed the operation 32 times, with a 25% mortality,- eight postoperative deaths. There were two deaths out of 14 anastomoses below the aortic arch. For anastomoses above the aortic arch, there were six deaths out of 18. Only three of the deaths were due to "sepsis", all in patients operated upon ". . . in 1944, before penicillin was available for civilian use. Since penicillin has been used routinely as a prophylactic measure, there have been no manifestations of infection of any kind in 29 consecutive cases."

Discussion

Harold W. Wookey, of Toronto, agreed that intrathoracic anastomosis was desirable when possible and that "The procedure of bringing the upper end of the esophagus over the arch of the aorta into the left side of the chest enables one to do an anastomosis which would be otherwise impossible." He showed a slide of a successful result from this, as well as another of a completed Torek operation with a good skin tube. He was nevertheless not confident of the ultimate solution, "The future, no doubt, will decide whether the intrathoracic reconstruction will eventually replace other methods. This will depend on the relative mortality rates and also on the function of the intrathoracic anastomosis over a period of years."

* * *

Gustaf E. Lindskog, of New Haven, Associate Professor of Surgery, Yale University, *Bronchiogenic Carcinoma,* analyzed the Yale experience with 100 consecutive primary pulmonary cancers seen in the five years ending, December, 1943. Sixty-five patients had hopelessly advanced tumors and were inoperable, three refused treatment, and exploration was performed in 32, of whom only 12 were found "suitable for resection at the time of exploration." There were no deaths among the patients merely explored. Of the 12 patients who underwent resection,- pneumonectomy in 10, lobectomy in two,- three died, a hospital mortality of 25%. Of the nine who survived operation, three were alive and apparently free of tumor two-and-a-half to five-and-a-half years later. One unoperated patient was alive and in good condition three-and-a-half years after radiotherapy alone.

Discussion

Evarts Graham, of St. Louis, opened the Discussion stating it was important to publicize the results to educate the medical profession, and said that, "I do not share the pessimism which some others have. The only aspect that I am pessimistic about is the fact that in most cases the condition is not recognized early enough to do something for the patient." In the last three years at the Barnes Hospital, they had seen 221 patients with bronchogenic carcinoma, 109 of them declared inoperable on the basis of the clinical examination and of the 112 operated upon, resection with a reasonable chance of cure was possible in only 39,- 18% of the total group. His first successful total pneumonectomy patient was still alive and well after 13 years and Graham had six others alive and well more than seven years. He was enthusiastic enough to say, "I think if patients can be obtained in larger numbers in an operable stage it will be possible in another decade for someone to report before this Association 50 to 60 per cent of five-year cures." Alton Ochsner, of New Orleans, was "astounded by the statements of Doctor Graham and Doctor Lindskog that so few are operable. We have had 267 primary carcinomas in which we

were able to do a resection in 103 cases, an incidence of 34.4 per cent" [actually 38%, one of the figures had to be wrong, but went on to explain the not very sound basis for his own operability rate], "I feel that inoperability means metastases. I think palliative resection is justifiable . . . I have one patient alive five years after resection of a tumor which had invaded the mediastinum, in which there was recurrent nerve paralysis . . ." Ochsner gave no other figures. Lindskog, in closing, said he had not meant to "leave a note of complete pessimism, but I do want to emphasize that our series is typical of the case material we are up against in general hospitals at the present time."

* * *

Arthur W. Allen, of Boston, Chief, East Surgical Service, Massachusetts General Hospital; Lecturer in Surgery, Harvard Medical School, and by invitation, Claude E. Welch, *Subtotal Gastrectomy for Duodenal Ulcer,* indicated pretty plainly that they thought the day of gastrectomy for ulcer might be over and the time had come to assess the results,- "Dragstedt and his coworkers [*Annals of Surgery,* 1945] have recently suggested the possibility of avoiding most of the operations upon the stomach itself by transthoracic vagotomy. Moore [Francis], Jones, *et al.,* in our clinic, have satisfactorily demonstrated in a carefully selected group of ulcer patients that this procedure is spectacular in its immediate results. It will require time and more extensive experience with this indirect attack on the problem to evaluate the ultimate outcome in these cases. In the meantime, it is essential that the accumulated experiences of surgeons who have treated duodenal ulcer by radical surgery be assembled." Allen and Welch surveyed the results of 136 elective gastrectomies for duodenal ulcer. Most patients had had the ulcer resected with the duodenum, a few had the ulcer turned in and there was a small number of antral exclusions with mucosal excision, and seven Finsterer operations in which the antral mucosa was left. The resection was stated to be a two-thirds gastrectomy. Their operative mortality was 5%, and, only a single death, in the last hundred gastrectomies. Allen mentioned the problem of operating for massive hemorrhage when the mortality rose with age and with the duration of the bleed, and that the five patients who died after several days of bleeding had been "uniformly operated upon after several days of bleeding as a final gesture." As far as long-term results were concerned, six out of the seven Finsterer operations gave bad results and of the remainder who had what were considered to be appropriate operations, 69% were entirely asymptomatic, considered "excellent", 18% "had trivial symptoms . . . about six per cent . . . were improved by the operation but still have symptoms requiring special diet or medical care . . . Definitely poor results occurred in about seven per cent of the group."

Discussion

Lester R. Dragstedt, of Chicago, opened the Discussion agreeing that a critical evaluation of the status of gastrectomy was required ". . . because, as Doctor Allen has so generously stated, we have now available an alternative method. During the past three years I have sectioned the vagus nerve to the stomach in 67 patients with peptic ulcers of various types—duodenal, gastrojejunal and gastric. The results so far have been so satisfactory that I think there is a real possibility that it will replace subtotal gastrectomy in the treatment of this disease." Subtotal gastrectomy, he had long thought, ". . . too disabling an operation for a benign lesion." Roscoe Graham, of Toronto [who performed an even higher gastrectomy], said Dragstedt's work was stimulating, but spoke of a technique for dealing with the difficult duodenum and, without using the term, spoke of the dumping syndrome ". . . the patient who, after a meal, usually breakfast, becomes nauseated, pale, sweating and weak . . . symptoms are relieved by recumbency, and rarely last longer than half an hour." He thought this was due to a large stoma with reflux into the proximal loop and had reduced the incidence by making a small stoma and suturing the proximal jejunal loop higher on the stomach than the efferent loop. Frank H. Lahey, of Boston, said that "Subtotal gastrectomy has . . . been such a satisfactory operation . . . over a period of years adequate to give it a thorough trial, that we must be careful not to relinquish it for one that is as yet really not demonstrated." He wondered about the effect of vagotomy on gastric motility and on the other viscera. As for the operation of gastrectomy, ". . . the technical problem . . . is not in the subtotal gastrectomy itself but in the removal of the ulcer. We have repeatedly said that we like to get the duodenal ulcer out because the patient is better off with it out, but particularly because it provides then a good flexible duodenum for safe inversion." Lahey said that Roscoe Graham had just described "the Hofmeister type of subtotal gastrectomy which we have employed over the years."

* * *

Edward J. Donovan, of New York, Attending Surgeon, St. Luke's Hospital, Babies Hospital; Associate Professor of Surgery, College of Physicians and Surgeons, Columbia University, *Congenital Hypertrophic Pyloric Stenosis,* reported a series of 507 Fredet-Rammstedt operations with a mortality of 1.8%. [Congenital hypertrophic pyloric stenosis had last been discussed before the Association in 1929 when Alfred Brown had reported 20 cases and no deaths.] The operation was not to be undertaken hurriedly and several days might be spent in preparing the baby with hypodermoclyses. "After operation, the baby is taken immediately to the 'Pyloric Room' where the temperature is kept constant and from which all visitors are excluded. These infants in particular must be protected from all sources of infection because of their low resistance." The tumor disappeared in about seven weeks after the operation but was known to persist throughout life in patients who had had a posterior gastroenterostomy. While the mortality since 1932 was 1.8%, in 1946, it was only 0.8% for 245 operations.

Discussion

William E. Ladd, of Boston, opened the Discussion, presenting his series at the Boston Children's Hospital which went back to 1915 and included many patients operated upon by the resident staff, "In that time we have had 1,145 cases . . . 1915 to 1935 . . . 588 cases, with 35 deaths, a mortality of 5.9 per cent. In the last ten years there were 557 cases, with five deaths, a mortality of 0.8 of one per cent. In the last three and one-half years, there have been 225 consecutive cases with no deaths."

* * *

John C. Burch, of Nashville, Associate Professor of Obstetrics and Gynecology, Vanderbilt University, formerly Chief of Surgical Service, Brooke General Hospital, and by invitation, H. C. Fisher, of Denver, Colorado, *Early Ambulation in Abdominal Surgery,* made the first presentation before the Association on this now popular subject. They cited the "Recent reviews by Leithauser and Newburger and articles by Powers, by Schafer and Dragstedt, and Elman . . . " Schafer and Dragstedt had claimed that atelectasis was much less common in those who were ambulant. Leithauser had shown that the vital capacity returns much more rapidly to normal. They cited Scandinavian and Russian authors as well. Their material covered 2,827 abdominal cases at the Brooke General Hospital, Fort Sam Houston, Texas, September 1, 1943 to August 1, 1945. Early ambulation at the hospital had been "inaugurated by Brigadier General James Bethea during his tour as Chief of the Surgical Service." Of the total operations, 918 were herniorrhaphies. One recurrence occurred in the hospital and two others were reported later by letter. They stated without comment "The policy of early ambulation in the treatment of inguinal hernia was discontinued by the Surgeon-General in a directive dated July 13, 1943." [It was employed in at least one general hospital in the European Theater, but when General Paul Hawley made an inspection the patients were drilled in the "appropriate" answer to the question he did in fact ask.] In general, they said things had gone well, that there had been only a single eventration, that there had been no cases of femoral or iliac phlebitis, but there had been two deaths from pulmonary embolism. There was essentially no statistical analysis, certainly no controlled study, and they summarized, "our experience, as well as the cumulative recorded experiences of many surgeons, testifies to the physiologic soundness of early postoperative ambulation. It is a proved procedure of great benefit to patients and is deserving of a much wider employment."

Discussion

The comments made by Herman E. Pearse, of Rochester, who had visited the unit at Brooke, were apropos, "We must admit to a certain amount of mental lethargy in not adopting this [early ambulation] for younger, healthier patients. The fear of wound disruption by early ambulation is a myth, handed down to us from the past. A wound may be disrupted by involuntary action such as coughing, sneezing, or vomiting, or by pressure from distention. It is not disrupted by voluntary effort, for a patient will not hurt himself. Any activity within the limits of comfort is safe. I am confident that venous complications begin soon after operation and that early ambulation alone will not be enough to prevent them. Early activity in bed must be added. In the first 24-hour period a patient is out of bed only a short time, so the percentage of time in bed, even with early ambulation, may permit venous stasis." He advised that the patient move in bed and exercise the legs at frequent intervals.

* * *

A new departure in the therapy of renal failure was presented by Jacob Fine, of Brookline, Massachusetts, Assistant Professor of Surgery, Harvard University; Head of Surgical Research, Beth Israel Hospital, and by invitation, Howard A. Frank and Arnold M. Seligman, *The Treatment of Acute Renal Failure by Peritoneal Irrigation.* They had already demonstrated in dogs that the peritoneum was an

effective dializing membrane which by irrigation "would provide 40–75 per cent of normal kidney function in terms of urea clearance, correct acidosis, and prevent death from uremia following bilateral nephrectomy." Now in four patients with renal failure, two from incompatible blood transfusions, one from sulfathiazole and one from bilateral renal obstruction, they showed substantial improvement in the uremia, and restoration of normal function. Three of the patients had developed positive cultures from the return fluid. Fine said that "The control of fluid and electrolyte balance is at least as important as the elimination of nitrogenous waste products, and is an integral part of this therapeutic method." They used Tyrode's solution, prepared in 20 liter pyrex carboys. In one patient, they also exteriorized a loop of bowel as a Thiry-Vella fistula and found that this, which would have eliminated the problems of peritonitis from peritoneal irrigation, was not a sufficiently efficient system. Fine claimed only "that a properly performed peritoneal irrigation can eliminate all clinical and chemical evidence of the uremic state . . . that significant improvement can be achieved within 36 to 48 hours . . . and that the efficiency did not decline with continued exposure of the peritoneum to the irrigating solution. A footnote added that the addition of 2% glucose to the irrigating fluid ". . . will prevent the production of edema from the absorption of water from the irrigating fluid" and would lead to some absorption of utilizable carbohydrate.

Discussion

Edward D. Churchill, of Boston, said that "despite all the optimistic reports on the successful management of shock in this war, renal shutdown was the stone wall against which we butted our heads many times. The reduced blood volume of shock could be corrected by transfusion, but the kidneys ceased to function and many wounded men died despite the most skilled surgical procedures . . . Doctor Fine's method represents one more procedure that may be applicable to men suffering from renal shutdown following severe trauma." Allen O. Whipple, of New York, considered it "a real advance." Alton Ochsner, of New Orleans, said that they had "been afraid of peritoneal lavage" and had used gastric lavage with very large amounts of fluid and with successful results. They had had two patients, with uremia after incompatible blood transfusions, who required two weeks and ten days, respectively, of gastric lavage before spontaneous renal function returned. Jonathan Rhoads, of Philadelphia, spoke of extracorporeal dialysis. They had

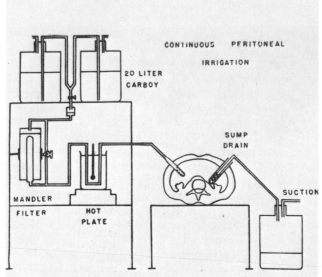

FIG. 1.—Diagrammatic representation of the circuit for continuous peritoneal irrigation.

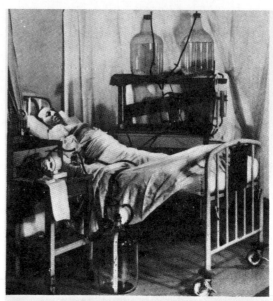

FIG. 2.—Photograph of apparatus for peritoneal irrigation.

The appropriate salts, except the sodium bicarbonate, were placed in 15 liters of sterile distilled water in the 20 liter carboy, the $NaHCO_3$, separately autoclaved in a liter of distilled water, added and, finally, heparin, penicillin and sulfadiazine were added to the solution. The fluid flowed by gravity through a bacterial filter and then through tubing in a water bath and into the steel peritoneal inlet tube and was sucked off through a stainless steel sump-drain. Fine and his associates reported use of the system in four patients with effective dialysis in all of them and a return to normal function. Jonathan Rhoads, in Discussion, spoke of his use in three patients of sausage casing for extracorporeal dialysis, a technique which Abel, Rowntree and Turner had employed in animals in 1913.

Jacob Fine, Howard A. Frank, and Arnold M. Seligman, *The Treatment of Acute Renal Failure by Peritoneal Irrigation*. Volume LXIV, 1946.

been experimenting clinically with that technique "in a much less thorough manner" since 1938; Abel, Rowntree and Turner, in 1913, had "set up a system of celloidin tubes through which the blood of animals was circulated", and Haas and Gantner, in Germany, had used peritoneal dialysis. Rhoads added that "It is now easier to employ the method of Abel, Rowntree and Turner, because suitable tubes for dialysis can be obtained in the form of sausage casing, which is available in lengths of 100 feet. About two years ago, Dr. Henry Saltonstall and I set up a system using 60 feet of this tubing in a bath of Ringer's solution with sufficient gelatin to counteract the osmotic pressure of the serum proteins, and by heparinizing the patient it was possible to allow his blood to flow out from an artery through this system and to reenter the circulation through the veins. This method, too, will reduce the urea nitrogen." Ralph Colp, of New York, had been supplied by I. Snapper [then in New York, but formerly of Holland] with an abstract "of a thesis by Doctor Kolff of Amsterdam, Holland, published in January,

1946 . . . " Kolff employed a cellophane tube, the tube wound around a cylinder which rotated in a dialysis exchange tank. Heparinized blood flowed through the tubing. Colp gave rather complete details without citing any experience. Jacob Fine, closing, reemphasized "Doctor Churchill's warning that this is still a highly experimental phase of the problem and is not presented as a satisfactory clinical method as yet." External dialysis might, he thought, prove satisfactory but required an arteriovenous anastomosis in patients already seriously ill. Continuous gastrointestinal irrigation, he thought was not sufficiently efficient.

* * *

The original paper by Blalock and Taussig in the *Journal of the American Medical Association* in May, 1945, had aroused tremendous interest, and now Alfred Blalock, of Baltimore, Professor of Surgery and the Director of the Department of Surgery, Johns Hopkins University; Surgeon-in-Chief, Johns Hopkins Hospital, *The Surgical Treatment of Con-*

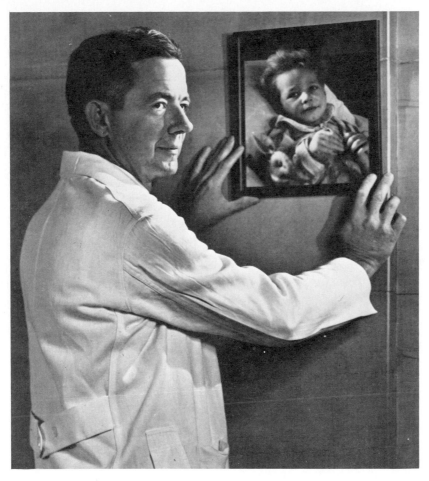

Alfred Blalock (1950,- the picture was sent him by a little French child upon whom he had done his operation for tetralogy of Fallot in 1947 at the time of his triumphal progress in London and Paris) 1899-1964. President, 1956 and President of ACS, 1954-55. M.D. Johns Hopkins, 1922. After two years at Hopkins in urology and in the laboratory, went to Barney Brooks' new Vanderbilt Service in Nashville as his resident, leaving Nashville in 1941, as Professor of Surgery, to accept the Chair at Hopkins. He had already established himself as a thoracic surgeon with an important series of pericardiectomies, and his work on traumatic shock had established that the fundamental basis was hypovolemia due to loss of fluid into the injured tissue. Within four years at Hopkins, he had pioneered thymectomy for myasthenia gravis, devised the first operative approach (subclavian turn-down) for coarctation, evolved and evaluated in the laboratory and applied clinically the subclavian pulmonary anastomosis for "pulmonic stenosis", which he had used at Vanderbilt as an experimental technique in the study of pulmonary hypertension. He established the pattern, for the future, of a laboratory for physiological evaluation of cardiac patients. He had an electrifying effect upon his medical school. He was demanding of his associates, took pleasure in recognizing their contributions, supported them strongly. The influence of the School of Surgery he created and of the men who took all or some of their training with him has been extraordinary both in terms of the scientific contributions of his disciples and of their acceptance of major academic and organizational roles. Always thoughtful, innately courteous, remarkably free of side, delighting in good company, he was superbly effective in his institution, and in the organizations he served.

Photography: Yousuf Karsh, Ottowa.

genital *Pulmonic Stenosis,* presented the results of his first 110 operations. "This figure includes all patients upon whom an incision was made and hence some in whom anastomosis was not performed. With one exception all operations were performed during the last 14 months." He had demonstrated in animals that the pulmonary blood flow could be increased by anastomosing a branch of the aortic arch to the side or distal end of a pulmonary artery in dogs and that in other dogs "after a high degree of chronic arterial unsaturation had been produced . . . the creation of an artificial ductus arteriosus resulted in an elevation in the oxygen saturation of arterial blood." It was not always possible to be sure whether they were dealing with patients in whom there was "an inadequate flow of blood to the lungs. Important in the diagnosis is the absence of visible pulsations in the lung fields as observed under the fluoroscope, and roentgenographic evidence that the pulmonary artery is small in size. The typical case of the 'tetralogy of Fallot' should not present great difficulties in diagnosis. There are, however, many borderline cases in which it is difficult or impossible to be certain of the true nature of the condition. If under such circumstances the patient has a hopeless prognosis without an operation, Dr. Taussig and I have taken the position that an exploration is indicated." The pulmonary artery pressure was usually measured at operation with a needle and a water manometer and "When the pressure is greater than 300 mm. of water, it is our opinion at present that an anastomosis is probably inadvisable." The patients operated upon successfully had ranged from five months in age to 21 years, two to ten years being considered the most desirable age period. Given the fact that most of these children had a ventricular septal defect, it was surprising, he said, how much clinical improvement and how much improvement in peripheral oxygen saturation was achieved by the operation. He had originally preferred to operate on the left, now he tended to operate on the side of the innominate artery so that he could use, as might be indicated, the innominate, the carotid, or the subclavian. The subclavian arising from the innominate made a 90 degree junction with its parent artery when anastomosed to the pulmonary artery, whereas the subclavian arising from the aortic arch tended to make a rather acute angle which tended to obstruct it. Of the 110 patients, 25 had died, an overall mortality of 23%. Of the 91 patients with an end-to-side systemic pulmonary anastomosis, 16 died, an 18% mortality. There were four deaths in the 46 patients in whom the subclavian artery was used, less than 10%, and 11 in the 36 patients in whom the innomi-

nate artery was used. "The commonest cause of death in this group was cerebral anemia or thrombosis." End-to-end systemic-pulmonary anastomoses had been employed in 10 patients, with four deaths. In six patients, an anastomosis was not performed, and in three, mistaken anastomoses were made, two to the right upper lobe pulmonary artery and one to the pulmonary vein. He had had no cases of empyema or mediastinitis or severe bleeding from the anastomosis. There had been no significant effect upon the arm from interruption of the subclavian artery. "Weakness or paralysis of the opposite side of the body in patients in whom the innominate or carotid artery was used either had cleared or was diminishing in all who survived the operation." They had not seen heart failure or streptococcus viridans endarteritis. "Although some of the operations were performed too recently to allow an evaluation, it appears that all of the patients with one exception who have survived the performance of an anastomosis are improved."

Discussion

Allen O. Whipple, of New York, spoke for the Fellows in paying "tribute to this magnificent presentation and to the outstanding leader in the new field of surgery of shunting operations, and I cannot express this too strongly . . . we shall always look back, those who have seen this, to this very remarkable presentation today." He emphasized, too, the "opportunity for studying the physiology of the patient with the shunting operation" [and as it turned out, Blalock set up such a laboratory for the physiological investigation of these problems,- under Richard Bing, Whipple's son-in-law]. Claude S. Beck, of Cleveland, with his wide knowledge of the literature of cardiac surgery, referred to the work of Jeger who had proposed shunting operations for aortic stenosis and for mitral stenosis. Of Blalock's operation, he said, "The operation does not cure this cardiac abnormality. The circulation is not restored to normal. It provides definite benefit. I think it is one of the nicest contributions to surgery made in my lifetime." Beck emphasized the magnitude of the health problem caused by cardiovascular disease and said that "progress in this field will be made by the direct approach to these structures. The Blalock-Taussig operation is based upon direct approach. There are funds available for cardiovascular research, and I hope that the internists who have charge of these funds will not forget that the direct surgical approach has something to offer and that surgical exploration should be encouraged." Elliott Cutler, of

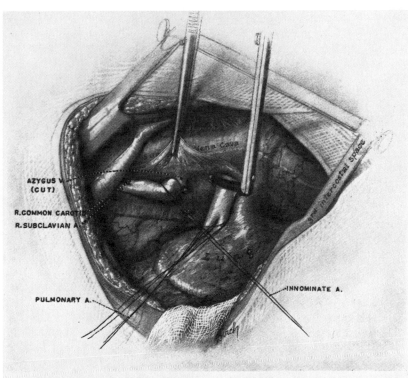

FIG. 1.—Showing the right pulmonary artery, the innominate artery, the right common carotid artery and the right subclavian artery prior to ligation and division.

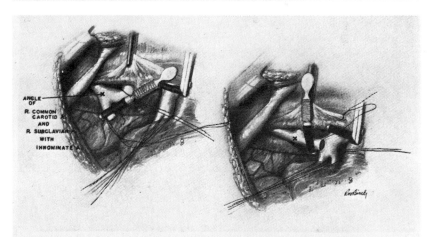

FIG. 2.—Showing the anastomosis of the proximal end of the right subclavian artery with the side of the right pulmonary artery. The transposed subclavian artery makes an angle of approximately 90 degrees with its parent vessel.

Blalock had done 109 operations in the 14 months after his first patient. He preferred to use the subclavian which came from the innominate because of the favorable angle which it formed with its parent vessel, as shown in the illustrations. The overall mortality for all patients operated upon was 23%. If the subclavian artery was used, it was less than 10%. He commented on the frequent difficulty in determining, clinically, whether the patient suffered from "an inadequate flow of blood to the lungs".

Alfred Blalock, *The Surgical Treatment of Congenital Pulmonic Stenosis.* Volume LXIV, 1946.

Boston, added his praise, and then the aged Rudolph Matas, of New Orleans, poured on his encomiums. He spoke, among other things, of Blalock's "fine, finished needle work in establishing lateral and circular anastomoses between the aortic and pulmonary branches . . . and Doctor Taussig's noted skill in the differential diagnosis of these congenital defects . . . " Emile Holman, of San Francisco, said that they had operated upon 15 dogs to perform subclavian pulmonary anastomses and had succeeded in half of them. He had undertaken the operation in two patients, one an 18-month-old patient who died, another a five-year-old child who did very well but developed a hemiplegia. In both of them, the blood was extremely thick. Had Dr. Blalock any comments to make about "what he does to improve the condition of the blood both before and after operation." Blalock answered that "the blood in practically all these individuals is thick; the red count may be eight, ten or 12 million; hematocrit readings as high as 95 percent. I do not think anything should be done about that preoperatively. If a great deal of blood is lost during operation I am confident that no blood should be removed after operation, but if the operation is bloodless . . . only a little is lost, we usually remove blood at the completion of the operation." He concluded with a caution that "I want you to realize that all these operations have been undertaken in a relatively short period of time. We can make no predictions as to the condition of these patients some years hence."

* * *

The paper by Lt. Col. Norman E. Freeman, of San Francisco, Associate Clinical Professor of Surgery, University of California Medical School, *Arterial Repair in the Treatment of Aneurysms and Arteriovenous Fistulae*. A Report of Eighteen Successful Restorations, was based on his experience at DeWitt General Hospital, one of the Army's three Vascular Centers in the Zone of the Interior. In 100 operations for aneurysm or arteriovenous fistulae, not a single case of gangrene had occurred. Paying tribute to the contributions of Matas before the Association in 1903, and of Bickham in 1904, in the techniques of vascular reconstruction in patients with arteriovenous fistulae, Freeman reported an experience with excision of the fistula, ligation of the vein, and end-to-end anastomosis of the artery in 23 cases. The suture of the artery was either longitudinal or transverse and end-to-end,- in the latter case preserving whatever fragment of normal wall remained. Normal pulsations and/or arteriography demonstrated complete success in 18 patients of the 23. The vein was sutured laterally in 18 of the patients, ligated in others.

Discussion

The indefatigable Rudolph Matas rose to present a long analysis of the problem, congratulating Freeman upon his good results and "high degree of technical skill" and after his full discussion said "With the kind permission of the Chair, I will now avail myself of a brief interval to exhibit lantern slides taken from patients of my own practice in which transvenous suture methods originally devised by Bickham and myself, 43 years ago, for the cure of arteriovenous aneurysms will be exhibited in their application to A-V aneurysms of the innominate, subclavian, carotid, external iliac, femoral and popliteal." [One's recollection is that those returning from the meeting said that Dr. Matas went on for an incredible length of time. The paper by Elkin and Harris on *Arteriovenous Aneurysms of the Vertebral Vessels,* which was presented later in the meeting, is not here mentioned, except to say that Rudolph Matas' discussion of that paper takes up two more pages of the fine type used for Discussions.]

* * *

Allen O. Whipple, of New York, Professor of Surgery, Columbia University; Director of Surgical Service, Presbyterian Hospital, who had been President in 1940, *Radical Surgery for Certain Cases of Pancreatic Fibrosis Associated with Calcareous Deposits,* said that it had now been demonstrated that total pancreatectomy was possible. Priestley had first done it, for an islet tumor, and now some 14 total pancreatectomies had been performed. Claggett in 1944 had performed the first successful total pancreatectomy for chronic pancreatitis, relieving the patient "of her unbearable pain. Ten weeks later, while in her home, she developed a severe hypoglycemic reaction which was not recognized, resulting in death. Her diabetes was controlled by a daily dose of eight units of protamin-zinc insulin and 30 units of regular insulin taken in one injection in the morning." Whipple was now reporting five radical operations for pancreatic lithiasis, two Whipple operations, one duodenectomy with resection of "all of the pancreas save a strip over superior mesenteric vessels" and two total pancreatectomies. Four of the patients were relieved of the pain and were doing well. One of the total pancreatectomy patients died of shock on the seventh day.

Discussion

Richard B. Cattell, of Boston, offered "a less radical procedure than total pancreatectomy . . . after division of the gastrocolic omentum, a long antecolic loop of jejunum is brought up and anastomosed to the duct in the midportion of the body of the pancreas over a T-tube." Alexander Brunschwig, of Chicago, had performed total pancreatectomy thus far only for carcinoma. Brunschwig asked why some patients with extensive calcification of the pancreas had severe pain and others had little or none. He commented on insulin sensitivity after total pancreatectomy, occurring in patients who required small doses of insulin. Dr. Whipple agreed that the symptoms bore an inconsistent relation to the calcification in the pancreas.

* * *

Herman E. Pearse, of Rochester, New York, Associate Professor of Surgery, University of Rochester, had previously [see page 852, Volume LX, 1942] presented before the Association his Vitallium tubes for reconstruction of the biliary tract and now, *Results from Using Vitallium Tubes in Biliary Surgery,* had written to Fellows of the Association and, combining their experience with his, had a total of 216 cases suitable for study. Of the 106 reconstructions of the bile duct preserving its continuity, 80% had good results. Using the tube to bridge a gap between the ends of the divided duct failed. In 79 cases of hepaticoduodenostomy over a Vitallium tube, there had been 58% good results and in 18 cases of hepaticojejunostomy with a tube, 15 or 83% had given a good result.

Discussion

I. S. Ravdin, of Philadelphia, said the important thing was an end-to-end mucosa-to-mucosa suture and it might not matter which type of tube was employed. Frank H. Lahey, of Boston, said flatly "We have implanted 41 Vitallium tubes. I have little faith in them. I think we have been under a misapprehension regarding them." There was no question but that Vitallium was well tolerated by the tissues, but "The important thing in my opinion is not how well they are tolerated by the tissues but whether or not they plug any less often than do other types of tubes. I do not think they do." Lahey made the first reference to a new synthetic material "called 'bouncing clay' [silastic], which we have obtained from the experimental laboratory of the General Electric Company. It is flexible, it will stretch, it will bounce like rubber and it can be cast in any shape. I am sure it has no advantages, as to whether or not it will plug, over either plain rubber or Vitallium tubes . . . its flexibility permits its introduction into the devious channels which one often meets in strictures of the bile ducts . . . it is easily handled." Lahey was still insisting on finding the lower end of the duct and anastomosing to it, "We have learned by splitting the lower end of the pancreas to find the common duct here and to demonstrate it well down to the point where it enters the duodenum . . . it is possible to so mobilize the duodenum that with this demonstrated portion of the duct, end-to-end anastomoses over tubes can frequently be accomplished." Lahey made the valid statement that "if a man injures the common and hepatic ducts during a cholecystectomy, he should seriously consider whether or not he has had enough experience to at-

tempt to repair it", and that certainly if he repaired it and failed, he should not attempt it once more.

The Business Meetings

The 1946 meeting, April 2, 3, and 4, was held at The Homestead, Hot Springs, Virginia, with William Darrach, who had been elected in 1944, in the Chair.

Among those who sent telegrams with regrets, because of their inability to participate in the meeting, was Dr. Leo Eloesser, from Peiping, China, where he was serving with the Communist Army.

The proposal, two years before, that the membership be increased to 200 by increments of five each year and that the Honorary membership be limited to 25 was accepted. The meeting " . . . scheduled for Philadelphia in the spring of 1945 had had to be postponed because of Government restrictions on travel. By the time these restrictions were lifted, it was too late in the year to prepare for a meeting. In order to maintain the continuity of the Transactions of the Association, the President and the Council decided to publish as many of the papers listed on the program as it was possible to obtain from the authors . . . nineteen papers . . . were published in the *Annals of Surgery,* and then bound together as the 63rd Volume of the Transactions of the American Surgical Association."

Dr. Firor, reporting for the Council, entered upon the experiment to " . . . accept all papers offered by members up to the deadline of December 15 . . . The number of papers received was more than could ordinarily fit into a three-day program." It was asked that speakers limit their talks to ten minutes. "It was also decided to do away with the selection of a person to open the discussions, because all too often that procedure resulted in practically a second paper."

The Development Committee, Arthur W. Allen, Chairman, Nathan Womack, Fred W. Rankin, Lester R. Dragstedt, and Alfred Blalock, considered a greater number of distinguished specialists should be taken into the Association and most startlingly criticized " . . . the present method for taking in new members" as unsatisfactory because they had to be proposed and supported by Fellows of the Association; and equally good men not so proposed could not be considered, and "Much pressure may be brought about by certain groups in support of men whose qualifications may be doubtful." They proposed the formation of a membership committee

" . . . to assist the Council in the investigation and selection of candidates." The committee " . . . to be composed of approximately 15 geographically distributed Fellows." The Development Committee had identified a large number of men throughout the country who might be seriously considered for membership and proposed that their qualifications be reviewed by this membership committee and further proposed that there be a standing membership committee. For the time being they did not propose any increase in the size of the Association.

President Darrach, speaking of the "qualifications for membership outlined in this report" said that " . . . the prestige of the Association will also be determined by the action of its members. For this reason the Council feels that the recent newspaper and magazine publicity to which several of our members have been subjected should not be allowed to pass without strong disapproval. We cannot criticise the younger men unless our skirts are clear." [This may well have referred to the publicity which had been the result of the intense national and world interest in Alfred Blalock's operations at Hopkins for relief of tetralogy of Fallot,- "The Blue Baby operation." The publicity was indeed great, and often generated in small towns as a method of raising funds to subsidize the trip of a child and parents to Baltimore. But at this time, there had been relatively little experience with intense press interest in medical developments.]

The war was over and the Committee on Problems Arising from the War asked to be dismissed.

Howard C. Naffziger, under New Business, recognized what was coming to pass in nursing, "I should like to speak of a situation which is urgent at the present time and has to do with nursing. We are all aware of the difficulty we are encountering in obtaining nursing help. The situation seems to be getting worse, and I do not know of any constructive steps that have been taken to remedy the shortage. This shortage may be accounted for in several ways: Many nurses who were engaged in administrative work during the war do not care to return to routine nursing and relatively few young women are interested in taking training. However, even before the war a policy was developing which is economically unsound. There has been an organized movement to give university education to those entering the profession; to require a five-year course, or a college degree. In the endeavor to elevate the standards of the nursing profession, attention has been centered on that rather than on improvement in the care of patients . . . We have learned a good deal during the past few years of what can be accomplished by women with little training."

At the Business Meeting on the third day, the Association did vote to accept the recommendation that an Adjunct Membership Committee be appointed, "to assist in the review and selection of candidates for membership; the size and composition of this Committee and the term of service of its members shall be determined by the Council."

The officers elected were Edward D. Churchill, of Boston, President; Thomas G. Orr, of Kansas City, and Edwin P. Lehman, of Charlottesville, Virginia, Vice-Presidents; and Warfield M. Firor, of Baltimore, Secretary.

LXV

1947

The 1947 meeting took place at The Homestead, Hot Springs, Virginia, March 25, 26, and 27, Dr. Edward D. Churchill, John Homans Professor of Surgery, Harvard University, in the Chair.

Among the memoirs of those deceased in the previous year, the volume contains those of Walter E. Dandy, John Staige Davis, John Shelton Horsley, and Howard Lilienthal.

* * *

The paper of Dallas B. Phemister, of Chicago, Professor and Chairman, Department of Surgery, The University of Chicago School of Medicine, and by invitation, Eleanor M. Humphreys, *Gastroesophageal Resection and Total Gastrectomy in the Treatment of Bleeding Varicose Veins in Banti's Syndrome,* stimulated a discussion which covered every phase of the subject. Phemister thought the only techniques "of much value" for esophagogastric hemorrhage in Banti's syndrome, were splenectomy, portocaval shunt and injection of the esophageal varices with sclerosing solutions. ". . . splenectomy, by removal of a large area of the portal bed, may ameliorate the hemorrhage for a variable length of time, but it usually recurs as the hypertension is built up again. Porto-caval shunt introduced by Whipple and co-workers is the ideal treatment . . . But in some cases of fibrous or cavernomatous transformation of the portal vein, it has been impossible to anastomose either the main trunk or one of its large tributaries with the inferior vena cava even when a vein graft was utilized . . . Previous splenectomy precludes splenorenal anastomosis . . . Moersch of the Mayo Clinic has recently made a follow-up study of 22 cases [of injection of esophageal varices with sclerosing solutions] for periods of three or more years after injection. Twelve have had no more bleeding, four are living with continued hemorrhages, three are dead of hemorrhages, and four are dead of unknown or unrelated causes." Resection of the bleeding segment of the alimentary canal was to be considered when all else had failed, and ". . . the recent mortality for both transthoracic esophago-gastric resection and total gastrectomy for carcinoma in experienced hands is under 15 per cent . . . The first reported case of one-stage, transthoracic esophago-gastric resection, performed by Adams and Phemister, is alive and well nine years after operation and the patients have lived for years after total gastrectomy with only mild anemia and slight impairment of nutrition." He had operated on two young adults with life-long history of splenomegaly and repeated hemorrhages, one by total gastrectomy and one by "Resection of the lower three and one-half inches of the esophagus and upper two inches of the stomach followed by esophago-gastrostomy . . ." Both patients had survived. The total gastrectomy patient had had some recurrent bleeding. The patient with a limited resection was perfectly well.

Discussion

Alfred Blalock, of Baltimore, introduced the Discussion mainly to show a motion picture of a "renal-splenic vein anastomosis as developed and popularized by Dr. Arthur Blakemore and Dr. Allen

897

Whipple" in a patient in whom he had previously exposed the esophagus through a left thoracotomy, planning to do an esophagogastrectomy, but removing only large plexuses of veins. The patient subsequently bled. Blalock's anastomosis was manual, a right-angled splenorenal anastomosis, after splenectomy. Owen H. Wangensteen, of Minneapolis, spoke at length of the importance of the acid-peptic factor in the causation of bleeding in patients with varices. Phemister had already pointed out that gross ulcerations were usually lacking. Wangensteen had done three, all but total, gastrectomies for bleeding esophageal varices. There was recurrent bleeding in the man who had only a 90% gastrectomy, no recurrence in the patients who had 95% and 98% gastrectomy and splenectomy as well. J. deJ. Pemberton, of Rochester, Minnesota, reinforced what Phemister had said about Moersch's experience with transesophageal injection of varices. With a diagnosis of Banti's disease, they were performing prophylactic splenectomy when possible and thought the results were much better than for splenectomy after hemorrhage had developed. Pemberton mentioned the fact that Moersch's work had been stimulated by that of Crafoord and Frenckner in 1939. Moersch's feeling was that injection was effective if the varices were in the esophagus but not if they had extended into the stomach. Arthur Blakemore, closing, said quite simply that any type of resection would involve reanastomosis of a portion of the gastrointestinal tract with a portal circulation to a portion with a systemic venous circulation "and, in the presence of portal hypertension, the subsequent development of varices is inevitable."

* * *

Frank Glenn, of New York, Associate Professor of Clinical Surgery, Cornell University Medical College, *Acute Cholecystitis following the Surgical Treatment of Unrelated Disease,* mentioned previous and infrequent reports of this condition and presented five patients of his own in whom acute cholecystitis had occurred shortly after an unrelated operation, not necessarily abdominal. One of the gallbladders contained no stones, and one of the gallbladders was found to be perforated. George Heuer, in 1934, had stressed the fact that perforation of the gallbladder was more frequent in acute cholecystitis than was generally realized, thought cholecystectomy should be performed promptly but that occasionally cholecystectomy might be performed as a preliminary procedure, in patients thought to be too ill for a cholecystectomy.

* * *

R. K. Gilchrist, of Chicago, Assistant Professor of Surgery, University of Illinois; Associate Attending Surgeon, Presbyterian Hospital, and Vernon C. David, of Chicago, Chairman, Department of Surgery, Presbyterian Hospital; Rush Professor of Surgery, University of Illinois, *A Consideration of Pathological Factors Influencing Five Year Survival in Radical Resection of the Large Bowel and Rectum for Carcinoma,* reviewed 200 patients operated upon more than five years earlier. The specimens had been cleared and the lymph nodes charted. They made the note that "The specimens used in this analysis were not always consecutive due to the work involved in the study of each one but were otherwise unselected except that the specimens from all fatalities were included. This results in somewhat higher mortality figures and lower five-year survival rates." These 200 patients represented 75% of those explored. There were 112 rectal tumors below the peritoneal floor, and 58 of these patients, 51.8%, were alive five to ten years after operation. There had been an operative mortality of almost 11%, positive lymph nodes in 60%. The presence of lymph node metastases lowered the five-year survival rate from 74% to 37%. Of carcinomas of the sigmoid and intraperitoneal rectum, there were 55, 65% of whom were alive five years after operation and 7% of whom had died of operation. The presence of positive lymph node metastases dropped the five-year survival from 90% to 51%. Six of the 200 patients had developed what were thought to be metachronous carcinomas of the colon. "The most striking finding . . . is in those tumors of the transverse colon, splenic flexure, and descending colon where there were involved nodes. All of these had obstruction resections and only three of the eight (37.5 per cent) were alive after five years. The widest possible resection is indicated here rather than the usual V-shaped wedge of mesentery resected. The favorable prognosis (77.7 per cent) seen in right colon lesions having involved nodes is undoubtedly due to the wide resection of mesentery (54 nodes per specimen) performed when doing an ileotransverse colon resection and anastomosis." As for the mode of spread of carcinoma of the colon they said, "The lymphatic spread of carcinoma of the colon is primarily embolic. The nodes where the emboli lodge prevent further spread until the node is completely overwhelmed by carcinoma. Further embolic spread is through the collateral channels, each new node involved tending to make a longer and more difficult channel for a new embolus to travel. Spread from one node to another does not seem to be common. Thus, the finding of a group of involved nodes within the field removable by surgery does not mean that a case is hopeless. However, it does indicate the need for the widest possible resection of lymph nodes draining the area of the carcinoma." Their five-year survival of patients without lymph node metastases, overall, was 78.5% and had they not included, as dying of carcinoma, those patients who died postoperatively of other causes and those patients lost to follow-up, their five-year survival would have been 90.9%. The overall five-year survival for the 125 with lymph node metastases was 44.8%. "Resection of fixed tumors and the structures to which they are adherent gives a better prognosis than might be expected, a 40 per cent five-year survival. Twenty per cent died postoperatively . . . Retrograde metastases to nodes one to five centimeters below the tumor occurred in seven of the 153 tumors below the promontory of the sacrum (4.6 per cent)." Their 140 abdominoperineal resections yielded an average of 55.3 nodes per specimen as apposed to 41.6 nodes per specimen with obstructive resection of the sigmoid or intraperitoneal rectum, "Lesions which are partially or completely below the peritoneal reflection have a high incidence of local and liver recurrence and pull through or sleeve resections are not much better than a local resection. The Miles operation seems to give the best chance of cure here . . . The point of the discussion about end to end anastomosis is missed, it seems to us. It should be, 'Can you remove all of the cancer?' and not, 'Can you sew two ends of bowel together?' Obviously in those intraperitoneal lesions below the promontory of the sacrum which are large or have palpably enlarged nodes, the abdominoperineal resection will give a greater chance of cure."

Discussion

The Discussion was opened by Fred W. Rankin, now of Lexington, Kentucky. He agreed with Gilchrist and David that ". . . radical extirpation of rectal malignancy with a widespread removal of gland-bearing tissue gives the highest percentage of long time freedom from recurrence." His own choice for cancer of the rectum ". . . has been for the past fifteen years the one-stage combined abdominoperineal resection after the technic of Miles." His own series of 167 patients operated upon 7 to 13 years earlier showed 55% of them alive and free of recurrence with an operative mortality of 5.3% and a resectability rate of 74%. He emphasized wider removal of the levator muscles to deal with lateral spread and occasional recurrence in the posterior vaginal wall [without recommending prophylactic resection of the posterior vaginal wall]. He decried

". . . the pull-through operation and the great emphasis placed by some surgeons on technical procedures which decry the sacrifice of the sphincteric mechanism of the rectum . . ." He agreed "with David and Gilchrist that the sphincter-saving operations are little more than local excisions for all cancers situated below the peritoneum." Thomas E. Jones, of Cleveland, agreed about the importance of Miles' operation. Richard B. Cattell, of Boston, reported an earlier study of patients with carcinoma of the rectum operated upon at the Lahey Clinic, 80% free of recurrence when there was no spread; 30%, alive and well five years later if there was lymph node involvement; 15% if there was blood vessel invasion. In a more recent study, in the absence of lymph node involvement, their five-year survival was 60%, and ten-year survival, 51.8% which dropped, with lymph node invasion, to 30.2% and 23.2%. Owen H. Wangensteen, of Minneapolis, rose to say that "Inasmuch as President Churchill has asked whether there is anyone here to speak for the more conservative operation in which continuity is reestablished, I come forward only in response to that request. Wangensteen admitted ". . . in low-lying rectal lesions less than 6 cm. from the external anal orifice, the sphincter-saving operation should not be done . . . in large ampullary lesions in juxtaposition to the levators, the conservative operation is out of order . . ." While the abdominoperineal was certainly the best operation for cure of cancer of the rectum, ". . . it is not a light matter to deprive a man of his rectal sphincter . . . surgeons cannot make a sphincter and one cannot be bought in any market at any price. Continence of feces without the internal sphincter does not exist and operations which destroy or remove the internal sphincter fail to preserve continence." They had done 60 or 70 of the "more conservative" operations but did not yet know the results. Nevertheless, "Despite the circumstances that I have a number of patients who are well without evidence of recurrence after excision of lesions lying 4 to 6 cm. from the anal orifice . . . I have learned the bitter lesson that it is unwise to attempt to salvage the sphincters in such low-lying lesions. If one does so, he compromises on the cure of the cancer. With reference to lesions in the rectosigmoid, however, I have the impression that as satisfactory an operation for cancer can be done for lesions here with restoration of continuity as with the more radical abdomino-perineal operation . . . I would suggest that, a tempered ambition to save the rectal sphincter as well as to cure the cancer, is a praiseworthy objective in *suitable* cases of cancer of the upper rectal ampulla and most, if not all remov-

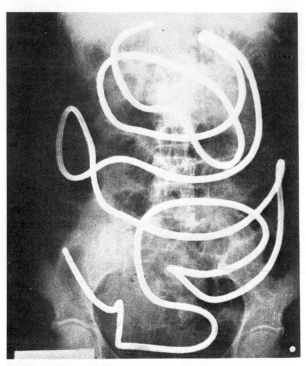

Fig. 3.—Miller-Abbott tube passed through the small intestine prior to resection of the colon.

Ravdin said that since 1938 they had been using the Miller-Abbott tube, passing the tube before operation and that as a result "two stage resections of the right colon have not been done in our clinic since 1938. We have since extended its use to the preparation of patients with lesions in the more distal segments of the large bowel . . . has frequently obviated the necessity of a proximal colostomy, except where acute obstruction or marked chronic obstruction was present."

I. S. Ravdin, Harold A. Zintel, and Doris H. Bender, *Adjuvants to Surgical Therapy in Large Bowel Malignancy,* Volume LXV, 1947.

able cancers of the rectosigmoid. Leo Eloesser, of San Francisco, offered "Just a small voice from the wilderness . . . to disagree with both Dr. Gilchrist and Dr. Wangensteen . . . I think one had to consider not only how *long* one's patients are going to live, but *how* they are going to live . . . I think that some of us might be inclined to forego this maximum . . . percentage of freedom from recurrence . . . and accept . . . a risk of living a few less years with a normally functioning anal sphincter, instead of eking out a few more years of life embarrassed by colostomy."

* * *

I. S. Ravdin, of Philadelphia, John Rhea Barton Professor of Surgery, Medical School, University of Pennsylvania; Surgeon-in-Chief, Hospital, University of Pennsylvania, and by invitation Harold A. Zintel and Doris H. Bender, *Adjuvants to Surgical Therapy in Large Bowel Malignancy,* spoke very generally of employing restorative measures for anemia, hypoproteinemia and hypovitaminemia. They stressed the preoperative use of an indwelling intestinal tube passed 48 hours before operation, which had essentially eliminated the use of colostomies in their patients, and commented that they had first reported this in 1940 with W. O. Abbott, and that Whipple, Newton, and Blodgett had adopted the practice as well. They were using oral antibiotic preparation, at first the sulfonamides and more recently streptomycin. Their mortality prior to 1938 for all operations of the colon was 18.4% and since adopting some or all of the precautions described, the mortality had dropped to 3.6%. "Resection with end-to-end anastomosis is supplanting Mikulicz types of resection in our clinic. One-stage procedures have entirely supplanted multistage operations except in the presence of perforation or obstruction."

There was no Discussion.

* * *

Rudolph N. Schullinger, of New York, Assistant Clinical Professor of Surgery, College of Physicians and Surgeons, Columbia University, *Observations on Mortality from Acute Appendicitis at a University Hospital, 1916 to 1946,* remarked on the appropriateness of the study at this point because ". . . 1946 marked the 60th anniversary of the first successful appendicectomy performed in this country (Richard Hall at Roosevelt Hospital, N.Y., on May 8, 1886) . . ." The mortality for acute appendicitis at the Presbyterian Hospital in the early years of the study was some 7%, and in the last years of the study 1.37%. There was a similar national trend. The mortality per 100,000 in the United States in 1930 was 15.3 and in 1945 was 5.1, although still representing in that figure 6,697 deaths from appendicitis in the country. There had been some decrease in delay by patients and a substantial decrease in the use of laxatives by the public. Improved anesthesia and sophistication of postoperative care permitted some of the profoundly ill patients to survive who had not earlier. The antibacterial agents had certainly had some effect, but they had not used them ". . . consistently or set down any rigid rules with reference to its use, but prefer to leave the decision with the surgeon . . ." Their review of large numbers of reported series during the same period showed an overall mortality for appendicitis varying from 1.6% (Roosevelt Hospital in New York, 1945)

TABLE VI

ACUTE APPENDICITIS AT THE PRESBYTERIAN HOSPITAL, NEW YORK CITY
January 1, 1916 to December 31, 1945

Classification	Mortality Rate 1916–1945	Last Five Year Average Mortality Rate	1945 Mortality Rate
All cases of acute appendicitis................	3.55%	1.37%	0.43%
Simple acute appendicitis...................	0.49%	0.39%	0.00%
Acute appendicitis with acute local peritonitis....	2.06%	1.35%	0.00%
Acute appendicitis with peritoneal (appendiceal) abscess................................	9.04%	4.16%	3.45%
Acute appendicitis with acute diffuse peritonitis..	15.48%	4.08%	0.00%
Acute appendicitis with progressive fibrinopurulent peritonitis..............................	82.35%	80.00%	*0.00%

* No cases for 1945.

FIG. I

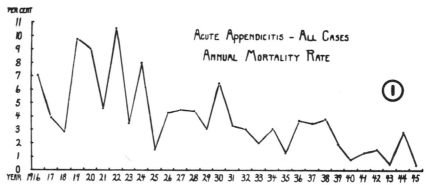

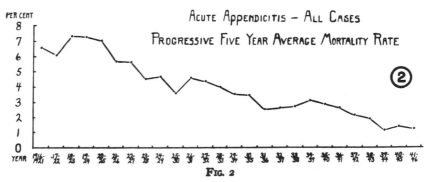

FIG. 2

Schullinger demonstrated the progressive decrease in mortality from appendicitis. The mortality of appendicitis with abscess was still 3.45% at Presbyterian Hospital, 2.38 at Johns Hopkins, 10% at Cincinnati General and at the Charity Hospital in New Orleans. [These figures represent a vast improvement from those presented in 1940 by Boyce and in the same year by Reid and Montanus.]

Rudolph N. Schullinger, *Observations on Mortality from Acute Appendicitis at a University Hospital, 1916 to 1946,* Volume LXV, 1947.

FIG. 1.—Graph showing total annual death rate from 1916 to 1945, inclusive, in 5405 cases of acute appendicitis with its associated lesions. Total number of deaths: 193; total mortality rate, 3.55 per cent. Mortality rate for 1945 was 0.43 per cent.

FIG. 2.—Graph for comparison with that in Figure 1, showing the total progressive five-year average death rate from 1916 to 1945, inclusive, for all cases of acute appendicitis with its associated lesions. Mortality rate for 1941 to 1946 was 1.37 per cent.

to 5.97% (Cincinnati General Hospital 1940). For simple acute appendicitis, the mortality was zero in many institutions,- Johns Hopkins, Baltimore City Hospitals, Lankenau, Jefferson, and Misericordia Hospitals,- rising to a high of 1.6% at Bellevue Hospital. With appendiceal abscess, the mortalities ranged from 2.38% at Johns Hopkins in 1939 to 1941, 7.06% at Johns Hopkins 1931 to 1939, 7.3% at the Peter Bent Brigham 1913 to 1940, 9.7% in the Cleveland Survey 1940 to 1941, 10% from the Cincinnati General Hospital 1934 to 1938, and 10.8% at the Charity Hospital in New Orleans 1930 to 1939. The table presented in their paper graphically shows the decreasing mortality from appendicitis in its various forms at the Presbyterian Hospital. Schullinger recommended prompt operation, taking if necessary, several hours for resuscitation in the most profoundly ill patients. They usually employed the McBurney incision, preferring either ligation or inversion of the stump of the appendix when feasible, but strongly condemned ". . . combined ligation and inversion of any appendix stump." They drained if there was an abscess, or necrotic tissue was left behind, if the appendix was not removed, if there was "gross contamination", if the closure of the appendiceal stump was insecure.

Discussion

Roy D. McClure, of Detroit, said they had looked up the Henry Ford Hospital statistics from 1937 to 1946, finding 13 deaths, 0.92% mortality, in 1,405 appendectomies for acute appendicitis. During the same period, they had simply drained 68 appendiceal abscesses with one death, a 1.5% mortality. They had had one death five years ago in acute appendicitis and none in 466 such appendectomies during the last four years. Penicillin had not been in use most of that time. "The Wangensteen principle of gastroduodenal decompression and drainage . . . and . . . the Miller-Abbott tube . . . have undoubtedly been of greatest help in the most recent years . . ." Better electrolyte and fluid maintenance had ". . . undoubtedly been a large factor. It is interesting to note, however, that the only probably helpful factor virtually restricted to the last five years is early ambulation." They favored the muscle-splitting incision, found the appendix by looking for it at its base rather than searching for its tip with a finger, and used soft drains. John S. Lockwood, of New York, now Professor of Surgery and Director of Surgical Laboratories, College of Physicians and Surgeons, Columbia University, said that all of the factors involved in preoperative and postoperative care had been instrumental in the lowered mortality, and that it had become "exceedingly difficult to evaluate in any mathematical way the relative significance of any one factor in treatment, and certainly that is true so far as chemotherapeutic agents and antibiotics are concerned." He thought an important effect of the antibacterial agents was their interruption of bacterial synergism, "Even though the drugs may not be active against all the flora involved, their ability to restrain growth activity of gram positive cocci seems to modify the tendency of the disease to spread." Grover C. Penberthy, of Detroit, reminded the Fellows that, at the 1942 meeting, the Children's Hospital of Michigan had reported 1,653 cases of appendicitis over the previous 15 years with a 4.2% mortality. In the period 1942 through 1946, they had had an additional 435 infants and children operated upon for appendicitis, 104 of them with a perforation and peritonitis. There had been no deaths in the entire group of 435.

* * *

D. W. Gordon Murray, of Toronto, Surgeon, Toronto General Hospital; Demonstrator of Surgery, University of Toronto, *The Pathophysiology of the Cause of Death from Coronary Thrombosis,* who had introduced the Association to the prophylactic use of heparin [see page 803, Volume LVI, 1938], now offered another in his series of startling and innovative proposals. He presented the results of a series of experiments in dogs ". . . which showed in my mind the following points: (1) Within a few minutes of tying a major branch of the coronary artery there is: (a) Blueness over the area of distribution of the vessel. (b) Dilatation of this segment of the heart muscle. (c) Lack of contraction over this area. (d) As soon as contraction of this area ceases there is paradoxical systole of the left ventricle. This probably is the most significant finding in relation to the signs under discussion. (e) This is accompanied by an immediate fall in blood pressure (f) and a diminished left ventricular output. If these effects are allowed to continue there is fibrillation and death. (2) If the ligature is released from the coronary artery before fibrillation sets in, then all these processes reverse themselves and everything returns to normal." He tried to prevent the paradoxical ventricular motion in the infarcted area by stitching "firm cloth" to the boundaries of the area which was to become ischemic, but produced only a diminution of the drop in blood pressure and in the fall in cardiac output; and quite simply said "The next part of the experiment has to do with an attempt at overcoming the effect of such a coronary occlusion. When the artery has been tied off and there is maximal dilatation of the area to be infarcted, with the fall in blood pressure, and the diminished cardiac output, then an attempt is made to resect the infarcted area of the left ventricle . . . This has been accomplished quite satisfactorily in 25 dogs . . . in the following way . . ." A continuous catgut suture was placed across the ventricle uniting the edges of the ischemic area to be excised, pulled tight, and "The infarcted area can then be excised quite neatly with a scalpel, taking care not to cut the suture which is vital at this time." The raw edges were then oversewn. They had sometimes done it all with catgut, sometimes added silk. "The results of removing this infarct produce an astonishing effect in the animal. The cardiac output increases considerably and the blood pressure rises moderately, although it does not return to the original level . . . the animal which one would judge, from control experiments, would die, survives quite satisfactorily and most of them have made quite a good recovery . . . I would think that practically all animals in whom we had resected this area, would have died of dilatation and finally fibrillation and heart failure. It is interesting, therefore, that many of these animals are alive and quite well for as long as one to two years later." In reconstructing the events following coronary occlusion, he said an infarct was produced; if it involved the conducting mechanism it produced one type of problem, if not it produced an area which ". . . is non-contractile. This area becomes dilated and acts as an expansion chamber. When the ventricle contracts, varying amounts of the blood of the ventricle, depending on the size of the infarct, are forced into this elastic chamber. The effectiveness of the contraction is partly lost because of this expanding chamber and consequently the amount of blood delivered into the aorta is much diminished. This paradoxical systole . . . probably accounts for many of the symptoms from which the coronary patient suffers, namely low blood pressure, signs of shock, lack of energy, and all the symptoms related to this lack of adequate peripheral circulation. It provides an explanation for the picture of shock which is evident in many of these patients . . . There are no drugs that have any effect on this." [We have no record of the actual terms in which he made his oral presentation, but the startling proposal in the published paper follows.] "While it is obviously facetious at this stage to make the following remarks, still I have a conviction that, as medical treatment is so ineffective, and is entirely helpless, except from a palliative point of view, the day may come when the best plan of dealing with a coronary thrombosis, would be an emergency opera-

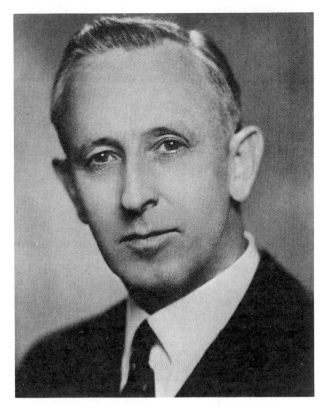

D. W. Gordon Murray 1897-1976, M.D. University of Toronto, 1921; spent his life at the Toronto General Hospital—Associate Professor of Surgery and Senior Surgeon, Toronto General Hospital. One of the most brilliantly imaginative Fellows of the Association, a surgeon of rare technical skill, he was a pioneer in the use of heparin to prevent thrombosis and embolism and to maintain patency in reconstructed vessels, successfully used vein grafts for arterial replacement decades before it became an accepted practice, experimented with fascia lata cardiac valve replacement, employed clinically a technique of blind, transcardiac closure of septal defects with fascial strips, performed arterial grafts to the coronary arteries and successfully treated aortic insufficiency by implanting a homograft valve in the descending aorta, and recommended excision of infarcted myocardium,- all long before the days of open heart operations. He devised his own external dialysis machine,- after Kolff,- for the treatment of renal failure and reported his clinical successes with it to,- as with many of his seemingly radical proposals,- a doubting medical world. The frequency with which his seemingly farfetched proposals proved to have merit may have led him,- and at least some others,- to be insufficiently critical when, late in his career, he was enthusiastic about repair of the transected spinal cord.

tion . . . undertaken before the patient gets a large expansion chamber . . . the right or left coronary areas could easily be excised and repaired with relative safety . . . It would overcome the immediate effect of the expansion chamber . . . it would remove the infarcted area, so that the coronary artery, which was occluded, would from then on, be of no significance. It would as well, remove the part of the heart in which a cardiac aneurysm may develop and which ultimately may rupture." He was realistic enough to say that "As this is making drastic inroads on the physician's territory, I have some doubts if my colleagues in medicine, will consider, that surgical treatment of this lesion is reasonable. Possibly I may not see a suitable case on which this could be done, but I feel at the present time, that in a properly selected case, this could be done with dispatch, with less danger than waiting for the unpredictable effects of the coronary occlusion to develop, and that ultimately the patient might be cured." [Murray, always somewhat outside the pale, was careful to state in a footnote "I acknowledge with pleasure the technical assistance of Mr. Newell Thomas and Dr. E. Delorme employed by the author, and Dr. Ray Heimbecker for his photography. This work was done without University or other assistance, apart from limited laboratory facilities in the Banting Institute."]

Discussion

The only Discussion which is published is that of Alfred Blalock, of Baltimore [always an admirer of Murray's originality], who committed himself quite firmly to the support of Murray's thesis, "I was sitting next to Dr. Rudolph Matas while Dr. Gordon Murray was presenting his paper and he stated to me that this work may be epoch-making. The lack of prolonged discussion is probably due to the fact that others are as amazed by these brilliant experimental observations as I am . . . It is only natural that Doctor Murray would hesitate to transfer immediately his experimental observations to the treatment of the patient. When one realizes that the average survival period of patients who survive the first attack of coronary occlusion is approximately five years, one hesitates to carry out what appears to be at this time a radical surgical procedure. I doubt if such a procedure appears to us to be more radical and bold than did the suture of heart wounds 50 years ago. The fact that Doctor Murray was able to prevent the death of animals following coronary occlusion by excision of the infarcted area is a magnificent accomplishment. I believe that there will ulti-

mately be a clinical application for his findings and it is to be hoped that Doctor Murray will continue and extend his studies."

* * *

Henry K. Ransom, of Ann Arbor, Associate Professor of Surgery, University of Michigan Medical School, *Subtotal Gastrectomy for Gastric Ulcer: A Study of End Results,* presented the results of a 20-year study during which 246 patients out of 1,356 with gastric ulcer, were operated upon,- 18.9%. During the last three years of the study, however, 30% of all patients with gastric ulcer were operated upon. The 20 patients requiring immediate treatment for a perforated ulcer were separately considered. The lesions had been thought to be benign at operation in every case, but 19 of them—10.1%—proved to have "malignant disease superimposed upon an old chronic ulcer." Most of the patients were operated upon because of failure of medical management and 28% because it was thought that malignancy might be present. In the 188 resections, there were 15 deaths,- a 7.9% mortality,- among them three due to peritonitis, one to pancreatitis, one to volvulus, one to wound disruption, and two to shock. Two patients with uremia were presumed to have had peritonitis also. Two of the 19 malignancies were lymphosarcomas. Eleven of the 19 patients were alive one to almost eight years, and one patient had died of a stroke almost eight years after operation and without recurrence. Both the lymphosarcoma patients were alive and well. In terms of the long term results, only 11 patients, 8%, had definitely unsatisfactory results in the 138 available for follow-up. 62% of the patients were absolutely well in every way with excellent results; in 30%, 41 patients, "For the most part the residual symptoms are related to the reduced capacity of the stomach and the altered mechanics of gastric emptying rather than simulating the original symptoms." Four patients had stomal ulcers, and seven other patients had poor results.

Discussion

Roscoe R. Graham, of Toronto, agreed that the difficulty in being certain about the absence of malignancy was a prime indication for operation and as opposed to the 10% error in Ransom's series, their own error was as high as 17%,- ulcers resected as benign actually proving to be malignant. Previously they had delayed operation until they had been forced, but "With the data which Dr. Ransom has presented, it becomes obvious that one should entertain very seriously the policy of advising early radical operative procedures for a patient with a gastric ulcer . . . advising patients suffering from what we believe to be a benign gastric ulcer to accept operation early in the course of the disease . . . the operation should be a radical gastrectomy. We have never accepted the Finsterer type of operation, in which a portion of the pyloric antrum was left in situ, even though a radical resection of the stomach was done." Frank H. Lahey, of Boston, said he wanted to ask "in which case we should apply and continue medical treatment, in which not to, and on what basis? I am well qualified to speak on this subject, since I have promoted over the years a set of criteria for applying medical measures to patients with gastric ulcers which I would like now to relinquish publicly [!] . . . I now believe that every patient with gastric ulcer should have a gastric resection, and for the following reasons: Our present mortality in the resection of 110 consecutive gastric ulcers is zero, compared with a mortality of 2.6 per cent in approximately 400 subtotal gastrectomies for duodenal ulcer and 2.2 per cent in approximately 100 consecutive subtotal gastrectomies for jejunal ulcer. I believe that all gastric ulcers should be resected because we have found it impossible in doubtful cases to be sure that patients come back often enough to be checked adequately against malignancy . . . in any lesion in which the pathologist himself, unless he makes serial sections, is often unable to determine whether or not malignancy is present . . . there are no methods by which surgeon, gastroenterologist or medical man can be sure that he is not carrying on medical treatment in one out of ten patients who may well have cancer of the stomach . . . there will be some ulcers resected which could have been treated medically, but the fatality percentage in this group from subtotal gastrectomy will, in my opinion, be infinitely lower than would be the case if some of these patients were treated medically and the malignancy overlooked until any prospect of cure by surgery was lost." In closing, Ransom spoke of the "syndrome sometimes referred to as the dumping stomach", which he attributed to a sudden elevation of the blood glucose from rapid absorption in the duodenum and then an overproduction of insulin with resultant hypoglycemia.

* * *

A long afternoon symposium on vagotomy was initiated by Arthur M. Schoen, by invitation, and R. Arnold Griswold, of Louisville, Professor and Head, Department of Surgery, University of Louisville, *The Effect of Vagotomy on Human Gastric Function*, A

Preliminary Report. The 30 patients had had vagotomy, 21 transthoracically, and nine infradiaphragmatically. Their studies permitted them to say that "The gastric secretory response to histamine, a humoral secretagogue, is not prevented by complete vagotomy . . . a vagotomized stomach is still capable of producing active digestive juice. Complete vagotomy reduces gastric secretion and emptying by abolishing the cephalic phase of gastric function . . . The basal secretory rate of six persons was reduced by an average of 36 per cent in response to vagotomy . . . The insulin test for complete vagotomy appears to be satisfactory when properly employed."

* * *

Francis D. Moore, of Boston, by invitation, *Vagus Resection for Ulcer: An Interim Evaluation*, was presenting the results of vagotomy in 84 patients performed two to 30 months earlier at the Massachusetts General Hospital. They had had poor results in 7%, fair in 18%, and good in 75%. In the five patients with poor results, two patients had pain, one patient had bleeding and pain, one had "ulcer without pain or bleeding." Diarrhea turned out to be a much more common side effect of the operation than they had realized. In their experience ". . . diarrhea is usually associated with poor gastric emptying", however, the 19 patients in the series who had a pre-existent or concomitant gastroenterostomy had as much diarrhea as the others. Transient sense of epigastric fullness was common—56%—but "Fulness with vomiting, constituting a major problem . . ." occured in only 8%. While stating that "Vagus resection for ulcer is at the crossroads", Moore indicated that with a 90% satisfactory result, "Vagus resection is an addition to the surgical armamentarium which may come to occupy a permanent and important place . . . A reserved attitude must be maintained until the present group of patients have been followed longer." He added that "The routine performance of posterior gastro-enterostomy coincident with vagus resection may so confuse results that in the future one will not know whether to assign the end-result, whether good or bad, to the gastroenterostomy or the vagus resection."

* * *

Waltman Walters, of Rochester, Minnesota, Professor of Surgery, The Mayo Foundation, and by invitation Harold A. Neibling, William F. Bradley, John T. Small, and James W. Wilson, followed with *A Study of the Results, Both Favorable and Unfavorable, of Section of the Vagus Nerves in the Treatment of Peptic Ulcer*. Walters was reporting on 40 patients operated on by himself at the Mayo Clinic, making reference to Dragstedt's 1946 report of 54 cases, Grimson's Duke report of 30 operations, and Moore's of 12 from the Massachusetts General Hospital. He preferred to call the operation "gastric neurectomy". He reminded the Fellows of Latarjet's 1922 operations. Walters preferred the transabdominal approach which allowed exploration of the abdomen. In 14 patients vagotomy alone was performed and 13 of these did well, the fourteenth died of a coronary occlusion immediately following operation. The operation was performed on patients with duodenal ulcers with or without previous operations, and on patients with anastomotic ulcers. They found reduction of the gastric acidity to be inconstant and the ". . . disturbance of motility of the stomach and small intestine are of frequent occurrence after operation." They had had at least one clear-cut recurrence, other ulcers had failed to heal, and they had had to reoperate on some patients to provide gastric drainage. Two of their three deaths were sudden cardiac accidents, the third was from "an unsuspected perforated duodenal ulcer with a subdiaphragmatic abscess" in a patient who had had a gastroenterostomy and a vagotomy.

* * *

The symposim was appropriately completed by the presentation of Lester R. Dragstedt, of Chicago, Professor of Surgery, University of Chicago, and by invitation Paul V. Harper, Jr., E. Bruce Tovee, and Edward R. Woodward, *Section of the Vagus Nerves to the Stomach in the Treatment of Peptic Ulcer,* Complications and End Results After Four Years. They had operated upon 212 patients, one of whom died of aspiration bronchopneumonia, and "there have been no deaths in the last 150 vagotomies . . . The clinical results of the operation have been excellent and have led us to the impression that a benign peptic ulcer may be regularly expected to heal if all the vagus fibers to the stomach are divided . . . best accomplished by exposure of these nerves along the

lower esophagus by either a transabdominal or a transpleural approach . . . Gastric vagotomy abolishes the nervous phase of gastric secretion and decreases very markedly the total amount of gastric juice produced. These effects appear to be permanent. Evidence of regeneration of the secretory fibers in the vagus nerves has not been observed even in the patients operated upon four years ago". They referred to intercostal pain, pleural effusion, pulmonary atelectasis, delayed gastric emptying, and diarrhea, for the most part mild and self-limited. Ulcer symptoms had persisted in five patients, who they thought had had incomplete vagotomy, and in two of them at reoperation "a residual vagus fiber was discovered and divided." Of the earlier work, he said, "It is probable that the poor results secured by the early workers in this field are due to the fact that attempts were made to section the vagus nerves in operations directed at the stomach instead of the esophagus and thus were in all probability incomplete." His preferred operation was transabdominal, and he once more described the operation, from below but through the esophageal hiatus.

Discussion

Keith S. Grimson, of Durham, North Carolina, opened the Discussion commenting that, with the 77 Duke cases, the afternoon panel had presented some 500 vagotomy operations. They had had considerable trouble with the need for secondary gastroenterostomies, ". . . one among each seven patients who did not already have enterostomy." In all they were satisfied, although the results upon gastric acidity were inconsistent and "At the present time we are employing subdiaphragmatic vagotomy with pyloroplasty, exclusion or gastrojejunostomy for duodenal ulcer, and reserving transthoracic vagotomy alone for stomach ulcer." Ralph Colp, of New York, began by saying that the results of vagotomy were "inconsistent, variable and in most cases unpredictable". In 20 patients who had duodenal ulcer,

Dragstedt stressed the need to divide the vagi in the mediastinum, and that "recurrence or persistence of ulcer ▶ symptoms may occur if even a small vagus fiber to the stomach has been overlooked." Complete vagotomy produced a permanent lowering of gastric acidity and volume of secretion. In 160 patients, they produced complete vagus section in 142, all of whom were well as were 13/18 of patients with incomplete section. The vagus did not regenerate. In the discussion, Grimson, of Duke, was supportive, Colp, of Mt. Sinai, was disappointed in vagotomy, adding gastroenterostomy for most cases and partial gastrectomy for those with high acid or bleeding without pain. Moore, of Boston, claimed fasting acidity and motility returned to normal in a year, doubted that vagal fibers in the esophagus affected gastric secretion much and thought gastroenterostomy confused the picture. He "shuddered" at the thought of adding gastrectomy to vagotomy. Wangensteen said Waltman Walters' poor results with vagotomy had had a discouraging effect in their area.

Lester R. Dragstedt, P. V. Harper, Jr., E. B. Tovee, and E. R. Woodward, *Secretion of the Vagus Nerves to the Stomach in the Treatment of Peptic Ulcer,* Complications and End Results After Four Years. Volume LXV, 1947.

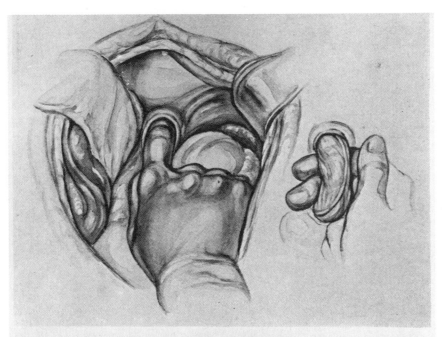

FIG. 3.—The finger is introduced over the esophagus into the mediastinum, the esophagus mobilized by careful finger dissection and pulled downward into the abdomen for a distance of 2 to 3 inches.

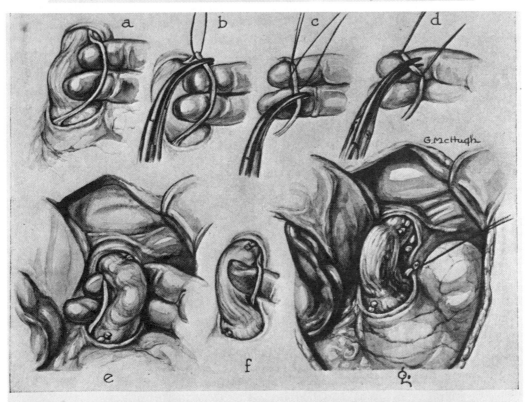

FIG. 4.—The vagus nerves are separated from the esophagus by finger dissection, ligated with nonabsorbable suture material, divided, and a segment 4 to 6 centimeters in length excised.

vagotomy was performed transthoracically and all but one were immediately relieved of pain, that one requiring a subtotal gastrectomy for an active ulcer in spite of a negative insulin response. Seven of 11 patients complaining of "epigastric fullness, gastric oppression, foul eructations and vomiting due to gastric dilatation with retention" were eventually relieved, but four of these and one other required operation, usually gastrectomy, the ulcer being found healed and the stomach atonic. "Twenty cases is admittedly a small series, but the fact that five of these patients required another surgical exploration, one for persistent pain and four for intractable motor disturbances, has convinced us that severance of the vagus nerves as a sole procedure should not be offered to patients with chronic duodenal ulcer without obstruction as a reliable therapeutic measure. We therefore have discontinued it for the present." They had also done 12 transthoracic vagotomies for anastomotic ulcers, six of those patients were well, two were improved, two had rebled, in three the ulcer had recurred, and one patient had died postoperatively. In their last 44 vagotomies, they had used the infradiaphragmatic approach. In 15 patients with a duodenal ulcer, vagotomy had been combined with a complementary gastroenterostomy, "From past experiences it is known that symptoms of a duodenal ulcer *per se* are invariably relieved by gastroenterostomy, and that the ulcer heals. The unfortunate disadvantage of this simple operation is the high incidence of gastrojejunal ulceration. Perhaps careful follow-up studies over the next five years will demonstrate the efficacy of combining gastroenterostomy with infradiaphragmatic vagotomy in either reducing or eliminating the incidence of gastrojejunal ulceration. Until then we shall continue to perform subtotal gastrectomy as the operation of choice for duodenal ulcer. We shall combine it with infradiaphragmatic vagotomy, especially in those patients whose preoperative free acid studies are high, and those in whom bleeding without pain was the outstanding symptom, two categories in which recurrent gastrojejunal ulceration occasionally occurs." They had done 26 such gastrectomies and vagotomies without any problems, "With the elimination of both the vagal and hormonal phases of gastric secretion, an anacidity is usually produced and, under such conditions, recurrent jejunal ulcer and hemorrhage should not occur." Colp thought his results with vagotomy for anastomotic ulcers were striking. Frank H. Lahey, of Boston, said he would not employ vagotomy for gastric ulcer because of the danger of overlooking a malignancy, and particularly favored a transthoracic vagotomy for ". . . jejunal ulcers which have occurred after subtotal gastrec-

tomy" and for duodenal ulcers close to the common duct. Edwin M. Miller, of Chicago, spoke of the widespread newspaper and magazine publicity and the awareness of the operation on the part of the lay-public, commenting that "There will be many doctors who will be carried away by the general enthusiasm, will be over-zealous in performing these vagus nerve operations, with unsufficient indications, without adequate preoperative study, without technical ability, and who have not the laboratory facilities for making careful postoperative follow-up studies." He was favorably impressed with an experience with 40 cases, the operation performed transthoracically to be certain that the vagotomy was absolutely complete. Harold M. Wookey, of Toronto, commented that if one wanted to be sure of dividing all of the fibers of the vagus, he had found ". . . that the esophagus and vagi are more easily reached by a rightsided approach through the thorax. The vagi may then be divided at a higher level and in this way one would be most certain that all fibers proceeding to the stomach are included. In my opinion, this is a simpler operation and less disturbing to the patient." Owen H. Wangensteen, of Minneapolis, while praising Dragstedt, said he thought vagotomy ". . . is a problem which should be threshed out in a few areas. Yet in my community, a number of surgeons in the Twin Cities who had never explored the possibilities of resection are performing vagotomies in large numbers. In January, Dr. Walters and his associates from Rochester presented their material on vagotomy. His results suggest definitely that vagotomy does not consistently afford patients with ulcer that degree of protection which one would like to find in an operative procedure. As a matter of fact, following Dr. Walters' talk on vagotomy for ulcer in St. Paul, it was to be noted that all the lobby telephones were busy. Internists and surgeons alike probably were already cancelling vagotomies that had been scheduled. In any case, in my area, the enthusiasm for vagotomy has been dampened perceptibly by the report of Dr. Walters and his colleagues." Wangensteen pointed out that vagotomy would not inhibit the humoral secretion of gastric acid as provoked by his histamine-in-beeswax preparation. Wangensteen cited the figures of anastomotic ulcer after gastrojejunostomy (40% at the University of Chicago Clinics) and concluded by stating that "The wisdom of adding gastrojejunostomy to vagotomy to thwart the ulcer diathesis in man is therefore a debatable matter." Francis D. Moore, of Boston, in closing, made the statement ". . . that one year after vagus resection the fasting acidity and motility of the stomach have readjusted themselves to denervation and returned to essentially normal values . . .

We should therefore not refer to vagus division as an operation which lowers gastric acidity. It produces a temporary change in fasting acidity, and doubtless a permanent change in acidity produced in response to cortical stimuli." He did not think that the vagal fibers found in the wall of the esophagus affected the gastric secretion, "I would not feel convinced that sectioning one of these small fibers had accomplished much change in the physiologic conduct of the rest of the organ. As for doing this operation with subtotal gastrectomy, I have shuddered when this has been mentioned as a routine procedure. It did not seem justified to subject a large group of patients to the side effects of vagus division when they were already having an operation carried out which has its own imposing list of by-products." The Massachusetts General Hospital group preferred to operate through the chest. Lester R. Dragstedt, of Chicago, closing, addressed himself in his gentle fashion to Wangensteen's comments. Histamine ulcers were due to the direct effect of histamine upon the ". . .neuroglandular apparatus in the stomach and not on the brain. Section of the vagus nerves, therefore, should not interfere with the secretory effect of the absorbed histamine . . . in patients with peptic ulcer, the excessive, continuous secretion of gastric juice is neurogenic in origin and is abolished by division of the vagus nerves to the stomach. The excessive, continuous secretion of gastric juice produced by the implantation of pellets of histamine and beeswax . . . is chemical in origin and should not be abolished by sectioning the vagus nerves to the stomach. The situation in the two cases is . . . not comparable." As for the statement that gastric acidity returned, "I was very much interested in Dr. Moore's statement that within a year following section of the vagus nerves to the stomach, the secretion of gastric juice and motility return to the preoperative level. In our experience, section of the vagus nerves has abolished permanently the nervous phase of gastric secretion . . . we have secured no evidence of regeneration of the secretory fibers in the vagus nerve to the stomach as determined by physiologic tests. The usual failure of the recurrent laryngeal nerve to regenerate following damage in thyroid surgery is of interest in this connection. While the period of clinical observation is still too short for us to know whether or not recurrence of these ulcers that have healed following vagus section will take place, the data from the experimental laboratory permit us to be quite optimistic. I do not believe that these ulcers will recur unless the vagus nerves regenerate and the excessive, continuous secretion of gastric juice of nervous origin is resumed. Since regenera-

tion of these nerves has not been seen even in the patients operated upon four years ago, it seems unlikely, on the basis of what we have learned about regeneration of nerves elsewhere, that this will take place."

* * *

Arthur H. Blakemore, of New York, Assistant Professor of Clinical Surgery, College of Physicians and Surgeons, Columbia University, *Restorative Endoaneurysmorrhaphy by Vein Graft Inlay,* reported his technique of inserting his vein-graft lined Vitallium tubes in the restoration of arterial continuity in the treatment of aneurysms. He reported four such successful operations. In one of them, a long segment of superficial femoral vein was used to replace a popliteal aneurysm, employing small Vitallium tubes at either end.

Discussion

D. W. Gordon Murray, of Toronto, admired ". . . the way he puts this damaged artery together. My own predilection would be for suture, but that is a weakness on my part . . . In my hands, by giving heparin I can be more certain to maintain the patency of the anastomosis. In one of the animals' hearts shown yesterday, removed from an animal in which we had done a vein graft in a carotid artery nine years previously, the vein graft was removed at this time. Its lumen was patent. It was slightly larger than the adjacent artery. The wall in some places was rigid so that it fractured when it was opened out. I am not sure whether it was calcium or bone . . . In a clinical case, a boy in whom a 2.5 inch graft of vein was placed in the femoral artery eight years ago, this has been working well ever since. There is no sign of aneurysm. On palpation it does not feel rigid or stiff . . . There probably is a place for venous grafts in arteries under suitable conditions . . ." As might be expected, Rudolph Matas, of New Orleans, rose in discussion [one-and-a-half pages]. He did more than comment on the past, "While great progress has been accomplished within the course of the half century since I began to utilize the suture as a conservative substitute for the ligature in the cure of aneurysms—so that now the repair of injured arteries and veins has become a sort of plastic art in which many of our younger contemporaries have become great artists—I believe that we are on the way to devise still simpler methods and more handy materials than venous grafts, to bridge over gaps in the arterial stream. The distance we have travelled on the road of progress, between the

Tuffier tube of the first world war and the venous lined Vitallium tube of the Blakemore pattern—is quite encouraging."

* * *

There were two papers on sympathectomy. Michael E. DeBakey, of New Orleans, Associate Professor of Surgery, Tulane University, George Burch, by invitation, Thorpe Ray, by invitation, and Alton Ochsner, William Henderson Professor of Surgery and Head of the Department, School of Medicine, Tulane University; Director of Surgical Section, Ochsner Clinic, *The "Borrowing-Lending" Hemodynamic Phenomenon (Hemometakinesia) and Its Therapeutic Application in Peripheral Vascular Disturbances,* spoke of the changing distribution of blood flow in accordance with physiologic need attributed to local changes in the vascular bed, and demonstrated what they thought was evidence of an increased flow in a limb with a sympathetic block, at the expense of flow in the opposite extremity and skin of the body. For peripheral vascular disease, they thought what was necessary was a method to produce local vasodilatation since drugs which produced general vasodilatation would be dangerous if administered to a degree which would be important in the affected extremity. Their arguments were largely theoretical and philosphical. The concept of peripheral vascular resistance does not appear.

* * *

Norman E. Freeman, of San Francisco, Associate Clinical Professor of Surgery, University of California Medical School, and by invitation, Frank H. Leeds, and Richard E. Gardner, *Sympathectomy for Obliterative Arterial Disease; Indications and Contraindications,* presented the thesis that sympathectomy had its effect by opening up pre-existing microscopic arteriovenous communications, and that it might bring about long lasting effects even though preoperative diagnostic tests,- paravertebral blocks, spinal anesthesia, etc., failed to show an adequate rise in skin temperature. On the basis of several patients with progressive gangrene after a sympathectomy, they concluded that "In advanced obliterative arterial disease . . . especially in patients without evidence of abnormal vasoconstriction, sympathectomy may result in gangrene. Although the total circulation may be increased after sympathectomy in these cases, much of the blood is probably shunted directly into the veins through the opening-up of numerous arterio-venous anastomoses. The nutrient capillary flow may actually be reduced. In the less advanced cases of obliterative arterial disease, sym-

pathectomy may promote the development of collateral circulation through permanent opening of these arterio-venous communications." He listed a number of patients with peripheral arteriosclerotic disease who had been improved by operation. In his outlined case reports, Freeman listed his indications for operation; cold, clammy extremities, venous constriction, improvement of claudication after lumbar sympathetic block, mottled, cyanotic skin, and Raynaud's phenomena. As contra-indications he listed, absent oscillations at ankle, pain due to ischemic neuritis, continued smoking, atrophy of soft tissues, and rapid blanching on elevation of the foot.

Discussion

Louis G. Herrman, of Cincinnati, who had been interested in passive vascular exercise [Pavex boot] suggested that ". . . sympathetic ganglionectomy should not be looked upon as an innocuous procedure, particularly in patients with extensive structural changes in the peripheral arteries . . .", accepting it as fact that "widespread denervation has been shown even to precipitate gangrene of the tissues." He thought sympathectomy did no more than to open arteriovenous communications in the skin, that this would ". . . divert large quantities of blood directly into the veins and thus reduce the nutrition of the tissues to an even lower level." I. Ridgeway Trimble, of Baltimore, agreed with Freeman that beneficial results had followed sympathectomy even in patients whose preoperative tests were not encouraging and went on to mention that he was ". . . investigating the possibility of lowering the incidence of postoperative thrombosis and thrombophlebitis by binding the lower extremities with elastic bandages during operation and by keeping these bandages in place after operation for a period of two weeks." Peter Heinbecker, of St. Louis, seemed to question whether the interference of sympathectomy with the local humoral sympathetic responses was necessarily good. Walter G. Maddock, of Chicago, said that sympathectomy "is a relatively simple procedure now and I place it under the heading of conservative treatment." Arteriosclerotics might be modestly benefited, and he doubted that the gangrene which was occasionally seen was necessarily caused by sympathectomy. Frederick L. Reichert, of San Francisco, felt similarly,- "That case of gangrene Doctor Freeman showed I think is due to thrombosis of the femoral vessels, and has nothing to do with sympathectomy . . . Sympathectomy has helped these people, up to the age of 80 or 90." In closing, Freeman made it clear that he still favored sympathectomy even in the face of arteriosclerosis, but that ischemia per se was not the indication for operation so much as ". . . evidence that abnormal constriction of the blood vessels exists."

The Business Meetings

The 1947 meeting, March 25, 26, and 27, was held at The Homestead, Hot Springs, Virginia, Edward D. Churchill in the Chair.

The Membership Committee, Arthur W. Allen reporting, had obtained the names of ". . . 300 surgeons in America who were thought to be worthy of consideration for Fellowship in this Association . . .", deleted half of them for a variety of reasons, "too immature", insufficient contributions, excessive age, and now were recommending 35 men to be proposed, in addition to the 70 whose nominations were under consideration, and the 47 men whose names were ready to be read out at this meeting for voting in subsequent years. The Committee recommended that the membership be gradually increased to 250, by 1952.

In the discussion, Dr. Frank Lahey said he thought the membership should be unlimited, "The decision as to selection of candidates is now in the hands of a small group. Such procedure tends to mitigate [a significant proportion of the distinguished Fellows confused mitigate and militate] against this association fulfilling its purpose as a representative group of American Surgeons." Evarts Graham favored more participation by the membership in the selection of candidates. Dr. Allen said that the Membership Committee functioned very well to represent the Association. Allen's report was accepted.

As a result of Howard C. Naffziger's comments about nursing the year before, he had been appointed Chairman of a committee to study the nursing problem. From questionnaires and other sources they concluded that ". . . at present in municipal and university and private hospitals the quantity of nursing was 55 to 60 per cent of that which was needed and the quality of that supplied was down to 75 per cent. The percentage of nursing requiremets which could be handled by 'nurses' aides' or by practical nurses was estimated at 60 per cent." There was general agreement that nurses' aides equal in experience to war-time volunteers, and under the direction of experienced nurses, would satisfy nursing needs satisfactorily, and a very guarded statement that "There was almost complete unanimity in the feeling of the surgical profession that the increase in the required training for nurses beyond the

three-year level had not improved their ability to care for the sick and that it had not promoted closer co-operation between doctor and nurse in the care of the sick . . . the professed aim of the nursing profession has been to elevate the nursing profession and to increase the educational content of training. They have lost sight of the need of the sick for adequate nursing care. As more of the nurse's time has been devoted to formal class instruction, the nursing care of the patients has become less satisfactory . . . the nursing schools no longer report on professional matters to the medical staff of the hospital but to a superintendent who may have no medical background . . . Schools of nursing have tended rapidly to center upon education of those who are to become supervisors, hospital and school administrators and public health nurses, and the direct care of the sick has become a minor interest." Naffziger decried the influence of the National League of Nursing Education and the American Nurses Association and the State Nursing Associations, speaking of their large financial resources from dues-paying members, ". . . able legal counsel and public relations advisors." The outcry for nursing help had forced the nurses' organizations to "acknowledge the need for subsidiary workers", but in many states and many hospitals the nursing profession had "not utilized this help. A closed shop practice has prevailed widely . . . The medical profession, the public, the hospitals and the sick patients demand adequate nursing care. It can be given. Years of higher education are not required to supply it, in spite of the unwise aims of national nursing bodies. There are opportunities for women who combine education at the university level with nurses' training. Such persons are entitled to appropriate compensation but they are not interested in bedside nursing, nor can the patient afford them. As a group they desire to retain the title of nurse but have devised their own definition of the word nurse. It does not agree with Noah Webster, nor can their definition be found in any available dictionary. The need for 'bedside' nurses at a reduced cost to the patient can be met at least in part by establishing one-year courses of training." Naffziger then proposed "that the American Surgical Association go on record as approving the use of personnel trained specifically for bedside care, and . . . immediate establishment of short courses for the training of bedside nurses." The resolution was unanimously accepted. In the discussion, Dr. McKittrick pointed out that the American College of Surgeons had circularized hospitals and their officers advising them "to admit and utilize the assistance of auxiliary nursing aid."

At the Second Executive Session, Fred W. Rankin, who had been a General, reported for the War Survey Committee. After some comments upon the conduct of matters during the war, they recommended unification of all the military medical services, "All who have studied this problem are in favor of total unification . . . ", and the setting up, in the Office of the Surgeon General, an Advisory or Consultant Board in Medicine or Surgery because of ". . . inevitable tendency of the Regular Medical Officer to think in terms of the Regular Army Medical Corps and not in terms always of what is best for the casualty or for the overall medical plan . . . " A Consultant in Medicine should be nominated by the Association of American Physicians and a Consultant in Surgery by the American Surgical Association, etc. Currently they thought the supply of physicians in the country was becoming inadequate, but made no recommendations. Within the armed forces, they advised rotation of medical officers from field installations back to hospital units.

The officers elected were: President, Elliott C. Cutler, of Boston; Vice-Presidents, William E. Gallie, of Toronto, and Warren H. Cole, of Chicago; Secretary, Warfield M. Firor.

LXVI

1948

The 1948 meeting was held at the Chateau Frontenac, Quebec, Canada, May 27, 28, and 29, President William E. Gallie, of Toronto, Professor of Surgery, Emeritus, University of Toronto, In the Chair, having succeeded to the Chair upon the death of Elliott Cutler. Among those who had also died in the previous year were: Arthur W. Elting, of Albany; and Roscoe Reed Graham, of Toronto.

President Gallie's untitled address was devoted to the problem of undergraduate education. He said the increasing number of specialties had led to more and more time for the teaching of surgery and the specialties in the medical school. "The result is that ten times as much space is given to the teaching of surgery as was given in 1903." He made the important statement that "The time has now come when the study of surgery must be established as a postgraduate course with not only the apprenticeship in hospital but also a special curriculum of studies covering surgery itself and all the appropriate basic sciences." He thought surgery should be principally a postgraduate discipline and that "the teaching of such subjects as peptic ulcer, carcinoma of the stomach, tumour of the brain, bronchiectasis and dozens of others should be conducted by the physicians or if by us, then as physicians and not as surgeons. Our time will come when the young graduate is definitely committed to the program which we have agreed is necessary for the training of a modern surgeon." The textbooks of surgery were too detailed for students and not sufficiently detailed for postgraduate students. He hoped the Association might appoint a committee to study the best points of undergraduate training in the schools of America and Europe.

He was a full-time Professor of Surgery and thought that was appropriate and enjoyed it, but emphasized that pensions had to be adequate, because after retirement from the Chair "there isn't a chance in the world, no matter how distinguished and accomplished the professor may be, of picking up private practice again in competition with the young men he has trained." As for the choice of the professor, he insisted that the professor "must be a first-class surgeon" and decried a tendency to appoint young men with no proven clinical record. He had no argument with the requirements that professors be biological scientists, "All I am doing is making the selection of the professor more difficult by demanding that he be also a good surgeon." In general, he thought the chairman of the department should be a general surgeon, and one with a particularly broad training in surgery. The full-time professorship worked best when the professor was also surgeon-in-chief of the hospital rather than merely the head of one of the surgical services. He reemphasized what he considered to be the weakness in the North American training of surgeons, the instruction in the basic Sciences.

* * *

Warren H. Cole, of Chicago, Professor and Head of the Department of Surgery, University of Illinois, College of Medicine, and by invitation, John T. Reynolds and Carl Ireneus, *Strictures of the Com-* **913**

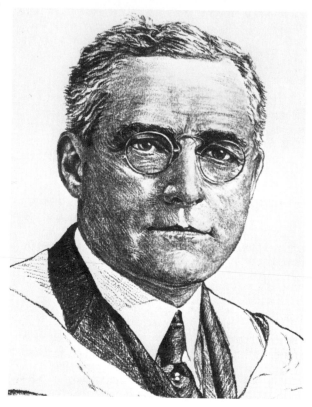

W. Edward Gallie, 1882-1959. President, 1948 and of the ACS, 1941-1946. M.D. Toronto, 1903. Trained at Hospital for Sick Children, Toronto; Toronto General Hospital, and Hospital for Ruptured and Crippled, New York. Ultimately Surgeon-in-Chief, Hospital for Sick Children [1921-1929], and Professor and Chief Surgeon at Toronto General 1929-1947. Life-long interest in bone and fascia healing, suture, and transplantation, used autogenous fascia (Gallie's suture) in hernia repair. A big man, of great warmth, charm and humor, he exerted great influence. Established the first planned training course for surgeons in Canada, which came to be known as The Gallie Course, and the men in training, inevitably, as "The Gallie Slaves".
Sketch courtesy of Imago Chirurgii, 1913-1963 (American College of Surgeons) Ethicon, Inc.

mon Duct, were speaking from an experience of 63 operations in 49 patients. Operative trauma was the cause of the strictures in 65%. They still preferred end-to-end anastomosis after resection of the stricture and had six good results out of seven, with one death in this group. They were particularly interested in the high strictures, at the liver. In spite of the fact that President Gallie, in the portion of his Address which he devoted to the rash introductions of large varieties of foreign bodies into patients, had said that "Murphy's button, McGraw's ligature, Vi-

tallium bile duct tubes, have all given place to more physiological procedures designed to imitate as closely as possible the normal", Cole, in reporting his experience with hilar duct to Roux Y anastomoses in 28 operations, three quarters of them with Vitallium tubes, was not prepared to abandon the Vitallium tube. More recently, he had been creating a mucosal tube at the end of his Roux Y, inserting that over a rubber stent well up into the duct in the liver, which he called a modified Hoag [1937] procedure and was encouraged by it. The first use of a Roux Y tube for biliary reconstruction, he attributed to Monprofit, 1908. Cole had performed 63 operations in 49 patients with four deaths and repeatedly stated that his operative mortality was 6% [although obviously 8% of the patients had died of operation].

Discussion

Alfred Blalock, of Baltimore, rose to present the still unpublished work of William P. Longmire, of Baltimore, in incising the left lobe of the liver to find a large duct to anastomose to a Roux Y loop in patients in whom no hilar operation was possible. Frank Lahey, of Boston, said all methods were difficult, all tubes plugged and all methods of reconstruction "are in general makeshift procedures", unless the ends of the duct were sutured together, "In any repair of an injured bile duct we have learned that one of the most important factors is the preservation of the sphincter of Oddi." In more than 200 cases, they had learned "that to get a satisfactory result one must have mucosa-to-mucosa anastomoses . . . the introduction of tubes is a truly makeshift procedure . . . while . . . many of them will work, in spite of what has been said about them, many will fail over a long period of time." He reemphasized the technique which he and Cattell employed of splitting the pancreas to find the distal end of the common duct, then mobilizing the duodenum so the distal end of the duct "can be approximated without tension to the lower end of the hepatic duct, and a direct mucosa-to-mucosa, end-to-end anastomosis can be done." They left a T-tube in place for several months, introduced through a separate opening in the common duct. He did not like "inflexible tubes such as Vitallium . . . they have no greater likelihood of maintaining patency than do rubber tubes and they have the greater disadvantage of producing pressure and not adjusting themselves to the tortuous tracts into which they must often be inserted. No matter what type of tube we have used, many of them have had to be taken out and another tube inserted within three years because of their becoming plugged with bile salts." Herman E. Pearse, of Rochester, New York, pointed out that Eliot's presentation of repair of common duct stricture [Volume LIII, 1935] showed 26% successful results, whereas now success was achieved approximately 80% of the time. He was "inclined to agree with Dr. Lahey that the best way to repair the damage is by direct end-to-end anastomosis . . . have no quarrel with the Roux type of procedure and use it when necessary." As for tubes "I have tested out most of the available materials and have found that Vitallium is the best for this purpose. It has faults and so I am searching for a better material." As for the length of the Roux loop, he thought it should be at least 12 inches to prevent regurgitation into the duct system.

* * *

Henry Doubilet, by invitation, and John H. Mulholland, of New York, George David Stewart Professor of Surgery; Chairman of Department, New York University College of Medicine, *Recurrent Acute Pancreatitis: Observations on Etiology and Surgical Treatment,* presented their experience with sphincterotomy of the sphincter of Oddi. Intraoperative cholangiography demonstrated the great frequency of a common channel for the bile and pancreatic ducts and they assumed that as a result of spasm of the sphincter of Oddi pancreatitis was caused by reflux of "bile which has been rendered noxious by concentration of its salts or some other change . . ." They did add that "An unsolved aspect of this problem is how the bile can enter the pancreatic duct against the secretory pressure of the pancreas itself." They attributed to Archibald the first deliberate division of the sphincter of Oddi [1919] in a patient with recurrent pancreatitis. T-tube cholangiograms demonstrated that when patients were given morphine or when N/10 hydrochloric acid was applied to the ampulla of Vater through a duodenal tube, the resultant constriction of the sphincter of Oddi raised the pressure in the common duct and allowed reflux of contrast material into the pancreatic duct. As for the technique of sphincterotomy, they preferred the transcholedochal insertion of a backward cutting hinged knife which cut a longitudinal sliver out of the ampulla [Colp, Doubilet, Gerber, 1936] or else a transduodenal incision of the sphincter over a probe passed down from the common duct. "The retraction of the sphincter muscle fibers prevents healing or regeneration of the muscle." They presented the details of 21 patients, most of them completely relieved by sphincterotomy, with one death from a mismatched blood

transfusion. In one patient with an external pancreatic fistula after a previous attempt at pancreatectomy, the fistula closed after sphincterotomy.

Discussion

Alton Ochsner, of New Orleans, opened the Discussion commenting upon Dr. Mims Gage's use of splanchnic block for pancreatitis. He also raised "the question of whether in these acute recurrent pancreatitis attacks, in which Dr. Mulholland has shown that section of the ampulla has so dramatically relieved them—it would not be better to perform a plastic procedure on the duct rather than trans-choledochal section. Only time will tell whether this will give rise to stricture later. We have had two patients in whom we have done plastics on the duct, making an incision transductally and then suturing the ductal mucosa to the duodenal mucosa." Evarts Graham, of St. Louis, asked "How long after cutting the sphincter does the paralysis last?" Mulholland, closing, was inclined to think that Ochsner's suggestion of a plastic operation might be inadvisable "I think it is vital to preserve the oblique passage of the common bile duct in the duodenal wall. The muscular intestinal wall containing the intramural portion of the common duct acts as a sphincter and is an effective bar to the reflux of duodenal contents in the biliary tract." In reply to Dr. Graham, Mulholland said that their longest follow-up was 18 months with "no evidence of sphincter spasm. Dr. Doubilet, who has done the basic experimental work concerned in this problem, has sacrificed dogs two years after the sphincter was cut and found it retracted and incompetent."

* * *

Laurence S. Fallis, of Detroit, Surgeon-in-Charge, Division of General Surgery, Henry Ford Hospital, and by invitation, D. Emerick Szilagyi, *Observations on Some Metabolic Changes after Total Pancreatoduodenectomy,* described their three patients with total pancreatectomy, one of them dying of recurrence 14 months after operation, one dying of intestinal obstruction three months after pancreatectomy, and one alive four months after operation. They could find "17 cases of total pancreatoduodenectomy mentioned in medical literature . . . seven lived long enough to allow postoperative investigations. . ." Their detailed studies allowed them to say "the characteristics of the diabetes in patients after total pancreatectomy are (a) a relatively low insulin requirement (20-60 daily units); (b) a sensitivity to insulin, and (c) frequent and often unpredictable fluctuations in the blood sugar level." Patients were best maintained "on the hyperglycemic side". They suggested that "the pathophysiology of total surgical diabetes is not identical with diabetes mellitus as understood in terms of the conventional clinical type." The replacement of the lost external pancreatic secretion was effective.

There was no Discussion.

* * *

Frederick A. Coller, of Ann Arbor, Professor of Surgery, University of Michigan Medical School; Chairman, Department of Surgery, and by invitation, Kenneth N. Campbell and Vivian Iob, *The Treatment of Renal Insufficiency in the Surgical Patient,* were speaking of "acute renal insufficiency of the low nephron type", which in their experience lasted seven to 14 days, during which the patient required support. The initial shock inducing the renal insufficiency having been treated, and renal insufficiency having become manifest, "the total fluid intake of the patient is immediately limited to the daily calculated insensible loss, (perspiration and respiration). This will vary between 1000 and 1800 cc. in the afebrile patient and consists of water given orally or 5% glucose in distilled water intravenously. The restriction of total fluid intake is enforced until adequate urine output ensues." Periodic determinations of a blood NPN and carbon dioxide combining power were "optional but at the same time desireable." If the CO_2 combining power dropped below 40 volumes %, patients were to be given sodium bicarbonate orally or one-sixth molar sodium lactate intravenously, although they recognized that "the use of these solutions leads to the introduction of sodium salts in the presence of renal insufficiency." The diet need not be a low protein diet, but the salt content should be restricted. During the diuresis in the recovery phase "abnormal water and electrolyte losses in this urine may place the life of the patient in jeopardy from acute dehydration or hypopotassemia . . . Therapy . . . is . . . directed at accurate replacement of urinary losses of sodium, potassium, and water." [This may be the first reference in the *Transactions* to the intravenous administration of potassium.] Decreasing the fluid intake did not decrease the diuresis in this phase and "When the urine output reaches a level of 5 liters or more daily, an equivalent amount of Ringer's solution intravenouly is given. Any difference between output and intake is paralleled by an oral intake of salt solution equivalent to the amount of urine passed with each urination."

Discussion

Everett Evans, of Richmond, Virginia, the only discusser, agreed that "one simply must not force the kidney to do work that it cannot do . . . we must let nature do what nature can do and, if nature cannot repair the damage, there is not much that one can do about tubular degeneration." He spoke about the necessity for treating shock promptly "to prevent the shocked kidney."

* * *

Howard Ulfelder and Ruth M. Graham, by invitation, and Joe V. Meigs, of Boston, Clinical Professor of Gynecology, Harvard Medical School, *Further Studies on the Cytologic Method in the Problem of Gastric Cancer* [citing in their bibliography only their previous paper of the same year and that of Papanicolaou, in 1942, and obviously seeking to extend the application of a technique they had found useful in cervical cancer], had done cytological studies in 48 patients with suspected gastric cancer. Specimens were unsatisfactory in five, 12 of 14 patients, proved at operation to have cancer, had been diagnosed correctly cytologically. One patient with a positive cytological report had "no detectable gastric lesion" and had not been operated upon, and a patient with a lymphoma of the stomach had not been diagnosed cytologically.

Discussion

There was no discussion from the floor and Dr. Meigs, closing, said that "Recently Mrs. Graham in our Vincent Hospital Laboratory has told me that within the last eighteen months any patient that she said had a positive smear for carcinoma of the cervix had carcinoma of the cervix. She has picked up between 25 and 30 unsuspected cancers of the cervix. It is wrong for us to think that as clinicians we can do this work. It should be done by experts."

* * *

Only the year before, Gilchrist and David and those who discussed their paper had all emphasized the need for the abdominoperineal resection for carcinoma of the rectum and lower sigmoid, but now Claude F. Dixon, of Rochester, Minnesota, Professor of Surgery, Graduate School at the University of Minnesota (Mayo Foundation), *Anterior Resection for Malignant Lesions of the Upper Part of the Rectum and Lower Part of the Sigmoid,* championed resection and low anastomosis. [He had not entered into the 1947 Discussion.] It had previously been

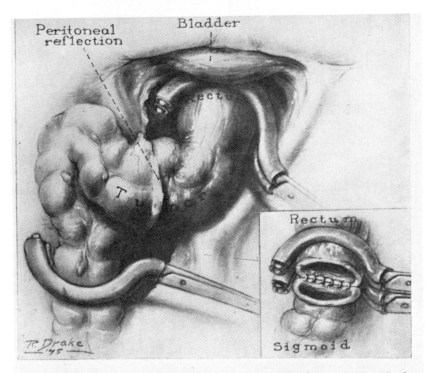

FIG. 3.—Curved intestinal clamps are placed beyond the lines of resection of the intestine. After the segment is resected the clamps are placed side by side and the open colorectostomy is performed as indicated in the insert.

At the 1947 meeting, but for a qualified reservation by Wangensteen, and Eloesser's sentimental preference for avoiding colostomy, the general tenor had been to accept abdominoperineal resection as the best operation for cancer of the rectum and lower rectosigmoid. Dixon held his peace then, obviously returned to Rochester and for the 1948 meeting, gathered together his experience of 18 years with preservation of the rectum in 523 patients. His mortality was now 2.6% and his five-year survival 64% for lesions at 6-10 cm. These superb results with this almost heretical operation stifled discussion.

Claude F. Dixon, *Anterior Resection for Malignant Lesions of the Upper Part of the Rectum and Lower Part of the Sigmoid*, Volume LXVI, 1948.

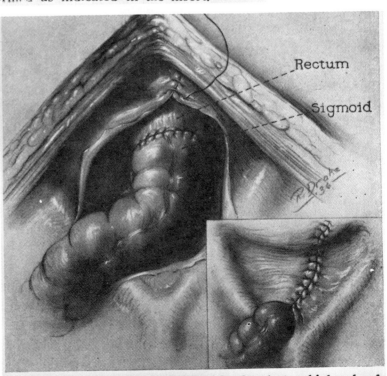

FIG. 4.—The pelvic peritoneum is closed at a higher level, which makes the anastomosis retroperitoneal. The drain has been omitted from the drawing.

Dixon's policy to perform a sigmoidostomy first and then in some cases to resect the lesion, leaving the distal rectum, reanastomosing the patients six to 12 months later if they were doing well, "The satisfactory survival rates, despite extensive lesions of high grade, suggested that the intestinal anastomosis could be performed at the second stage of the operation . . . the rectal stump can survive if supplied by the inferior hemorrhoidal vessels alone, regardless of the fact that the textbooks have denied this . . . Sudeck's point is not as critical as described and . . . it is possible to excise sufficient tissue in the mesocolon and distal portion of the sigmoid and to obtain good clinical results. Apparently it sufficed to remove only 3 or 4 cm. of bowel distal to the lesion . . . the occasional distal spread of carcinoma to lymph nodes beyond 2 cm. is due to proximal blockage. In such instance it is possible that no surgical procedure is sufficiently radical . . ." From 1930 to 1938, he had performed the operation in three stages, and since 1938, in two stages unless obstruction required a preliminary colostomy. He was using sulfasuxidine or sulfathaladine before operation and "In addition, 5 Gm. of sulfathiazole is scattered intraperitoneally at the close of the operation." Appropriate manual delivery of the rectum and division of the lateral stalks permitted one to place a clamp 3 to 4 cm. below the lesion, even when the lesion was a measured 6 to 8 cm. from the dentate line. He performed an open anastomosis with interrupted sutures, one layer posteriorly, two layers anteriorly. "Any so-called aseptic anastomosis in this region is a gymnastic feat attended by difficult clamp maneuvers deep in the pelvis, danger of tearing the rectum, the hazard of catching the opposite mucosa to create a persistent diaphragm, or of perforating the rectum in forcing the anastomosis open, and finally the possibility of a poor anastomosis. A valuable extra centimeter or more of rectum may be consumed in the process." A Penrose drain was placed in the hollow of the sacrum. Colostomies were closed intraperitoneally and they had now only two deaths from colostomy closure, a 0.6% mortality, one of those from coronary occlusion, one from peritonitis. A "temporary defunctioning loop type of tranverse colonic stoma" was the safest effective decompression and "the mortality rate is considerably higher when colostomy is omitted than when it is included", particularly when the lesion was at or below the pelvic floor. Since 1930, Dixon had performed the operation in 523 patients. In 447 cases, the lesion was 20 cm. or less from the dentate line. In an analyzed group of 426 cases of anterior resection of lesions between 6 and 20 cm., there were 35 deaths,- 5.9%. In 1934 at the

Mayo Clinic, the mortality for all operations on the colon was 16% and in the past four years, it had been less than 5%, "I attribute a large part of the success in reducing the mortality rate to the use of sulfonamides." Mortality for anterior resection had been 8.5% from 1930 to 1935, rose to 12.8% in 1936 to 1940, when the operation was made more radical, and dropped to 2.6% in 1941 to 1947. His five-year survival rate was 67.7% in 272 cases, 63.7% for lesions 6 to 10 cm. from the dentate line. All patients had sphincter control. Eight males with low lesions volunteered that there was no emission during ejaculation, "it is probable that the seminal vesicles or ducts were detached in the course of the dissection." During the same period of time, 185 Miles combined abdominoperineal resections were performed and the five-year survival rates were 40.7% for lesions 0 to 4 cm., 43.6% for lesions 5 to 9 cm., and 57.9% for those 10 to 14 cm. He concluded that the "operation is sufficiently safe and radical for lesions of the upper half of the rectum . . . The survival rate after resection of low rectal lesions is poorer than that following resection of lesions higher in the bowel."

[One may speculate upon the reason that no Discussion is recorded. The proposal at the time was regarded as nearly heretical, yet Dixon's survival figures supported his thesis, which, of course, has since been accepted.]

* * *

Ralph Colp, of New York, Clinical Professor of Surgery, Columbia University; Attending Surgeon to the Mount Sinai Hospital, and by invitation, Percy Klingenstein, Leonard J. Druckerman, and Vernon A. Weinstein, *A Comparative Study of Subtotal Gastrectomy with and without Vagotomy,* presented an extension of the experience to which Colp had alluded in the discussion of vagotomy the previous year. There had been an earlier experience at the Mount Sinai Hospital with left vagotomy and gastric resection, going back to 1929. In their recent series, subtotal gastrectomy and simultaneous bilateral infradiaphragmatic vagotomy had first been undertaken for special indications, principally bleeding or an excessively high acid. More recently they had been encouraged to broaden the indications. They were now comparing gastrectomy alone in 54 patients, with gastrectomy plus vagotomy in 46. Three of the gastrectomy-vagotomy patients had "A temporary duodenal fistula.". There were no deaths. The incidence of postoperative achlorhydria was increased by the addition of vagotomy. In the vagotomy patients, "The reaction to operation was somewhat more severe, and the pulmonary complications were more frequent." Gastric atony was not a problem in patients who had a resection in addition to vagotomy. Thus far, the postoperative results at four to 28 months were equivalent, except that there had been one anastomotic ulcer in the gastrectomy without vagotomy series.

Discussion

Lester R. Dragstedt, of Chicago, opened the Discussion. It would appear that in his spoken remarks, Colp had said that vagotomy or vagotomy and gastroenterostomy had not been satsifactory, and Dragstedt was "somewhat surprised that Dr. Colp and his associates have apparently been unable to secure satisfactory results in the treatment of peptic ulcer by vagotomy alone or by vagotomy combined with gastroenterostomy, in those cases that have obstruction at the pylorus. In our clinic this operation has made its way until at the present time all the surgeons in our hospital prefer the operation of vagotomy alone or vagotomy plus gastroenterostomy to subtotal resection." They had done 430 of these operations and the results were "more satisfactory than we have seen from subtotal gastrectomy. It would seem to me that a combination of the two procedures is unwarranted at the present time . . . It is true that postoperative management is a little more difficult with vagotomy alone than if the operation is combined with gastroenterostomy. That is due to the necessity for controlling the postoperative decrease in tonus and motility of the stomach. In our clinic, however, we are successful in doing this, and at the present time we have no difficulty on this score." Owen H. Wangensteen, of Minneapolis, emphasized the difficulty in achieving a complete vagotomy. He now found that vagotomy protected dogs against a histamine-induced ulcer and believed that it was "owing largely to delay in gastric emptying." When a gastrojejunostomy was added, the protective effect of vagotomy against histamine ulcer seemed to disappear. Wangensteen devoted most of his very long discussion to the observation he had recently made that, in patients with esophageal stricture, a gastric resection had relieved the stricture and the necessity for repeated dilatations, and felt "justified in suggesting that esophagitis and esophageal stricture may be manifestations of ulcer disease and may be relieved by an effective gastric resection" [and with his usual enthusiasm, had also attempted to see whether the operation would relieve a patient with cardiospasm]. Ralph Colp, closing, said "Subtotal gastrectomy as the procedure of choice has been used in our clinic for about twenty-five years. We are satisfied with the procedure. What worries us is the incidence of recurrent jejunal ulceration . . . we thought perhaps we might diminish the incidence of jejunal ulceration by combining it [infradiaphragmatic vagotomy] with subtotal gastrectomy." He was willing to say that "none of the operations we are doing for ulcer are ideal . . . If the secretion of acid . . . could be controlled medically, all these procedures we are doing at present will probably go into the discard."

* * *

George H. Yeager, of Baltimore, Clinical Professor of Surgery, University of Maryland, and by invitation, R. Adams Cowley, *Studies on the Use of Polythene as a Fibrous Tissue Stimulant,* had been struck by the fact that some investigators had been using cellophane, with success, in conditions requiring the generation of a massive inflammatory reaction, and that others had been using it to replace dura, etc., where a reactionless material was required. Investigation had disclosed the fact that du Pont introduced di-cetyl phosphate into the manufacturing process of its cellophane and this was the irritating material which aroused so much fibroplasia. Yeager and Cowley had applied a polythene sheet about a carotid artery aneurysm with success, and to the surface of a lumbar aortic aneurysm, with a decrease in size of the mass and in the patient's awareness of throbbing. They had used the material in two aneurysms, for 11 inguinal hernias and four ventral hernias and were thus far satisfied after periods of observation ranging from three to eight months.

Discussion

Herman E. Pearse, of Rochester, New York, commented that some years before he had wrapped vessels with cellophane with ultimate occlusion and that repetition of the experiments had been unsuccessful. He now understood why. Daniel C. Elkin, of Emory University, said he was experimenting with aortic occlusion by placing a cuff of polythene about the aorta under a clamp, hoping that the fibroplasia would prevent the necrosis usually produced by an occluding band. Amos R. Koontz, of Baltimore, thought "the irritating type of polythene . . . which causes an increase in fibrous tissue, should be of great value in reinforcing suture lines when weak structures are sutured together." Doctor Gallie had inveighed against the use of tantalum in his Presidential Address, but Koontz was still enthusiastic about it for ventral and groin hernias, and was im-

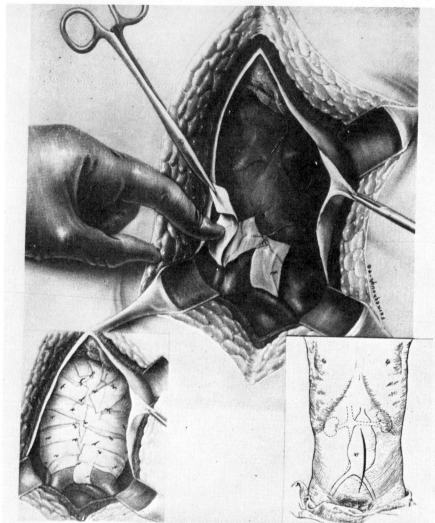

FIG. 6 (G. F. 36376).—Aneurysm of the abdominal aorta, secondary in arterio-sclerosis, extending from L 1 to its bifurcation into the common iliacs. Peritoneum reflected from aneurysmal sac, and polythene-du Pont being plicated onto its wall.

Yeager and Cowley discovered that the fibroplastic response produced by polythene depended upon the use of di-cetyl phosphate in its manufacture, explaining the fact that some polythenes were reactionless and others produced an intensive fibroplasia. In the aneurysm shown, two months after operation, the mass seemed to have become smaller and the patient was relieved of his symptoms. In a recurrent inguinal hernia, strips of polythene were placed about the neck of the sac, under the conjoined tendon-Poupart's ligament suture line, and over it. In five months, the repair was solid. For a period of time, this "wrapping" of aneurysms was widely investigated, until it was found not to prevent enlargement of the aneurysm, and rupture.

George H. Yeager and R. Adams Cowley, *Studies on the Use of Polythene as a Fibrous Tissue Stimulant*. Volume LXVI, 1948.

pressed by the amount of fibrous reaction it produced.

* * *

John D. Stewart, of Buffalo, Professor of Surgery and Chairman of the Department, University of Buffalo, and by invitation, Sidney M. Schaer, William H. Potter, and Alfred J. Massover, *Management of Massively Bleeding Peptic Ulcer*, set out to evaluate "the merits of rapid blood replacement and early surgical operation" for massively bleeding peptic ulcer. Acute hemorrhage meant "vomiting of blood or passage of blood by rectum with attendant signs of cerebral anoxia within one week of admission to the hospital" and severe enough to produce a hemoglobin of 2.5 million or less and to reduce the circulating red cell volume to 6% of normal or less. They had a total of 54 patients who met these criteria, 33 of whom were operated upon. Twenty-one other patients who declined operation or whose physicians declined operation served as controls, without operation. Of the 54 patients, 24 showed signs of hemorrhagic shock on admission, and of these 24, 15 were in the operative group "and the operation was not postponed but resuscitation and operation were carried out concurrently." Eighty percent gastrectomy and Hoffmeister reconstruction was performed within 24 hours of admission to the hospital. Patients operated upon received an average of 3600 cc. of blood, those not operated upon, 2040 cc. of blood, although the average measured operative blood loss was 360 cc. Sixteen of the patients had a previous diagnosis of peptic ulcer. When, as in five patients, no lesion was detected in the stomach or duodenum, "extensive gastric resection is performed without hesitation". All five showed "shallow ulcers with open vessels". Four patients had lesions other than peptic ulcer of the stomach and duodenum,- esophageal varices, hiatal hernia and esophageal ulcer, carcinoma of the cardia, lymphosarcoma of the stomach. All four survived. There were five deaths in the 33 operated patients who underwent gastric resection,- 15%,- and six deaths in the 21 patients who had no operation,- 29%. Stewart was puzzled by the fact that the hemoglobin and serum proteins so frequently dropped fairly strikingly several days after operation although the patients never bled after operation and showed no hemoglobinemia. He proposed "early restoration of hemoglobin values and gastric resection as the method of choice in the management of acute massive hemorrhage from peptic ulcer", as controlling the hemorrhage directly, lowering the mortality, providing definitive treatment for the underlying ulcer disease, establishing the diagnosis in doubtful cases and frequently requiring much less blood than nonoperative treatment.

Discussion

Allen O. Whipple, of New York, opened the Discussion. He did not commit himself on the point of the presentation, except to say that Stewart's paper "emphasizes the importance of not delaying surgery too long in the care of the severely bleeding gastric or duodenal ulcer", and devoted much of his discussion to warning against overtransfusion. Edward D. Churchill, of Boston, discussed the vulnerability of patients who stopped bleeding after a massive transfusion and then rebled, "I have heard it pointed out repeatedly by Dr. Allen that such a patient cannot tolerate the crises of further hemorrhage and surgical operation." Stewart's demonstration of the disappearance of much of the transfused hemoglobin interested Churchill greatly, although he offered no good explanation. Jonathan E. Rhoads, of Philadelphia, agreed that such patients should not be transfused indefinitely and turned over to the surgeons only in extremis, however, he obviously preferred to try a vigorous program of transfusion before operation, "It seems to me there is a good deal of experience to show that large numbers of these patients will stop bleeding spontaneously, and that they can be operated upon more safely after they have recovered from the immediate effects of hemorrhage. For that reason, many of us have felt it better to give most of them a chance to stop bleeding on a medical regimen." Gavin Miller, of Montreal, said that "For 20 years I have advocated 'immediate' operation; that is, if bleeding does not stop within 24 hours, on patients past 45 years of age who are admitted with massive hemorrhage. In this group of patients—who number 8 or 9—no fatality has occurred when the stomach was resected." Stewart, closing, said "There is need . . . for early decision as to definitive treatment of these cases and that is one of the main points I want to bring out . . . I do not believe it is possible to tell with any degree of assurance which patients will stop bleeding. I am particularly opposed to a 'wait and see' policy, for during the period of procrastination irreversible changes in vital organs may occur and the opportunity to perform effective surgery may be lost." As for separating the patients according to age, "some young patients die and some old patients survive. Our approach to date has been more in the direction of setting up an active plan of treatment which offers the best prognosis regardless of age."

* * *

The paper of Blalock and Park, suggesting an operative technique for coarctation of the aorta, had appeared in 1944 and the clinical successes of Crafoord and of Gross had been published in 1945. Now R. J. Bing, J. C. Handelsman, J. A. Campbell, H. E. Griswold, all by invitation, and Alfred Blalock, of Baltimore, Professor of Surgery and Director of the Department of Surgery, Johns Hopkins University, *The Surgical Treatment and the Physiopathology of Coarctation of the Aorta*, presented the Hopkins experience. Blalock agreed that the direct

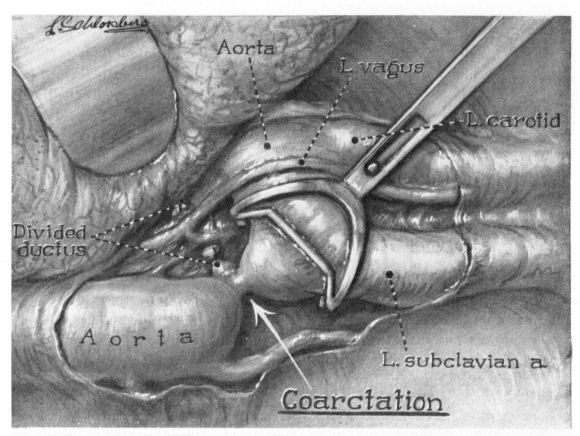

FIG. 1.—Illustrates the modified Potts clamp in position. It may be seen that while it occludes the aorta completely, it permits blood to flow through the subclavian artery.

Blalock's use of a modified Potts partial aortic occlusion clamp [devised for tangential aortic occlusion at the mouth of the patent ductus] for proximal aortic occlusion in the presence of a short proximal segment, proceeding to resection and end-to-end anastomosis. Blalock and Park in 1944 had described the experimental development of the technique of turning down the divided subclavian to bypass a coarctation. In 1945, both Crafoord and Gross reported clinical successes with direct end-to-end aortic anastomoses. In Blalock's 22 attempted anastomoses now reported with 2 deaths, 17 were end-to-end, which he considered the ideal procedure. Crafoord at this meeting presented, in Discussion, 32 operations, one of the Blalock type, and one death. Gross did not attend the meeting.

R. J. Bing, J. C. Handelsman, J. A. Campbell, H. E. Griswold, and Alfred Blalock, *The Surgical Treatment and the Physiopathology of Coarctation,* Volume LXVI, 1948.

approach of Crafoord and of Gross was "a better method", to be used whenever possible. He now followed "the advice of Crafoord" in trying to spare the intercostals distal to the coarctation, whenever possible. Blalock had modified Potts' aortic partial occlusion clamp so that it could be placed over the aortic-subclavian juncture to occlude the proximal aorta beyond the subclavian while permitting circulation through the subclavian. He used a single layer of sutures through the full thickness of the aortic wall as opposed to Crafoord who "attemped to

avoid inclusion of the intima of arteries in his anastomoses." Blalock preferred an everting anastomosis with 5-0 silk. He had thus far operated upon 23 patients, varying in age from seven to 31 years, 13 of them over 20. Anastomosis was attempted in 22 and completed in 21. The patient in whom the anastomosis was not attempted, had a long hypoplastic segment. The anastomosis could not be completed in a patient in whom the proximal clamp slipped off with immediate and permanent cardiac arrest even though the bleeding was almost instantaneously controlled. Seventeen of the 21 anastomoses were end-to-end. The only death in these was in a 13-year-old boy who died of cerebral thrombosis. The left subclavian artery was swung down by the technique of Blalock and Park in four patients early in the series, with one death, in a child who had proved at autopsy also to have "Mitral stenosis, thickening of the tricuspid valve, pulmonary arterio- and arteriolar scleroses, and pulmonary edema." One of the three surviving patients with the Blalock-Park procedure had a partial paraplegia, probably "due to an occlusion of the anterior spinal artery". They observed that when headache had been prominent preoperatively, it was conspicuously absent postoperatively, and "the systolic blood pressures in arm and leg require some five to ten days to stabilize", as Gross had already indicated. They studied the preoperative and postoperative hemodynamics in 22 patients. Cardiac output appeared to be within normal limits before and after operation. Preoperatively the blood flow through the left forearm was substantially elevated and postoperatively declined toward normal. Arterial pressure in the lower extremities and the blood flow rose postoperatively. The preoperative hypertension in the upper part of the body and hypotension of the legs was corrected by operation. Given the normal cardiac output, hypertension had to be due to an increase in vascular resistance and it had been suggested that either the resistance was in the aortic stricture and collateral vessels or else was generalized, "Such a disturbance exists in renal and in essential hypertension." He interpreted their studies of peripheral vascular resistance as "evidence for the absence of a renal mechanism in the pathogenesis of hypertension in coarctation. . ." The final statement was "It is probable, therefore, that the hypertension in coarctation of the aorta is not attributable to a renal pressor mechanism, but is due to the resistance of the stenosis and collaterals." [The subsequent work of H. W. Scott and H. T. Bahnson from Blalock's department did much to contradict this thesis and to establish the renal nature of the hypertension in coarctation of the aorta.]

Discussion

Clarence Crafoord, of Stockholm initiated the Discussion. He had now operated upon 32 patients with 31 resections and anastomoses and one Blalock, subclavian to distal aortic, anastomosis. There had been two deaths, one from bleeding on the day of operation, the other from a dissecting aneurysm which ruptured into the bronchial tree. In five additional patients, an anastomosis had proved to be impossible, patients between 25 and 35 with "arteriosclerotic changes of the walls of the arteries". Blalock had mentioned angiography. Crafoord "introduced an ordinary cardiac catheter through the radial artery, pushing it forward down into the aortic arch. With a rapid injection of 50 to 70 cc. diodrast we can get an excellent X-ray picture of the first part of the aorta and the coarctation . . . we may be able to exclude most of the unsuitable cases from exploratory thoracotomy . . ." Twenty-seven of Crafoord's patients had been followed three months to three-and-a-half years and in 13 of these, the blood pressure had returned to normal with higher pressures in the legs than in the arms. In six, the blood pressure was equal in the legs and in the arms, and in eight, it was still slightly higher in the arms than in the legs. He thought in those eight that the anastomosis had not been sufficiently wide. Three of the 30 survivors had developed small dissecting aneurysms. One of these was growing and "we are discussing the possibility of reoperation". He did not use the everting suture which Blalock and Gross did, because he tried to resect as much of the constricted areas as possible and avoiding eversion spared two to three millimeters of length. He apparently thought that his end-to-end suture would be less likely to produce aneurysms than the everting suture. Norman E. Freeman, of San Francisco, discussed the technique of Fariñas, of Havana, Cuba, "for catheterization of the abdominal aorta through the femoral artery", which he gradually modified to a simple forceful retrograde injection into the femoral artery outlining the abdominal aorta. The technique which Freeman had adopted for demonstrating coarctation involved exposure of the left common carotid artery, inserting a needle into the carotid toward the aorta and injecting 70% diodrast. This had given very good visualization. John C. Jones, of Los Angeles, had operated upon 13 patients for coarctation of the aorta and completed an anastomosis in all, end-of-the-subclavian to side-of-the-distal aorta in two, end-of-the-subclavian to end-of-distal aorta in two, direct aortic anastomosis in the remainder. There were two deaths, one from dissection and exsanguination on the ninth day in a 31-year-old male, and one four hours after operation in a 17-year-old male who appeared to have had an unremarkable operation. The end-to-end aortic and subclavian-aortic anastomoses gave excellent results. The blood pressure results were not quite as good in the end-of-the-subclavian to side-of-the-aorta patients. They had operated upon three children, five years or younger and the easiest operation and the smoothest course was in a two-and-a-half-year-old

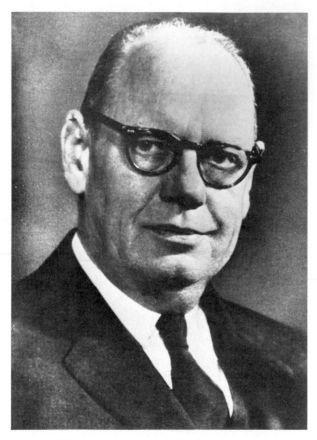

Arthur H. Blakemore, 1897-1970. M.D. Johns Hopkins, 1922. House officer training, Johns Hopkins, Henry Ford and Roosevelt Hospitals. His entire surgical career was at Columbia Presbyterian Medical Center. At the time of retirement he was Associate Professor of Clinical Surgery. For aneurysms of the aorta, refined the wiring technic, tried and abandoned polyethylene wrapping, and when in his laboratory Voorhees made the observations which led to the use of synthetic vascular prostheses, he was the first, in 1953, to implant such a prosthesis in the human aorta. With J. W. Lord, he developed the Vitallium tube non-suture vascular anastomotic technic. First using that technic, then the suture technic, he pioneered the application of porto-systemic anastomoses to the problem of portal hypertension and introduced balloon tamponade of esophageal varices. He was ruggedly honest and unassuming, to the point of emphasizing his failures and bad results.

Portrait courtesy of the College of Physicians and Surgeons of Columbia University, New York, N.Y.

child. "Since the collateral circulation is well developed early in life in these individuals, the indications are to operate upon them early." H. B. Shumacker, Jr., of New Haven, had studied arterial anastomoses by the Crafoord and Blalock techniques. "Histologi-

cally, one gained the impression that the direct anatomic repair [Crafoord] resulted in nicer repair, but functionally there was no doubt that the everting mattress technic was superior", showing fewer strictures, dehiscences, small ancurysms, etc. There was no difference in the incidence of thrombosis in the two methods.

* * *

Arthur H. Blakemore, of New York, Assistant Professor of Clinical Surgery, College of Physicans and Surgeons, Columbia University, *The Portacaval Shunt in the Surgical Treatment of Portal Hypertension,* was now presenting 58 patients in whom portacaval shunts had been established, 48 of them by Dr. Whipple or by Blakemore beginning in 1943. There had been 11 deaths in the entire series, three of "Cholemia", two of cerebral damage, one of cardiac failure, three of mesenteric thrombosis, one of shock from intra-abdominal hemorrhage, and one from gastrointestinal hemorrhage. One of the liver failure patients had active viral hepatitis and should not have been operated upon, they thought, and another was a severe cirrhotic who had not been sufficiently nursed before operation. Blakemore presented, in the frankest way, each of the deaths and analyzed the factors. Of 35 patients who had had severe bleeding before their operations, 11 had had one or more subsequent attacks of hemorrhage. Five of them had had previous splenectomies, and four of them were patients with extrahepatic portal block in whom the shunts performed were, in three cases, between the inferior mesenteric vein and the vena cava, in two cases the superior mesenteric vein to the vena cava and in one the inferior mesenteric vein to the vena cava. They had swung over very largely to the suture method, abandoning the Vitallium tube anastomoses. They had employed the direct portacaval anastomosis in nine of the 58 patients and for this recommended a thoracoabdominal approach. Recently Blakemore, seeing through this approach how closely the vena cava and the portal vein lay to each other, had performed a side-to-side anastomosis. He thought the side-to-side anastomosis would permit portal blood flow through the liver if the pressure relations were appropriate and that there would be less likelihood of thombosis of the hepatic end of the portal vein up into the liver. "Fear of this more than any other single factor deterred us from using the end to side portal vein to vena cava type of portacaval shunt more frequently. This fear was not unfounded, because the one postoperative death in the eight cases in which end to side anastomosis was

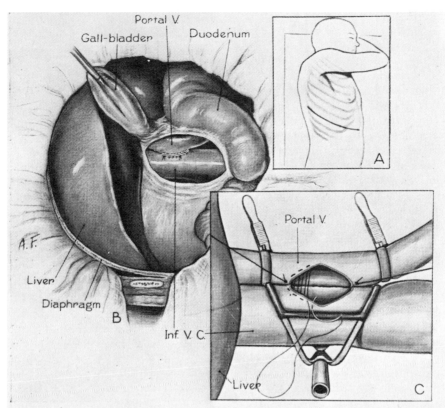

Fig. 1 (A.)—Shows the position of the patient on the operating table with the right side up. Note the incision over the ninth rib starts slightly beyond the posterior axillary line and continues obliquely downward and forward to cross the right rectus muscle to the midline of the abdomen. (B.) Illustrates a distinctly lateral approach to the hepato-duodenal ligament. The completed side-to-side anastomosis of the portal vein to the venacava is finally covered by suturing the cut edges of the peritoneum with a few interrupted sutures of fine black silk. (C.) Shows rubber covered clamps in place with the portal vein and venacava being anastomosed. The posterior half of the anastomosis has been completed employing a running everting mattress suture of #00000 braided silk. The posterior running suture is interrupted by tying to three stay sutures, two of which are illustrated. Note, that the transverse incision across the portal vein should extend two or three millimeters beyond the middle. This affords an anastomosis, which when completed, is slightly larger than the cross section area of the portal vein.

"After employing the thoracoabdominal approach for the end to side anastomosis of the portal vein with the vena cava and observing that the two vessels, after mobilization, touched one another, I have recently done one case anastomosing the portal vein side-to-side with the vena cava. The designing of clamps that now permit one to do side-to-side suture anastomoses of the portal vein to the vena cava on humans without the necessity of closing off entirely the flow of blood through the vena cava, at long last makes the true Eck fistula procedure clinically practical." In the same report, he also described anastomosis of the superior or inferior mesenteric veins to the vena cava.

Arthur H. Blakemore, *The Portacaval Shunt in the Surgical Treatment of Portal Hypertension.* Volume LXVI, 1948.

done did have thrombus extension from the ligated portal vein."

The brief Discussion was peripheral.

* * *

Once more, Gordon Murray, Surgeon, Toronto General Hospital; Demonstrator of Surgery, University of Toronto, startled the Association with an imaginative proposal, this time, with clinical application, *Closure of Defects in Cardia Septa.* Murray said he was concerned with moderately large but not excessive septal defects before the heart had enlarged enormously and before maturity. He was speaking entirely of isolated septal defects. He made the observation [precocious for the time] that "In the few cases I have operated on, I was impressed with the high pressure in the pulmonary artery . . . about equal to that of the pressure in the aorta. Whether that high pressure is the result of the septal defect or whether it is accounted for by some congenital anomaly in the pulmonary vascular tree, I do not know. Neither do I know whether this high pressure is reversible if the hiatus in the septum is closed . . . I have a suspicion that there is some abnormal physiology in the pulmonary vascular tree which may not be remedied by closure of the septal defect alone." In animal experimentation, "With practice, we were able to locate the position of the septum, from the surface markings on the anterior and posterior surfaces of the heart. Using this information we were able to pass needles and probes through the heart anteroposteriorly in the plane of the septum, and place ligatures, crossing artificially formed defects, in the interventricular and interauricular septa." His objective "was to pass a suture, of considerable size on cross section, through the heart from front to back so that it would pass across the defect in the septum. It was hoped that by slight compression of the heart from before backwards, by this suture, the hiatus could be diminished somewhat in size . . . that the substance of the fairly massive living suture would in itself obstruct the hiatus to a degree . . . then perhaps two or more could be passed in such a way as to interweave them and give fairly complete occlusion of the hiatus. This, accompanied by some local thrombosis, and healing of this area might, with good luck, cause sufficient obstruction of the hiatus to improve the function of the heart and relieve the patient of symptoms." In dogs, with artificially created interatrial septal defects, they had been able to pull the sutures taut, completely obliterating the defects. He reported three patients with ventricular septal defects attacked in this way. The first was a 17-month-old infant with a huge heart, cyanosis, and clubbing who withstood the operation. This child died with what was thought to be atelectasis, no fatal defect being found in the heart or at the site of operation. The other two were patients of 11 and 13 years of age who did very well after operation with relief of symptoms, decrease in size of the heart, etc. One child with an atrial septal defect had a very good result. Two children were explored, but found to have transposition and not operated upon.

Discussion

Once more, Alfred Blalock, of Baltimore, arose to express his admiration for Murray. "You all remember the amazing paper on coronary occlusion presented by Dr. Gordon Murray at the last meeting of this Association, and now he comes forward with an even more amazing presentation. Certainly it never would have occurred to me to place sutures blindly in this manner." He asked the nature of the sutures and whether embolism had occurred. He assumed that a good part of the occlusion was from thrombosis occurring about the suture material. Experimentally, of course, Murray had employed a number of techniques for creating an interatrial septal defect and Blalock arose to mention a method "devised by Dr. [C. R.] Hanlon and myself and the advantage of it is that is can be done under direct vision and without excessive blood loss . . . the right auricle, together with the pulmonary vein immediately posterior to the auricle, is occluded by an especially devised clamp. An opening is made in the pulmonary vein and a similar opening in the right auricle. The posterior segment of the auricle is adherent to the anterior wall of the pulmonary vein, so one can simply excise this segment of the two walls; in fact, one can pull an additional quantity of this septum out and excise it. The closure consists simply of suturing the anterior part of the auricle to the anterior segment of the pulmonary vein." They had created an atrial septal defect in a child with transposition just ten days earlier and "The post operative result is good thus far, although it is too early to know the eventual outcome." Murray, closing, replied to questions from Arthur Blakemore about the needles, which he said were skin needles, the point removed, and passed in reverse. For interventricular septa, they used fascia lata of the thigh. For the interauricular septal defect, they used linen, cotton, or silk. They gave heparin on the second or third day to prevent embolism. Local thrombosis had caused no problem and they had had no peripheral embolism.

* * *

Claude S. Beck, of Cleveland, Professor of Neurosurgery, Western Reserve University School of Medicine, *Revascularization of the Heart,* between 1932 and 1942, demonstrated revascularization of the heart by extracoronary anastomoses and by coronary-coronary anastomoses, produced by creating inflammation on the surface of the heart. "These methods were effective to the extent of reducing by

50 per cent the mortality that occurred after ligation of the descending ramus of the left coronary artery at its origin. Thirty-seven patients with severe coronary artery disease were operated upon using these methods and the clinical results confirmed the experimental studies." For the past three years, he had been working on attempts "to revascularize the heart by converting the coronary sinus into an artery" [by a remarkable feat of timing, the report appeared in the *JAMA* for May 29, 1948, the very day Beck's paper was presented]. In dogs, after ligations of the carotid sinus, he performed left carotid artery to coronary sinus anastomoses, and aortic-coronary sinus anastomoses with free graft of vein or artery, "It appears that a vein is preferable to artery and we are using vein grafts at the present time." Whereas, in control dogs, seven out of ten animals died within 24 hours of ligation of the descending ramus of the left coronary artery, in ten dogs with patent carotid coronary sinus anastomoses, descending ramus ligation resulted in no early deaths and only two late deaths,- eight and 13 days. The control dogs had large infarcts, the experimental animals had little or no infarction. He thought the reversed arterial circulation of veins was effective, but asked, "Does this arterial blood in the venous system have the same functional possibilities in reference to oxygen-exchange as does blood in the arterial system? Does any of the arterial blood from the venous side bypass the capillary bed and escape into the chambers of the heart without giving up its oxygen? We have no studies on this subject." They had attempted operation in one 45-year-old man with disabling angina pectoris. A segment of the left brachial artery was used for the aorta-to-sinus graft. The anastomosis was completed, the sinus having been ligated on the side toward the ostium. The patient awoke, but died of circulatory failure in 24 hours with what autopsy showed to be a recent infarct. The anastomosis was patent. The patient had had a period of hypotension during operation and it was assumed that that was the cause of the infarct.

Discussion

B. N. Carter, of Cincinnati, commented on the wide variety of Beck's contributions to experimental cardiac surgery. Carter had been experimenting with the production of anastomoses between the lung and the heart and had found such anastomoses could be produced. He asked Beck how to regulate the flow into the sinus so that it was neither too much nor too little, how venous drainage from the sinus was "affected if the venous bed is filled with arterial

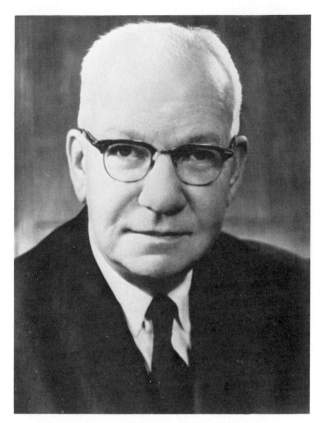

Claude S. Beck (c. 1965) 1894-1971. M.D. Johns Hopkins, 1921, Fellow in Surgery at Harvard, went to Western Reserve with Elliott Cutler, became Professor of Neurosurgery 1940-52, and Professor of Cardiovascular Surgery 1952-65, the first such in the U.S. Associated with Cutler in the development and application of their closed, punch valvotomy, he devoted his life to the problems of cardiac arrest and fibrillation, and the restoration of the coronary circulation. The operations for coronary artery inadequacy,- constriction of the coronary sinus and aorto-coronary venous anastomosis and various attempts at stimulating ingrowth of new circulation through the epicardium,- represented a lifetime of laboratory and clinical effort to solve a problem before the tools were available. His insistence on the feasibility of reversing circulation in the veins led to his undertaking carotid jugular anastomoses for epilepsy and for mental deficiency which resulted in the academic imbroglio which plagued him. Yet he demonstrated the clinical feasibility of defibrillation of the human heart, argued everywhere for the installation of defibrillators in emergency rooms and elsewhere, and his evangelistic efforts convinced physicians and laymen that a "fatal" cardiac attack need not be fatal, and laid the ground for the wide acceptance and effectiveness of cardiopulmonary resuscitation when the closed chest method of cardiac resuscitation was developed.

Portrait courtesy of William D. Holden, M.D., Cleveland, Ohio.

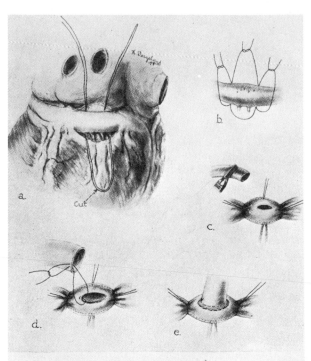

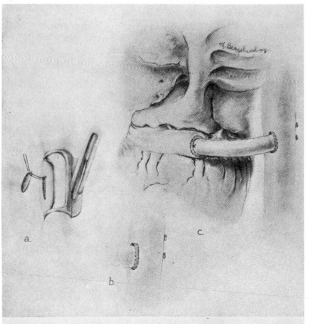

FIG. 3.—Free graft of vein between aorta and coronary sinus of the dog. The aorta is dissected free for a distance of about 3 cm. Two intercostal arteries are cut. The special clamp is placed on aorta as in (a.) allowing some blood to pass the clamp. The aorta is opened by incision about 5 mm. in length. An everting mattress suture is placed between garft and aorta at each end of this incision. Anastomosis is completed by a continuous everting suture as in (b.) (c.) shows the complete operation.

FIG. 2.—Anastomosis of left common carotid artery to coronary sinus in the dog. (a) and (b) show method for isolation of segment of sinus so that it can be opened without hemorrhage. The sinus is partially dissected free. A carrier with two silk sutures is passed beneath the sinus at two points as indicated. One piece of silk is cut. A proximal and a distal ligature and a mattress suture are thereby provided. These are tied as in c and the sinus is opened. Four cardinal everting mattress sutures are placed between sinus and artery as shown in (d). The anastomosis is completed by a continuous everting suture as in (e). Trauma to sinus is minimal to prevent thrombosis. (J. A. M. A.).

Beck, in the laboratory, had demonstrated the protective effect against coronary occlusion, of artificially created inflammation of the cardiac surface, and had employed the procedure clinically. Moving on to direct vascular procedures, he ligated the coronary sinus and implanted autogenous vein or artery grafts between the aorta and the coronary vein. In dogs, this protected against death from ligation of the descending ramus of the left coronary. In a single patient death supervened from a fresh myocardial infarct.

Claude S. Beck, *Revascularization of the Heart,* Volume LXVI, 1948.

blood?", what would be the result of such an A-V fistula close to the heart, and how would patients with myocardial damage tolerate the operation? Alfred Blalock, of Baltimore, commented that "since Dr. Beck pioneered in this field", a number of laboratories were pursuing the work and that Blalock and [Vivien] Thomas had anastomosed the carotid to the coronary sinus in 53 experiments, sometimes end-to-end, sometimes end-to-side. He thought that "most of the animals die unless thrombosis occurs. In other words, as Dr. Carter has intimated, it may be that the carotid transports too much blood." He tended to be pessimistic, "one must conclude that even if this type of shunt or bypass operation is proved to be sound from a physiologic viewpoint, one should hesitate to use it clinically because of the technical difficulties and the associated high mortal-

ity." Samuel A. Thompson, of New York, said that stimulated by Beck's earlier work, he had been injecting talcum powder into the pericardium to produce pericardial adhesions, and new circulation. Results were good to excellent in 70% of 30 patients. Claude S. Beck, closing, replied to Carter's question that "it does seem possible to deliver too much blood to the heart and the vein graft had to be "constricted so that its inside diameter is about 3.5 cm." [sic! mm.] As for the escape of venous blood from the perfused sinus, "It seeps through the various channels in the heart and escapes into the four chambers of the heart." In dogs, it was possible to ligate the sinus several days before the anastomosis was performed. He did not think that the arteriovenous fistula aspect of the problem would cause physiologic difficulties. As for whether the patients could tolerate the operation, Beck said, "I can only say that a patient with coronary artery disease is not a good risk for any operation. Some of our patients have died without operation. Once we get arterial blood into the sinus I think there will be improvement of the heart and that this improvement will, indeed be significant." As for thrombosis of the anastomosis, that was a matter of operative technique, "We know when we make a satisfactory anastomosis and when we make an unsatisfactory anastomosis. The incidence of thrombosis is directly proportional to the amount of operative trauma. I think a solution of this problem is possible."

The Business Meetings

The 1948 meeting, May 27, 28, and 29, was held at the Chateau Frontenac, Quebec, Canada. Elliott Cutler was known to have been suffering from carcinoma of the prostate and widespread metastasis at the previous meeting when he had been elected President, with the words ". . .we have nominated a man who has been a brilliant investigator, an inspiring teacher and a skillful surgeon, who had had a brilliant military record in both wars, and who at present is showing great courage and energy in his most difficult battle of all . . . Dr. Elliott Cutler." He had died in the interim and the First Vice-President, Dr. W. Edward Gallie, of Toronto, had succeeded to the Presidency.

Since the 1946 meeting, papers had been limited to ten minutes and were still so limited, 35 of the 53 papers submitted having been accepted.

The Committee studying the nursing problem made another report indicating that the problem was as great as ever and as far from being solved.

The Amendment to the Constitution raising the membership to 250 was moved and carried at the Second Business Meeting. Dr. Graham had been pressing for several years for distribution to the

membership of details concerning all the new members, but finally withdrew his motion, "I have discussed this motion with Dr. Firor, and in view of the exceedingly fine work being done by the Membership Committee, it has been decided that this will prove to be unnecessary."

The American Society of Anesthesiologists had gone on record as disapproving ". . .the training of persons other than doctors of medicine in the science and art of anesthesia. . .", an attack upon nurse anesthetists who had given devoted and skilled service in the hospitals of many of the Officers and Fellows of the Association. Council now recommended "A statement of adverse comment relative to a Resolution adopted by the Board of Directors of the American Society of Anesthesiologists, Inc., relating to the training of personnel for the administration of anesthesia", with instructions that this be sent to that Society, to the A.M.A., and to the American College of Surgeons," and such other organizations as may be determined by the Secretary."

The nursing problem was discussed once more. Dr. Lahey urged that any report be couched in tactful terms ". . .to eliminate any part of it that might be irritating to the nurses. . ." Dr. McKittrick said that it was an enormously complicated problem, the training schedules had to be revamped, hospitals which had been using student nurses for patient loads would have heavy financial obligations, state laws would have to be changed, etc. There had been great activity in the A.M.A. and in the American College of Surgeons. The A.M.A. was handling the job beautifully, and "The A.M.A. has got to be the body that carries the responsibility for American medicine." He urged the Association not to inject itself into the fray.

The officers elected for the following year were Fred W. Rankin, of Lexington, Kentucky, President; Vice-Presidents, Wilder Penfield, of Montreal, and Emile Holman, of San Francisco; and Secretary, Nathan A. Womack, of Iowa City.

LXVII

1949

The 1949 meeting took place in St. Louis at the Jefferson Hotel, April 20, 21, and 22, President Fred W. Rankin, of Lexington, Kentucky, Clinical Professor of Surgery, Louisville School of Medicine, in the Chair. Among those who had died in the previous year were Stuart McGuire, of Richmond, whose father, Hunter McGuire, had been President in 1887, and George Tully Vaughan, who had been a Fellow since 1902.

* * *

H. Glenn Bell, Professor of Surgery and Chairman, Department of Surgery, University of California, San Francisco, *Cancer of the Breast,* reviewed their experience with 819 cases. In their overall group, 264 patients were living and well after five years, a survival rate of 32.2%, excluding operative deaths and deaths of intercurrent disease. In 470 operations there was a mortality of 0.85%. In 101 patients without axillary involvement, radical mastectomy alone yielded a 70% five-year survival; the addition of preoperative X-ray therapy in 22, a 54% five-year survival; and both preoperative and postoperative X-ray in 22, a 68% survival. If there were positive nodes in the axilla, the survivals were 40%, 42% and 24%, respectively. He posed the problem,- "One of the puzzles of the problem of cancer of the breast is why we fail to obtain a 100 per cent cure in patients with a localized lesion without evidence either clinically or pathologically of axillary spread. It must mean that there is already extension of cancer cells that we are unable to detect at the time of surgery, or that some cells are spread during the surgical procedure. It is also curious that some of these patients have a recurrence after many years of apparent cure. We wonder where the malignant cells have been all the time and why they wait 10, 20, or even 30 years before becoming evident . . . Is there such a thing as cancer immunity that in some patients holds the growth in check and then for some reason is lost, allowing the cells to grow? " He discussed McWhirter's simple mastectomy followed by roentgen therapy and commented that "One would like to know how many of his cases were really stage I, since with simple mastectomy there is no microscopic examination of lymph nodes, and we know from experience that our judgment of the presence or absence of cancer in the axilla on clinical examination alone is wrong 30 per cent of the time. McWhirter's views are so contrary to the teaching in this country that one would hesitate to adopt this course without further proof that it is the procedure of choice." He concluded by stating "From our study so far, roentgen ray therapy as an adjunct to the surgical treatment of carcinoma of the breast has not significantly increased the five year survival rate. The study will be continued."

Discussion

Grantley W. Taylor, of Boston, said that Bell's results were in agreement with those of most others.

930

They had been unable at the Massachusetts General Hospital to ascertain that postoperative and preoperative radiation conferred any advantage. [William Crawford White had preceded him in the Discussion urging wide skin excision to prevent local recurrence], and Taylor said they had not been able to see that that had any advantage. He emphasized the complications of postoperative irradiation, particularly the swollen arm. Owen H. Wangensteen, of Minneapolis, said he was not "an experienced breast surgeon, but I have been interested in the aggressive therapy of cancer . . . I believe that our only hope is for the surgeon to be more aggressive . . . I submit that one of the weaknesses of the present so-called Halsted operation is our inability to get cancer out of the brachial plexus. I believe that by dividing the clavicle and putting it together again, and removing the first rib, in Stage II cases one can dissect the components of the brachial plexus just as well as one can the axillary vein . . . Careful stripping of the adventitia of the axillary vein and artery as well as the brachial plexus over long lengths, I believe should come to be standard practice in the conventional radical breast operation." [See Halsted's discussion of the supraclavicular operation, Volume XXV, 1907, Page 367, and Volume XVI, 1898, Page 214.] He had done five such operations, repairing the clavicle with a Kirschner wire. He mentioned also Sampson Handley's removal of the intercostal lymph nodes. In apparent answer to one of Bell's questions, he said "There is an advantage in removing the *entire* lymphatic drainage area for a cancer because failure to demonstrate lymph node involvement is not synonymous with absence of small microscopic deposits. Our failure to cure 100 per cent of Stage I breast cancers is owing in part to the circumstances that there are now and then microscopic lymph node deposits beyond the site of lymph node removal, and in part to the occurrence of direct venous invasion." Robert M. Janes, of Toronto, said that they had felt ". . . increasingly convinced that preoperative radiotherapy plays an important part", but confined himself to the mention of individual patients.

* * *

William S. McCune, of Washington, D.C., by invitation, *Malignant Melanoma,* Forty Cases Treated By Radical Resection, examined the question of resection of the regional lymph nodes. In 25 cases with palpable lymph node enlargement and radical dissections, lymph nodes with metastases were found in 23 of the patients and only two of the 23 were alive and well. In 12 patients, who had pro-

phylactic node dissections in the absence of palpable involvement, seven patients were found to have microscopic involvement and all seven were alive and well one to six years after operation. He considered that this ". . . demonstrated conclusively the importance of early radical resection of regional lymph nodes, whether or not they are enlarged, whenever a diagnosis of malignant melanoma is made."

Discussion

Robert H. Kennedy, of New York, agreed with the concept of prophylactic lymph node dissection, "although all too commonly what one thinks is a prophylactic dissection is proved by the pathologist

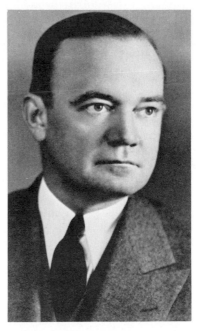

Fred W. Rankin, (c. 1949), 1886-1954, President 1949, also of the American College of Surgeons 1953-1954, and the American Medical Association 1942-1943. M.D. University of Maryland 1909, trained at the Mayo Clinic, went to Louisville, Kentucky, as the first full-time Professor of Surgery, returned to the Mayo Clinic for a distinguished career, particularly in colon and rectal surgery and went back once more to Kentucky in private practice. During World War II, was Chief Consultant in Surgery to the Armies of the United States, with particular responsibility for assignment of surgical personnel. He represented the type of expert clinician, almost antagonistic to academia, with the kind of charm, vigor and intelligence which naturally leads to selection for high office.

(Portrait courtesy of Hiram C. Polk, Jr., (University of Louisville School of Medicine, Louisville, Kentucky.)

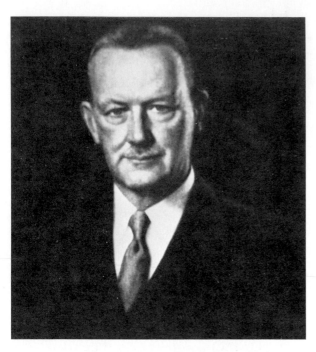

Willis J. Potts, (c. 1949) 1895-1968. M.D. Rush Medical College of the University of Chicago 1924; Intern Presbyterian Hospital, Surgeon-in-Chief, Children's Memorial Hospital and Professor of Surgery, Northwestern University 1946-1960. Some astute person, before Potts returned from World War II, engineered his appointment as Surgeon-in-Chief at Children's Hospital (he had been Clinical Associate Professor of Surgery at Rush and was unknown in pediatric surgery). In Baltimore, he observed Blalock's performance of the operation for tetralogy of Fallot, very shortly, in Chicago, with a specially devised partial occlusion clamp for the aorta, presented, with Sidney Smith, his aorto-pulmonary anastomosis. His instrument maker, Richter, produced the multitoothed vascular clamps which permitted gentle but secure compression of vessels. Potts' ingenious expanding knives and dilators for transventricular relief of valvular pulmonic stenosis, represented a great advance over Brock's knives and dilators of graduated sizes. Tall, lanky, sandy-haired, with a marvelous wit and an elegant use of language, able to jest at himself, he was a great contributor to all fields of pediatric surgery. His extraordinarily personal book, *The Surgeon and the Child,* is a classic of sympathetic writing and a precise record of one man's interest and performance in a broad range of pediatric surgical problems in 1959, and as such is a historical document as well as a literary classic.

(Portrait courtesy of Lowell R. King, Chicago.)

to show one node with a few melanotic cells, or even a number of small involved nodes which were not large enough for anyone to palpate." Grantley W.

Taylor, of Boston, had studied 176 cases from the State Cancer Hospital and the Massachusetts General Hospital. He thought "The principal problem is to be sure that the primary disease is controlled, and therefore we invariably defer our regional dissection, if we can, until at least . . . two or three weeks have elapsed . . . " and then could be sure that there had been an adequate local extirpation. Ralph F. Bowers, of Memphis, Tennessee, had become "convinced that one must not touch the local lesion except for the necessary biopsy, and must not manipulate or cut across lymphatic channels or its first main nodal barrier, and therefore we devised a more radical procedure in the treatment of melanoma, particularly in those cases below the umbilicus, which all of us know to be prompt killers." At the Kennedy Veterans Administration Hospital for melanoma, they had done two forequarter amputations, and four hindquarter amputations, two of the latter in patients without palpable lymph node enlargement, who were shown microscopically to have such involvement. He admitted the operation was both radical and mutilating, but a recent series of 34 cases of melanoma in three years, with disastrous results, had led to this approach. Mims Gage, of New Orleans, was in agreement with McCune. He emphasized the necessity for excision rather than cauterization of the local lesion, and the propensity for late distant hematogenous and lymphatic metastases.

* * *

Willis J. Potts, of Chicago, Associate Professor of Surgery, Northwestern University Medical School; Surgeon-in-Chief, Children's Memorial Hospital, a new Fellow, *Surgical Treatment of Congenital Pulmonary Stenosis,* was reporting on his experiences, since his publication three years before, with anastomosis between the pulmonary artery and the aorta as an alternative to Blalock's subclavian or innominate artery to pulmonary anastomosis. His anesthetist, William O. McQuiston, had been using controlled hypothermia induced by ice bags or cold water mattress to decrease the metabolic demands of the sickest and most cyanotic infants. This controlled hypothermia had been used on 71 patients with pulmonary stenosis, "No deleterious effects have been noticed. There has been no increase in postoperative respiratory complications. We believe . . . that the mortality and morbidity from severe anoxia has been lessened by the use of hypothermia." They had originally insisted on the aorta-pulmonary anastomosis whether the aorta descended on the right or left, but now found that the wisest course was to enter the chest always from the left to perform an aortic-pulmonary anastomosis, if there was a left aortic arch, and a subclavian pulmonary anastomosis if there was a right aortic arch. In in-

fants below one year of age, the subclavian artery on the left they thought, ". . . is apt to be too small for a satisfactory anastomosis and the approach is on

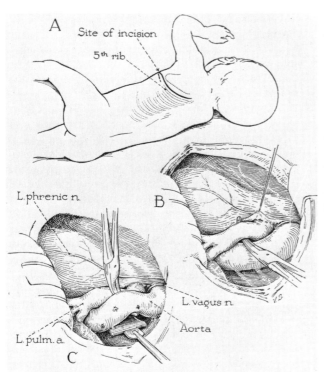

Fig. 1.—Technic of aortic-pulmonary anastomosis.
A. Lateral incision through the left fourth interspace.
B. The pulmonary artery is thoroughly freed from surrounding structures.
C. The aorta is elevated with a cystic duct forceps as the aortic clamp is slipped beneath it.

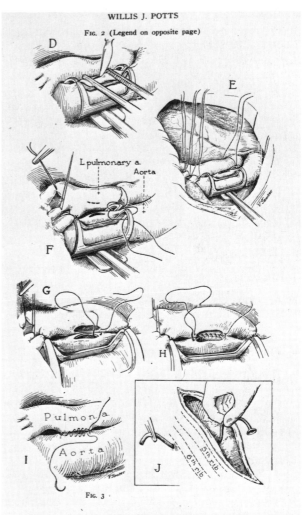

WILLIS J. POTTS

Fig. 2 (Legend on opposite page)

Fig. 2.—Technic of aortic-pulmonary anastomosis continued.
D. Incision in the aorta must be in exactly the right place (see text).
E. Ligatures of heavy oiled silk are placed around the left pulmonary artery and its branches.
F. The lower branch of the pulmonary artery is tied to the lower edges of the clamp first, then the main vessel is tied to the upper part of the clamp.

Fig. 3.—Technic of aortic-pulmonary anastomosis continued.
G. The first stitch is so placed that the knot is outside the lumen of the vessel.
H. The posterior row of stitches, as well as the two at the lower angle, coapt the edges of the vessels adventitia to adventitia.
I. The anterior row of sutures is left loose until all the stitches have been placed. The entire anastomosis is done with one continuous suture.
J. The chest is routinely drained with a de Pezzer catheter through the sixth interspace.

For tetralogy of Fallot, Potts freed up the aorta by dividing bronchial and intercostal arteries as needed. The Potts-Smith partial occlusion clamp was applied to the aorta and the double-throw ligatures around the pulmonary artery tied to the clamps, approximating the two vessels. He stressed precise size of the anastomosis and the danger of cardiac failure from an excessively large anastomosis. The incision for the anastomosis was to be exactly 4/16 of an inch long, measured with a caliper. He had a 9.7% mortality in 165 anastomosed patients and a series of 41 without a death in the five months before the meeting.

Willis J. Potts, *Surgical Treatment of Congenital Pulmonary Stenosis,* Volume LXVII, 1949.

the right side for an aortic-pulmonary anastomosis." He was reporting 165 patients with 16 operative deaths, mortality of 9.7%. In 16 additional patients who were explored, without anastomosis, there were seven deaths, 42.8%. The mortality was 20% in 59 children under three years of age undergoing an anastomosis and 3.8% in 106 children three to 16 years of age at the time of anastomosis. Almost all of the children had shown immediate enlargement of the heart, excessive in some of them, and two had gone into heart failure because, Potts thought, the anastomoses were too large. In the last 149 anastomoses, he thought only a single anastomosis had closed.

Discussion

H. William Scott, Jr., of Baltimore, agreed that "cardiac anoxia" accounted for the majority of deaths and that hypothermia might well be helpful. At Hopkins they still preferred anastomosis of the subclavian branch of the innominate artery to the side of the pulmonary and, when the pulmonary was very small, they preferred an end-to-end anastomosis rather than a side-to-side aortic-pulmonary anastomosis. Robert M. Janes, of Toronto, rose to present work which was being done in his department by Dr. W. G. Bigelow, on hypothermia, showing the relation of fall in temperature to fall in oxygen consumption. Potts, closing, commented upon the fallibility of statistics, and the fact that operative mortality ". . . depends upon a number of factors: choice of patients, age and coincidence, or more frankly, on runs of good or bad luck. During the terrible month of February 1948, our mortality was 50 per cent. During the past five months, there has been no mortality in a continuous series of 41 patients in the surgery of pulmonary stenosis." He thought from infancy to 16 years of age, operating on all comers, the overall mortality should be no more than 10%. In children from three to 16 it should be 5% or less.

* * *

Richard H. Sweet, of Boston, Visiting Surgeon, Massachusetts General Hospital; Associate Clinical Professor of Surgery, Harvard Medical School, and, by invitation, Edward F. Bland, *The Surgical Relief of Congestion in the Pulmonary Circulation in Cases of Severe Mitral Stenosis,* Preliminary Report of Six Cases Treated by Means of Anastomosis between the Pulmonary and Systemic Venous Systems, mentioned the early attempts of Cutler to relieve mitral stenosis and the recent [1948] work of Harken with valvulotomy with "somewhat better results." He alluded to the fact that Lutembacher [1916] had sug-

gested that patients with a tight mitral stenosis, who had interauricular septal defects, were protected against paroxysms of pulmonary edema and that Blalock had developed an experimental approach to the creation of interauricular septal defects. Sweet attacked the problem by way of decompressing the pulmonary circulation, creating an end-to-end anastomosis between the pulmonary end of the superior branch of the right inferior pulmonary vein and the cardiac end of the divided azygos vein. He now reported six such operations, the anastomoses performed with Blakemore-Lord tubes, in patients with severe long-standing mitral stenosis and repeated attacks of pulmonary edema. One patient died with tachycardia, pulmonary edema and high fever on the 11th day. [His figures show a striking pulmonary hypertension in this patient, 110/30, at rest, 145/65 mm. of mercury after exercise, although he makes no comment about the significance of this.] The others were all doing well. On the operating table, pressure in the left auricle was shown to drop significantly, 8.2%, 28.4%, and 19.5% in three cases.

Discussion

Alfred Blalock, of Baltimore, opened the Discussion. He mentioned the 1922 attempts at cutting the stenosed mitral valve by Graham and Allen in St. Louis, the work of Cutler and Beck with the valvulotome, and more recently the work of the late Horace Smithy [of Charleston, South Carolina]. Of the current work, he said, "Harken uses a valvulotome. He has operated on five patients, with two survivals. Bailey uses a curved knife inserted alongside the finger, and attempts to cut the valve at the commissure. He has operated on approximately a dozen patients, with four survivals." Blalock mentioned the Blalock-Hanlon procedure for creating an atrial septal defect, to which Sweet had made reference, saying, "We have not attempted to use this in patients with mitral stenosis thus far. We have used it on approximately a dozen patients with transposition of the aorta and the pulmonary artery, and in one patient with a tricuspid atresia." He felt that an interauricular defect was a little more likely to stay open than a venous anastomosis. Finally he mentioned by-passing procedures, that of "Jeger in Germany in 1913, in which he suggested that one attempt to by-pass the stenotic mitral valve by using a vein graft connecting either the auricle or the pulmonary vein with the left ventricle . . . More recently Rappaport has suggested the anastomosis of the left auricular appendage to the left ventricle. I am quite confident that this anastomosis will thrombose. I understand that Dr. Robert Gross is now using (at least experimentally) a graft of aorta connecting the auricle and the ventricle. From a theoretical point of view this method would seem to be the best of all. As to whether the technical features can be worked out, I don't know." Henry Swan, of Denver, Colorado, had been studying the effect of pulmonary venous anastomosis in the laboratory using the "Vitallium tube technic." Neither Sweet nor Blalock had made the point which Swan now brought up, "As Dr. Sweet pointed out, the purpose underlying the operation is a reduction in the pressure of the pulmonary system by making the shunt from the high pressure area, that is, the pulmonary veins, to a low pressure area—the vena cava. One hopes thereby to prevent or delay the right-sided heart failure. It must be admitted, however, that in so doing one substitutes a marked increase in the blood flow through the right side for the decrease in pressure . . . a certain amount of blood . . . must continuously pass through the right side of the heart. This can be accomplished only by diminution in the output on the left side of the heart. Whether in the long run it is better for the right ventricle to have an excessive output against a somewhat diminished pressure, in contrast to a smaller output against a high pressure, only time will be able to tell." Swan also raised the question of pulmonary hypertension, as to whether it would be relieved or conceivably worsened by the operation. Frederick E. Kredel, of Charleston, South Carolina, spoke for Dr. Horace Smithy [who had himself just died of aortic stenosis]. Smithy had used his valvulotome on seven patients who had mitral stenosis and had five survivors, two of them were now a year after operation ". . . the stenosis has been relieved clinically, and there has been no trouble from mitral insufficiency." Richard H. Sweet, in closing, said that having no experimental preparation for mitral stenosis, they had been unable to try the operation on animals. He appeared a little uncomfortable in responding to Swan's questions about pulmonary hypertension and ended by saying that this had been ". . .nothing but a preliminary presentation, and it is a procedure which may ultimately not be of any value; but I am absolutely certain, on the basis of clinical observation, that at least four of these patients are for the moment completely rehabilitated."

* * *

Daniel C. Elkin, of Atlanta, Whitehead Professor of Surgery, Emory University; Surgeon-in-Chief, Emory University Hospital, and by invitation, Frederick W. Cooper, Jr., *Surgical Treatment of Insidious*

Thrombosis of the Aorta, Report of Ten Cases, had found in William H. Welch's 1909 paper on the subject, a citation of a paper from Paris by Barth in 1848 describing "insidious obliteration of the aorta". Elkin and Cooper were aware of Leriche's 1923 and 1940 papers in French, and finally Leriche's 1948 paper, which appeared in the *Annals of Surgery*. They had seen at Emory, in 20 months, ten instances of the condition and commented on the pain in the hips and legs, easy fatigability, weakness in the thighs and legs on walking, and loss of sustained erection. The diagnosis was easily made by the absence of pulsations in the lower extremities, and the "trophic changes, such as thickening and roughening of the nails, and loss of hair . . ." They quoted Leriche as stating, ". . . that the ideal treatment would be to resect the obliterated zone and to bridge the vascular defect by a graft", and regretted that "Unfortunately, the thrombosis frequently is present in the iliac arteries as well as the aorta, and surgical technics for such a procedure have not been perfected." The available procedures were bilateral lumbar sympathectomy and resection of the bifurcation of the aorta and the thrombosed area, which "removes the thrombosis, and prevents the continuation of its formation, which otherwise would be fatal. It also removes the area of irritation which is the site for excitatory vasoconstrictor impulses which produce vasospasm in patent peripheral channels [obviously Leriche's theory]. Either or both of the above procedures are indicated in the treatment of this disease, and when both are utilized they may be performed simultaneously." Despite the fact that they found at sympathectomy in four of the patients that the aorta was completely thrombosed, they resected the aorta in none of these patients. In a single patient who presented with gangrene requiring amputation of one limb, they performed sympathectomy on the other side and performed "terminal aortectomy", resecting the bifurcation of the aorta. They said not a word about the technique. Their operated patients showed at most modest improvement.

Discussion

Emile Holman, of San Francisco, had had four patients with this syndrome, all substantially relieved by sympathectomies, so that "It is our opinion that resection of the calcified aorta, as advocated by Leriche and his co-workers, is too hazardous for the gain obtained, and that bilateral lumbar sympathectomy will provide as much improvement as can be expected." Mims Gage, of New Orleans, Louisi-

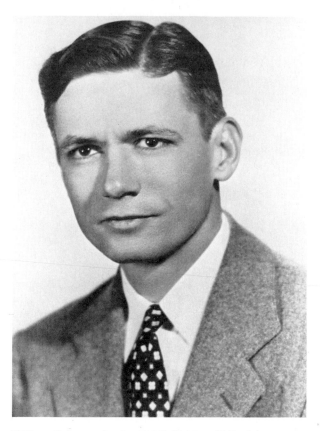

William P. Longmire (c. 1950) 1913—. M.D. Johns Hopkins 1938. President 1968, and of the American College of Surgeons 1964. Went through residency at Johns Hopkins, rose to Associate Professor and went to University of California at Los Angeles as the first Professor of Surgery in the new school in 1948. Apart from early contributions to coronary endarterectomy, and experimental and clinical work in transplantation, his contributions have been largely in gastrointestinal surgery,- usually in fields where his superb technical skill was most advantageously employed,- his operation of hepatojejunostomy for the destroyed common duct, evaluation of the role of total gastrectomy for gastric cancer, operative approaches to chronic pancreatitis, hepatic resection. At the new Medical School in California, he built an outstanding department of surgery, starting alone, in wooden World War II barracks buildings. His has been a major, measured voice in the national affairs of surgery.

ana, used the term, "Leriche's syndrome". He had operated upon one patient, planning to do an aortic division, but "The aorta was not ligated because of the extensive arteriosclerosis. A bilateral sympathectomy was done." Frederick L. Reichert, of San Francisco [who usually tended to disagree with what had been said], commented that "This claudication

business in the thigh might well be due to shutting off the lumbar segmental artery. In cutting out the coarctation of the aorta, the segmental arteries are divided. It might be well to preserve them . . . I think sympathetic denervation would be much more to the point."

* * *

W. P. Longmire, Jr., Chairman, Department of Surgery, University of California at Los Angeles; Chief of Surgical Service, Wadsworth Veterans Hospital, Sawtelle, California, a new member, and by invitation, M. C. Sanford, of Baltimore, *Intrahepatic Cholangiojejunostomy for Biliary Obstruction—Further Studies,* discussed the new operation to which Alfred Blalock had alluded the previous year in the discussion of bile duct strictures [and which had been developed at Hopkins before Longmire accepted the California chair]. In patients with benign obstructions of the extrahepatic biliary ducts not amenable to direct reconstruction, a portion of the left lobe of the liver was cut away exposing a large dilated branch of the left duct which was further exposed by curetting away the surrounding sclerotic liver substance. Mucosa-to-mucosa, Roux Y anastomosis was then performed between this duct and the jejunum. Of their four patients, three were alive and relieved of jaundice, the fourth had died of homologous serum hepatitis which occurred after her jaundice had cleared. It had proved relatively uncomplicated to find a satisfactory duct, bleeding from the liver had not been a problem, and the ducts had been large enough for anastomosis. They had attempted the operation for congenital biliary atresia without success.

Discussion

Richard B. Cattell, of Boston, commenting upon "Dr. Longmire's beautiful presentation of his ingenious operation of intrahepatic anastomosis of the left hepatic duct to the jejunum . . .", nevertheless suggested that if the left duct was draining the entire liver, there must have been a stump of common hepatic duct sufficient for an anastomosis, and if this were not true, then only the left lobe of the liver was being drained. However, he had had two patients, in whom one hepatic duct had been drained at the liver, who had done well and he would wait "until we have autopsy findings on these cases to show that we are actually draining both ducts by the operation which Dr. Longmire proposes." Warren Cole, of Chicago, said he had already used Longmire's operation successfully. Waltman Walters, of

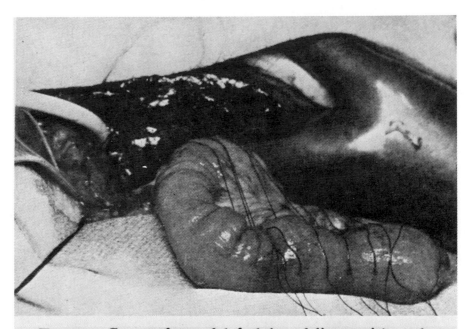

FIG. 1.—Cut surface of left lobe of liver with catheter in intrahepatic duct. Roux type jejunal segment mobilized for anastomosis. Note position of duct opening immediately beneath the level of the anterior abdominal wall.

Longmire transected the left lobe of the liver in patients with irremediable common duct strictures, curetted away the liver substance around the dilated duct exposed in the cut liver surface, brought up a Roux-Y loop of jejunum, performed a mucosa-to-mucosa duct-to-jejunum anastomosis over a rubber tube left in place and sutured the jejunum to the liver. He had performed the operation, with relief of jaundice in four patients. In infants with bilary atresia, no suitable dilated ducts could be found in the cut surface of the liver.

W. P. Longmire and M. C. Sanford, *Intrahepatic Cholangiojejunostomy for Biliary Obstruction—Further Studies*, Volume LXVII, 1949.

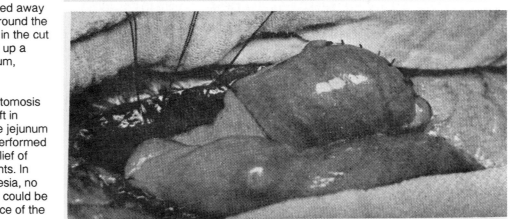

FIG. 2.—Anastomosis completed. Antimesenteric border of jejunum being sutured to superior surface of liver. End of catheter, which passes through the anastomosis, can be seen protruding into wall of jejunum.

Rochester, enthusiastic about Longmire's operation, showed a cholangiogram which demonstrated communication between the right and left ducts, and was "of the opinion that permanent results of duct-to-duct anastomosis are not going to be as good as those following anastomosis of the duct to intestine because of the danger of contracture on anastomosis of the ends of the ducts. Results were excellent in 82

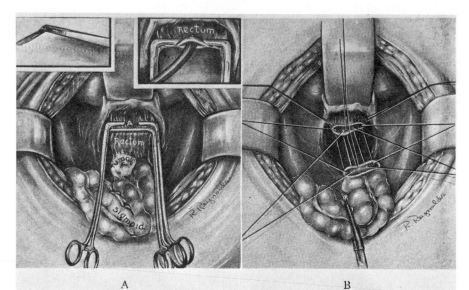

FIG. 4.—Anterior dissection, resection and anastomosis. (A.) Special clamps** applied below the tumor mass permit transection at least one inch below the tumor margin. Catheter suction introduced into lower segment between clamps removes contents. (B.) Short nosed lower clamps removed and replaced by guy sutures to steady lower segment. Five long posterior catgut guide sutures inserted to direct correct apposition of posterior walls; knots will be on mucosal side.
** By V. Mueller Company, Chicago, Illinois.

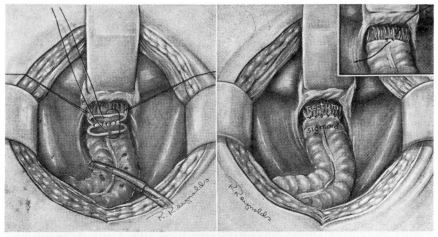

FIG. 5.—Anterior dissection, resection and anastomosis. (A.) The five posterior guide and inversion sutures have been tied. One similar inversion catgut suture is placed on the anterior wall, knot on mucosal side. (B.) The anastomosis is completed with a layer of figure of eight silk sutures on anterior and lateral walls and insofar as possible on the posterior wall. A penrose drain is placed in the hollow of the sacrum, peritoneum of pelvic floor is sutured over the drain and around the rectum. A Gibson type cecostomy is accomplished and after closure of abdomen, the patient is turned on the left side and the drain delivered posteriorly through a small incision alongside the coccyx.

Best made a reasoned plea, based on the adequacy of a 3.5 cm. distal margin, for three different restorative operations. I. Anterior dissection, resection, and anastomosis (Fig. 4 and 5) for lesions above 10 cm. II. Anterior dissection, posterior resection and anastomosis for lesions below 10 cm. III. Entirely posterior operations for low lesions in feeble patients. He reserved abdominoperineal resections for extensive tumors, and tumors below 5 cm. He had no survival figures as yet. His presentation was roughly handled by Vernon David and Tom Jones.

R. Russell Best and James B. Blair, *Sphincter Preserving Operations for Rectal Carcinoma as Related to the Anatomy of the Lymphatics*, Volume LXVII, 1949. (Figure continues on facing page.)

per cent of my first series of cases in which the duct was anastomosed to the duodenum, in contrast to 55 per cent in which the ends of the duct were joined."

* * *

R. Russell Best, of Omaha, Professor of Surgery, University of Nebraska, School of Medicine, and by invitation, James B. Blair, *Sphincter Preserving Operations for Rectal Carcinoma as Related to*

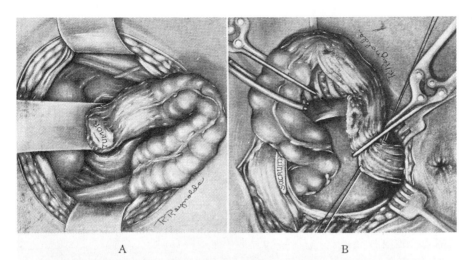

A   B

Fig. 6.—Anterior dissection with posterior resection and anastomosis. (A.) Through an abdominal incision, pelvic structures have been dissected and freed. The tumor mass which has been freed is replaced in the hollow of the sacrum and the pelvic floor peritoneum sutured around the rectum loosely enough to permit drawing the sigmoid downward through the posterior incision. A Gibson type cecostomy is accomplished and the abdomen closed. (B.) With the patient on his left side, an incision has been made along the coccyx and sacrum, coccyx is removed, wide dissection of levator ani structures is accomplished, and the rectum and sigmoid delivered and resected.

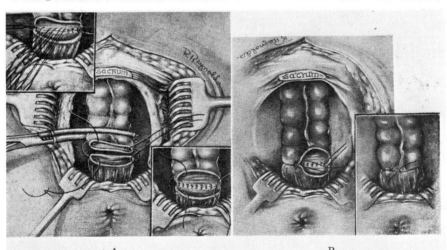

A   B

Fig. 7.—Anterior dissection with posterior resection and anastomosis. (A.) Traction sutures of catgut are placed at both angles of the anastomosis in such a manner that knots will be on the mucosal wall. A layer of interrupted catgut sutures is inserted on the anterior wall with knots on the mucosal side, inverting the margin of anastomosis. All of these sutures are inserted before any of them are tied. (B.) Several similar sutures, with knots on mucosal side, are inserted on the posterior wall. The anastomosis is completed by inserting a layer of figure of eight silk sutures on the posterior wall, lateral walls, and insofar as possible on the anterior wall. The incision is closed and a penrose drain is placed in the hollow of the sacrum and brought out at upper angle of incision.

the Anatomy of the Lymphatics, pointed out many confirming reports attesting to the infrequency of metastasis to lymph nodes below the level of the tumor. For the past decade, Best had been convinced that if a margin of three-and-a-half centimeters below the tumor could be given, every effort should be made to restore continuity. Three basic operations were, (1) A low anastomosis done entirely from the abdomen for lesions at or above 10 cm. (2) For lesions below 10 cm., an abdomino-sacral operation freeing the tumor from above and performing the lower part of the resection and the anastomosis transsacrally. He pointed out that this permitted a more radical local operation than was possible from an entirely intra-abdominal operation. (3) Finally in some poor risk patients, the entire operation might be done transsacrally. They had tried the modified pull-through methods of Hochenegg, Babcock and Bacon, and had been dissatisfied. In their series of 51 consecutive cases of rectal cancer, there had been an operability rate of 86% and a resectability rate of 74%. [No survival figures were given.] In those with resectable lesions a sphincter-preserving operation was accomplished in three-quarters and the abdominoperineal resection in one-quarter. The mortality for the anastomosed cases was 6.8%, for the abdominoperineal resections, zero. One advantage of the operation, he thought, was that the rectal examination permitted earlier diagnosis of recurrence in the pelvis. He had no information on the survival rates. He pointed to the fact that in Waugh's Mayo Clinic statistics, the five-year survival rate of 52.4% for the abdominoperineal resection, was poorer than Dixon's personal series from the Mayo Clinic of 67.7% in patients who had anastomoses. "This is most difficult for those surgeons who are strong advocates of the Miles procedure in all cases of rectal carcinoma to appreciate, or for the surgeon who believes the sphincter preserving operation is only indicated in selected cases, because the five year survival rate is better in the group where a sphincter preserving procedure was accomplished."

Discussion

As might be expected, Best's thesis was not very kindly received. Vernon C. David, of Chicago, pointed to the difficulties of wide resection for low-lying tumors, the involvement of the levators and of the vagina so that "In my judgment this adds up to the necessity of performing the most widespread removal of soft parts possible in low-lying carcinoma of the rectum. The technical ability to do an end-to-end anastomosis deep in the pelvis or preservation of the continuity of the bowel, no matter how desirable, should always be considered secondary to permanency of cure of the patient." Thomas E. Jones, of Cleveland, Ohio, referring to some of Best's studies of the lymphatics, rather sharply, said, "Dr. Best's experiments were on animals. Mine have been on humans. I have a report to make today on ten-year survival rates which might be of interest." He

had a complete follow-up on 92 abdominoperineal resections out of 102 done in 1938 and 1939. With fewer than five nodes involved, 60% were alive at five years and 50% at ten years. With more than five nodes involved, 22% were alive at five years, and 11% at ten years. Without venous involvement, the five-year survival was 60% and ten year 50%. With venous invasion, the five-year survival and ten-year survival were both 30%. His overall five-year survival was 52.5% and ten year 43.7%. He concluded that ". . . if these are the best results we can obtain with the more extensive operation, I do not see much use in fiddling around with smaller or so-called sphincter-saving procedures." Claude F. Dixon, of Rochester, Minnesota, limited his remarks to ". . . cancerous lesions which occur in the lower half of the rectum." Whereas in his paper of the previous year, alluded to by Best, he had emphasized anastomotic procedures for higher rectal and sigmoid lesions, he now emphasized a wide abdominoperineal resection for low rectal lesions. At the second portion of the operation, ten to 12 days after the first, ". . . a radical perineal operation is carried out, at which time portions of the gluteal muscles, the levator muscles and pelvic fascia are removed. The peritoneum is opened and the rectum and remaining segment of sigmoid and mesosigmoid are removed." He criticized the pull-through procedure, although that was not what Best had recommended. R. Russell Best, in closing the Discussion, agreed that pull-through operations ". . . do not seem radical enough in the region of the levator ani muscle", and he pleaded for ". . . more and wider dissection of tissues in the region of the levator ani muscles . . . Theory and emotion must be replaced by experience in sphincter preserving operations and a final tabulation of the end results. Personally, I do not believe that sufficient experience has been had by a sufficient number of surgeons in a sufficient number of cases over a long enough period of time to unequivocally make a statement."

* * *

Harvey Cushing, who had championed the intracapsular extirpation of acoustic tumors, and Walter Dandy, whose enthusiasm for total removal of these tumors had been one of the foci of their mutual enmity were both now dead, as Gilbert Horrax, of Boston, Head to the Neurosurgical Service, The Lahey Clinic, and James L. Poppen, by invitation, *The End Results of Complete versus Intracapsular Removal of Acoustic Tumors,* presented a masterful analysis of the situation. Cushing's intracapsular extirpation had been introduced in 1917 reducing the operative mortality from prohibitive figures to some 10%. Nevertheless, the five-year mortality in the patients surviving the operation was on the order of 56%, the reason for Dandy's 1922 operation for complete removal of the tumor, and by 1925 Dandy had done five such without a death. [Neither Cushing nor Dandy had presented his operation before the Association.] The very large Swedish experience of Olivecrona of 185 complete extirpations was accompanied by a five-year mortality,- including operative mortality,- of 25% and for intracapsular operations, a mortality of about 54% over five years. Sixty percent of the patients whose tumors were totally removed and only 34% of those with intracapsular extirpation were leading useful lives. Harvey Cushing's patients were practically all operated upon by the intracapsular procedure. An analysis of the several reports of Cushing's patients indicated that in the subsequent five-year period only 77 of 176 patients had survived. Dandy's last report in 1943 listed 46 patients with complete removal of acoustic tumors and five operative deaths,- 10.87%. Two patients had died within a year. It was difficult to know what the postoperative recovery was of the others, but Horrax assumed that it would ". . . at least be as good as others who have made similar studies." Horrax and Poppen had operated upon 72 patients by complete extirpation with eight deaths, an operative mortality of 11.1%. There had been no further deaths. There was a useful life survival of 65% of the total group. Their unequivocal statement from review of the literature and of their own experience vindicated Dandy's stand, "There can be no question that any operation on an acoustic tumor is a difficult and somewhat hazardous procedure, but with patience and care they can now be removed completely in the vast majority of instances. If this is done, the patient will not only have as good a chance of coming through the operation as by the old intracapsular method, but will also have an infinitely greater chance of living a permanently useful life." Facial paralysis was a frequent concomitant of the complete operation, ". . . but this can be improved to some extent by an anastomosis, and in our experience every patient with one exception has preferred this disability rather than to be faced with a recurrence of the tumor and a far more serious secondary operation."

Discussion

Francis C. Grant, of Philadelphia, agreed with the conclusions of Horrax and Poppen, "The mortality is lower after complete extirpation, and all chances of recurrence are avoided," Howard C. Naffziger, of San Francisco, also agreed but commented on the extraordinary skill of both Horrax and Poppen. Cobb Pilcher, of Nashville, suggested that in old people who were poor risks and had a shortened life expectancy, an intracapsular removal might well be preferable. Gilbert Horrax, in closing, agreed with Pilcher and said that it was Poppen who had ". . . urged me to take up the complete enucleation of these tumors . . ."

* * *

Bronson S. Ray, of New York, Attending Surgeon, New York Hospital; Professor of Clinical Surgery, Cornell University Medical College, and by invitation, A. Dale Console, *Evaluation of Total Sympathectomy,* proposed to test the dictum that ". . . the degree of success is proportional to the extent of the sympathectomy . . . The earlier types of limited operation came to be largely supplanted by the thoracolumbar resection from the eighth or ninth thoracic to the upper lumbar levels proposed by Smithwick ten years ago. Peet changed to a higher resection of the thoracic sympathetics in his supradiaphragmatic operation. More recently others (Poppen, and Hinton and Lord) have extended the resection of the thoracic chain up to the third or fourth thoracic ganglia, and have implied that blood pressure lowering effects were better. A logical conclusion would seem to be that consistently good results might be expected if total sympathectomy were performed, providing, of course, the patient could tolerate the operation and not be left a 'homeostatic cripple' ". Eight years earlier Grimson had reported before the Association three patients with total paravertebral sympathectomy and Ray assumed that Grimson's numbers had increased since. Ray and Console were reporting operations on 30 patients, 17 having angina pectoris, and many of them having retinopathy. Six of the patients had previously had a T8-L3 sympathectomy with little improvement, and 24 had the total sympathectomy as a primary procedure, the two sides done separately, two or four weeks apart in some, the operation performed in three stages in others. The complete operation removed the chain from the stellate to the third lumbar ganglion. The operative approach was retroperitoneal and retropleural. In several patients the celiac ganglia were removed as well. There were two operative deaths,- 6.3% both in patients with angina pectoris, one of coronary infarction, one of cardiac failure. One patient died suddenly at home 11 months after operation, having been relieved of angina pectoris and otherwise improved. The extension of the sympathectomy to include the stellate ganglia bilaterally, abolished cardiac pain and slowed the cardiac rate. The complete sympathectomy totally or substantially relieved the pain of angina pectoris in the chest and arms and increased the capacity for exercise, but three patients ". . . had occasional and moderate pain in the neck and jaws on exertion." The 21 patients with advanced retinopathy ". . . all showed a subsidence of these changes within one to three months after the completion. . ." of the bilateral operation. They had seen this as well with the less extensive thoracolumbar operation. The improvement in headache was no better than that with less extensive sympathectomy. "All but two of the patients who survived operation were rehabilitated to the degree that they either resumed wholly or in large part their former occupations and activities, or else led a fairly active existence within moderate restrictions." The one-year mortality in the 21 patients with "advanced hypertension" and severe retinopathy was 9.5% combined, substantially better than the 14% achieved with thoracolumbar sympathectomy and very much better indeed than the reported 69% one-year mortality with nonoperative treatment. Although the blood pressure fell after each stage of the operation, in the patients with three stages there was still a diastolic fall of 20 mm. of mercury after the third stage. Of 20 surviving patients with initial total sympathectomy nine,- 4.3%,- had diastolic pressures consistently below 100 mm. of mercury, and the remaining 12 all had some lowering of their diastolic pressure, usually ". . . to a much safer level than originally existed." In general they were able to state that ". . . the evidence indicates that total sympathectomy has a greater effect in lowering blood pressure than a lesser resection of the sympathetics in some patients. In this series a poor or mediocre result after thoracolumbar operation was improved in 50 per cent of the patients by adding the excision of the remaining sympathetics." Nevertheless, a total sympathectomy, even performed as the initial procedure, did not always lower the resting blood pressure significantly and sometimes lowered it not at all. Because of the inability to sweat in these sympathectomized areas, "In the early period after completion of the operation, extremes of temperature are not well tolerated . . . The hypotension and its symptoms of giddiness and weakness that accompany change in posture and exercise may be profound soon after operation, and are often of greater degree than that seen following thoracolumbar sympathectomy." The patient might be distressed by the Horner syndrome as well, "Yet within a relatively short time the degree of these symptoms and signs begins to subside and somehow the body makes a progressive adjustment." They were inclined to agree ". . . to the likelihood that the partial return of homeostasis after total paravertebral sympathectomy is due to the presence and augmented activity of residual sympathetic nerves, already present, which do not traverse the paravertebral ganglionated chains, splanchnic nerves or celiac ganglia." The special advantage of total paravertebral sympathectomy lay not on its somewhat greater blood pressure lowering effect but in the relief of angina pectoris, tachycardia, and vasospastic states in the extremity.

Discussion

Reginald H. Smithwick of Boston, was in general agreement. He had been performing thoracolumbar sympathectomy for ten years, having found it superior to either subdiaphragmatic or supradiaphragmatic splanchnicectomy and had additionally done some 16 total sympathectomies. However, four of those patients ". . . were totally disabled for long periods of time because of their inability to stand, having lost both their capacity to constrict the splanchnic bed and to accelerate the heart rate . . . total sympathectomy should never be performed as a primary procedure in hypertensive patients. The morbidity and mortality will be great, aside from the probability that it is unnecessary. Specifically, the patients with coronary heart disease and angina pectoris and those with postural tachycardia were not to be treated with thoracolumbar splanchnicectomy, but by transthoracic sympathectomy "removing the chains bilaterally from the inferior cervical to the twelfth thoracic ganglia in the former, and from the second thoracic to the twelfth ganglia in the latter group." He personally did not feel ". . . that it is necessary to do a total sympathectomy as a primary procedure in patients with hypertension and angina pectoris or tachycardia." He, too, had compared his patients with the unoperated patients of Keith, Wagener and Barker from the Mayo Clinic, finding the results all to the advantage of operation.

* * *

Sidney C. Werner, David V. Habif, H. T. Randall, all by invitation, and John S. Lockwood, of New York, Professor of Surgery, College of Physicians and Surgeons, Columbia University, *Postoperative Nitrogen Loss:* A Comparison of the Effects of Trauma and of Caloric Readjustment, discussed the older theories of a specific antianabolic, or catabolic effect of trauma, "toxic destruction of protein . . .

alarm response attributed to activation of the adrenal cortex . . ." used to explain the demonstrated negative nitrogen balance after trauma. Werner had already demonstrated a similar nitrogen loss in healthy subjects on diets with sharply reduced caloric and protein intake. They now reported preoperative and postoperative studies in vigorous patients admitted for elective cholecystectomy or herniorraphy, performing careful intake and output metabolic studies. They concluded that there was no significant increase in nitrogen output after the operation except as justified by the decreased caloric intake and "The concept is proposed that simple caloric lack explains the postoperative nitrogen loss found following operation uncomplicated by infection."

Discussion

Oliver Cope, of Boston, reminded the Fellows of ". . . the observations of Dr. John Howard at Johns Hopkins, who showed that the nitrogen balance, or metabolic reaction of the patient to operation and trauma, varied according to the size of the trauma, and also to the health of the patient." In reply, Dr. Werner thought it not unreasonable "to suspect that if the body reacts to trauma in a given way for one degree of injury, that the reaction will be the same with more severe traumata." Even in burns where infection increased the protein loss, Hirschfeld had been able to restore nitrogen equilibrium.

* * *

Robert Elman, of St. Louis, Professor of Clinical Surgery, Washington University School of Medicine, and by invitation Richard A. Lemmer, Theodore E. Weichselbaum, James G. Owen, and Richard W. Yore, *Minimum Postoperative Maintenance Requirements for Parenteral Water, Sodium, Potassium, Chloride and Glucose,* said about the study of the daily minimum requirements of the patient taking solely intravenous alimentation,- ". . . a series of observations were made on surgical patients given daily 2000 cc. of fluid containing glucose with and without added sodium chloride for four postoperative days. The findings suggest that a smaller intake of both water and salt than is usually given seems to be adequate." In all they studied 40 patients. There was usually an oliguria in the first 24 hours in patients given two liters of 10% glucose intravenously with no salt of any kind, a conservation of salt was shown "by a gradual decrease in the amount of sodium and chloride excreted on each consecutive day during the four day postoperative

study period." With an intake of nine grams of salt a day there was increased salt retention and they ultimately thought that ". . . an average of between 2 and 4 Gm. of sodium chloride a day would probably produce balance in the average patient. The need for adding potassium rests on the assumption that losses in this element should be replaced. On such a basis about one to 2 Gm. of potassium salt should be added to the daily intake." To avoid adding an excess of chloride, the potassium might be given as lactate or gluconate. Elman was foresighted enough to say that "This does not take into account other electrolytes such as magnesium and perhaps the anions sulfate and phosphate." [He also pointed out what is so often forgotten ". . . for short periods of time it is unlikely that serious physiological impairment will follow small deficits in these electrolytes, such as might follow their deprivation. Thus it might be argued that simple fluids without salt might be adopted as routine." Nevertheless, he thought exact replacement was preferable.] Gamble had shown that in normal human beings, 100 Gm. of glucose a day produced a maximal protein sparing effect and an increase to 200 Gm. did not decrease tissue protein loss and their findings were in accord. They concluded that with an intake of two liters of fluid a day there was "adequate urinary output during the four postoperative days of about one liter except for a moderate oliguria during the first postoperative day . . . accompanied by a decreased creatinine excretion with no change in specific gravity . . . With no electrolyte intake, the body rapidly conserves sodium and chloride, but not potassium and phosphate . . . No changes in plasma levels of sodium, potassium, CO_2, proteins or in red cells volume were observed . . . an intake of 2 liters of water plus 2 to 4 Gm. of a mixture of sodium and potassium chloride (or gluconate) would meet the minimum requirements for these elements in the postoperative patient . . . The nitrogen sparing effect of 200 Gm. of glucose was not significantly greater than 100 Gm. of glucose."

There was no Discussion and Elman, in closing, said, "In spite of the published warnings of Dr. Coller and many others, it had been my observation that too much intravenous fluid is still being given in many hospitals. I would include in this plasma and whole blood transfusions."

* * *

Leland S. McKittrick, of Boston, Clinical Professor of Surgery, Harvard Medical School; Visiting Surgeon, Massachusetts General Hospital, and by invitation, John B. McKittrick, Thomas S. Risley,

Transmetatarsal Amputation for Infection or Gangrene in Patients with Diabetes Mellitus, had fifteen years earlier before the Association reported a mortality of 13.7% in amputations of the lower extremity in diabetic patients. They had done their first transmetatarsal amputation for gangrene of a toe in a diabetic patient in 1944,- a lesion ". . . for which we had previously considered amputation through or above the mid-lower leg as the operation of choice." They had now done 215 transmetatarsal amputations at the New England Deaconess Hospital. The indications were gangrene of one or more toes, which had become *stabilized,* stabilized infection or ulcer in the distal portion of the foot, and an open infected lesion in a "neurogenic foot". The operation was performed under low spinal anesthesia, and a long plantar flap employed. There had been two hospital deaths, a mortality of 0.9%, and complete healing in 155 patients at the time of discharge. Sixty patients failed to heal and reamputation was ultimately undertaken in 27, 26 of them healing promptly. Both the deaths were from coronary thrombosis, whereas 10% of the patients in the previous series had died from infection. The functional result was good, "Most patients with unilateral amputations use lamb's wool in the toe of their own shoe."

Discussion

Louis G. Herrmann, of Cincinnati, said that they had been using "conservative amputations through the foot for gangrene of the toes due either to arterial disease or to infection" since 1934, and preferred the transmetatarsal amputation. They usually left the stump open, allowed it to granulate and then grafted it. Michael E. DeBakey, of Houston, Texas, was struck by the ". . . salvage of functioning extremities, and . . . the strikingly low mortality . . . Only about ten years ago the case fatality rate in the surgical management of such cases was as high as 30 to 40 per cent, with emphasis being placed on amputation above the knee." DeBakey asked if there was any difference between the diabetics and the nondiabetics with arteriosclerosis, his own observation being that, if anything, better results were obtained in diabetics. What had been the effect of combining the operation with sympathectomy?, "In our experience, sympathectomy has appeared to be a valuable adjunct in the treatment of this particular group of patients." Reginald H. Smithwick, of Boston, indicated that ". . . the advent of chemotherapy and antibiotics have made it possible to consider conservative amputations in in-

creasing numbers of patients." He thought it important to estimate the degree of collateral circulation. The temperature of the skin at the site of amputation should be ". . . 75 degrees Fahrenheit or more after exposure of the extremities to a room temperature of 68 degrees Fahrenheit for one hour . . . Secondly, when, after blanching of the foot on elevation, flushing in the dependent position begins in twenty seconds or less, in all probability the collateral circulation is adequate." He did use skin flaps, avoided trauma, etc. McKittrick agreed with the comments about atraumatic technique, had not used Herrmann's technique of an open amputation with secondary skin graft. Most of their patients had been diabetics. They had performed sympathectomy in a few and thought occasionally it obviated amputation, occasionally added to the security of amputation.

* * *

The Business Meetings

The 1949 meeting, April 20, 21 and 22, was held at the Jefferson Hotel, St. Louis, Missouri, Fred W. Rankin, Clinical Professor of Surgery, Louisville School of Medicine, in the Chair.

Thirty-seven papers had been accepted out of the 46 abstracts submitted.

The Council was "gravely disturbed" by the action of the American Board of Obstetrics and Gynecology in stating, "If gynecology is classified in a given hospital as a subdivision or subservice of surgery, approval cannot be granted for resident training in gynecology."

Arthur W. Allen, for the "Committee on Membership", pointed out that it was "purely advisory" to the Council, and "only the Council can approve men for election to this Association", and reminded the Fellows that "The members of this Association do not realize that it is their duty to place on the so-called master list any young, promising surgeons that he may know about." There were at the time "125 names on the master list beside those that are up for consideration for election by the Council."

The officers elected were Thomas G. Orr, of Kansas City, President; John J. Morton, of Rochester, New York, First Vice-President; B. Noland Carter, of Cincinnati, Ohio, Second Vice-President; and Nathan A. Womack, of Iowa City, Secretary.

In the early days of the Association, there had been difficulties in the election of Fellows because of the requirements for near unanimity, and the requirement had been substantially relaxed. Now, in a reverse move, it was proposed that election, instead of being by three-fourths of the ballots, be by nine-tenths of the ballots. There must have been some dissatisfaction with the list of candidates proposed, because another proposed amendment stated, "The Secretary shall make available, upon request of any Fellow of the Association, the list of the candidates passed by the Council for membership." The two proposed amendments were to lie over until 1950.

1950s

THE NEW YORK TIMES - WEDNESDAY, APRIL 19, 1950 - THE FIRST DAY OF THE MEETING OF THE AMERICAN SURGICAL ASSOCIATION IN COLORADO SPRINGS, COLORADO

The first commercial jet plane, Canadian built, touched down at Idlewild; the Postal Service was in trouble and planning to reduce residential mail deliveries to one per day; there was concern about the need of international "atomic controls"; the Communization of Czechoslovakia was proceeding; a United States Navy patrol plane "on a routine training flight to Copenhagen" had been shot down by Russian fighters; Senator Joseph McCarthy was pursuing Owen Lattimore and attacking Senators Tydings and McMahon.

(Copyright 1950 by the New York Times Company. Reprinted by permission.)

"All the News That's Fit to Print"

The New York Times.

LATE CITY EDITION
Cloudy with showers later today
Fair and cooler tomorrow
Temperature Range Today-Max.,68; Min.,55
Temperatures Yesterday—Max.,73; Min.,55
Full U. S. Weather Bureau Report, Page 25

VOL. XCIX. No. 33,688.
Entered as Second-Class Matter, Post Office, New York, N. Y.
NEW YORK, WEDNESDAY, APRIL 19, 1950.
Times Square, New York 18, N. Y. Telephone Lackawanna 4-1000
RAG PAPER EDITION
SEVENTY-FIVE CENTS

U. S. CHARGES RUSSIANS DOWNED PLANE OVER BALTIC AND DEMANDS AN APOLOGY; TRUMAN ASKS G. O. P. AID FOREIGN POLICY

ONE MAIL DELIVERY A DAY IN HOMES SET IN POSTAL ECONOMY

Donaldson Cites Budget Slash, Deficit—Service Is Also Cut on Parcel Post

LETTER PICK-UPS REDUCED

Commercial Areas Lose Trip on Saturdays—10,000 Jobs May Go—Union Protests

By W. H. LAWRENCE
Special to The New York Times.

WASHINGTON, April 18—In a sweeping economy move, Postmaster General Jesse M. Donaldson today ordered residential mail deliveries restricted to one a day and other reductions in postal service.

Mr. Donaldson said the action was essential to curtail a mounting deficit in the operation of the Post Office Department. He also said he acted after cuts in the Post Office budget were made by a House committee.

His action was assailed at once by the Association of Letter Carriers, A. F. L., as "a rape of the postal service." The association said it would protest to Congress.

Mr. Donaldson's order was spelled out in a thirty-six-point directive in today's issue of The Postal Bulletin, which most postmasters will receive tomorrow. The orders are effective immediately.

10,000 Jobs Probably Lost

Officially the Post Office Department declined to estimate how many jobs would be lost as a result of the economy order, but an informed source said tonight that he would regard 10,000 as a "good guess." The reductions will be made in first and second class post offices, of which there are about 8,000 in the country. Some probably will not be affected, one official said.

Following are the main points of the economy program:

City delivery routes are to be readjusted to provide one delivery daily Monday through Saturday in residential areas, instead of two as at present. Most persons will get their mail in the afternoon instead of in the morning, as at present.

Neighborhood stores and professional offices also are to receive one delivery daily. However, in mixed business and residential areas, where a second delivery is necessary to provide for other businesses and concerns dependent upon the mail service, efforts should be made to consolidate delivery to those areas to the minimum number of carriers required to make a second trip, according to the order.

On Saturdays, there will be one delivery less in business areas. Districts that received three deliveries will get two, and one trip will be made where there have been two deliveries.

Collection of mail from street letter boxes is to be reduced to a minimum, with the last pick-up getting mail to post offices not later than 8:30 P. M.

One Parcel Post Delivery

Parcel post deliveries are to be restricted to one delivery weekdays in both business and residential areas. Exceptions may be made only in business areas where the volume of parcel post exceeds storage capacity of the post office.

Window service at main post offices is to be provided between 8 A. M. and 6 P. M., and at branch offices between 8 A. M. and 5:30 P. M. Local postmasters receive authority to close at 5 P. M. wherever possible. Saturday window service is to be limited to 8 A. M. to 12 noon in branch offices, and to the minimum period necessary in main offices. Local offices are to close on Saturdays where possible.

Post offices are to discontinue from 6 P. M. to 6 A. M. the dis-

Continued on Page 24, Column 3

Dry Day Tomorrow; Save for Children

Water officials again yesterday urged the public to "give us all possible cooperation" in cutting water use to a minimum tomorrow, the sixteenth water holiday of the present conservation campaign. Cutting down on water use at this time of year, it was argued, is no hardship. Furthermore, it was emphasized, reduced consumption now may mean some water for children's swimming and wading pools in the public parks this summer.

First Jet Liner Seen Here Flies From Toronto in Hour

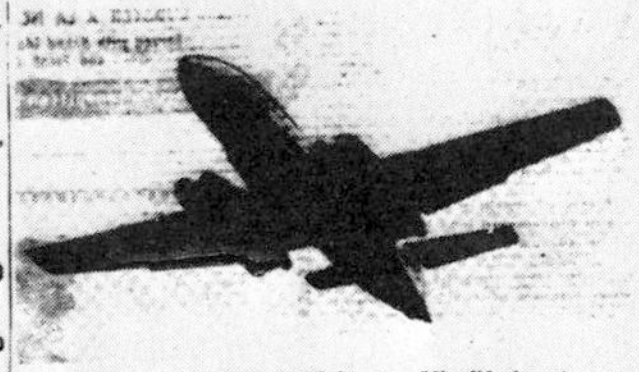

The Avro jet liner in flight over Idlewild airport
The New York Times (by Sam Falk)

The Avro jet liner, the first turbojet transport plane ever flown in the United States, arrived yesterday at New York International Airport, Idlewild, Queens, after a flight from Toronto that took slightly less than one hour.

The sleek new air liner received a prolonged welcome from the several hundred spectators who gathered at the airport to witness its first landing outside of Canada, where it was built by a company formed only four years ago.

Carrying three crew members, three passengers and the world's first "jet-borne" airmail, the four-engined plane set a record for the 365-mile flight from Moulton Airport, Toronto, to Idlewild.

Piloted by Donald H. Rogers, chief test pilot for A. V. Roe Canada, Ltd., manufacturer of the sixty-passenger airliner, the jet liner's departure from Toronto was clocked at 9:30:04 A. M. It arrived at Idlewild at exactly 10:30 A. M., making its flight time fifty-nine minutes and fifty-six seconds.

Mr. Rogers said he spent the first twelve minutes in the air climbing to a cruising altitude of 20,000 feet. From that point on his average speed was 400 miles an hour. For a short time he was making 425 miles an hour, aided by a tail wind.

One of the passengers, Gordon R. McGregor, president of Trans-

Continued on Page 23, Column 2

M'CARTHY SUBMITS 2 MORE WITNESSES

Former F.B.I. Undercover Man and Ex-Agent Are Named to Testify on Lattimore

By WILLIAM S. WHITE
Special to The New York Times.

WASHINGTON, April 18—Senator Joseph R. McCarthy announced today that he was handing in to Senate investigators the names of two additional witnesses in connection with his "case" against Prof. Owen Lattimore.

These witnesses, Mr. McCarthy, a Wisconsin Republican, told reporters, were respectively a former under-cover agent for the Federal Bureau of Investigation who had joined the Communist party in order to do his work, and a former F. B. I. agent who had been active in counter-espionage.

Senator McCarthy added that, as in the instance of Prof. Louis F. Budenz, he would ask that the two former agents be subpoenaed by the Senate subcommittee that is investigating his charges of heavy Communist infiltration of the State Department.

As to the announcement of yesterday by the subcommittee chairman, Senator Millard E. Tydings, Democrat of Maryland, that the group was going to conduct inquiries running beyond the McCarthy accusations, Mr. McCarthy observed: "I won't believe it until I see it, but it is a good sign."

"It is the first sign we have had," he added, "that Tydings and McMahon (Senator Brien McMahon, Democrat of Connecticut, a member of the subcommittee) are not completely dedicated to the proposition that the truth about Communists and perverts must not come out."

Apart from the two witnesses he now proposes to call, Senator McCarthy said:

"I will also have other witnesses in the next few days who will

Continued on Page 2, Column 3

'NEW THINKING' SEEN ON ATOM CONTROLS

McMahon Says Congressional Restudy of U. S. Plan Spurs Administration to Ponder

Special to The New York Times.

WASHINGTON, April 18—Senator Brien McMahon said today that Congressional restudy of the United States plan for international atomic controls had prompted the Administration to take a "more intensive look-see at the whole situation."

The Connecticut Democrat, chairman of the Joint Congressional Committee on Atomic Energy, declared he was "glad to see the committee's action has initiated some new thinking on the subject in the Executive Department." He did not elaborate beyond saying that no new plan had been "stimulated."

He issued this somewhat enigmatic statement just after his committee, opening its own reexamination of the nation's present proposal for control "in the light of projected hydrogen weapons," heard its first witness, Gen. Omar N. Bradley, chairman of the Joint Chiefs of Staff.

The general, according to Mr. McMahon, reported to the committee "on the state of a resurvey of the military implications of the hydrogen bomb." The Senator added that the testimony, given behind closed doors, was in the nature of a general discussion.

Others high in the Administration, including Dean Acheson, Secretary of State, will be heard during the three months the committee expects to spend on the job, the Senate said. He indicated that John D. Hickerson, Assistant Secretary of State for United Nations Affairs, would be the next witness. No date was set for the next hearing.

While details of the Bradley testimony were withheld, the General

Continued on Page 4, Column 6

Stray Shot Kills Woman Passer-by In Central Park West Thief Chase

An off-duty detective, firing at two thugs caught looting a parked car last night on Central Park West near Eighty-sixth Street, accidentally killed a woman pedestrian. One of the men was wounded; the other escaped.

The dead woman was identified from papers as Mrs. Carrie James, 50 years old, of 46 West 120th Street. Frightened by a warning shot fired by Detective Nicholas F. Adrizzo of the Pickpocket Squad, she had jumped up from a bench on which she was sitting and run into the path of Mr. Adrizzo's second shot at the fleeing bandit. The bullet struck her left eye.

A third shot by Detective Adrizzo caught the theft suspect in the back, lodging near his spine. The thug had pulled a switch-blade knife on the detective when caught looting the car, the police said. His companion got away by running to the other side of the street.

The wounded man identified himself as Vincent Cordero, 40, of 144 West 103d Street. While in an ambulance en route to Knickerbocker Hospital, he allegedly told police that he had a criminal record of ten previous arrests. At the hospital his condition was reported serious.

Detective Adrizzo said his suspicions had been aroused when he saw the two men approach the parked automobile. He boarded a southbound bus, but, glancing back, saw the men were prying open the side window of the car.

The detective got off the bus and started to run toward the car. He saw Cordero take a topcoat and his companion a suit of clothes and a pair of shoes from the auto. As the detective approached, Cordero pulled a knife. When they saw Mr. Adrizzo draw his revolver, the thugs separated and ran north on Central Park West, on opposite sides of the street.

The detective said he fired a warning shot. Then, he said, Mrs. James rose from her seat and

Continued on Page 32, Column 1

CRIPPS DASHES HOPE OF TAXATION RELIEF IN BRITISH BUDGET

Only Lowest Income Bracket Gets Slight Concession—No Industrial Palliative

WELFARE COSTS LIMITED

Food Subsidies Are Reduced—Gasoline Doubled, Price Up—Better Beer Promised

By RAYMOND DANIELL
Special to The New York Times.

LONDON, April 18—Once more Sir Stafford Cripps, Chancellor of the Exchequer, hammered home the lesson today that the welfare state meant sacrifice as well as benefits. He announced that its whole cost must be met out of revenue, or, in other words, that the taxpayers must foot the bill.

This dashed all hope of substantial tax relief although Sir Stafford, presenting his new budget to the House of Commons, did manage to lower the burden slightly on income taxpayers in the lowest income brackets.

His budget, calling for revenue of £3,897,800,000, however contained no palliatives for industry, the middle class or the harassed housewife.

[The £3,897,800,000 figure is equivalent to $10,913,840,000 at the current exchange rate of $2.80 to £1, but in terms of the British internal economy £1 (20 shillings or 240 pence) represents more than $2.80 in purchasing power.]

Some Save Shilling a Year

The relief that Sir Stafford granted to the long-suffering British income taxpayers fell upon all in accordance with the Labor party doctrine. Every one of the country's 14,500,000 taxpayers benefited in theory, according to his need.

Some among the higher income brackets saved one shilling a year but the luckiest—those earning a net income of £250—henceforth will pay £11 5s a year less in income tax. Private motorists and truckmen in competition with the nationalized transport services will make up the difference to the Treasury.

The budget for the coming year, although larger than last year's—largely as a result of the increased cost of the health service and national defense—provided for a smaller surplus as a guard against inflation.

Yet Sir Stafford warned that the

Continued on Page 12, Column 3

World News Summarized

WEDNESDAY, APRIL 19, 1950

This country accused the Soviet Union yesterday of having shot down "an unarmed American plane over the open" Baltic and called on Moscow to apologize, pay for the "unprovoked destruction of American lives and property," punish the men involved and avoid any repetition of the incident. A note contradicting the Soviet charge that a United States plane had violated Russian territory and opened fire on Soviet fighters said the "only American military aircraft" in the air in that area on April 8 was an unarmed Navy Privateer that has been missing with its crew of ten. A State Department spokesman said the Soviet action belied Moscow's "oft-proclaimed" peaceful aims. He commented acidly that Russia had not helped seek the missing plane. [1:8.]

Strong support for the note came from Congressmen, who felt it was "high time" to be firm with the Russians. [1:6-7.]

"New thinking" by the Administration on international atomic control was disclosed by Senator McMahon. General Bradley warned the nation not to succumb to the "temptation to relax" efforts to win the "cold war." [1:3.] This warning was also voiced by retiring Air Secretary Symington, who said the Russians had the air power for a surprise atomic attack against any part of this country and we had no adequate defense. Defense officials revealed that the Air Force was buying 1,250 planes and the Navy 798 at a cost of nearly $1,750,000,000 out of their current budgets. [5:1.]

President Truman announced a plan to keep Republicans "currently informed" on foreign policy and to "solicit their views" on its formulation and implementation. [1:5.]

Washington showed little enthusiasm for French Premier Bidault's proposal of a "high council" to unify North Atlantic political and economic policies with defense. [10:1.]

A £3,897,800,000 budget bringing the British little relief was presented to the Commons. [1:4.]

Chancellor Adenauer of West Germany demanded control over foreign policy and protested the Western powers' "distrust" of his Government and then led Berliners in singing "Deutschland Ueber Alles." [1:6.] Outbursts of anti-Semitism in Germany were denounced by High Commissioner McCloy. [15:1.]

Czechoslovakia will convert monasteries into hospitals and workers' apartments, it was announced. Two persons of sixteen charged with spying for the United States were sentenced to die. [1:7.]

Conflicting accounts surrounded the reported invasion of Hainan by Chinese Communists. [17:3, with map.] The Soviet representative in the United Nations refused to transmit to Moscow Nationalist charges of Soviet military aid to the Communists. [17:1.]

Mail deliveries to homes will be cut to one a day and those to business addresses sharply reduced in changes ordered into immediate effect to meet budget cuts and a departmental deficit. [1:1.] Congressional fiscal experts forecast a combined deficit of $14,000,000,000 for the 1950 and 1951 fiscal years, $3,100,000,000 more than the President's estimates. [25:4-5.]

Senator McCarthy said he would call two former F. B. I. agents to prove his "case" against Owen Lattimore. [1:2.]

Governor Dewey signed bills creating a state civil defense agency [8:1], fixing minimum retail liquor prices [25:6] and exempting school and hospital construction in this city from "down-payment" requirements of state law. [24:5.]

Index to other news appears on Page 30.

SENATORS INVITED

Bridges Sees President and Acheson, Reveals Collaboration Plan

ARCH-CRITIC IS CAUTIOUS

He and Others Want to Know More Facts—Connally Says Minority Already Sits In

By ANTHONY LEVIERO
Special to The New York Times.

WASHINGTON, April 18—President Truman announced today an unprecedented plan to summon Republican Senators to White House conferences to help in making and carrying out the nation's foreign policy.

By a turn of irony the plan was disclosed by Senator Styles Bridges, Republican of New Hampshire, an arch-critic of the Administration who has started a Republican movement to force the resignation of Secretary of State Dean Acheson. At Key West recently President Truman denounced Mr. Bridges as one of the Kremlin's greatest "assets."

Yet it was Senator Bridges who walked into the lobby of the executive offices of the White House, a little before noon, and gave the first word after a conference with the President and Secretary Acheson. He said they had summoned him there to outline the new plan to him as the senior Republican Senator in the absence of the ailing Senator Arthur H. Vandenberg of Michigan, who is the acknowledged Republican leader in foreign affairs.

Soon afterward Charles G. Ross, the President's press secretary, issued a formal statement by President Truman in which he said:

"It will be my purpose as well as that of Secretary Acheson not only to keep the members of the minority currently informed, but to solicit their views and take them into serious account in both the formulation and implementation of our foreign policy."

The President's latest action to

Continued on Page 22, Column 2

Most Congressmen Hail Note As Effective Reply to Russia

Republicans and Democrats Say Soviet Must Not Be Appeased—'High Time' Such a Stand Was Taken, Many Feel

By C. P. TRUSSELL
Special to The New York Times.

WASHINGTON, April 18—Congress appeared today to stand solidly behind the State Department's stern note to Russia, charging that her airmen had shot down a "wholly unarmed" United States Navy plane over the free waters of the Baltic and demanding that she pay and punish for the act.

Seldom has a checking on reaction through the usually widely differing segments of Senate and House membership on scores of questions indicated such unity.

The situation created by the disappearance of a Navy Privateer with ten men aboard on April 8, and Russia's allegations that the plane had been flying over Latvian territory and that its crew had fired first, was conceded to be delicate and serious. It was concluded almost generally, however, that the State Department had found convincing evidence in refutation before it dispatched its findings through Ambassador Alan G. Kirk at Moscow this morning.

A repeated reaction was that it was "high time" for the United States to take a firm, unyielding stand with Russia, that a positive position was now forced upon this Government, and that the note and demand sent today be treated as more than "merely a formal protest."

The new American-Russian development crashed into the day when the baseball season opened. Both Senate and House were cutting loose from work early—it is a tradition—to be on hand at Griffith Stadium to watch the Washington Senators and the Philadelphia Athletics slug it out after President Truman had thrown the first ball onto the diamond. It was

Continued on Page 3, Column 2

INDEMNITY IS ASKED

Washington Also Calls on Moscow to Punish All Fliers Involved

FINDS PEACE ENDANGERED

Officer of State Department Assails Soviet Neglect to Aid Hunt as Inhuman

Texts of note to Moscow and McDermott statement, Page 3.

By WALTER H. WAGGONER
Special to The New York Times.

WASHINGTON, April 18—The United States charged flatly today that the Navy patrol plane missing since April 8 with ten persons presumed lost had been shot down over the open Baltic Sea in an unprovoked attack by Soviet fighter aircraft.

A note to this effect, sharp and unequivocal, was delivered to the Soviet Ministry of Foreign Affairs in Moscow this morning by Admiral Alan G. Kirk, United States Ambassador. Ambassador Kirk was further instructed by the State Department to protest "in a most solemn manner against this violation of international law and the most elementary rules of peaceful conduct between nations."

On the assumption that the aircraft and ten airmen were lost in the Baltic Sea, over which the plane was due to pass on a routine training flight to Copenhagen, Denmark, the United States demanded that the Soviet Government pay "appropriate idemnity for the unprovoked destruction of American lives and property."

The note also said this Government was expecting an apology from the Soviet Union and prompt and severe punishment of the persons responsible for the attack.

Charge Based on Inquiry

The United States took this uncompromising position after a week-long investigation had been completed by the Defense Department and a final report of its findings sent to the State Department over the week-end.

The Defense Department began looking into the matter last week after the Soviet Union, in a note April 11, had protested to the United States that a B-29 bomber had passed over Soviet-controlled Latvia, fired upon a Soviet fighter plane, and then had fled after one of the Soviet planes had returned the fire.

An investigation, said the State Department in its note handed to Andrei A. Gromyko, Soviet deputy Foreign Minister, proved all these allegations false: the plane was unarmed and it was not over Soviet or Soviet-controlled territory. Rather, it was "fired upon" by the Soviet planes over the open Baltic Sea, and is now considered lost, the statement added.

The note positively identified the plane involved in the attack as a Navy Privateer, a disarmed and converted B-24 bomber, which had been missing over the Baltic area since April 8, en route from Wiesbaden to Copenhagen. A week-long search for the plane ended at sundown last Sunday.

McDermott Assails Russians

The public release of the United States note at 10:40 o'clock this morning, shortly after Ambassador Kirk had been due to deliver it, was accompanied by an oral statement by Michael J. McDermott, the State Department's chief press officer.

Mr. McDermott's remarks, minus the conventional niceties of diplomatic language, were harsher even than the formal note. Neglect of the Soviet Union to take part in the search for the missing plane, he declared, or to exhibit the "slightest evidence of concern," showed "an astonishing lack of common international courtesy and an unusual disregard of the loss of human life."

Mr. McDermott accused Moscow of "using an aggressive tone," having made "impossible allegations," and having confused the issue with "false propaganda claims and diatribes against the United States in the Soviet-controlled press."

"This attitude of the Soviet Government shows clearly the inhu-

Continued on Page 3, Column 6

BONN CHIEF LEADS DEUTSCHLAND SONG

Adenauer Calls On Berliners to Sing Unity Verse After He Asks Foreign Rights

By MICHAEL JAMES
Special to The New York Times.

BERLIN, April 18—Chancellor Konrad Adenauer asked today that his Western German Government receive control over its own foreign policy. In a speech here he also suggested that the Western powers drop what he called their "distrust" of the Bonn Government.

At the end of his address Dr. Adenauer asked his audience to sing the third verse of the old German Imperialist anthem, "Deutschland Ueber Alles ("Germany Over All"). "The audience lustily complied, but Socialist leaders on the rostrum walked out and the three Western Allied commandants pointedly remained seated during the singing. [The third verse deals with German unity, rights and freedom.]

Later Dr. Kurt Schumacher, head of the Social Democrats, said his party opposed "bringing in a kind of national anthem in a dictatorial manner which is against the expressed wishes of the great majority of Berliners."

"This party sees in the conduct of the Federal Chancellor a complete lack of understanding of the idea and practice of democracy," Dr. Schumacher added.

Repercussions to the singing of a verse of the old national anthem came quickly. Maj. Gen. Geoffrey K. Bourne, British Commandant in

Continued on Page 16, Column 5

PRAGUE TO CONVERT MANY MONASTERIES

Buildings to Be Made Hospitals and Workers' Homes—16 Convicted as U. S. Spies

Special to The New York Times.

PRAGUE, Czechoslovakia, April 18—Many Czechoslovak monasteries will be converted into hospitals, social institutions and workers' apartments while the monks and nuns have been "concentrated in a smaller number of monasteries," the official news agency announced tonight.

The move was presented as a sequel to the trial of ten leading members of Roman Catholic Premonstratensian, Jesuit, Dominican, Franciscan and Redemptorist orders who were convicted on April 5 on charges of espionage in the service of the Vatican.

The announcement said the move had been ordered to stop the hostile activity of the orders that had sheltered "agents, spies and even murderers," concealed weapons and broadcasting apparatus and served as bases for espionage.

The text of the announcement follows:

"It has been proved at the recent trial of monastic priests that many monasteries were being used to shelter hostile agents, spies and even murderers. In some monasteries weapons and secret broadcasting apparatus were discovered and many monasteries served as bases for espionage and disruptive activity.

"To stop this hostile activity of the Catholic orders measures have been taken which will bring those

Continued on Page 11, Column 3

Rockefeller Donates $1,000,000 To Barnard's Development Fund

A gift of $1,000,000 in securities has been made by John D. Rockefeller Jr. to Barnard College's Development Fund, it was announced jointly yesterday by Mrs. Ogden Reid, chairman of the college's Board of Trustees, and Mrs. Frank Altschul, national chairman of the fund, which has a goal of $10,800,000.

Mr. Rockefeller's gift was made "for the over-all development program, to be used in such ways as the trustees of the college may in their discretion, think best." However, he expressed the hope that it would be applied ultimately to a contemplated new building "when the necessary monies therefor are available."

Mr. Rockefeller commented that he had refrained generally from entering the educational field, "except in an occasional instance where the unique character of an institution, its outstanding service, its location or some program or personality have made me feel justified in contributing to it as an exception to the policy I have followed."

The cost of the proposed new building, which would be erected on a block of college-owned land fronting on Riverside Drive between 119th and 120th Streets, has been estimated at $3,500,000, but the trustees have indicated that $4,500,000 in endowment for scholarships, faculty salaries and strengthening of the curriculum must be raised before the building program can be undertaken. The building would house the science departments, the library and a theatre.

Mrs. Reid said that the income from Mr. Rockefeller's gift, plus the income from a $100 tuition increase approved by the trustees on April 5 would eliminate an estimated $105,000 operating deficit for 1950-51, and would give the institution a balanced budget for the first time since 1944.

Mr. Rockefeller said he felt that through the establishment of the General Education Board and its

Continued on Page 23, Column 3

LXVIII

1950

The Association met at the Broadmoor Hotel, Colorado Springs, Colorado, April 19, 20, and 21, 1950, with Thomas Orr, of Kansas City, Professor of Surgery and Chief of the Second Surgical Division, University of Kansas Medical Center, in the Chair.

During the preceding year, Walton Martin, who had earlier been so active in the meetings, had died at the age of 80, and the inimitable Thomas E. Jones, of the Cleveland Clinic, had also died.

* * *

Frederick A. Coller, of Ann Arbor, had long been campaigning against the excessive use of fluids after operation ". . . I feel the principal function of my afternoon round is to separate the patient from the bottle that is hanging over his head, by pulling out the needle." Coller had demonstrated the retention of sodium and now Henry T. Johnson, Jerome W. Conn, Vivian Iob, by invitation, and Frederick A. Coller, Professor of Surgery, University of Michigan Medical School; Chairman, Department of Surgery, *Postoperative Salt Retention and Its Relation to Increased Adrenal Cortical Function,* set out to analyze the cause. It had already been demonstrated from Albright's laboratory ". . . that a major surgical procedure elicits a sharp increase in adrenal cortical function, as indicated by increased amounts of urinary excretory products which reflect steroids of the 11-oxysteroid and androgenic types", and the elevation of the 11-oxysteroids was inversely propor-

tional to the peripheral eosinophil count. "No direct measurement of changes in endogenous production of such electrolyte-regulating steroids is available" so that they employed a determination of the electrolyte composition of sweat, the concentration of sodium and chloride being inversely proportional to desoxycorticosterone activity. The administration of desoxycorticosterone to normal persons produced reduction of urinary excretion of sodium, chloride and water, as George Thorn had shown, with associated increased extracellular fluid and blood volume. At the same time, there was an increased renal excretion of potassium. They had demonstrated, by having postoperative patients sweat in a hot room and analyzing the sweat, that sweat sodium fell for several days and then rose to preoperative levels and much the same was true of sweat chloride. However, sweat potassium rose very sharply immediately after operation and returned to normal levels after four or five days. The eosinophil count dropped very sharply within hours of operation and was back to normal by the second day. The sweat effect in their patients appeared to be similar to that produced by the 11-oxycorticosterone-like steroids. The disappearance of eosinophils from blood right after operation appeared to be an 11-oxysteroid effect. They concluded that "Since the entire metabolic picture exhibited by the postoperative patient can be duplicated in healthy individuals by injections of anterior pituitary adrenocorticotrophic hormone (ACTH) it

948

is now evident that a major surgical procedure constitutes an 'alarming stimulus' [Selye] in man."

Discussion

Jonathan E. Rhoads, of the University of Pennsylvania, said that they had puzzled over the transitory oliguria of the first day or two after a major operation and that Dr. James Hardy [a future President, but not yet a member] had been correlating ". . . adrenal cortical activity with the change in fluid balance following extensive surgical operations." Hardy's data were in agreement with those just presented and Rhoads said "It seems clear that the adrenal cortex plays a significant and important role in the postoperative retention of salt and water." Francis D. Moore, of Boston, agreed with Coller's conclusions and said "We find that 100 to 150 mg. of ACTH over a two-day period corresponds roughly to the alarm reaction of a subtotal gastrectomy." The eosinophil count returned to normal before the sodium-potassium balance had been restored, ". . . interesting evidence of the disassociation of these two actions of two of the adrenal hormones." Bernard Zimmerman, of Minneapolis, had made the same observations of the drop in sodium and chloride concentrations of the serum after operation, although he thought that levels returned to normal about as quickly as the eosinophil counts did.

* * *

Alfred Blalock, of Baltimore, Professor of Surgery and Director of the Department of Surgery, Johns Hopkins University, School of Medicine; Surgeon-in-Chief, Johns Hopkins Hospital, and by invitation, Richard F. Kieffer, Jr., *Valvulotomy for the Relief of Congenital Valvular Pulmonic Stenosis with Intact Ventricular Septum,* Report of Nineteen Operations by the Brock Method, mentioned Doyen's unsuccessful 1913 operation and the 1948 reports of Russell Brock and of Holmes Sellors, in England, of direct transventricular valvotomy for isolated valvar pulmonic stenosis. Blalock said that Brock had been attacking the infundibular stenosis in the tetralogy of Fallot, but indicated that since there was a ventricular septal defect for decompression, "In such a situation the mixed blood of the left ventricle can be shunted to the lungs by an anastomosis between a systemic and a pulmonary artery, with great improvement in arterial oxygen content and relatively little danger of right-sided heart failure." The patient with an isolated valvar pulmonic stenosis had no such safety valve. [Blalock was convinced of the cor-

rectness of the direct approach to isolated valvar pulmonic stenosis and in this paper and elsewhere gave Brock full credit, but disagreed with Brock's attempt to resect the infundibular stenosis in tetralogy of Fallot and seemed to take offense at it.] The transventricular incision of the valve was performed by Brock's technique and, in fact, seven of the operations had been performed at the Johns Hopkins by Brock ". . . while he was serving as an Exchange Professor in The Johns Hopkins Medical School and Hospital." In all they had operated upon 19 patients. Only five of them squatted whereas most of the patients with tetralogy of Fallot squatted. All of the patients had a valvar pulmonic stenosis, "Three of the patients, however, had previously been thought to have the tetralogy of Fallot and had had an artificial ductus created", two at Hopkins and one elsewhere. There had been two deaths in the series of 19, the first in one of the children who had had a Blalock-Taussig anastomosis at Hopkins two-and-a-half years earlier and had been in right heart failure ever since. The second patient became comatose two days after operation and had a frontal lobe abscess drained, but went on to die. [She had had headaches for several weeks before operation and leukocytosis, but the incidence of brain abscess in congenital heart disease was not yet appreciated.] The other 17 patients all did well.

Discussion

Willis J. Potts, of Chicago, opened the Discussion. At this point he was using a cataract knife blade ". . . soldered to a rounded shaft of such size that it will fill the hole made in the ventricle by the blade." Charles P. Bailey, of Philadelphia [whose operations for mitral valve disease Blalock had mentioned the year before], said that by this technic he had operated upon the stenotic pulmonary valve of six babies with tetralogy of Fallot and in two children, had used a specially devised rongeur to remove the infundibular obstruction, with dramatic results. He had had five good results out of six and no deaths. Blalock, closing, agreed with the remarks the others had made that the differential diagnosis between tetralogy of Fallot and valvar pulmonic stenosis might be difficult. At operation one should feel for the "dome-shaped valve" in the pulmonary artery, and one might feel the jet of blood in the distal pulmonary artery.

* * *

The year before, Robert Janes, of Toronto, alluded to the work of W. G. Bigelow on hypothermia

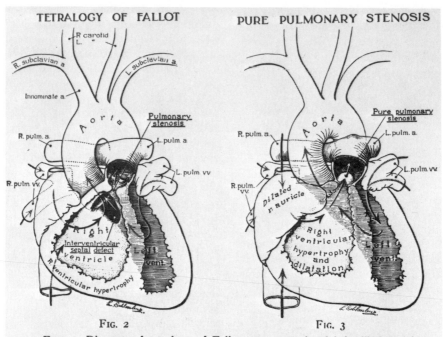

TETRALOGY OF FALLOT

PURE PULMONARY STENOSIS

FIG. 2

FIG. 3

FIG. 2.—Diagram of tetralogy of Fallot—note stenosis of infundibulum with the infundibular chamber lying between the point of stenosis and the essentially normal pulmonary valve. There is a high interventricular septal defect with overriding of the aorta.

FIG. 3.—Diagram of "pure" pulmonic stenosis—note fusion of valvular cusps to form diaphragmlike structure with small central perforation. The interventricular septum is intact and the main pulmonary artery beyond the valve is dilated. There is a greater degree of hypertrophy of the right ventricle and right auricle than is seen in the tetralogy of Fallot. Patency of the foramen ovale is not indicated, but is usually present.

The familiar drawings by Leon Schlossberg, which in sometimes more stylized form, have been classically employed ever since. In tetralogy of Fallot, where the ventricular septal defect permitted decompression of the right ventricle, Blalock preferred a systemic pulmonary anastomosis. For isolated valvar pulmonic stenosis, he agreed with Brock's direct approach. He was using Brock's knives. Potts had not yet devised his ingenious sheathed, expandable knife and dilator.

Alfred Blalock and Richard F. Kieffer, Jr., *Valvulotomy for the Relief of Congenital Valvular Pulmonic Stenosis with Intact Ventricular Septum.* Volume LXVIII, 1950.

and now, by invitation, W. G. Bigelow, J. C. Callaghan, and J. A. Hopps, *General Hypothermia for Experimental Intracardiac Surgery,* The Use of Electrophrenic Respirations, and Artificial Pacemaker for Cardiac Standstill, and Radio-Frequency Rewarming in General Hypothermia, presented their experimental material in the dog. The animals were cooled between blankets containing coils of circulating refrigerant. For artificial respiration when spontaneous respiration ceased, they employed Sarnoff's [1948] electrophrenic respiration. The cardiotomy performed was termed "a token operation". Nevertheless, the fact was that in 23 of 39 dogs a cardiotomy was performed "It has been possible at a body temperature of 20°C to exclude the heart from

the circulation for periods of 15 minutes with survival. In some of the animals during the period of exclusion the heart has been opened and then sutured." The cardiotomy was no more than an opening of the right auricle. Twenty animals, including 11 with cardiotomy, were revived to normal body temperature, and six of those survived indefinitely, the others ". . . developed a state of shock which appeared in two to 12 hours . . . characterized by a progressive fall in blood pressure with cyanosis." The cause of death was not explained. Fibrillation when it occurred, they had treated by the defibrillating technique of Hooker, Kouwenhoven, and Langworthy. They had four cases with unresponsive standstill. They used a "stimulator, with rotating potentiometer . . . to deliver impulses at any desired rate. An indifferent electrode is clipped onto the chest wall and the stimulating electrode placed in the region of the S-A node. Normal appearing heart action is observed and the heart rate is varied within limits by adjusting a dial. In two experiments the artificial pacemaker was used for ten to 15 minutes, and when it was discontinued the heart returned to standstill. In the other two animals following electrical control of the heart beat for ten and 30 minutes, normal spontaneous heart beats returned." They had used defibrillation after cardiac massage but said of their pacemaking that ". . . the possible advantages in hypothermia where the stimulating wire could be left in place during closure of chest and rewarming are obvious. Should such a technic prove worthwhile, its extension to other clinical conditions with cardiac arrest might be considered." They had used radio-diathermy rewarming.

Discussion

William L. Riker, of Chicago, rose to speak about the hypothermia at the Children's Memorial Hospital in Chicago, to which Potts had referred the year before. The patient was on a mattress filled with cold or hot water as needed. In cyanotic patients, they had attempted to keep the patient's temperature at 96° and occasionally, down to 93° for poor risk patients. Clarence Dennis, of Minneapolis, rose to mention his extracorporeal circulation, "With considerable misgivings, Mr. Chairman, in the presence of pioneers like Dr. Crafoord and Dr. Bjork and Dr. Gibbon . . ." He could pump 2800 cc. of blood per minute and, "We have been successful in opening the right ventricle of the heart, closing the ventricle, carrying the dog for half an hour on the machine, and having the dog recover", but the dogs died subsequently,- ". . . late death, such as Dr. Bigelow has observed." He seemed to think this was an enzymatic problem. Bigelow, closing, was not sure that Dennis was dealing with the same problem except that Dennis mentioned a low pH and some of Bigelow's dogs had a pH as low as 6.6.

* * *

Frank H. Lahey, of Boston, Surgeon-in-Chief, New England Baptist Hospital; Surgeon-in-Chief, New England Deaconess Hospital, and Samuel F. Marshall, Surgeon, Lahey Clinic, *Should Total Gastrectomy Be Employed in Early Carcinoma of the Stomach"*; Experience with 139 Total Gastrectomies,

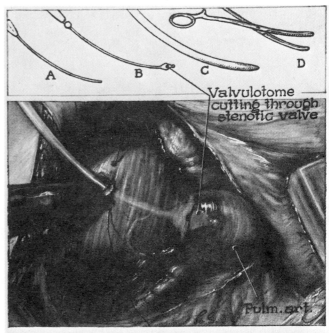

FIG. 8.—Transparency to demonstrate cutting of pulmonary valve with the flat Brock valvulotome.

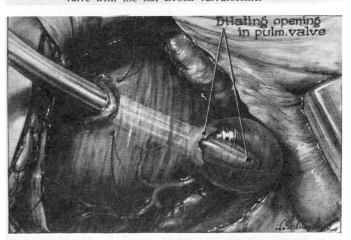

FIG. 9.—Transparency to demonstrate dilatation of previously divided pulmonary valve by passage of curved sound.

The tip of the valvulotome having found the opening in the valve, the knife was forced through. As first the knife and then the dilators were withdrawn from the heart, the operator's finger was placed over the small cardiotomy. Blalock reported 19 operations with two deaths. Three of the 19, under mistaken diagnosis of tetralogy of Fallot, had previously had systemic-pulmonary anastomoses, two at Hopkins, one elsewhere.

Alfred Blalock and Richard F. Kieffer, Jr., *Valvulotomy for the Relief of Congenital Valvular Pulmonic Stenosis with Intact Ventricular Septum.* Volume LXVIII, 1950.

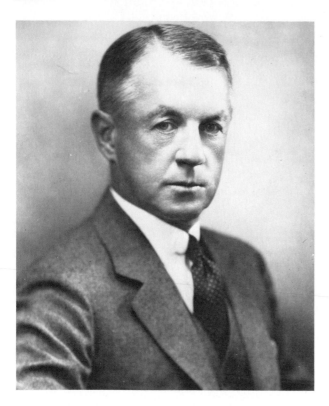

Frank H. Lahey (c. 1950) 1880-1953, President of the AMA, 1941-42. M.D. Harvard, 1904. Hospital training at the Long Island (Massachusetts) Hospital, Boston City Hospital and Haymarket Square Relief Station, four years in all. He held teaching positions at Harvard for brief periods wide apart and was Professor of Clinical Surgery, 1923-24; holding ranks up to Professor at Tufts. He had a huge experience in surgery and great skill,- with a particular interest in surgery of the thyroid, the common duct and the gastrointestinal tract. A forceful, dogmatic, colorful speaker, backed up by impressive statistics, and clear exposition, he could be remarkably convincing. The very successful Lahey Clinic, one of the great private clinics, he created in Boston in an atmosphere that was at the least not supportive of his efforts. The *"Surgical Practice of the Lahey Clinic"* was a resident's bible of surgery in its day.

Portrait courtesy of the Lahey Clinic Foundation, Boston, Massachusetts.

said that until recently total gastrectomy had been performed ". . . in cases in which the cancer of the stomach was too advanced to be completely removed by partial gastrectomy." The first total gastrectomy at the Lahey Clinic had been done in 1927. In 1938, Lahey had reported eight, with three postoperative deaths, and in 1944, a total of 73, with a 33% mortality. They had now done 139 total gastrectomies, 127 for malignant tumors of the stom-

ach, and 12 for benign gastric ulcer. From January, 1944, to March, 1950, they had done 64 total gastrectomies with six deaths,- 9.4% operative mortality, and one death in a group of 12 total gastrectomies for ulcer,- 8.3% mortality, so that ". . . the mortality of total gastrectomy can be brought within the same range as partial gastrectomy . . . The mortality of partial gastrectomy for malignant disease of the stomach from 1937 to July 1949 was 9.2 per cent." Welch and Allen had reported only a 20% five-year survival rate after subtotal gastrectomy for cancer, and Lahey's survival was 22.3%. Marshall thought ". . . total gastrectomy for cancer, when compared with other radical operations for cancer, does more satisfactorily fulfill the requirements of radical removal of the lesions and the adjacent nodes than does subtotal gastrectomy." As to whether the approach was to be transthoracic or transabdominal, if there was any argument about extension above the diaphragm, the approach should be transthoracic, ". . . and when the esophagus can be demonstrated as free, we prefer the abdominal route." The tumor was rarely operable if the total gastrectomy could not be done from below. The duodenum was to be resected well down toward the common duct because of the frequency of submucosal spread of the cancer. All of the gastrohepatic omentum was to be removed, the spleen and frequently a portion of pancreas. They preferred anastomosis of the esophagus to a jejunal loop with a long entero-enterostomy. In their total of 127 patients they had 31 postoperative deaths, 12 patients were alive five years or longer, and 21% had lived three years or longer.

Discussion

Arthur W. Allen, of Boston, thought the mortality of Lahey and Marshall in their most recent cases would not soon be matched by ". . . the average surgeon in this country . . ." In addition, he was concerned about the postgastrectomy state in the patients who succumbed a year or two after operation without recurrence of tumor. As for recurrence, when he and Claude Welch had reviewed the figures quoted from Massachusetts General Hospital, looking to see whether total gastrectomy might be indicated, they found the patients died of recurrence which occurred in areas which would not have been touched by total gastrectomy. So that in the main, their message was one of caution, "Although the salvage rate in this group of patients is only 21 per cent of those who could be subjected to resection—and it might very well be elevated to some extent by total gastrectomy—we feel at the moment that the morbidity and mortality associated with total gastrectomy may offset this radical attack." Owen H. Wangensteen, of Minnesota, mentioned his second-look operation for lymph node metastases which might have escaped unnoticed at the first operation. He had mentioned this the year before at the meeting of the Association, "The extirpation of cancer is very much like the eradication of quack grass. You cannot do a complete and thorough job in one sitting. When the field is surveyed a few weeks after the initial effort, surviving quack grass sprouts can be seen here and there still. And so it is, too, in the lymph node positive cancer cases." They had done second-look operations in 16 colon and rectal cancer patients, and third-looks in two patients, "One of these now is negative; I regard her as cured; the other is still positive. We already have her permission for a fourth 'second-look.' The residual cancer in both these patients was finally concentrated in a few peri-aortic lymph nodes." Joseph E. Strode, of Hawaii, with his large experience with gastric carcinoma in the Japanese, was aggressive about cancer of the stomach. In his series "the subtotal gastric resections had a mortality of 16.5 per cent, and in 21 total gastrectomies the mortality was 10.5 per cent." Philip R. Allison, of Leeds, England, spoke of the anatomy of the lymphatics and the necessity for removing as well "The cellular tissue between the viscus and the lymphatic glands . . . the body of the pancreas and the spleen with the retro-peritoneal tissue on the under aspect of the diaphragm . . ." He preferred reconstruction by the Roux principle to avoid pancreatic and bile reflux and resultant esophagitis, and because it could be done at any height in the mediastinum. Lahey closed. Dr. Allen was "largely right regarding difficulties in feeding these patients . . .", but Lahey did not feel quite as pessimistic. They had still been performing the operation only for patients too far advanced for subtotal gastrectomy, "It is probably going to require courage to do a total gastrectomy in the case of small gastric malignancies. On the other hand, we are never going to find out . . . whether or not this more aggressive and radical surgical approach to the problem is a wise one until we accumulate some data as to whether or not these procedures will improve on the one which is now so unsatisfactory, subtotal gastrectomy."

* * *

Lester R. Dragstedt, of Chicago, Professor of Surgery and Chairman, Department of Surgery, University of Chicago, and by invitation, Edward R. Woodward, Edward H. Storer, Harry A. Oberhelman, Jr., and Curtis A. Smith, *Quantitative Studies on the Mechanism of Gastric Secretion in Health and Disease,* presented one of the classic papers on gastric secretion with which Dragstedt and his laboratory had begun to enrich the surgical literature. They concluded from many experiments with vagotomy, with innumerable techniques of transplanting or extrapolating the antrum, etc., that "Complete division of the vagus nerve supply to the isolated stomach of dogs reduces the output of hydrochloric acid by an average of 76 per cent . . . Complete removal of the antrum of the stomach in Pavlov pouch dogs decreases the output of hydrochloric acid from the pouch by an average of 86 per cent . . . Removal of one-half or two-thirds of the antrum does not decrease the secretion of gastric juice in Pavlov pouch dogs, but subsequent removal of the remnant produces a marked decrease in secretion. Exclusion of the antrum of the stomach in Pavlov pouch dogs, by a method resembling that of Finsterer and Devine, produces no reduction in pouch secretion in 50 per cent of cases . . . Exteriorization of the antrum of the stomach so that it does not come in contact with food produces a decrease in secretion comparable to that secured by antrum resection . . . Transplantation of the antrum of the stomach into the colon as a diverticulum causes a persistent hypersecretion of gastric juice from the Pavlov pouch . . . the antrum of the stomach accounts for the gastric phase of secretion . . . its mucous membrane is highly specific in function and differs in this respect from that of the fundus or intestines. The data are in harmony with the view that the antrum is an internal secreting organ which elaborates a powerful gastric stimulant (the gastrin of Edkins) when it comes into contact with food or products of digestion . . ."

* * *

The symposium on peptic ulcer disease was continued by J. William Hinton, of New York, Professor of Surgery, New York University (Postgraduate Medical School); Chairman, Department of Surgery, Postgraduate Medical School of New York University, *The Evaluation of End Results in Physiologic versus Pathologic Operative Procedures for Chronic Duodenal Ulcer during the Past Two Decades.* Hinton reviewed his changing view of the operative treatment of ulcer from the 1920's when "it was our feeling that gastroenterostomy was a very satisfactory operation for a chronic duodenal ulcer, even though Lewisohn had reported 34 per

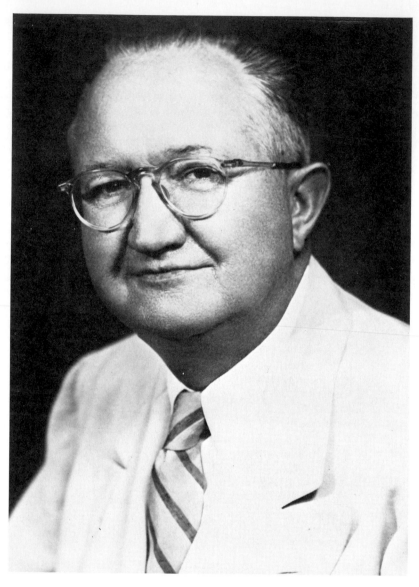

Lester Dragstedt (c. 1950) 1893-1975. M.D. Rush, 1921. Dragstedt was Professor and Chairman of the Department of Pharmacology and Physiology at Northwestern University, when in 1925 at the age of 32, he went with Phemister to the new Department of Surgery at the University of Chicago as Associate Professor of Surgery, receiving his surgical training "on the job" eventually succeeding Phemister in the chair and continuing the tradition of a Department of Surgery with a heavy orientation toward laboratory investigation. It is not likely that any surgical contemporary made more, more lasting or more important contributions to the physiological understanding of pancreatic function and gastric secretion. His innumerable experimental preparations with gastric pouches, transplanted antral pouches, rearrangements of sequence of entrance of secretions into the alimentary canal have all become standard. His written and oral presentations were models of lucidity and simplicity and his personality that of "a man too nice to be a surgeon." His clear separation of antral-gastrin and vagal stimulation of gastric acid secretion and the numerous overlapping, dove-tailing, reinforcing experiments led him to laboratory and clinical demonstration of the value of vagal resection in the treatment of duodenal ulcers, which produced a major revolution in gastric surgery. He "retired" from Chicago to join E. R. Woodward, his old resident, pupil, and collaborator, at the University of Florida in Gainesville, directing a productive laboratory until his death 16 years later and stimulating another generation of students, house officers and research fellows.

Portrait courtesy of Edward R. Woodward, Gainesville, Florida.

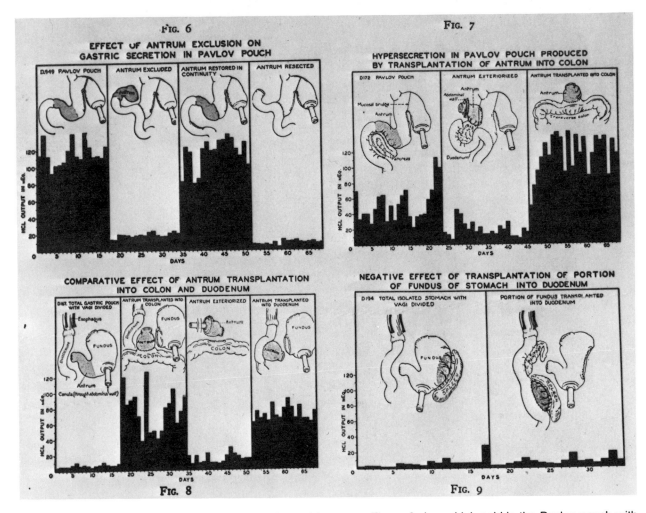

FIG. 6

EFFECT OF ANTRUM EXCLUSION ON
GASTRIC SECRETION IN PAVLOV POUCH

FIG. 7

HYPERSECRETION IN PAVLOV POUCH PRODUCED
BY TRANSPLANTATION OF ANTRUM INTO COLON

COMPARATIVE EFFECT OF ANTRUM TRANSPLANTATION
INTO COLON AND DUODENUM

NEGATIVE EFFECT OF TRANSPLANTATION OF PORTION
OF FUNDUS OF STOMACH INTO DUODENUM

FIG. 8

FIG. 9

Illustration characteristic of those which Dragstedt used for years. Figure 6 shows high acid in the Pavlov pouch with the antrum intact, low with the antrum by-passed, high again when the antrum was restored with gastroduodenal continuity, and finally low again when the antrum was completely resected. Figure 7, showing in the third compartment the extreme hypersecretion in the Pavlov pouch produced by the transplantation of the antrum into the colon, was one of Dragstedt's classic preparations.

Lester R. Dragstedt, Edward R. Woodward, Edward H. Storer, Harry A. Oberhelman, Jr., and Curtis A. Smith, *Quantitative Studies on the Mechanism of Gastric Secretion in Health and Disease.* Volume LXVIII, 1950.

cent gastrojejunal ulcers in 1925 and Berg of the same hospital [Mount Sinai] was advocating subtotal resections exclusively for chronic duodenal ulcer." However, in 1935, Hinton had found, with a four-and-a-half-year follow-up of 79 patients, a 16.5% incidence of anastomotic ulcer, and by 1940, with a 7.1 year follow-up, in 106 gastroenterostomies, the incidence was 24.5%. They had abandoned gastroenterostomy in January, 1933, and from 1933 to 1945 they had performed subtotal gastrectomy. As the title would suggest, he distinguished between the benefits of operation conferred by "altered phys-

iology" and those achieved by "correcting the pathology". This latter meant to him resection of the ulcer, "To us it seemed essential to remove the duodenal ulcer from the adherent viscus, in most instances, the pancreas." Resection of the ulcer was important to prevent ". . . continuation of the disease process in the pancreas . . ." In 162 cases of chronic duodenal ulcer undergoing subtotal gastrectomy, all of them with removal of the ulcer, his mortality was 3.7%. One gastrojejunal ulcer was proved, and two suspected, and 90% of the patients had excellent results over an average follow-up of 3.8 years.

956

Vagotomy had entered into their operative plans from 1945 to 1948, being performed as the sole operation in 35 patients with chronic duodenal ulcer, and in association with subtotal gastrectomy in 58 cases. They had performed 35 transthoracic vagotomies for duodenal ulcer, with four deaths, all from cardiorespiratory problems. The results were considered satisfactory only in 11,- 35%,- with six failures because of continued or recurrent ulcers sometimes requiring gastrectomy. Since July, 1948, they had "reverted to sub-total resection with removal of the ulcer in toto in all chronic intractable ulcers." They performed an antecolic Polya, shortloop anastomosis. Dumping and diarrhea, common after vagotomy in their hands, were essentially not seen without vagotomy. In further discussing the advantage of resection of the ulcer, Hinton discussed the question of the massive bleeder uncontrolled by transfusions of 2,500 to 5,000 cc. of blood. He had operated on 27 such, one gastric ulcer, two gastrojejunal ulcers, and 24 posterior duodenal ulcers with six deaths, a mortality of 22%, none of the survivors having bled again.

* * *

Francis D. Moore, of Boston, now Surgeon-in-Chief, Peter Bent Brigham Hospital; Moseley Professor of Surgery, Harvard Medical School, and five associates, *The Effect of Definitive Surgery on Duodenal Ulcer Disease,* A Comparative Study of Surgical and Non-Surgical Management in 997 cases, presented a rather unusual statistical analysis of 1,246 patients seen over four years at the Massachusetts General Hospital. Although stating that "it is common knowledge that duodenal ulcer is a life-long recurrent disease, and although this statement is repeatedly made in the literature, there are surprisingly few facts available which prove that any form of treatment has altered this life-long history", they nevertheless were analyzing patients with a maximum follow-up of four years and with useful follow-up data in only 80%. The thrust of their study was that "The concept of 'progressive' or 'virulent' duodenal ulcer disease emerges as expressing the outstanding feature of that fraction of the ulcer population who do poorly without definitive surgery . . . The occurrence of a past perforation with present symptoms, and acute hemorrhage, progressive pain under a physician's care at home, or onset at the extremes of life in male patients are clues to this diagnosis. The mortality from hemorrhage, perforation and late obstruction in non-operated patients appears to balance the intrinsic hospital mortality of

definitive surgery . . . Following definitive surgery only half as many patients have an unsatisfactory result in symptomatic or economic terms as do those managed without surgery." In the face of what they termed " 'progressive virulent ulcer disease'. . . Our data indicate that subtotal gastrectomy should be undertaken" [although Moore had recently been writing enthusiastically about vagotomy]. They recognized that this course could be followed conscientiously ". . . only when the surgical skill and facilities are available to permit performance of subtotal gastrectomy with an acceptable mortality."

* * *

John D. Stewart, of Buffalo, Professor of Surgery and Chairman of the Department, University of Buffalo; Head of the Department of Surgery, and three associates, *The Definitive Treatment of Bleeding Peptic Ulcer,* reported again on the study which had been presented at an earlier stage two years previously. They had now had 65 patients with massive bleeding, ". . . of such severity as to lower the total circulating red cell mass to less than 60 per cent of normal." They had operated upon 65 such patients now with seven deaths, 10.7%, and another 42 had refused operation, with nine deaths, 21.4%. Just as they were becoming more and more convinced of the need for operations so were referring physicians who ". . . are coming to share our viewpoint, for fewer and fewer cases are available to us for control study without operation." In the last 50 cases operated upon, the mortality rate was 6%. While their protocol described almost immediate operation, in fact "The average interval between admission and operation for the group as a whole was 12 hours, but in some instances operation was begun within two hours." The case material, the findings, and the results were much as they had been in the earlier report, and they ended with ". . . the conviction that early gastric resection offers the best results in the treatment of acute massive hemorrhage from peptic ulcer, provided proper surgical and transfusion facilities are at hand. The method is definitive in that anemia can be corrected, bleeding can be arrested, and the tendency to form new peptic ulcers can be controlled." The operation was an 80% gastrectomy. They always removed a gastric ulcer and removed about two-thirds of the duodenal ulcers, performing a Hofmeister short loop antecolic anastomosis.

* * *

Ralph F. Bowers, Chief of Surgery, Veterans Administration, Medical Teaching Group; Chief,

Surgical Service, Kennedy VA Hospital, Memphis, and by invitation, N. E. Rosett, *Bleeding Peptic Ulcer*, Favorable Results by Conservative Treatment, treated 171 patients with bleeding ulcer, 150 "proved", by combined medical and surgical therapy. The patients were put to bed, sedated, given a Meulengracht-type diet, alkali, psychotherapy, and transfusion, and decision for early operation made in the first 48 hours. Twenty-four were operated upon in all, only two in the first day, the others nine days to four months later. Bowers [who might have seemed radical in his proposal a year earlier for hindquarter and forequarter amputations for melanoma] was much less agressive in the treatment of bleeding ulcer. A considerable number of the patients bled massively, but they had only two deaths in the entire group, one patient who bled for six days and died as operation was being arranged for her, and the second patient after operation on the 27th day for a large gastric ulcer, who died of peritonitis, "Suture lines were intact." They considered their version of combined therapy ". . . as a satisfactory method of treatment—at least for the type of patients presently being admitted to Kennedy Hospital."

Discussion

The Discussion of the papers on ulcer disease was begun by Constantine J. MacGuire, of New York, whose experience was in another division of Bellevue Hospital than that in which Hinton's work had been done. They had over the years modified their philosophy much as he had, ". . . but we disagreed very strongly with him on one feature of his work, and that was the removal in toto, of a duodenal ulcer. We have not found this practical . . . The resident surgeons . . . are doing almost all of these operations on the general service, and I think our advice to them must be carefully considered. To advise them to resect all duodenal ulcers would be very disastrous. Incidentally, our mortality at Bellevue, as gone over by Dr. [Robert] Wylie recently, showed that in the last ten years it has been 2.6 per cent. In the early years it was 18 to 20 per cent." Howard A. Patterson, of the Roosevelt Hospital, said their experience was more like that of Dr. Stewart than that of Dr. Bowers. They operated in about "one massive bleeder in three . . ." and felt that "the age of the patient has been emphasized too much, and that the age of the lesion has not been emphasized enough . . . an old lesion in a young person will bleed about as stubbornly as a young lesion in an older person." In the last 31 promptly undertaken operations, they

had had two deaths, one of them in a known hemophiliac. Warren H. Cole, of Chicago, agreed with Bowers that as far as the mortality rates in the literature were concerned, the nonoperative treatment was better than the operative treatment, but in spite of Bower's ". . . very convincing presentation, I am still not quite convinced, and up to date I am operating on at least some of the patients with massive bleeding from duodenal ulcers." He operated if a patient's blood pressure was still not restored in six to ten hours. He warned against mere ". . . ligation of an adjacent large artery . . ." to stop the bleeding without formal gastrectomy. He cited no overall figures from his experience. John R. Paine, of Buffalo, added the factor of blood matching and the Rh factor, pointing out that if a patient had not been previously transfused one could give him Rh positive blood, as much as one wished for 72 hours, when the patient became sensitized, "Try to have the issue settled, the surgery over, or, if the medical people insist on keeping the patient, make them promise to have the patient stop bleeding within 72 hours." Frank H. Lahey, of Boston, returned to the question of resection of the duodenal ulcer which he insisted upon, ". . . not because leaving the ulcer does any harm, but because in so many of the cases it is not possible to do a safe inversion of the duodenum without removing the ulcer." Nevertheless, the duodenal stump might create difficult problems and "The mortality of subtotal gastrectomy for duodenal ulcer is not related to the subtotal gastrectomy. It is related to the duodenum, particularly in the technical difficulties of removing duodenal ulcers and obtaining good closure of the duodenal stump when the duodenal ulcer is not removed." He devoted most of his long discussion to describing the difficulties with the duodenal stump, problems with the common duct, etc. No one had discussed Dr. Dragstedt's paper. In his closing, Dragstedt returned to one of his preparations in which ulcers could be produced in animals with totally isolated stomachs with the vagus intact, never with the vagus divided. He was persuaded of "the old dictum, 'No acid, no ulcer'. . . Does that also mean, 'Some acid, some ulcer'? Obviously, it does not." Dragstedt was obviously upset, having misunderstood [he was hard of hearing and wore a hearing aid] Hinton as having called subtotal gastrectomy a "physiologic" procedure. "I think it is clear now that the secretory abnormality in duodenal ulcer patients is a hypersecretion of gastric juice in the fasting stomach, and an excessive response of the fundic mucosa to the normal stimuli of gastric secretion, gastrin, food, alcohol, or histamine . . . Since the major pathogenic factor in duodenal ulcer is hypersecretion, and since this hypersecretion is of cephalic or nervous origin—it is not of antrum origin, nor of intestinal origin—then the argument is clear that the physiologic operation for duodenal ulcer is either a vagotomy or the administration of a drug like Banthine, which depresses the nervous phase of secretion. Gastroenterostomy should be coupled with vagotomy to simplify postoperative management and lessen gastric stasis. I cannot imagine how one can call resection of the stomach a physiologic procedure." Hinton, closing, reemphasized the need for resecting the ulcer. Francis D. Moore on the other hand said ". . . there is no correlation whatsoever in our group between the result and whether or not the duodenal ulcer is left in, but there is a very high correlation between the result and whether or not all of the antral mucous membrane has been taken out. We believe that there is confusion in the literature on this important point [translation: "We believe Dr. Hinton is confused on this point"]." John D. Stewart, in closing, thought it not unreasonable that there were different approaches and almost certainly there were different spectra of case material. He pointed out that the careful measurements which he made of blood volume, hemoglobin, etc., ought to be matched in other series, if they were to be compared with his.

* * *

John C. Hawk, Jr., and Walter F. Becker, by invitation, and Edwin P. Lehman, of Charlottesville, Virginia, Professor of Surgery and Gynecology, University of Virginia School of Medicine; Chief Surgeon, University of Virginia Hospital, *Acute Appendicitis—III*, An Analysis of One Thousand and Three Cases, reviewed their experience from 1943 to 1948 comparing it with the experience from 1933 to 1937 when they had 1,069 cases of acute appendicitis. They divided their cases into those with simple acute appendicitis, those with a contaminated pertoneum, those with localized peritonitis, and those with diffuse peritonitis. For simple appendicitis their mortality was 0.24%, as it had been in the earlier period. In localized peritonitis, mortality had dropped from 5% to zero. For diffuse peritonitis it had dropped from 40.6% to 7.5%. The mortality for the entire group had dropped from 3.27% to 0.8%. So far as their numbers went, the mortality in diffuse peritonitis with the conservative treatment, operation being withheld, the patient being treated expectantly, given antibiotics, etc., was 13.3%, and with immediate operation was 6.15%, but only 13 patients had been treated conservatively.

Discussion

Thomas H. Lanman, of Boston, presented the Children's Hospital series of 836 cases of acute appendicitis still running 50% or 60% ruptured. Since 1944 they had had 588 consecutive cases of appendicitis with no deaths, all operated upon soon after admission. "We, therefore, feel it is important that we discard in our teaching the so-called 'waiting policy,' and we think it is particularly important to discard that teaching in . . . cases . . . in which there is a diffuse peritonitis."

* * *

Henry Doubilet, by invitation, and John H. Mulholland, of New York, George David Stewart Professor of Surgery, Chairman of Department, New York University College of Medicine; Director, 3rd Surgical Division, Bellevue Hospital, *Surgical Treatment of Calcification of the Pancreas,* returned to the subject which they had discussed before the Association two years before. Of the 73 patients with proved pancreatitis, whom they had treated by section of the sphincter of Oddi, four had roentgenographic evidence of calcification of the gland. A sphincterotomy was performed in each, with relief of symptoms. Their conclusions were simple and reassuring, "Calcification of the pancreas occurs as an occasional incident in the development of chronic pancreatitis. Pain, if present, will be abolished, and recurrent severe attacks of pancreatitis prevented, by section of the sphincter of Oddi. This simple procedure will arrest the progress of the disease, and salvage the residual external and internal pancreatic function."

Discussion

Lester R. Dragstedt, of Chicago, opened the Discussion. He, too, referred to the work of Opie and Archibald and the effect of the reflux of bile into the pancreas upon the production of pancreatitis. Dragstedt had performed transduodenal spincterotomy twice for recurrent attacks of acute pancreatitis, with relief, and he agreed "In all probability, in most—possibly not all—cases of pancreatitis, there is a reflux of bile into the pancreas, and the favorable results reported by the earlier surgeons from external drainage of the common bile duct, it seems to me, are in harmony with that point of view." Ralph F. Bowers, of Memphis, said that he had achieved the same results in four cases of pancreatitis, one with calcification, by transecting the common duct and performing a choledochojejunostomy en Roux-Y. "All four patients have had brilliant recoveries . . ." Robert Elman, of St. Louis, had also performed transduodenal sphincterotomy several times with satisfaction. Owen H. Wangensteen, as he said, rose ". . . only to relate the observations and thinking of some of my associates on this problem." Logan Leven had ". . . described the observation of regurgitation of Lipiodol into the pancreatic duct during cholangiography . . ." Dr. Carter Howell had demonstrated with a T-tube in the common duct, that if contrast medium was injected into the pancreatic duct, an elevation of the blood amylase resulted in 35 patients, but never when the pancreatic duct was not demonstrated. Dr. Lyle Hay had in two cases "implanted the severed duct of Wirsung into the duodenum at a lower level. These people have had complete relief of their pain and have not had recurrent attacks of pancreatitis."

* * *

Howard K. Gray, of Rochester, Professor of Surgery, Mayo Foundation; Head of a Section in Surgery, Mayo Clinic, and by invitation, Frank B. Whitesell, Jr., *Hemorrhage from Esophageal Varices, Surgical Management*, in three patients added truncal vagotomy to another operation for portal hypertension. There were three principal techniques available to deal with portal hypertension, splenectomy which reduced the portal flow by 25% to 40% and interrupted some of the collateral circulation, destruction of the varices by injection or by distal esophagectomy, and finally ". . . decompression of existing varices by shifting the circulatory burden to the inferior vena cava or one of its tributaries (portacaval shunts, Talma-Morison operation, and so forth)." They added vagotomy in three patients,- whose anatomical situation was unsuitable for a splenorenal anastomosis,- in one, also stripping the veins from the lower end of the esophagus, in another, performing a splenectomy and devascularizing eight centimeters of the esophagus, in this patient adding posterior gastroenterostomy to the vagotomy, and in the third, performing splenectomy, devascularizing the esophagus and adding posterior gastroenterostomy to the vagotomy. The patients had not bled in the succeeding 14, 11, and five months, respectively. They thought this the first attempt, ". . . to prevent the possibility of mucosal erosion in the region of varices caused by regurgitation of gastric acid chyme . . ."

Discussion

Louis M. Rousselot, of New York, [who had been a member of Dr. Whipple's spleen clinic] said that since hypersplenism was present ". . . in nearly all the cases . . . It is our opinion that any surgical procedure which does not include splenectomy as a part of the procedure is, therefore, irrational. Furthermore, all cases will not necessarily need a shunting procedure." Nathan A. Womack, the Secretary, then at the University of Iowa, had operated upon five cirrhotic patients with massive variceal hemorrhage, performing esophagogastrectomy and splenectomy. One patient died in the hospital of cirrhosis; another, a child with juvenile cirrhosis died a year later of hepatic insufficiency; the other three had been well 14 to 23 months. Mr. Philip R. Allison, of Leeds, said that ". . . try as I may (and it isn't from lack of endeavor), I have never yet heard at a meeting or seen in any literature a description of esophageal varices seen through the esophagoscope before operation, and described as seen through the esophagoscope after operation." Diagnosis and further course were so variable that the mere fact that a patient was alive a year or two after operation proved nothing. He had "been working along the lines of devascularizing the esophagus from the upper end of the stomach, taking great care to leave intact the vast network of collaterals extending up the mediastinum outside the esophagus . . . I find that it is quite possible to divide every vessel going in and out of the esophagus from the left main bronchus down to the cardia, and to divide every mesenteric vessel going in and out of the upper half of the stomach, and to divide the muscle layers of the esophagus and sever the longitudinal submucous veins going into it, and suture the muscle wall again, and all this without sloughing of the esophagus . . . and as far as my esophagoscopic observations go, up to now, that is the only thing which has produced any really appreciable diminution in the size of these varices . . ." Emile Holman, [in what may have been the first mention of an operation for splenic transposition] said "Several years ago it was demonstrated that we could ligate the portal vein in dogs completely only if we first provided a collateral circulation. This collateral circulation was developed by implanting the spleen, following scarification of its surface, in the lateral abdominal wall in a small peritoneal pocket, and by completely dividing the splenic artery. This reversed the flow of blood in the splenic vein, shunting portal blood into the spleen and thence into the collateral bed of the abdominal wall. This operation has been applied successfully in two patients, one with ascites, and in a patient of 27 who had had many hemorrhages from esophageal varices. The spleen, twice normal size, was implanted in the lateral wall four years ago and the splenic artery ligated. There have been no hemorrhages since." Gray, in closing, referred to the fact that Rienhoff had been ligating the hepatic artery for portal hypertension [as had Berman, of Indianapolis], as close to the celiac axis as possible" and had done it in three cases which had no bleeding since, and in four cases for ascites with clearance of the ascites in all four.

The Business Meetings

The 1950 meeting, April 19, 20, and 21, was held at the Broadmoor Hotel, Colorado Springs, Thomas G. Orr in the Chair.

The Advisory Membership Committee, still reviewing the "master list of possible candidates." (there were 95 men on their list who had not yet been proposed for membership) were fearful that there were other names which should have been on the master list. [It is quite clear that Arthur W. Allen, Chairman, and his consultants had taken the initiative to seek out the names of promising candidates.]

In 1948, there had been appointed a committee on the role of the surgeon in undergraduate medical education consisting of Oliver Cope, Chairman, M. E. DeBakey, Daniel C. Elkin, Robert M. Janes, Carl A. Moyer, and Philip B. Price. The Committee thought there had been very little change in the undergraduate medical curriculum in 50 years except for ". . . the accretion of a number of specialty departments." They thought there was ". . . a need for experimentation in medical education." The present curriculum was too rigid, there was insufficient exchange between preclinical and clinical science, the curriculum was too crowded, "Special interests occupy too much of the time . . . Emphasis in teaching should be more on the human and less on the experimental animal. Increasing use of men trained in restricted fields of laboratory science as teachers of medical science is to be regretted." There were too few surgical teachers and the budgets of surgical departments needed support, "Intellectual opportunities must be afforded the younger surgeons to entice them into teaching careers."

The reports of the representatives to the various Specialty Boards, often routinely accepted, were spiced this time by Isaac A. Bigger's report that the American Board of Obstetrics and Gynecology had disqualified GYN residency programs in those hospitals in which gynecology was a subservice or subdivision of surgery.

Leo Eloesser asked for a fuller discussion of Specialty Boards, complaining of the likelihood of "certification for an external hemorrhoidal specialist, or for a superior rectal specialist . . ."

Deryl Hart said that the Boards were being used "for political propagandizing, or pressures to be brought on people", speaking particularly of anesthesia.

At the Second Executive Session, the Secretary reported that the Council had expressed itself in opposition to both the proposed amendments,- requiring a nine-tenths favorable vote for new members and requiring the Secretary to make available the list of candidates passed by the Council for membership. It was explained in the discussion "These two amendments were suggested . . . to decrease the number of men necessary to blackball a candidate, with the provision that immediately after the Council meeting, the names of the candidates the Council is going to suggest to the Fellows to vote upon, be passed around indiscriminately to all the members." [It was explained that the "member who submitted these two changes in the Constitution and By-Laws is not at the meeting today, and cannot describe them himself."] The measures were vigorously discussed and defeated.

At the previous meeting, Frank L. Meleney had suggested that the Association go on record as favoring international control of the atomic bomb. The Council recommended this be recorded in the Minutes ". . . with the recommendation that no action be taken at the present time."

The officers for the following year were Samuel C. Harvey, of New Haven, President; Warfield M. Firor, of Baltimore, First Vice-President; John M. Foster, of Denver, Second Vice-President; and Nathan Womack, of Iowa City, Secretary.

A motion by Willis D. Gatch was approved decrying ". . . the formation of so many separate and independent boards as being contrary to the best interests of the community at large . . ."

LXIX

1951

The 1951 meeting took place in Washington, D.C., April 11, 12, and 13 at the Shoreham Hotel, in the Chair, Samuel C. Harvey, of New Haven, Professor of Surgery, (Oncology) Yale University School of Medicine; Associate Surgeon, New Haven Hospital [he had retired as Chairman of the Department of Surgery in 1947].

Among the members who had died in the preceding year were John S. Lockwood, Fred B. Lund, George J. Heuer, William DeW. Andrus, and Roy McClure.

The Korean War was in full swing, President Truman had recalled General Douglas MacArthur the day before the meeting started, and President Harvey addressed himself to *Medical Education in the Present Emergency*. The philosophy of this thoughtful man is expressed. "We consider ourselves a peaceful nation and are astonished rather than resentful at being called 'war-mongers' and 'aggressive imperialists', yet in the 175 years since the Declaration of Independence we have been engaged in seven major conflicts. Of these, two—the Spanish and Mexican wars—may have been at their inception tainted with 'imperialism' but the eventual outcome of each scarcely conforms to this description. Three—the Revolution, the War of 1812, and the War Between the States—were in a sense internecine and fought on basic issues of a constitutional nature; they would not have been totally destructive of our safety and welfare had they been decided other than

was the case. Only World Wars I and II, and this cold conflict—all three historically will probably be considered as one—involve such fundamental values that defeat would mean a total disaster, not only to our civilization but also to that of the world as a whole . . . comparable to the fall of the Roman Empire together with the disintegration of the Greek civilization, followed by one thousand years of barbarian unenlightenment and disorder—the so-called Dark Ages." He predicted correctly of the cold war, that the "conflict is not one that can be brought to a conclusion by a decisive battle or campaign, for neither side will commit itself to the issue unless it be reasonably sure of success, or is forced in desperation by an impending collapse to take the risk . . . in all probability it will be one of attrition, accompanied by limited explorations in force, both diplomatic and military . . . a prolonged contest in which the rival forms of government, of societal organization and economics, and of civilizations will be put to a lengthy and searching test." In a short and desperate war, "the deviation of all manpower and material resources" could be made up for after the war. "In a war of prolonged attrition . . . a balance must be maintained between the requirements of the armed forces and those of civilian life . . ." There was a danger that for the "production of more physicians to meet the needs of military and civilian defense . . ." medical schools might be called on to increase enrollment and reinstitute "the highly unde-

961

TRUMAN FIRES M'ARTHUR

Woman Tells Of Soliciting 'Gifts' From Job-Seekers

Senators Question Committeewoman In Mississippi Truman Faction

JACKSON, Miss., April 10 (P)—A member of the pro-Truman State Democratic Executive Committee told Senate investigators today that persons she recommended for Federal jobs were required to make "contributions" to insure their appointments.

Another former member of the State committee admitted that every contribution she party received for 18 months came from persons getting Federal jobs and that he could recall only two persons who received jobs without making contributions.

Mrs. C. A. Murphy's case members of the Senate investigations subcommittee a detailed account of patronage in Mississippi which led Senator Karl Mundt (R-S. Dak.) to remark, "This is one of the most vicious of our leaders I have ever heard of."

Another highlight witness was B. F. Beasley, former acting secretary-treasurer of the State committee who denied that the organization demanded the contributions in payment for jobs, but he admitted ...

Delay Denied In Sawyer Contempt Case

By Joseph Paull
Post Reporter

Secretary of Commerce Charles Sawyer and nine others were formally charged yesterday with civil and criminal contempt of the United States Court of Appeals.

The court action taken in the long and bitter Dollar Line litigation charges the defendants with contemptuous and contumacious acts in refusing to deliver effective possession of 92 percent of the voting stock of the American President Lines Ltd. to the Dollar interests.

Court hearing on the contempt charge is scheduled for 10:30 a.m. Thursday with all those cited instructed to be in court. Among them are Assistant Attorney General Peyton Ford, Solicitor General Philip B. Perlman and Assistant Commerce Secretary Philip J. Fleming.

The Appeals Court refused to grant a Justice Department motion to postpone the contempt action so that the case could be taken to the Supreme Court. The motion may be renewed on Thursday if it appears justified, the court said.

Allied Fire Wipes Out Chorwon

Enemy Still Holds Hwachon Reservoir Despite Furious Ground, Air Blows

TOKYO (Wednesday), April 11 (P)—Allied planes and artillery were reported today to have wiped out Chorwon, the rallying center of three Chinese Red armies in west-central Korea.

The ruined western base of the big communist triangle is 17 miles north of the 38th parallel. Its destruction was reported in a field dispatch.

But Chinese defenders of the huge Hwachon power dam at the eastern base of the triangle still clung to that hydroelectric plant today. The Reds opened some of its flood gates Monday in a futile attempt to swamp advancing American forces.

AP Correspondent Tom Bradshaw reported from the front that Allied troops last night pushed closer to the dam—third largest in Korea.

Texts of Statements On MacArthur Firing

Text of President Truman's statement that he has to relieve Gen. Douglas MacArthur of his commands:

"With deep regret I have concluded that General of the Army Douglas MacArthur is unable to give his wholehearted support to the policies of the United States Government and of the United Nations in matters pertaining to his official duties. In view of the specific responsibilities imposed upon me by the Constitution of the United States and the added responsibility which has been entrusted to me by the United Nations, I have decided that I must make a change of command in the Far East. I have, therefore, relieved General MacArthur of his commands and have designated Lieut. Gen. Matthew B. Ridgway as his successor.

"Full and vigorous debate on matters of national policy is a vital element in the constitutional system of our free democracy. It is fundamental, however, that military commanders must be governed by the policies and directives issued to them in the manner provided by our laws and Constitution. In time of crisis, this consideration is particularly compelling.

"General MacArthur's place in history as one of our greatest commanders is fully established. The Nation owes him a debt of gratitude for the distinguished and exceptional service he has rendered his country in posts of great responsibility. For that reason I repeat my regret at the necessity for the action I feel compelled to take in his case."

The text of President Truman's order to MacArthur relieving him of his commands:

Order to General MacArthur from the President

"I deeply regret that it becomes my duty as President and Commander in Chief of the United States military forces to replace you as supreme commander, Allied Powers; Commander in Chief, United Nations Command; Commander in Chief, Far East, and commanding general, U. S. Army, Far East.

"You will turn over your commands effective at once, to Lieut. Gen. Matthew B. Ridgway. You are authorized to have issued such orders as are necessary to complete desired travel to such place as you select.

"My reasons for your replacement will be made public concurrently with the delivery to you of the foregoing order and are contained in the next following message (See attached statement by the President).

The text of Secretary of Defense George C. Marshall's orders naming Ridgway to succeed MacArthur:

"Order to Lieut. Gen. Matthew B. Ridgway

"From Gen. George C. Marshall, Secretary of Defense

"The President has decided to relieve Supreme Commander and appoint you as his successor as Supreme Commander, Allied Powers; Commander in Chief, United Nations Command; Commander in Chief, Far East, and Commanding General, United States Army, Far East.

"It is realized that your presence in Korea in the immediate future is highly important, but we are sure you can make the proper distribution of your time until you can turn over active command of the Eighth Army to its new commander. For this purpose, Lieut. Gen. James A. Van Fleet is enroute to report to you for such duties as you may direct."

Wheeler, Niles Say They Tried To Aid Dawson

By The Associated Press

White House Aide David K. Niles and former Senator Burton K. Wheeler identified themselves yesterday as the men who made moves interpreted by Senator Tobey (R., N. H.) as an effort to interfere in the RFC investigation.

Each of the two interviewed separately, said all that really happened was that word went to Tobey through Wheeler that Donald Dawson another White House official is a good guy and the Senatorial investigators ought to go easy on him. Both denied there was any effort to apply pressure.

Senator Tobey said at a news conference last night however that the way he interpreted it—the White House palace guard tried to interfere in a Senate investigation.

He said he considers Wheeler's remark "simply that of a man relaying a message" that he is not resentful against the former Senator.

But he said of the reported role of Niles in arranging the call from Wheeler:

"I thought the thing irregular and improper, so I went before the subcommittee and told the story."

Senator Fulbright (D. Ark.) chairman of the Banking subcommittee said that Wheeler had told this story at a secret meeting Monday.

Wheeler said the "go easy" suggestion was meant to apply to the way Dawson should be dealt with as a witness. The inquiry on the assumption that he would testify.

President Cites Three Phases Of Gen. M'Arthur's Non-Support

By Alfred Friendly
Post Reporter

Concurrently with the President's order relieving General MacArthur of command in the Far East the White House issued early this morning a series of documents that then hitherto of the highest secrecy throwing light on the background of steady and growing conflict between Washington and Tokyo.

They were of three main categories.

The first beginning with a presidential directive of last December 6 had to do with the White House orders for a minimum of public statements on the policies. The message to MacArthur bluntly reminded him of the December directive the implication that he had breached it was clear.

The second series related to efforts by Washington to MacArthur that the Administration did not support his desire to permit an enlargement of the war in Korea beyond the 38th parallel. MacArthur this time was cleared for any advance north of the 38th parallel.

McFarland Signals Speedup Hoping for August Recess

By Robert C. Albright
Post Reporter

Senate Democratic leaders today recommended an extension of all Price Control Act which expires at the end of June. Legislation to permit it in ...

Failure to Support Policy Given as Reason for Action; Ridgway, Van Fleet Named

President Truman has relieved Gen. Douglas MacArthur of his commands in the Far East for being unable to give his full sympathy to the Government's foreign policy.

He has named Lieut. Gen. Matthew B. Ridgway to succeed him.

The sensational announcement was made at the White House at 1 o'clock this morning by Press Secretary Joseph Short.

Col. S. H. Huff of MacArthur's Staff said in Tokyo the general had no prior knowledge of the Truman announcement.

President Truman notified MacArthur that the fact been believed in a direct message to the Far East commander sent over the military network.

It was daylight in Tokyo when the announcement was made here.

"Deep Regret" Expressed

Mr. Truman in his statement "with deep regret" that "General of the Army, Douglas MacArthur is unable to give his wholehearted support to the policies of the United States Government and of the United Nations in matters pertaining to his official duties.

The President said that in view of the responsibilities imposed upon him by the Constitution and the added responsibility entrusted to him by the United Nations.

"I have decided that I must make a change of command in the Far East. I have, therefore, relieved General MacArthur of his commands and have designated Lieut. Gen. Matthew B. Ridgway as his successor."

Secretary of Defense Marshall's orders to Mr. Truman, directed General Ridgway to turn over his command of the Eighth Army to Lieut. Gen. James A. Van Fleet.

Mr. Truman said that full and vigorous debate on national policies was a vital element in our free democracy. But it was fundamental he said that military commanders must be governed by the policies and directives issued to them in the manner provided by our laws and Constitution.

"In time of crisis" he said "this consideration is particularly compelling.

One of Greatest

Mr. Truman concluded his statement by saying that MacArthur's place in history as one of our greatest commanders is fully established. He said the Nation owed him a debt of gratitude and reprinted his feeling of regret that he had to relieve him.

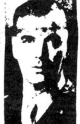

DOUGLAS MacArthur
... loses command

MATTHEW B. RIDGWAY
... succeeds MacArthur

J. A. Van Fleet
... succeeds Ridgway

News Strikes Tokyo Like Thunderclap

TOKYO (Wednesday), April 11—President Truman's removal of General MacArthur struck this headquarters like a thunderclap today.

The news broke here in a broadcast over the Armed Forces radio.

MacArthur himself was at his luxurious Embassy residence for his customary afternoon rest. He was not immediately available.

Officers received it with evident bitterness and sadness. MacArthur's staff has been working to lead to him and his views.

"If the President does that," said one officer "he will lose the men too and then some."

There was no indication whether the general himself would issue a statement on his removal.

See CONGRESS, Page 3, Column 3   See HISTORY, Page 5, Column 1   MacARTHUR, Page 8, Col. 4   See NILES, Page 11, Column 4

Congress Behind Schedule

Today's Index

sirable and accelerated program adopted in the late war." At the same time that the military were clamoring for more physicians, there were to be taken into consideration "those who have seen in the provision of more doctors, a method for lowering the cost of medical care, the thesis being that as practice becomes more competitive more services will be provided at lower cost . . . one of those economic generalizations which disregards the factor of quality and the psychology of the producer and consumer alike." He thought it was interesting that in World War II "Around 25 per cent of the physicians were in the armed forces. There is no statistical evidence that the health of the civilian population suffered perceptively . . . Undoubtedly there was a certain amount of delay and unpleasantness . . . and less consideration of trivial and inconsequential complaints, but in the serious illnesses seen in hospital practice there was no memorable depreciation of medical care." The fact that the present war was a limited one, that the physician-troop ratio could be lower because there were not so many theaters of operation and such masses of troops in long journeys, should make the present military requirements lower and it had been an experience of World War II that "there came about a 'stock-piling' of physicians, a very considerable number of whom were not active or engaged in professional work." He thought the ratio of physicians to troops could be dropped from the 6.5 per thousand of World War II to 3.3 per thousand for this time and the National Security Resources Board had, in fact, recommended a ratio of 3.7 per thousand. In spite of that, increased medical school enrollment and acceleration of the teaching program were being strongly recommended. He pointed out the problems in civilian life as well, of assigning adequate numbers of doctors to rural areas, to central cities and, for that matter, to medical school faculties. "The primary objective of this address has been to call to your attention as forcefully as possible the impending degradation of medical education by reason of inadequate financial resources, and of pressure from those responsible for budgets in the universities, as well as by the weight of governmental agencies, to the end of increasing enrollment, thus seriously lowering the quality of the teaching, and of undertaking again the three years' accelerated program which, with scarcely any exception, has been condemned on the basis of experience as materially impairing medical education . . . under the present circumstances where, over a long time, a careful balance must be maintained between civilian polity and armed defense, it is essential that education, particularly at the higher levels where it is most vulnerable to interference, be maintained secure as regards its quality. What the citizens of this country need is more good doctors of medicine, not more poor ones; more well-qualified specialists, and fewer of limited knowledge, experience and judgment; and to come closer to home, more surgeons and fewer surgical technicians . . . we need not more mediocre or deficient schools of medicine, but the elevation of the standards of a considerable number of those that we have, and assurance that new schools shall be of adequate quality."

* * *

Owen H. Wangensteen, of Minneapolis, Professor of Surgery and Surgeon-in-Chief, University of Minnesota Hospitals, *A Physiologic Operation for Mega-Esophagus: (Dystonia, Cardiospasm, Achalasia)*, in a rather rambling paper pointed out the extreme susceptibility of the esophagus to injury by acid-peptic juice and for that matter by bile and pancreatic juice, and went on to state that cardiospasm was not an acid-peptic disorder. He commented upon the demonstration of the absence of Auerbach's plexus in the esophageal wall, by Rake, in 1927, and made comparisons between this disease and Hirschsprung's disease of the colon. He referred many times to the work of Brazilian investigators with both diseases [without commenting on the association in Brazil of these conditions, acquired and not congenital, with South American trypanosomiasis]. He described the numerous previous operations.

THE WASHINGTON POST - WEDNESDAY, APRIL 11, 1951 - THE FIRST DAY OF THE WASHINGTON MEETING.

◀ The Korean war had gone badly. The Chinese had swept down from the North putting to rout the United Nations Forces who had advanced almost to the border of Manchuria on the assumption that the Chinese would not involve themselves. The massive Chinese attack had been halted and our troops were once more on the offensive. It was apparent that MacArthur wished to pursue the Chinese across the Yalu River and carry the offensive to them. He appeared to be ignoring or rejecting contrary orders from Washington and President Truman firmly took the bold action of dismissing one of the greatest military strategists,- and heroes,- in United States history.

(Newspaper courtesy of the Library of Congress, Washington, D.C.)

The Gröndahl, Finney type esophagoplasty, and the Heyrovsky lateral esophagogastric anastomosis all invited esophagitis and were unacceptable. The Heller extramucosal myotomy, he considered "Functionally satisfactory—fails to reduce size of esophagus materially." He had now, in seven patients performed a resection of all but the gastric antrum, a resection of the distal five to ten centimeters of esophagus, esophagogastrostomy and pyloroplasty. The earliest operation was in August of 1949. He had four excellent results. The esophagus had been markedly reduced in size in all patients. One patient had some narrowing at the anastomosis. The operation was done through a midline incision, splitting the distal sternum to provide access to the mediastinum. He commented that it was Barrett of London, in 1950, who had pointed out that reflux after all of the operations but the Heller procedure invited severe esophagitis and had been supported in this view by Allison. [Wangensteen's comments about the Heller procedure, are for the most part, favorable except for the comment "the esophagus usually remains dilated, a circumstance which is somewhat unsatisfying to both radiologist and surgeon . . . the surgical result is often more satisfying to the patient than is the fluoroscopic evidence to the surgeon."] His own operation, he believed, "relieves the dysphagia . . . is followed by a considerable reduction in size of the atonic esophagus . . . does not invite erosion of the esophagus . . . an operation satisfying to patient, radiologist and surgeon." The operation was not to be undertaken unless dilatation failed to provide relief. He apparently did do the Heller procedure, and through the same mediastinal approach, ". . . it would appear that the Heller myotomy would suggest that all patients needing repeated dilatations should be subjected to operation. Why make an invalid of a patient who can be relieved of a serious functional disturbance by a procedure as simple as the extra-mucosal Heller myotomy?" Referring again to the parallel with Hirschsprung's disease of the colon, he said that he understood that "an extra-mucosal myotomy is considered the operation of choice for megacolon in Brazil. Correia-Neto (1934) . . . described extra-mucosal myotomy at the narrowed rectosigmoidal juncture for megacolon several years ago . . . Perthes of Tuebingen (1905) widened the narrow rectosigmoidal segment in one patient with megacolon by an open plastic procedure but failed to observe any improvement."

Discussion

Evarts A. Graham devoted himself to the remarks about megacolon. A little over a year earlier,

stimulated by Swenson's reports of a segment of constriction in Hirschsprung's disease, he had done a myotomy of the rectosigmoid in a six-year-old girl with "a pretty good result", in a baby with a moderately good result, and in a boy of seven with a brilliant result, and finally in an infant with a less satisfactory result. Barium enema showed prompt evacuation by x-ray in the successful cases. Nathan A. Womack, of Iowa City, preferred for achalasia "the U-shaped plastic procedure" [Gröndahl]. He had done some 12 such and had been very pleased with them until the past year when four patients had returned with hemorrhage, severe in three, one of whom died. None of these four had any free hydrochloric acid in their stomachs. Richard H. Sweet, of Boston, said that at the time when he had discussed the condition with Barrett the year before, he had had no difficulty with the Wendel [Heineke-Mikulicz plasty] type procedure which he had done, but since then, he had seen four patients with bleeding. He had in some 26 patients done an operation much like Wangensteen's ". . . a very radical operation, including a large segment of the stomach and of the esophagus as well" and had trouble with hemorrhage in four. He corrected the substance of Wangensteen's comparison to Hirschsprung's disease by stating "It seems to be different, in our experience in that the lack of ganglion cells seems to exist not only in the lower atrophic segments particularly, but in the hypertrophic upper esophagus, as well. It is my understanding that this is not true in megacolon." Wangensteen, closing, seemed to recommend the Heller procedure rather than the operation he had been at pains to describe, "If one makes an attempt or two at effecting a bloodless rupture of the muscle fibers of the distal end of the esophagus by use of a hydrostatic dilator and does not succeed, I would say the Heller operation of myotomy is in order. It must not be forgotten either that a bloodless myotomy, achieved by use of the hydrostatic dilator, is not without risk." In his closing remarks, he discussed the vulnerability of the esophagus to peptic ulceration, but never so much as mentioned the resection operation.

* * *

Douglas A. Farmer, Chester W. Howe, William J. Porell, all by invitation, and Reginald H. Smithwick, of Boston, now Surgeon-in-Chief, Massachusetts Memorial Hospitals; Professor of Surgery, Boston University School of Medicine, *The Effect of Various Surgical Procedures upon the Acidity of the Gastric Contents of Ulcer Patients,* had studied the gastric acidity of volunteers and of patients with duodenal ulcer, with anastomotic ulcer, and after gastrectomy, after vagotomy and gastrectomy, and vagotomy and gastroenterostomy, measuring the pH and milliequivalents of acid per hour, basal, and after insulin broth and histamine stimulation. They concluded that the "quantity of acid in the gastric contents of duodenal ulcer patients was found to be greater than in normals" particularly after fasting conditions. Patients with gastrojejunal ulcers were like those with untreated duodenal ulcers. Fifty percent gastrectomy and vagotomy "resulted in a marked reduction in both the quantity of free acid and hydrogen ion concentration of the gastric contents" and was more striking than the result following vagotomy and gastroenterostomy. A greater than 50% gastrectomy did not still further decrease the acid secretion. "Thus far the clinical results following removal of approximately 50 per cent of the stomach combined with vagotomy seem superior to those following more radical resections with or without vagotomy." They thought the operation might be as good as radical subtotal resection alone, or better. Vagotomy plus gastroenterostomy frequently did not produce a striking reduction in acid. "The greatest drawback to procedures involving resection of the vagus nerves is the hazard that the denervation may not be complete in a small but definite per cent of the cases. Also, the possibility of regeneration of the vagus nerves has not yet been excluded."

* * *

Lester R. Dragstedt, of Chicago, Professor of Surgery and Chairman, Department of Surgery, University of Chicago, and by invitation, Harry A. Oberhelman, Jr. and Curtis A. Smith, *Experimental Hyperfunction of the Gastric Antrum with Ulcer Formation,* enlarged upon one of the experimental preparations discussed in their paper the previous year. If the antrum of the dog's stomach was transplanted into the side of the transverse colon as a diverticulum there was a profound increase in gastric secretion and the development of stomal ulcers in the jejunum or duodenum. Most fascinating of all, "When the entire stomach is isolated from continuity with the intestinal tract, and its vagus innervation interrupted, a meager secretion of gastric juice is produced . . . When the antrum is removed from the isolated stomach . . . transplanted into the colon as a diverticulum, gastric secretion is markedly increased, and ulcers regularly develop in the isolated stomach, progress, cause hemorrhage, or perforate, in a relatively short time . . . While it is probable that these antrum hyperfunction ulcers and the histamine beeswax ulcers of Hay, Varco, Code and

Wangensteen are both dependent upon a hypersecretion of gastric juice, some objection has been voiced to the latter [histamine in beeswax] procedure in that it involves the administration of a foreign toxic agent." He discussed in considerable detail the implications of the secretion of acid by the stomach as a result of antral stimulation. The introduction to the paper contains what must have been the substance of Dragstedt's thoughts at this time about clinical application, "These data suggest that the vagus nerves and the antrum of the stomach contain the key to the activity of the gastric glands, and since the effects of both can be easily removed by the surgeon, it is unnecessary to sacrifice the storage function of the body and fundus of the stomach in order to reduce the secretion of gastric juice to a small fraction of its normal level."

Discussion

Ralph Colp, of New York, initiated the Discussion, presenting the acid studies in 253 patients, 148 treated by subtotal gastrectomy, 105 by subtotal gastrectomy and vagotomy. In the subtotal gastrectomies, there had been a 5% incidence of gastrojejunal ulceration, there had been none when vagotomy was added, ". . . but statistically, according to our biometrician" the figures were not significant. The addition of vagotomy to subtotal gastrectomy increased the incidence of postoperative anacidity, overnight and stimulated. They had had no deaths in 329 consecutive subtotal gastrectomies. They still did an occasional gastroenterostomy and vagotomy in a poor risk patient. Waltman Walters, of Rochester, Minnesota, said that it had been their experience that as time passed, the gastric acidity after vagotomy alone returned to preoperative levels, as often as 26% of the time. Walters asked "What does vagotomy, alone, do for duodenal ulcer? It reduces the acidity in 42 per cent, in our experience. That contrasts unfavorably with the 72 per cent reduction of free hydrochloric acid after resections of half or more of the stomach for duodenal ulcer." Smithwick now went back over his figures to show that there was in fact no increase in gastric acidity with time after vagotomy, "As you can see, so far, there is no definite evidence of regeneration on the basis of the secretory studies." J. Albert Key, of St. Louis, although an orthopedic surgeon, asked a key question "I want to ask Dr. Dragstedt if the prolonged administration of extract of the antrum would produce these ulcers in normal animals, and in vagotomized animals, and in animals which had had gastroenterostomy. In other words, is he able to get something out of the antrum which will work on the stomach

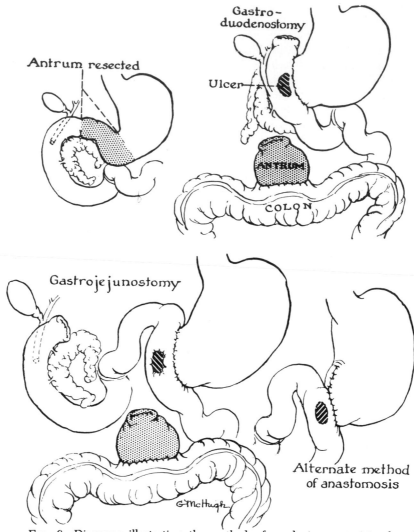

Fig. 6.—Diagrams illustrating the method of producing gastrojejunal and gastroduodenal ulcers by transplantation of the antrum of the stomach into the transverse colon.

In addition to these preparations, if the entire stomach was isolated from the intestinal tract and its vagus interrupted, that gastric pouch produced very little acid and ulcers never developed. But when the antrum of that isolated stomach was implanted into the colon as a diverticulum, gastric secretion occurred and ulcers developed in the isolated stomach, and bled or perforated.

Lester R. Dragstedt, Harry A. Oberhelman, Jr., and Curtis A. Smith, *Experimental Hyperfunction of the Gastric Antrum with Ulcer Formation*. Volume LXIX, 1951.

like secretion on the pancreas?" Farmer agreed in general with Colp. They had as yet had no gastroje-junal ulcers. Like Colp, their incidence of achlorhydria, if anything, rose with time following subtotal gastrectomy, and after gastrectomy and vagotomy. Dragstedt, in closing, answered Dr. Key's question, ". . . potent extracts of the mucous membrane of the pyloric antrum have been prepared by Professor Uvnas, of Lund, Sweden, and also by Komarov and Thomas of Philadelphia. The active principle in these extracts is not histamine, and is in all probability the hormone of the gastric antrum." He commented again that "We are indebted to Varco, Code, and Wangensteen of Minnesota for the demonstration that a hypersecretion of gastric juice can be regularly produced in experimental animals by the implantation of pellets containing histamine and beeswax into the subcutaneous tissues" and thought it probable "that a hypersecretion of gastric juice could also be produced with gastrin if injected in a similar manner." As for the clinical problem of vagotomy, they had now operated on some 740 patients and their results were better than at first, just as the more recent results with subtotal gastrectomy were better than they had been at first. Dragstedt emphasized that even operating through the abdomen, the vagotomy was supradiaphragmatic,- "the operative procedure that we employ is quite different from the one described by Dr. Colp and also the one employed by Dr. Walters. Although our approach is by way of the abdomen, the vagus nerves are divided at a point from two to three inches above the diaphragm. This is accomplished by opening the diaphragm and pulling the esophagus downward into the abdomen. I believe that it is impossible to do a complete vagotomy in any larger proportion of cases by an operative procedure directed to the vagus nerves along the stomach and beneath the diaphragm." As for regeneration, neither in animals nor in man had there been any evidence of regeneration so that "the situation here resembles that in recurrent laryngeal nerve damage, where we have learned, to our sorrow, that regeneration does not occur if this nerve is cut or severely damaged." He emphasized the importance of performing gastric acid output studies as Smithwick's group had done, measuring not merely the acidity but the volume as well, reminding the Fellows that Pavlov had pointed out that "whenever gastric juice is secreted it always contains a constant concentration of acid. Variations in the acidity of the gastric content are due to variations in the amount of neutralizing material present . . . It is only when you measure both the concentration of free acid and the volume of secretion that the total output of hydrochloric acid from the stomach in a measured period of time can be determined."

* * *

Arthur H. Blakemore, Associate Professor of Clinical Surgery, College of Physicians and Surgeons, Columbia University, and by invitation, Hugh F. Fitzpatrick, *The Surgical Management of the Post-Splenectomy Bleeder with Extra-Hepatic Portal Hypertension,* had now performed 148 portosystemic shunts and addressed the problem of dealing with the patient who bled after he had had a splenectomy for extrahepatic portal block. They had had

40 patients with extrahepatic block and had been able to perform anastomoses in all of them, with only three postoperative deaths. Fourteen of the patients had previously had splenectomy. They had given up the Vitallium tube method of anastomosis because of "gradual fibrotic occlusion in the anastomosis of veins" and resorted to direct suture. In the post splenectomy bleeders, they had usually been able to find and use the central stump of the splenic vein but is was difficult to get enough length to reach the renal vein. Earlier in their experience, he and Dr. Whipple "employed superficial femoral vein grafts in two cases: One portal vein to vena cava anastomosis and one splenorenal anastomosis." The post splenectomy bleeder provided "an essential role for the vein graft" between the splenic vein and the left renal vein. They had been persuaded by the work of Gordon Murray and Norman Freeman that local heparinization was effective and they had employed it by constant injection of heparin through a fine plastic catheter placed in the vessel close to the shunt. They gave no figures of patency, total numbers of shunts used of each kind, etc.

Discussion

Allen O. Whipple, of New York, mentioned Dr. Blakemore's "use of the balloon in the patients who are bleeding profusely and are going to have a fatal outcome unless the hemorrhage is controlled. The use of the balloon, as he has developed it and used it, has tided over a number of these patients, so that they are able to undergo a shunt procedure later on." Louis M. Rousselot, of New York, in the previous 12 months had used autogenous vein grafts in seven splenorenal shunts with one death 13 days after operation from hemorrhage due to hypoprothrombinemia, the graft intact and open. One patient had a single subsequent hemorrhage, the other five had been well for three to 12 months. Norman Freeman, of San Francisco, attributed to Best and Murray the development of regional heparinization in 1938, Freeman, in 1949, having reported its use in arterial surgery. He had been using it recently in thromboendarterectomy.

* * *

Robert R. Linton, of Boston, Visiting Surgeon, Massachusetts General Hospital; Chief of the Peripheral Vascular Clinic, Massachusetts General Hospital; Assistant Clinical Professor of Surgery, Harvard Medical School, *The Selection of Patients for Portacaval Shunts.* With a Summary of the Results in 61 Cases, was reporting the results in 61 pa

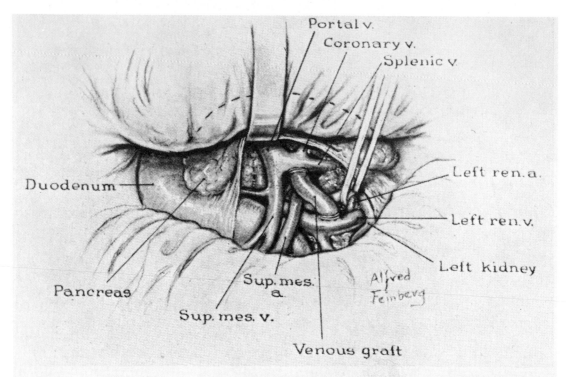

Portal v.
Coronary v.
Splenic v.
Duodenum
Left ren. a.
Left ren. v.
Left kidney
Alfred
Feinberg
Pancreas
Sup. mes. a.
Sup. mes. v.
Venous graft

FIG. 1.—This illustrates a completed shunt. A segment of superficial femoral vein has been used to bridge the distance from the splenic vein, near its junction with the superior mesenteric vein, to the left renal vein. Note the large size of the splenic vein at its junction with the coronary vein.

Whipple and Blakemore had previously employed grafts of superficial femoral vein in two cases and, in the post-splenectomy bleeders it was obvious that grafts were required. The central stump of the splenic vein was usually available. The anastomosis was either to the renal vein or to the vena cava. The superior mesenteric vein was considered too fragile to use. They had occasionally used very large collateral portal veins connecting them to the vena cava with femoral grafts which they called "H-grafts".

Arthur H. Blakemore and Hugh F. Fitzpatrick, *The Surgical Management of the Post-Splenectomy Bleeder with Extra-Hepatic Portal Hypertension*, Volume LXIX, 1951.

tients operated upon at Massachusetts General Hospital in the previous six years for portal cirrhosis and for "the so-called Banti's syndrome with an extrahepatic block." In 65 operations in 61 patients for bleeding esophageal varices, they had had 11 deaths,- one death in the 24 patients with extrahepatic blocks and 10 deaths in the 37 patients with intrahepatic blocks. Of 26 shunts done in 24 patients with extrahepatic blocks, 19 were splenorenal, of 39 shunts done in 37 patients for intrahepatic blocks, 27 were splenorenal. He preferred the splenorenal anastomosis because it reduced the portal hypertension without bypassing the liver completely, as in the case of the end-to-side portal shunt. In "a few cases" after splenectomy the superior mesenteric vein had been anastomosed to the inferior vena cava or the inferior mesenteric vein to the left ovarian vein. Of the 23 surviving patients with extrahepatic block, four had subsequent major bleeding and two had minor bleeding. Two of the patients with major bleeding underwent secondary portacaval shunts with relief. Of the 27 surviving patients with intrahepatic blocks, two subsequently had major bleeding and both underwent secondary shunts, with relief. Of the total group of 50 patients surviving operation, 47,- 94%,- were alive from one month to six years after operation and no patient died of esophageal hemorrhage.

Discussion

Arthur H. Blakemore, emphasized the importance to the prognosis, of the state of the liver. In 108 shunts for cirrhosis of the liver, he had a 20% postoperative mortality. In the 58 good risk patients there were only six deaths. Alfred Blalock, of Baltimore, expressed some reservations, "I would like to repeat that the shunting procedure is the best method that has been devised thus far in the treatment of bleeding esophageal varices, but that the subject is not a closed one." Blalock had said that varices often persisted, but Linton, in closing, remarked that this should not be used as a criterion of cure since some of his patients who had not bled for four or five years had persistent varices. He was aware of the feeling that enthusiasm for shunts was waning and was "glad to have had this opportunity this evening to present these statistics. They demonstrate, I believe quite clearly, that anastomoses of this type do function satisfactorily in the majority of our patients." He agreed with Blalock that the direct portacaval shunt reduced portal hypertension more satisfactorily, but thought it might reduce it too much and sometimes the vascularity in the region made exposure of the portal vein dangerous. He was inclined "to do direct portacaval shunts only in those patients with portal cirrhosis who have a relatively small spleen."

* * *

Julian Johnson, of Philadelphia, Professor of Surgery, School of Medicine and Graduate School of Medicine, University of Pennsylvania, and by invitation, Charles K. Kirby, *The Surgical Treatment of Ventricular Fibrillation,* had attempted cardiac resuscitation in 20 patients over a four-year period. Half of the patients had cardiac arrest and half had ventricular fibrillation. Three of the four with ventricular fibrillation who recovered were cardiac surgery patients,- one intraoperative patient was defibrillated electrically, the other two patients, undergoing cardiac catheterization, had the chest opened, the heart massaged, lungs ventilated mouth-to-mouth, the patients intubated, transported to the operating room, where defibrillation was successful. The fourth recovery was in a patient undergoing a Rubin test, who had 25 minutes of cardiac massage followed by electrical defibrillation and ultimate recovery. The six fibrillating patients who died probably had gone more than six minutes before resuscitation was begun. They emphasized the need for establishing artificial circulation by cardiac massage, and artificial respiration at the mouth or through a tube. Defibril-

lation was not to be undertaken until the heart had been well oxygenated. Procaine or Pronestyl should be administered intravenously to decrease myocardial irritability. They had not yet had an instance of successful resuscitation on the ward but looked forward to it.

Discussion

R. K. Gilchrist, of Chicago, said they had been "plagued with this problem" for the last five years at the Presbyterian Hospital, in Chicago. He attributed it to the increasing use of Pentothal. In only one of their "13 serious cardiovascular complications" had a life been saved by massage. He thought the problem was "sensitivity to Pentothal, rather than the anoxia". Frank H. Lahey, of Boston, said that they had had 19 cardiac arrests, that "things go wrong easily in the hot excitement of a time limit of four minutes." Procaine, epinephrine, and needles for them, and heart needles were always to be available. He was not sure that a shock apparatus was necessary. All of their 19 arrested hearts were revived, seven patients subsequently died in the hospital, 12 recovered with normal mentality, but one of these subsequently had a coronary occlusion. There were thus 11 patients living and well. Seven of the last ten were alive and well. There was still a certain amount of inertia "To strip off the chest drapes, to incise in the fourth interspace and put one's hand into the chest requires the overcoming of a not inconsiderable number of inhibitions, and if one delays in overcoming these inhibitions, the procedure will have been wasted." Alfred Blalock, of Baltimore, with his heavy schedule of cardiac surgery, was able to open his remarks by saying that "the only thing I can report which we have had more of than has Dr. Lahey—and this is a very doubtful distinction—is cardiac standstill." Blalock said it was important to open the pericardium as well as the chest, something Johnson and Lahey had not mentioned. The fibrillating heart should be massaged for a minute or two before being defibrillated. Dr. Jerome Kay, in Blalock's laboratory, had been successful in defibrillating the heart with Procaine only 50% of the time, so that they preferred not to use it. Ten percent calcium chloride [Claude Beck in 1937, Volume LV, mentioned its use by Prevost and Batteli in 1899, and Beck found it useful in dogs once the heart had been defibrillated] was extraordinarily effective in restoring cardiac action and he employed both that and dilute epinephrine. Henry Swan, of Denver, mentioned a patient who sustained a cardiac arrest during aortography. His heart was massaged for 65

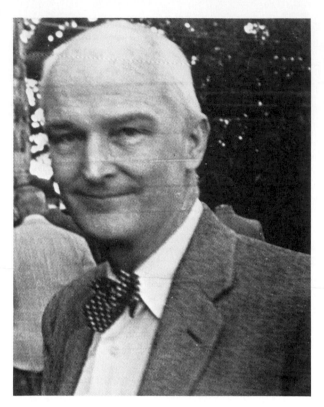

John H. Gibbon, Jr. 1903-1973, M.D. Jefferson 1927. President 1955, Recorder 1947-52, Vice-President 1953. Interned at Pennsylvania Hospital. Research for two years at Massachusetts General Hospital in Churchill's laboratory. Conceived the idea for a heart-lung machine for extracorporeal circulation and with his wife, Maly (Mary Hopkinson), who had been Churchill's research technician, spent twenty years on the problem at Harvard, the University of Pennsylvania and after 1946 at Jefferson where he became the Samuel D. Gross Professor and Chairman of the Department. On May 6, 1953, he performed the world's first successful open heart operation under cardiopulmonary bypass,- closure of an atrial septal defect,- a rare example of a man's seeing a problem and its solution, working on it for a lifetime, and carrying out the initial successful clinical application. An ardent tennis player (he suffered his first major coronary occlusion on the tennis court and his fatal one playing tennis). He was an accomplished portrait painter.

(Photography: Henry T. Bahnson, M.D., Pittsuburgh, Pa.)

minutes before spontaneous respirations were resumed and the heart began to beat after 82 minutes; the patient recovered. D. W. Gordon Murray, of Toronto, said that if a heart had gone into fibrillation, it could not recover until it was emptied and agreed with Blalock that opening the pericardium

for massage was the most effective way. Emile Holman, of San Francisco, pointed out that with a dilated adult heart, one massaged it by compressing it upward against the chest wall. He thought rather than massage, it should be called "intermittent compression of the heart." Robert S. Dinsmore, of Cleveland, contributed a marvelously humorous and very long Discussion, describing the complex pharmacological manipulations of the anesthetists, the fact that arrests were new to surgeons, "Everyone says that they have been occurring from time immemorial, but neither Dr. Crile nor I ever had one in a thyroidectomy." It was insistence by surgeons and anesthetists alike on deep anesthesia and profound relaxation which was responsible.

* * *

Bernard J. Miller, by invitation, John H. Gibbon, Jr., of Philadelphia, the Recorder, Professor of Surgery and Director of Surgical Research, Jefferson Medical College, and by invitation, Mary H. Gibbon [Mrs. Gibbon had collaborated on the work since it had first begun in Dr. Churchill's department at the Massachusetts General Hospital many years before], *Recent Advances in the Development of a Mechanical Heart and Lung Apparatus,* presented the single paper, of those presented at this meeting, which was to have the greatest impact on surgery. Gibbon said that there was a "dual purpose in developing a mechanical heart and lung apparatus. The first is to maintain a part of the cardiorespiratory functions temporarily in patients with a failing heart or lung, or both . . . The second purpose is of surgical interest. It consists in the maintenance of the entire cardiorespiratory function by an extracorporeal circuit for periods of time long enough to permit precise operative procedures under direct vision within the open chambers of the human heart." To procure rapid and complete saturation of blood with oxygen had proved to be one of the most difficult problems, "The problem briefly consists of converting a stream flow of blood into a thin film exposed to an atmosphere of oxygen, and then reconverting the film flow into a stream flow. This must be accomplished without the production of foam and with minimal damage to the cellular elements of the blood." It was necessary to produce some turbulence to achieve this end. They had come to use a stainless steel screen over which the blood flowed to provide the turbulence necessary. Their first screen oxygenator had been a vertical cylinder with a bullet-shaped top on which a jet of blood was streamed. The principle was sound, but for human use would have required

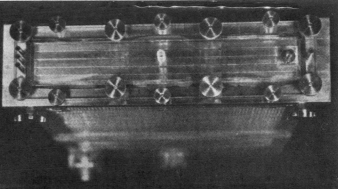

B

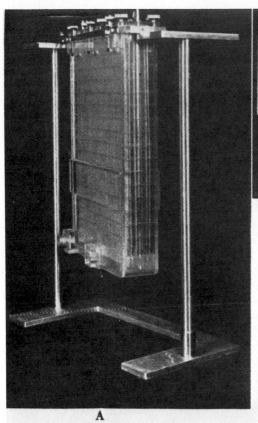

A

FIG. 3.—Photographs of the side (A), and the top (B), of the battery-type oxygenator.

Gibbon had come to the choice of metal screens on which to pass the blood and provide the turbulence necessary for oxygenation. A vertical cylinder of stainless steel wire worked very well, but an enormous cylinder would have been required. Shown are the six flat stainless steel screens suspended inside a clear lucite box. This is, in fact, very nearly the finished oxygenator which Gibbon first employed clinically and successfully in 1953 for the repair of an atrial septal defect.

Bernard J. Miller, John H. Gibbon, Jr., and Mary H. Gibbon, *Recent Advances in the Development of a Mechanical Heart and Lung Apparatus,* Volume LXIX 1951.

an enormous cylinder, so that they changed "to a series of six flat screens suspended in parallel from a distributing chamber and enclosed in a clear plastic case." The entire cardiorespiratory function of 21 dogs had been maintained by the machine for periods of 20 minutes to one hour and 36 minutes and seven of the dogs that survived were normal. Seven dogs died of easily explainable causes, but for seven, the cause of death was not obvious. The venous drainage from the dogs was by two catheters, one through the stump of the azygos vein into the superior vena cava, the other into the inferior vena cava through the tip of the right auricular appendage. The blood was returned through a cannula in the femoral artery. The venae cavae were occluded by ligatures around the cavae over the cannulae, thus directing the entire venous return into the extracor-

poreal circuit. They said that "If successful experiments of this type can be consistently performed, the next logical step is to demonstrate experimentally that operations can be performed within the opened heart under direct vision. This step will involve the additional difficulty of keeping the cardiac chambers clear of the venous blood returning to the heart through the coronary sinus and the cardiac veins. It seems to us that the demonstration of the ability to perform such operations on animals should precede attempts to use the apparatus in operations on human patients." [Perhaps an allusion to the next paper.]

* * *

Gibbon's paper was followed by a second attack on the same problem, *Development of a Pump-*

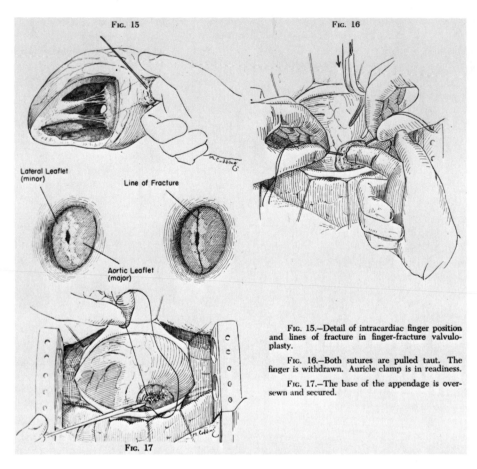

Fig. 15.

Fig. 16.

Lateral Leaflet (minor)

Line of Fracture

Aortic Leaflet (major)

Fig. 15.—Detail of intracardiac finger position and lines of fracture in finger-fracture valvuloplasty.

Fig. 16.—Both sutures are pulled taut. The finger is withdrawn. Auricle clamp is in readiness.

Fig. 17.—The base of the appendage is oversewn and secured.

Fig. 17

In 86 operations for mitral stenosis, Harken had done 71 finger-fracture valvuloplasties, nine valvulotome valvuloplasties and two of Sweet's azygos-pulmonary vein bypasses. He considered the finger-fracture technique "vastly superior to the others."

Dwight E. Harken, Lewis Dexter, Laurence B. Ellis, Robert E. Farrand, and James F. Dickson, III, *The Surgery of Mitral Stenosis,* Volume LXIX, 1951.

Oxygenator to Replace the Heart and Lungs: An Apparatus Applicable to Human Patients and Application to One Case, by Clarence Dennis, of St. Paul, Professor, Department of Surgery, University of Minnesota; Richard L. Varco, of Minneapolis, Associate Professor of Surgery, University of Minnesota, and, by invitation, six co-authors. Dennis achieved his oxygenation by filming the blood on a large rotating disk in an oxygen chamber. They had previously used the Gibbon rotating vertical cylinder oxygenator in a good many dogs and found its effects deleterious. They had used their new pump in nine dogs, three died after perfusion "because of failure to maintain pulmonary exchange." One died of air embolism "from faulty rubber tubing to the caval cannulae". One died of surgical error in not recognizing the [atrial] septum, another died from faulty closure of the atrium, one died when a faulty connection

failed during perfusion. However, two dogs survived for several days and one was kept for 15 months. They undertook operation on a patient with a large atrial septal defect. The patient was found to have a persistent ostium primum. Closure was not successfully achieved and the patient succumbed on the table. They thought the apparatus was superior and behaved very well and did not see in the patient the metabolic acidosis that they had seen in dogs.

Discussion

Russell M. Nelson, of Minneapolis, one of the co-authors, commented on the two papers on extracorporeal circulation. Some of the dogs in the early perfusions had died of metabolic acidosis which proved to have resulted from contamination of the apparatus with gram-negative organisms. Alfred

Blalock, of Baltimore, commended "Dr. Gibbon and Dr. Dennis for the epoch-making work which was presented in the first two papers. I know that John Gibbon started this work many years ago, when he was with Dr. Churchill, and he has shown persistence which is so necessary in developing a difficult field, which is beginning to bear fruit. One of his best collaborators in this difficult task is Mrs. Gibbon. I hope Dr. Gibbon and Dr. Dennis and others will shortly be in a position to attack problems such as congenital transposition of the great vessels in patients, a condition in which only moderately successful results have been obtained thus far by methods which do not utilize the artificial circulation." No one else commented on the presentation which Blalock correctly described as epochal and neither of the essayists said anything further.

* * *

This was the day of the exploration of the limits of cardiac surgery without cardiopulmonary support, and now Dwight E. Harken, Lewis Dexter, Laurence B. Ellis, Robert E. Farrand, and James F. Dickson, III, all by invitation, *The Surgery of Mitral Stenosis*. III. Finger-Fracture Valvuloplasty, were reporting on their experience with 86 patients. As they said "Initially, it was our feeling that it was morally right to accept only those patients who were dying of their disease. We felt the technical failures would inevitably account for the loss of a number of the earlier patients . . ." A group of 19 patients selected for operation refused or did not come to operation and 17 of them were dead within a year, 15 of those within six months. The chest was entered through a third left anterior intercostal incision, the third and fourth costal cartilages divided, procaine injected into the pericardium, double purse-string sutures of 0 braided black silk placed around the base of the auricular appendage, the appendage seized with a clamp, the tip amputated and the finger inserted as the clamp was released. There was no need for haste; as the finger was inserted, the anesthetist was asked to compress the carotid arteries to decrease the likelihood of cerebral embolism from dislodged clot. Finger-fracture could split apart a rigid fusion of the valves. If the fusion was fibrous and elastic, the finger was withdrawn and one or another type of knife inserted with the finger to cut the commissures, "*the surgeon must not use force but, rather, gently retreat in order to resort to incisional valvuloplasty* (Bailey's 'commissurotomy')." When the procedure was completed, the opposing purse-string sutures were pulled taut as the finger was

withdrawn and the base of the appendage oversewn. Twenty of the 71 patients who had had finger-fracture valvuloplasty were dead, 18 of the deaths associated with the operation and two unrelated to it. Dividing patients into four classes very much like the American Heart Association Classifications, they noted that in their Group III patients with progressive disability, hemoptysis, pulmonary edema, etc., they had operated upon 21 patients with one operative death "due to a technical error incident to forcing hastily a Type II [elastic fusion] valve following cardiac arrest." There were 16 deaths in the 34 Group IV patients essentially terminal and completely incapacitated with right ventricular failure, enlarged liver, etc. "Furthermore, the clinical improvement of Group III is far more dramatic than Group IV." Four of the deaths in Group IV were associated with emboli and five with poor valvuloplasties which could now be done better. Thirty-five of the 55 Group IV patients were fibrillating. Hemorrhage during operation had ceased to be a problem with the development of auricle clamps. For the future, it seemed clear that operation would continue to be offered to Group III patients and might now, perhaps, be offered to Group II patients who were somewhat handicapped by moderate dyspnea or infrequent attacks of acute dyspnea. Valvuloplasty in the desperate risk Group IV, "must continue until such time as we have established conclusively which patients are benefitted and, conversely, which patients have no salvage in life or comfort." They calculated "that the estimated valve orifices are doubled or trebled in size." Pulmonary artery resistance dropped strikingly after operation, particularly in patients where it was high before operation. As for whether the "leaflets seal back together?" they expected they would not, but could not answer the question except to say that patients had continued to improve clinically and that one patient who died late, of cirrhosis, showed no recurrent stenosis. [In this paper, no details were presented of intraoperative or postoperative complications, or subsequent course.]

Discussion

Alfred Blalock, of Baltimore, was the single discusser, "Our experience in the surgery of mitral stenosis has not been so great as that of Dr. Bailey and Dr. Harken and, probably, of others. My work has been in connection with my medical colleague, Dr. E. C. Andrus, a twin of our recently deceased and beloved member, Dr. William Andrus." Most of his cases had been Group III. They had operated on 26 patients. The single death was in a patient probably Group IV. "The improvement in most of the patients has been very gratifying." An additional patient died in whom the atrium was obliterated by thrombi and the pulmonary vein too small for insertion of the fingers so the operation was abandoned, the patient dying of a cerebral embolus. Blalock felt "very strongly that finger fracture or tear can be used in doing the commissurotomy in something like 90 per cent of the cases. I believe I can determine the point at which the commissure is being torn or fractured more accurately with my finger than I can with a knife. But I thoroughly agree with you and with Dr. Bailey and others that a knife should be available, in case it is impossible to tear or fracture the commissure region." Blalock had discussed the contraindications to operation,- "active rheumatic activity, endocarditis, extreme mitral regurgitation, intractable right-sided heart failure and left ventricular enlargement of a marked degree. We do not consider auricular fibrillation or a history of peripheral arterial embolism as contraindications to operation." Harken added to these, "severe aortic valvular disease" which would place a great burden "on the newly restored mitral flutter valve." Harken stressed [without commenting on the attempts of Cutler and others to produce a controlled insufficiency for mitral stenosis] "the importance of the restoration of the flutter valve and the correction of stenosis without the production of regurgitation."

* * *

There followed a series of three papers on the use of arterial grafts. Conrad R. Lam, of Detroit, Associate Surgeon, Henry Ford Hospital, and by invitation, Hartley H. Aram, *Resection of the Descending Thoracic Aorta for Aneurysm.* A Report of the Use of a Homograft in a Case and an Experimental Study, reported a tour de force in the bypassing of a syphilitic aneurysm of the thoracic aorta. They had experimented with Hufnagel's lucite tubes for replacing the aorta and, like him, had found them untrustworthy for replacement of the aorta, but useful as a temporary conduit during reconstruction along the lines originally suggested by Carrel, in 1908. In his patient, Lam clamped the aorta below the subclavian and above the diaphragm, transected the aorta and inserted into the two ends a lucite tube on which a cadaver homograft had been placed, tying the lucite tube in place at both ends to restore the aortic flow. [Of the homograft, he said "After

several trips to a public morgue, one of us was permitted to take the descending thoracic aorta of a 55-year-old man who had died three weeks after severe burns. It was removed approximately ten hours after death, the body having been refrigerated during most of this time. After its aseptic removal, it was placed in sterile Tyrode's solution to which had been added penicillin, 100 units per cubic centimeter. It was refrigerated at 5° C until the next day, when the specimen was trimmed and 17 intercostal and 3 esophageal vessels were ligated. The specimen was 5 days old when it was used as a graft." He said nothing about cultures and did not suggest that the eventual disaster from infection was related to the graft.] The upper anastomosis was performed, the posterior row of the lower anastomosis performed, the clamps reapplied, the lucite tube withdrawn and the anastomosis completed. The patient recovered well but for a partial paraplegia. There had been periods of occlusion of the aorta of 24 minutes and of 15 minutes. On the basis of animal experiments subsequently performed, Lam thought the paraplegia probably due to interruption of aortic circulation rather than to the division of intercostal vessels. The patient was febrile for several days after operation "until 36 hours before discharge from the hospital" and had a constant leukocytosis. He did well for six weeks, then deteriorated very rapidly and died shortly after readmission to the hospital. Autopsy disclosed that the original aneurysm, which had been left in situ, was filled with pus connecting to a rupture of the distal anastomosis.

* * *

Robert E. Gross, Ladd Professor of Children's Surgery, Harvard Medical School; Surgeon-in-Chief, Children's Hospital, Boston, Massachusetts, *Treatment of Certain Aortic Coarctations by Homologous Grafts.* A Report of Nineteen Cases, had now operated upon 180 patients for coarctation and had had only four deaths in the last 100. Eighty percent of their patients had had blood pressure restored to normal. Some of the failures had resulted because of incomplete resection of the coarcted segment, leading to too small an anastomosis. In addition, they were now facing the problem, particularly in adult patients, of associated aneurysms of the aorta or the intercostal arteries. "In the effort to develop methods for correcting those malformations which were previously thought to be inoperable and also to improve the results in that group for whom we were obtaining only partial relief of hypertension, grafting of aortic segments has been adopted as a method for

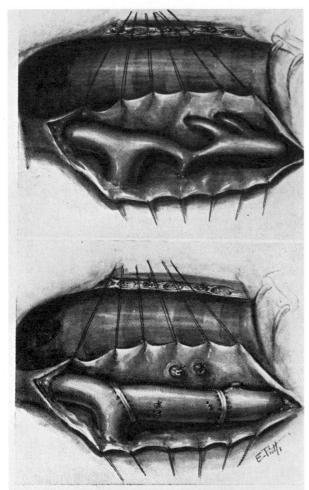

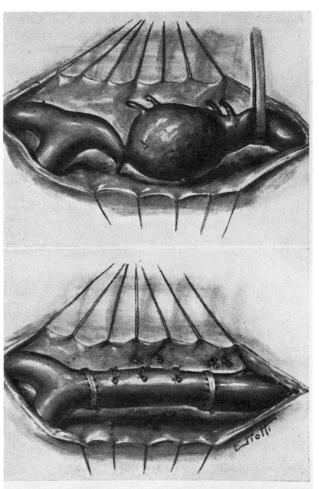

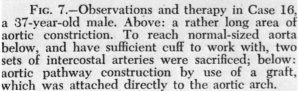

FIG. 7.—Observations and therapy in Case 16, a 37-year-old male. Above: a rather long area of aortic constriction. To reach normal-sized aorta below, and have sufficient cuff to work with, two sets of intercostal arteries were sacrificed; below: aortic pathway construction by use of a graft, which was attached directly to the aortic arch.

FIG. 8.—Treatment in Case 17, a 34-year-old man. Above: coarctation, below which is a thin-walled aneurysm of the aorta (there had been previous *Streptococcus viridans* infection). Below: removal of narrowed and dilated portions of aorta and replacement by graft.

Gross was reporting the use of homografts in 19 patients for the replacement of long segment narrowing (12 cases), inelasticity of the aorta preventing direct anastomosis, one case, aneurysm of the aorta, five cases, operative injury to the aorta, one case. Two patients died of renal failure on the fourth day (massive transfusion), one patient had a moderate relief of hypertension, one patient had no relief of hypertension. The others all had excellent results.

Robert E. Gross, *Treatment of Certain Aortic Coarctations by Homologous Grafts,* A Report of Nineteen Cases, Volume LXIX 1951.

constructing an aortic pathway." They had done extensive experiments [reported two years earlier] with homografts in the laboratory "and while marked histologic changes are known to occur in the walls of such vessels, it is quite clear that in an extremely high percentage of animals a grafted segment can form a channel which is very satisfactory for carrying blood." The graft did not persist, but formed "a scaffolding or mold along which the host builds a new intima, adventitia, and possibly a rudimentary media." They had now implanted aortic homografts in 19 patients. In the first 16 patients, they had used autografts, obtained from fresh autopsies under sterile conditions, preserved in modified Tyrode solution and stored at 2° to 4° C. In the last three patients, they used grafts which had been "frozen in carbon dioxide snow and stored in a carbon dioxide refrigerator at −50°C . . ." for 21 and 72 days. The first graft had been obtained under sterile conditions, the other two had not been. Both had been "given high-voltage cathode-ray irradiation, to the extent of 2,000,000 'Roentgen equivalent physical units' ". Animal experiments had demonstrated that this sterilized contaminated grafts satisfactorily, and no infection had resulted in the two patients in whom this technique had been used. There were two deaths, both of renal shutdown and uremia on the fourth day, both patients having excessive blood loss and massive transfusion during the operation. "The long-term blood pressure levels have been classified as *unsatisfactory* in one case, *fair* in one, *satisfactory* in one, and *excellent* in 14." In the "*unsatisfactory*" case, the pressures in the arms had been normal for six months when quite suddenly, leg pressures fell and arm pressures rose, suggesting "that thrombosis may have occurred within the graft, though at no time has there been anything to indicate embolism in the legs or abdominal viscera." The patients had been followed up to three years and as yet, there had been no rupture or aneurysm formation in any, but one already showed calcification in the graft. Gross concluded by saying that "There can be no doubt that the ideal therapy for aortic coarctation is that in which the stricture is removed and an aortic anastomosis is made which establishes a lumen of completely normal size." When this was otherwise impossible, the use of grafts made reconstruction feasible, but "No final conclusions should be made until these patients have been followed for several decades."

* * *

William S. McCune, by invitation, and Brian Blades, of Washington, D.C., Professor of Surgery, George Washington University School of Medicine; Chief of Surgery, George Washington University Hospital, *The Viability of Long Blood Vessel Grafts*, investigated the relationship between the length of the homograft and its survival. They removed entire aortas from 22 dogs, implanting them in other dogs either by end-to-end anastomosis to the thoracic and abdominal aorta, or end-to-end anastomosis to the divided descending aorta and end-to-side to the abdominal aorta. They concluded that "The length of the transplants had no effect upon their viability". Six of the 18 animals with end-to-side anastomoses with the thoracic aorta had thrombosed their grafts.

None of the four end-to-end anastomoses had thrombosed and they said that "viability of preserved blood vessel grafts is not related to length, and within the limits of this experiment long arterial grafts are feasible for the replacement of blood vessel segments damaged by injury or disease."

Discussion

Earl B. Mahoney, of Rochester, New York, had hoped to use lucite tubes in the replacement of aortic aneurysms and although they had learned to insert the tubes securely into dogs, their studies, now with follow-up to a year-and-a-half, showed gradual thrombosis beginning between six months and a year. Dr. Frank Gerbode, of San Francisco, had been "testing the feasibility of transplanting a large vein autograft to the thoracic aorta, believing that, if one of the patient's own vessels could be used, one might avoid the degenerative changes which occur in homografts." In dogs, the vena cava served very well for the replacement of a portion of the descending thoracic aorta. Thus far, there had been no aneurysm formation, bursting, or leakage. After months, the vein simply thickened. ". . . these preliminary results indicate that one might safely utilize a vein, such as the internal jugular, to bridge a defect in the aorta, particularly in children." Henry Swan, of Denver, discussed the use of homografts in peripheral arterial lesions, citing a resection of the femoral artery in a man with a neurogenic tumor of the groin, inserting a homograft brachial artery. Swan's second patient had an external iliac arteriovenous fistula, which was excised, the vessel reconstructed with a homograft. Finally, he mentioned the question of acute trauma in war wounds, citing a man with a bullet wound injury of the superficial femoral artery which was successfully repaired with a graft. "In the face of our limited experience so far with this technic, we feel it should be given a further try. We think arterial ligation is probably seldom indicated, and that most peripheral lesions involving arteries can be better handled by either an insertion of homografts or, as Dr. Gerbode suggests, the use of autogenous venous grafts." D. W. Gordon Murray, of Toronto, had "applied three grafts of aorta in the abdominal aorta in patients for aneurysms." He mentioned that one patient had lived three months and died of other causes. He had experimented with venous grafts "many years ago", and grafts survived and functioned for as long as nine years, without aneurysm formation, but with some sclerosis and calcification. He had replaced a popliteal aneurysm in a patient, with a vein graft, 17 years before "and it is still working well",- in a lumberjack! "He is still functioning with his external jugular vein in place of his popliteal aneurysm." He had put a venous graft in the femoral artery of a newsboy who had cut his femoral artery with a knife,- with a good result, the man having been accepted for military service. A third venous graft in the brachial artery had been functioning well for 15 years. "Veins make good grafts. We heparinize them all, to make sure they remain patent. Perhaps the aorta graft is as good. The difficulty with aorta is that it is not autogenous, and I think autogenous grafts are probably better." Lam, closing, was surprised that no one had commented upon the reason for the ultimate failure in his case. He should have tried to reduce the occlusion time of the aorta and he should have resected the sac of the aneurysm [he still did not question the sterility of his graft]. Gross, in closing, agreed with Murray "that it is probably much more desirable to use autografts when possible", that was feasible and desirable in peripheral arteries, but there was no vein of the proper size for the aorta, to be taken from the same subject. He emphasized what his illustrations had shown, the preservation of pleural flaps to wrap around the graft. McCune, closing, said that "one vein graft and three or four homografts" had been used at Walter Reed Hospital for femoral and brachial artery war wounds. [The signature of Michael E. DeBakey, of Houston, Texas, appears in the Registration Book at this meeting, but no discussion by him is recorded.]

The Business Meetings

The seventy-first meeting of the American Surgical Association was held April 11, 12, and 13, 1951, at the Shoreham Hotel, Washington, D. C., Samuel C. Harvey in the Chair.

The Program Committee reported that 42 out of 63 submitted titles were accepted for presentation. Dr. Arthur W. Allen, for the Advisory Membership Committee, felt ". . . that the innovation, last year, of sending advance information to the fellows, for their comments on prospective fellows, was very successful." He warned the Membership that in about two years the quota of 250 active members would be reached, ". . . and the fellows must begin to consider whether that is a limit which should be continued. Undoubtedly, in the near future (certainly, within two or three years), this is going to become a very serious problem."

Warfield M. Firor, saying that "One of the great evils in the practice of surgery in this country is the performance of unnecessary operations", moved that the President appoint a Committee to evaluate the problem and recommend corrective action. The motion was passed.

Lord Alfred Webb-Johnson, President of the Royal College of Surgeons, was introduced as an Honorary Member, relatively few Honorary Members having been elected in recent years.

At the Second Executive Meeting, all 16 of the new members proposed were elected, as well as Clarence Crafoord of Stockholm, as an Honorary Member.

An official letter had been sent to Stuart Symington, Chairman of the National Security Resources Board; General George Marshall, Secretary of Defense; General Lewis Hershey, Selective Service System; and a number of others, protesting the fact that "During the past few weeks, a number of residents receiving surgical training in teaching hospitals have been called to duty with the armed forces [the Korean War]. As far as can be determined, no over-all provision has been made for deferment of residents until they finish their education, on the basis of residency training alone. That this situation will affect adversely both civilian and military surgery is so apparent . . . " they requested, in what was rather a long letter, that "In order to prevent unnecessary deterioration of surgical care, not only for the present but for the future, and in order to prevent the residency program for the training of surgeons from being badly damaged, perhaps irreparably, we request respectfully that you direct the restoration and continuance of the deferment from military service of resident surgeons in teaching hospitals throughout the United States", and if still greater surgical quotas were required so as to make compliance with this request difficult ". . . we urgently ask that some men responsible for the training of these men be adequately consulted." [Times had not changed, and, like previous attempts of the American Surgical Association to offer its advice to the National Government, nothing resulted. The Secretary, Dr. Nathan A. Womack commented "Replies to this letter were most cordial and gracious, and most innocuous and ineffective."]

Officers elected for the following year were Daniel C. Elkin, of Atlanta, President; Owen Wangensteen, of Minneapolis, First Vice-President; James F. Mitchell, of Washington, D. C., Second Vice-President; and Nathan Womack, of Chapel Hill, Secretary.

LXX

1952

The 1952 meeting was held April 16, 17, and 18, at The Greenbrier, White Sulphur Springs, West Virginia, President Daniel C. Elkin, of Atlanta, Whitehead Professor of Surgery, Emory University; Surgeon-in-Chief, Emory University Hospital, Atlanta, Georgia, in the Chair.

In the previous year Alfred W. Adson, Barney Brooks, Dallas B. Phemister, and Honorary Members Henri Hartmann and George Grey-Turner had died.

Elkin, a marvelously engaging man with a delightful sense of humor, *A Case for the Study of the Humanities in the Making of a Doctor,* pointed to the progressive deterioration of the scholarly preparation of physicians in the nonscientific, humanistic disciplines. Greek and Latin had disappeared. "The colleges have said requiem over Greek, which is as dead as the dodo, and Latin is rapidly on the way to join the passenger pigeon and the New England heath hen. What we have substituted is a bauble of practicality–not just the practical but what appears to be the *immediately* practical." The study of history had become a two-quarter survey, and the students had usually had ". . . a comprehensive course, one quarter, in English literature from Chaucer to Ogden Nash." Medical school catalogues listed chiefly the prerequisites in the sciences for entrance, skimping or ignoring the general education foundation, and admissions committees, in any case, concentrated on preparation in the sciences. In addition, he questioned the repetition of science courses in secondary school, and college, and then again in medical school. He complained about ". . . the pov-

erty of the humanities in the college curriculum of students who express a desire to enter medicine", and indicated that as busy as medical students were, they were not beyond redemption in terms of broadening their outlook in the humanities but ". . . will hardly be inclined to lend their support in that direction if we, having obtained what to them is professional success, do not convince them of its value . . . Our students observe our actions and our thinking as interpretation of our values, our maturity, our education, and draw their own conclusions." He made no specific recommendations, feeling that a detailed study of preprofessional education would first be in order. The nub of his feeling was that,- "I am in complete agreement with those who believe that we should eliminate in deed and truth the word 'premedical' from the curriculum. If 'premedical' meant a sound and inspiring education in scientific and humanitarian thinking and an acquaintance with cultural achievements, so combined and so offered that the student is inspired to recognition of his own potentiality, then there would be no lost time and crossed-purpose for the students who *do not* get into medical school; and those who *do* would have acquired a proper background of education. But I have just described what does not exist." [It is of some interest that he made no mention of proficiency in foreign languages.]

* * *

D. Emerick Szilagyi, Arthur B. McGraw, and Nicholas P. D. Smyth, by invitation, *The Effects of*

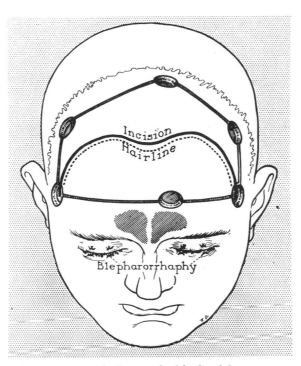

Fig. 4.—The line of scalp incision and the single block of bone removed in approaching the orbits. The lids of both eyes have been closed temporarily by peripheral two-point blepharorrhaphy. (Reproduced with permission from Winchell McK. Craig, and Henry W. Dodge, Jr.: The Surgical Treatment of Malignant Exophthalmos. Surgical Clinics of North America.)

Craig substantiated the value of Naffziger's (Vol. XLIX, 1931; Vol. LVI, 1938) approach, had modified the incision and in addition, withdrew spinal fluid at the beginning of the operation and replaced it at the end, and did not unroof the optic nerve canal. In 28 patients he had one death, lost one eye, and in one patient exophthalmos progressed.

Winchell McK. Craig and Henry W. Dodge, Jr., *Surgical Treatment of Progressive Exophthalmos.* Volume LXX, 1952.

Adrenocortical Stimulation on Thyroid Function, Clinical Observations in Thyrotoxic Crisis and Hyperthyroidism, commented on the long-time feeling that there was an interrelationship between the thyroid gland and the pituitary-adrenal endocrine system. As far back as 1897 Solis-Cohen had described ". . . a protective action of crude adrenal extract against thyroid intoxication . . ." and others over the years had made similar observations. In three patients with thyrotoxic crisis before operation, ACTH had had a remarkable effect and the patients had gone on to successful thyroidectomy. This led them to study the effect of ACTH in five patients with severe hyperthyroidism which ". . . had presented unusual difficulties in preoperative preparation." In only one of these cases did the laboratory indices of thyroid function show significant decrease. They concluded that "Corticotropin does not seem to offer any useful addition to the current methods

of medical treatment of hyperthyroidism", although they were not quite willing to say that corticotropin or cortisone might not be a helpful additional medication in some patients.

* * *

Winchell McK. Craig, of Rochester, Minnesota, Head of Section on Neurologic Surgery, Mayo Clinic, and by invitation, Henry W. Dodge, Jr., *Surgical Treatment of Progressive Exophthalmos,* presented their experience with 28 patients operated upon since 1934 by a modification of the operation which Howard C. Naffziger had presented before the Association in 1931 and in 1938. The concealed hair-line incision exposed both orbits by a single massive bone flap. Fifty centimeters of spinal fluid was drawn by the anesthetist through a previously placed lumbar needle, ". . . the dura and brain fall away to such a degree that only minimal retraction is necessary to visualize the sphenoid wing and region of the optic canal." At the beginning of closure, the withdrawn spinal fluid was reinjected by the anesthetist. Like Naffziger, they found the orbital pathologic changes to consist of "Marked increase in size and weight of the intra-orbital contents, hypertrophy of the ocular muscles, edema, lymphocytic infiltration and fibrodegenerative changes." They had a single operative death in a man of 76. In eight of the patients ". . . it had been thought advisable to do the orbital decompression during the toxic phase of their goiter, although they were under Lugol therapy at the time." One eye was lost postoperatively. In one patient progressive exophthalmos was not affected by the operation ". . . in all others but this one case the progression of the protrusion was arrested . . . diplopia, once experienced, has proved troublesome and persistent . . . the operation is not a cure but a means of retarding the progress of the disease."

Discussion

Howard C. Naffziger, of San Francisco, found a similar female preponderance in his patients. He had not routinely used spinal puncture, and agreed now with Craig that ". . . unroofing of the optic nerve canal, which was first advised, is now unnecessary." The etiology was still not completely elucidated, and [like some of Craig's cases] ". . . 17 per cent of our cases with bilateral progressive exophthalmus and with the characteristic pathology have shown no discernible relationship to thyroid disease", and in those with thyroid disease the eye problems might become obvious before evidence of thyrotoxicosis or might first appear after thyroidectomy. He spoke in percentages and did not indicate the total number of patients he had operated upon. He had performed the operation for cosmetic reasons only in an actress who had become unemployable ". . . because of her startling appearance . . . This procedure was primarily devised as a lifesaving procedure for those cases which frequently went on to extreme protrusion, panophthalmitis, and finally death from meningitis and brain abscess. When, in these patients with increasing proptosis, impaired vision appears, operation should be considered before the stage of extreme edema and protrusion of the mucous membrane." Robert S. Dinsmore, of Cleveland, said that in the face of acute hyperthyroidism and developing exophthalmos, early thyroidectomy improved the chances of recession of the exophthalmos. After three or four months it was not likely that the exophthalmos would recede after thyroidectomy. In

children with exophthalmic goiter, the recession of the proptosis was rapid and striking. Retrobulbar edema he thought was the initial factor, "The edema, as I see it and believe, occurs first in the retrobulbar spaces. There is a surgeon in Cleveland, Dr. Frank Gibson, who had a patient, a man who developed an acute exophthalmic goiter. He had a glass eye, and he had to be operated upon because he couldn't keep his glass eye in place, and the edema in his retrobulbar space was almost unbelievable. As soon as the gland was removed, that edema in the retrobulbar space disappeared, and he was able to wear his glass eye."

* * *

Louis T. Byars, of St. Louis, Assistant Professor of Clinical Surgery, Washington University School of Medicine, *Preservation of the Facial Nerve in Operations for Benign Conditions of the Parotid Area,* referred to Blair's 1912 technique of finding the main nerve trunk ". . . at its emergence from beneath the upper aspect of the posterior belly of the digastric muscle", Adson's 1923 technique of picking up ". . . the inframandibular filament of the nerve in the face anterior to the parotid gland, tracing this back to its junction with larger branches . . .", and J. Barrett Brown's 1950 recommendation for ". . . a direct approach to the tumor with dissection of nerve fibers as they are encountered." Byars' recommended technique depended upon the identification of the posterior facial vein, "The identification of the lower division of the facial nerve is readily accomplished by taking advantage of its position relative to the posterior facial vein. This division is large enough to be recognized from appearance alone, without the use of mechanical or electrical stimulation. The posterior facial vein arises superior to the parotid gland and courses downward through its substance, leaving the gland near the anterior central point of its lower tip, terminating in the common facial vein. This vein may be located by freeing the lower pole of the gland from its attachment to the fascia of the sternomastoid muscle . . . On dissecting within the gland immediately anterior to the vein, toward the chin, a sizeable division of the facial nerve is encountered almost immediately, paralleling the vein." As far as the operation was concerned, "The object of the conservative operation is total removal of the tumor without facial nerve injury. No effort is made to enucleate the tumor at the level of its false capsule; where feasible, a thin layer of adjacent normal gland is excised with the tumor. Nor is any attempt made to remove the en-

Byars' description of the stages immediately prior to Figure 5 reads, "As the lower pole of the parotid gland is separated from the sternomastoid muscle, the posterior facial vein is encountered emerging from the anterior central portion of the tip of the lower pole of the gland . . . The lower division of the facial nerve is easily located by searching immediately in front of the posterior facial vein within the substance of the parotid gland."

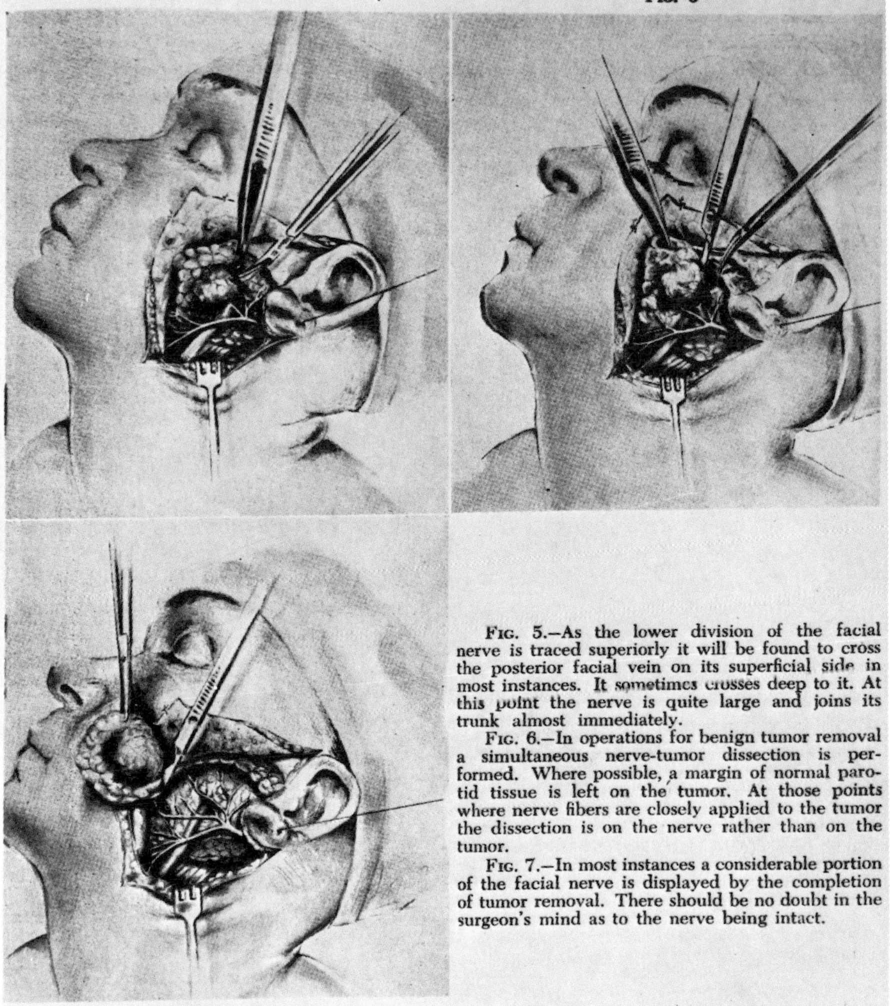

Louis T. Byars, *Preservation of the Facial Nerve in Operations for Benign Conditions of the Parotid Area.* Volume LXX, 1952.

FIG. 5.—As the lower division of the facial nerve is traced superiorly it will be found to cross the posterior facial vein on its superficial side in most instances. It sometimes crosses deep to it. At this point the nerve is quite large and joins its trunk almost immediately.

FIG. 6.—In operations for benign tumor removal a simultaneous nerve-tumor dissection is performed. Where possible, a margin of normal parotid tissue is left on the tumor. At those points where nerve fibers are closely applied to the tumor the dissection is on the nerve rather than on the tumor.

FIG. 7.—In most instances a considerable portion of the facial nerve is displayed by the completion of tumor removal. There should be no doubt in the surgeon's mind as to the nerve being intact.

tire parotid gland except in radical operations for malignancy." Byars provided no statistics of any kind.

Discussion

Robert M. Janes, of Toronto, Canada, said he long since described a technique of identifying the trunk of the nerve posteriorly, and then following it into the gland.

* * *

Lester R. Sauvage, by invitation, and Henry N. Harkins, of Seattle, Professor of Surgery and Executive Officer, Department of Surgery, University of Washington, *An Experimental Study of the Effects of Preservation on the Fate of Aortic and Vena-Caval*

Homografts in the Growing Pig, studied the fate of grafts in 50 young pigs who grew from 30 pounds to 237 pounds at the time of slaughtering, an average weight increase of 690%. The duration of the period of preservation had no effect upon the incidence of thrombosis or the growth of the pig. Nor did it seem to be related to degenerative charges in the grafts. Short aortic homografts in the abdominal aorta of the growing pig, ". . . increase in dimensions but at a slower rate than does the aorta of the host." Vena caval grafts similarly implanted ". . . remain stationary or actually decrease in diameter following implantation . . ."

Discussion

Henry Swan, II, of Denver, was encouraged by the enlargment of the aorta grafts with the growth of the pigs. They had tried a variety of preservation techniques and recently turned to the "technic of dehydration. In this technic the vessels are first quick-frozen and then dried under vacuum, then just stored at room temperature in a test tube. They are used by placing them in Ringer's solution." Grafts stored thus for nine months, had been used successfully. J. Albert Key, of St. Louis, commented that Nageotte "About 30 years ago . . . claimed that the connective tissue elements persisted, and the cells died, and that these grafts were then repopulated by living cells from the host." Key had studied the matter in Boston and in Baltimore,- "We speak of 'creeping substitution' in bone replacement. I think you have 'creeping substitution' in these vascular grafts and in tendon grafts, and that they are replaced not by normal tissue but by scar tissue. They act as temporary prostheses and the whole graft is gradually removed and replaced by scar tissue, and this may exhibit a tendency to contract and a tendency to give way. This demonstration of the persistence of the elastic tissue [by Sauvage and Harkins] is the first good evidence I have seen that the graft really persists."

* * *

Ormand C. Julian, William S. Dye, John H. Olwin, and Paul H. Jordan, of Chicago, by invitation, *Direct Surgery of Arteriosclerosis*, referred to the history of blood vessel grafting,- Carrel's 1907 technique of vascular anastomosis, Bernheim's 1913 suggestion of the use of autogenous vein grafts reversed and shorter than the precise defect, Binnie's 1910 suggestion that vein grafts could replace an obstructed and diseased artery. From France, Kunlin, in 1949, and Fontaine, in 1951, had reported clinical experience with venous grafts in arteriosclerotic disease. dos Santos, 1947, had performed endarterectomy through incisions at either end of the obstruction, using a specially designed instrument. Rebout, in 1949, had made an arterial incision the length of the obstruction, lifted out the atheroma and closed the vessel longitudinally. A number of important clinical reports had now appeared, Freeman having added continuous regional heparinization, and Wiley, after thromboendarterectomy of the aorta having reinforced the aortic wall with fascia lata. They chose their patients for evidence of segmental ob-

struction, with lack of ischemic changes in the foot, with intermittent claudication but with no rest pain and no neuritic pain. Pulses were to be absent and the arteriogram, made either by translumbar aortic injection or percutaneous femoral puncture, determined operability. A normal artery, abruptly blocked, and communicating by demonstrated collaterals to a good vessel below, was operable no matter what the length of the occluded area. A proximal artery, with many irregular filling defects above and below was usually operated upon but not with the same degree of success. If the principal channels distal to the obstruction were not filled by the arteriogram, the operation usually failed. In patients with diffuse disease and irregularity of the arterial tree and no complete obstruction, operation was not undertaken. In many cases rather than sacrifice a potential collateral vessel, usually the profunda femoris, ". . . the elastic outer coats were everted to form a cuff and then slowly stripped back, the cuff being threaded onto the vessel while a clean cleavage plane was carefully separated. When the collateral vessel was reached, its ostium from within the major channel could then be visualized and freed of partially occluding material. This process seemed to leave a relatively smooth surface free of remaining shreds of atherosclerotic material." Intimectomy alone had been done in six iliac arteries and one superficial femoral, from the common femoral bifurcation to the popliteal bifurcation. They had placed 19 vein grafts in the superficial femoral artery with successes in 12 as judged by return of pulses at the ankle, increase in the oscillometric index in the calf, and relief of intermittent claudication. There had been six failures, one death, and two amputations,- the death from coronary occlusion. The intimectomy of the superficial femoral artery was successful for the three months before the patient suicided. Three of the other vessels treated by intimectomy were demonstrated by aortography to be open and two to have occluded. A single resection of the aortic bifurcation and replacement with an aortic homograft, in a young woman, had been successful thus far for two months. They expressed a certain pessimism, "Except in unusual instances, the value to the patient of such procedures cannot be thought of as extending over a very long period of time. Most patients although they have operable distinct segments

---

The saphenous vein was reversed, the femoral artery excised and the anastomoses performed end-to-end. Twelve of 19 grafts, all performed for intermittent claudication, were considered to be successful. They were often combined with "intimectomy" as shown in their Figure 9, commonly superiorly, to permit opening the orifice of the profunda femoris. In one patient, the entire femoral artery was successfully opened by this technique, without vein graft. ▶

Ormand C. Julian, William S. Dye, John H. Olwin and Paul H. Jordan, *Direct Surgery of Arteriosclerosis*. Volume LXX, 1952.

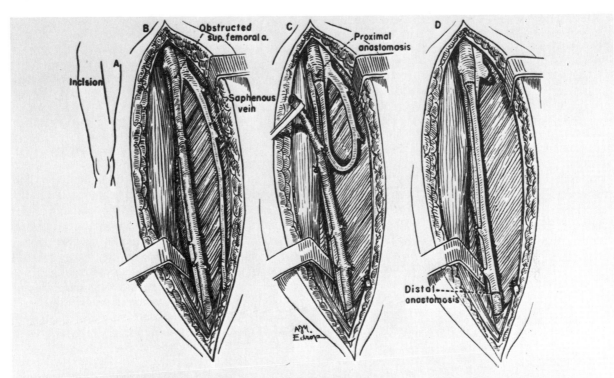

FIG. 6.—Steps in technic of placing saphenous autograft to replace superficial femoral artery.

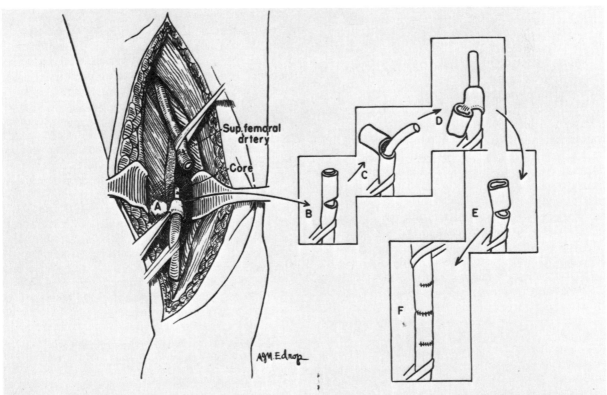

FIG. 9.—Diagram showing everting method of intimectomy when applied to long arterial segments as in case shown in Figure 8.

of arteriosclerosis, also have arteriosclerotic involvement outside the resected area. They are, therefore, subject to other arterial obstructions elsewhere and to re-obstruction of the vessel above and below the site of surgical treatment."

Discussion

Norman E. Freeman, of San Francisco, congratulated Dr. Julian and his associates saying, however, that ". . . surgery hasn't got very much to offer in the treatment of arteriosclerosis, *per se.* Arteriosclerosis is a widespread, generalized disorder . . ." Freeman presented the case of a man with an aortic thrombosis in whom the thrombus was removed from the renal artery down, with relief, and a patient in whom a lumbar aortic aneurysm was bypassed, turning down the splenic artery to the iliac [the aneurysm ruptured three weeks later]. In another patient he brought the left superficial femoral to the right common femoral with success.

* * *

Harry W. Fischer, of St. Louis; Harold Albert, of New Orleans; William L. Riker, all by invitation, and Willis J. Potts, of Chicago, Associate Professor of Surgery, Northwestern University Medical School; Surgeon-in-Chief, Children's Memorial Hospital, *Successful Experimental Maintenance of Life by Homologous Lungs and Mechanical Heart,* had previously demonstrated that adequate respiration could be maintained in dogs by pumping a dog's blood through homologous lungs, and Mustard and Chute, also in 1951, had made similar experiments. Potts and his colleagues now reported ". . . that life of a subject animal can be maintained by homologous lungs and a membrane pump while the heart and lungs of that animal are excluded from function for short periods of time and that such an animal will survive the experiment without evidence of organ damage." The superior and inferior venae cavae of the subject dog were cannulated from the jugular and femoral veins respectively. The caval blood was then pumped into the pulmonary artery of the donor lung from which it emerged through a tube in the attached left atrium. The donor lung's trachea was connected to an anesthesia machine. The blood was returned to the subject animal's femoral artery. Complaining that "It hardly seems possible that so many pitfalls could present themselves in the performance of these seemingly simple experiments", they presented the results in four animals surviving complete occlusion of the venae cavae from 32 minutes to 40 minutes, showing very satisfactory maintenance of pH and arterial oxygen saturation. The animals survived and remained in good health, and they concluded that "Homologous lungs serve as a satisfactory mechanism for the respiratory exchange of gases."

Discussion

Clarence Dennis, now of Brooklyn, opened the Discussion with a statement that "Dr. Claude Beck suggested to our group in 1949 that we undertake to try to carry out oxygenation by means of the lungs of a dog" and they had succeeded, but fearing ". . . that in practical clinical application, it would not be possible to get lungs at times when lungs were needed", and after experimenting with perfusion of a single lung of the subject dog, had abandoned such efforts, "At the present time I think Dr. Gibbon and his group, and our group, are satisfied that the exchange of gases in mechanical oxygenators is no longer a serious bulwark in the way of the solution of the problem." Robert M. Janes, of Toronto, said he had ". . . watched the work of Mustard and Chute for the last four or five years, and their attempts to use what they call a biological oxygenator. I thought perhaps the Association would be interested in knowing that they have recently applied this method to several young infants, using a monkey lung to oxygenate the blood. I watched them on one occasion, and it was very striking, indeed, to see the saturation of 50 to 60 per cent quickly change to a saturation of over 90 per cent. On one occasion recently they have carried the patient . . . for as long as three hours. They have been balked by the congenital defect they encountered, but it seems to me the oxygenator, despite the tremendous mechanical difficulties, seems to have worked." John H. Gibbon, Jr., of Philadelphia, agreed with Dennis ". . . that probably it would be quite difficult to get a nice, fresh human lung that is going to serve as an oxygenator, and that we had better stick by the methods which we have been working with, in order to accomplish the gas exchange in the blood." Since the previous year, Gibbon had a completely new apparatus of the vertical screen type and had 12 dogs alive and well following dependence upon the artificial circulation for periods of over an hour, "I think we are all on the borderline of using these apparatuses on human patients. Dr. Dennis, as you know, has used them on two patients." [At the 1953 meeting, in the Discussion of the paper by Geoghegan and Lam on air embolism during cardiac operations, Dennis mentioned the fact that his second patient had a satisfactory closure of an atrial septal defect on extracorporeal circulation, but had subsequently died because the blood level in the oxygenator fell and oxygen was pumped into the patient's arterial system.] Gibbon had used his apparatus for the partial support of a woman dying of cardiorespiratory failure, introducing the venous catheter through the jugular vein and the arterial catheter through the radial artery. The head and the arm had become pink and they had learned that they should have used the subclavian artery and that the venous catheter should have gone down into the heart. Willis J. Potts appropriately said, "It has been about 15 years since Dr. Gibbon presented his paper, and so he is actually the father–I should say the youthful father– of all of this whole story of extracorporeal circulation." After they had been working in Chicago for a couple years, "I heard of the work of Mustard and Chute up at Toronto . . . Their apparatus is beautiful compared to ours. Ours is really primitive . . . I am interested to hear that the monkey lungs work." Potts made no comment on the relative advantages of heterologous lungs and artificial oxygenators, saying only, "It appears that the respiratory epithelium of the lungs is a nonspecific membrane, and that the lungs are primitive structures serving only for the exchange of gases."

* * *

William H. Muller, Jr., and J. Francis Dammann, Jr., of Los Angeles, both by invitation, *The Surgical Significance of Pulmonary Hypertension*, presented an analysis of the problem of pulmonary hypertension, which was beginning to be appreciated as a serious consequence of long continued high pulmonary artery flow, and thought to be a particular problem in patients with Eisenmenger's complex. They pointed out that "A significant group of patients with pulmonary hypertension is that in which the communication between the systemic and pulmonary circulations is intracardiac. This group includes patients who have a single ventricle without pulmonic stenosis, large ventricular septal defects, and the Eisenmenger's complex. In each of these abnormalities the heart functions physiologically as a single ventricle in that there is a common ventricular ejectile force . . . At the present time there is no satisfactory surgical procedure for treatment of these deformities. Correction of the septal defect is logical and has been attempted, but will probably not be practical until the extracorporeal pump can be used satisfactorily. It has been suggested by Civin and

Edwards [1950] that pulmonary hypertension and blood flow might be diminished by surgically creating pulmonary stenosis in these patients and thus affording protection to the small pulmonary arteries. The case which they reported lent support to this suggestion." Blalock [1951], and Goldberg [1951], had discussed the possibility of creating pulmonary stenosis. Muller and Dammann employed Hufnagel's [1951] technique for creating pulmonary stenosis by excising a portion of the pulmonary artery with a partial occlusion clamp, in addition narrowing the pulmonary artery by 80% and wrapping the narrowed portion with "reactive polyethylene film and cotton tape" to prevent subsequent dilatation, a technique which Clatworthy [1950] had employed for producing experimental aortic coarctation. The technique proved to be satisfactory in producing pulmonic stenosis in dogs. They had performed the procedure on three patients,- with great success in a four-and-half-months-old infant thought to have a single ventricle, a postoperative death in a nine-month-old infant with a two-chambered heart and rudimentary left ventricle and a good result in a five-year-old boy who had a large ventricular septal defect and coarctation as well, simultaneously corrected. In these, and other patients, they studied the pulmonary arteries by biopsy and pointed out that it was, as yet, unknown whether the pulmonary vascular disease associated with pulmonary hypertension was reversible or not (see illustration on p. 986).

* * *

Chester E. Herrod, Russel H. Lee, W. H. Goggans, R. K. McCombs, all by invitation, and Frank Gerbode, of San Francisco, Associate Clinical Professor of Surgery, Stanford University School of Medicine, *Control of Heart Action by Repetitive Electrical Stimuli*, said that acute ventricular fibrillation was treated by electrical defibrillation with intracardiac procaine or potassium. Cardiac standstill was treated by injection of epinephrine or calcium into the heart and rhythmic manual compression, "The frequent failure of such measures has been a stimulus to investigate methods which supply an artificial pacemaker for the heart." Some work had been done [Bigelow, See page 950, Volume LXVIII, 1950] and Sweet in 1947 had reported clinical stimulation of the sino-atrial node for intraoperative standstill. Their instrument was a combination defibrillator and pacemaker. "The electrodes were applied to the sino-atrial node at the junction of the superior vena cava and the right auricle, to the auricular-ventricular junction anteriorly, and to the surface of

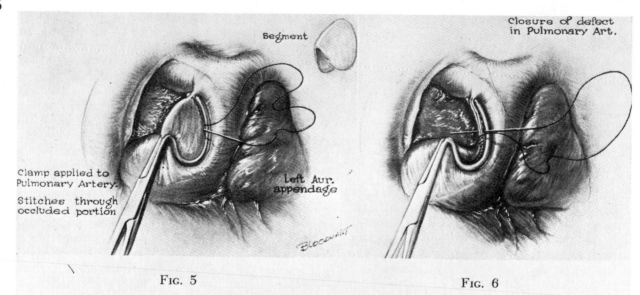

FIG. 5   FIG. 6

FIG. 5.—The partial occlusion clamp has been applied to the mid-portion of the pulmonary artery and a continuous mattress suture is being placed in the portion of the vessel occluded by the clamp. The segment to be excised is in the upper right corner.

FIG. 6.—The segment of vessel wall within the occluding clamp has been excised and a continuous over-and-over hemostatic suture is being placed along the cut edge. (By permission of Surgery, Gynecology and Obstetrics.)

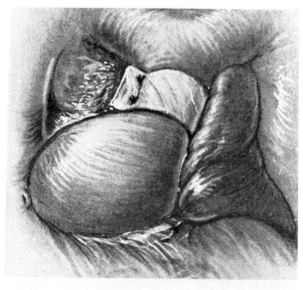

FIG. 7.—Drawing showing the band made of reactive polyethylene film and cotton tape which has been sutured about the area of narrowing in the main pulmonary artery. (By permission of Surgery, Gynecology and Obstetrics.)

the heart over the interventricular septum." Repetitive electrical stimuli of two to three volts, 0.04 to 0.06 amps. of 0.02 to 0.10 seconds duration superimposed beats on the normally beating heart and domi-

Technique employed by Muller and Dammann for narrowing the pulmonary artery in three children with severe pulmonary hypertension associated with ventricular septal defect, successfully in two. To Hufnagel's excision technique for narrowing the pulmonary artery, they had added the banding with reactive polyethylene film and cotton tape. Banding alone soon became, and for a time remained, a standard preliminary treatment for children with excessive flow to the lungs, and in inoperable situations, the only treatment.

William H. Muller, Jr., and J. Francis Dammann, Jr., *The Surgical Significance of Pulmonary Hypertension,* Volume LXX, 1952.

nated the rhythm,- if large doses of procaine amide were given. More intense or longer stimulation caused ventricular fibrillation. After fibrillation and defibrillation, the pacemaker was effective if the anoxia had not been of such long duration as to damage the heart, and after standstill, "Rhythmic manual compression is more effective than repetitive electrical stimuli in reviving the heart . . ." They suspected that the method had not much clinical application for use in cardiac arrest, except perhaps ". . . in vagal asystole . . . and perhaps in certain instances of drug depression." [No mention is made of the use of pacemakers in patients with heart block.]

* * *

Charles Huggins, of Chicago, Professor of Surgery (Urology), the University of Chicago; Director, Ben May Laboratory for Cancer Research, [who was to be the second member, after Alexis Carrel, to receive the Nobel Prize in the first 100 years of the Association] and Thomas Ling-Yuan Dao, by invitation, *Adrenalectomy for Mammary Cancer,* discussed the application of adrenalectomy to breast cancer [Huggins having in 1945 reported his celebrated first successful total adrenalectomy for prostatic cancer in man]. They had performed bilateral adrenalectomy on six women with cancer of the breast, recurrent several months to five years after mastectomy, and in one patient with a far-advanced primary tumor. Four patients had had satisfactory results with "Relief of pain. Healing of fracture. Partial sclerosis of osseous lesions. No new ones"; "Pain-free. Resorption of pleural fluid. Actively at work"; "Remarkable regression of local recurrence . . ."; "Complete relief of pain and return to active work." One patient with pulmonary metastases had no relief and died 34 days after operation, another had remarkable regression of pulmonary and cerebral metastases for six months but was dead within eight months. The patient with a far-advanced primary tumor showed no effect and died in six months. In all, they had done bilateral adrenalectomy in 42 patients for a variety of indications, with no deaths in the last 38 bilateral adrenalectomies. In four of the women cited, they had also removed the ovaries, and the others were postmenopausal. They had also performed adrenalectomy in a man with carcinoma of the breast who had a good remission for six months, from pulmonary and cerebral metastases. They preferred the posterior approach through the bed of the 12th rib, and after operation maintenance on cortisone had proved not to be difficult.

Discussion

Lester R. Dragstedt, of Chicago, said that it was interesting that patients could get along without their adrenal medulla, the secretions of which were not replaced by Huggins, adding that "We know, however, that chromaffin tissue resembling that found in the medulla is present elsewhere in the body. Is it possible that after removal of the adrenal glands, this extra-adrenal chromaffin tissue takes over the function of the medulla and restores the former concentration of epinephrine in the blood? ", and asked whether Huggins had any data on this. Oliver Cope, of Boston, commented further on the total removal of an endocrine gland. "We all recall the era of total thyroidectomy for heart disease, where a decreased load on the heart of hypothyroidism was balanced against a myxedematous heart, a heart less able to carry on. Another example of total resection of a gland is total resection of all the parathyroid tissue for Paget's disease . . . I am guilty of having practiced it twice under the aegis of Dr. Albright, another adventurous endocrinologist, and in that case the osteolytic process of Paget's disease was balanced off against tetany. The Paget's disease got better, but the patient suffered at least as much, if not more, from tetany. There is another example of total removal of a normal gland and that is the total removal of the adrenal, recently recommended by the Brigham group for essential hypertension. It is true that hypertension occurs in Cushing's disease, and that the normal adrenal has something to do with the maintenance of blood pressure. It can readily be realized that if the adrenals are resected, producing hypocortinism, the hypertension wouldn't be so severe . . . I have found what one would suspect, that you can lower the blood pressure but you have a patient with Addison's disease, and he is exceedingly sick. When you make them better by giving them an adequate dose of cortisone, their hypertension comes back. This is true of essential hypertension. It is not true of the Cushing's disease hypertension which is due to hyperfunctioning adrenals." Huggins, he said, had referred to ". . . the double function of the adrenal cortex . . . the sex-like or sex-supporting activity in the adrenal, which is really what he is getting rid of with cortisone. He replaces completely that aspect of the cortex which has been called the life-maintaining aspect—the aspect related to hypertension . . . His idea looks solid, for it appears that the body can dispense with sex . . . Sex, at least as the adrenal makes it, isn't essential for life." F. L. Reichert, of San Francisco, said that ". . . years ago the pituitary gland was thought to be essential to life, and now it isn't. They found in this gland one hormone, then two, three, and it's up to six or eight now. There are more than just two hormones in the adrenal cortex. I'm not

988

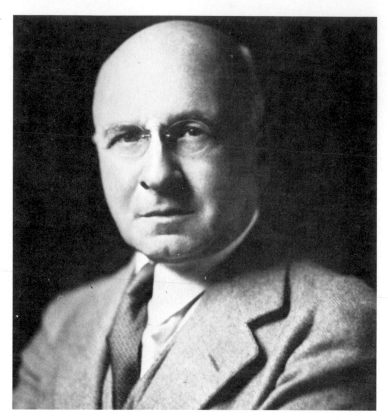

Alexis Carrel 1873-1944, Nobel Prize 1912, French born.   M.D., Lyons 1900, hospital training Lyons 1900-1904. A man of brilliant imagination, great energy and always a great gift for self-promotion. Emigrated to the United States in 1904, securing a post at the University of Chicago in the Hull Physiological Laboratory, where he was assigned to work with the junior C. C. Guthrie. Carrel had already worked on vascular anastomoses in France and the two began a productive collaboration. From Chicago, Carrel went to the Rockefeller Institute as one of its original members, creating the Department of Experimental Surgery. He was brilliantly creative and imaginative, marvelously dextrous. This history records his contributions to vessel suture and repair, grafting, prosthetic replacement, intracardiac surgery, coronary vascularization, organ replantation, most of these technics long before their time of clinical application. Tissue culture was his creation. During World War I, he introduced the hypochlorite (Carrel-Dakin solution) treatment, a great contribution at the time to the treatment of infected wounds. With Charles Lindbergh, he worked on an extracorporeal circulation. His memory is tainted by reports of his pro Nazi sympathies and actions during World War II.

   (Portrait courtesy of Falk Library of the Health Professions, University of Pittsburgh, Pa.)

THE NOBEL LAUREATES

The Nobel Prizes in Medicine have generally not been awarded to surgeons and most of the few surgeons receiving the award (viz. Ross for his work in malaria, Banting for the discovery of insulin) were honored for work not in the domain of surgery. The great unfolding and development of abdominal surgery, neurosurgery, thoracic surgery,

(Continues on facing page.)

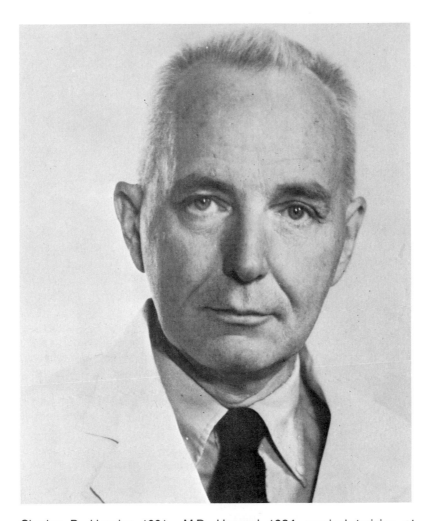

Charles B. Huggins 1901-, M.D. Harvard 1924, surgical training at University of Michigan. Joined Phemister at Chicago in 1927, turned to urology and became Professor in 1936. Nobel Prize in 1966 for his "discoveries concerning hormonal treatment of prostatic cancer". A tireless, endlessly inquisitive investigator, (still active as he approaches his ninth decade), mentor of a series of physiologically-minded urologic surgeons and numerous other investigators who have come through his laboratory. Invited by Blalock to the Chair at Hopkins,- long before the Nobel Prize,- he accepted, arrived, tested the waters for a day, resigned, and resumed his work and position in Chicago.

cardiac surgery, and transplantation have gone unrecognized in Stockholm. In endocrine surgery, only Theodore Kocher (Honorary Fellow of ASA, 1894) received the Nobel Prize in 1909 for his contribution to "the physiology, surgery and pathology of the thyroid gland." Nor have the contributions of surgery to the biologic sciences in these areas and in the understanding of shock, infection, gastrointestinal and endocrine physiology, cardiac function, neurophysiology, etc., received the Stockholm accolade. Clearly there is often disagreement over who merits an award in a given area, but whole fields of endeavor seem to have been considered not worthy of recognition by the conferring of this award. The Prize was awarded to Fellows of the Association in 1912 and 1966 for work recognizably surgical.

saying that you shouldn't take the adrenal cortex out and make an Addisonian individual, or even superimpose—as Dr. [W. W.] Scott has—taking out the pituitary and making a pituitary-less individual and an adrenal-less individual in an attempt to free him of his metastases. I simply want to point out that since we know so little about these various portions of the adrenal cortex and of the pituitary, and their relations to the metabolism and the function and the resistance in the body, just a few of the individuals in surgery should continue this work." Huggins, in closing, reemphasized the necessity for a meticulous and total removal of the unbroken adrenal. "I have the great advantage of having a Chinese assistant, and—in emphasizing the necessity for avoiding blunt dissection (with which I thoroughly concur)—Dr. Dao expressed it in a typical classical form of Chinese aphorism, 'Too much dissection with fingers tears gland.'" "Certainly, in these patients, the adrenal stress factor has been eliminated by adrenalectomy [he had apparently not measured the catecholamines in patients after adrenalectomy, but] . . . After adrenalectomy, people maintained on a constant amount of cortisone, given by mouth, state that they are rather calmer mentally than before, that they can get angry, that fear, pain, hunger and rage still operate; they can get angry, but it doesn't hold over . . ." Blood pressure was totally unaffected and patients whether hypotensive or not retained the same pressure after operation that they had had before. He did point out that people on cortisone after the operation did have a darkening of the coloring of the hair, "We believe that cortisone acetate prevents pigmentation of the skin, but cortisone acetate apparently is not able to prevent pigmentation from occurring in the hair, and this occurs, to the surprise and quite often the delight of the patient." He agreed with Oliver Cope that "the benefit that accrues after adrenalectomy is through the elimination of sex steroids." He agreed with Dr. Reichert ". . . that this is rather thin ice on which we skate . . . However, through adrenalectomy, one can relieve suffering and prolong life . . .", and finally cautioned that "In endocrine control I wish to emphasize once more that no one speaks of this in terms of cure. All we consider is a decrease in activity, a decrease in size of the tumor . . . but never do we consider this in terms of cure."

* * *

[There had been considerable interest in the early years of the Association in the operative treatment of epilepsy by simple trephine, or by excisions

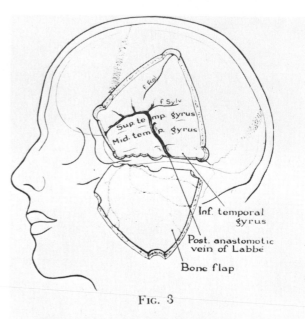

Fig. 3.

FIG. 3.—The bony opening designed to expose the fissures of Rolando and Sylvius as well and the frontal operculum.

Under local anesthesia, including injection around the middle meningeal artery and often injection into the Gasserian ganglion, the epileptogenic focus was identified by reproducing the symptoms with cortical stimulation and by the detection of abnormal cortical electrical activity. Penfield insisted on the necessity for finding abnormal and scarred tissue and for deep excision,- by the sucker,- of the epileptogenic focus. If one did not go more than 5.5 cm. back from the tip of the temporal lobe, visual field defects were not produced. Fifty percent of the patients were completely relieved.

Wilder Penfield and Maitland Baldwin, *Temporal Lobe Seizures and the Technic of Subtotal Temporal Lobectomy.* Volume LXX, 1952. (Figure continues on facing page.)

of the cortex (W. T. Briggs, 1884, W. W. Keen, 1888; D. Hayes Agnew, Nancrede, Park, 1891; P. S. Conner, 1892) and the general attitude had become one of discouragement.] Now Wilder Penfield, of Montreal, Professor of Neurology and Neurosurgery, McGill University; Director, Montreal Neurologic Institute; Attending Surgeon, Royal Victoria and Montreal General Hospitals, and by invitation, Maitland Baldwin, of Montreal, *Temporal Lobe Seizures and the Technic of Subtotal Temporal Lobectomy,* presented their second paper before the Association on the treatment of epilepsy. Five years earlier, they had presented "a discussion of the treatment of focal epilepsy in general by cortical excision . . . pointed out that although the history of the en-

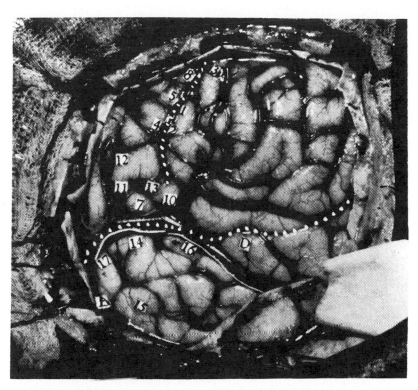

Fig. 4.—Case F. D. Operative photograph showing stimulation tickets on the brain. The intended line of excision is shown by white thread parallel to the vein of Labbé. Dotted white lines are placed in the fissure of Rolando and in the fissure of Sylvius.

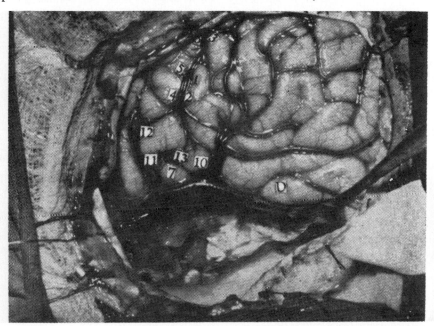

Fig. 5.—Case F. D. Partial excision of the temporal lobe has been carried out along the vein of Labbé. The white matter of temporal stem and the insula can be seen in the depth of the operative cavity.

trance of surgery into this field had been filled with records of disappointment, the time had come when wise clinical analysis of the history of each case checked by electroencephalographic localization and roentgen ray analysis made it possible for the surgeon to stand on firm ground in his approach to the radical treatment of selected patients." Gibbs, Gibbs, and Lennox, in 1938, had identified by electroencephalography a type of epilepsy to which they gave the name "psychomotor". Jasper, in 1941, had "pointed out that discharge was localizable in the temporal regions, and that in the majority of cases the originating focal discharge was present in one temporal lobe." Penfield and Flanigan, in 1950, reported 55% success in 68 cases of temporal lobe epilepsy treated by "excision of a larger or smaller portion of one temporal lobe". Half the patients had had no further attacks and half had three attacks before seizures disappeared. In 1951, Bailey and Gibbs and Green, Duisberg, and McGrath reported resections of the anterior part of one temporal lobe for epilepsy. Penfield insisted that, as in removal of an epileptogenic focus in the cortex elsewhere, it was necessary to remove "cortex which is abnormal by gross and microscopic standards" the focus being found "as indicated by E.E.G., seizure pattern, electrical stimulation and the assistance of a conscious patient." The bone flap was elevated under local anesthesia. The cortex was stimulated with a unipolar electrode, a square wave generator supplying a current of 1 to 2 volts with 2 milliseconds wave duration and 60 pulses per second. When the epileptogenic focus was stimulated, the patient's seizures were simulated and recording electrodes from the same area showed abnormal discharges. The portion of the brain was removed with a sucker. In most cases "the anterior portion of the first temporal convolution is found to be tough in the depth of the removal, and this tough tissue extends into the uncus and hippocampal gyrus mesially and posteriorly." If the inferior horn of the ventricle was opened into, it was then usually sealed with a bit of gelfoam sutured into place. In addition to scalp anesthesia, anesthetic was injected about the middle meningeal artery and often into the Gasserian ganglion. Appropriate excision of the anterior portion of the temporal lobes did not produce visual field defects. Resection more than 5.5 cm. from the anterior tip produced permanent homonymous upper quadrantic defects. The gross and histologic changes found in the excised brain,- astrogliosis, patchy demyelinization,- they agreed was the effect of anoxia, probably neonatal. Penfield said nothing more about complications and nothing about mortality.

Discussion

William Jason Mixter, of Boston, the only discusser, expressed his gratitude to Penfield for his contributions, "He has shown us where the lesion lies, and I think most of us have had the feeling—I know I did—up to a short time ago that the lesion lay much more on the surface of the temporal lobe rather than deeply, and that it could be picked up by electro-encephalography in the absence of any appearance of scar tissue. That is important, because partial operations in this region, with removal of the surface focus—I know from my own experience—do not give relief."

* * *

N. Logan Leven, of St. Paul, Clinical Professor of Surgery, Department of Surgery, University of Minnesota; Richard L. Varco, of Minneapolis, Associate Professor of Surgery, University of Minnesota; and by invitation, Bernard G. Lannin, and Lyle A. Tongen, *The Surgical Management of Congenital Atresia of the Esophagus and Tracheo-Esophageal Fistula,* since Leven's world's first successful case of management of tracheo-esophageal fistula in 1939, had seen 103 cases. They favored an extrapleural right-sided approach removing the fourth rib. The distal end of the esophagus was divided from the trachea and the trachea closed with interrupted sutures, over some of the mediastinal fat and areolar tissue. Esophageal anastomosis was with a row of interrupted 5-0 silk sutures reinforced by a second row of sutures in the muscularis. Gastrostomy was usually performed the next day, and oral feedings on the tenth day, after radiologic confirmation of anastomotic integrity. Seven patients were not operated upon for a variety of reasons, and five patients died after preliminary gastrostomy. Thirteen of 23 patients survived the completion of a multiple-stage operation and 43 of 68, 75%, survived primary anastomosis. Anastomotic leaks occurred in 16 patients and contributed to the death of ten, three of them with a recurrent tracheo-esophageal fistula. In the last half of the series they had had only three anastomotic leaks.

Discussion

Conrad R. Lam, of Detroit, initiated the Discussion, showing follow-ups on two patients with successful multiple stage operations,- closure of the fistula, cervical esophagostomy, exteriorization of the distal end of the esophagus, connection of the two ends with a chest wall skin tube. Cameron Haight, of Ann Arbor, who had reported the first successful direct anastomosis of the esophagus in this condition in 1943, had now performed 94 anastomoses, ". . . early in our series, we assumed the all-or-none position of trying to obtain an anastomosis, rather than attempting the multiple-stage plan", explaining his less satisfactory overall recovery rates than those of Dr. Leven. He had 57 survivors in a total of 131 patients, 43.4%. In the last three years, he had again undertaken some multiple-stage operations. Since 1947, he had had a 62.9% survival. Mark M. Ravitch, of Baltimore, said that in those cases ". . . in which the most desirable method of operation—Dr. Haight's—is unsuccessful . . . it is now possible to reconstruct the esophagus . . . by a secondary method, very quickly, without the trouble that brought it into ill repute for several years." In patients with failed anastomoses and a cervical esophagostomy, an antethoracic loop of jejunum could be brought to the neck in one stage, and anastomosed to the esophagus a few days later in the second. He pointed out that he had twice seen ". . . peptic ulceration of the jejunal loop in such patients . . ." and that perhaps it was preferable not to insert the distal end of the jejunal loop into the stomach but to leave it attached to the bowel in Roux-Y fashion. I. A. Bigger, of Richmond, preferred a preliminary gastrostomy particularly if there was much abdominal distention. N. Logan Leven, in closing, expressed pleasure that Dr. Haight had now agreed that multiple-stage operations were appropriate in some patients. As to the matter of peptic ulcer in the jejunal loop. ". . . in all likelihood we might get more duodenal ulcers if we do not attach it to the stomach, because we will have pure gastric juice passing through the pylorus into the duodenum without any mixture of food; so you're in a dilemma as to whether you get regurgitation into the jejunum, with jejunitis, or duodenal ulcer. In his reconstructions, Dr. Varco has put the jejunum on the antrum, so that if we should get ulceration of the duodenum, we could go in there transthoracically and resect the cardiac end of the stomach to reduce the acid."

* * *

John D. Stewart, of Buffalo, Professor of Surgery, University of Buffalo; Head of the Department of Surgery, Edward J. Meyer Memorial Hospital, and by invitation, George M. Sanderson, and

Charles E. Wiles, Jr., *Blood Replacement and Gastric Resection for Massively Bleeding Peptic Ulcer*, presented the third report on their continuing study of immediate operation for bleeding peptic ulcer. They now had 110 patients with massive bleeding ulcer, 94 of them operated upon within one to 24 hours after admission, the average being 7.5 hours. Nineteen of the patients proved to have bled from ". . . acute superficial gastric or duodenal ulcer, single, or more commonly, multiple . . . Even at laparotomy . . . there may be no palpable induration and no visible serosal change. At operation, if there is blood in the stomach and if no other cause for bleeding can be found, it is our practice to proceed with subtotal gastrectomy." Their program of immediate blood replacement and subtotal gastrectomy in a consecutive series of 110 cases, resulted in 12 deaths.

Discussion

Michael E. DeBakey, of Houston, agreed that if when operating for massive hemorrhage there is blood in the stomach and yet no obvious lesion ". . . the most effective operative procedure is probably gastric resection." DeBakey considered most of such hemorrhages to be due to diffuse gastritis. Claude E. Welch, of Boston, ". . . preferred to reserve operation for the group of patients that demonstrate continued or recurrent massive hemorrhage, under observation . . ." He maintained that there was ". . . no question but that interval operation is safer for this group of patients if it can be obtained", and that frequently hemorrhage was not as massive as the surgeon feared. At the Massachusetts General Hospital, the surgical mortality rate in the previous three years from massive bleeding duodenal ulcer ". . . as Dr. Stewart has defined it, has been 6 per cent under the age of 70, but it is still about 30 per cent above that age." Ralph F. Bowers, of Memphis, said that bleeding ulcer must be different in Memphis than in Buffalo, where ". . . he [Stewart] handles more elderly people, and has a higher percentage of gastric ulcers . . .", and more of the patients admitted with ulcer disease bled in Buffalo than in most reports. Nevertheless, "For the kind of patients treated by Dr. Stewart, the mortality rate is excellent, his results are very good, and I congratulate him on this splendid record." Calvin M. Smyth, of Philadelphia, agreed absolutely with Dr. Stewart that he could not tell which patients were going to stop bleeding and which were not. He agreed with DeBakey's comment that ligation of all of the arterial supply to the stomach was not sufficient. They were unable to operate as early as Dr. Stewart, but liked to operate within 24 hours.

The Business Meetings

The 1952 meeting was held April 16, 17, and 18, at The Greenbrier, White Sulphur Springs, West Virginia, President Daniel C. Elkin in the Chair.

Dr. Frederick A. Coller made the first report of what was to be a series of annual reports on what he correctly informed the Association was the Committee on " 'Unnecessary Operations', not unnecessary surgery. Surgery implies methods of thinking." The Committee consisted of Calvin Smyth, John Goode, Joe Meigs, Robert Dinsmore, and F. A. Coller as Chairman. [One had the impression, each year in fact, that the work on the report was entirely Dr. Coller's.] He informed the Association that from the School of Public Health, University of Michigan, he learned that in the year 1949 there had been 10,000,000 operations, 4,500,000 of them carried out by general practitioners, 2,000,000 by surgeons, 1,800,000 by ear, nose and throat specialists, and the remaining 1,700,000 by all other specialists; 1,900,000 of the operations were performed in "doc-tors' offices, patients' homes and in out-patient departments." One of the problems, of course, was that they could evaluate the operations which were being done "in the hospitals where you gentlemen work", but operations to twice that number were being performed by general practitioners. Coller had asked ". . . 80 or 90 younger surgeons scattered throughout the country—many of them in smaller towns—to give us evaluations of the work going on in hospitals in their communities, small hospitals." He promised a fuller report the following year.

The old custom, of having the President introduce to the Membership all of the invited guests, had been honored in the breach for some years, and now an Amendment to the Constitution was proposed, for action the following year, to recognize the changing times.

The new President was Robert S. Dinsmore, of Cleveland; Vice-Presidents John H. Gibbon, of Philadelphia, and R. Kennedy Gilchrist, of Chicago; Secretary, Nathan A. Womack, of Chapel Hill.

LXXI

1953

The 1953 meeting was held at the Statler Hotel, Los Angeles, April 1, 2, and 3, Robert Scott Dinsmore, of Cleveland, Chief of Surgery, Cleveland Clinic Hospital, in the Chair.

At the Washington meeting, Dinsmore had been emotional in his acceptance of the office, indicating by expression of gratitude to the Fellows that, as a purely clinical surgeon, he must have owed his election to friendship rather than to scientific merit. In the sentimental peroration of his Presidential Address, he said, "It is not in me to write or read such scholarly addresses as have been given by my predecessors", and commented on the "invisible presence of a group of former members here on the stage", mentioning, among others, "Fred T. Murphy, George Crile, Starr Judd, Dr. Roscoe Graham and Dr. Tommy Jones . . . Most of these men had a real sense of humor, and all of them had surgery in their souls. They are a bit disillusioned and highly amused that I should be doing this, but deep in my heart I in turn am amused at them, because they just think they are dead." In point of fact, his address, *Trends of Surgery in the Last Decade,* is a model of common sense review from the perspective of an enormously experienced surgeon. He spoke of surgery of the thyroid, a consuming lifelong interest of his,-"There is little doubt that the severity of the disease has greatly changed, and I actually think we are treating a mild type of the disease as measured by former standards. In the late 20's and early 30's, 50 of our patients died preoperatively. All of these patients died in the acute crises of the disease, and most of them were admitted with high temperatures, high pulse rates, delirium, and severe gastrointestinal symptoms . . . None of my residents in the last decade has seen a true crisis of hyperthyroidism . . . we do not see patients of this type admitted; in fact, few of them even use a wheel chair." Thiouracil, "enthusiastically hailed as the clinical cure for hyperthyroidism . . . proved to be a most unsatisfactory and dangerous drug . . . propylthiouracil has proved to be the most satisfactory . . . [but] long time remissions of all types of hyperthyroidism have not been much above 50 per cent, and the real advantage of the thiourates has been in the preparation of patients for operation." He had been initially dubious of the value of radioactive iodine, but "now can simply state that the patients who have a diffuse goiter with hyperthyroidism treated with I^{131} are the only ones I have ever seen who at the end of eight weeks are comparable to those who have had subtotal thyroidectomy." He seemed to suggest that the decrease in thyroid disease was not due alone to the correction of iodine deficiency, and suggested that it was due to "nutritional factors . . . The eating habits have changed during the past four or five decades, the principal change being a year-round, widely-diversified diet . . . progress in the transportation and processing of foods . . . refrigerated freight cars and trucks . . . the giant canning industry . . . air transportation and the freezing of foodstuffs." There had been a striking change in the nature of malignant goiters, "Adenocarcinomas formerly represented 85 to 90 per cent of our cases . . . highly maligant, angio-invasive in character, and metastasized through the blood stream. About 15 years ago we began to see what appeared to us to be an increasing number of papillary tumors in children and young adults . . . 65 per cent of all malignant cases are of this character . . . a much lower degree of malignancy, and metastasize through the lymphatics . . . the cause of this change presents the same enigma as the decrease in the severity of hyperthyroidism." He found that "the most spectacular development in all surgery of the last decade has been that accomplished by the men doing cardiac surgery." The country and the American Surgical Association could take pride "because so many of these men have presented their initial work before the Association. These same men are grateful for the real contributions of Crafoord, Brock and Sellors." He referred to the radical change in the "personality quotient of the Cardiologist", who saw previously hopeless patients restored to life, referring to the pioneer work of "Doctors Gross and Blalock", and recalling Sir Thomas Lewis' severe criticisms "of the initial efforts of Cutler, Levine, Beck, Graham, and others, to open the mitral valve . . . stating that it was the damaged myocardium which was the real problem." He mentioned Forssman's first catheterization of the human heart, and that "Cardiac surgery following the suggestions of Cournand, Dexter, Warren, Stead, and Bing has given us the best example of applied physiology of the last decades". But Dinsmore could not resist commenting that "two young members of our cardiac catheterization team became so adept that they actually tied the catheter in a figure of eight knot in the right ventricle. As yet they have not explained to me the intracardiac dynamics which untied the knot, except that I gained from them the impression that whatever it was, it took too long." He was heartened by the insistence of Blalock and of Potts on light anesthesia, and impressed by the "painstakingly, meticulous and accurately" technical performance of cardiac surgery, and insistence of cardiac surgeons upon "dissecting with the sharp end of a Bard-Parker knife." He commented upon the technical, physiological jargon "introduced to hospital corridors and staff rooms", and again could not resist the gentle dig that, "Of course, if a patient has a constriction in the urethra or the common duct, it is called a stricture, but in this field if it occurs in the aorta it is a coarctation." He mentioned Whipple's pancreatico-duodenectomy, with an obvious emphasis upon the brief survival of so many of the patients, was impressed by the increasing success with operation for hyperinsulinism, and attributed to Whipple, and then to "Paxton and Payne from the County Hospital in Los Angeles", the demonstration that operative intervention

for acute pancreatitis substantially increased the mortality. He remained cautious about vagotomy, only going so far as to say "vagotomy is based upon sound physiologic principles, and everyone doing gastric surgery will upon occasion find that a useful procedure." He was dubious about the enthusiasm for total gastrectomy, "I do not believe that surgeons will ever agree that a total gastrectomy is indicated for all carcinomas of the stomach. The overall mortality, morbidity and metabolic effects will be greater." Dr. Brunschwig, he thought, was owed a debt "for at least exciting our imagination" about "the excision of multiple organs for eradication of cancer." He suggested that the principal benefit might be if it led "to doing wider operations in the upper abdomen, and the pelvis, with sacrifice of the expendable organs . . .",- the transverse colon, spleen, and a part of the stomach could be spared. "The organ in the upper abdomen which causes us the most difficulty is the pancreas; in the pelvis, the expendable organs are the uterus, ovaries and tubes, and part of the large bowel, but there is real difficulty when the bladder is invaded." Lower morbidity and mortality of mechanical intestinal obstruction resulted "from the teachings of Wangensteen and Coller on the pathophysiology of the small intestine and on the electrolyte and fluid balance" but "the mortality remains too high in strangulation obstruction of the small intestine," for the long tubes frequently failed to pass, "and when they do there is a tendency toward complacency and a feeling of false security." There had been a progressive decline of the mortality and morbidity of colon surgery, and the better physiological support of the patients and the addition of the "slightly soluble sulfonamides, penicillin and the mycin drugs . . . has led to the almost complete disappearance of stage operations of any kind, resulting in less mortality and morbidity . . ." Sometimes he thought "the factors of preoperative preparation with the correction of all nutritional deficiencies, fluid balance and antibiotics, are overemphasized . . . men like Miles, Rankin, David, Jones, Dixon and some of the other pioneers, did not have these advantages in doing their colon work . . . Dr. Thomas Jones, until the last three weeks of his life, did not use any antibiotics in his colon surgery." Nonetheless, Jones' mortality for abdominoperineal resections for carcinoma of the rectum had dropped from 37 deaths in 329 cases to 30 deaths in 1,000 "and in the last two years of his life he performed 736 colon resections with 18 deaths, a mortality of 2.4 per cent." Dinsmore paid particular tribute to "Unquestionably, the most significant contribution to colon work in the last decade . . . that of Orvar Swenson, who in 1948 introduced the concept that the contracted and normal-appearing rectum and sigmoid were the abnormal portions of the colon in Hirschsprung's Disease. He modified Maunsell's procedure [Maunsell, of New Zealand, see comments by Gerster, Volume XIII, 1895, p. 165 and C. H. Mayo, Volume XXIV, 1906, p. 348] in such a way as to remove these areas of myenteric agenesis and restore intestinal continuity . . . the first surgical procedure introduced in this disease that has restored these children to normal life . . ." Dinsmore commented upon modern anesthesia and the polypharmacy involved in the same vein as he had in his marvelous discussion at the Washington meeting the year before, ". . .surgeon and anesthetists . . . have created a tetralogy of their own, in which too much preoperative sedation is given, and too many drugs and agents are administered at an operative procedure . . . in turn act too fast . . . cause too deep anesthesia; and then, too many reasons are given for the resulting anoxia . . . oftentimes a substance is injected into the vein and the patient is told to count to ten, if he says eleven, he is sure to get something else." He spoke about the acute shortage of nurses and complained that "we have seen the rise of per diem costs in hospitals reach unprecedented rates, and in the four large Cleveland hospitals this morning the per diem cost is $23.00 per bed. Here in Los Angeles it is $28.00." [The cost of a bed today, November 12, 1979, at the Hospital of the University of California at Los Angeles is $238. The cost of a bed at the Cleveland Clinic Hospital is $166. The cost of a day in the surgical intensive care units of those institutions is $547 and $454 respectively.] He spoke warmly of the efforts of the American College of Surgeons, the dedication of its Regents, of the American Board of Surgery and of the quality "of the appraisal meetings at the completing of these [Part II-oral] examinations. For sheer honesty of purpose and fairness, these meetings are a stimulus to any surgeon who attends them."

* * *

Richard H. Sweet, Visiting Surgeon, Massachusetts General Hospital; Associate Clinical Professor of Surgery, Harvard Medical School, *Total Gastrectomy by the Transthoracic Approach. A Subsequent Report*, had accumulated a great deal more experience and radically modified his operative practices since his 1942 presentation with E. D. Churchill before the Association. He was now reporting total gastrectomy in 84 patients. Five times he had performed the operation for benign lesions,-

two huge penetrating ulcers of the posterior wall of the stomach, thought to be carcinomas, two cases of multiple polyps, and one of cirrhosis with variceal bleeding. The original approach had been purely transthoracic but "Beginning in 1946 . . . following the suggestions of Garlock and Humphreys" he had increasingly used a thoracoabdominal approach beginning with the abdominal incision to determine operability, then extending it across the costal arch. He had employed that approach in 24 of the last 30 patients. From the first, he had removed the entire omentum, he had removed the spleen for injury or because of involvement in the cancer in 50 of the 77 patients with carcinoma, had performed partial pancreatectomy in 18, partial colectomy in four and a resection of a portion of the liver in three. Analysis of the pattern of lymphatic extension lent "support to the contention brought forth by Longmire, [*Surgery, Gynecology,* and *Obstetrics* 84:21, 1947] and supported by Lahey and Marshall [Volume LXVIII, 1950, page 951] and others, that total gastrectomy should be employed in all cases of carcinoma of the stomach". [It must have been a source of some discomfiture to him to have had President Dinsmore precede him with a directly contrary statement.] Allison and Borrie had "advocated the inclusion of splenectomy and partial pancreatectomy in all patients with carcinoma involving fundus or cardia . . . this suggestion should be adopted in the performance of the operation of total gastrectomy as well." He had performed his reconstruction by esophagoduodenostomy in 14 patients and by esophagojejunostomy in 70. Of these, eight were Roux-en-Y and 59 end of the esophagus to side of a loop of jejunum, with an enteroenterostomy between the jejunal loops, which were usually of considerable length. Patients with esophagoduodenostomy or with a Roux-type anastomosis "experienced no delay in swallowing at any time", whereas the patients with an end-to-side anastomosis had difficulty in taking fluid "During the first few days after operation." Thereafter, the advantages were "in favor of the patient with an end-to-side esophagojejunostomy, especially if a long entero-enterostomy was made between the two arms of the loop. These patients seem to tolerate larger meals than the others." There was no difference in dumping. Dividing one or more jejunal arteries, it was possible to bring even such a jejunal loop well up into the thorax, otherwise a Roux-en-Y loop was used for that purpose. A considerable length of esophagus was usually resected so that in 47 patients, the anastomosis was above the diaphragm. Analyzing the mortality by the availability of antibacterial agents,- mortality in

998

the sulfadiazine era was 12%, all from sepsis, and the mortality in the penicillin and streptomycin era was 13%, none from sepsis. Fifteen patients died of the operation, 90% of the series. One patient died of shock, six patients died of "sepsis" [the term anastomotic leak is not mentioned anywhere in the text], and one patient died of disruption of a duodenal stump closure. As for survivals, there were nine in the 44 operated upon three years or more, and two in the 28 operated upon five years or more before. He concluded by recommending the abdominothoracic approach, a wide resection of tissue,- "include the removal of a long segment of the esophagus, the paracardial and left gastric lymph nodes, the spleen, the left half of the pancreas, a sufficient cuff of duodenum, the lymph nodes in the duodenal area, and the great omentum."

Discussion

George Humphreys who attended the meeting did not discuss Sweet's paper [Longmire and Lahey are not recorded as having attended, and Garlock, to whom Sweet had referred, was not (and never became) a Fellow of the Association. Nor did any representative from the hospitals of these men rise in discussion]. Owen Wangensteen, of Minneapolis, did discuss Sweet's paper at length, emphasizing his preference for a Roux-Y anastomosis, citing references to its use in total gastrectomy by "Goldschwend . . . 1908 . . . Tom Orr . . . 1950 . . . Mont Reid . . . 1925". For carcinoma of the stomach, he preferred his "extrapleural sternal split into the left fourth interspace", although admitting that it was not adequate for carcinoma of the esophagus. James T. Priestley, of the Mayo Clinic, Rochester, Minnesota, commented, "I think that one can do virtually as radical a removal of lymph-node-bearing area if a small amount of stomach is preserved as if total gastrectomy is performed. From our point of view, at least, we have not as yet been convinced that total gastrectomy is the operation of choice in all cases of cancer of the stomach." Sweet, closing, said that, of course, high in the chest, the Roux-Y anastomosis had to be used and that the 56% involvement of the esophagus by cancer was a matter of bias in the referral of cases, which came to him because of dysphagia.

* * *

J. M. Emmett, of Clifton Forge, Virginia, Chief Surgeon, Chesapeake and Ohio Railway Company, and by invitation, E. T. Owens, *Gastrectomy as a Treatment for Perforated Peptic Ulcers,* referred to the initial papers of Judin, of Moscow, in 1937 and 1939, the previous American papers by Graves, and the subsequent publications of Strauss, Bisgard, DeBakey and others. General experience was that simple closure of a perforation resulted in persistent ulcer symptoms in some 80% of patients, and the experience in the published reports indicated that mortality was not increased by immediate resection. They had performed 33 resections, apparently with no mortality, 16 of the ulcers were malignant and two of these were small perforations not suspected of being cancer. They agreed that emergency gastrectomy did not increase the mortality and concluded "gastrectomy for perforated ulcer is indicated in any case of perforation which is remedial to surgical treatment."

Discussion

J. Dewey Bisgard, of Omaha, who had been referred to by Emmett, had done 36 such resections in selected cases with a single death, from coronary thrombosis on the sixth day. He thought that no more than 30 to 50% of patients who had simple closure would subsequently require laparotomy and restricted the indications for emergency resection to perforated carcinoma, recurrent perforation, perforations with obstruction, and the rare cases of combined hemorrhage and perforation. Joel W. Baker, of Seattle, agreed, with respect to gastric ulcers but "was not certain that Dr. Emmett wished to justify sacrifice of the stomach in all cases of *duodenal* perforation." For perforated duodenal ulcers, he reserved resection for those patients "with a convincing past history". Michael E. DeBakey, of Houston, said, "On the basis of the concept that perforation of a peptic ulcer constitutes good evidence of intractability or virulence of the lesion, we began doing immediate gastric resection as the preferred method of treatment in such cases, unless it was felt that this type of surgery would cause undue risk to the patient." In two years, they had done 55 such operations with a single death. Three quarters of the patients were operated upon within 12 hours of perforation but 10% more than 24 hours after perforation. The single operative death was cardiac. Henry N. Harkins, of Seattle, reserved immediate resection for perforated peptic ulcer in 16 selected cases in the previous three years, attributing the first use of the technique to Keetley, of London, 1902. He thought that approximately one-third of cases of perforated peptic ulcer, those who had a previous perforation, multiple ulcers, a history of bleeding or history of intractability, should have immediate gastrectomy. One of his patients had been perforated for 72 hours and did well. Carleton Mathewson, Jr., of San Francisco, performed primary gastric resection in only five of 202 perforated duodenal ulcers. In his experience, 72% of patients remained well after simple closure, and only 9% subsequently required operation. Eighty percent of the perforated gastric ulcers remained asymptomatic after simple closure and only 9% required subsequent operation. He could not agree that immediate gastrectomy was indicated "in more than a small group of selected patients. Once the stomach has been removed, it cannot be replaced". Emmett, closing, mentioned emphasis of his initial presentation ". . . we are of the opinion that any patient, regardless of the length of time since perforation occurred, who is a candidate for surgical treatment of any sort, may be resected without fear of added complications from the resection."

* * *

Henry T. Bahnson, of Baltimore, by invitation, *Considerations in the Excision of Aortic Aneurysms,* presented the first paper to be given before the Association on the truly curative treatment of aortic aneurysms. He had not been impressed in animal experiments with the effective contraction of the fibrous reaction produced by polyethylene film with dicetylphosphate, nor with Osler Abbott's published results with this treatment in 33 patients. Controlled heating of coils of wire fed into the aneurysm [Blakemore] in 63 patients had resulted in 27% success. Bahnson [*Surgery, Gynecology,* and *Obstetrics,* April, 1953] had reported excision of thoracic aneurysms and, "Only Tuffier, in the early part of this century, and recently Cooley and DeBakey, have advocated this as a method of choice when possible." He clearly separated syphilitic aneurysms, usually saccular, almost invariably thoracic, occurring in younger patients and with erosion of bone, from arteriosclerotic aneurysms, usually below the renal arteries, fusiform, in older individuals and rarely producing erosion of bone. Estes' 1950 report of 102 patients with such arteriosclerotic aneurysms, showed 67 dying in one year, only 10% surviving for eight years, as against the expected survival of 67% in a control population. In the preceding 14 months, Bahnson had operated upon 17 patients "with the intention of excising the aneurysm." Operations were completely successful in 12 patients, six of whom had thoracic aneurysms, five of them syphilitic and one traumatic. Five were classical lumbar aortic aneurysms.

A final patient had an enormous abdominal aneurysm, apparently traumatic, requiring a thoracoabdominal approach, "The mouth of the aneurysm appeared to extend from posterior to the origin of the celiac axis to the level of the renal arteries, a distance of 12 to 15 cm." The thoracic aneurysms were all treated by tangential excision, and suture of the aortic wall, as was the one enormous thoracoabdominal aneurysm. One of the successful lumbar aortic arteriosclerotic aneurysms was "operated upon as an emergency because of recent rupture". Four of the lumbar aortic aneurysms were replaced by arterial homografts,· one preserved in tissue culture medium, the other three frozen and dried. In one of the reconstructions, the tubular graft was placed end-to-end from the aorta to the right common iliac, the left common iliac being implanted in the side of the graft, "The latter procedure is similar to that which was done by Dubost and associates in the first reported case of excision of aortic aneurysm and replacement by homograft [1952]." The single death from an arteriosclerotic aneurysm, a ruptured one, occurred before the aneurysm had been removed. "Excision of aortic aneurysm with preservation of aortic continuity is a procedure which has much to recommend it . . . allows removal of the tumor, restores the lumen of the aorta to as nearly normal size as possible, and removes the weakest link in the vascular system."

* * *

Ormand C. Julian, of Chicago, Clinical Assistant Professor of Surgery, University of Illinois; Associate Attending Surgeon, St. Luke's and by invitation, William J. Grove, William S. Dye, John Olwin, and Max S. Sadove, *Direct Surgery of Arteriosclerosis. Resection of Abdominal Aorta with Homologous Aortic Graft Replacement,* reported five more resections of the aorta and bifurcation with replacement by homologous bifurcation grafts, three of the operations for thrombosis and two for aneurysm, without a death. Julian mentioned Wylie's successful thromboendarterectomy for the Leriche syndrome, in 1951, and Oudot's successful resection and replacement by preserved homologous grafts in three such patients (1951). Resection for aneurysm and replacement by vessel grafts he attributed to Dubost (March, 1951), Lam (1951), and Brock (1952) and discussed the temporary use of shunts in resection of thoracic aneurysms as reported by Swan (1950) and by Schafer (1952). He had been aided by "The use of hypotensive drugs by the anesthetist . . . during the time of application of the proximal aortic clamp. This has reduced the forcefulness of the pulse

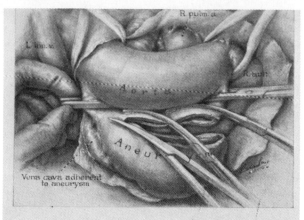

FIG. 2-B

FIG. 2-B. (Case 1.) Operative exposure of the aneurysm on the ascending aorta. The sac partially obstructed the superior vena cava and left innominate vein. The mouth of the aneurysm was dissected free and temporarily occluded with an intestinal clamp. The aneurysm was opened and the edges grasped with three curved Potts coarctation clamps.

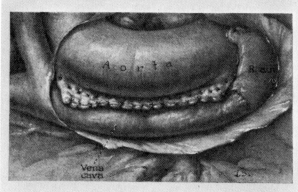

FIG. 2-C

FIG. 2-C. (Case 1.) The aneurysm has been excised and the opening in the aorta closed by two rows of interrupted fine silk sutures.

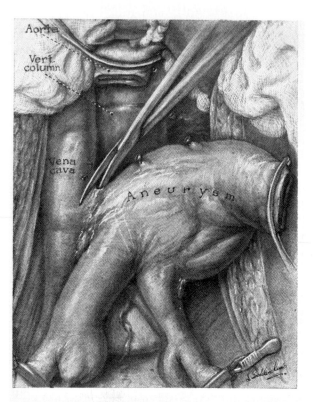

FIG. 4-C

FIG. 4-C. (Case 3.) The aorta and external iliac arteries have been occluded and the aneurysm is being removed. Adherence to the vena cava has been intimate in all such patients and several tears are usually sutured.

Bahnson had successfully resected six saccular thoracic aneurysms, five luetic, one traumatic, reconstructing the aortic lumen, as in his Fig. 2B and 2C, employing the perilous appearing sequential application of strong clamps. He presented also, successful resection and homograft replacement of four lumbar aortic aneurysms excising the entire aneurysm as in his Fig. 4C and 4D. During the same period of time he had five unsuccessful cases, four aneurysms of the thoracic aorta and one ruptured abdominal aneurysm.

Henry T. Bahnson, *Considerations in the Excision of Aortic Aneurysms,* Volume LXXI, 1953. (Figure continues on facing page.)

pounding against this clamp, and has minimized trauma to the diseased vessel." Anticoagulants were not used in any of the patients.

Discussion

Conrad R. Lam, of Detroit, presented a case operated upon by Emerick Szilagyi, successful resection of a lumbar aortic aneurysm, agreeing with Bahnson that the old aneurysm should be "removed, or it will become infected". Denton A. Cooley, of Houston, congratulating Bahnson, agreed that "The removal of the involved portion of the aorta, with preservation of aortic continuity or restoration of continuity by aortic graft, should always be considered the method of choice in such lesions." His first

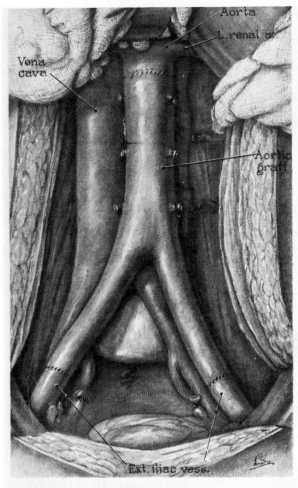

FIG. 4-D

FIG. 4-D. (Case 3.) The aortic homograft has been sutured to the aorta just below the renal arteries and to the two external iliac arteries.

an aortic tube of normal caliber." He pointed out that by the formula of LaPlace, restoration of the normal radius of the aorta reduced the lateral pressure upon the aneurysmal wall. Of his results, Lillehei said only that "successful clinical experience has convinced us of the soundness of this approach to the problem of the treatment of arteriosclerotic aneurysms of the abdominal aorta". Michael E. De-Bakey, of Houston, said his group had resected and replaced with homografts eight aneurysms of the lower thoracic and abdominal aorta with a single death. DeBakey said that "In order to avoid injury to the vena cava, which is often intimately adhered to the right posterior lateral wall of the aneurysm, it may be desirable in excising the aneurysm to leave a thin portion of the posterior wall of the aneurysm that is adherent to vena cava." [It has become standard practice to leave a large part of the posterior wall of the lumbar aortic aneurysm.] Robert R. Linton, of Boston, thought he "should get up in the defense of the intrasaccular wiring method", which might be useful when resection was not feasible, and showed slides of dramatic successes. Bahnson commented of Lillehei's procedure that LaPlace's formula had been developed in rigid-walled systems "and the situation is different in elastic structures", commented at some length about the danger of infection from retained aneurysmal wall. In response to Linton, Bahnson stated that his cases had been consecutive and unselected, taking all comers and finally that "excision with replacement by homograft of the distal aortic aneurysms oftentimes is much easier than some of the other apparently simpler, but actually more complicated procedures." Julian, closing, predicted that since arteriosclerosis would progress "these patients will, in the end, develop aneurysms proximal to the graft." In his two operations for aneurysm, he had left a strip of posterior aneurysmal wall and thought this presented not too much danger."

* * *

successful case had been in July, 1951, "a massive saccular aneurysm . . . which involved the arch of the aorta at the base of the innominate artery." He cited five patients without indicating the results or the total experience. C. W. Lillehei, of Minneapolis, championed "restorative aneurysmectomy . . . excision of nearly all of the aneurysm sac, leaving only enough remaining to reconstruct an aortic lumen of normal caliber . . . carried out by carefully dissecting out the entire aneurysmal sac until it lies free of all attachments." After cross-clamping the lumbar aorta above and below the aneurysm, "The arteriosclerotic debris is cleared out by an endarterectomy, then the major portion of the sac is excised, leaving only enough remaining wall so that closure results in

J. Garrott Allen, of Chicago, Professor of Surgery, University of Chicago, and by invitation, Henry S. Inouye and Carolyn Sykes, *Homologous Serum Jaundice and Pooled Plasma—Attenuating Effect of Room Temperature Storage on Its Virus Agent,* pointed up the problem of homologous serum jaundice from transfusion of blood products. Experimental transfusion with plasma drawn from donors sick with homologous serum jaundice had been reported to produce jaundice in 30 to 70% of human volunteers. Storage of that icterogenic plasma in liq-

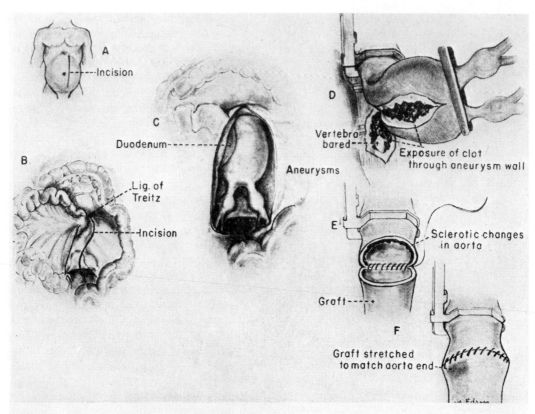

A ---Incision

B.

C

Duodenum---

Lig. of Treitz

---Incision

Aneurysms

D

Vertebra bared---

Exposure of clot through aneurysm wall

E

Sclerotic changes in aorta

Graft----

F

Graft stretched to match aorta end---

FIG. 6. Operative stages in Case 4. The aneurysms of the common iliac arteries necessitated resection down to external iliac artery on each side. The area of impending free rupture is shown.

Ormand Julian reported five successful homograft replacements of the lumbar aorta,- three for occlusion and two for aneurysm. At this point, Oudot had reported three homograft replacements for occlusion of the abdominal aorta, and abdominal aneurysms had been successfully resected by Dubost, Lam, Schafer, Swan and Brock. In the combined Discussion of Bahnson and Julian's papers, Cooley discussed a successful resection of an innominate aneurysm and mentioned five operations for aneurysm; Lillehei discussed "restorative endoaneurysmorrhaphy" for lumbar aortic aneurysm; DeBakey had reported eight resections of aneurysm of the lower thoracic and abdominal aorta, with one death and Linton defended the wiring when resection was "not feasible"; Lam seconded Bahnson's advice to excise the aneurysm in toto, but DeBakey suggested it was wise to leave behind the strip of aneurysm on the vena cava, and Julian agreed.

Ormand C. Julian, William J. Grove, William S. Dye, John Olwin, and Max S. Sadove, *Direct Surgery of Arteriosclerosis:* Resection of Abdominal Aorta with Homologous Aortic Graft Replacement, Volume LXXXI, 1953.

uid state at room temperature for six months led to jaundice in only one volunteer out of ten. Such plasma stored for only three months produced jaundice in two out of five volunteer recipients. The incidence of homologous serum jaundice from blood alone had been reported to be from 3 to 6%. At the University of Chicago, plasma in pools from 25 to 30 donors had been stored at room temperature in liquid state for six months or more over the previous 11 years. During this time, in patients who received only blood, the attack rate of hepatitis was one for every 189 patients transfused; in patients receiving blood and plasma in combination, it was one for every 155 patients transfused. In the 294 patients receiving only the liquid plasma stored at room temperature, there were no cases of homologous serum jaundice. The four patients who became jaundiced after receiving blood and plasma had received

A Century of Surgery

plasma, portions of which had been given to 38 other patients, none of whom developed jaundice. It seemed certain, therefore, that the jaundice had been the result of the blood the patients had been given, not the plasma. "Attack rates for pooled *dried* plasma have been reported to range between 5 and 20 per cent of the patients transfused", and this was in blood drawn from apparently well donors. Allen concluded that, "The room temperature storage procedure as used at the University of Chicago Blood Bank offers a practical and simple method for preparing plasma pools in community blood banks."

Discussion

Warren H. Cole, of Chicago; I. S. Ravdin, of Philadelphia, and Everett I. Evans, of Richmond, all spoke enthusiastically of the importance of Allen's data. Evans said that in his burn unit, they used no plasma, depending entirely upon plasma substitutes and that in somewhere between 1,500 and 2,000 burn patients "who got no pooled plasma, but who did receive many blood transfusions, only one patient developed clinical evidence of virus hepatitis. During the same time, almost 10% of patients received from other hospitals, where they had been treated with pooled plasma, developed hepatitis. Allen, in closing, said that storage of liquid plasma at room temperature for six months might solve the problem of jaundice from plasma, but there was still the very difficult and totally unsolved problem of making whole blood safe, with respect to transmission of hepatitis.

* * *

John H. Gibbon, Jr., of Philadelphia, Professor of Surgery and Director of Surgical Research, Jefferson Medical College; Frank F. Albritten, of Philadelphia, Assistant Professor of Surgery, Jefferson Medical College; and by invitation, John Y. Templeton, III, and Thomas F. Nealon, Jr., *Cancer of the Lung—An Analysis of 532 Consecutive Cases,* had followed 100% of their patients. Of the total, 380 were accepted for operation, and of these, 20 died following exploration alone, and 45 died after extirpation of the cancer, a mortality of 11% for exploration and 22% for extirpation. Of the entire group of 532 patients, 30% left the hospital alive with the cancer resected. Thirty-four of the 45 deaths after resection were due to "obvious" errors,- bronchopleural fistula, hemorrhage, tension pneumothorax, empyema, retained secretions, cardiac arrest, inadequate blood replacement, resection of superior vena cava,

etc. In 117 cases, the tumor extended beyond the lung and the mortality here was 28%, whereas in 88 cases, in which the tumor did not extend beyond the lung, the hospital deaths amounted to 14%. Five-year survival in the patients with the cancer extirpated was 22%,- representing 9% of the entire group of patients. If the tumor was not removed, all patients were dead within two years. Tumors extending beyond the lung but extirpated yielded a 6% five-year survival. Tumors not extending beyond the lung and removed provided a better than 40% five-year survival. Forty-three patients had a vocal cord paralysis and not one had a resectable tumor. The mortality in tumors requiring chest wall resection was twice that in the rest of the group and no patient requiring chest wall resection survived longer than 18 months. The emphasis of Gibbon's talk was on vigorous attempts at resection, "Analysis of this and other reported series appears to indicate that the proportion of the total number of patients leaving the hospital alive with the cancer removed is directly related to the proportion of the total number of patients in whom extirpation of the cancer is attempted."

Discussion

John C. Jones, of Los Angeles, had seen 633 patients with carcinoma of the lung over ten-and-a-half years, all private patients. Forty-five percent were operated upon, only half of these proved to have resectable lesions,- 23% of the entire group, and some of these were "the so-called 'palliative resections' with cancer left behind at the completion of the operation. If the latter were eliminated, our resectability would be significantly lower." Michael E. DeBakey, of Houston, had analyzed 1122 cases and agreed with almost everything Gibbon said, except that DeBakey had found some resectable tumors in patients with recurrent laryngeal nerve palsies. The reported five-year survival of all patients with carcinoma of the lung fluctuated from report to report between 5 and 8%. Otto C. Brantigan, of Baltimore, on the basis of 280 private patients, reported similar results. Contraindications to operation, in addition to distant metastases, were cytologically positive pleural fluid, the Pancoast Syndrome and recurrent nerve palsy. His longest survival with chest wall resection was 27 months. In his series, 27% of those surviving operation lived four years or longer. Brian Blades, of Washington, D.C., quoted Veterans' Administration figures to show "a terrifying increase of this disease . . . far ahead of carcinoma of the stomach and rectum. Carcinoma of the stomach is a little more frequent than carcinoma of the rectum." Herbert D. Adams, of Boston, said "These very pessimistic results . . . are closely paralleled by our own cases". They had begun using preoperative super voltage irradiation. Evarts A. Graham, of St. Louis, said they had not recently reviewed their figures but he thought they would be not very different from Gibbon's. Gibbon had not defined resection as to whether it meant pneumonectomy or lobectomy, and Graham was critical, as he was also of a recent report of Churchill, Sweet, and Soutter which indicated that "simple lobectomy had as high an incidence of five-year recovery or survival as total pneumonectomy . . . in my own opinion, those figures are so few in number . . . that they do not have any statistical significance . . ." He discussed the question of lung function and the need for "more simple and reasonably accurate tests for respiratory function. The genito-urinary surgeons are ahead of us chest surgeons in this respect. They can tell us easily whether or not it is safe to remove a kidney . . . but at the present time it is very difficult for us to know whether it is safe to remove an entire lung . . . without very serious respiratory embarrassment later . . ." He, too, stressed the fact that cancer of the lung had become more common than cancer of the stomach and was the number one cancer in men and that "this disease is progressing constantly at an alarming pace, most alarming pace . . . in the last 25 years, both in this country and in England and Wales, it has increased fifteenfold in incidence . . . 1500 per cent. Cancer of the stomach is not increasing, nor is cancer of the colon increasing to amount to anything." In closing, Gibbon said that of the 205 patients in whom the cancer was removed, 190 had pneumonectomy and only 15 had a lobectomy, bilobectomy, or local excision. The nine patients surviving more than five years had all had pneumonectomy, two of the 15 patients with lesser excisions were still alive at three-and-a-half years. Like all of the speakers, he emphasized the seriousness of the problem of delayed diagnosis.

The Business Meetings

The 1953 meeting was held at the Statler Hotel, Los Angeles, April 1, 2, and 3, President Robert S. Dinsmore, of Cleveland, in the Chair.

The Program Committee, for the first time meeting as a group to draft the final program, had selected 33 of the 68 abstracts submitted.

Dr. Oliver Cope reported for the Committee on Graduate Surgical Education, which had been set up at the Washington Meeting in 1951. In general, the effect of the Boards had been to improve surgical training, although there was a tendency to fragmentation into specialties. The technical training of surgeons and specialists was in general good, but some of the broader educational aspects of surgery were being neglected, particularly in some of the specialties. Large numbers of hospitals had undertaken residency training programs and in many of these the programs were padded to fit the presumed desires of the Boards. There was concern about the diminishing number of charity patients, and the report stated [in characteristic Cope language] "The care of private patients fits well with apprentice schemes, particularly in group practice. We had better be about developing such schemes. In planning, we should heed the need for flexibility." The report returned several times to the problem of the Specialty Boards, "Members of some of the boards are known to have turned to colleagues in other fields of medicine to compose questions for their examinations. Such questions are dishonest, since the examiners do not know enough about the subjects to evaluate the answers. Such questions are window dressing. The number of boards should be ruthlessly cut back." The report proposed a rather sweeping change, "A central authority must be set up combining the American College of Surgeons, the American Board of Surgery, and the existing specialty Boards. Eventually all of the Boards should be dissolved in this authority. Candidates should be examined for competence in special fields only after passing a basic examination in surgery." Not content with that, they made an even more far-reaching proposal, "Two standards of performance should be recognized, the lower standard to legitimize as many surgeons as possible, the higher standard to set a more ambitious goal . . . the American College of Surgeons should have two levels of membership. By a title such as Licentiate the College would welcome as many as possible to attend its regional and annual meetings . . . By Fellowship the College would recognize greater achievement." The concern was about the "pariahs", men who had taken training, were practicing surgery and had not been able to be certified by an appropriate Board.

The Minutes carried no note of any discussion, nor of any move toward implementation.

Fred A. Coller now gave the second report of his Committee on Unnecessary Operations. It was still difficult to get facts and figures, "It is almost unbelievable, but true, that it is impossible to find out the number and kind of the operations that are carried out in this country, and what is more important, who does them." Dr. Coller thought that as a result of his representations a question about operations would be introduced into the next Census. Exclusive of the Federal Service, there were 179,000 physicians in 1949. From 1940 to 1949 the number of surgeons had gone from 6,600 to 12,000. In 1950 there were 11,000 Osteopathic Physicians in the United States, and in only 14 states was major operative surgery by osteopathic physicians not permitted. Many small hospitals had recently been constructed through local effort or Federal aid or both. "There are not enough nurses, pathologists, roentgenologists and competent physicians to staff them, and we are not training enough surgeons to make all hospitals efficient areas in which to care for the sick." He said that about half the hospitals in 8,000 surveyed had "no connection with the pathologist in any way, shape or form, either in his physical presence or by mail." From published reports in the surgical literature, Coller found statements that a third of the hysterectomies analyzed were without indication or contraindicated, that in one study, 47% of the ovaries removed in Los Angeles were normal. In another, 44% of 10,000 appendices removed in and around Minnesota were normal. Appendectomy was performed with greater frequency in nonteaching hospitals in Rochester, Minnesota, than in teaching hospitals. "It seems evident that the chief sites of unwarranted surgical operation lie in those anatomical areas in which the operative attack is without great risk, and in which the removal of certain organs may not do immediate appreciable harm. Notably, the appendix, the gallbladder, the organs in the female pelvis, and in those easily visualized areas, the vagina and the anal canal." He had analyzed medical audits in ten nonteaching hospitals of "middle size" which regularly undertook ". . . scrutiny of performance, careful analysis of deaths and of complications" and found little evidence of inappropriate operating. ". . . this is the situation that exists in a great majority of our well conducted middle size and large hospitals. There is as yet no way of scrutinizing the medical performance in many small hospitals since records and the opportunity to study them, if they exist, are seldom available." He had come to the conclusion that ". . . unnecessary operations are uncommon if they ever occur in the fields of neurosurgery, orthopedic surgery, thoracic surgery and urology." This situation was equally true in plastic surgery, "but there are still a few so-called specialists who insist upon the validity of the correction of certain defects which, in the opinion of many, might better be managed by the psychiatrist." He divided unnecessary operations into three groups: 1. When there are "Honest differences of opinion", 2. "Operations carried out with honest intent, but the indications based on ignorance and on lack of diagnostic facilities", and 3. "Operations carried out in an unscrupulous fashion for gain and for venal reasons . . . a comparatively small number of our total performance . . . it is this dark area that we should attack most forcibly, knowing that these abuses are usually associated with the pernicious custom of fee-splitting." Abuses were best combatted by: 1. Improved training including emphasis on "our heritage of mortality, religion and integrity . . ," 2. Insistence upon the development in every hospital of medical and surgical audits, Tissue Committees, and developing "some way of placing 'guts' in the hospital staff", and training more pathologists and urging them to maintain "courageous attitudes" 3. It was necessary to "Develop a method by which a force could reach into the small hospital to scrutinize their performance with power to criticize, educate and advise."

Ormand C. Julian, H. W. Scott, Jr., and Orvar Swenson were among the Fellows elected.

The elected President was Howard Naffziger, of San Francisco; First Vice-President, J. Stewart Rodman, of Philadelphia; Second Vice-President, Lawrence Chaffin, of Los Angeles; and Secretary, to succeed Dr. Womack, R. K. Gilchrist, of Evanston, Illinois.

LXXII

1954

The 1954 meeting was held at the Hotel Cleveland, Cleveland, Ohio, April 28, 29, and 30, President Howard C. Naffziger, of San Francisco, Professor of Surgery, University of California Medical School; Surgeon-in-Chief, University of California Hospital, in the Chair. During the previous year, there had died, of a coronary occlusion, Everett I. Evans, of Richmond, who was only 46 years old; Samuel C. Harvey, of Yale, and Frank H. Lahey, of Boston had also died.

Dr. Naffziger spoke generally about the influence of medical societies on a surgeon's education, of the change in medicine which had occurred so that surgeons took more postgraduate education and training than internists. He expressed concern that so many medical students were indicating a desire to go into general practice, ". . . there has never been a time when there is less need for general practitioners than today", citing the decreased number of sparsely settled areas, the great improvement in transportation, the greater efficiency resulting from concentration of physicians in groups. At this meeting, there was to be a symposium dealing with the cost of medical education. "The wisdom of accepting federal funds, the development of foundations to supplement our budgets and the influence of grants from other sources are some of the pressing problems before us", an example of the kind of problem with which he felt the Association should be concerned.

* * *

Michael E. DeBakey, of Houston, Professor of Surgery and Chairman of the Department of Surgery, Baylor University College of Medicine, and by invitation, Oscar Creech, Jr. and Denton A. Cooley, *Occlusive Disease of the Aorta and Its Treatment by Resection and Homograft Replacement,* indicated the rapid rate at which operations upon the aorta were increasing in frequency. In the previous year, in the Discussion of the papers of Bahnson on aortic aneurysm and Julian on distal aortic thrombosis and aneurysm, DeBakey had mentioned eight replacements of the aorta with grafts for thoracic aneurysm and had not mentioned occlusive disease. He now reported 22 resections and homograft replacements of the aortic bifurcation for occlusive disease. The ten patients, who presented the fairly classical Leriche syndrome, but were younger, did not have diffuse arteriosclerosis, although intermittent claudication in the hip, and sexual impotence were common. The 12 patients presenting partial aortic occlusion were older, the arteriosclerosis frequently extended proximally, and usually into the iliacs from which the atheroma had to be cored out and there was less fibrosis and periaortic inflammation than in the Leriche types. Nevertheless he considered this a continuum in which the Leriche disease was the completed process. There were no hospital deaths. One patient died subsequently of mitral valvular disease, another died at home a week after discharge from rupture of the left common iliac artery distal to the anastomosis,- a patient who had had a thomboendarterectomy of the iliac artery. Results in the ten patients with complete occlusion were uniformly good with restoration of pulses, often with restoration of sexual potency, essentially relief of all symptoms. Nine of 12 of the patients with incomplete aortic occlusive disease had good improvement in the circulation in the extremities, but two required a subsequent amputation, DeBakey remarking that "It appears significant that these three patients with partially occlusive disease also had appreciable degree of associated peripheral arteriosclerosis." (See p. 1008.)

Discussion

Emerick Szilagyi, of Detroit, properly separated the two groups of patients DeBakey had described, agreeing with the French that the Leriche disease was an inflammatory one and that the "partial occlusive disease" of DeBakey was ". . . advanced atherosclerosis . . . part of a systemic disease." Resection was appropriate for Leriche's syndrome and he had done it in four patients, but in the arteriosclerotic type he thought endarterectomy was the appropriate procedure [DeBakey had discussed endarterectomies performed by Wiley and others but evidenced only restrained enthusiasm for it]. Robert R. Linton, of Boston, said that at the Massachusetts General Hospital, they had resected the aorta and inserted bifurcation homografts in 20 patients for a variety of lesions, and stressed the importance of having ". . . at least two bifurcation grafts in the bank, and in addition, several iliac and femoral arteries in case it is necessary to replace these vessels, as we have had to do in several cases. I have had to insert a graft from the bifurcation of the aorta down to the popliteal artery, a distance of 45 cm. Without such a long graft being available, the circulation of the extremity would have been seriously endangered." The injection of heparin into the distal arteries, which he employed, had been suggested by several the year before and he warned ". . . you should be prepared for long operative procedures, since some have required as long as nine to ten hours to complete." Ormand C. Julian, of Chicago, said the homograft of the longest known duration was that placed in France four years before. One of his patients was now 25 months after resection and replacement for thrombotic occlusion. Like DeBakey

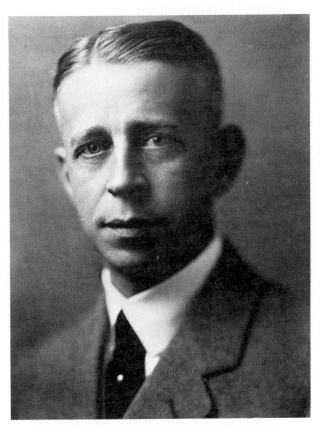

Howard C. Naffziger (c. 1940) 1884-1961. President 1954 and of the American College of Surgeons 1938-39. M.D. University of California 1909. Professor and Chairman, Department of Surgery, University of California 1929-47; Chairman, Department of Neurological Surgery, 1947-51. Tall, handsome, distinguished with impressive bearing and a rich voice. Like Cushing, under whom he trained at Hopkins, a neurosurgeon well founded in general surgery, who headed a major university department of surgery, and there established a formal residency plan. His major neurosurgical contributions, like the operation for progressive exophthalmos, dealt with the technical aspects. He was a major force in the great expansion of the Medical Schools at the University of California.
(Portrait courtesy of Mrs. Howard C. Naffziger)

he had operated on some patients with occlusion of only one iliac.

* * *

Arthur H. Blakemore, of New York, Associate Professor of Clinical Surgery, College of Physicians and Surgeons, and by invitation, Arthur B. Voorhees, Jr., *The Use of Tubes Constructed from Vinyon "N" Cloth in Bridging Arterial Defects—Experimental and Clinical,* the year before had demonstrated

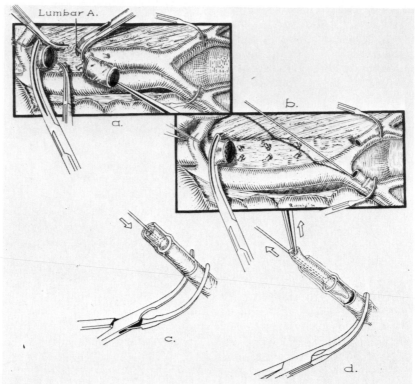

Fig. 5. Drawing of operative technic continued from Figure 4. (a) The diseased segment of aorta and bifurcation is excised between occluding clamps applied to aorta above and iliac arteries below. Lumbar arteries are clamped, divided and ligated individually. (b) The lumen of iliac arteries is restored by performance of thromboendarterectomy, which is facilitated by use of wire loop similar in design to Mayo vein stripper. (c and d) By threading thrombotic process through wire loop it can be easily peeled away and lumen thus restored.

Aortic resection and homograft replacement was performed in 22 patients. Ten with the typical Leriche syndrome, 12 with incompete obstruction and much associated distal arteriosclerosis. Involved aorta and iliacs were removed in all cases as shown. In the patients with arteriosclerosis, distal endarterectomy and sometimes proximal endarterectomy were performed. Freeze-dried aortic homografts were inserted with continuous through-and-through sutures of 4-0 silk and a lumbar sympathectomy usually performed. The ten "Leriche" patients all had good results, as did 9/12 of the patients with arteriosclerosis. One patient died at home of rupture of the endarterectomized iliac artery. The bifurcations were inserted into the proximal iliacs and two of the patients with arteriosclerosis and "partial occlusion of the aorta" subsequently required amputation.

Michael E. DeBakey, Oscar Creech, Jr., Denton A. Cooley, *Occlusive Disease of the Aorta and Its Treatment by Resection and Homograft Replacement*. Volume LXXII, 1954. (Figure continues on facing page.)

that arterial defects could be bridged by tubes of synthetic cloth. [That publication and word-of-mouth information from Presbyterian Hospital stimulated some interest in the problem, but there was no hint of the explosion in blood vessel replacement which was to come as a result of their work.] They referred to the work of Levin and Larkin, 1908, demonstrating "that devitalized homografts will function over brief periods of time in the experimental animal", the 1919 publication of Guthrie [with whom Carrel had collaborated previously] concluding from experiments with formalinized venous grafts as arterial replacements that ". . . to restore and maintain function, an implanted segment need only temporarily restore mechanical continuity and serve as a scaffolding or bridge for the laying down of an ingrowth of tissue derived from the host." Blakemore said tubes of prosthetic material previously reported, glass, paraffined metal, methyl methacrylate, polyethylene, thrombosed too frequently to

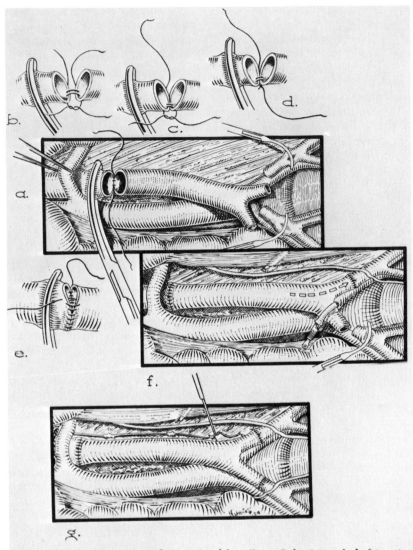

FIG. 6. Drawing of operative technic continued from Figure 5 showing method of inserting aortic bifurcation homograft. (a-c) Anastomosis is accomplished with a simple continuous through-and-through suture of 0000 arterial silk. (f) After completing aortic and left iliac anastomosis, occluding clamps to these vessels are removed permitting blood flow through graft into left lower extremity while remaining iliac anastomosis is being done. (g) After graft anastomosis has been completed bilateral lumbar sympathectomy, L 2–4, is performed.

be acceptable clinically. Their prostheses were hand-fashioned from sheets of Vinyon "N" cloth. Vinyon "N" implantations in 31 dog vessels, for the most part in the aorta, resulted in three complete thromboses and three partial thromboses, all in the first half of the series, and a single anastomotic disruption resulting from excessive tension. Performance of the grafts for more than two years in the dogs had suggested no deterioration or dilatation. Blood loss through the interstices of the graft was significant

for 15 to 30 seconds, and ". . . was circumvented by using cloth of a tighter weave, by allowing blood to clot in tube *in vitro*," and by releasing the distal clamp first, "allowing low pressure retrograde flow to seal the interstices". They described the almost immediate deposition of ". . . a uniform coat of fibrin and blood cells, which ranges from 1/2 to 1 mm. in thickness", migration of fibroblasts in the ensuing weeks from the surrounding tissues through the interstices, and by the fourth week into the inner coat. "By the seventh week, flattened islands with polished grey surfaces appear on the surface of the granulating coat. Endothelial proliferation at either end of the prosthesis never produces a pannus of more than a few millimeters in width. Between the seventh and the fourteenth weeks the islands become confluent, and form a uniform, polished surface, indistinguishable from the endothelial coat of the adjacent artery." Thereafter there was essentially no histological change. A review of 365 aortic aneurysms treated at the Presbyterian Hospital of which 118 were arteriosclerotic abdominal aneurysms, convinced them that "Therapeutic measures other than excisional therapy in our hands have brought symptomatic relief to some, temporary alleviation of symptoms to a larger group, and no overall measurable change in symptoms or added life expectancy to the majority." [Blakemore had been the prime exponent and the most skillful practitioner of the refinement of intrasaccular wiring which had been described, and had been a pioneer in the application of synthetic materials to the outer surface of aneurysms.] Since the spring of 1953, they had resected and replaced with Vinyon "N" prostheses, 18 arteriosclerotic aneurysms,- 17 of the abdominal aorta, and one of the popliteal artery. There were ten survivors, all symptom free and well, the longest ten months after operation. Two of the survivors had straight-tube replacements of the abdominal aorta. Six had Y-tube implantations. In one, the proximal end of the Y-tube was attached to the abdominal aorta above the celiac axis, the distal aorta being sutured closed below the renal arteries. Two of the deaths resulted from rupture of the aorta by the proximal clamp, one from cardiac arrest at the time of release of the clamp after reconstruction of the aorta, two from shock after operation, and three, later in the postoperative period, from renal insufficiency, two of these brought on by prolonged hypotension from hemorrhage and one from occlusion of the left renal artery by thrombus. They had learned to protect the proximal aorta when it seemed diseased by wrapping it with Vinyon "N" cloth before clamping and to protect suture lines by wrapping a Vinyon "N" cuff about them as indicated. They excised ". . . the major portion of the aneurysm . . . leaving only a shell attached to the adherent structures." They usually attached the "Y" graft to the left iliac artery first, then to the aorta, allowing the aorta to empty into the left iliac, and then performed the right iliac anastomosis. They said that ". . . the versatility and functional result of the prosthesis has been gratifying." The deaths were due ". . . either directly or indirectly to our inability to deal successfully with arteries in which advanced degeneration was present", and felt that they had learned how to deal with that problem, but made no recommendations or predictions.

Discussion

Harris B. Shumacker, of Indianapolis, spoke for many in stating that when the original paper by Voorhees, Jaretzki, and Blakemore had appeared, "most of us . . . paid entirely too little attention to it and did not attribute to it the significance that this work merited." He had found that thin sheets of nylon functioned very much like the Vinyon and had done experiments similar to those of Voorhees. Shumacker had trouble with the nylon because of ". . . bleeding through the graft . . ." and had rendered the tubes impervious either by coating them with methyl mythacrylate or fusing them to a sheet of nonreactive polyethylene. He stated that they had employed these impervious grafts to replace the lumbar aorta and bifurcation in six patients ". . . and in all cases patency has been maintained". Conrad Lam, spoke of the use of Betapropiolactone to sterilize homografts, but commented prophetically, "If the work of Drs. Blakemore and Voorhees turns out to be as good as it looks, my discussion here will be entirely superfluous." Edgar J. Poth, of Galveston, had used multiple layers of relatively open mesh, wrapping an impervious material around it for three to five minutes. He appeared to think that the grafts became lined by true endothelium and thought ". . . there is a very good possibility that it might arise from the capillary buds which grow into the organized clot within the wall of the material." Linton asked how small a diameter graft had been employed. Arthur B. Voorhees, Jr., closing, answered that grafts in the dogs' femoral and carotid arteries had been as small as four millimeters in diameter and had functioned well.

* * *

Hugh F. Dudley, Eldon A. Boling, Leslie P. LeQuesne, all by invitation, and Francis D. Moore, of Boston, Surgeon-in-Chief, Peter Bent Brigham Hospital; Moseley Professor of Surgery, Harvard Medical School, *Studies on Antidiuresis in Surgery: Effects of Anesthesia, Surgery and Posterior Pituitary Antidiuretic Hormone on Water Metabolism in Man,* presented one of the careful physiologic studies of the control of fluid and electrolyte balance, which were becoming a hallmark of Moore's laboratory. Diminished urinary output following operation or other trauma had been remarked upon many times since Pringle's observation in 1905. Intraoperative depression of renal blood flow and the gradual development of sodium conservation by the kidney under hormone influences had been offered as the explanation by J. D. Hardy in his presentation before the Association in 1950. Evidence had gradually accumulated, implicating the antidiuretic hormone of the pituitary, and they set about studying this by the infusion of single doses of 600 ml. to 800 ml. of 5% glucose in about 40 minutes to patients who had undergone gastrectomy or cholecystectomy, and to unoperated volunteers. They concluded that the response suggested ". . . posterior pituitary antidiuresis", and warned that "If electrolyte-free fluid is administered during this phase of diminished renal excretory capacity, reduction in serum sodium concentration occurs . . . Serum potassium is usually also reduced, but paradoxical changes may occur which are similar to the sodium-potassium inversion seen after trauma in depleted patients. The diminished excretory capacity for water should be borne in mind in prescribing postoperative fluids . . . Except under special circumstances, maintenance of, or increase in weight [post-trauma] indicates a retention of water."

Discussion

William D. Holden, of Cleveland, demonstrated that antidiuretic factors could be ". . . recovered from the urine of patients who have been subjected to major surgical procedures", and raised the question whether this represented an increased production of antidiuretic substance or a failure of inactivation, in the liver or elsewhere, of normally produced antidiuretic hormone. Carl A. Moyer, of St. Louis, reviewed the development of the knowledge of this antidiuresis, referring to the studies of Theobald and Verney, found that the acute fall in urine flow accompanying trauma was not prevented by removing one kidney and denervating the other, so that a renal reflex mechanism was excluded. Theobald also found that after hypophysectomy in dogs trauma no longer produced antidiuresis. Francis D. Moore, in the Discussion of the paper, which had apparently been presented by Dudley, emphasized what he called the "post-traumatic sodium-potassium shift" or "serum electrolyte inversion", ". . . in response to some forces within the patient which we do not as yet understand . . . a very regular feature of post-traumatic metabolism."

* * *

Henry N. Harkins, of Seattle, Professor of Surgery and Executive Officer, Department of Surgery, University of Washington, and by invitation Everett J. Schmitz, Lloyd M. Nyhus, Edmund A. Kanar, Ralph K. Zech, and Charles A. Griffith, *The Billroth I Gastric Resection: Experimental Studies and Clinical Observations on 291 Cases,* concluded that ". . . gastrojejunostomy following partial gastrectomy results in a higher level of gastric secretory activity (hormonal phase) than does gastroduodenostomy. Marginal ulceration occurs earlier and oftener after gastrojejunostomy than after gastroduodenostomy in these experiments. [The anastomotic ulcers referred to were in experimental animals given histamine in beeswax and in dogs stimulated by antral transposition into the colon, by Dragstedt's technique.] The Billroth I gastric resection as performed by us in clinical practice permits an adequate and satisfactory resection in the great majority of conditions for which gastric resection is indicated, and is productive of a high yield of good results. There were seven deaths, only one from suture line leakage. Average measured gastric resection in 120 of the patients was 71.9%. When direct end-to-end gastroduodenostomy was not possible—17 cases—they employed the Finney-von Haberer terminolateral anastomosis, which had ". . . made possible the virtual abandonment of the Billroth II operation on the author's service during the past three years." Seven percent of the patients gained weight, 21% maintained their weight, and 32% lost weight. Thirty-four percent of the patients had some dumping, but only a third of these had dumping at the end of one year, and dumping was severe and incapacitating in only two patients. Eight patients had postoperative diarrhea, severe and disabling in only one. Seven patients were suspected of having recurrent ulcer, proved in only three. They had also performed a series of 33 hemigastrectomies with transabdominal vagotomy. One patient developed pancreatitis and one developed a pancreatic cyst requiring operation. There were no deaths.

Discussion

Robert M. Zollinger, of Columbus, Ohio, opened the Discussion. He thought most surgeons would agree that "gastroduodenostomy is technically much easier than the more complicated Billroth II operation . . ." It had been his experience that with a 75% resection and Hofmeister reconstruction, three-quarters of the patients had difficulty maintaining their weight. He had employed vagotomy and hemigastrectomy in 120 patients. He was inclined to think that the postoperative weight trend was related to the patient's state of nutrition before the operation and the amount of stomach that was removed, ". . . two out of three patients above their ideal weight at the time of operation maintained their ideal weight, regardless of how much stomach had been removed and no matter what type of operation had been employed." Patients who were well below their ideal weight did not do as well, and he had taken to leaving such patients more stomach, performing a vagotomy and hemigastrectomy. In patients who were exceedingly thin ". . . and unable to maintain satisfactory nutrition with an intact stomach . . . vagotomy and gastroenterostomy is the operation of choice." If gastric resection and Billroth I required a 75% resection, he thought it ought to be limited to individuals above ideal weight. Owen H. Wangensteen, of Minneapolis, said that leaving a bit of antrum behind in animals was not as deleterious if it were left in the intestinal stream as if it were excluded, and ". . . one great advantage in the Billroth I over the Billroth II . . . is that you can not exclude the antrum." [As he said, he had been ". . . partial . . . to retention of the antrum in segmental gastric resection . . ."] Lester R. Dragstedt, of Chicago, confirmed Harkins' experimental work. His animals with antrum transplant into the colon developed a stomal ulcer 80% of the time with the Billroth II reconstruction, and 20% of the time with a Billroth I reconstruction, ". . . the duodenum has a greater resistance to the digestive action of the gastric content than is the case with the jejunum." Tilden Everson, of Chicago, reported animal studies of nutrition after Billroth I and Billroth II anastomoses, concluding, in support of Harkins, that ". . . the efficiency of assimilation of both fat and protein was noted to be better following types of gastric resection which maintained the normal continuity of the gastro-intestinal tract, *i.e.,* Billroth I and segmental gastric resections." They were employing Billroth I in 90% of their patients with duodenal ulcer with results similar to those of Harkins. Edgar J. Poth, of Galveston, introduced a disturbing note, stating that while "I have always been enthusiastic about the Billroth I procedure . . . I should like to report that at the present time I have four patients who have developed duodenal ulcers following the Billroth I procedure. None of them has been done for duodenal ulcer. Two were done for carcinoma of stomach and two were done for gastric ulcer." Harkins, closing, said that if the duodenum was adequately mobilized, just as radical a gastrectomy could be done for reconstruction by gastroduodenostomy as by gastrojejunostomy. His mortality was explained by the fact his were elderly patients on the charity service at King County Hospital. In very difficult duodenal stumps, he closed the duodenal stump and did a Finney-von Haberer end-to-side gastroduodenostomy.

* * *

Arnold J. Kremen, of Minneapolis, Associate Professor of Surgery, University of Minnesota; Director, University Surgical Service, Mt. Sinai Hospital, and by invitation, John H. Linner, and Charles H. Nelson, *An Experimental Evaluation of the Nutritional Importance of Proximal and Distal Small Intestine,* presented a paper which was destined to produce an enormous interest in intestinal short-circuiting procedures to provide weight loss in the pathologically obese [and the value of which was still being discussed at the 1979 meeting, 25 years later, q.v.]. They divided the bowel of dogs proximally and distally, prepared the intervening segment as a Thiry-Vella fistula, restored the continuity of the bowel by end-to-end anastomosis, and then did nutritional balance studies on the animals over a period of months. The fecal fat losses were approximately the same in Groups II, III, IIIA, and V, and the fecal nitrogen losses similarly. They concluded that, "The proximal 50 to 70 per cent of the small intestine of dogs can be removed with no apparent ill effects. Weight is maintained, and protein and fat absorption are not significantly altered. Sacrifice of the distal 50 per cent of the small intestine produces a profound interference with fat absorption associated with loss of weight. The ileocecal valve appears to have an important effect on the nutritional adjustment to sacrifice of the distal small bowel, but appears less important in sacrifice of the proximal small bowel."

Discussion

Herbert Willy Meyer, of New York, mentioned a soldier injured in the Battle of the Bulge [World War II] who required resection of ". . . the small intestine except the upper 18 inches of the jejunum, all of the cecum, ascending colon, and a portion of the transverse colon" upon whom he performed a jejuno-transverse colostomy. Now nine years later, the patient weighed 125 pounds as opposed to his preoperative weight of 138 pounds and was fully employed, had three or four soft bowel movements ". . . suffers from avitaminosis . . . has developed

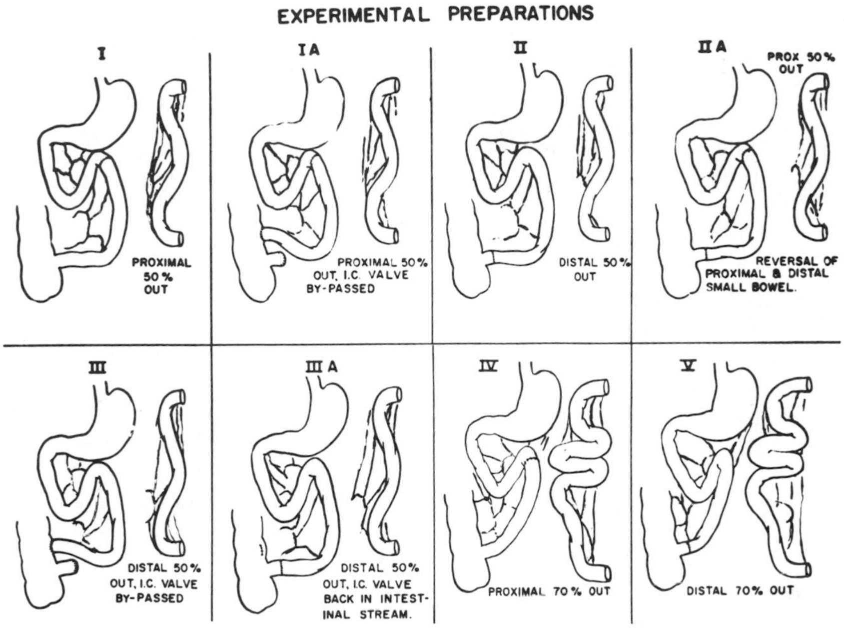

EXPERIMENTAL PREPARATIONS

FIG. 1. Experimental animal preparations. (I) The proximal 50 per cent of small intestine removed from intestinal continuity as a Thiry-Vella fistula. Anastomosis at ligament of Treitz. (IA) Group I animals reoperated upon after 24 weeks with bypass of ileocecal valve. Distal two centimeters of ileum inverted and closed. (II) The distal 50 per cent of small intestine removed from intestinal continuity as a Thiry-Vella fistula. Anastomosis two to three centimeters proximal to ileocecal valve. (IIA) Group II animals reoperated upon after 24 weeks of observation. The previously excluded distal bowel replaced into the intestinal stream and the proximal 50 per cent of small bowel excluded as a Thiry-Vella fistula. (III) The distal 50 per cent of small intestine removed from intestinal continuity as a Thiry-Vella fistula. The terminal three centimeters of ileum closed and inverted. Anastomosis end-to-side to right colon. (IIIA) Group III animals reoperated upon after 24 weeks. The anastomosis to the right colon taken down with reanastomosis to the previously closed three-centimeter stump of terminal ileum. (IV) The proximal 70 per cent of small intestine removed from intestinal continuity as a Thiry-Vella fistula. Anastomosis at ligament of Treitz. (V) The distal 70 per cent of small intestine removed from intestinal continuity as a Thiry-Vella fistula. Anastomosis two to three centimeters proximal to ileocecal valve.

Group I animals lost 15% of their weight by seven weeks and had regained it by 24 weeks. Conversion to Group IA made no difference. The Group II animals lost 15% of their body weight by 15 weeks, then stabilized but did not regain their weight. Conversion to Group IIA restored their weight. Group III animals lost weight steadily and progressively, without compensating. Restoring continuity through the ileocecal valve stopped the progressive weight loss. Extending the by-pass to 70% instead of 50%, Group I to Group IV and Group II to Group V increased the weight loss without deleterious effects.

Arnold J. Kremen, John H. Linner, and Charles H. Nelson, *An Experimental Evaluation of the Nutritional Importance of Proximal and Distal Small Intestine.* Volume LXXII, 1954.

some anemia, and has had to have liver injections." Philip Sandblom, of Lund, Sweden, said that Dr. V. Henrikson of Gothenburg "tried to control obesity in a woman whose appetite was better than her character, by resection of an appropriate amount of the small intestine. He found that although the lady lost very much weight, it was difficult to keep her in balance. After this beautiful study by Dr. Kremen *et al,* this questionable method of controlling obesity will have the necessary experimental foundation." Arnold J. Kremen, closing, "had hoped that nothing would be mentioned along the lines that Dr. Sandblom discussed. We have seriously thought about that problem, and as a matter of fact, I recently operated on a very obese woman for just that reason. However, we didn't take out all of the bowel, Dr. Sandblom. We left the defunctionated segment with its blood supply preserved, so that if we overreached ourselves we could replace it in the intestinal stream." They had left 36 inches of jejunum and

ILEOSTOMY

MATURATION OF ILEOSTOMY

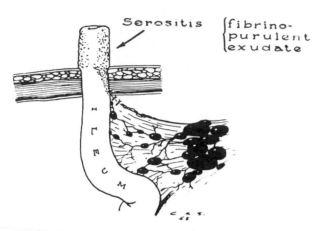

FIG. 3. Serositis of the exposed ileostomy.

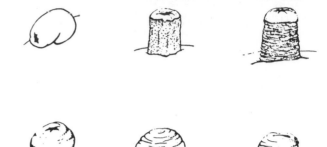

4th TO 6th WEEKS

FIG. 4. Maturation of the ileostomy.

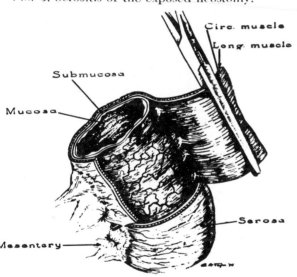

FIG. 5. Technique of removing the seromuscular coats of the ileostomy.

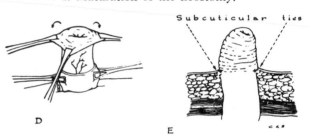

FIG. 6. Eversion of the submucosal-mucosal layers over the ileostomy.

Figures 3 and 4 indicate events occurring in a standard ileostomy, the bowel simply pulled through the abdominal wall. Crile and Turnbull compared it to ". . . a peritonitis of the protruding segment" which persisted until the serosal surface had healed to the abdominal skin. They performed their "mucosal-grafted ileostomies" in 13 patients in a group of 28 undergoing ileostomy. The 13 patients required less parenteral fluid than those with the classic ileostomy, and ". . . ileostomy dysfunction has been notably absent, and except for the two patients with staphylococcal enteritis, there was no diarrhea of the ileostomies." In classic ileostomy "Dehydration, hyponatremia, hypochloremia and hypokalemia were common occurrences."

George Crile, Jr., and Rupert B. Turnbull, Jr., *The Mechanism and Prevention of Ileostomy Dysfunction.* Volume LXXII, 1954.

18 inches of terminal ileum in the alimentary stream, emptying the by-passed bowel into the colon, "It has not been very long since we did this operation, but she is free of diarrhea, eating whatever she wants and is slowly losing weight."

* * *

George Crile, Jr., of Cleveland, Member of the Staff of Cleveland Clinic Foundation, and Rupert B. Turnbull, Jr., by invitation, *The Mechanism and Prevention of Ileostomy Dysfunction,* spoke of the intractable diarrhea and disturbances of fluid and electrolyte balance frequently seen for a time after the establishment of an ileostomy. This had been thought to be due to the loss of the water-absorbing function of the colon, which was then gradually taken over by the ileum. The 1940 paper of Cave and Nickel before the Association had reported a 33% mortality for ileostomy [See page 823, Volume LVIII], "in no small measure has the high mortality been due to a rapid and excessive loss of fluid and chlorides from the ileostomy immediately after operation." Warren and McKittrick's 1951 report of 210 patients undergoing ileostomy indicated dysfunction of the ileostomy with increase in discharge, and fluid and electrolyte deficiencies in 62%, accounting for seven of the 37 deaths. Crile and Turnbull thought the excessive fluid loss might be due to partial obstruction in the exteriorized bowel, "There is little wonder that the newly constructed ileostomy does not function as efficiently as normal small intestine. A naked, unprotected segment of ileum is suddenly brought into the septic environment of its own discharges. Serositis with fibrinopurulent exudate is noted by the third or fourth day. This is in reality a peritonitis of the protruding segment. Edema, rigidity, and loss of peristalsis of the exteriorized segment soon follow, just as they do in any peritonitis. Although a tube or finger can be passed easily, functional obstruction is present and can be demonstrated by roentgenogram." The sequence of healing of this inflamed ileostomy they referred to as "maturation", and varying degrees of dysfunction could be expected to persist until maturation was complete. Dragstedt had achieved the effect of maturation by split-thickness skin grafting the surface of the ileostomy ". . . but this was done to protect the abdominal skin . . . No mention was made of the role of the graft in preventing inflammation of the ileum." B. M. Black and J. F. Thomas from the Mayo Clinic performing four skin-grafted Dragstedt ileostomies, had indeed stated that "in none of the cases was there the profound upset in fluid and electrolyte balance so frequently observed after performance of the

usual ileostomy." Brooke, in England in 1952, had described a complete eversion of the ileal stoma suturing the mucosa to the skin. Turnbull, in 1953, had suggested stripping the serosa and muscularis from the exteriorized bowel and turning back a mucosal cuff to be sutured to the skin. They had compared a series of 13 patients with this ileostomy to 15 performed during the same period with a classic ileostomy and found a sharply decreased need for fluids, a disappearance of electrolyte imbalance, and of ileostomy dysfunction.

Discussion

Clarence Dennis, of Brooklyn, said that suturing the ileostomy closed and keeping a catheter in it for 48 hours permitted the bowel to be unsoiled, "With this technic there is no dysfunction, no late prolapse, and no dilatation of the ileum proximal to the ileostomy . . . Mr. Bryan N. Brooke, of Birmingham, England, visited New York two years ago . . ." and demonstrated his everting technique which Dennis had used repeatedly since then, with complete satisfaction. Richard Warren, of Boston, said he had used a technique similar to Turnbull's ". . . for about two years, and agree that this is an excellent maneuver."

* * *

Charles Huggins, of Chicago, Professor of Surgery (Urology), The University of Chicago; Director, Ben May Laboratory for Cancer Research, University of Chicago, and, by invitation, Thomas L-Y. Dao, *Characteristics of Adrenal-Dependent Mammary Cancers,* continued the report which they had made the year before. They now had performed bilateral adrenalectomy in 100 women with far-advanced mammary cancer with a 5% operative mortality. There had been remissions of varying duration in 38 cases and profound regression had persisted for over 36 months, in soft-tissue, pleural, peritoneal, hepatic, and osseous metastases. The results were best in women between the ages of 40 and 65 with a prolonged interval between radical mastectomy and onset of the metastasis, best in women with adenocarcinoma, and best in women who had a high titer of estrogenic substances in the urine. Patients with appearance of metastases in less than a year following mastectomy rarely responded to adrenalectomy.

* * *

The discussion of this subject was continued by Maurice Galante, J. Max Rukes, Peter H. Forsham,

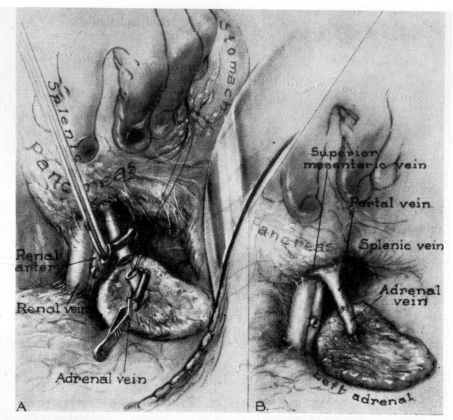

Fig. 15. End-to-end anastomosis between the left adrenal and splenic vein as performed in patient I. C.

Three weeks after right adrenalectomy, the left adrenal vein was anastomosed to the left splenic vein and the largely mobilized adrenal surrounded with omentum to minimize the likelihood of systemic venous drainage. In the first of four patients so operated upon, there was a striking remission in symptoms and regression of metastases, and all four patients showed no significant amounts of estrogens in the urine after the operation, and required no substitution therapy. The assumption was that the adrenal estrogens were inactivated in the liver.

Maurice Galante, J. Max Rukes, Peter H. Forsham, David A. Wood, and H. Glenn Bell, *Bilateral Adrenalectomy for Advanced Carcinoma of the Breast with Preliminary Observations on the Effect of the Liver on the Metabolism of Adrenal Cortical Steroids.* Volume LXXII, 1954.

David A. Wood, all by invitation, and H. Glenn Bell, of San Francisco, Professor of Surgery and Chairman Department of Surgery, University of California Medical School, *Bilateral Adrenalectomy for Advanced Carcinoma of the Breast with Preliminary Observations on the Effect of the Liver on the Metabolism of Adrenal Cortical Steroids.* They performed adrenalectomy and oophorectomy on 31 women with advanced metastatic carcinoma, unresponsive to roentgen ray, androgens or estrogens. They had had one postoperative death from asphyxia and one from hepatic failure, in a patient with extensive liver metastases, and ten patients had subsequently died,

all of their carcinoma. At variance with the report of Huggins and Dao, although the best results had been shown in two patients with adenocarcinoma, there had been ". . . objective evidence of improvement in five cases of predominantly undifferentiated carcinoma . . ." As a purely experimental procedure, in four patients they had performed a right adrenalectomy and anastomosed the left adrenal vein to the splenic vein, diverting the adrenal blood through the liver where the estrogens could be inactivated. In fact, ". . . estrogen assay in daily urine samples . . . failed to reveal any significant amounts of estrogens." The first patient underwent a striking remission, they did not mention the course of the other three. The patients required no substitution therapy. Of their 100 patients with bilateral adrenalectomy 22 showed objective improvement and 45 more claimed subjective benefit. Their final word was that "The transitory nature of the arrest of the metastatic spread makes this a palliative procedure only."

Discussion

Charles Huggins, bestowed encomiums upon Dr. Galante, ". . . for showing resourcefulness, great technical ingenuity, and great promise for the future" [but said not a word about his thoughts concerning the adrenal-splenic venous anastomosis].

* * *

Frank Glenn, of New York, Lewis Atterbury Stimson Professor of Surgery and Surgeon-in-Chief, New York Hospital, Cornell Medical Center, and by invitation, John Evans, Malcolm Hill, and John McClenahan, *Intravenous Cholangiography,* said that of the agents available for intravenous injection for demonstration of the extrahepatic biliary system in the previous six years, iodopanoic acid and triiodeothionic acid had certain deficiencies. Now 30 years after the introduction by Graham and Cole of opacification of the gallbladder, they were reporting on ". . . Cholografin, made available to us and others by E. R. Squibb and Sons . . ." They had administered it 88 times to 80 patients who after subcutaneous injection of two drops, had shown no hypersensitivity, then a small dose injected intravenously, after which if no untoward symptoms occurred, the full dose was injected slowly over five to ten minutes. They had seen nausea 19 times, flushing 11 times, vomiting 8 times. The common duct had been demonstrated in 66% of the patients, and in 76% of those who had had a previous cholecystectomy. In 25 patients without a gallbadder and free of jaundice or other signs of liver failure, the common duct was demonstrated in 23,- 92%. Intravenous cholangiography was particularly advised preoperatively to show possible stones in the common duct, in patients in whom oral cholecystography was not feasible or had failed, and in children, and in emergencies. "Body-section radiography" [laminograms] combined with intravenous choledochography had produced strikingly clear pictures.

Discussion

Evarts A. Graham, invited by the Chairman to initiate the Discussion, had never seen the material used. He reminded the Association "that in our early publications on this subject, Dr. Cole and I stated specifically that although we had experimented with more than 60 different substances, most of which were products of our own brains, we felt that there would always be additional substances found which would visualize the gallbladder and perhaps the bile ducts, and would be much better than anything we had discovered ourselves up to that time." Warren H. Cole, of Chicago, said that what little experience with the drug they had supported Dr. Glenn's observations. Leon Goldman, of San Francisco, asked whether the test had been used in the diagnosis of acute cholecystitis in which he would expect the gallbladder not to be visualized. Glenn, in closing, agreed that acute cholecystitis might be a specific indication for the use of intravenous cholecystography. They had had two such cases.

The Business Meetings

The 1954 meeting was held at the Hotel Cleveland, in Cleveland, Ohio, April 28, 29, and 30, President Howard C. Naffziger in the Chair.

Thirty-four of 71 abstracts were accepted by the Program Committee, meeting again all together with the President, a practice which they recommended be made a regular one.

Once more Dr. Frederick Coller reported for the Committee on Unnecessary Operations. It had occurred to Dr. Coller to consult the Michigan Blue Shield, which covered the surgical fees of 3,000,000 of the 6,000,000 people in Michigan; 5,200 physicians and 900 osteopaths had received fees from Blue Shield [Coller's report refers to slides, in most cases indicating the figures shown on the slides]. An interesting fact emerged about the charges made for operations. Board surgeons charged $188 for cholecystectomy, non-board surgeons $170, and men not known to be surgeons by training charged as much or more than the Board certified surgeons. The same was true for hysterectomy. Of the tonsillectomies, 9% were done by osteopaths, 16% by Board members, and the other 75% by practitioners. On the other hand, of subtotal gastrectomies, 51% were done by specialists (men certified by the Board or members of the College) 28% by nonspecialists, and

11% by osteopathic physicians; appendectomy, however, 26% by specialists, 59% by non-specialists, 8% by osteopaths; cholecystectomy, 41% by specialists, 44% by nonspecialists, 10% by osteopaths. Given the relatively small number of osteopaths, Coller said "If you multiply this by five you will see that the osteopaths are really getting their share." The specialists did 37% of the herniorrhaphies; nonspecialists, 50%; and osteopaths, 7.8%. Suspension of the uterus,- specialists did only 20%; nonspecialists did 46% and the osteopaths did 33%, Coller commenting that "I am glad to see that at the University Hospital we either have no business or we are not suspending uteri." "You and I both know that the suspensions of the uterus . . . probably were unnecessary in a large number of cases." The specialists did 52% of the thyroidectomies; the nonspecialists, 33%; and the osteopaths, 7%. Salpingectomy, the specialists did 18%; nonspecialists, 61%; and the osteopaths, 20%, "They are running high on this and high on suspension of the uterus."

The 1954 meeting was the first at which the Fellows sat at a reserved front section behind tables. This popular innovation became a fixed feature of future meetings.

During the Business Meeting, Dr. Francis Moore rose to state that he had not marked his ballot "because three distinguished anesthetists, who have been proposed for membership, have not been presented to us for vote. I feel strongly that one of the ways in which the very difficult problems of professional relationships with anesthesia in this country is going to be solved is to recognize that the anesthetist is a brother surgeon and is practicing a subspecialty of surgery, and that he should be a member of our Society." The propriety of nominating an anesthetist had been agreed upon several years before. [It was hardly coincidence that the following year in Philadelphia, John Adriani, of New Orleans, Henry Knowles Beecher, of Boston, and Robert Dunning Dripps, of Philadelphia, were all duly elected to membership!]

The new officers were John H. Gibbon, Jr., of Philadelphia, who had been Vice-President in 1953, President [his father, John H. Gibbon, who had been President in 1926, was in the room at the time]; Robert Moore, of Galveston, First Vice-President; D. M. Glover, of Cleveland, Second Vice-President; and R. K. Gilchrist, of Evanston, Illinois, as Secretary.

LXXIII

1955

The 1955 meeting was held at the Hotel Warwick, Philadelphia, April 27, 28, and 29, President John H. Gibbon, Jr., of Philadelphia, Professor of Surgery and Director of Surgical Research, Jefferson Medical College, in the Chair. The previous year had seen the deaths of Isaac A. Bigger, of Richmond; David Cheever, of Boston; Fred W. Rankin, of Lexington, Kentucky, as well as John Alexander, after an extraordinarily productive career and the founding at Ann Arbor of a great school of Thoracic Surgery, in spite of a continuing illness from a variety of manifestations of tuberculosis.

* * *

Richard L. Varco, of Minneapolis, Associate Professor of Surgery, University of Minnesota, and by invitation, Lloyd D. MacLean, Joseph B. Aust, and Robert A. Good, *Agammaglobulinemia: An Approach to Homovital Transplantation,* proceeded from the assumption that the evidence was that homograft rejection was an immunological phenomenon as indicated by the fact that "The time required for rejection of homotransplants is approximately the same as that required for antibody formation . . . the rate of transplantation rejection becomes a function of the dose of 'antigen' . . . Circulation . . . without a barrier to antibody contact is essential for the rejection of homotransplants . . . Evidence for an anamnestic reaction towards homotransplants exists . . . An agent decreasing antibody

formation (cortisone) prolongs the survival time of homotransplants . . . rejection of skin transplants is accompanied by the appearance in the blood of antibodies against donor cells." They tested this hypothesis on two patients with congenital agammaglobulinemia "an immunological paralysis associated with secondary inability to create gamma globulin" and on two patients with acquired agammaglobulinemia which they termed "immunoparesis". Split thickness and full thickness homografts survived indefinitely in the two patients with congenital agammaglobulinemia and survived only temporarily in the two patients with acquired ,agammaglobulinemia. They hoped that "inquiring workers will be keenly aroused by these immunological challenges, and by virtue of greater interest bring sooner to successful practice, clinical, homovital organ grafting. Such an accomplishment represents a maturation of surgery that is a bright vista to contemplate."

Discussion

Bradford Cannon, of Boston, congratulated MacLean and his colleagues as having provided "the first evidence in the human that the absence of circulating antibodies in the recipient alters the reaction to the homotransplant." No one said anything of the future of transplantation.

* * *

1019

Hypothermia in Surgery. Analysis of 100 Clinical Cases, illustrated the vigorous investigation of this method which was being undertaken in Denver by Henry Swan, Professor and Head of the Department of Surgery, University of Colorado School of Medicine and his associates, by invitation, Robert W. Virtue, S. Gilbert Blount, Jr., and Lorence T. Kircher, Jr. The prime indication for the use of hypothermic anesthesia was "to perform an operation in a bloodless field during temporary occlusion of the blood supply to or through the organ . . . to prolong the time-tolerance to ischemia . . . by . . . reduction in tissue metabolic rates". Intracardiac surgery under direct vision was still competing with indirect techniques [viz., R.E. Gross' atrial well] and Swan said "That the blind but educated finger is capable of accomplishing much within the heart, is to be freely admitted, and much admired; that it should be considered as the best method in the long run is absurd." Hypothermia also improved the operative risk in patients with severe congenital or acquired heart disease. "A deeply cyanotic child with a pulse rate of 150 to 175 may achieve an almost normal color with a pulse rate of 100 at 30° C." Air embolism was a prime hazard of intracardiac surgery. To prevent it, they employed the transverse incision across the sternum to provide access to all chambers of the heart, appropriate tilting of the table to put the cardiotomy uppermost, filled the heart with Ringer's solution before the last suture in a septal defect was tied and filled it again before the atrium was clamped shut. They had recognized air embolism twice and had been able to salvage both patients by reclamping the aorta and massaging the heart until air disappeared from the coronaries. Hypothermia was induced by placing the child in a tub of cold water after anesthesia had been induced and anesthesia maintained deep enough to prevent shivering. At 31 degrees, anesthesia could usually be discontinued. The temperature continued to drift downwards after removal of the patients from the ice water. Through a transverse sternum-dividing bipleural incision, the aorta and pulmonary artery were occluded at their bases "with a non-crushing clamp". They had no deaths in 12 patients with pulmonary valvar stenosis, no deaths in two patients with pulmonary infundibular stenosis, one death in 22 with a secundum auricular septal defect, 19 of them cured, two deaths in three children with a primum septal defect and four deaths in five patients with a ventricular septal defect. In the tetralogy of Fallot, they achieved partial relief of valvar stenosis in four children with no deaths, partial relief of infundibular stenosis in six children with two deaths.

In four children with pulmonary stenosis and an atrial septal defect, they had had two deaths, and one child with both atrial and ventricular septal defects died. They had thus 12 deaths in 59 open cardiac procedures. In 21 closed cardiac procedures under hypothermia they had had seven deaths, two in three operations for tricuspid atresia, two in two operations for aortic regurgitation, one in two operations for aberrant pulmonary veins and one in the one patient with a single ventricle and one in a patient with pulmonary hypertension. Ventricular fibrillation had been a problem. They were under the impression that coronary perfusion with prostigmine reduced the hazard of fibrillation. With occlusion times of eight minutes or less at body temperatures not lower than 26° C, the technique was "both effective and safe in congenital lesions which can be repaired through a right heart approach . . ." and considered it "the method of choice in the treatment of isolated valvular or infundibular pulmonary stenosis and of interatrial septal defect." They had had no recognized brain sequellae but had had peripheral neurological lesions in 12 patients "possibly due to increased susceptibility of the cold nerve to pressure . . ." of the encircling rubber band holding the electrocardiographic electrodes.

* * *

Hypothermia was similarly under investigation at the University of Minnesota and F. John Lewis, Associate Professor of Surgery, University of Minnesota; Mansur Taufic, by invitation; Richard L. Varco, Associate Professor of Surgery; and by invitation, Suad Niazi, *The Surgical Anatomy of Atrial Septal Defects: Experiences with Repair under Direct Vision*, reported an experience with 35 operations. [The first successful closure of an atrial septal defect under hypothermia and inflow occlusion had been reported by Lewis in 1953.] They employed hypothermia, a transverse incision across the sternum, bilateral thoracotomy, digital exploration of the heart through the right auricular appendage, occlusion of the cardiac inflow and outflow, and a wide atriotomy. The length of inflow occlusion had been between three to seven-and-three-quarter minutes. They had closed 23 foramen ovale defects with three deaths, five high defects above the foramen ovale with no deaths. Of three patients with persistent ostium primum defects, one died of heart block on the third day, the other two surviving but with permanent heart block. There were thus four deaths in 33 patients. Results were excellent in all survivors except the patients with persistent ostium primum.

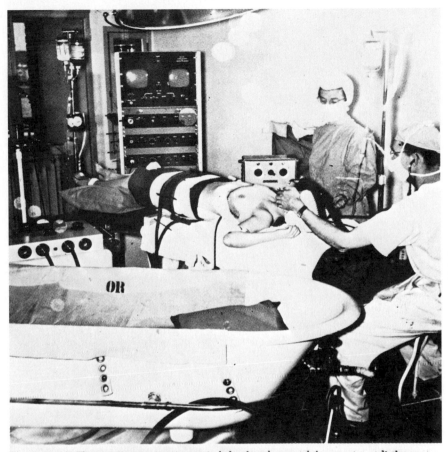

Fig. 1. The operating room equipment includes the tub, a rectal thermometer, a diathermy unit, a multi-channel electronic recording device, the defibrillator, a direct writing EEG, and a standard anesthesia machine. At least two intravenous plastic cannulae are in place. The patient is in the operating position immediately after wound closure.

After anesthesia had been induced, the child was placed in the tub and anesthesia continued until body temperature was at 31° C. The temperature continued to drift downward after removal of the patient from the tub. The temperature was maintained at 26° or above by diathermy coils about the abdomen and rewarming begun with this as soon as the "surgical manipulation of the heart" was completed. Of the duration of occlusion, Swan said only that operations undertaken must be those which could be performed in eight minutes. He was reporting his experience with 100 patients.

Henry Swan, Robert W. Virtue, S. Gilbert Blount, Jr., and Lorence T. Kircher, Jr., *Hypothermia in Surgery*. Analysis of 100 Clinical Cases, Vol. LXXIII 1955.

Ventricular fibrillation occurred in 11 patients, all of whom were successfully defibrillated.

Discussion

H. T. Bahnson, of Baltimore, said that they had operated by closed methods on 14 patients with secundum type defects without a death. They had lost three of three patients with ostium primum defects. Conrad R. Lam, of Detroit, said he had operated also with closed techniques, upon 13 patients with septum secundum defects without a death and without ventricular fibrillation. Both Swan and Lewis indicated, in closing, that the open method permitted a better visualization of atrial defects. Lewis had catheterized 12 patients after operation, and the defect was completely closed in ten.

* * *

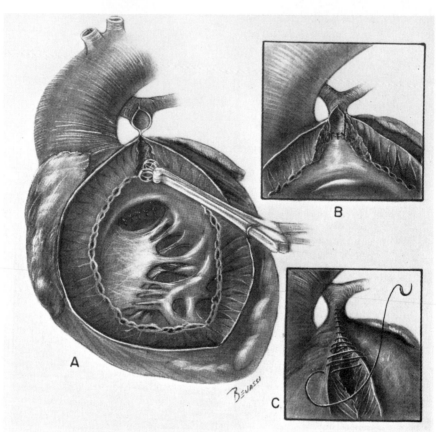

Fig. 13. Pulmonary atresia correction. The method utilized in correcting the outflow tract obstruction in patient L. K. (A) A new outflow channel is being cut through the solid infundibular muscle. The main pulmonary artery has been opened distally for orientation. (B) The opened pulmonary artery has been pulled down and anastomosed to the newly created outflow tract. There was no pulmonary valve present in this patient. (C) The cardiotomy incision closed by a continuous 000 silk stitch sewn superficially to further enlarge this outflow channel.

In A, the ventricular septal defect is shown already closed by direct suture. In two patients, the sutures were tied over a compressed Ivalon sponge. In one patient, an atrial septal defect was simultaneously closed. Six of the ten patients survived and were symptomatically well after definitive repair, relying on "controlled cross circulation" with a donor connected to the patient by tubing through which the blood was propelled by a finger pump.

C. Walton Lillehei, Morley Cohen, Herbert E. Warden, Raymond C. Read, Joseph B. Aust, Richard A. DeWall, and Richard L. Varco, *Direct Vision Intracardiac Surgical Correction of the Tetralogy of Fallot, Pentalogy of Fallot, and Pulmonary Atresia Defects.* Report of First Ten Cases, Volume LXXIII, 1955.

The most dramatic of the papers on cardiac surgery which created such a stir at the meeting was certainly *Direct Vision Intracardiac Surgical Correction of the Tetralogy of Fallot, Pentalogy of Fallot, and Pulmonary Atresia Defects.* Report of First Ten Cases, C. Walton Lillehei, Morley Cohen, Herbert E. Warden, Raymond C. Read, Joseph B. Aust, Richard A. DeWall, all by invitation, and Richard L. Varco, Associate Professor of Surgery, University of Minnesota. They were employing controlled cross circulation with human volunteers serving as "oxygenators", propelling the blood by a "finger" pump [a technique which had startled the world when presented by the Minnesota group the year before]. They had previously put forward the hypothesis of the "azygos flow" technique, suggesting that a flow equivalent to that returned by the azygos vein, "1/6 to 1/4 of the resting cardiac outputs for normal individuals of comparable size and weight" was sufficient for the purposes of operation under brief exclusion of the heart from the circulation, six to 21-1/2 minutes in this series. [The presentation concentrated on the ten patients with variants of Fallot's tetralogy.] They had mentioned in passing that they had operated "on 47 additional individuals with other types of intracardiac lesions" under "total cardiac and pulmonary by-pass for corrective intracardiac surgery at comparable rates of perfusion and at normal body temperature without a single instance of cerebral, hepatic, or renal dysfunction attributable to these low flow rates." They attempted to preserve normothermia, placing the patient on a heat blanket. Low flow rate minimized return to the heart during inflow occlusion, and they further maintained the field dry by occluding the aorta as needed by a cotton tape held in a Rumel tourniquet. Three of the cross circulation donors had their discharge from the hospital delayed one or two days for unexplained fever, the others were said to have totally uncomplicated recoveries. The tetralogy of Fallot repair consisted in direct suture of the ventricular septal defect through a right ventriculotomy, carrying the incision into the pulmonary artery if necessary, and infundibulectomy with a modified tonsil punch. In one instance, a concomitant atrial septal defect was closed by direct suture. In two instances, the sutures in the ventricular septal defect were tied down over pledgets of compressed Ivalon sponge. Six of the children survived, were asymptomatic, and their systemic atrial oxygen saturations were now in the normal range. Two children had been recatheterized, one had a persistent small left-to-right shunt high in the right ventricle, the other had "oxygen content and pressure measurements demonstrating unequivocally that complete anatomical and physiologic restoration to normal can be achieved in a patient born with these tetralogy defects." They concluded by saying "As a result of these gratifying successes, together with the four instructive failures, the curative operation has been adopted in our clinic as the method of choice for all patients with the tetralogy of Fallot defects who are in need of surgical treatment at this time. For the lesser degrees of disability, we recommend temporary postponement of any surgical operation . . . and periodic re-evaluation . . . For the patient currently in need of surgical treatment and for whom an intracardiac procedure is not available, we recommend an anastomotic operation without the opening of the pericardium. This operation provides significant palliation, and does not interfere with the intracardiac operation should it be deemed necessary subsequently." [In their opening paragraphs, they were less charitable to the anastomotic procedures,- "Since our initial experience in 1954 with the curative procedure for the tetralogy defects, we have come to adopt that plan for all patients with this lesion currently in need of surgical treatment."]

Discussion

The Discussion was appropriately opened by Alfred Blalock, of Baltimore. "I must say that I never thought I would live to see the day when this type of operative procedure could be performed. I want to commend Dr. Lillehei and Dr. Varco and their associates for their imagination, their courage and their industry." Nevertheless, he guessed "that the ultimate answer will be the artificial heart lung as developed by our President, Dr. Gibbon, and as it is being used now by more and more people. Dr. Gibbon has used it successfully for intracardiac surgery. [Gibbon, in 1951 (see Volume LXIX) had presented his all but final version of the pump oxygenator on which he had been working for so many years. At the 1952 meeting Gibbon said he had 12 dogs alive and well after "dependence upon the artificial circulation." At the 1953 meeting, Dennis mentioned his two human attempts with his oxygenator. In 1954 Gibbon (Application of a Mechanical Heart and Lung Apparatus to Cardiac Surgery. Minnesota Medicine 37:171–180 and 185, 1954) reported the first successful intracardiac operation,- closure of an atrial septal defect,- in a human, with the use of an artificial pump oxygenator.] I have heard that Dr. Kirklin, of the Mayo Clinic, has now used it successfully in closing several ventricular septal defects." The direct attack was ultimately the ideal one but "the mortality rate at the present time with the anastomotic procedures in the treatment of the tetralogy of Fallot is considerably less than that with the open operative procedure . . . we have had two groups of 45 consecutive survivals following anastomotic operations . . . the results are very gratifying . . ." He was astonished that direct suture could "close an interventricular defect where the aorta is overriding this defect. From the many specimens that I saw postmortem, I would not have dreamed that this could have been done, because this aorta straddles the defect, and there is nothing between the defect and the aorta. So, to me, that, perhaps, is the most important part of their contribution . . . Will the defect remain closed? . . . Is there some concern about the myocardial scar that results from a big incision such as this? . . . will this small pulmonary artery be able to carry the blood if the ventricular defect is closed?" Clarence Dennis, of Brooklyn, said that they had been working for sev-

1024

eral years on the problem of air embolism with his heart-lung machine and showed a motion picture of its use in the dog. [An addendum written after the meeting reports "the repair of a septal defect in most gratifying manner in an 18-year-old girl. Both the right atrium and the right ventricle were opened while on perfusion. She has completely recovered."] D. W. Gordon Murray, of Toronto, was "amazed at what has happened . . . since reporting to this Association nine or ten years ago on perhaps the first closure of septal defects [Vol. LXV, 1947]." He agreed with Blalock that the open method was better if it could be done safely, but "until the mortality rate is reduced a bit, perhaps there is still a place for the closed method of doing these things. I have done 32 septal defects, 17 auricular, 15 ventricular, and in the last ten there has been no mortality. I quite agree that they aren't all closed." He did want to add [in an allusion that aroused much laughter and some ribald remarks] "speaking for the Canadians, but not speaking for the Americans, who are much more enlightened people, and speaking also for a good number of the British, if you will recall, there may be one very important biological function where direct vision is not a necessity." H. W. Scott, of Nashville, said that a year before under inflow occlusion and hypothermia, they had, in a child with a tetralogy, closed a ventricular septal defect and excised the infundibular diaphragm. However, in several other children, they had only been able to do the infundibulectomy, "We were unable to close the accompanying associated defect in the short period of time available by this method." Hypothermia and inflow stasis did not provide the time which was required. President Gibbon expressed delight over the papers presented, congratulated the authors, said that he had supplied the Mayo Clinic with the plans for his oxygenator. "Dr. Kirklin isn't here today, but I understand they have done eight cases, with four successfully, with the use of this machine." C. W. Lillehei, of Minneapolis, closing, acknowledged a debt to "the epochal contribution of Doctors Blalock and Taussig in 1945". Autopsy room study had convinced the Minnesota group ["For several years prior to the availability of any satisfactory method for intracardiac surgery, it had been and continued to be our policy to be present at every autopsy upon a patient succumbing with a known or suspected congenital heart defect. With the heart still *in situ,* these defects have been exposed by a surgical cardiotomy, and a corrective procedure carried out."] that the lesions in tetralogy of Fallot were, in fact, directly correctable and they had set about finding the least complicated technique for total cardiopul-

monary bypass. He thought controlled cross circulation had satisfied the requirements and said they had no donor mortality. He mentioned as other techniques the "continuous arterial perfusion from a reservoir of arterialized-venous blood" and "the use of an excised heterologous (dog) lung". He was willing to "predict a bright future in this field of surgery for the role of artificial oxygenators, but not for the complex types that have been described to date . . . The essence of wide applicability is simplicity, and we look forward to the clinical use within this year of an artificial oxygenator so simple that it costs only a few dollars to construct, has no moving parts, and is disposable after each use. Such an oxygenator, which has been developed in the laboratory by Dr. Richard DeWall, is combined with the same simple cross circulation pump." [A footnote added after the meeting indicated they had successfully corrected the tetralogy in a 22-month-old infant, no longer with a volunteer donor and cross circulation, but "utilizing a simple inexpensive disposable artificial oxygenator assembled from materials available in the average hospital supply room."] As for the question about the healing of the cardiotomy scar, he could only say that "in the experimental animals these invariably heal very well . . ." In regard to the problem of the overriding of the aorta and the pulling out of the closure stitches, he said the proper insertion of the stitches had not proved to be a problem.

* * *

K. Alvin Merendino, of Seattle, Professor of Surgery, University of Washington, School of Medicine, and by invitation, David H. Dillard, *The Concept of Sphincter Substitution by an Interposed Jejunal Segment for Anatomic and Physiologic Abnormalities at the Esophagogastric Junction,* With Special Reference to Reflux Esophagitis, Cardiospasm, and Esophageal Varices,- disputed the thesis that there was an "increased inherent sensitivity of the small bowel [to gastric juice] as one progresses distally from the pylorus, at least as far as the midjejunum." They attributed the increased susceptibility to anastomotic ulcers with distance from the pylorus "to the fact that the buffering capacity of the intestinal contents has been so altered in transit that at lower levels of the intestine it is quantitatively inadequate to neutralize acid delivered at the stoma." Merendino had already shown [1954] that his jejunal interposition operation protected against esophagitis and that the interposed jejunum "exhibited greater resistance to acid-peptic trauma than either (Text continued on p. 1029.)

CARDIAC SURGERY - THE FIRST WAVE

Even among the Fellows of the American Surgical Association, there is some arbitrariness in grouping contributors to a field in this way, and others are pictured elsewhere,- Gross, Blalock, Bahnson, Cooley, DeBakey,- and still others in later years. After Gross pointed the way with the patent ductus, and Crafoord and Blalock with coarctation, Blalock demonstrated with his systemic-pulmonary shunts that patients with abnormal hearts could tolerate anesthesia, and manipulation of the great vessels and that physiologic derangement could be compensated for by rearranging the circulation. The field of cardiac surgery exploded. Harken, and Bailey [neither of whom ever became a Fellow] established closed mitral valvotomy; Blalock and Hanlon created interatrial defects to benefit children with transposition of the great arteries; Varco corrected pulmonic stenosis under inflow occlusion; Potts developed his ingenious knives for pulmonic stenosis and his fine multi-toothed clamps; Lewis—after Bigelow's studies in Toronto on hypothermia—corrected atrial septal defects by open cardiotomy under hypothermia, the first "open heart" operations, Lillehei corrected tetralogy of Fallot under cardiopulmonary bypass with controlled cross circulation using human volunteers as the oxygenators; Potts, Campbell, Mustard and Bigelow experimented with animal lungs as oxygenators; Gibbon introduced his screen oxygenator and performed with it the first successful open heart operation with a mechanical pump oxygenator, and DeWall established the practicality of the much simpler bubble oxygenator. Each of those mentioned and portrayed was involved in and made multiple contributions to cardiovascular surgery.

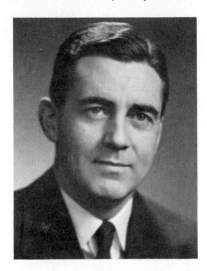

Wilfred Gordon Bigelow - (c. 1954) 1913-. M.D. University of Toronto, 1938, Residency Toronto General Hospital. Research Fellow Johns Hopkins, 1946-47; Professor of Surgery, University of Toronto; Head, Division of Cardiovascular Surgery, Toronto General Hospital. Suave, urban, thoughtful. Introduced the concept and developed the technique,- 1950-65,- of hypothermia for open heart surgery after prolonged and detailed physiological studies, beginning with the hedgehog. In 1950 (Volume LXVIII) suggested leaving a percutaneous cardiac electrode at the conclusion of cardiac operations to deal with heart block and in 1951 developed the first electrical pacemaker for the heart.

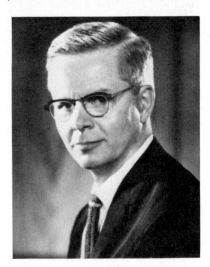

Clarence Dennis 1909- . (Vice-President 1972) M.D. Johns Hopkins 1935, University of Minnesota, intern to Professor 1935-1952. Professor and Chairman, State University of New York, Downstate Medical Center, 1952-1972; National Heart and Lung Institute, 1973-1975; Professor of Surgery, State University of New York, Stony Brook 1974-. Began his work on an extracorporeal pump oxygenator while still in Minnesota, twice attempted, before Gibbon, an open heart procedure under cardiopulmonary bypass. In his oxygenator, a jet of blood was directed against a single large disk, the rotation of which filmed the blood—in an oxygen atmosphere. Contributions in bowel surgery, ulcerative colitis, intestinal suture.

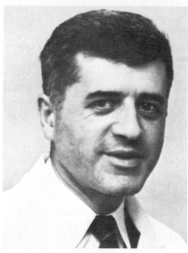

Johann L. Ehrenhaft, (c. 1950) 1915- . M.D. University of Iowa 1938, Training, Johns Hopkins and the University of Iowa; Thoracic Surgery, Barnes Hospital, St. Louis, with Evarts Graham. Chairman, Division of Cardiothoracic Surgery and Professor of Surgery at the University of Iowa. Record of unusually good results in every phase of surgery for congenital heart disease, and reputation for blunt directness and accuracy. Demonstrated that in tetralogy of Fallot in most cases enough of the obstructing muscle could be resected from within the heart to obviate the need for outflow patches.

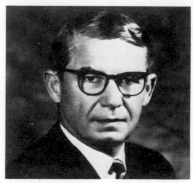

Frank Gerbode, (c. 1950) 1907- . M.D. Stanford 1936; Intern, Highland Hospital, Oakland; Assistant in Pathology, Munich; Residency, Stanford 1937-40; Instructor to Clinical Professor, Stanford 1945-71. Remained in San Francisco when the medical school moved to Palo Alto. Since 1959, President of the Institute of Medical Sciences, Director of the Heart Research Institute, Pacific Medical Center. Early leader in developing techniques of closed and open cardiac repairs. Devised a transventricular mitral dilator, introduced the transverse ventriculotomy for repair of tetralogy of Fallot. Massive effort in computer monitoring of critically ill and postoperative patients. Developed one of the first practical membrane oxygenators. An international surgical ambassador, his laboratory and clinical service have trained men from overseas who have become world leaders.

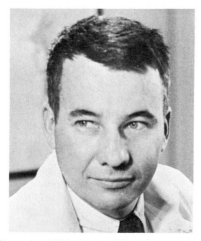

W. W. L. Glenn, (c. 1959) 1914- , M.D. Jefferson 1938. Training, the University of Pennsylvania and Massachusetts General Hospital. Best known contribution, the Glenn shunt—superior vena cava right pulmonary artery anastomosis for tricuspid atresia. Introduced deliberate intraoperative cardiac fibrillation as a measure of preventing air embolism, introduced implantable radio frequency cardiac and phrenic stimulators.

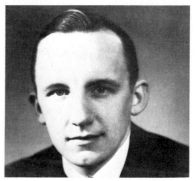

C. R. Hanlon, (c. 1955) 1915- . M.D. Johns Hopkins, 1938. Unique distinction of having been The Resident both with Mont Reid at the University of Cincinnati and Alfred Blalock at Johns Hopkins. Associate Professor at Hopkins. Established the fact of increased longevity in transposition patients with large atrial defects, the Blalock-Hanlon closed atrial septostomy evolving as the solution. Went to St. Louis University in 1950 as Professor and Chairman. With T. Cooper and V. Willman, in preparation for cardiac transplantation, conducted a series of systematic pharmacologic, histologic and physiologic studies of cardiac function in surgically denervated and autotransplanted hearts in dogs and anthropoids. Secretary of the Association, 1969, when he resigned to become Director of the American College of Surgeons. A surgical scholar and humanist, with a forbidding mastery of language, he has made an immense contribution at the College in that post,- the first "academic" surgeon to hold it,- by virtue of his highly developed political antennae, great administrative skill, and his unimpeachable integrity and devotion to principle.

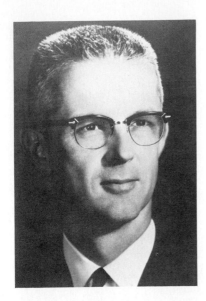

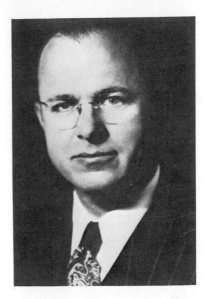

J. W. Kirklin, 1917- . M.D. Harvard 1942. Training, University of Pennsylvania, Mayo Clinic, and Children's Hospital, Boston. Mayo Clinic 1950-1966, Professor of Surgery and Chairman of Department 1960-1966; University of Alabama, Professor and Chairman 1966-. Innumerable technical and conceptual contributions to cardiac surgery for both congenital and acquired lesions. Early modified and simplified Gibbon's oxygenator. Consistently produced results matching or bettering others reported. It may be that his major contribution has been using the operating room and intensive care unit as sophisticated laboratories to demonstrate the value of systematic measurements and construction of formulae and nomograms to indicate when in the course of a given cardiac lesion operation is to be undertaken, and which operation under which circumstances. Extended the concept and design of computer management of the patient after operation to indicate automatically what was to be done, how much and when. His superb technical performance and excellent results in large numbers of patients have permitted his units to make substantial contributions to each developing phase of cardiac surgery.

Conrad R. Lam, (c. 1950) 1905- . M.D. Yale 1932. Training and career all at Henry Ford Hospital. Surgeon-in-Charge of the Division of Thoracic Surgery 1946-1970. Studies on prevention and treatment of trapping air in the heart, contributed to many phases of operative cardiac surgery (viz., 30 successive transarterial pulmonary valvotomies under normothermic inflow occlusion) as it was developing, reporting his results with a pleasant directness. The international symposium on cardiac surgery, which he organized in Detroit in 1955 at the height of the excitement over the explosion of cardiac surgery, was a signal event.

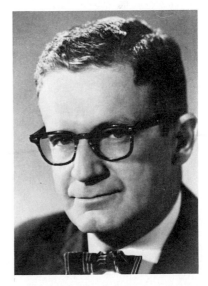

F. John Lewis, (c. 1955) 1916- . M.D. University of Minnesota 1942, Associate Professor of Surgery 1957, to Northwestern University as Professor of Surgery 1957-1976. Member of the bustling brood of cardiac surgeons in Wangensteen's department and technically one of the most brilliant. His initial major contribution to the field was the demonstration of the feasibility of the closure of atrial septal defects under hypothermia and inflow occlusion,- subsequently interested in computer applications to medicine.

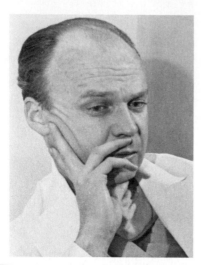

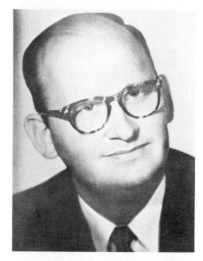

C. Walton Lillehei, (c. 1958) 1918-. M.D. University of Minnesota 1942. Graduate of Wangensteen's prodigious, somewhat unorthodox school, which developed so many competitive, innovative, laboratory-oriented surgeons. Brilliant, imaginative, unorthodox, his major initial contribution,- of many,- was certainly the demonstration in patients cross-circulated with human volunteers who thus served as the oxygenators, that one-stage complete correction of intracardic defects could be performed, tolerated by the heart and by the patient, and could produce a healthy organism with an effective heart. Professor of Surgery at Minnesota 1956-1967, and Director of Surgery, New York Hospital, Cornell Medical Center, 1970-74.

W. H. Muller, (c. 1955) 1919- . (President, 1975; Recorder 1962-1967; President, American College of Surgeons, 1980). M.D. Duke 1943. Trained at Hopkins, 1944-49, and joined Longmire at the new UCLA medical school,- Assistant Professor to Associate Professor, 1949-54; 1954—Professor and Chairman, Surgery, University of Virginia School of Medicine; 1976—Vice President for Health Affairs. At U.C.L.A. with F. Dammann studied the natural history of pulmonary hypertension and demonstrated that constriction of the pulmonary artery offered protection to patients with pulmonary hypertension and the then untreatable ventricular septal defect. Contributed a technique for instrumental dilatation of aortic stenosis, and a total replacement of aortic valve with a tricuspid teflon prosthesis.

H. B. Shumacker Jr., 1908- . Secretary, 1965-68; Vice-President 1961. M.D. Johns Hopkins 1932, training Johns Hopkins and Yale. After World War II, from Hopkins to Yale to University of Indiana as Professor and Chairman 1948-1968. Contributions from the laboratory and the clinic to many phases of surgery of the heart and aorta, including his ingenious 1953 closed technique of closure of septum secundum atrial defects by inversion and suture, to the edges of the defect, of a diverticulum of pericardial tissue fashioned in the atrial wall. He made a major effort in the artificial heart program.

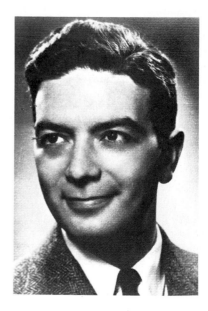

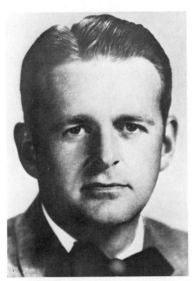

Henry Swan, (c. 1955) 1913- . M.D. Harvard 1939. Training, Peter Bent Brigham, Children's Hospital, Boston; to University of Colorado 1946, Professor and Chairman 1950-1961. Initial major contribution was the vigorous investigation of the limits of open heart surgery under hypothermia induced by external cooling.

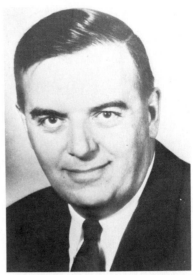

Richard L. Varco, (c. 1955) 1912- . (Vice-President 1968) M.D. University of Minnesota, 1937 and entire career there, Professor of Surgery 1950-. One of the major factors in the productivity and intellectual ferment in the Wangensteen clinic and the outstanding technical surgeon in the group. In cardiac surgery, with Payne early reported enviable experiences with Blalock's operation, demonstrated feasibility of normothermic inflow occlusion in operating for pulmonic stenosis. Colossal corpus of seminal work in cardiac surgery, duodenal ulcer (histamine in beeswax preparation) immunology, transplantation, oncology. Blunt, uncompromising, frighteningly brilliant, demanding of associates, a major force in a major clinic for his professional lifetime.

the stomach or duodenum". In the basic experimental preparation now, the esophagogastric junction was excised, the stomach closed, the vagus divided and an isoperistaltic segment of jejunum interposed between the esophagus and the anterior surface of the gastric fundus, adding a Ramstedt pyloromyotomy in some animals and a Finney pyloroplasty in others. The animals were tested with daily injections of histamine in oil and beeswax. Ulcers of the esophagus developed in no animal, and minimal inflammation in one, but "severe gastric and duodenal ulceration was produced in all groups". The Finney pyloroplasty reduced the incidence of jejunal reaction from 40 to 50% in the other groups, to 10%. In three animals with either an intact pylorus or a py-

loromyotomy, the ulceration of the jejunal segment was more severe than that in the stomach or duodenum. It had become apparent from clinical observation that when the cardiac sphincter was destroyed by incision or excision, esophagitis frequently resulted. They had performed the interposition procedure on 12 patients, with one death, in a 75-year-old woman with a hiatus hernia and severe reflux esophagitis with stricture, who died apparently of a leak from erosion of the gastric wall by an indwelling nasogastric tube. Of the seven patients with hiatus hernia and reflux esophagitis, in addition to the one death, one patient whose esophagus was resected through a zone of intense inflammation, developed a stricture in the retained portion of the esophagus.

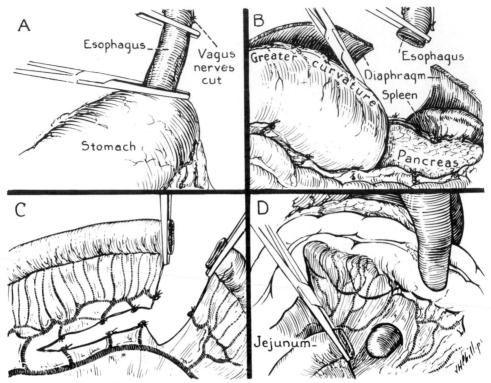

Fig. 9. (A) A bilateral vagotomy has been performed. The lesion is excised, making sure that all of the squamous epithelium of the esophagus has been removed with the cardia. (B) The gastro-splenic ligament is divided, as well as the attachments between the dorsal wall of the stomach and posterior peritoneum and pancreas. This maneuver makes the lesser omental sac and posterior mediastinum contiguous. (C) Development of the jejunal segment. (D) An opening is made in an avascular area of the transverse mesocolon and the jejunal segment, with blood supply intact, is delivered in retrocolic fashion into the lesser omental sac.

Merendino employed a thoraco-abdominal incision, splitting the diaphragm, extrapolated a 15 to 20 cm. segment of jejunum, comfortably below the ligament of Tretiz, bringing it up through the transverse mesocolon. Cardia and diseased distal esophagus were excised and the jejunal loop interpolated between esophagus and stomach. Jejunal continuity was restored and a Finney pyloroplasty performed. There was one death in 12 cases, due to perforation of the stomach by an indwelling nasogastric tube. The other 11 patients with reflux esophagitis, esophageal stenosis or bleeding varices were considered to have good or excellent results.

K. Alvin Merendino and David H. Dillard, *The Concept of Sphincter Substitution by an Interposed Jejunal Segment for Anatomic and Physiologic Abnormalities at the Esophagogastric Junction,* Volume LXXIII, 1955.

One operation was performed for esophagitis after a cardioplasty for achalasia. Two patients had jejunal interposition for extrahepatic portal block with esophageal varices, both of whom had had a previous splenectomy and one a partial gastrectomy. "The clinical results to date have been so encouraging that this operation has become standard procedure for some diseases unsatisfactorily treated in the past, and the indications for its use are being extended." The operation was performed through a thoraco-abdominal incision, upper midline extended into the sixth or seventh intercostal space with a long diaphragmatic incision, to the left of the pericardial attachment.

Discussion

Stanley R. Friesen, of Kansas City, thought that his own experimental work suggested "that if one is going to interpose a segment of jejunum between the esophagus and the stomach it must be more than a conduit. It must be a functioning sphincter." George H. Humphreys, II, of New York,

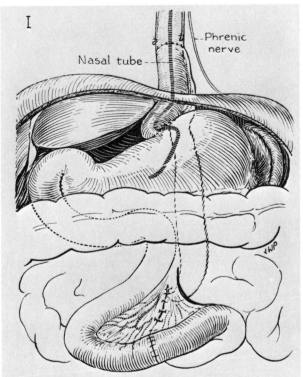

FIG. 11. Any excess jejunum is delivered below the transverse mesocolon and a jejunojejunostomy is performed. The opening in the mesocolon is closed loosely, taking care not to impinge on the pedicle to the interposed segment. Ordinarily, these steps are taken prior to the Finney pyloroplasty (Fig. 10G) and partial closure of the diaphragm (Fig. 10H).

agreed that the jejunum was resistant to gastric juice. He had substituted a jejunal loop for the entire thoracic esophagus, in four patients for esophageal varices, one for esophagitis following hiatus hernia, one for lye stricture, one for esophageal atresia, one for achalasia. None had developed ulceration of the jejunum. Richard H. Sweet, of Boston, was not sure that the susceptibility of the dog's esophagus to peptic erosion could be transferred to humans. He emphasized the importance of "the relief of gastric obstruction by doing a Finney-Von Haberer pyloroplasty to ensure prompt emptying of the stomach." In his own clinical experience "with a very large number of esophagogastric anastomoses done for various conditions" he had had more difficulty with the stomach and an apparent gastritis, than with the

esophagus and had found this to be relieved by pyloroplasty. David Watkins, of Denver, Colorado, agreed with the principles enunciated by Merendino and had for several years been constructing "a baffle type valve from the esophagus itself in the performance of esophagogastrostomy . . . The results over this period of time have been very encouraging. The portion of the esophageal baffle which comes in contact with the acid peptic gastric juice early in the postoperative course ulcerates, heals and becomes lined with an undifferentiated types of gastric epithelium . . ." Merendino, in closing, did not think that Dr. Friesen's observations contradicted his own work. He indicated uncertainty as to the necessity for vagotomy, but thought that the combination of vagotomy and the Finney pyloroplasty gave the best

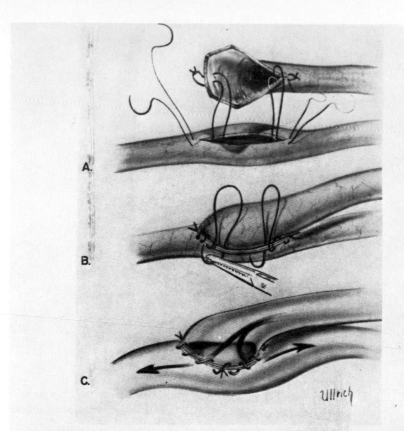

FIG. 4. The End-to-Side Technic (continued). (A) The two mattress sutures have been placed. Note that the needles have gone through the host artery from inside to outside, to prevent loosening and fragmenting the atheromatous intima. (B) The mattress sutures are tied, then commencing at each end they are used to continue the anastomosis with a simple running over-and-over type of stitch. This everts the edges to give an intima-to-intima approximation, and it is also hemostatic. (C) To complete the anastomosis the two ends of each are tied together where they meet in center of the suture line on each side. As indicated by the arrows, the blood will flow both proximally and distally in the host artery with this type of anastomosis.

The distal end of the homograft has been split and the resultant sharp corners excised. An everting intima-to-intima anastomosis is secured with a continuous suture. In femoral homografts, Linton attributed his increase in patency from 50% to 87% to the abandonment of distal end-to-end anastomoses and adoption of end-to-side anastomoses. He attributed the technique to J. Kunlin, of France, 1951.

Robert R. Linton and Charles V. Menendez, *Arterial Homografts: A Comparison of the Results with End-to-end and End-to-side Vascular Anastomoses,* Volume LXXIII 1955.

results. He emphasized the point that "our concept in the use of this operation involves not esophageal substitution, but sphincteric substitution."

* * *

Robert R. Linton, of Boston, Visiting Surgeon, Massachusetts General Hospital; Assistant Clinical Professor of Surgery, Harvard Medical School, and by invitation, Charles V. Menendez, *Arterial Homografts: A Comparison of the Results with End-to-End and End-to-Side Vascular Anastomoses,* spoke of the re-establishment of the circulation in the lower extremities by use of vascular grafts as "without ques-

tion, one of the outstanding developments in vascular surgery in recent years." Julian, Kunlin, Rob, and dos Santos had pointed to the segmental nature of the occlusive process in the femoral artery. Kunlin, and Julian, had recommended the use of autogenous venous grafts, whereas Rob had preferred homologous arterial grafts. Kunlin had employed "a parallel shunt utilizing the end-to-side type of anastomosis, thereby preserving the collateral branches, and the main arterial channels. Rob, and Julian, recommended the resection of the diseased artery . . . and the insertion of an autograft or homograft by the end-to-end technic . . .", the method Linton had employed until June, 1954. Cockett had given up the end-to-end operation in favor of the end-to-side because of the high incidence of late thromboses with the former. Linton had initially performed end-to-end anastomoses, excising the diseased vessel "until a good calibered lumen was found both distally and proximally." Later, resection was almost entirely abandoned, except for the length necessary to permit anastomosis. The end-to-end anastomosis was given up because of the high percentage of early and late failures,- 60% in from one hour to six months. Two of those patients had already been salvaged by second grafts with end-to-side anastomoses. With end-to-side femoral grafts, they had 16 grafts with three failures,- from sepsis not from thrombosis,- leaving 81% open grafts. They employed the same technique in the distal anastomoses in aortic bifurcation homografts. Twenty-nine of 30 distal anastomoses by the end-to-side technique remained open, as against 11 out of 14 by the end-to-end technique.

Discussion

Ormand Julian, of Chicago, had not been employing end-to-side anastomoses and he thought it might explain "a rather high proportion of initial failures in substitution therapy in the small vessels", but was not as pessimistic about the end-to-end anastomosis as was Linton. Richard Warren, of Boston, reviewed 24 femoral reconstructions, two-thirds with autogenous veins and one-third with homologous arteries, found only six of the 24,- 25%,- still open, 22 of the 24 patients having left the hospital with open grafts. He had employed end-to-end anastomoses but was optimistic about the possibilities of the end-to-side anastomosis, particularly because "with the end-to-side technic, if the graft closes, there has been no loss of limb as a result of closure." Linton, closing, said the end-to-side anastomosis was more effective than the end-to-end because "there is a funneling effect both of the end of the homograft and of the site of the longitudinal incision in the host artery . . . in contradistinction to the end-to-end type of anastomosis, since no matter how you construct the latter, there will always be a slight stenosis . . . With the end-to-side type there is a widening both of the end of the graft and the host artery itself . . . greatly reducing the chance of stenosis and secondary thrombosis." He rinsed the graft frequently in heparin while preparing the host vessel and injected heparin in the host arteries proximal and distal to the occluded area. He thought it was "unnecessary to continue heparinization, and in fact, I believe with

these extensive dissections, it is a dangerous procedure . . . because of the danger of postoperative hemorrhage."

* * *

Surgical Considerations of Dissecting Aneurysm of the Aorta, Michael E. DeBakey, Professor of Surgery and Chairman of the Department of Surgery, Baylor University; and Denton A. Cooley, Associate Professor of Surgery, Baylor University College of Medicine, Houston, and Oscar Creech, Jr., by invitation, was another in the avalanche of startling displays of virtuosity in aortic surgery which had begun to appear from Houston. Dissecting aneurysm was "rapidly fatal in from 75 to 90 per cent of the cases" and had never been successfully operated upon before. DeBakey and his colleagues had now operated upon six patients with dissecting aneurysm, five of them chronic, of varying durations, from three weeks to two years. In all of the patients, they transected the aorta completely and a portion of the inner wall of the proximal segment was excised to permit reentry of the blood into the true lumen. The inner and outer walls of the distal segment and the remaining portion of the proximal segment were whipped over. [One of the patients, in fact, had simply a saccular aneurysm of the aortic arch which was tangentially excised and proved to have a dissection in its wall but not into the aorta proper.] In one patient they performed a resection of a sigmoid aneurysm of the thoracic aorta with an end-to-end anastomosis after whipping the two layers of the proximal and distal segments together before the anastomosis. In two they performed a resection of the aneurysm, again obliterating the proximal and distal false lumina, and implanted a homograft. In one patient, they whipped over the false lumen proximally and distally in the thoracic aorta, reanastomosing the aorta and then did the same thing in the distal aorta, the patient dying some days subsequently of rupture into the pericardium from the original dissection of the proximal aorta. In one patient, they transected the thoracic aorta, resected a portion of the internal wall of the aorta, whipped over the remaining portion of the false channel in the distal end, and reanastomosed the aorta. The second death apparently resulted from an unrecognized pneumothorax.

Discussion

[It was obvious that the membership had not much experience with the treatment of the lesion.]

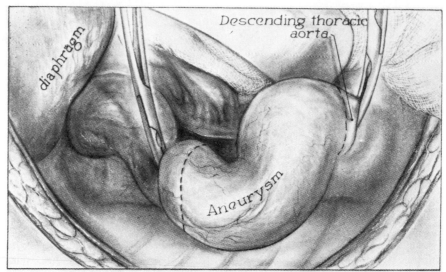

FIG. 5. Drawing made at operation in Case 1, showing occluding clamps applied above and below the aneurysm and the levels of transection of the aorta.

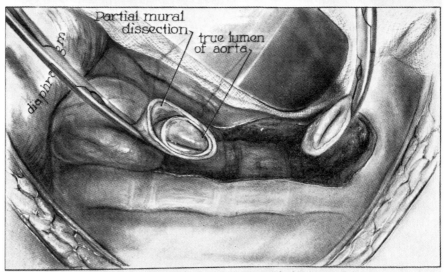

FIG. 6. Drawing made at operation in Case 1, showing double lumen in distal segment of arota and single lumen proximally.

The patient had a sigmoid aortic aneurysm and it was possible to resect the aneurysm, to whip over the inner and outer aortic walls proximally and distally, and perform a direct reanastomosis, with recovery.

Emerick Szilagyi, of Detroit, presented an instance of an arteriosclerotic lumbar aortic aneurysm which he had resected and demonstrated to have been an aneurysm dissecting into both common iliac arteries. Herbert C. Maier, of New York, had operated on a ruptured dissecting aneurysm of the ascending aorta, "we were able to stop the hemorrhage by the use of Vinyon mesh . . . Unfortunately the patient suc- cumbed in the postoperative period from a cerebral hemorrhage, such as his brother also had." De-Bakey, closing, said that the patients who survived had all done well, the first now for nine months, and added the significant comment that "one important point is control of hypertension, both during and following the operation, because hypertension is a very common associated condition, and probably

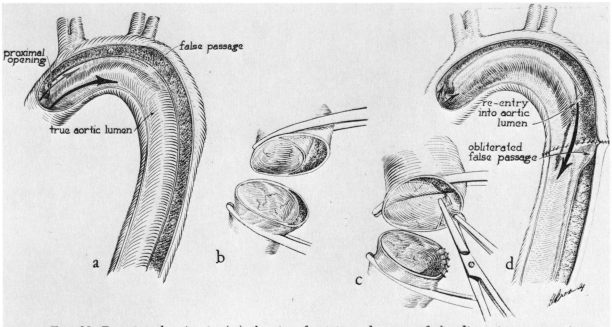

Fɪɢ. 23. Drawing showing in (a) the site of origin and extent of the dissecting process in the thoracic aorta in Case 5. In (b) the aorta has been divided. In (c) the false lumen has been obliterated distally, and proximally a segment of the inner layer is being excised to create a re-entry passage. In (d) the anastomosis is completed.

Technique applied in one case to decompress the dissection into the lumen by excising a portion of the inner layer, permitting the proximal outer channel to flow into the single distal channel constructed by oversewing the distal cut edges. The Houston group reported six operations for dissecting aneurysm (one was actually a saccular aneurysm, tangentially excised). Four of the six patients survived.

Michael E. DeBakey, Denton A. Cooley, and Oscar Creech, Jr., *Surgical Considerations of Dissecting Aneurysm of the Aorta,* Volume LXXIII 1955.

contributes to the pathogenesis of the disease." He urged early operative intervention.

* * *

Resection of Ruptured Aneurysms of the Abdominal Aorta, Hushang Javid, William S. Dye, William J. Grove, all by invitation, and Ormand C. Julian, of Chicago, Associate Professor of Surgery, University of Illinois, had resected and replaced the ruptured aneurysm in four patients with survival in two, both operated upon relatively late. It was interesting that in the first patient, no homograft being available, a graft of the patient's dermis was prepared and sutured in place. There was no bleeding in the short postoperative period that the patient survived. The other three patients all had frozen homologous grafts inserted. In the two fatal cases of the four, bleeding was temporarily controlled by a clamp on the aorta above the diaphragm and in one of the suc-

cessful cases, in which the aneurysm ruptured freely shortly after operation was begun, a clamp was placed on the abdominal aorta above the renal arteries.

Discussion

Frank Gerbode, San Francisco, had successfully operated two years earlier upon a ruptured aortic aneurysm and had operated upon "at least three patients whom we thought were rupturing, but found instead a very remarkable inflammatory response around the aneurysm, no doubt due to the perhaps little tears and dissections within the wall . . . " Gerbode thought it was not necessary to enter the chest to control the aorta and perhaps not even to clamp the aorta above the renals, "Perhaps finger control, with a good assistant, above the renals, can

RESECTION OF ANEURYSM

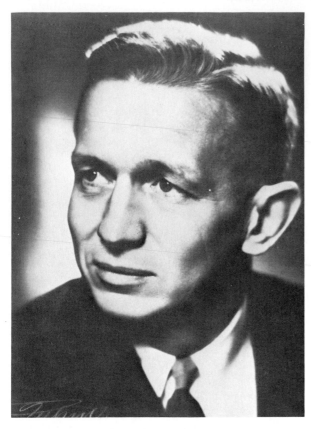

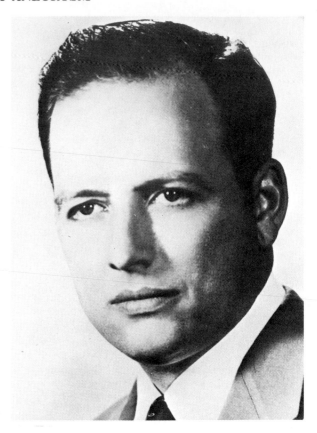

H. T. Bahnson, 1920- (c. 1962). M.D. Harvard 1944; Johns Hopkins, Intern to Professor 1944-1962; Professor and Chairman, University of Pittsburgh 1962—. His 1953 paper,- he was 32,- presented a series of tours de force of aortic surgery, including resection with frozen-dried homograft replacement, and tangential excision and aortic reconstruction for thoracic and thoracoabdominal aneurysms. Developed teflon aortic valve leaflets, with Spencer introduced postoperative monitoring of cardio-pulmonary function employing catheters placed intraoperatively. Major contributions in surgery of congenital defects. Single cardiac transplantation early on resulted in six-month survival and death from complications of excessive immunosuppression. Skier, mountain climber, white water enthusiast. Extraordinary breadth of interests and abilities, inexhaustible energy.

Denton A. Cooley, 1920- (c. 1955). M.D. Johns Hopkins 1944. Trained at Johns Hopkins 1944-1950; Brompton Hospital, London, 1950-1951; joined DeBakey in Houston in 1951, to Professor of Surgery, parting in 1969 to form his own Texas Heart Institute. Despite his major role in the early Houston aneurysm experience, progressively concentrated on cardiac surgery, particularly congenital lesions. Handsome, debonair, a versatile athlete and a surgeon of extraordinary facility, flair and speed, his claim to having performed, by 1978, "over 30,000 open heart operations, more than any other surgeon in the world" is not likely to be challenged. He quickly followed Barnard's cardiac transplantation with a substantial series, the results in which soon led him to abandon the effort. A single, unsuccessful cardiac replacement with an implanted artificial heart was the occasion of a bitter controversy.

RESECTION OF ANEURYSM

Michael E. DeBakey, 1908- (c. 1955), M.D. Tulane 1932. Trained at Charity Hospital, New Orleans, and abroad with Leriche in Strasbourg and Kirschner in Heidelberg,- in the tradition of an earlier day. Instructor to Associate Professor at Tulane 1937-1948 as associate and collaborator of Alton Ochsner; to Houston in 1948, first Professor and Chairman of Baylor College of Medicine in Houston, successively also President and Chancellor. With Cooley in 1954, published the first Houston experiences with resection of aneurysm. The Houston reports covered progressively larger and larger series of more and more complex aneurysms, involved and ingenious reconstructions. As DeBakey conducted the extraordinary expansion of his Baylor enterprise and his association with Cooley was severed, other technically brilliant surgeons, Morris, Crawford, contributed to the development of techniques and amassing of staggering statistics. DeBakey abandoned cardiac transplantation after a brief, intensive and unsuccessful clinical effort. Long an international figure, a high level Washington consultant, he had a major role in developing the artificial heart program and mounted a major laboratory effort of his own in it. A prodigious worker with legendary operating lists, writing and administrative schedules, he has wide interests and innumerable publications in various phases of clinical and experimental surgery.

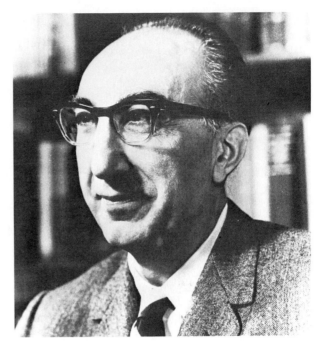

control the bleeding temporarily while the clot is removed, and the clamp applied lower." Harris B. Shumacker, of Indianapolis, had treated five patients for ruptured aneurysm, four of whom survived the operation itself, two of them dying of uremia and two recovering completely. Two of the patients had been operated on previously, in one, the aorta had been wrapped with an Ivalon sponge and the other had had internal wiring. Ben Eiseman, of Denver, mentioned rupture of the aneurysm into the duodenum,- "We have had such a case temporarily repaired by *en bloc* resection of the involved duodenum with the diseased aorta",- also rupture into the vena cava, successfully operated upon. Denton A. Cooley, of Houston, indicated that they had had 18 patients with ruptured aneurysm of the abdominal aorta and a 38% mortality. One of the survivors had the rupture into the vena cava which Eiseman had already mentioned. Cooley thought the retroperitoneal hematoma surrounding the homograft produced "local conditions . . . not favorable for support of the homograft" and sutured the omentum around the homograft as a pedicled graft. Julian, closing, said that it had been technically impossible, because of the huge hematoma, to control the aorta within the abdomen in the two patients in whom

they clamped the thoracic aorta, and thought in those patients that the thoracotomy had played no part in the patients' death.

* * *

At the 1954 meeting Arthur Voorhees had presented the Columbia Presbyterian experience in arterial replacement with tubes of Vinyon "N" cloth. *The Use of Plastic Fabrics as Arterial Prostheses,* Edgar J. Poth, of Galveston, Professor of Surgery, University of Texas Medical Center, and by invitation, Joseph K. Johnson and John H. Childers, suggests that the intervening year had not shown as widely escalating an application of the Blakemore-Voorhees technique as one remembers. Poth had studied a considerable variety of synthetic fibers and had found a very specific DuPont nylon suited the requirements best and his group were still using the multilayered prosthesis which they had mentioned the year before. Dimensions required were to be taken from the exposed recipient vessel segment before it was excised. Poth added the novel suggestion that the ends of the prosthetic tube have cuffs turned back which could be flipped over the completed anastomoses to reinforce them. They thought "Arterial prostheses made from inert synthetic fabrics

1038

have definite advantages over arterial homografts . . . readily available . . . inexpensive . . . can be tailored to fit the vessels of the host". Thromboses in their hands did not occur in animals whose prostheses were larger than 5 mm. in diameter. They mentioned no clinical experience.

Discussion

Brian B. Blades, of Washington, D.C., said that they had used some Vinyon-N tubes obtained through Dr. Blakemore. In his laboratory, stainless steel mesh had been employed in the aortas of dogs "and it appears to behave very much the same as Vinyon-N behaves." Oscar Creech, of Houston, reported two types of prostheses used by them. The first, "fashioned on the sewing machine, and then rendered impervious by the application of a liquid vinyl plastic" which avoided leakage but made the tube difficult to sew. They had implanted that in 12 patients, 11 of whom were doing well and one of whom died of erosion of the prosthesis into the duodenum. The second type of orlon prosthesis was a knitted one "constructed at the North Carolina State Textile School at the instigation of Dr. Paul Sanger . . . made of three seamless tubes joined by a circular seam to form a bifurcation prosthesis." They had employed this successfully in three patients. Poth, in closing, made the observation [presently to be proved valid and controlling] that the inert implants had to be "pervious, permitting each small fiber to become walled off individually by the ingrowth of fibrous tissue. An impervious implant would become encapsulated as a single, large foreign body and be poorly tolerated."

* * *

Gustaf E. Lindskog, of New Haven, Professor of Surgery, Yale University School of Medicine; Surgeon-in-Chief, New Haven Hospital, and by invitation, Warren J. Felton, II, *Considerations in the Surgical Treatment of Pectus Excavatum,* reported their treatment of 16 patients, in all of whom the defect had been recognized at birth, and in seven of whom there were associated abnormalities. Six of the patients had cardiorespiratory symptoms,- precordial pain and disabling dyspnea in one, and varying degrees of exertional dyspnea in five others. All had poor posture, some degree of dorsal kyphosis, 11 had a cardiac murmur. Cardiac catheterization was carried out in five cases and in the oldest patient, there was an "elevation of right atrial pressure, and a decrease in the cardiac output." They excised the

cartilages subperichondrially, divided the lower intercostal bundles, performed a transverse sternal osteotomy and maintained the sternum in corrected position by percutaneous traction with steel wire, removed on the twelfth and fourteenth day. There were no deaths. The result was "disappointing in only one patient, who was operated upon too late at age 27." Ten of Lindskog's patients were operated upon for cosmetic reasons and six for cardiorespiratory symptoms. Lindskog thought operation should be postponed till after the third or fourth year.

Discussion

Rollin A. Daniel, of Nashville, had operated upon 18 patients since 1947 and after the first two, had used no external fixation, employing the Ravitch technique until two years earlier when after excising the cartilages subperichondrially, he had divided the intercostal bundles laterally, lifted them up over the intact ribs and sutured them there suspending the sternum in that way. Daniel felt "the functional aspects of this deformity are perhaps of more importance than Dr. Lindskog gave emphasis to . . ." Several of the children had had repeated severe respiratory infections before operation, not after, and two of their three adults "had early heart failure which was promptly and completely relieved after correction of the chest deformity." Conrad R. Lam, of Detroit, announced the frequency of "keloid scars which result very frequently when skin over the sternum is incised for any purpose." He had operated upon some 20 patients "the prime indication in all was cosmetic and psychological, and we did not feel there was serious pulmonary or cardiac disability in any." Mark Ravitch, of New York, thought "Dr. Lindskog and some of the discussers have done themselves an injustice in saying that the sole indication in so many of the cases was cosmetic", pointing out the long published record of patients with cardiorespiratory difficulty and his own experience in that regard. Ravitch emphasized earlier operation, even in infancy, and stressed the frequency with which increased vigor and appetite and weight gain occurred in children who had not been thought deficient in these respects before operation. He had now, by his technique, operated upon 47 patients ranging in age from three months to 39 years, with one death, previously reported, in the second patient operated upon. Felton, closing the Discussion, defended the use of external traction and repeated that six of their patients had had cardiorespiratory symptoms, but that on the other hand, ten of them had not. He emphasized leaving the xiphoid process, which they had formerly resected, and "perhaps postoperative roentgen radiation of the wound to minimize keloid formation, and close attention to postural re-education in the postoperative period." [The carcinogenic effect of irradiation upon the thyroid was only just being realized.]

* * *

Ralph F. Bowers, of Memphis, Chief of Surgery, Veterans Administration Medical Teaching Group; Chief of Surgical Service, Kennedy VA Hospital, *Choledochojejunostomy—Its Ability to Control Chronic Recurring Pancreatitis,* had previously presented the operation as a technique for complete diversion of the biliary stream, to prevent pancreatitis, from possible regurgitation into the pancreatic duct. He now had a series of 14 patients, in whom he could say there had been no operative deaths, that common duct stricture and cholangitis had occurred in only one patient, who had had a very small common duct at the time of the original operation, and in him a second choledochojejunostomy with the now dilated common duct had been successful. No patient had been demonstrated to have developed a peptic ulcer. One patient developed a pseudocyst a year after choledochojejunostomy and was relieved by a cyst gastrostomy. Twelve of the 14 patients "can be stated to have received perfect control of pancreatic attacks" and the only two deaths were in two heavy drinkers who died in traffic accidents, "Neither had the slightest pain, but accelerated their drinking activities because pancreatitis was controlled. As a matter of fact, the main deterrent to the operation from this study reveals acceleration of alcoholic consumption, because the G. I. tract will 'take it.' " There had been two failures, neither in a drinker, one was in the man who had a subsequent pseudocyst and was improved but not well. The second patient classified as a failure, was so classified only because he insisted on having small doses of codeine for the relief of pain. "Most observers, including the patient's wife, family physician and several Kennedy physicians, do not believe that the pain, if any, is the result of pancreatitis. Nevertheless, a codeine addict before operation has not been rid of his habit after operation for pain, and the patient must be classified as a failure." Bowers said that diversion of the biliary stream by a shunting procedure had been previously recommended by Maingot, Poth, Cole, Trimble and others.

Discussion

James T. Priestley, of Rochester, Minnesota, opened the Discussion. A recent review from the Mayo Clinic showed that for pancreatitis the results of biliary drainage, internal or external, were superior in the group of patients who had disease of the biliary tract. In such patients, they had "used the direct biliary intestinal anastomosis rather than the Roux-Y type." Clarence Dennis, of Brooklyn, rose to mention the new technique for relief of pancreatitis of Dr. Merlin K. DuVal,- amputating the tail of the pancreas and anastomosing the tail of the pancreas to a Roux-Y intestinal loop. Results thus far had been satisfactory, but his longest follow-up had been only a-year-and-a-half. Edgar J. Poth, of Galveston, said he had had about as many cases as Bowers for the same period of time [up to six-and-a-half years] and had considered the results of internal drainage and decompression of the common bile duct good in most instances, with one frank failure. He demonstrated a variety of possible anastomoses and seemed to prefer the side of the common duct to the end of the Roux-Y limb.

* * *

The paper by Robert M. Zollinger, of Columbus, Professor and Chairman of the Department of Surgery, Ohio State University College of Medicine, and by invitation, Edwin H. Ellison, *Primary Peptic Ulcerations of the Jejunum Associated With Islet Cell Tumors of the Pancreas,* was destined to have almost as large an impact on gastrointestinal surgery as the several papers on cardiac and vascular surgery were to have in their areas. In the previous two years, they had observed two "problem cases of benign ulceration of the upper jejunum associated with extremely high gastric acid production over a 12-hour period." They reported the "findings of islet cell adenomas associated with almost unbelievable levels of 12-hour nocturnal gastric secretion despite complete vagus section and radical gastric resection . . ." [The diagrams here reproduced indicate the course of their two patients.] They were able to find reports of four similar cases with gastric hypersecretion, peptic ulceration and noninsulin-secreting islet cell adenoma of the pancreas. Three of the patients were dead, one of recurrent ulceration, one of malignant islet cell tumor, one of pulmonary embolism, and one patient was alive and well a year after removal of the adenoma. They postulated, "An ulcerogenic humoral factor of pancreatic islet origin"

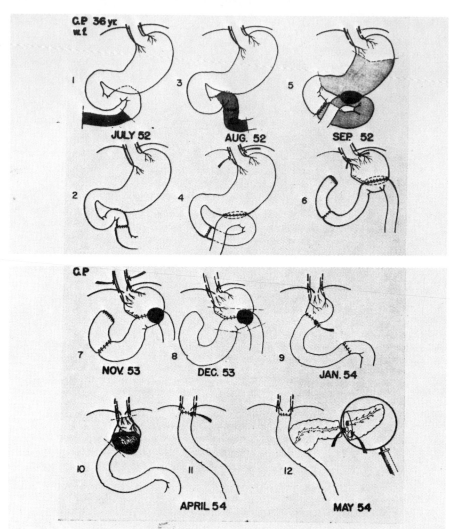

FIG. 1. Schematic representation of clinical course of Case 1 (C. P.), including sites of recurrent ulcerations and operative procedures through total gastrectomy. The pertinent autopsy findings are indicated in Diagram 12.

Zollinger and Ellison reported two patients with what they recognized to be a new syndrome. Both patients underwent the sequence of multiple operations which for a few years thereafter continued to characterize the course of patients with beta cell adenomas of the pancreas and gastric hypersecretion. Patient 2 continued to have abnormally high amounts of free hydrochloric acid until total gastrectomy was performed.

Robert M. Zollinger and Edwin H. Ellison, *Primary Peptic Ulcerations of the Jejunum Associated with Islet Cell Tumors of the Pancreas*, Volume LXXIII, 1955.

tended to implicate glucagon, and "suggested . . . A clinical entity consisting of hypersecretion, hyperacidity, and atypical peptic ulceration associated with non-insulin-producing islet cell tumors of the pancreas."

Discussion

Hilger Perry Jenkins, of Chicago reported the case of a woman of 30, who died of a perforated jejunal ulcer, and was found to have ulcerations of the duodenum as well, and an islet cell tumor of the pancreas. Lester Dragstedt, of Chicago, had found a "remarkably similar" case, a sequence of subtotal gastrectomy, anastomotic ulcer, transthoracic vagot-

omy, gastrojejunocolic fistula, subdiaphragmatic vagotomy, fatal hemorrhage from gastrojejunal ulcer and "a small islet-cell carcinoma of the head of the pancreas with one small metastasis in the liver." He thought that "in these patients the repeated ulceration was due to a hypersecretion of gastric juice of humoral origin" and that it was "quite likely that the humoral stimulant has had its origin in the pancreatic tumors." [He came remarkably close to the ultimate nature of the humoral substance], "It is quite possible that a study of these pancreatic cells may provide clues to the type of cell in the gastric antrum that produces gastrin." Edgar J. Poth apologized "for arising again this morning, but this pre-

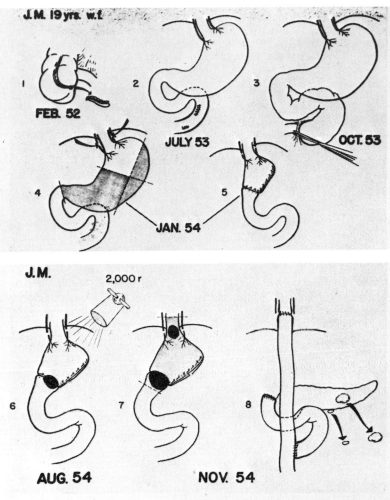

FIG. 4. Schematic representation of clinical course of Case 2 (J. M.), including operative procedures from time of initial symptoms through total gastrectomy. Complications of the primary jejunal ulcerations and sites of recurrent ulcer are indicated. Radiation of the gastric pouch is indicated in Diagram 6. The location of the pancreatic islet tumors excised at the time of total gastrectomy are shown in Diagram 8.

sentation interests me beyond my restraint." He reviewed his experimental studies with intravenous glucagon and the stimulation of gastric secretory activity, concerning which, the essayists had spoken and added, "I have a patient under observation after four gastric resections and a vagotomy because of recurrent ulcerations. Probably less than 5 per cent of the stomach remains, but gastric secretory activity corresponding to that observed following glucagon administration continues unusually elevated." Carl A. Moyer, of St. Louis, presented two patients with the same dismal sequence of repetitive operations for ulcer and death with autopsy evidence of islet cell tumor of the pancreas, in both cases malig-

nant. Zollinger, closing, attributed to Dr. Hilger P. Jenkins, of Chicago, the suggestion, when he saw the motion picture of the extensive gastric resection in the second patient, that an islet cell tumor might be found. "This certainly made us aware of the possibility long before the islet cell tumor was actually found." He said "We feel that a new clinical syndrome can be supported, and we hope you will review your problem cases of peptic ulcer to determine if it is a definite syndrome and, if so, how frequently it occurs." He did not indicate what the appropriate operation was and seemed a little defensive about having done a total gastrectomy on his 19-year-old surviving patient.

The Business Meetings

The 1955 meeting was held at the Hotel Warwick, Philadelphia, April 27, 28, and 29, John H. Gibbon, Jr. in the Chair.

Frederick A. Coller reported again on unnecessary operations complaining again that ". . . thousands of our smaller hospitals in this country . . . have no connection with pathologists . . . have itinerant roentgenologists, if any, and a low intellectual level in every field of specialization." He now had a more detailed report of the operations performed in Michigan and paid for by the Michigan Medical Service, which insured 46% of the 6,3000,000 people in Michigan. There were 1,800 men having Boards of any kind, surgical or nonsurgical, and additionally 1,824 Fellows of the American College of Surgeons who were not certified by a Board, but were for the most part, Coller thought, qualified competent surgeons. There were 1,185 osteopaths in actual practice in Michigan. Salpingo-oophorectomies were done, 170 by Board men; 104 by F.A.C.S. men, both groups considered trained; 475 by general practitioners; 117 by osteopaths. Subtotal hysterectomy was much the same,- 104 by the Board men; 98 by F.A.C.S. men, 353 by general practitioners; and 32 by osteopaths. Total hysterectomy: Board members 1,458; other surgeons, 675; general practitioners, 1,885; and osteopaths, 742. Uterine suspensions: 170 were done by Board men; 141 by non-Board surgeons; 739 by general practitioners; and 755 by osteopaths. Appendectomy "Competent people", 2,371; F.A.C.S., l,553; general practitioners, 6,709; and osteopaths, 1,867. Herniorrhaphy: Board men, 2,798; non-Board men, 1,716; general practitioners 4,000; and osteopaths, 782. Hemorrhoidectomy: Board men, 1,094; non-Board men, 829; general practitioners, 3,997; and osteopaths 1,5000. Tonsillectomy: 8,936 by Board men; 2,230 by non-specialists; 23,361 by general practitioners; and 5,650 by the osteopaths. Gastrectomy: Board men, 613; non-Board surgeons, 230; general practitioners, 314; and osteopaths, 157. Thyroidectomy: Board men, 744; non-Board, 318; general practitioners still the high number of 452; and osteopaths, 106.

The ten Board Certified surgeons, who had done the most operations paid for by Blue Shield, had averaged $45,500 in payments. The Fellows of the American College averaged $37,400. The ten general practitioners averaged $35,000. The osteopaths averaged $55,000. Two osteopaths in that year had been paid over $100,000 each by Blue Shield. He concluded that "More than half of the operations are performed by operators who are not acceptable operating in surgery. The ratio between operations done by the untrained and trained surgeons . . . is shifting. The more surgeons we train, the more they will get to do, and the less the other man will do." With respect to operations which the untrained men did in larger numbers, "I pointed out the uterus field, which is a notable one . . . perhaps the appendix and perhaps the gallbladder." It was Coller's "impression that most of these unnecessary operations are carried out through ignorance. The man does not have training; he does not know; his judgment is not good; and I think that is the cause for this type of surgical attack, rather than anything else." As fee splitting disappeared, and it had almost disappeared in Michigan, he thought that operating for profit would cease. The answer was "education of more and more competent surgeons in all fields, the training of more pathologists, more roentgenoligists—in short . . . the improvement of the training of those in every medical and surgical specialty" as well as education of "the public to the value of being treated by one with known skills . . ." Coller requested that his "Committee on Unnecessary Operations" be discharged, but President Gibbon simply ignored his plea.

The problem of invited guests and their requests to participate in the discussions continued to concern the Officers and now, given that there were some 200 guests at the meeting, President Gibbon said ". . . the Chair would like to restrict the privilege of the floor to non-members who are co-authors of papers presented at this meeting, and to certain foreign guests."

Among those elected to Fellowship were W. G. Bigelow, D. A. Cooley, J. W. Lord and W. H. Muller.

The officers elected were Alfred Blalock, of Baltimore, President; Stuart Harrington, of Rochester, and Julian Johnson, of Philadelphia, Vice-Presidents; and R. Kennedy Gilchrist, of Chicago, Secretary.

LXXIV

1956

The 1956 meeting was held at The Greenbrier, White Sulphur Springs, West Virginia, April 11, 12, and 13, Alfred Blalock, of Baltimore, Professor of Surgery and Director of the Department of Surgery, Johns Hopkins University, School of Medicine; Surgeon-in-Chief, Johns Hopkins Hospital, in the Chair. There was a long list of Members whose deaths had been memorialized in the *Transactions,* among them John Alexander, of Michigan (who had died in 1954), Vilray P. Blair, of St. Louis, John H. Gibbon, Sr., who had been President in 1926 and whose son, John H. Gibbon, Jr., had been President in 1955; John Albert Key, of St. Louis; Thomas G. Orr, of Kansas City; and the distinguished Honorary Member René Leriche.

Blalock spoke on *The Nature of Discovery,* one of the few Presidential Addresses which repays reading for its own merit rather than as a reflection of the times in which it was given. In a series of delightful vignettes, he illustrated in some detail examples of *"Discoveries by Chance or Accident", "Discoveries by Design or Intention",* and *"Discoveries by Intuition, Imagination or Hunch".* His own philosophy emerged clearly. In commenting upon "The important discovery by Enders, Weller and Robbins that the poliomyelitis virus can be cultivated in tissue cultures of non-nervous origin . . .", he commented "The prepared minds seized the opportunity, performed the appropriate experiments, and drew the correct conclusions." In regretting that space did not permit his dwelling ". . . upon scores of other discoveries . . . A number . . . made by members of the American Surgical Association", he said that

"If I attempted this, I would be writing a history of medicine, and as all my friends know, my main interest is not in the past, of which I often fear I am a part, but in the future." [In point of fact, like any master of his discipline, he was well versed in its history, and although he often stressed the importance of looking forward rather than looking back, he was not unappreciative of the efforts of his colleagues in medical history. I am confident that he would have enjoyed this history of the American Surgical Association, and would have used it as a resource. I know that he would have questioned the expenditure of effort involved in recounting what is already known, when so much remains to be discovered.] He was clearly speaking biographically when he said "The keen observer who is willing to work will likely make important, even if not monumental, discoveries and in so doing he will have a great deal of pleasure. I agree with Henderson that the important contributor to advances in medicine will experience the contentment that comes from work well done, the pleasure of masterly performance, the satisfaction that comes from aiding the sick and stimulating others in the same endeavor, the appreciation of the value of science for its own sake, the answer to his curiosity, and the exhilaration that comes at the conclusion of the hunt or the chase . . . No satisfaction is quite like that which accompanies productive investigation, particularly if it leads to better treatment of the sick. The important discoveries in medicine are generally simple and one is apt to wonder why they were not made earlier. I believe that they are made usually by a dedicated person who is will-

1043

ing to work and to cultivate his power of observation rather than by the so-called intellectual genius. Discoveries may be made by the individual worker as opposed to the current practice of large team research; simple apparatus may suffice; all of the analyses need not be performed by technicians; large sums of money are not always necessary. Important basic ideas will probably continue to come from the individual. Whether by accident, design or hunch, the diligent investigator has a fair chance of making an important discovery. If he is unwilling to take this chance, he should avoid this type of work as well as horse races, the stock market and Las Vegas." [Las Vegas was a gambling center in the state of Nevada.] He reminded the Fellows, representing the Establishment in American Surgery of their responsibilities, "It is incumbent on you and me to try to provide favorable conditions under which the young surgeon interested in research may work. He should be encouraged but not spoon-fed. He should be given adequate laboratory facilities but they need not be palatial. Claude Bernard laid the foundation of modern physiology in a 'sepulchre-like cellar.' An attempt should be made to see that the young surgeon does not have financial worries, which unfortunately is not always possible. Freedom of action should include the right to choose his own project and an absence of pressure to produce definite results in a short time. He should have access to pertinent literature. It is important that he should be free of excessive routine clinical and administrative duties which too frequently interrupt his research program. The person who provides good opportunities for young associates derives great pleasure from it."

* * *

William V. McDermott, Jr., Joan Wareham, Athol G. Riddell, from the Department of Surgery, Harvard Medical School and Massachusetts General Hospital, all by invitation, *Bleeding Esophageal Varices,* A Study of the Cause of the Associated "Hepatic Coma", presented McDermott's continuing work on the problem of ammonia intoxication on which he had first published two years before. Sanguinetti, in Argentina [1934], had defined the concept of alimentary azotemia and H. N. Harkins and others had studied it experimentally. Davidson, in America in 1952 and Stahl, in France, in the same year, had described "The syndrome of intolerance to nitrogenous materials introduced into the gastrointestinal tract of a patient with cirrhosis of the liver . . ." McDermott and his colleagues had demon-

strated in normal dogs that administration of a large mass of human blood by gastric tube produced a sharp elevation in the serum urea nitrogen and little or no elevation in the blood ammonia, whereas in previously well-maintained dogs with an Eck fistula, the elevation of urea nitrogen was substantially less and the elevation of blood ammonia very great. Eighteen patients with bleeding esophageal varices had neurological symptoms ranging from mild confusion and disorientation to coma. The blood ammonia levels bore a direct relation to deaths from all causes, and four of the patients were thought to have died from "hepatic coma". The patients who survived all had blood ammonia levels below 300 micrograms. While emphasizing the multi-factorial causes of death in patients with cirrhosis and hemorrhage, they felt they had demonstrated that ammonia intoxication existed, that it resulted from the absorbed blood and that even in the absence of a threat from exsanguination this indicated the need to control hemorrhage by the evacuation of blood by cathartics and enemas and the administration of antibiotics, because "By depressing the bacterial count in the gastro-intestinal tract, the sources of urease and amino-acid oxidase can be controlled." They stated, without discussing the problem that *"L-glutamic acid* has proved to be a valuable adjunct to therapy . . . orally or parenterally . . ."

Discussion

C. Stuart Welch, of Albany, had done similar animal experiments and made observations in humans with the same results and conclusions. In his patients ". . . only five of 20 survived when the ammonia was elevated, in contrast to ten survivals out of 16 when there was no elevation of blood ammonia. So, the coma which ensues and the ammonia intoxication are very significant in the causation of death." None of his patients died of coma after the hemorrhage had been stopped. Champ Lyons, of Birmingham, Alabama, said that they had been unable to demonstrate "bacterial production of urease in the gastro-intestinal tract . . ." the presumed mechanism of the production of absorbable nitrogenous products. Ben Eiseman, of Denver, reported a clinical experience similar to McDermott's and pointed out that "cases of hepatic coma precipitated by exogenously administered ammonia salts usually have a good prognosis . . . this had not been our experience in patients thrown into hepatic coma following massive gastro-intestinal bleeding." While sodium glutamate would lower the blood ammonia levels, the effect was only temporary so that they

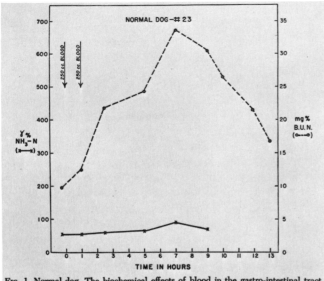

Fig. 1. Normal dog. The biochemical effects of blood in the gastro-intestinal tract.

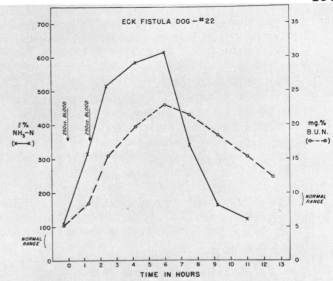

Fig. 2. Eck fistula dog. The biochemical effects of blood in the gastro-intestinal tract.

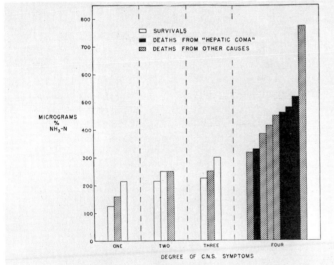

Fig. 5. Diagrammatic correlation of ammonia levels, central nervous system symptoms and mortality in 18 patients with bleeding esophageal varices.

McDermott and his colleagues demonstrated the great increase in blood ammonia produced by instillation of large amounts of human blood in the stomachs of well-maintained dogs with Eck fistula as compared to the effect in normal dogs, and the substantially smaller rise in the blood urea nitrogen. The hyperammonemia was associated with neurological symptoms and coma which proceeded in one dog to death. In patients, there was a direct relation between the blood ammonia level and mortality from all causes, and four patients died of "hepatic coma". All of the surviving patients had ammonia levels under 300 micrograms.

William V. McDermott, Jr., Joan Wareham, Athol G. Riddell, *Bleeding Esophageal Varices.* Volume LXXIV, 1956.

employed "a slow infusion over a 24 hours period." Animal experiments with extracorporeal hemorrhage demonstrated that "the portal blood ammonia concentration is markedly elevated, but simultaneous portal blood flow measurements indicate that this is . . . a reflection of decreased blood flow and that there is no increased endogenous production of ammonia in the portal bed . . . The patient with a liver bordering on failure will go into coma . . . when the insult of diminished hepatic blood flow resulting from gastro-intestinal hemorrhage is added to the injury of an ammonia load resulting from the absorption products of blood within the intestinal tract." Alfred Blalock, the President, asked whether

McDermott's observations led him to prefer an end-to-side or a side-to-side anastomosis. McDermott, replying to Champ Lyons concerning "the question of bacteria in the gastro-intestinal tract as the source of amino acid oxidase and urease . . . presumably . . . the enzymatic pathway by which ammonia is produced", said that Dr. Baird Hastings in the Department of Biochemistry at Harvard was "quite convinced that it is intestinal bacteria which is the source of these enzymes that lead to the production within the lumen of the gastro-intestinal tract of ammonia from any source of pooled nitrogenous material." L-glutamic acid, McDermott thought, acted by "a binding mechanism in the peripheral blood", acted only when it was being given, and it was important to stop the bleeding. With regard to the type of shunt to be employed,- the "end-to-side portacaval shunt is the most effective type of decompression for portal hypertension . . . without any question the greater the decompression you get, the more metabolic problems you have associated with the absorption of ammonia and very probably of other materials from the gastro-intestinal tract bypassing the liver . . . with the increasing knowledge of the metabolic changes associated with a direct end-to-side portacaval shunt, and our increasing ability to control these metabolic derangements, I think we can utilize the more successful type of hemodynamic decompression."

* * *

J. Garrott Allen, at the 1950 meeting, had reported the prevention of homologous serum jaundice from plasma by the storage of the plasma for six months at room temperature. Now, Paul I. Hoxworth, of Cincinnati, Associate Professor of Surgery and Director, University of Cincinnati Blood Transfusion Service, Cincinnati General Hospital, and Walter E. Haesler, Jr., by invitation, *Safety of Stored Liquid Plasma—A Clinical Study,* confirmed Allen's observations. In 370 followed recipients, who had received both plasma and whole blood, there were four cases of hepatitis; in 164 followed patients who had received stored plasma only, there were no cases of hepatitis.

Discussion

Joel W. Baker, of Seattle, said that the King County Blood Bank had processed its plasma liquid and stored it six months, and had not been able to find a single instance of homologous serum jaundice from plasma alone in a ten-year follow-up. During the same period, there had been 48 cases of homologous serum jaundice in patients who had received blood alone, or blood and plasma. J. Garrott Allen, of Chicago, said that they had now had "some 80 cases of hepatitis following the transfusion of blood and have had none following the administration of six-month-old pooled plasma totaling some 20,000 donor units." He emphasized that "the effectiveness of six months' temperature storage is greatly influenced by the temperature at which storage is carried out." He recommended that the temperatures range between 80° and 100° F. for six months. If lower temperatures were used, the duration of storage had to be increased.

* * *

J. Garrott Allen, of Chicago, Professor of Surgery, University of Chicago, and by invitation, Edward Stemmer and Louis R. Head, *Similar Growth Rates of Litter Mate Puppies Maintained on Oral Protein with Those on the Same Quantity of Protein as Daily Intravenous Plasma for 99 Days as Only Protein Source,* had undertaken the study to answer the question, "Can the daily intravenous administration of homologous plasma to litter-mate puppies support growth and body weight when no other source of protein is available?" The intravenously-fed animals, the orally-fed animals with a protein diet and the animals fed a non-protein diet all received 1000 calories a day. George H. Whipple, of Rochester, New York, had maintained for years that whole protein given intravenously as plasma could be utilized for nutrition, but "several workers in this field have been unwilling to concede that the transfusion of whole protein, plasma in particular, could be utilized at a rate sufficient to meet body needs [Albright 1946, Elman 1947]". Allen's studies demonstrated that his pups fed intravenously achieved "a gain in height and weight equal to, if not exceeding, that of their litter fellows receiving the same quantity of horsemeat and liver by mouth. Nitrogen balance studies under these conditions disclose a positive nitrogen balance. Intravenous plasma appears to be an excellent source of protein nutrition."

Discussion

Owen Wangensteen, of Minneapolis, was delighted by the experiment, "his criteria of measurement are very simple; they are the camera and the weighing scale. I think some of us who affect to do research may take heart that these simple yardsticks have proven so useful and crucial in an important experiment." He thought Allen's dogs received more glucose intravenously than a human could receive, "Today, to give even 2,500 calories to a person intravenously is quite a task." William D. Holden, of Cleveland, was inclined to believe that the utilization of plasma proteins was delayed, "I am quite sure that Dr. Allen did not imply that intravenously injected protein is immediately available, metabolically speaking, or that it is rapidly degraded and rapidly re-synthesized into the patient's own protoplasm", and emphasized the dangers of producing an osmotic effect with plasma administration. Allen, closing, demonstrated that his dogs had indeed begun gaining weight at once and quoted Whipple's studies which "demonstrated within a matter of hours, by radio-autographic techniques", the distribution of transfused homologous plasma within the body cells. Allen had limited the plasma administration to achieve a serum protein concentration level of between 6.5 and 8 to 8.5 grams percent. Wangensteen had asked whether Allen had tried amino acid hydrolysates, and Allen replied that such studies were underway.

* * *

Thomas Taylor White, of Seattle, by invitation, and William Crawford White, of New York, Consulting Surgeon, Roosevelt Hospital, St. Luke's Hospital, [son and father], *Breast Cancer and Pregnancy,* Report of 49 Cases Followed 5 Years, had operated upon 11 women during pregnancy, upon 14 women during nursing, whose cancers had been discovered during pregnancy, upon 12 patients during nursing, the tumor first having been discovered then, and reported 12 further patients who had become pregnant at varying intervals after a radical mastectomy. They concluded that in the absence of axillary spread, pregnancy at the time of radical mastectomy did not affect the prognosis, that those of their patients with axillary spread were neglected cases with a bad prognosis, that the outlook of patients becoming pregnant after radical mastectomy was "unusually good . . . the interval between operation and pregnancy does not appear to be important."

Discussion

Stuart W. Harrington, of Rochester, Minnesota, thought that his own results were somewhat "less good in pregnant patients without axillary node spread than in non-pregnant patients without axillary spread. Twenty years ago [See page 794, Volume LV, 1937] his own analyses had shown that the survival rates in patients becoming pregnant subsequent to a mastectomy were "very good". In this respect, he thought that one could only "observe that it is possible for patients to bear children after radical mastectomy and to live for many years without recurrence of the carcinoma of the breast." Alson R. Kilgore, of San Francisco, found the Whites' conclusions in accord with his own experience, but raised the question of the social wisdom of having a woman, with a treated carcinoma of the breast, undertaking to raise a child, "A woman who is found to have axillary metastases, and who later becomes pregnant, is highly likely to leave her child for somebody else to raise", and even in the absence of axil-

lary metastases, such a woman would do well to wait two or three years before becoming pregnant.

* * *

Bronson S. Ray, of New York, Professor of Clinical Surgery, Cornell University Medical College; Attending Neurosurgeon, Memorial Hospital, and by invitation, Olof H. Pearson, *Hypophysectomy in the Treatment of Advanced Cancer of the Breast,* reported their experience with 74 women, operated upon March, 1954—December, 1955, and followed three to 24 months. Their first publication had been in 1954, and they had now performed hypophysectomy for various types of advanced cancer in 130 patients. "The results of hypophysectomy in the treatment of malignancies other than breast cancer, and possibly prostatic cancer, have not been encouraging. One of two males with breast cancer and one of five with prostatic cancer were benefited." Not benefited were patients with melanoma, choriocarcinoma, hypernephroma, thyroid carcinoma, pancreatic carcinoma, and reticulum cell sarcoma. He was particularly disappointed with the failures in seven melanomas and three choriocarcinomas, "since these two types of tumor are thought to have some link to the endocrine system." They operated only when "any beneficial effect of previous radiation or endocrine treatment has ended", and excluded only patients with "gross evidence of intracranial metastases, serious impairment of vital capacity from intrapulmonary disease, or extensive liver metastases with jaundice or identifiable hepatic failure." They operated by a frontal approach, divided the hypophyseal stalk with "enlargement of the opening in the diaphragm sellae; removal of the pituitary gland by curettement and suction followed by exposure of the sella turcica to Zenker's fluid . . ." Patients were given large doses of cortisone prior to operation and the doses gradually tapered to maintenance doses by the end of the week. Most patients developed diabetes insipidus in the first 24 hours after operation which sometimes required pitressin [no statement was made as to the duration of the diabetes insipidus]. Thyroid deficiency became manifest in four to six weeks and then patients were given thyroid replacement therapy. Removal of the gland was demonstrated to have been incomplete in five of the 74 patients, one of whom had a second operation to complete the removal. Seven of the patients died within 30 days, three certainly from direct effects of the intracranial procedure and one from pulmonary embolism. Two patients had "important visual loss" and two patients had "minor visual loss",- quadrantic visual field defects. Three patients had a transient hemiparesis and two patients developed intracranial hematomas which required evacuation,- both recovered. Five percent of patients had seizures immediately after operation, none thereafter. The left olfactory nerve was usually damaged by retraction in half the patients, with resultant impairment or loss of smell function. Objective remission was demonstrated in 36 patients, of whom in eight the disease was arrested and in 28, there was regression and they pointed out that "New remissions can be obtained by hypophysectomy in patients who have been temporarily benefited by castration or by a combination of castration and adrenalectomy . . . if hypophysectomy is not employed as the initial ablative operation in altering endocrine influence on the disease, it is probably preferable to adrenalectomy as a second operation following castration." The survival period was more than twice as long in those patients who obtained a remission after hypophysectomy as in those who did not, and they expected this difference to increase with prolongation of the period of observation.

Discussion

Nathan Womack, Chapel Hill, North Carolina, discussed the activity of estrogen as a stimulus to the growth of breast cancer and the effect of castration and hypophysectomy upon this. He had been fearful of a formal hypophysectomy, but "one of our men in neurosurgery, Dr. Gordon Dugger" had developed a technique for simply sectioning the hypophyseal stalk and inserting "a small bit of tantalum foil between the severed ends so that the vascular system could not regenerate." The operation was short, easily tolerated, and six patients had shown immediate reduction in the hypophyseal function. The followup was still too short to discuss the effects upon the cancers. Francis D. Moore, of Boston, said "Dr. [Donald] Matson of our group performed his first hypophysectomy only three years ago, and we have now carried the procedure out on 15 patients with carcinoma of the breast." There had been a single early death and they were very much encouraged about the results. He cautioned that partial interference with the hypophysis gave varying results, "The gonadotropic and thyrotropic functions are the first to go, and the ACTH function is the last to go." He cautioned with respect to the enthusiasm for irradiation of the pituitary, that the pituitary was "a remarkably radio-resistant organ." They thought that in advanced cancer of the breast they had had better results with hypophysectomy than from other endo-

crine ablative operations, and that the postoperative care was simpler if there had not been a previous adrenalectomy. Harris B. Shumacker, Jr., of Indianapolis, said that in 1933, he and W. M. Firor, "in the Hunterian Laboratory in Baltimore", then working on the pituitary, performed a hypophysectomy on a bitch with a large fungating carcinoma of the breast which melted away, although [in those pre cortisone days] they were unable to keep the dog alive. James C. White, of Boston, indicated appreciation of the operative technique which Ray had developed, said they had performed only a few hypophysectomies at the Massachusetts General Hospital and wanted to stress, as Olivecrona had in Sweden, ". . .the fact that this operation relieves the pain of bony metastases. Pain from cancer of the breast is the variety we have had the greatest difficulty with in relieving by chordotomy." Bronson Ray said he had not tried the operation Dr. Womack referred to and reinforced the "caution Dr. Moore offered us . . . something less than a total hypophysectomy will sometimes produce a beneficial effect." He made sure that the Fellows understood "The difference between adrenalectomy and hypophysectomy . . . when the hypophysis is removed there is no disturbance in salt balance. Aldosterone produced in the adrenals seems not to be under the influence of the hypophysis." He agreed with Dr. White's observations about pain, ". . .it is remarkable how often the patients with painful skeletal metastases are relieved. It is hard to believe (and I hesitate to mention) that often the patients wake up and the first thing they comment on is their relief of pain . . . There have been some patients who have been relieved of pain yet in whom we cannot prove an objective remission."

* * *

Michael E. DeBakey, of Houston, Professor of Surgery and Chairman of the Department of Surgery, Baylor University College of Medicine, and Oscar Creech, Jr., and George C. Morris, Jr., by invitation, *Aneurysm of Thoracoabdominal Aorta Involving the Celiac, Superior Mesenteric, and Renal Arteries. Report of Four Cases Treated by Resection and Homograft Replacement,* frankly startled the Association by the presentation of four instances of resection of the abdominal aorta with restoration of circulation in the celiac, superior mesenteric, and both renal arteries. All four of the patients survived the immediate operation, two of them dying days later, and two leaving the hospital well. The patients were operated upon under general body hypother-

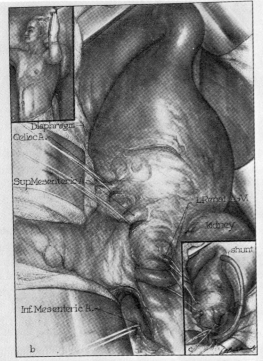

Fig. 11. Drawings made at operation in Case 2. (*a*) The patient is placed in the supine position with left shoulder slightly elevated and left arm supported overhead. Left thoracolumbar incision is employed. (*b*) The aorta above and below the aneurysm has been exposed and the celiac, superior mesenteric, and left renal arteries and the left renal vein have been isolated and tapes passed about them. The right renal artery lies behind the superior mesenteric artery and is not seen. (*c*) A shunt made of compressed polyvinyl sponge has been attached as an end-to-side anastomosis to the descending thoracic aorta above the aneurysm and to the abdominal aorta below the aneurysm.

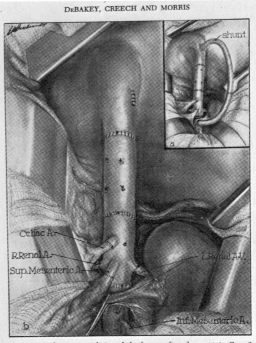

DeBAKEY, CREECH AND MORRIS

Fig. 13. Drawing showing completion of the homograft replacement in Case 2. (*a*) All anastomoses have been completed and blood flow through the aorta has been restored although the shunt is still in place. (*b*) The shunt has been removed and the openings in the aorta repaired.

In DeBakey's first patient, an attempt to resect the aorta, implant the graft and re-establish visceral arterial flow without a bypass resulted in death from uremia. In the next three patients, a compressed polyvinyl sponge shunt was used as shown in the small drawing *c.*, the graft inserted above the left renal artery, which was anastomosed to it, restoring circulation to that kidney very rapidly, the remainder of the vessels clamped, the aneurysm resected, the graft anastomosed distally and the visceral branches anastomosed seriatim to the corresponding branches of the aortic homograft. Two of these patients went home well, one died of massive hemorrhage from gastrojejunal ulcer on the thirteenth day when recovery had seemed assured.

The illustration suggests that the aortic graft was a composite one made of two grafts sutured together, but this is not explained in the text.

Michael E. DeBakey, Oscar Creech, Jr., and George C. Morris, Jr., *Aneurysm of Thoracoabdominal Aorta Involving the Celiac, Superior Mesenteric, and Renal Arteries. Report of Four Cases Treated by Resection and Homograft Replacement.* Volume LXXIV, 1956.

mia induced with the cooling mattress. In the first patient, the aneurysm was excised, all the arterial branches anastomosed to the graft seriatim, the renal arteries having been occluded for 105 minutes each. The patient died in uremia on the seventh day. To minimize the period of flow interruption to the viscera, in the second patient "a temporary shunt made of polyvinyl sponge, with an internal diameter of 14 mm. and approximately 40 cm. in length, was utilized. The shunt was attached to the descending thoracic aorta above the origin of the aneurysm by an end-to-side anastomosis and then similarly implanted into the abdominal aorta just above the level of the inferior mesenteric artery." The aorta was transected proximally, an aortic graft attached proximally, the left renal artery attached to the graft, the remaining arterial branches clamped, the aneurysm resected, the aortic graft anastomosed to the distal aorta, and the right renal, celiac, and superior mesenteric vessels reanastomosed. The occlusion time of the kidneys was stated to be 23 and 27 minutes. There was depressed renal function for several days, the patient was discharged well, after two-and-a-half months. The third patient similarly had a polyvinyl shunt inserted and essentially the same operation performed except that the right renal artery was not involved. He left the hospital a little more than a month after operation. A very similar procedure was performed on the fourth patient who had previously had a subtotal gastric resection for a peptic ulcer. The patient was up and about, taking a soft diet, and asymptomatic, when on the thirteenth day, he had massive hematemesis, became hypotensive and was found at operation to have an anastomotic ulcer from an old gastrojejunostomy, and died during the operation. The use of the shunt had obviously been more successful than the use of hypothermia alone. In the three successful cases the period of occlusion of the renal arteries had ranged from 15 to 46 minutes with a resultant depression in renal function for the first four of five days after operation and return to normal in ten days to two weeks. The 44 to 116 minute occlusions of the celiac artery had produced no recognizable alterations in hepatic function nor had the 36 to 102 minutes of occlusion of the superior mesenteric artery caused any recognized disturbances in gastrointestinal function.

Discussion

[There was no need for DeBakey to say that this was the first time these feats had ever been performed.] John H. Gibbon, Jr., of Philadelphia, arose to proclaim one long hosannna to DeBakey's skill, modesty, brilliance, and tremendous achievements, and Henry T. Bahnson, of Baltimore, continued in like vein, although pointing out that in some patients these aneurysms were eccentric, did not involve the mouths of the vessels and could be tangentially excised. Arthur H. Blakemore said that just before leaving New York for the meeting, he had operated upon a man with a threatened rupture of a huge abdominal aneurysm distal to the renal arteries. The technical problem was that the transected aorta just below the renals was 9 cm. in diameter and the distal aorta 6 cm. in diameter, but, "Doctor Arthur Voorhees produced a braided tube of orlon measuring 4 centimeters in diameter, the largest diameter that was leakproof to blood that the present braiding machine will fabricate . . . the ends of the braided tube dilated to accommodate the suture line. Thus, with this special feature of the braid, the prosthesis became evenly streamlined toward the ends compensating to form even junctions at the sites of anastomosis." The patient had done well, even though the proximal suture line was really in the upper end of the aneurysm. He joined in the enthusiastic applause for DeBakey, but did not suggest that prosthetic replacement might be employed in the resection of thoracoabdominal aneurysms involving portions of the aorta giving rise to the visceral branches. DeBakey, in closing, said that the sort of aneurysms they had been treating had so much of the aneurysm above the renals that Blakemore's type of operation could not have been performed.

* * *

D. Emerick Szilagyi, John G. Whitcomb, Roger F. Smith, from the Department of Surgery, Henry Ford Hospital, Detroit, all by invitation, *The Causes of Late Failures in Grafting Therapy of Peripheral Occlusive Arterial Disease,* presented one of the careful, long-term evaluations of the results of peripheral reconstructive arterial surgery, which Szilagyi was to make intermittently over the next 20 years. They were analyzing 120 consecutive grafting operations in 80 patients with an observation of from one to 33 months, and in their analysis gave no different value to second operations than to primary operations. "If the symptoms were severe enough to interfere with the patient's mode of life and in particular with his earning of a living, and, further, if the arterial image demonstrated by angiography showed a suitable pattern, grafting therapy was recommended." Operation was abandoned if there was no outflow from the lowest explored distal vessel. In aorto-iliac disease they excised the diseased segment with end-to-end or, less commonly, end-to-side distal anastomoses. In the femoral artery, they excised the diseased segment and performed end-to-end anastomoses, later abandoning the resection of the diseased original artery, and in the latter cases, the distal anastomosis was end-to-side. End-to-end anastomosis was easier proximally, end-to-side anastomosis easier distally. Arterial homografts freshly preserved or lyophilized were used in all cases except two in which seamless woven teflon prostheses were employed. Graft patency was determined by the unequivocal return of peripheral pulses and by angiography. Most patients had angiography two to four weeks after operation and subsequently at six to 12 month intervals. Early success or failure was judged by patency at the time of discharge. Late failures or successes were assessed at the last follow-up visit. Out of the 120 anastomoses, 23 were early failures, 21 were late failures, and 76 were long-term successes. The early failure rate of 19.1% ranged from 7.7% in the aorto-iliac anastomoses to 21.6% in the iliacs and 22.5% in the femoropopliteals. Seven of the patients with late failure of the grafts were re-explored, the grafts biopsied and ". . .the most common cause of late graft failure was the extent and severity of the pre-existing arterial disease either through postoperative progression or owing to incomplete excision . . . the technical superiority of procedures utilizing end-to-side distal anastomosis was confirmed . . . this type of anastomosis may delay narrowing near the suture line . . . in a considerable number of cases (17 per cent) progressive angiographic changes were noted in the arterial substitutes that may in time lead to occlusion."

Discussion

Richard Warren, of Boston, said they had been "struggling with the problem of whether it is graft reaction or progress of the arteriosclerotic process which had caused a high percentage of late closure in our patients. . ." Late closure in their femoral cases was 70% and they had seen either "creeping thrombosis in the graft on one hand, or actual arteriosclerosis of the graft on the other." William P. Longmire, Jr., of Los Angeles, commented upon "the work of two members of our department, Dr. Jack Cannon and Dr. Wiley Barker, who for several years now have been interested in the subject of thromboendarterectomy . . . about the only grafts used for vascular work in our department are applied to patients with aneurysm." Endarterectomy permitted the re-establishment of circulation "to certain of the collateral vessels that are bypassed by grafts." The immediate failure rate was less than 10% and in 80 cases followed for a year or more, there had been less than 1% of late closures. "Drs. Cannon and Barker attribute part of this result to the fact that they were able to treat extensive disease by this method. It is not unusual for them to remove the thrombus and perform an endarterectomy of the distal aorta, both iliac arteries, and one or both femoral arteries at the same operation." Jere W. Lord, Jr., of New York, reported the use of 21 autologous vein grafts for peripheral arterial reconstructions "below the inguinal ligament and the axillary artery." Nine of these were for arteriosclerotic disease. The 12 done for arterial injury or aneurysm were all patent. Only four of the nine vein grafts inserted for arteriosclerotic disease were patent. His view was "perhaps the disease itself is the problem at fault, the narrowed vessel above and below or the extensiveness of it. . ." Ormand Julian, of Chicago, said they had had about 40% of early failures and six late failures in 30 vein grafts, one of which was due to threatened rupture of the graft. Szilagyi, in closing, emphasized that progression of the occlusive disease was in the host vessel, proximal or distal to the graft. The finding of late degenerative changes in the arterial grafts was disturbing, although there was considerable variability. He admitted that the work of Cannon and Barker, which Longmire had quoted, had resulted in a "remarkable success rate" and in spite of the "cumbersome complexities of operative technique", if their results were maintained, the situation would have to be reviewed.

* * *

Thomas H. Burford, of St. Louis, Professor of Thoracic Surgery, Washington University School of Medicine, and Carl E. Lischer, Assistant Professor of Clinical Surgery, Washington University, *Treatment of Short Esophageal Hernia with Esophagitis by Finney Pyloroplasty*, provided one of the frequent examples of a paper made valuable chiefly by the Discussion. Reasoning that reflux into the esophagus after esophagogastrectomy was obviated by a pyloroplasty, they performed Finney pyloroplasty on 16 patients with gastric reflux, "Esophagograms in all cases were considered characteristic of short esophageal hernia with shortening of the esophagus, and concentric herniation of a gastric pouch through the hiatus." Fifteen of the patients had had "virtually complete relief of symptoms" and esophagitis had been proved to clear in the three who had been endoscoped. The patient who was not improved was demonstrated subsequently to have a paraesophageal hernia.

Discussion

Herbert C. Maier, of New York, questioned the existence of the short esophagus. ". . .thus far in our experience we have not encountered one in whom we could not draw the esophagus to below the diaphragm unless long-standing esophagitis had produced fibrosis and secondary shortening . . . I know of no way of clearly differentiating such [short esophagus] from a sliding hiatus hernia, either radiologically or endoscopically, prior to operation." He thought that was what the patients had and that diaphragmatic herniorrhapy would have been the preferable operation. O. T. Clagett, of Rochester, Minnesota, took the same view, "It is my feeling that these for the most part are sliding types of hernias with an acquired short esophagus, and I would agree with Dr. Maier that many of them can be brought below the diaphragm for repair. . .", unless there was a stricture. Clagett mentioned the procedure of his associate, Dr. Henry Ellis, which they had employed in ten patients, consisting of "a transthoracic operation to resect the stricture of the esophagus and to mobilize the cardia, bringing it up and anastomosing it to the esophagus, and then doing a resection of the antrum of the stomach with a gastroduodenostomy." William M. Tuttle, of Detroit, in his characteristically direct manner, continued the attack, "I do not believe there is any person in this room who has seen fifteen patients with a short esophagus . . . some of these individuals in this series could have been treated by other types of operative procedures which would have benefited them more than the ones used."

* * *

Herbert R. Hawthorne, of Philadelphia, Professor of Surgery and Chairman of the Department of Surgery, Graduate School of Medicine, University of Pennsylvania, and by invitation, Alfred S. Frobese and Paul Nemir, Jr., *The Surgical Management of Achalasia of the Esophagus,* reported their experience in 35 patients, all operated upon by a modified Heller extramucosal esophagocardiomyotomy extending two-and-a-half inches above the gastroesophageal junction and one-and-a-half inches below, usually through a transabdominal approach. There was one immediate death from a cerebrovascular accident and three late deaths from carcinoma of the mid-esophagus, pneumonia, and tuberculosis. All patients had complete relief of dysphagia immediately after the operation but two returned with dysphagia. Four who were relieved of dysphagia developed reflux and esophagitis, two of these being patients with duodenal ulcers. Three other patients had repeated upper gastrointestinal tract bleeding. The addition to the operation of pyloromyotomy had failed to protect the patient against reflux and esophagitis.

Discussion

William M. Tuttle, of Detroit, described a technical modification of "Heller's operation by sewing the muscular layer of the esophagus to the serosa of the stomach, thereby giving a valve-like result which, we feel, has prevented regurgitation. Twenty-one patients have been operated upon and there has been no regurgitation in 19." Owen H. Wangensteen, of Minneapolis, referred candidly enough to the Association's meeting five years before when he had described "complete excision of the acid-secreting area together with the lower 7 to 10 cm. of the dilated esophagus . . . The predominant opinion at the time of my earlier presentation rather favored the idea of a return to the extramucosal cardiomyotomy of Heller." In performing the Heller operation now, after having begun the cardiomyotomy,

he had the anesthetist pass a tube into the stomach and pulled back on the tube a large Foley catheter, the balloon of which was distended so as to stretch the esophagus and either break the remaining strands of esophageal musculature or throw them into relief for easier division by the surgeon. Alton Ochsner, of New Orleans, arose to retract a proposal that he and DeBakey had made earlier for treating achalasia by esophagogastrostomy. "I have come to believe (and I think Mike believes the same way) that this is not the best procedure." He had returned to performing the Heller operation and "Since we have now been doing a longer length of incision through the circular musculature, our results are much better." Orvar Swenson, of Boston, said that "A few years ago I had a visitor from South America who came to discuss megacolon . . . his patients were much older than our group. As a matter of fact, he was talking about the aged [Swenson did not mention the term Chagas' disease]. . ." The sections showed degenerative lesions of Auerbach's plexus and absence of ganglion cells, but "20 per cent of these aged patients with a degenerative lesion in the ganglion cells of the colon also have an esophagus very similar to those we have been discussing this morning . . . there is a degenerative lesion of Auerbach's plexus . . . Careful study of cases of achalasia of the esophagus may reveal this same degenerative lesion of the ganglion cells . . . would support the contention that this condition is due to a parasympathetic dysfunction."

* * *

William P. Longmire, Jr., of Los Angeles, Chairman, Department of Surgery, University of California, and by invitation, Paul H. Jordan, Jr., and John D. Briggs, *Experience with Resection of the Pancreas in the Treatment of Chronic Relapsing Pancreatitis,* discouraged with the results in their hands of "indirect and less radical surgical procedures" had undertaken pancreaticoduodenectomy in five patients and total pancreatectomy in three more. Clagett, in 1944, had performed the first total pancreatectomy for pancreatitis and Whipple, in 1946 [See page 894, Volume LXIV, 1946] had reported five cases of pancreatitis treated by radical resection. The UCLA group, prior to their recent experience, had performed 41 procedures,- sphincterotomy, "gastric" procedures, pancreatic duct ligation [five cases], neurectomy, caudal pancreatectomy and pancreaticojejunostomy, choledochojejunostomy, etc., with 31 poor results and only three known good results. They had been led to consider the resectional technique because of the "superior results obtained in two cases of chronic relapsing pancreatitis treated by pancreaticoduodenectomy for the presumptive diagnosis of carcinoma. . ." The operations for pancreatitis were indicated by frequency and severity of the recurrent attacks together with suggestions that the pancreas had been partly or largely destroyed, as evidenced by the absence of amylasemia during attacks when formerly it has been present, calcification in the pancreas, onset of diabetes, change in character of the stools. There were no operative deaths in their five pancreaticoduodenectomies and three total pancreatectomies. One patient died four months after a total pancreatectomy "presumably as a result of complications from diabetes". The patient had first had a distal pancreatectomy with failure to obtain relief. Longmire concluded that ". . .removal of the architecturally destroyed pancreas with its distorted and obstructed ductal system is a more satisfactory surgical approach than indirect measures designed to influence the patho-physiology of the disease. The nutritional and metabolic changes associated with total pancreatectomy are so marked compared with those following pancreaticoduodenectomy that the former procedure should not be performed unless the functional capacity of the entire gland has been severely involved in the destructive process."

Discussion

John M. Waugh, of Rochester, Minnesota, thought that it was advisable to perform transduodenal sphincterotomy and "retrograde drainage of the tail of the pancreas" before undertaking resection. They employed resection for localized abscess in the tail or body, for large inflammatory masses that "overlie the pancreas and will cause quite a bit of destruction of the pancreas", for cutaneous fistulae, rather than performing anastomosis of some kind, and finally for localized calcification in the head of the pancreas with severe pain "if the less radical procedures fail". He warned the Fellows of the difficulties of pancreatectomy except in totally burned out calcified pancreases, and said that in the two total pancreatectomies performed by Clagett and himself, death had resulted a year to a year-and-a-half later from the diabetes. Ralph F. Bowers, of Memphis, Tennessee, [who had reported his satisfactory results with choledochojejunostomy en Roux-Y, see page 1037, Volume LXXIII, 1955] was "at a loss to understand why he [Longmire] had not obtained better results with indirect procedures. . ." Bowers continued to employ choledochojejunos-

tomy en Roux-Y and "Sixteen of 17 patients have had their pancreatic attacks controlled and well controlled by this operation. The one failure occurred in a patient who has received great benefit and who works three-fourths of the time during the year." He cited two cases of persistent acute pancreatitis which finally responded, one to T-tube drainage and the other to choledochojejunostomy. Nevertheless, he thought that in the "burned out" phase, which perhaps Dr. Longmire was attacking, resection might be useful. John H. Mulholland, of New York, said "It seems somewhat defeatist to extirpate the gland as treatment for its attempts to regenerate", commented on Doubilet's demonstration with a catheterized pancreatic duct, that distension of the duct reproduced the pain, and said that they had observed "relief of pain in patients of this type after sphincterotomy or after a decompressing procedure such as proposed by Dr. DuVal [caudal pancreatojejunostomy en Roux-Y]. . .Extirpation involves the production of two other diseases, sprue and diabetes. In only rare instances is this a fair exchange for some relief of pain." Richard B. Cattell, of Boston, said that to some degree the differences of opinion represented discussion of different phases of the disease, that "obstruction of the pancreatic duct is the most important factor in the production of symptoms and in the continuation of the inflammatory process." A variety of operations had been designed to relieve or bypass the obstruction, but "When multiple points of obstruction are present . . . the pancreas has become fibrotic, usually with associated pancreatolithiasis, resection becomes necessary." At the Lahey Clinic, he and Dr. Kenneth W. Warren had 104 patients operated upon for chronic relapsing pancreatitis, ten had transduodenal sphincterotomy, 25 had spincterotomy plus dilatation of the main pancreatic duct, 15 had distal pancreatectomy, and 20 had pancreatoduodenectomy "with anastomosis of the pancreatic duct to the jejunum" and one patient had total pancreatectomy. Cattell agreed with Longmire that it was well to save some pancreatic tissue if possible. In sum, one-third of their patients required resection. Of the 20 patients with pancreatoduodenal resection, 15 had a satisfactory result. Jonathan E. Rhoads, of Philadelphia, had a successful total pancreatectomy of eight years' duration, although the operation had been exceedingly difficult. The various nerve-cutting operations had relieved pain in only half of their cases. He congratulated Longmire ". . .because if the procedures that he has used can be carried on with as little mortality as he has had, they certainly deserve much wider use." Merlin K. DuVal, Jr., of

Brooklyn, after three years of experience with caudal pancreatectomy and pancreatojejunal drainage, said that three criteria were necessary in the choice of cases. One was documented weight loss, the second was a dilated pancreatic duct, and third ". . .the more 'burned out' the pancreas, the more eager we are to do this procedure". They had done 19 of the operations and thought the results were highly satisfactory in 17. Alfred Blalock, of Baltimore, asked whether the residual stump of the pancreas was of any value except in preventing diabetes. Paul H. Jordan, Jr., of Los Angeles, closed. He agreed with Dr. Waugh's "admonition about the difficulty with diabetes in totally depancreatectomized patients". The one death they had had "was in a patient who was not intelligent enough to manage his diabetes." They thought it possible that if they had used their "indirect" operations earlier in the course of disease, the results might have been more favorable. Alfred Blalock had asked about the purpose of saving the tail of the pancreas and Jordan demonstrated figures from his patients indicating that preservation of the tail of the pancreas prevented the massive loss of fat in the stool which appeared after total pancreatectomy. "Therefore, the absence of diabetes and the greater efficiency in the absorption of nutrients from the gastro-intestinal tract in a partially depancreatectomized patient compared with a totally depancreatectomized patient are the reasons we feel that it is so important to leave the tail of the pancreas unless there is incontrovertible evidence that its functional capacity has been lost by virtue of the pathologic process."

* * *

Isidore Cohn, Jr., by invitation, and James D. Rives, of New Orleans, Professor of Surgery, Louisiana State University School of Medicine, *Protection of Colonic Anastomoses with Antibiotics,* presented their experiments in animals upon the effect of systemic, oral, and intraluminal antibiotics administered during and after an operation in which a colonic anastomosis was performed and segments of 5, 7, or 10 cm. of colon on one side of the anastomosis devascularized. With no preoperative bowel cleansing and a 5 cm. devascularization, all control dogs died of perforation in the devascularized bowel, not at the suture line. Six of seven experimentally protected dogs with a 5 cm. devascularized segment survived and one animal died of kidney failure with intact bowel. With a 7 cm. devascularized segment and preoperative castor oil and enemas, six out of ten control dogs died of peritonitis and all five dogs

protected with antibiotics survived to be explored and to be found to have no difference between the vascularized and the devascularized bowel. When a 10 cm. segment of bowel was devascularized, there was no difference in the mortality between the treated and untreated groups, although the peritonitis was odorless in the treated group and the necrosis of the bowel much more localized. The technique, including the intraluminal installation of antibiotic through a fine polyethylene catheter inserted into the bowel just proximal to the anastomosis and brought out through the abdominal wall, was employed in 21 patients but without controls. One of the two deaths was associated with profound diarrhea. There was no autopsy. They were able to assert that "Antibiotic therapy limited to postoperative intraluminal administration will protect a devascularized colonic anastomosis . . .", and that preoperative mechanical cleansing and antibiotic use improved results, and the addition of intraluminal antibiotics after operation still further improved the results.

Discussion

Herbert R. Hawthorne, of Philadelphia, was impressed with the applicability to the clinic of the polyethylene tube-intraluminal administration technique of antibiotic administration. William A. Altemeier, of Cincinnati, said there were a good many who "believed preoperative and postoperative antibiotic therapy were useless in the majority of intestinal resections . . . the experiments we have just heard are indicative of the definite value of preoperative and postoperative antibiotic therapy in preventing septic or infectious thrombosis of the vessels within the wall of a 'devascularised' segment of bowel . . . there is a definite intramural circulation of the bowel itself, and this has remained intact in the authors' experiments . . . The real value of this experiment has been the demonstration that the bacterial growth within this segment of bowel is minimized to the point that thrombosis of the vessels within the wall is prevented by bacterial enzymes . . . a fascinating experiment, and should answer for all of us the question of whether or not pre- or postoperative antibiotic therapy is important." [Neither Cohn nor Altemeier had made any mention of the extensive published work of Poth, Blaine, Harkins, and many others on the protection of devascularized bowel by the use of oral or systemic antibiotics and now this omission was to be corrected.] Alfred Blalock, of Baltimore, said "When I moved back to Baltimore in 1941, Dr. Poth . . . had rigged up a beautiful device by which he would place sulfaguanidine or some such agent in meatballs. The dogs would be fed throughout the 24-hour period without Dr. Poth having to lose too much sleep. The surgeons at first would not accept his findings, but I think they do now." Edgar J. Poth, of Galveston, now rose to document some of the earlier studies, "In 1941, Dr. [Stanley] Sarnoff, who was then a senior medical student at Johns Hopkins, showed that sulfasuxidine would protect a 50 cm. loop of distal ileum from necrosis after it had been made ischemic by ligation of the blood supply. The protection was demonstrated to be due to the prevention of thrombosis of the small caliber vessels in the wall of the bowel . . ." Poth then showed slides of an experimental preparation of 10 cm. of ischemic distal ileum with an anastomosis in the middle of the ischemic segment and showed the effect of the protection by preoperative, intraoperative, and postoperative antibiotics of various kinds. "Large doses of penicillin and streptomycin parenterally protected all of the animals, but they were ill during the immediate postoperative period. The administration of neomycin at the time of operation and postoperatively resulted in 100 percent survival without a stormy postoperative course. Preoperative, 20-hour preparation with neomycin and sulfathalidine protects all animals, and they experience practically no postoperative anorexia . . . The bacteria disappeared [from the stool] in about one and one-half hours after the first oral administration." He cited clinical series to show the effectiveness of the antibiotic regimen and the results favoring the neomycin-sulfathalidine combination. Cohn's experimental regimen had included achromycin and neomycin orally and into the bowel and penicillin systemically and Cohn concluded now "some of our studies with the combination of neomycin and sulfathalidine, as recommended by Dr. Poth, have given results very closely similar to those obtained with neomycin and achromycin."

* * *

Two papers on colectomy followed. Charles W. Mayo, of Rochester, Professor of Surgery, Mayo Foundation Graduate School, University of Minnesota, and by invitation, Orceneth A. Fly, Jr., and Michael E. Connelly, *Fate of the Remaining Rectal Segment after Subtotal Colectomy for Ulcerative Colitis,* found that in the years 1949 through 1953, 241 patients had undergone subtotal colectomy and that in 45 of these "a rectal segment which varied in length from case to case remained for more than 90 days." The original plan, in 30 of the cases, had been

to complete the colectomy; in nine of the cases, to perform an ileoproctostomy; and no definitive plan was recorded for six of the cases. In point of fact, 21 of the 30 planned proctectomies had ultimately been performed, 13 of these demonstrating active chronic ulcerative colitis, two demonstrating malignant disease and five demonstrating severe submucosal scarring, contraction or strictures. One patient had had the abdominoperineal resection done elsewhere "because of peritonitis secondary to rupture of a rectal abscess." Of the nine patients with a retained rectal stump, in two the stump was at the level of the levators despite which one had continued "activity" on proctoscopic examination and the other a persistent draining perineal fistula. In one case, the abdominoperineal resection had to be abandoned because of carcinomatosis. Of the nine patients in whom it had been originally planned to perform a subsequent ileoproctostomy, one had undergone abdominoperineal resection within five months for severe clinical activity of the disease and five patients after intervals of as long as 11 years still had proctoscopic evidence of activity of the chronic ulcerative colitis. In two patients, the rectum appeared to be free of disease. One patient had had an ileoproctostomy with a stormy postoperative course too recent for evaluation. In the six patients in whom there had been no fixed plan after the initial colectomy, three had undergone abdominoperineal resection, one for malignancy, one for stricture and one for profuse rectal discharge. Two of the remainder had severe symptoms from the retained rectum. Mayo concluded that "if ileoproctostomy is not possible at the time of colectomy, the colon should be resected to as low a level as possible, with preservation of only a segment that can be removed later by a minor procedure . . . the major portion of the rectum should be removed in all cases. The hazard of malignancy is real, and continuation of the disease (for a period of 11 years in one case) . . . all too frequently requires later resection."

* * *

The argument was carried a step further by Mark M. Ravitch, Associate Professor of Surgery, Johns Hopkins University; Surgeon-in-Chief, Baltimore City Hospitals, *Total Colectomy and Abdominoperineal Resection (Pan-Colectomy) in One Stage.* The increasing aggressiveness of the surgical attack on ulcerative colitis was cited, from the initial colostomies to permit irrigation, through the period of ileostomy performed earlier and earlier in the disease, to total abdominal colectomy performed in

fewer and fewer stages. Crile, Cave, Miller, and Rip-
stein, had proposed subtotal resection at the time of
ileostomy. Ravitch, in 1948; Goligher, in 1953;
Hughes and King, in 1955; Nickel, in 1955, had all
performed one-stage proctocolectomies. Pointing out
the sometimes increased difficulty of a second-stage
abdominoperineal resection, and the complications
of fatal hemorrhage from the retained rectum in the
immediate postoperative period or of necrosis of the
distal bowel, Ravitch advocated "performing a total
colectomy with abdominoperineal resection . . . at
the time of the ileostomy, even in the most profoundly ill patients . . . moderately debilitated patients, with intractably diseased colons, will usually
tolerate the definitive one-stage procedure . . . patients with fulminating disease: septic-suppurative,
perforative, or hemorrhagic, stand a better chance of
survival, if all the diseased bowel is removed." To
the consideration of pancolectomy for ulcerative colitis, he added the consideration of one-stage pancolectomy for familial polypoid adenomatosis of the
colon. For polyposis, he preferred the operation of
anal ileostomy [endorectal submucosal stripping and
ileal pull-through]. He now reported from the Johns
Hopkins Hospital and the Mt. Sinai Hospital, of
New York, 27 one-stage pancolectomies with one
death. In all the nine for polypoid adenomatosis,
anal ileostomy was performed. In the 18 for ulcerative colitis, anal ileostomy was added in four. The
one death was in a woman profoundly ill with ulcerative colitis at the time, who had a Noble plication
of the ileum at the time of pancolectomy and developed intestinal obstruction of which she died. He
concluded that "Pancolectomy (one-stage total
colectomy and abdominoperineal resection of the
rectum) is the preferred procedure for patients requiring operation for ulcerative colitis and for patients with polypoid adenomatosis of the colon not
denied operation because of advanced age or overriding additional disease. Anal ileostomy should be
added in all cases of colectomy for polyposis and in
suitable instances of colectomy for ulcerative colitis."

Discussion

Discussion of the two colectomy papers was
initiated by Ian Todd, of St. Mark's Hospital, London, who said that his aim was "to preserve the anal
sphincteric mechanism when possible." The difficulty in predicting which patients would have further trouble from the retained rectum led them to

perform the operation in two stages bringing the rectum out as a mucous fistula at the first stage. He
cited no success rate. Total proctocolectomy in one
stage had a higher mortality in their hands than the
operation done in stages, and he agreed "with Dr.
Mayo that one should leave a very short rectal
stump if one decides upon 'total' proctocolectomy,
but that it should be done in two stages if this is
done." In polyposis, he tended to do very low anastomoses and fulgurate the rectal stump finding that
occasionally the polyps did not recur. "I believe it is
possible that there is some agent completely unknown that tends to make the polyps grow in the
rectum and in the colon, and that having removed
the greater part of this organ in some people, they
will lose the tendency to form polyps." L. K. Ferguson, of Philadelphia, agreed with Mayo that in some
patients "it would appear unwise to remove the
lower rectal segment" and that some patients would
not give consent for this. In four cases, they had ultimately performed an ileorectal anastomosis. He did
not cite the outcome, and he had had two carcinomas in the rectal segment in 60 patients. Clarence
Dennis, of Brooklyn, when at Minnesota, had found
only six patients in whom the colon had been left
behind because of the patient's refusal and four of
the patients had died of carcinoma arising in the retained segment of colon. He had published a Minnesota series of 55 primary colectomies of which 13
were pancolectomies with one "surgical death" and
had done 12 more proctocolectomies in New York
with one death. He reported nine ileo-anal anastomoses, all of which had failed. In 42 patients with
ileoproctostomy, the functional results were poor
and the complications numerous and two patients
developed carcinoma in the retained rectal segment.
The Brooke ileostomy and the Koenig-Rutzen bag
had made ileostomy less of a problem and "a logical
favorite to me over an ileo-anal or ileo-rectal anastomosis." He did "heartily agree with Dr. Ravitch that
primary removal of the entire large bowel carries but
a fraction of the risk of ileostomy alone." Laurence
S. Fallis, of Detroit, agreed with the philosophy of
one-stage proctocolectomy, carrying it "a step further by continuing the dissection down through the
levators so as to include the entire anal canal and
perianal skin in the specimen [removed from a
purely abdominal approach]." George Crile, Jr.,
asked Dr. Mayo how he handled the problem of infection when transecting the rectum low in the pelvis
in the first stage, a problem which had caused them
always to leave enough distal segment for a mucous
fistula. He asked Dr. Ravitch what the effect was of
the intermittent obstruction produced by a continent

anal sphincter in the patients with anal ileostomy. Charles W. Mayo, closing, said that the dissection was much closer to the rectum than the dissection for carcinoma and therefore, in answer to L. K. Ferguson's question about resultant sterility, there were fewer effects. With respect to Dr. Crile's question about the infection in the subperitoneal retained rectum, "I swab with tincture benzethonium (phemerol) and, strangely enough, I still use about 5 gm. of sulfanilamide powder. I put in a sump drain and bring it out through the anus . . . I have had no difficulty with this procedure to date." For polyposis, he still preferred resection with end-to-end ileorectal anastomosis and proctoscopic examination every six months. He had no personal experience with anal ileostomy but had taken down two such operations "although Dr. Ravitch had not done the primary operations." Ravitch stated, in closing, in regard to the question about the effect on sexual function "our male patients have had perfectly satisfactory sexual powers." As for "Dr. Crile's suggestion that one is producing intestinal obstruction in the ileum with a continent anal ileostomy", that was entirely valid, "Of course you produce it, otherwise it would not work. The bowel does dilate, sometimes tremendously . . Some . . . have very severe cramps for months . . ." The patients with anal ileostomy remained in good state of nutrition. As for the operation for ulcerative colitis, he did not believe that "there really is a great deal of difference between Dr. Mayo's suggestion that everything but the last little bit of rectum be removed at one stage, and ours, that all of it be removed at one stage."

The Business Meetings

The 1956 meeting was held at The Greenbrier, White Sulphur Springs, West Virginia, on April 11, 12 and 13, Alfred Blalock in the Chair.

President Blalock appointed the Nominating Committee, John Gibbon, Chairman; Howard Naffziger, Robert Dinsmore, Dan Elkin, and William E. Gallie, all, of course, Past Presidents, commenting, "Fortunately, we have most of the Past Presidents of this Association at this meeting. I understand Dr. Churchill is here. Fred Coller is here. I think Vernon David is not here. Dr. Stone [Harvey] is not here. Seated near the front, I see Dr. Allen Whipple and Dr. Evarts Graham. Dr. Matas, of course, could not be here. Our Senior Past President is Dr. Rudolph Matas, who was President of this organization in

1909. I am so pleased that at the last meeting of our Association, Dr. John Gibbon, Sr., the late Dr. Gibbon, could be present with his son, who was standing where I am standing now. Dr. Gibbon was President in 1925. Now there is no one between Dr. Matas, President in 1909, and Dr. Evarts Graham, President in 1936, a period of 27 years. Dr. Matas must have very, very good genes." [Blalock is known to have commented, "given the age at which they elect Presidents, there are seldom very many around".]

William Altemeier reporting for the Program Committee had a number of recommendations to make: that the practice of printing titles and abstracts of papers submitted but not selected for the program be discontinued "In the interest of economy and prevention of delay in getting the program to the printer"; that a brief memorandum of instructions be sent out with invitations requesting abstracts, rather than the detailed letter which was now sent and probably was not read; "that the length of abstracts submitted not exceed the maximum . . . that the established practice of not considering papers from the Department or immediate group of associates of any member of the Program Committee should be questioned. It is the feeling of the Program Committee that many good papers on new subjects are eliminated by this practice."

President Blalock explained that the problem with publishing abstracts of papers not on the final program was that there was a long delay involved, in writing to people whose papers had not been accepted, asking whether they wanted their abstracts to appear. "Most of them write back and say that unless the paper is accepted for the program, they do not wish the abstract to appear."

The proposals were accepted by the Association.

Fred Coller again reported on the problem of unnecessary operations. He said, "I have been able to get all of the facts beautifully from Oklahoma, which is a rural community in contrast to General Motors and Ford. Thanks to Dr. McKittrick and Dr. Hayden, we almost got Massachusetts. I got one month, and I am hoping for the other eleven months, but I will give you that one month as a matter of interest. I tried California, but apparently I saw the wrong people, and failed. Dr. Zollinger tried to get Ohio for us, but they had no interest in it." In Michigan, 51% of the appendectomies were carried out by general practitioners; in Oklahoma, 71% of them. General practitioners carried out 41% of the herniorrhaphies in Michigan and 61% in Oklahoma. "We [Michigan] have more Doctors of Osteopathy than any other state, except California." In Michigan, general practitioners did 38% of the cholecystectomies and 9% were done by osteopaths. In Oklahoma, 44% of the cholecystectomies were performed by general practitioners. Gastric resections were performed 33% of the time by general practitioners in Michigan and 35% in Oklahoma. 33% of the radical mastectomies in Michigan were done by general practitioners in that year, and 39% in Oklahoma, but the figures for hysterectomy were 50% general practitioners in Michigan and 60% in Oklahoma, rising for subtotal hysterectomy to 64% in Michigan and 81% in Oklahoma. 80% of the uterine suspensions in Oklahoma were done by "untrained men" and 80% in Michigan. "It is fine to talk about our boards, but they are not the ones who are doing the majority of the operations . . . You can see that the generalist does 68 per cent and the osteopaths 5 per cent in Oklahoma, and in Michigan we have 52 and 12 per cent." Even in Massachusetts for the one month in which the figures were available, 25% of the thyroidectomies were done by "generalists", 36% of the simple mastectomies, 15% of the radical mastectomies, 40% of the subtotal hysterectomies, 25% of the total hysterectomies, 50% of the uterine sus-

pensions, and even 23% of the gastric resections. As he did every year, Coller, concluded, "Mr. President, I suggest that the Committee under this title be discontinued; I also suggest that it is a matter of real interest to you gentlemen as teachers of surgery to follow through, but I would get a different title for the Committee and select a different Committee. Thank you very much", to which his good friend, President Blalock, promptly answered, "Thank you, Dr. Coller. I am sure the membership would prefer that we continue with our present Committee, and I hope you will give us another report next year."

At the Executive Meeting on the third day, all 15 new members proposed were elected, among them John M. Beal, Jr., of New York; James D. Hardy, of Jackson, Mississippi, who was to be elected President in 1975; C. Walton Lillehei, of Minneapolis; and Honorary Members Sir Gordon Gordon-Taylor and Sir James Paterson Ross, both of London.

Officers elected were Loyal Davis, of Chicago, President; Vice-Presidents, Brian Blades, of Washington, D.C., and Oliver Cope, of Boston; Secretary, Richard K. Gilchrist, of Chicago. Dr. Davis was overseas and could not be led to the platform.

LXXV

1957

The 1957 meeting was held in the Palmer House, in Chicago, May 8, 9, and 10, Loyal Davis, of Chicago, Professor of Surgery, Chairman Department of Surgery, Northwestern University Medical School, in the Chair. Among those who had died in the previous year were Carl Eggers, of New York; Robert Elman, of St. Louis; and notably, Evarts A. Graham, of the Graham-Cole test for visualization of the gallbladder, contributor to the physiology of pneumothorax and empyema, prime mover in the creation of the American Board of Surgery, first successfully to perform a planned one-stage pneumonectomy. He died, ironically, of a carcinoma of the lung which was hopelessly far advanced when first discovered. His own land-mark patient, a Pittsburgh obstetrician, who had had a carcinoma of the lung resected by Dr. Graham in the first successful deliberate one-stage planned resection in 1933, was still alive.

* * *

The problems of injury from exposure to atomic radiation were discussed by John J. Morton, Jr., of Rochester, New York, Professor of Surgery, Emeritus, University of Rochester, *Radiation Burns Due to Atomic Explosions,* and by J. Garrott Allen, Professor of Surgery, University of Chicago (and four associates by invitation), *The Causes of Death from Total Body Irradiation,* An Analysis of the Present Status after Fifteen Years of Study. Morton reported the available information and his own personal observation concerning the radiation injuries resulting from the hydrogen bomb test at Bikini in March of 1954, as it affected American Servicemen, the Marshallese islanders, and the Japanese fishermen on the ill-fated Fukuryu Maru which was covered by ". . . a fall of powdery material like snow . . ." which they did not clean off for the two weeks it took them to return home. The severity of symptoms apart from the cutaneous burns, was directly related to the effectiveness of the victims in washing off the radioactive material and protecting themselves from further contact with it in the environment, or inhalation of particles. Allen reviewed the published material on the Hiroshima and Nagasaki exposures and reported his own extensive animal experiments with dogs, exposed to a 250-kv. machine for varying doses of irradiation, from 175r, which gave a 100% survival, through 250r which gave a 50% survival, and 450r which gave a 100% mortality,- all at thirty days. His conclusions were pessimistic in the extreme. "Despite all efforts and the generous support in this field, there is no evidence that mortality has been materially reduced by any procedure, including blood and platelet transfusion, plasma, antibiotics, fluids and electrolytes and many other agents, once radiation exposures in the range of the LD50 or greater have been encountered." Blood, blood products, and antibiotics made little difference in these people and were best saved for those with lesser injuries in whom they might affect the outcome. Irradiated animals operated upon within the first three to five days showed unimpaired healing of their wounds [laparotomy, thoracotomy, compound fractures]. Once the delayed symptoms of radiation appeared, between the fifth and 50th day, operative wounds tended to heal very poorly. Similarly, anesthesia was well tolerated in the first three or four days and very poorly thereafter.

Discussion

Frank B. Berry, now Assistant to Secretary of Defense, in Charge of Surgical Manpower, spoke at length and while he mentioned ". . . a disaster which we devoutly hope will never occur . . ." neither he nor any of the other discussants mentioned the inadmissibility of the concept of another major international conflict with the certainty of atomic warfare. He spoke hopefully of the possibility of storing large volumes of red cells by a freezing technique. Herman Pearse, of Rochester, New York, one of the active investigators in the field, pointed that in fact ". . . in Japan, about 85 per cent of the lesions from the atomic bombing were thermal burns and blast injuries, particularly from flying missiles . . . most people are on the periphery where they have sublethal or no ionizing radiation." He emphasized Allen's remarks about the intolerance of animals to operative procedures once radiation sickness had become manifest, ". . . we have lost animals by just doing a biopsy, or by giving an intravenous anesthetic, and yet, prior to the onset of their irradiation sickness, they would tolerate major surgery." Pearse said that the fallout from an atomic bomb exploded in air was not as hazardous as that of a hydrogen bomb exploded on the ground, as at Bikini, "This fusion bomb was detonated on the ground, so disintegrated much material that was carried up in the convection cloud only to fall out later. Fall out from conventional atomic bombs is not particularly dangerous. I have been in a fall out. It scared me, but it didn't hurt me. If we have accurately visualized what atomic warfare would be like, then it is my opinion that the surgeon will be called upon to treat the traditional lesions of burns and wounds in the vast majority of the casualties."

* * *

1956 and 1957 were the apogee of what amounted to a world-wide pandemic of staphylococcal infections affecting infants, nurseries, complicat-

ing respiratory disease in other patients, and apparently causing wound infections as well. Chester W. Howe, from the Department of Surgery, Massachusetts Memorial Hospital and Boston University School of Medicine, by invitation, *The Problem of Postoperative Wound Infections Caused by Staphylococcus Aureus,* described this rapid increase in the awareness of staphylococcal infections, and the concomitant observations,- "The percentage of antibiotic-resistant staphylococci in large hospitals throughout the world has increased steadily so that now nearly three-fourths of all strains are resistant . . . Bacteriophage typing studies on organisms from patients and staff indicate that infections of the same type are acquired by cross-infection from other patients and hospital personnel . . . It is not uncommon at present to find strains resistant to all of the commonly used drugs . . . in some hospitals postoperative sepsis caused by this organism [staphylococcus aureus] has reached serious proportions. Blowers in England was the first to report the closing down of a hospital for reorganization for this reason [1955] . . . The staphylococcus has been incriminated for endocarditis following mitral valve surgery, and other serious sepsis both postoperative and unrelated to operation in patients and in personnel . . . The frequency of furunculosis as a posthospitalization complication . . . an over-all postoperative infection rate . . . on a university hospital service . . . of 10 per cent over a four-month period. The incidence of sepsis following gastric surgery was 40 per cent, largely due to the staphylococcus . . . there is reason to believe that small epidemics or outbreaks are occurring sporadically in hospitals in certain specialized situations including surgical wards." He raised the question as to whether the problem was new or just indicated increased awareness, or whether there had been an initial decrease in infections with the advent of the antibiotics and all that had happened now was a return to the former infection rate as organisms became resistant to the antibiotics. He believed there was actually a true increase in the total number of infections, but hard data were scanty. Although accepting the possibility that carriers could be the responsible sources for the infection, he suggested that the carrier rate in ward personnel must necessarily rise when there were wound infections about and the most important thing was the maintenance of careful techniques, at least in the handling of the wound. Studying the wound infections occurring at the Massachusetts Memorial Hospital from 1949 through 1956, he concluded in fact, that gram-negative bacteria were involved in the problem as well as gram-positive bacteria. Most of the infections proved to be caused by antibiotic-resistant organisms. He thought the percentage of infections caused by the staphylococcus had increased with the advent of antibiotics, but felt the statistical base, for earlier times, was not satisfactory for a judgment. Either staphylococci today had greater virulence than they had formerly or there was a concentration in the hospital of the virulent strains. There was a divergence, in their material, between infection rates and carrier rates. Antibiotics, he was convinced, would not solve the wound infection problem, which would be solved by ". . . meticulous wound management and surgical technic . . . emphasis upon rigid antiseptic and aseptic methods . . . The routine use of prophylactic antibiotics in clean surgery may be more harmful than beneficial . . . housekeeping cleanliness and environmental disinfection are important."

Discussion

Champ Lyons, now of Birmingham, Alabama, opened the Discussion. Because penicillin was so specific for streptococcal infection, he urged its use in wounds in which the streptococcus was one of the invaders, agreed with the importance of operative technique and concluded by saying "I personally depend, as Dr. [Hans] Zinsser taught me, quite heavily on thorough saline irrigations of wounds prior to closing." William R. Sandusky, of Charlottesville, Virginia, cited [Maxwell] Finland's 1956 Boston City Hospital survey showing staphylococcal infections ". . . in 15 per cent of hospitalized patients, 62 per cent of whom acquired the infection in the hospital." He was not convinced that there was evidence ". . . that the staphylococcus of today is producing a more virulent disease than was the case before antibiotics; nor that drug-resistant strains are more virulent than non-resistant ones . . . there is reason to believe that organisms from an active lesion are more important in initiating infection in a new host than are strains from a persistent nasal carrier." He stressed the emergence of resistant strains, ". . . with the introduction of each new drug, there are relatively few staphylococci resistant to it, but as use of the drug continues, an increasing number of resistant strains emerge", and suggested ". . . withdrawing from general use certain agents and reserving them for serious infections." Like Lyons and Howe, he emphasized good surgical technique. Deryl Hart, of Durham, took the opportunity to discuss the use of ultraviolet radiation in the operating rooms at Duke which, introduced after a study of

wound infections in 1930 to 1936, had convinced them that ". . . in the absence of gross contamination of the skin of a member of the surgical team or patient with virulent staphylococci, the clean wound was contaminated largely by the organisms floating in the air, after being given off from the noses and throats of the occupants of the room." Ultraviolet radiation could ". . . with an exposure of one minute, kill over 99 per cent of the organisms present in the air at the site of operation." Since 1936 he did not know of a single death from a wound infection following a clean operative procedure when they had used the ultraviolet irradiation. ". . . the slight inconvenience of wearing protective covering or shading was a small price to pay for the assurance that the patient's postoperative course will not be complicated by an 'unexplained' wound infection." William A. Altemeier, of Cincinnati, noticed the fluctuating incidence of clinically derived hemolytic staphylococcus aureus sensitive to penicillin, and suggested that it might have accounted for the fluctuations in the curve of infection which Dr. Howe had shown.

* * *

Henry T. Bahnson, of Baltimore, Associate Professor of Surgery, The Johns Hopkins University, and, by invitation, Frank C. Spencer, and Ivan L. Bennett, Jr., *Staphylococcal Infections of the Heart and Great Vessels Due to Silk Suture,* had a series of five patients,- ligated ductus arteriosus (two), resected innominate aneurysm, closure of an atrial septal defect, and transventricular pulmonary valvotomy, all of whom had developed staphylococcal septicemia, in all of whom antibiotics were ineffective until the silk sutures in the blood vessel or heart were removed. All the patients survived.

Discussion

Frank Gerbode, of San Francisco, with Dr. Emile Holman, had had a similar instance, in a patent ductus recurrent after ligation, similarly cured by removal of a single suture. Bahnson, closing, responded to a question from the floor about sutures, "At the second operation, the [innominate] aneurysm was repaired with 6.0 stainless steel wire. In the 2 cases of patent ductus, we closed the aorta in one with stainless steel wire and in the other, closure was with 5.0 arterial silk."

* * *

Leon Goldman, of San Francisco, Professor of Surgery, Chairman Department of Surgery, University of California Medical School, and, by invitation, Gilbert S. Gordan, and E. L. Chambers, Jr., *Changing Diagnostic Criteria for Hyperparathyroidism*, had seen during the previous 23 years ". . . 33 cases of surgically proved hyperparathyroidism, of which 23 were seen during the last two years . . ." In the first 21 years all but one of the patients had skeletal disease. Of the 23 patients seen in the last two years, only two had bone disease, whereas 18 had nephrolithiasis, one had nephrocalcinosis, and two patients had no symptoms at all. "Seven per cent of all patients with nephrolithiasis associated with hypercalcuria who were studied in our laboratory have been found to have hyperparathyroidism." The evaluation of these patients who now frequently did not have very high serum calciums, usually did not have hypophosphatemia, was helped by frequent determinations of the serum calcium, and by a simplified technique for determining tubular reabsorption of phosphate which always showed subnormal reabsorption and was diagnostic ". . . in those patients with minimal hypercalcemia and normal phosphate levels."

Discussion

Henry Royster, of Philadelphia, asked what the parathyroid glands showed in the chemically borderline cases. Oliver Cope, of Boston, echoed Dr. Goldman's appraisal of the need for a more accurate test for hyperparathyroidism and emphasized the fact that Goldman's figures showed no overlap between the calcium blood levels of his patients and of the normal patients, whereas there was a considerable overlap in the phosphate values. He hoped that there would be very little overlap in the tubular reabsorption of phosphate test. William Anlyan, of Durham, said that at Duke they had similarly been seeing an increased number of parathyroid hyperplasia patients, having removed 26 adenomas in the last two-and-a-half years. The tubular reabsorption of phosphate was studied ". . . in the last 16 cases and was low in 15 of the 16; it was low-normal in the 16th case." Periodic chemical re-examination of patients with borderline values was essential he thought. Goldman, closing, said that hyperparathyroidism was a special case since ". . . we depend more on the laboratory for diagnosis than we do for other diseases." He replied to Dr. Royster that all but three of his patients had adenoma, some of them multiple.

* * *

Fred C. Collier, W. S. Blakemore, R. H. Kyle, H. T. Enterline, and C. K. Kirby, all by invitation, and Julian Johnson, of Philadelphia, Professor of Surgery, School of Medicine and Graduate School of Medicine, University of Pennsylvania, *Carcinoma of the Lung: Factors Which Influence Five Year Survival with Special Reference to Blood Vessel Invasion*, presented a second large series, 600 patients with carcinoma of the lung, [344 explored, 226 resected] from Philadelphia just four years after Gibbon's large study [see Page 1003, Volume LXXI, 1953]. They pointed out that radical pneumonectomy at Memorial Hospital in New York had shown a 27% five-year survival "or essentially the same as obtained by less radical surgery . . . the most important factor in survival is the removal of the lung before the tumor has extended beyond the lung." Seventy-three percent of their resections were lobectomies. [That factor was not discussed.] They concentrated on the significance of histologically demonstrated invasion of the blood vessels. Five-year survivals were 6% with blood vessel invasion, and 75% without it, and if there was blood vessel invasion the addition of lymph node metastases did not affect the survival. The five-year survival overall was 26.8%. "In the absence of blood vessel invasion or lymph node invasion, the five-year survival rate was 83 per cent."

* * *

Conrad R. Lam, of Detroit, Surgeon-in-Charge, Division of Thoracic Surgery, Henry Ford Hospital, and, by invitation, Thomas Gahagan, Charles Sergeant, and Edward Green, *Clinical Experiences with Induced Cardiac Arrest during Intracardiac Surgical Procedures*, presented the first discussion before the Association on the use of cardioplegic agents. Björk in Stockholm had worked with acetylcholine, and Hooker and Wiggers long before had employed potassium chloride. In 1955, Lam had attempted correction of transposition of the great vessels by revision and transposition of the arterial trunks under hypothermia, with potassium chloride. The arrested heart could not be restarted. Although the experimental results of the potassium chloride had been good they returned to the laboratory to investigate acetylcholine and were pleased with it. "The reservoir source of oxygenated blood was of course soon replaced with a pump-oxygenator, which not only provided the ideal way of resuscitating the heart but permitted an apparently unlimited operating time while the heart and lungs were out of the circulation. We chose to use a pump-oxygenator of the bubble

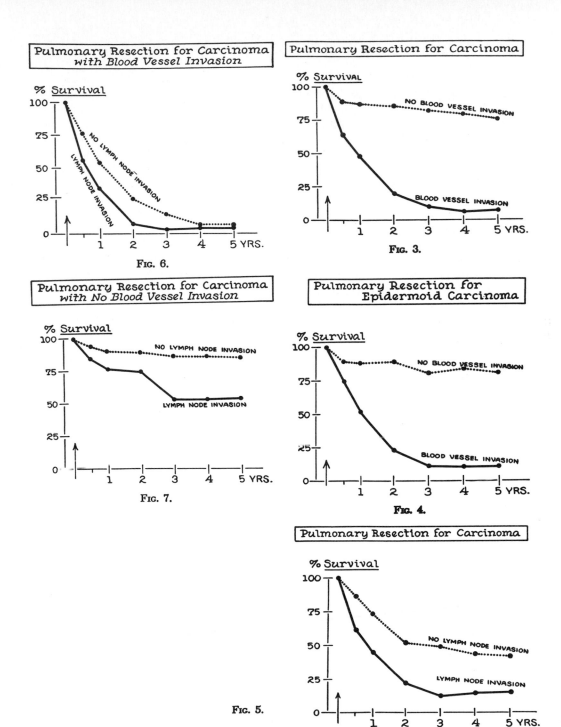

Pulmonary Resection for Carcinoma with Blood Vessel Invasion

% Survival

Fig. 6.

Pulmonary Resection for Carcinoma

% Survival

NO BLOOD VESSEL INVASION

BLOOD VESSEL INVASION

Fig. 3.

Pulmonary Resection for Carcinoma with No Blood Vessel Invasion

% Survival

NO LYMPH NODE INVASION

LYMPH NODE INVASION

Fig. 7.

Pulmonary Resection for Epidermoid Carcinoma

% Survival

NO BLOOD VESSEL INVASION

BLOOD VESSEL INVASION

Fig. 4.

Pulmonary Resection for Carcinoma

% Survival

NO LYMPH NODE INVASION

LYMPH NODE INVASION

Fig. 5.

In the total series of 600 patients with carcinoma of the lung, 226 underwent pulmonary resection with a 7% operative mortality, 100% of them followed more than five years. The overall survival was 25% at five years. With blood vessel invasion, the five-year survival was 6%, without blood vessel invasion the five-year survival was 75%. If there was lymph node invasion and no blood vessel invasion, the five-year survival was 50%. If there was no lymph node invasion and no vessel invasion, the five-year survival rate was 83%.

Fred C. Collier, W. S. Blakemore, R. H. Kyle, H. T. Enterline, C. K. Kirby, and J. Johnson, *Carcinoma of the Lung, Factors Which Influence Five Year Survival with Special Reference to Blood Vessel Invasion,* Volume LXXV, 1957.

type devised by DeWall, Lillehei and their associates [1956]." They had then heard of the [1955] work of "Melrose of London who had stopped hearts in the laboratory by intra-coronary perfusion with potassium citrate." In animals they did not think that the Melrose technique was superior to the acetylcholine technique. Effler [at the Cleveland Clinic, 1956] employed the Melrose method clinically and Moulder [University of Chicago] had employed acetylcholine clinically in addition to hypothermia. Lam had now employed induced cardiac arrest with acetylcholine 10 mg./K gm. body weight in 80 cardiac operations, 54 of them for ventricular septal defects. "In the perfectly dry and quiet field, suturing can be done with great accuracy." Atrioventricular block had been ". . . the most vexing problem in the septal defect cases. It was present in nine of the ventricular septal defect operations . . . in five, the persistent block seemed to be the chief factor in the death of the patients . . . the same complication plagues those surgeons who repair the defects without stopping the heart and the answer cannot be had until after an analysis of a considerable number of cases done by both methods." The overall mortality in the septal defect patients was 35%, 65% in those under one year and 5% in those over three years,- one out of 19.

Discussion

Denton Cooley, of Houston, said they had used cardiopulmonary by-pass 150 times ". . . in treatment of various cardiac and aortic lesions and have used cardioplegics in approximately half of these cases. We reserve induced cardiac arrest for cases of ventricular septal defect, aortic stenosis, and A-V communis but rarely use induced cardioplegia for other less difficult lesions." They tried acetylcholine and were not satisfied with it nor were they with potassium chloride and expressed a preference for potassium citrate [so briefly after the introduction of pump-oxygenator and cardiopulmonary by-pass, Cooley did not even mention the type of pump or oxygenator he was using].

* * *

Denton A. Cooley, of Houston, Associate Professor of Surgery, Baylor University College of Medicine; Michael E. DeBakey, Professor of Surgery and Chairman of the Department Surgery, Baylor University College of Medicine, and, by invitation, George C. Morris, Jr., *Controlled Extracorporeal Circulation in Surgical Treatment of Aortic Aneurysm*, went a step beyond the presentation of the previous year and now for aneurysms of the ascending aorta or aortic arch, employed total extracorporeal circulation with a pump-oxygenator and for aneurysms of the descending aorta, employed a by-pass with a pump, between the left atrium and the femoral artery. In the previous year they had operated upon ". . . 32 patients with aneurysms of the thoracic aorta . . ." by these techniques and 16 had died. Of the ten patients with aneurysm of the ascending aorta and arch, two patients were surviving and well, and eight were dead, three of them having died more than a week after operation. In the ten fusiform aneurysms of the descending thoracic aorta, there were two deaths from heart failure in the first week, all of the surviving patients had neurologic sequelae, and two of the surviving patients were patients with traumatic aneurysms. Of nine patients with dissecting aneurysms of the thoracic aorta, four died during the first week after operation, but the last five patients operated upon had all survived. Three patients with aneurysms of the lower thoracic and proximal abdominal aorta were operated upon with a temporary pump shunt, one died of heart failure, and one of bleeding. They considered the method technically preferable to that of the Ivalon shunt which they had reported the previous year.

* * *

Eastcott, Pickering and Rob in *Lancet* in 1954 reported resection of the obstructed carotid bifurcation and the restoration of continuity, and a number of reports had since appeared of individual cases, some operated upon successfully. Now Champ Lyons, still listed as Associate Professor of Surgery, School of Medicine, Tulane University, though he had gone to his Chair at the University of Alabama, and, by invitation, Garber Galbraith, *Surgical Treatment of Atherosclerotic Occlusion of the Internal Carotid Artery*, had six operations ". . . with five successful shunts and four patients surviving without significant neurologic signs or symptoms." In four cases a nylon prosthesis from the subclavian artery to the internal carotid by-passed the obstruction. In a fifth, the unsuccessful case, the prosthesis went from the common carotid to the internal carotid. One patient proved to have a complete occlusion and no anastomosis was made. Of the reported cases, Lyons said that only the original case by Eastcott, Pickering, and Rob, and the second case of that group reported by Edwards and Rob, had been successful.

Discussion

Michael E. DeBakey, of Houston, said that their experience with segmental occlusive disease, of which this was an example, was more extensive in the lower extremities where they had more than 500 cases. He cited a case, operated by Cooley, of incomplete obstruction of the carotid bifurcation treated by thromboendarterectomy over a temporary shunt in a patient illustrating ". . . the more proximal type of occlusive disease (which, incidentally, has been termed by various designations such as 'aortic arch syndrome', 'pulseless disease', and 'Takayasu's disease')." This patient had a pulseless arm and was not able to use his arm because of cramping pain. A bifurcation graft was employed, the stem attached to the aorta, and the limbs to the subclavian and common carotid arteries after endarterectomy of the cranial end of the carotid artery. William McCune, of Washington, described the removal by endarterectomy of a short one centimeter block, with considerable improvement in a patient with paralysis of the right arm and leg, and aphasia. Lyons, in closing, emphasized the frequency of the condition and described, the "little stroke syndrome".

* * *

W. G. Waddell, H. B. Fairley, by invitation, and W. G. Bigelow, of Toronto, Assistant Professor of Surgery, University of Toronto Medical School, *Improved Management of Clinical Hypothermia,* Based upon Related Biochemical Studies, had first presented their work on hypothermia for cardiovascular surgery before the Association seven years earlier. The technique had been substantially modified and now there were three surgical teams at the University of Toronto employing hypothermia,- Dr. W. T. Mustard, 151 cardiovascular cases in children; Doctors Botterell and Lougheed, 88 neurosurgical cases; and Bigelow's group of 85 adult cardiovascular cases. In the entire series there were 78 open heart operations performed under hypothermia and inflow occlusion. Patients were cooled with cooling blankets and ice packs except for the small children who were placed in a cold water bath. When the temperature had reached a level 1° to 4°C. above the desired temperature, the upper blanket was removed and the lower blanket switched to rewarming. There was a continued downward drift of body temperature of 1° to 4°C., "The average rate of cooling in adults has been a reduction of 6°C. in one hour and 30 minutes", permitting one to operate at the desired temperature. By the end of the operation the lower blanket was up to 36° or 37°C. and the patient

began to rewarm. They warned of acidosis during rewarming and after,- a problem in their early cases,- 21% of the overall series. The evidence was that they were dealing with a combined respiratory alkalosis and a metabolic lactate acidosis. As a result of their studies they maintained the temperature of adults between 28° and 31°C. To prevent the acidosis, they maintained strict control of pH during the cooling period, eliminating alkalosis, and prevented shivering to reduce lactate production. At the conclusion, spontaneous respiration was instituted as rapidly as possible. The incidence of symptomless acidosis now was about 12%. They had been concerned about the effects of the citrate in large amounts of blood and now attempted to use heparinized blood exclusively. They had employed elective acetylcholine cardiac arrest in five patients up to 11.5 and 12 minutes without any detectable residual mental effect. In hypothermia, total interruption of the circulation was certainly tolerated for seven or eight minutes at 28°C., "This has allowed correction of the simpler congenital defects with satisfactory results." By-pass operations had become simpler in the past two years and there were those who suggested the employment of by-pass for even the simpler cardiac defects, because it permitted better assessment of the defects, even though the risk was still higher. Bigelow's statement [ambitious for that day] was that "The real problem is to obtain knowledge that will allow us to cool patients, without mechanical aids, to low body temperatures of the order of 10° to 15°C. which would allow circulatory interruption of 30 to 40 minutes." He reported 11 early and late deaths including some in salvage operations for such things as ruptured thoracic aneurysms. In six of the deaths hypothermia might have been a factor. Five of the deaths occurred in the first 30 cases, and there had only been one death in the last 15. Of the 21 open heart operations among those patients studied biochemically, there were two deaths, one in a patient with cardiac failure and one in a patient with pulmonary hypertension. Mustard during the same period had operated upon 54 children with atrial septal defect, pulmonary stenosis, or aortic stenosis with two deaths. "Thus our combined figures for open heart surgery in such cases is 75, with four deaths or a mortality rate of 5.3 per cent."

Discussion

Henry Swan, of Denver, Colorado, also used heparinized blood and agreed that ". . . hypothermia has become very safe." He used both hypothermia and pump-oxygenator systems, reserving hypothermia for those requiring eight minutes or less of intra-cardiac operating time. In his first 100 hypothermic patients, 15 fibrillated, and 12 died. They had had a single fibrillation in their last 41 patients, and that from coronary air embolism, and with a successful outcome. In their first 44 patients with atrial septal defect, they had lost seven, and in the last 35, they had lost none. "Therefore, although we feel that the pump-oxygenator offers tremendous potential, we agree with Dr. Bigelow that because of its simplicity and its current safety, we will continue to use hypothermia for those procedures that fit within its limitations." F. John Lewis, now of Chicago, was in general agreement with Bigelow, particularly about the necessity for maintaining a constant pH, and like Bigelow and Swan, his figures had improved from 11 instances of ventricular fibrillation in the first 33 patients with atrial septal defect, to two out of the last 31, mainly due to changing from manually assisted respiration to an automatic respirator. Conrad Lam, of Detroit, supported closed techniques. He had operated upon 60 atrial septal defects ". . . cured by a closed operation with our two-pointed needle", and without ventricular fibrillation in any. If the atrial septal defect proved to be a complicated one, he clamped the atrium shut and resorted to hypothermia. For pulmonic stenosis, he was still using the Brock operation, monitoring the

cardiodynamic results by operative pull-back pressures. Julian Johnson, of Philadelphia, employed hypothermia, and suggested that if the occlusion time did not permit complete correction of a complicated defect, the atriotomy could be clamped closed, the circulation restored for ten or 15 minutes, after which another period of arrested circulation could follow safely, "In one complicated defect we had the heart open for a total of 16 minutes in four periods of four minutes each without the slightest difficulty." Earle Mahoney, of Rochester, New York, spoke up for protecting the heart by perfusion of the coronary artery with heparinized oxygenated whole blood during inflow occlusion under hypothermia. His experience had been entirely with dogs. Bigelow, closing, said that he, too, always used an automatic positive-negative respirator ". . . instead of adding or taking away CO_2 . . . we install or take away the CO_2 absorber or vary the rate or depth of respiration."

* * *

George E. Moore, of Buffalo, Director and Chief of Surgery, Roswell Park Memorial Institute; Associate Professor of Surgery, University of Buffalo School of Medicine, and, by invitation, Avery Sandberg, and Jean Rae Schubarg, *Clinical and Experi-*

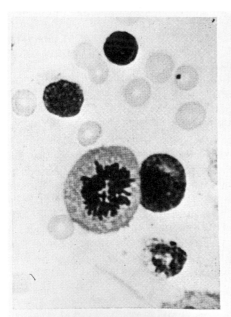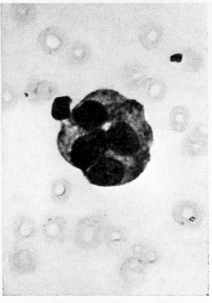

Fig. 3. #76578. Carcinoma of the pancreas. Tumor cells undergoing mitosis are not uncommon. Polyploid numbers of chromosomes and abnormal configuration of the spindle are frequent. Blood sample obtained after surgical manipulation; premanipulation specimen was negative.

Fig. 4. #77914. Carcinoma of sigmoid colon with metastases. A multi-nucleated tumor cell from a blood sample obtained before surgical manipulation from a mesenteric vein.

Moore and his colleagues, making smears of cellular concentrates, from the blood of 179 patients both with operable and with advanced lesions, found recognizable tumor in the peripheral circulation in 93 instances. Veins draining tumor sites, aspirated at the beginning or end of the operative procedure yielded tumor cells in 60 of 109 patients.

G. E. Moore, A. Sandberg, and J. R. Schubarg, *Clinical and Experimental Observations of the Occurrence and Fate of Tumor Cells in the Blood Stream*, Volume LXXV, 1957.

mental Observations of the Occurrence and Fate of Tumor Cells in the Blood Stream, recounted the studies of Engell in Scandinavia in 1955, and earlier studies showing tumor cells in the peripheral blood of patients with cancer. In his own work, 5 ml. blood samples were withdrawn, heparinized, sedimented, the plasma removed, centrifuged and the sediment stained. Tumor cells were found both in the peripheal blood and in the regional vein draining a malignancy at operation. Peripheral blood samples taken immediately after operation did not differ significantly from those taken immediately before operation, and Moore was not inclined to think that surgical manipulation disseminated tumor. In general, tumor cells in blood were more frequently found with advanced lesions and those which had already metastasized, but ". . . several small gastric and lung malignancies judged to be 'curable' had many tumor cells in blood from regional veins." Patients with early lesions rarely had tumor cells in their peripheral blood. The significance of circulating tumor cells in the peripheral blood was unclear. Some patients with such tumor cells and metastatic disease seemed no more ill than other patients with metastatic disease and few tumor cells in the circulating blood. Engell's follow-up studies, six months to four years, in patients with colorectal carcinoma showed that the presence of tumor cells in the peripheral blood initially was equally common in survivors and non-survivors. Human tumors, in which Moore's colleagues had found tumor cells in the blood, were various malignancies of the gastrointestinal tract, of the breast, lung, "sarcoma", and pharyngeal malignancies as well as a miscellaneous group of "Kidney, thyroid, pancreas, malignant melanoma, testes . . ." In 179 patients with tumors of all kinds and all stages, they found tumor cells in the peripheral blood in 93, the blood in the veins draining tumor sites contained tumor cells in 60 out of 109. The significance in respect to survival was yet to be determined.

Discussion

W. D. Gatch, of Indianapolis [then 79 years of age], described in very modern terms ". . . a necessary characteristic of metastasizing cancer . . . was first described by Virchow and . . . recently . . . thoroughly studied by Coman. It is a lack of cohesion of cancer cells. It permits their easy detachment from the parent growth. It has been shown that they then have amoeboid motility. They crawl into blood and lymph vessels, and by way of these, travel to far destinations. The common notion that the chief characteristic of a cancer is a lawless and rapid multiplication of its cells is, therefore, not entirely correct. If its cells stuck firmly together, it could spread by direct extension only . . . some cancers which the pathologist regards as very malignant have undetachable cells. Perhaps nearly all the cancers we really eradicate are of this kind. There is also good reason to believe that nearly all cancers of major forms, with few exceptions, spread early in their course by veins . . . it may explain why some metastases lie dormant for many years. Perhaps this is because their cells, in a new environment in the body, acquire a firm cohesion." Charles Lund, of Boston, referred to a demonstration some 25 years before by Eugene Pool and George Dunlop of the presence of cancer cells in the peripheral blood. He warned against undue pessimism because of the demonstration of cancer cells in the peripheral blood in patients operated upon for cancer for "They have been getting loose for the last hundred years in all the operations that have been done", yet the results were improving. He quoted Engell again to indicate that there appeared to be no correlation between recovery of cancer cells in the blood and the prognosis. George Moore, closing, once more repeated the apparent inconsistency between positivity and survival, and concluded by saying that "The significance of these studies to the rationale of adjuvant chemotherapy at the time of surgery when the minimal amount of established tumor remains, and the maximum number of 'free' cancer cells occurs, should be obvious . . . only a highly effective chemotherapeutic agent is lacking."

* * *

That phase of the problem was next addressed by Francisco Morales, Millar Bell, Gerald O. McDonald, by invitation, and Warren H. Cole, of Chicago, Professor and Head of the Department of Surgery, University of Illinois College of Medicine, *The Prophylactic Treatment of Cancer at the Time of Operation.* It was their feeling that the limits of extirpative surgery were being reached, that a number of agents were effective against animal tumors, that cancer cells were disseminated by operation, and they wished to try the combination of operation and chemotherapy ". . . in the supposition that cancer cells might be very vulnerable to the action of anticancer agents if they are given on the day of operation, before these 'loose' cells developed a blood supply." Wound washing, from a variety of tumor operations, yielded cancer cells. They had in 1954 showed that cancer cells were present in the venous blood draining tumors of the large bowel. Cole and his group had shown in rats with portal vein injection of Walker carcinosarcoma 256 that nitrogen mustard and thiotepa given shortly after inoculation sharply decreased the number of takes, the animals lived longer and died with smaller tumors than the controls. Experiments with animals suggested that four daily doses might be more preferable than a single immediate postoperative dose although even with this regimen, animals were not cured of cancer, but simply lived longer. "This would suggest that although nitrogen mustard may not destroy a tumor, it might nevertheless damage it so that life of the host would be prolonged." They had, since March 1956, treated 65 patients with nitrogen mustard at the time of operation for cancer of the gastrointestinal tract and breast. Patients with intraperitoneal tumors were given their first doses intraperitoneally, at the time of operation. There was only one operative death, a patient who received the nitrogen mustard in the peritoneal cavity at the time of the completion of an abdominoperineal resection, the patient dying of fulminating staphylococcal enterocolitis, thought not to be related to the nitrogen mustard. Early in the series, they had lost a patient following a radical mastectomy who had received rather large doses of nitrogen mustard, developed a leukopenia, wound infection and died of septicemia. Apart from these cases, four patients showed slight bleeding tendencies, four showed transient leukopenia below 3,000, some patients showed nausea and vomiting, or diarrhea. They were tending to increase the size of the first dose "Since our experiments indicate that the effect of nitrogen mustard diminishes as time elapses after inoculation of cells . . ." They had nothing yet to say about results except that "Nitrogen mustard appears to destroy these circulating [tumor] cells temporarily . . ."

Discussion

The paper had been presented by Millar Bell and the only Discussion addressed to the paper was Dr. Cole's lengthy comment, of which the most interesting part was the statement that "I am very glad to know that the National Cancer Institute, through the National Cancer Chemotherapy Center, under the supervision of Doctors Endicott and Ravdin, is going to organize a clinical project using this plan in ten or 15 clinics throughout the country. This project making several hundred cases available in a year or two will allow us to get an answer in a much shorter time than if only one clinic were con-

ducting it. Dr. [George] Moore . . . did not tell you, but he is the chairman of this committee which is preparing protocols for this project."

* * *

As President Dinsmore had indicated in his 1953 address, the establishment of a rational basis for the treatment of Hirschsprung's disease had been one of the outstanding advances in the preceding decade and now Orvar Swenson, Surgeon-in-Chief, Boston Floating Hospital for Infants and Children; Clinical Professor of Pediatric Surgery, Tufts College Medical School, who had been responsible for this advance, *Follow Up on 200 Patients Treated for Hirschsprung's Disease during a Ten-Year Period*, gave his results of the first decade of his operation. There had been six deaths in the 200 patients who had had the completed operation. This did not include deaths of patients who died in spite of a preliminary colostomy. Four out of the six deaths were in infants ". . . this has prompted us to postpone resections until the children are 12 to 18 months of age, maintaining the patients with colostomy until this age." The most serious complication was the slough of the pulled down rectum, which nevertheless was converted to final success after a number of operations. Patients with early gross anastomotic leaks required colostomy as did one patient whose massive hematoma became infected and produced a fecal fistula, and another with a pelvic abscess which drained into the colon and required a colostomy. One girl had a small and temporary rectovaginal fistula. Stricture of the anastomosis occurred in nine patients, eight responding to dilatation, one requiring resection. There had been five cases of enterocolitis. The follow-up covered 196 of the 200 patients. In 73 patients followed from five to ten years, all but one were perfectly normal, this boy having recurrent attacks of enterocolitis, still eight years after operation but otherwise being in general good health. "Incontinence has not been a problem." It occurred early in the postoperative course in some children but cleared in all. In the 64 patients followed two to five years, all but one were perfectly normal, a child who for the first year after operation had chronic diarrhea and slight distention but was now improving. Of the 52 patients operated upon in the past two years, all sustained good results except three,- one had some constipation, and two had recurrent diarrhea. There was a cloud in the sky "The most distressing finding in this follow up study is that one to five years from operation seven children have died suddenly following illnesses of less than 24 hours'

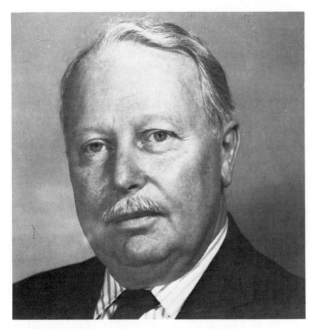

Orvar Swenson (c. 1970) 1909 (Helsingborg, Sweden)—. M.D. Harvard 1937; Intern, Ohio State; Residency, Children's Hospital—Peter Bent Brigham, 1938-1945; Instructor to Associate in Surgery, Harvard, 1944-1950; Associate Professor to Professor of Pediatric Surgery, Tufts, and Surgeon-in-Chief, Floating Hospital, Boston, 1950-1960. Professor of Surgery, Northwestern, and Surgeon-in-Chief, Children's Memorial Hospital, Chicago 1960-1973. Perhaps the most brilliant and productive of the Ladd-Gross School. A thoughtful and ingenious investigator, a meticulous and masterful surgeon, early achieved enviable results with esophageal atresia and other problems. Established in 1948, the seat of the problem in Hirschsprung's disease as the distal, narrow segment [his paper made no mention of aganglionosis] and adapted the Maunsell operation for its cure. His operation, thirty years later, slightly modified, retains its validity and is one of the three standard operative approaches. His detailed, exhaustive long-term follow-ups are a model of objectivity. Unequivocally the discoverer of the curative procedure for Hirschsprung's disease, his aggressive disinterest in alternative procedure is understandable. Manufacturer of archery equipment and an inveterate salt-water sailor. (Portrait courtesy of: William Kiesewetter, M.D., Childrens Hospital, Pittsburgh, Pa.)

duration. In all but one a postmortem examination was performed, and infection with severe dehydration has proved to be the cause of death." Swenson was inclined to attribute this to ". . . some defect in the normal mechanism to combat infection . . .

there may be abnormalities in the autonomic control of water balance and electrolytic concentrations to account for the extreme dehydration observed in the patients after illnesses of less than 24 hours." [It would appear that these children had a fulminating enterocolitis, well-known before and after operation for Hirschsprung's disease.] He also mentioned seven who had come under his care after ". . . segmental resections of the left colon with anastomosis of the transverse colon to the rectosigmoid at the level of the pelvic peritoneal reflection" [State's operation, 1952]. Eight of Swenson's male patients had married and fathered children, none of the other six men over 20 claimed a defect in ejaculation. "Since removal of the pathologic colon down to within two centimeters of the mucocutaneous margin can be accomplished without disturbance of ejaculation or fecal continence, and since failure to accomplish this fails to relieve the patient's symptoms, it seems that resection of the aganglionic segment to within two centimeters of the anal canal is the operation of choice."

There was no Discussion.

The Business Meetings

The 1957 meeting took place May 8, 9, and 10, at the Palmer House, Chicago, Illinois, President Loyal Davis in the Chair.

Dr. Richard H. Sweet reporting for the Program Committee of Sweet, H. William Scott, and Richard Varco, said the 81 papers submitted were the most in the last five years. They had chosen 34 based on "1) The timeliness or current interest of the subject; 2) The general interest of the subject considering the diversification of special interests of the membership; 3) The originality of the subject; and, 4) The relative excellence of the presentation as given in the abstract which was submitted." Those factors covered the intrinsic merit of the paper. They considered also the relation of the subject to that of each of the other papers available for the construction of a diversified program, and considered "the probability on the basis of previous experience that the presentation would be well given and within allotted time", and finally some papers were rejected because they had been given previously at other meetings by the same author. [A complaint heard again and again for the next 25 years. On occasion such a paper accepted and on the printed program was deleted from the program at the meeting.] This was the first year that, by vote of the membership, material from the departments of the members of the Program Committee had been considered [only one paper from the three departments was accepted,- from Minnesota, on Surgical Treatment of Ruptured Aneurysms of the Sinus of Valsalva]. The Program Committee thought that two other older precedents should be broken [as they had been for the past two years], the precedents that a given author or clinic should not be allowed to repeat in successive years, and that no more than one paper should be accepted in any one program from any one hospital group or clinic. "It is our firm belief that these considerations have no validity and that each contribution should be considered on its own individual merits regardless of the other aspects." The Committee also believed it to be the preference of the majority of the Members "that in cases of multiple authorship the paper should be presented by the member or senior author or, if none is a member, by the author who has actually done the work."

Dr. Dwight Clark, the Chairman of the Committee on Local Arrangements, in the course of his announcements said "The Association's annual cocktail party will be held in this room tomorrow evening beginning at 6:30 p.m., and as is the custom, wives of the Fellows are invited. Starting at 7:30 p.m. tomorrow evening, the annual dinner of the Association will also be held in this room. Again as is the custom, only the members of the Association are to attend the dinner."

Dr. Coller again reported for the Committee on Unnecessary Operations. He appeared to be saying that in Massachusetts the 18% of physicians who were qualified carried out over 95% of the operations, and in Michigan the 25% of the men who were qualified carried out 40% of the operations. The osteopaths were 18% of the physicians and carried out 12% of the operations in Michigan. "The unqualified carry out still, certainly about half of the operations." In Oklahoma, as the year before, 18% of the men were qualified and they carried out less than 30% of the operations, "while a much larger number of operations is performed by those who have no special qualifications." Forty-five percent of the hemorrhoidectomies in Massachusetts were carried out by qualified men, 50% "by the so-called generalist". In Massachusetts, 60% of the tonsillectomies were done by trained men, and less than 40% by the generalists. In Michigan the generalists and osteopaths did 70% of the tonsillectomies, and the generalists did over 80% in Oklahoma. In Massachusetts only 20% of herniorrhaphies were carried out "by those who are not skilled", and the corresponding figure in Michigan was 50%, and in Oklahoma, 60%.

Seventy percent of the salpingo-oophorectomies performed in Massachusetts were done by men with training, whereas in Michigan 70% were carried out by the osteopaths and the generalists, and in Oklahoma the percentage was even higher than in Michigan. He concluded, "As a result of this rather superficial study, extending over five or six years, I can state, and I think I have given the evidence, that in all probability, some operations of a comparatively minor magnitude (I'm talking about the suspensions and oophorectomies and so on) have been performed that were not necessary, but these were usually performed by those without orthodox surgical training, done in ignorance. In those states where cults are allowed to practice surgery, it is not our fault. That is the fault of the legislature . . . the sick patient will be better cared for when we have trained surgeons, physicians, roentgenologists, internists and general practitioners . . . The market is not glutted for good surgeons. There still are many areas where they are needed and where they should practice."

At the Second Executive Session, the Council offered a resolution by Dr. Blalock [which does not seem to have been acted upon], "The title, 'resident,' as now used in American surgery, identifies a surgeon, usually in full-time hospital practice, who is expanding his experience and perfecting his skills under conditions which make available and assure the ready consultation and assistance of colleagues already qualified as experts in the general and special fields of surgery. Since its foundation, over seventy-five years ago, the American Surgical Association has concerned itself with the establishment and maintenance of the highest standards in the surgical care of the American people. The Association takes this opportunity to assure governmental and private agencies which are bearing an increasing responsibility, both direct and indirect, in relation to the care of patients suffering from injury or surgical disease that the nature and quality of surgical care, including the performance of operations, provided by residents in approved programs, meet in full the high standards desired by its members." The resolution was to be transmitted to the Council on Medical Education and Hospitals of the American Medical Association, clearly in a move to protect the status of residents in performing operations upon insured patients.

Among new members elected were Oscar Creech, Jr., Edwin H. Ellison, and David Hume. Elected as officers were President, John H. Mulholland, of New York; Vice-Presidents, Richard Gilchrist, of Chicago, and Henry Harkins, of Seattle; and as Secretary, William Altemeier, of Cincinnati.

LXXVI

1958

The 1958 meeting was held at the Waldorf Astoria Hotel, in New York, April 16, 17, and 18, President John H. Mulholland, George David Stewart Professor of Surgery, Chairman of the Department, New York Unversity College of Medicine, in the Chair. The previous year had seen the deaths, among others, of Sterling Bunnell, the distinguished hand surgeon, Robert S. Dinsmore, who had been President in 1953; the venerable Rudolph Matas at the age of 97, who had been President of the Association 48 years earlier and had last participated in a meeting as recently as 1947 when he was 87. Gilbert Horrax, W. J. Mixter, and Arthur Allen had also died in that year.

* * *

The Program Committees, with the President to advise them, sometimes seemed to vary their techniques, at times saving the most exciting and the newest papers for the last, to keep the attendance maximal up to the last hour, at others choosing to start the meeting with the greatest excitement on the program. The tempo of peripheral vascular surgery had been accelerating and in their presentation now at the third consecutive meeting, Michael E. DeBakey, of Houston, Professor of Surgery and Chairman of the Department of Surgery, Baylor University College of Medicine; E. Stanley Crawford, by invitation; Denton A. Cooley, Associate Professor of Surgery, Baylor University College of Medicine; and

by invitation, George C. Morris, Jr., *Surgical Considerations of Occlusive Disease of the Abdominal Aorta and Iliac and Femoral Arteries: Analysis of 803 Cases,* rather overwhelmed the Association with their numbers, their techniques, their results, and the elegance of their illustrations. They continued to reemphasize the ". . . frequently well localized and segmental . . ." nature of chronic arteriosclerotic occlusive disease of the lower extremities, which their operative experience continued to demonstrate. The two major clinical problems were aorto-iliac occlusion, and femoral occlusion. In 448 cases of aorto-iliac occlusion the high proportion of 44% showed complete occlusion of the aorta. In 18% there was in addition some peripheral arterial occlusive disease, more often in those with partial aortic occlusion. The aorto-iliac occlusive disease was treated by thromboendarterectomy, by excision with graft replacement, or by bypass graft. In the 448 cases of aorto-iliac occlusion they had slightly better than 94% successful results whether the occlusion had been complete or incomplete. Lumbar sympathectomy was added to the procedure in almost half these cases. After their earliest grafts, freeze-dried homografts, they tried Orlon, nylon and Dacron synthetics, and had finally come to use ". . . a specially devised tube of knitted Dacron made flexible by proper crimping . . . developed in cooperation with the Philadelphia Textile Institute." The knitted Dacron had been used exclusively for the past year,

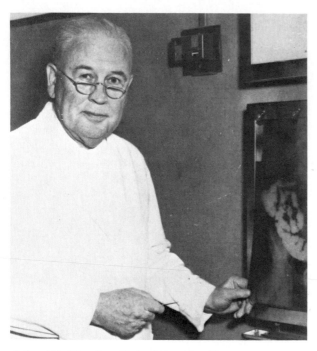

Arthur W. Allen (c. 1951) 1887-1958. [Allen was never an officer of the American Surgical Association, although his stature is indicated by the fact that he had been President of the Boston Surgical Society, the Society of Vascular Surgery, the American College of Surgeons, the Massachusetts Medical Society, and of the Pan-Pacific Surgical Society, and Chairman of the Surgery Section of the AMA. Then, as now, great figures, whom one would deem obvious candidates for the President's office, have been passed over. W. S. Halsted, L. Dragstedt, Frank Lahey, and surgeons still among us, come to mind.] Allen, a graduate of the Johns Hopkins Medical School, spent his entire surgical life at the Massachusetts General Hospital, becoming Chief of the East Surgical Service, and Lecturer in Surgery, Harvard Medical School. His contribution to surgery was as a superb clinician, a demanding and beloved postgraduate teacher, and a sound and thoughtful evaluator of progress in surgery. The last paper he presented before the Association, in 1954, was on Primary Malignant Lymphoma of the Gastro-Intestinal Tract. He had been diagnosed as having malignant lymphoma in 1941 and died of it in 1958, a month before the New York meeting.

(Portrait courtesy of Claude E. Welch, M.D., Boston, Massachusetts)

with great satisfaction. There were 12 operative deaths in the aorto-iliac series,- due to coronary thrombosis in five, renal failure in four, hemorrhage in two, and pulmonary embolism in one. In the femoral occlusions, they were bothered by the frequent occurrence of diffuse distal disease. They had oper-

ated upon 353 femoro-popliteal occlusions, bilateral 27% of the time. Initially they had often employed endarterectomy, or excision and graft replacement ". . . these procedures were associated with a relatively high morbidity and failure rate, presumably as a result of the more extensive nature of the operative procedures, the greater likelihood of destroying collateral channels and the frequent occurrence of incomplete removal of the occlusive lesion." Such procedures had now been almost entirely abandoned in favor of a bypass procedure, "At the present time endarterectomy is employed only when the lesion is quite discrete and localized to a short segment not exceeding a few centimeters in length." For the bypass graft, they had variously employed arterial homografts, tubes made of compressed Ivalon sponge, the Edwards-Tapp tube, and were now using their flexible knitted Dacron tube. Long-term results were not known, but they had not seen the aneurysms and degenerative changes which had occurred in homografts, nor the delayed false aneurysms seen with the use of the Edwards-Tapp tube. Eighty-four percent of the patients were discharged from the hospital with palpable distal pulses, a much better result than the 52% they had achieved with endarterectomy.

* * *

This paper was followed by that of Edwin J. Wylie, by invitation, and Leon Goldman, of San Francisco, Professor of Surgery, Chairman, Department of Surgery, University of California Medical School, *The Role of Aortography in the Determination of Operability in Arteriosclerosis of the Lower Extremities.* Translumbar aortography, in order to show the peripheral vessels and collaterals in the extremity, required the injection of a relatively large volume of concentrated radiopaque material. They accomplished this by the simultaneous translumbar insertion of two 17 gauge needles, into the aorta, and having tried Diodrast, Hypaque, Urokon and Renografin, had settled on 70% Urokon combining good opacification with minimal toxicity, and injected 20 to 50 cc. They performed translumbar aortography for the elucidation of peripheral arteriosclerosis in 500 patients. In 202 patients with aorto-iliac disease, 36 were demonstrated to have such advanced distal disease, extending beyond the popliteal arteries that no operation was undertaken. In 199 patients with femoro-popliteal disease, 121 or 61% had either diffuse proximal and distal disease or diffuse distal disease contraindicating operation. Depression in renal function was common after supra-

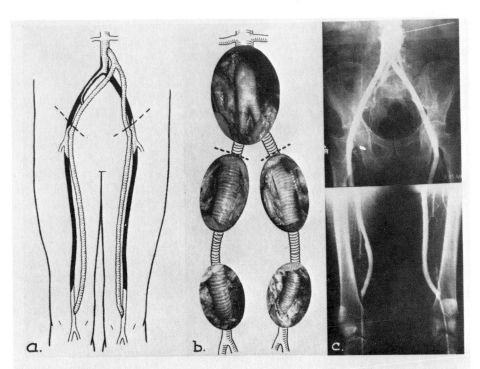

FIG. 13. Illustrations in case of aorto-iliac occlusion associated with segmental occlusion of both femoral arteries showing application of bypass method of treatment. (a) Diagrammatic drawing showing extent of occlusive lesion (in black) and bypass graft. (b) Photographs made at operation showing end-to-side anastomosis of graft to abdominal aorta above occlusion, side-to-side anastomosis of graft to common femoral arteries, and end-to-side anastomosis of graft to popliteal arteries. (c) Post-operative aortogram showing restoration of circulation through graft.

DeBakey's Figure 5 shows diagrammatically the types of operations employed. His Figure 13 is characteristic of some of the elaborate compound illustrations he used,- the projections at meetings being usually in color. There were 448 such aorto-iliac lesions (Figure 5) and satisfactory pulses resulted from operation in 95% by whatever operative method. Complete lumbar sympathectomy, performed routinely at first, was now replaced by resection of the fourth and fifth ganglia in most cases.

For the 353 femoro-popliteal operations, after an earlier experience with a variety of techniques, they had settled on the femoro-popliteal bypass graft with their crimped Dacron tube. Their Figure 13 shows a patient, a portion of whose common femoral artery was open on each side so that the bypass goes side-to-end at the aorta, side-to-side at the common femoral, end-to-side at the popliteal, employing their now one-year old crimped Dacron graft. Bypass in 317 femoro-popliteal occlusions was considered successful in 86%. Michael E. DeBakey, E. Stanley Crawford, Denton A. Cooley, George C. Morris, Jr., *Surgical Considerations of Occlusive Disease of the Abdominal Aorta and Iliac and Femoral Arteries: Analysis of 803 Cases.* Volume LXXVI, 1958.

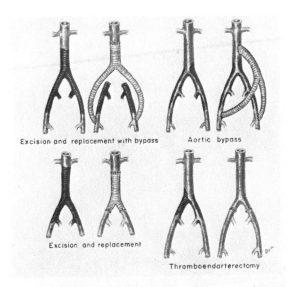

Excision and replacement with bypass

Aortic bypass

Excision and replacement

Thromboendarterectomy

FIG. 5. Drawing illustrating principal types of operative procedures employed in occlusive disease.

renal aortic injections. One patient developed thrombosis of the renal arteries and died, the only death from aortography. One patient developed a transient Brown-Séquard syndrome as a result of injection at the level of the diaphragm, and recovered after four months. Three patients developed bloody diarrhea.

Discussion

Robert R. Linton, of Boston, opened the Discussion, saying that he did not agree with all that had been said but that it was true that his own opinion kept changing in this rapidly moving field. He hoped that ". . . in the next few years, Dr. DeBakey will be able to tell us what has happened to these 800-odd cases that he has reported with an initial success of 95 to 97 per cent." In his own patients, only 60% of arterial homograft replacements were patent two to three years and he did not think that was good enough,- ". . . and as yet I have not seen a prosthesis to bypass obliterative disease of the femoral artery, which is even as good as these arterial homografts." Linton doubted whether the type of synthetic made much difference. He implanted 12 artificial prostheses in the lower limbs with initial success, but only one was still open. Prostheses were probably safer for the aorta and iliac than for the femoral and popliteal arteries [although he seemed to be concerned principally about the possibility of peripheral embolism from ". . . fibrinous coagulum becoming dislodged . . ." from the neo-intima]. His own preference in treatment of ". . . obliterative disease of the femoral arteries . . . first, without question, a saphenous vein autograft, put in by the end-to-end bypass technic . . . To my knowledge no patent saphenous vein autograft in a discharged patient has become occluded . . . next best . . . thromboendarterectomy . . . advocated by Cannon and Wylie . . . third choice . . . arterial homografts . . . fourth choice . . . synthetic prostheses." Linton could not agree with Wylie's enthusiasm for aortography because in 300 aortograms, his complications had included one death, one hemiplegia, and one complete renal shutdown, and he had ". . . abandoned this method of study, except in a very rare instance." Femoral arteriography by percutaneous injection into the femoral artery he thought was absolutely necessary. Richard Warren, of Boston, also emphasized the importance of waiting for late results. With thromboendarterectomy a constriction occurred but the vessels frequently remained open, ". . . the late results being better than the arterial homografts." H. William Scott, Jr., of Nashville, referred to the work in his laboratories of Killen and

Lance on the nephrotoxicity and neurotoxicity of the various injection media. Hypaque was substantially less toxic than Urokon. DeBakey, in closing, said that late occlusion seemed not to be a problem in the aorto-iliac reconstructions, but in the femoral artery "Over a three-year period, the rate of recurrence in our cases, where femoral bypasses were employed, was about 14 per cent." They were convinced of the importance of both ". . . a good proximal inflow as well as a good peripheral outflow." DeBakey stressed that none of the patients were made worse as a result of recurrent subsequent thrombosis, and in half the patients with occlusions, a second operation successfully restored circulation. Edwin J. Wylie, closing, referred to the long-term results of his endarterectomy procedure performed on 165 patients for aorto-iliac lesions. "Of the approximately 150 patients who had a satisfactory early result in terms of restoration of luminal patency, there has been only one instance of late thrombosis in the operated segment" [a footnote inserted at the time the galleys were corrected indicates that there had since been one more late thrombosis]. Endarterectomies in the femoral area were not quite as successful. Their early results with arterial homografts showed 18% occlusion after two years.

* * *

Joseph E. Murray, John P. Merrill, by invitation, and J. Hartwell Harrison, of Boston, Clinical Professor of Genito-Urinary Surgery, Harvard Medical School; Urologic Surgeon, Peter Bent Brigham Hospital, *Kidney Transplantation between Seven Pairs of Identical Twins,* presented the brilliant record of these transplantations at the Peter Bent Brigham Hospital. In 1945 at the Brigham, Landsteiner and Hufnagel had attempted without success to provide renal function by vascularizing a cadaver kidney through the recipient's upper extremity vessels. That problem was reinvestigated in 1951 and some 15 such temporary kidney transplants were performed, four of them showing measurable function and temporary clinical improvement for a period of time and one of them functioning for five-and-a-half months. The first patient for intra-abdominal transplant was admitted to the hospital in October 1954. They had now seen 15 pairs of monozygotic twins and had undertaken transplant in seven. The result had been brilliantly successful in four, one patient had "albuminuria and facial and ankle edema . . . Slight blood pressure elevation

PERIPHERAL VASCULAR SURGERY

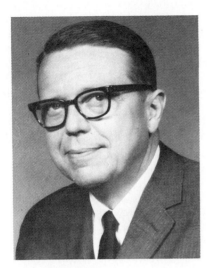

Ormand C. Julian, 1913- . M.D. University of Chicago, 1937; Intern, St. Luke's Hospital, Residency Training, University of Chicago; Instructor to Professor, University of Illinois 1947-59; Professor of Surgery in the reactivated Rush Medical College at Presbyterian–St. Luke's, 1971-79. Contributed importantly from the first to every phase of vascular and cardiac surgery, probably the first in the U.S. to perform an aortic bifurcation graft (1952), and to perform a series of saphenous vein femoral bypasses. Warm, genial and witty, with an incisive instinct for the direct road to surgical progress.

   (Portrait courtesy of H. Javid, Chicago, Illinois)

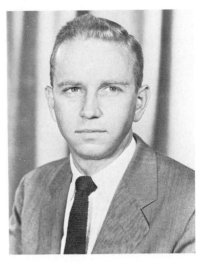

E. J. Wylie, (c. 1957) 1918- M.D. Harvard 1943. Intern, New York Hospital, residency at University of California, San Francisco to 1948. Instructor to Professor and Chief of Vascular Surgery Service. Emphasized the need for complete arteriographic studies, long preferred meticulous endarterectomy to prosthetic replacement, was one of the first to describe fibromuscular hyperplasia of the renal arteries as a correctable cause of hypertension. Prominent in discussions at the national level on the degree of training and experience required for those holding themselves out as vascular surgeons. His own specialized training program has populated the West with qualified vascular surgeons.

D. Emerick Szilagyi, 1910- (1960). M.D. University of Michigan 1935. Trained at University of Michigan, Ann Arbor and at Henry Ford Hospital, where he spent entire career, Chairman, Department of Surgery 1966-1975. Meticulous, precise, pedantic, obsessively detailed evaluator of his own results and those of others, contributed a series of model long-term follow-ups. Emphasized the effect of the progressive nature of the underlying arteriosclerosis, the progressively poorer results with more distal lesions, preference for endarterectomy in aorto-iliac disease, preference for long rather than short bypass in distal disease, restriction of operation for femoral disease to those with disabling claudication or rapid progression, and encouraged operation for femoropopliteal lesions with rest pain and incipient gangrene. His series demonstrated the excellent long-term results with saphenous vein grafts, the minimal pathologic changes in those and the relation of such changes to imperfections of technqiue.

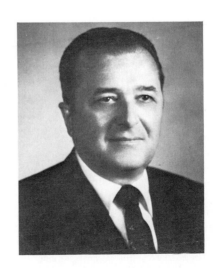

and recurring symptoms of the nephrotic syndrome make his prognosis poor." One patient died 12 days after operation because of technical failure caused by arterial anomalies in the donor kidney, and one patient died four months after transplant from the occurrence of subacute glomerulonephritis in the transplanted kidney, manifested seven weeks after transplant. Citing their animal experiments, they preferred implantation in the iliac fossa to replacement in the renal fossa, placing the left kidney in the right iliac fossa, the right kidney in the left iliac fossa. Early removal of the nonfunctioning diseased kidneys was required to reduce the threat of infection, hypertension, or the occurrence of the original disease in the transplant."

Discussion

The Discussion was initiated by David M. Hume, who had earlier been involved in the transplantation work at the Brigham and was now Professor of Surgery, Chairman of the Department, Medical College of Virginia, Richmond, Virginia. Hume mentioned the series of unsuccessful renal homografts at the Brigham, in which he had participated, and reported a recent identical twin transplant at Richmond, in a profoundly ill patient who was feeling better by the next morning. William P. Longmire, of Los Angeles, presented the work in his laboratory performed together with Dr. Jack Cannon and Dr. Paul Terisake [who was shortly to play such an important role in the development of histocompatibility testing for organ transplantation]. They were studying the factors of host resistance to the graft and had demonstrated by syringe crosstransfusion between chick embryos, that they were able to make the recipient of the blood transfusion subsequently receptive to a skin graft from the donor of the blood. Francis D. Moore, of Boston, now offered an over-view of the problem, which was to achieve a functioning whole-organ transplant in the recipient. The twin transplants had permitted solution of the portion of the problem which did not deal with genetic differences. He could see that in attacking the problem of genetic differences [the word rejection was not employed] one might attempt to treat the donor, or the tissue,- "Extracorporeal perfusion may alter tissue. Cooling it or freezing it may alter its antigenic properties",- or attempt to affect the recipient, "Changing the recipient is an interesting area now. This is where a lot of work is going on, producing immunoparalysis (usually with irradiation, sometimes with toxins) and then replac-

ing the immune tissue with a more 'tolerant' immune system, usually bone marrow, from the prospective tissue donor." J. Hartwell Harrison, in closing, wished to ". . . mention the wholehearted and continuous support of Dr. George Thorn and of Dr. Benjamin Miller, whose arrival at the Peter Bent Brigham Hospital along with Dr. David Hume rejuvenated the interest in renal transplantation. They initiated the beginning of this study which Dr. Murray has described in such detail for us today."

* * *

It was 26 years since Cushing's initial public presentation of his syndrome and now Frank Glenn, of New York, Professor of Surgery and Head of the Department, Cornell Medical College; Surgeon-in-Chief, New York Hospital, and by invitation, Richard C. Karl, and Melvin Horwith, *The Surgical Treatment of Cushing's Syndrome,* presented the experience at the New York Hospital with 32 patients with proven Cushing syndrome, ranging in age from nine to 52 years. Muscular weakness and fatigue were the commonest symptoms, amenorrhea occurred in 24 of the 28 women at risk, a moon facies was noted in 25, and truncal obesity with tapered extremities in 19. Nineteen patients were obviously emotionally disturbed. Urinary 17-hydroxycorticoid excretion was the most useful laboratory diagnostic test and the excretion was elevated in 19 of the 22 patients. The urinary 17-ketosteroids were elevated in 15 of 28 patients. In 25 of the 32 patients, the primary pathologic finding turned out to be adrenal hyperplasia, and in seven, there was an adrenal adenoma. They preferred the twelfth rib approach, except for patients with severe osteoporosis ". . . who cannot be placed in the lateral position without risking a compression fracture of a vertebral body and possible damage to the spinal cord." They had operated on 30 of the 32 patients, and performed a bilateral adrenalectomy in 20, unilateral resection for adenoma or hyperplasia in nine, biopsying normal adrenals in one. There were no operative deaths. They considered that the danger of recurrent disease from hypertrophy of an adrenal remnant, if less than total adrenalectomy was performed for hyperplasia, was greater than the risks of adequately managed operatively produced Addison's disease.

Discussion

Waltman Walters, of Rochester, Minnesota, who had presented a paper on this subject before the Association in 1934 at Toronto when he had ten cases, said that at last tabulation at the Mayo Clinic

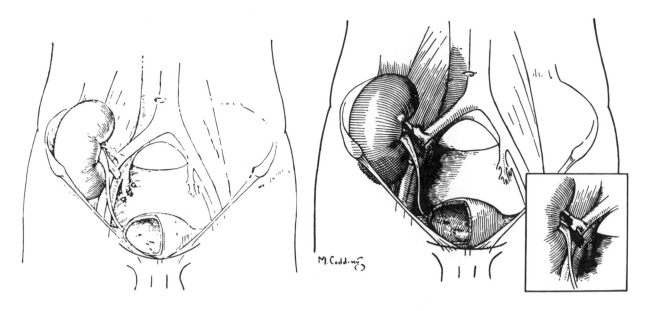

FIG. 11a (left) (originally published in J. A. M. A., Jan. 28, 1956)

Anatomic details of kidney transplant in four instances with only one renal artery anastomosis. End-to-end arterial anastomosis, end-to-side venous anastomosis; ureter led through muscular tunnel to bladder mucosa. (B) Anatomic details in three transplants where donor kidney had two or three individual arteries. Where three renal arteries are present, the largest is cut obliquely and anastomosed to a branch of the hypogastric end-to-end, and a polar artery implanted end-to-side to the external iliac. (Right lower inset) After successful anastomosis surgical failure occurs in Case 6 (J. F.) because of kinking and subsequent thrombosis.

Murray, Merrill and Harrison had two years before published the report of their first successful renal transplant between identical twins. They had now transplanted kidneys from an identical twin in seven patients. One was a "surgical failure . . . because of anatomical anomalies" and one developed "her original disease" in the transplanted kidney and died, and one had developed nephrosis. The other four were all well and one had been delivered of a healthy baby. No immunosuppression was employed [or known]. They recognized that the technical details learned would stand them in good stead "should the individually specific genetic barrier between individuals be overcome in the future."

J. E. Murray, J. P. Merrill, and J. H. Harrison, *Kidney Transplantation Between Seven Pairs of Identical Twins*, LXXVI, 1958.

three years earlier, they had had 100 cases of Cushing's syndrome,- 14 with adenomas, five with carcinomas. Eleven tumors were so small they would not have been demonstrated radiologically or even by transabdominal palpation, and required direct surgical exposure. He, too, preferred the lumbar incision. He still stood by his 1951 recommendation to the Association for ". . . 90 per cent removal of adrenal tissue, total removal of one gland and subtotal of the other." In ten patients in whom total adrenalectomy had been performed, pituitary tumors had subsequently become obvious. Was the tumor present initially or did it arise in response to replacement therapy? James Hardy, of Jackson, Mississippi, asked whether the fact that patients could be maintained in good health after total adrenalectomy meant ". . .

that one can send a patient back 100 miles to the local practitioner and not have him get in trouble?" Howard C. Naffziger, of San Francisco, who had been President in 1954, had operated for pituitary tumor in a woman with Cushing's syndrome a year after Cushing's original paper, ". . . I operated upon her and removed several fragments of her pituitary. The change in her was very striking and reached its peak in about one year after operation." Her symptoms recurred and she subsequently had an adrenalectomy. The histologic findings from the pituitary were disputed. He apparently mentioned this simply as ". . . the first case . . . that was operated upon for what is called Cushing's syndrome." Edwin H. Ellison, of Columbus, Ohio, said that in seven years they had had 15 patients with Cushing's syndrome, ten with adrenal hyperplasia, one with a malignant adrenal cortical tumor, and two with primary pituitary tumors. He preferred the abdominal route so that he could examine both adrenals before either one was removed, and resected all of one adrenal and 70% of the other for hyperplasia. William E. Abbott, of Cleveland, said it was their custom to operate simultaneously on both sides through the posterior approach, with two teams. Oliver Cope, of Boston, was concerned about performing total adrenalectomy ". . . I have stubbornly resisted it for the reason that the adrenal cortex secretes not one but several compounds, and the substitution therapy is complicated . . ." He had carried out subtotal adrenalectomy in 54 patients with Cushing's disease and had had to reoperate on eight,- two of them had had three operations,- for recurrence. J. Hartwell Harrison, of Boston, had employed total adrenalectomy in 18 out of 25 patients and subtotal adrenalectomy ". . . in young patients having hyperadrenocorticism of short duration." One of his patients for a time had been substantially relieved by total adrenalectomy, but after three years had suddenly become deeply pigmented and that pigment disappeared again after hypophysectomy removed a large pituitary tumor. Harrison commented, "It seems that we have traveled the full cycle back to Dr. Cushing, and it is necessary to study our patients with bilateral adrenalectomy with this possibility of primary pituitary origin of hyperadrenocorticism in mind. The trigger mechanism in the pituitary need not be a basophilic adenoma."

* * *

D. Emerick Szilagyi, Richard T. McDonald, and Lloyd C. France, all by invitation, *The Applicability of Angioplastic Procedures in Coronary Atherosclerosis*, An Estimate through Postmortem Injection Studies, said that the good results in peripheral angioplastic procedures suggested that ". . . direct surgical operative methods ought to be applicable to the correction of the occlusive process in coronary atherosclerosis as well." To determine whether this was so or not, required angiographic study of the nature of coronary atherosclerosis and this they had now provided from a study of 190 human hearts obtained at autopsy. Of the 114 hearts which showed occlusive lesions, 34 came from patients with no history of coronary atherosclerosis, 79 from patients with clinical atherosclerotic heart disease of whom 23 had had angina pectoris, almost alone. "The earliest and most sharply localized occlusive lesions were found in the subclinical group; the most ad-

vanced and widespread involvement occurred in the clinical group with angina . . . it appeared that coronary atherosclerosis when clinically manifest tends to be generalized." Taking into consideration also the technical problems which would be involved in getting at the location of the obstruction, 43% of the hearts in the "subclinical" group were judged inoperable, and 44% in the "clinical" group, while "curability" applied to only 13% of the clinical group. "The importance of a safe and reliable clinical method of coronary angiography for the realization of the potentialities of angioplastic procedures in the treatment of these lesions were emphasized."

Discussion

William P. Longmire, of Los Angeles, tended to differ because,- ". . . numerous autopsy observations of Dr. Jack Cannon in our Department, and Dr. Blalock and Dr. Sabiston, in Baltimore, have led us to believe that localized occlusions of the major coronary arteries with a patent distal arterial tree occur frequently in a patient without myocardial infarction." Since December 1, 1957, he had operated upon five patients for ". . . severe, incapacitating angina pectoris, without evidence of myocardial infarction." At operation, employing a binocular magnifying loupe, one or more, usually two, of the major coronary arteries, were found occluded and were opened by direct arterectomy. The second patient died of asystole after removal of the atheromatous core from the second major artery but the other four patients all survived and were thus far all free of anginal pain and showed increased exercise tolerance. Claude S. Beck, of Cleveland, rose to expound his theory of red and blue areas of the heart as causing ventricular fibrillation and his fear that the sudden opening of a coronary artery might produce just exactly this result. As for endarterectomy, "My experience with this disease, and I have operated on about 500 patients, is that almost always arterial disease is widespread, involving primary, secondary, and tertiary coronary arteries. To me it seems quite impossible to accomplish very much with such widespread disease. You surgeons know that endarterectomy has not been successful with such small arteries elsewhere in the body and the experiences with the coronary arteries should be very much the same . . . The important problem in the treatment of coronary heart disease is to produce an even distribution of the blood that is available in the substance of the heart and this can be accomplished by surgical operation by the creation of intercoronary communications." Szilagyi, closing, said he would await, with

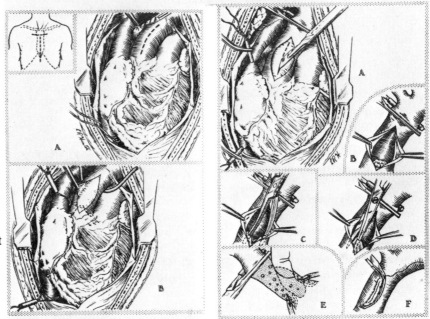

FIG. 2 (Left). A. Exposure of the heart, vena cavae and aorta through a median sternal incision. B. Superior and inferior vena cavae encircled with tapes. Adventitial tissue over anterior aspect of aorta dissected.

FIG. 3 (Right). A & B. Superior and inferior vena cavae occluded, aorta cross-clamped and incised just distal to the base of the aorta. C. Calcified stenotic valve being opened by heavy hemostat. D. Congenital stenosis being opened by incisions with scissors releasing aorta and vena cava occlusion, then closing arteriotomy with curved Potts coarctation clamp. E. Mechanism by which coronary air embolism was produced in only patient exhibiting this disaster. Occlusion of the arterotomy wound with finger must be avoided because air-fluid mixture will be forced into coronary arteries by ventricular contraction. F. Aortotomy wound excluded in jaws of curved Potts' coarctation clamp in preparation for closure.

Julian and his group performed aortic commissurotomy under direct vision with hypothermia and inflow occlusion in 23 patients, 18 acquired lesions, and five congenital, two of those subaortic. In acquired cases, they had nine excellent results, in the congenital, three excellent results. They had three operative deaths in the acquired group, and none in the congenital group.

William S. Dye, Ormand C. Julian, Hushang Javid, William J. Grove, Donald E. Morehead, and Oldrich Prec, *Aortic Commissurotomy Under Direct Vision.* Volume LXXVI, 1958.

interest, the further progress of Longmire's patients, but his own forecast was not bright for operative relief of arteriosclerosis of the coronary arteries.

* * *

William S. Dye, by invitation, Ormand C. Julian, of Chicago, Associate Professor of Surgery, University of Illinois; Hushang Javid, William J. Grove, Donald E. Morehead, and Oldrich Prec, by invitation, *Aortic Commissurotomy under Direct Vision,* supplemented Julian's 1956 report of two cases of aortic commissurotomy under direct vision using hypothermia and inflow occlusion, with 21 cases for a total of 23. [It was still possible to list all of the people who had worked on the problem, Tuffier, Smithy, Brock, Bailey, Harken, Swan, Swann, Pearl, Fell, Muller, Lewis, and Kaiser.] The first actual visualization of an aortic valve for operation in a human was by Clowes in 1954, in that case with a pump-oxygenator. The patient succumbed. Julian's 18 patients with acquired lesions suffered three operative deaths, but nine of them were excellent and two of them were improved after operation. There were no deaths in the congenital lesions, of which two were subaortic and three valvar, and the results were excellent in three. They pointed out that cardiopulmonary bypass might be better but that hypothermia gave all the time that was required for these simple procedures, the valve being forced open with ". . . a heavy curved hemostat separating as many commissures as is possible. One subaortic valve ring was removed with a small rongeur . . . In one congenital valvular stenosis no commissural lines could be visualized, and the valve was cut in two places producing a bicuspid valve without resulting regurgitation." They thought they enlarged the valve openings relatively little but that that was all that was required to relieve physiologically embarrassing stenosis.

Discussion

Conrad R. Lam, of Detroit, had operated, by a variety of techniques, on 90 patients for aortic stenosis. The last 12 patients had all survived. He wanted also to say a word about pulmonic valvulotomy. Since the last meeting, when he had still favored the operation of Brock [transventricular valvotomy], he had done that operation for pulmonic stenosis only once ". . . while 30 patients have been operated on by the trans-arterial route with direct vision of the valve, without hypothermia, allowing one minute of occlusion of the cavas [a procedure first performed by Varco] . . . the time needed for the valvotomy is so short that hypothermia is not necessary." Will C. Sealy, of Durham, North Carolina, said the operative treatment of the aortic valves required time for ". . . deliberate, precise, surgical manipulation. Hypothermia alone, does not permit this, nor does it allow time for correction of technical mishaps that can occur, such as a torn aorta or air emboli." He employed an extracorporeal circuit with a heat exchanger in it to induce hypothermia. Denton A. Cooley, of Houston, said that "Among the 346 patients operated upon in Houston using temporary cardiopulmonary bypass were 34 in whom operation was performed for disease of the aortic valve." In one patient with aortic insufficiency, ". . . a small tear-drop shaped piece of tissue was excised from the aortic annulus in the non-coronary cusp. This reduced the circumference of the annulus when the aortotomy was repaired, permitting apposition of the aortic leaflets." Henry Swan, of Denver, Colorado, said that since his ". . . first successful open procedure on the aortic valve in November of 1955, we have had an opportunity to observe approximately 20 patients with various types of stenosis . . ." He did not give his results but thought that hypothermia and inflow occlusion gave all the time that was required. J. Gordon Scannell, of Boston, had done postmortem aortic perfusions of two patients in whom he had operated and thought the residual aortic stenosis was quite "reasonable" nor was there much regurgitation, "This prompts us to continue with the open repair of aortic stenosis until, of course, some better method is known." Frank C. Spencer, of Baltimore, said that the Hopkins group had operated upon 15 patients with congenital aortic stenosis with a pump-oxygenator without any fatalities, having produced some aortic insufficiency in perhaps a quarter of these patients. They attempted with a knife to split the commissure so that a portion of the commissural tissue would be on the cusp

on each side. In subaortic stenosis, they had found it necessary to cut away some of the adjacent muscle. "Because of the absence of mortality and the low incidence of insufficiency, we are at the present time recommending operation in children with congenital stenosis in all instances, if they show signs of increasing evidence of left ventricular hypertrophy, or strain."

* * *

It was a long time since the gloomy assessments of the hernia problem at the early meetings of the Association [Volumes VII, 1889 and VIII, 1890] and now Chester B. McVay, of Yankton, Clinical Professor of Surgery, University of South Dakota; Chief of Surgery, Yankton Clinic, and by invitation, John D. Chapp, *Inguinal and Femoral Hernioplasty,* The Evaluation of a Basic Concept, discussed in considerable detail McVay's Cooper's ligament repair of groin hernias, McVay pointing out that he wished to ". . . acknowledge the paper of Lotheissen [1898], who first used Cooper's ligament in inguinal and femoral hernioplasty . . ." McVay's thesis was that "Since the posterior inguinal wall inserts into Cooper's ligament (ligamentum pubicum superius) and has only a contiguous relationship to the inguinal ligament, we have always maintained that the repair of the groin hernias that compromise the posterior inguinal wall (large indirect, direct and femoral hernias) should use Cooper's ligament in the hernia repair and not the inguinal ligament." He was now reporting 580 hernioplasties in which the inguinal ligament had not been used once. The type of operation depended upon the individual hernia "For the small to medium size indirect inguinal hernias we do nothing more than excise the hernial sac and tighten the abdominal inguinal ring to normal by suturing the transversalis fascia to the anterior layer of the femoral sheath, medial to the cord . . . For large indirect inguinal, direct inguinal, and femoral hernias we reconstruct a new posterior inguinal wall . . . excising all attenuated aponeurotico-fascial structures . . . relaxing incision, and a 'slide' of the rectus sheath into the position of a new posterior inguinal wall. This new posterior wall is sutured to Cooper's ligament as far laterally as the femoral vein and after the *transition suture,* the transversalis fascia is sutured to the anterior layer of the femoral sheath far enough laterally to make a snug abdominal inguinal ring . . . the spermatic cord is replaced in its normal position and the external oblique aponeurosis closed to make a snug subcutaneous inguinal ring in the normal position." Of his 580 herni-

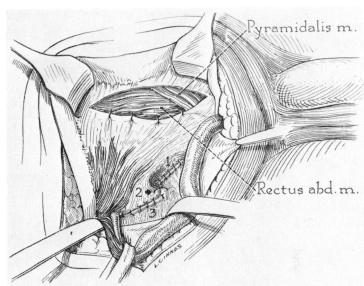

Fig. 2. Reconstruction of the posterior inguinal wall. 1. Rectus sheath sutured to Cooper's ligament. 2. Transition suture. 3. Transversalis fascia sutured to anterior femoral sheath. (From Hernia, by C. B. McVay, Courtesy of Charles C Thomas, Publisher, Springfield, Illinois.)

McVay's standard operation for "large indirect inguinal, direct inguinal, and femoral hernias . . ." is shown in his Figure 2. It involved the vertical paramedian rectus relaxation incision, and the suture of the medial structures to Cooper's ligament until the femoral vein was reached when the transition suture was placed, the closure stepped up, and the transversalis fascia then sutured to the anterior femoral sheath. The aponeurosis was closed over the cord. For small indirect inguinal herniae, he excised the sac and repaired the abdominal ring as in his Figure 3. In 580 hernias, he had a 2.24% recurrence rate, that for the Cooper's ligament repair being 0.85%, and that for the abdominal ring repair being 3.2%.

C. B. McVay, John D. Chapp, *Inguinal and Femoral Hernioplasty:* The Evaluation of a Basic Concept. Volume LXXVI, 1958.

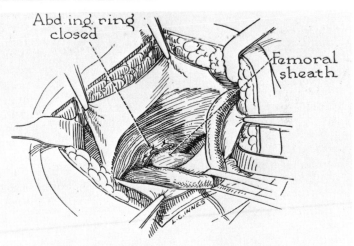

Fig. 3. Abdominal inguinal ring repair. (From Hernia, by C. B. McVay, Courtesy of Charles C Thomas, Publisher, Springfield, Illinois.)

orrhaphies, 467 were for indirect inguinal hernias of all kinds, 74 were for direct inguinal hernias, and 39 for femoral hernias. The total recurrence rate was 2.24%. He strongly emphasized the importance of the relaxing incision, and never used fascial sutures, fascial grafts, or dermal grafts, had four times used stainless-steel wire mesh. In the entire series of 580 herniorrhaphies, there had been three deaths, two of pulmonary embolism, and one of uremia and congestive heart failure on the fourth day. The recurrence rate in 236 reconstructions of the posterior inguinal wall by the McVay method was 0.85%.

Discussion

Henry Harkins, of Seattle, said he had been persuaded by McVay long since, but recently he had been using the Cheatle-Henry transabdominal preperitoneal approach to groin hernias in which, in any case, ". . . the thickened transversalis fascia at the superior margin of the defect is sutured to Cooper's ligament at the inferior margin . . ." Amos R. Koontz, of Baltimore, pointed out that a few years ago Estes had reported 500 herniorrhaphies with a recurrence rate of less than 1%, that he had had about the same size series himself two years before with a similar recurrence rate "Now Chester McVay has done the same thing, and all of us used different methods." Koontz said that whatever repair was used, if it did not appear strong enough, he reinforced it with tantalum mesh [invariably, the house staff thought]. He asked whether the recurrence rate of 2.2% in the smaller inguinal hernias in McVay's series did not mean an inadequate operation. William L. Estes, Jr., of Bethlehem, Pennsylvania, said he sutured ". . . the conjoined tendon to both Cooper's Ligament *and the inguinal ligament* because there seemed to be a dead space left between the conjoined tendon and the inguinal ligament when only Cooper's ligament was used." The five-year follow-up of 400 cases of herniorrhaphy had shown a 1.5% recurrence rate, 1.18% in indirect hernias, 1.6% in direct hernias, and 4.8% in recurrent hernias. McVay made the curious statement in closing that ". . . we always replace the cord in its normal position,- the Bassini position."

* * *

William E. Abbott, of Cleveland, Associate Professor of Surgery, University Hospitals, and by invitation, Harvey Krieger, and Stanley Levey, *Technical Surgical Factors Which Enhance or Minimize Postgastrectomy Abnormalities,* had studied some 85 patients who had undergone various gastric procedures, and 15 normal volunteers, by detailed barium-food X-rays. They agreed about the ". . . importance of a small stoma in the prevention of dumping symptoms and undernutrition." Gastric mucosal folds might alter the effect of stoma size. The internal diameter of the stoma they thought should not exceed 2 cm.

Discussion

Ralph F. Bowers, of Memphis, opened the Discussion stating that they had compared a series of 100 gastrectomies with Hoffmeister reconstructions with a small stoma,- 1.5 cm. to 2.5 cm.- with 100 similar patients in whom the stoma measured 2.5 cm. to 4.5 cm. in length. In an average follow-up of three years, 53 of the 100 small stoma patients, had ". . . absolutely no symptoms". Thirty-one of the small stoma group demonstrated "mild atypical symptoms while 40 of the control group experienced these mild symptoms." There were 16 instances of dumping in the small stoma group, and 32 in the control group. Average weight loss in the small stoma group was 3.84 pounds, in the control group,

9.83 pounds. In a patient who had lost 66 pounds and had marked dumping, narrowing the stoma ". . . from 4.5 cm. to 1.75 cm. produced excellent results promptly. He gained 7-1/2 lbs. in 3 months, dumping symptoms have disappeared, weakness has disappeared and for the first time since his gastrectomy he has returned to work and a useful life." Henry N. Harkins, of Seattle, said that his anastomoses were 3.2 cm. external diameter, possibly too large since he had an undesirable incidence of dumping. He wondered whether the size of the gastric remnant affected dumping. H. William Scott, Jr., of Nashville, claimed personal expertise because he himself was a "large stoma dumper". In the last ten years at Vanderbilt, beginning with the work of Dr. Leonard Edwards, they had been employing truncal vagotomy and antrectomy, in almost 600 patients, with only two ulcer recurrences thus far. He had been impressed by ". . . the good postoperative status of the patient who has the Shoemaker-Billroth I gastroduodenostomy. It provides a large gastric reservoir, a small stoma . . . the transit time is very close to normal." There was much less dumping in the Billroth I group than in the 167 patients with a Billroth II, and there was no severe dumping at all in the Billroth I group. He converted two Billroth II patients who were severe dumpers to Billroth I with good results. Robert M. Zollinger, of Columbus, Ohio, was inclined to agree that a small stoma made dumping less likely. He had been performing vagotomy, hemigastrectomy, and a small stoma gastroduodenostomy—Billroth I. William E. Abbott, in closing, said they had not yet had to reoperate on any patients for obstruction of the small stoma, but had had some five patients who took a week or two ". . . to open up . . ." He did not believe the size of the gastric remnant played any part in the dumping syndrome.

* * *

Karl E. Karlson, and Irving F. Enquist, by invitation, and Clarence Dennis, of New York, Professor and Chairman of the Department of Surgery, State University of New York College of Medicine, and Sidney Fierst, by invitation, *Results of Three Methods of Therapy for Massive Gastroduodenal Hemorrhage,* A Statistically Valid Comparison, separated their patients with massive hemorrhage, rated according to Stewart's criteria [Volume LXX, 1952], into three therapeutic groups "1) non-operative regimen, 2) immediately operative regimen, and 3) selectively operative regimen." The non-operative regimen consisted of "Bed rest, gelatin-milk mixture every two hours, and mild sedation. Transfusion only for air hunger, and evidences of cerebral or myocardial hypoxemia or for blood pressure below 80 mm. of mercury systolic, and then in 250 cc. amounts only." These patients were to be followed and supervised by the medical consultant. In the immediately operative regimen "Three-quarter gastrectomy will be undertaken in every patient in this group as soon as the patient is completely evaluated and proper preoperative preparation accomplished . . . Preoperative preparation should not require more than 12 hours." In the selectively operative regimen, they operated within 12 hours on all patients 50 years of age or over, all patients with severe arteriosclerotic changes ". . . in eye grounds, films of the aorta, or peripheral arteries . . .", all patients with a history of a previous massive hemorrhage, all patients in whom transfusion failed to correct shock. If 1,500 ml. of blood promptly administered did not bring the patient out of shock, transfusion was to be continued and operation undertaken. If after restoration to normotensive levels with 1,500 ml. of blood, more than 500 ml. was required every eight hours, operation was to be undertaken. Of the 239 patients seen with upper gastrointestinal hemorrhage, 130 were found to meet the criteria for admission to the study. Mortality in each group was exactly 14%. One of the by-products of their study was the observation that none of those patients excluded from the protocol, because they had lost less than 40% of the calculated normal total circulating red cell mass, died of gastrointestinal bleeding. But, of course, the patients who survived the massive hemorrhage without operation, still had their ulcer disease to contend with. One of the patients in the immediate operative group actually died before operation could be undertaken so that the mortality of those actually operated upon was 11%.

Discussion

John D. Stewart, of Buffalo, thought this was the first study of its kind,- prospective and controlled, and with a patient population evaluated for standard hemorrhage. Stewart pointed out that there were 58 cases in the non-operative group, 37 in the immediate operative group, and 35 in the selective operative group, so that the study should be continued until the groups were larger and equalized. Just how rapidly, in fact, were the "immediate" operations undertaken? How many of the patients had diffuse superficial ulcerations? Dr. Stewart reported that in his own patients, still all treated under the plan of immediate operation, there were presently over 250 cases ". . . the operative mortality rate is

approximately what he [Dennis] reports in this present study." J. E. Dunphy, of Boston, said that indeed at the Brigham from 1933 to 1945, patients were treated by the modified Andresen regimen,- Dennis' non-operative regimen,- with a 15% mortality. He, too, thought Dr. Dennis needed larger numbers to achieve statistical validity "If I get anything from this study, it is that in Group I [no operation] the cause of death was exsanguination primarily, and so I would conclude by saying that until more data is available, I think we should regard bleeding ulcer in general as an exsanguination syndrome best treated in the selected patient by operation." Claude E. Welch, of Boston, was concerned about the factor of selection of the patients and thought the series would have to be expanded to take varying ages of patients into account. He agreed that the patients who recovered without operation were still subject to the risk of their disease, and said that "We have found that the results are so poor afterwards that our main question with a massive hemorrhage is not whether or not to operate, but when to operate. That is the only question." He expressed the hope that the study would be continued and that the results would not show that the mortality was the same whether the patients were operated upon or not. Stanley Hoerr, of Cleveland, pointed out that the first two groups might have been random groups but the third one, those patients selectively operated was, of course, not random. Dennis, closing, replied to Dr. Stewart that the patients were operated upon within 12 hours. Dennis was concerned that the numbers did not quite jibe but drew the conclusion that "there is no statistically significant difference among the 3 types of therapy which were employed." As far as follow-up of the individual patients who were not operated, Dennis despaired of that in the New York City Municipal Hospital system.

* * *

Oscar Creech, of New Orleans, William Henderson Professor of Surgery and Chairman of the Department of Surgery, Tulane University School of Medicine, and by invitation, E. T. Krementz, Robert F. Ryan, and James N. Winblad, *Chemotherapy of Cancer:* Regional Perfusion Utilizing an Extracorporeal Circuit, said that the limiting factor of chemotherapy for malignant disease was systemic toxicity, even when the agent was introduced directly into the arterial supply of the tumor. It had occurred to Creech that the heart-lung apparatus could be employed to isolate and maintain ". . . a tumor-bearing area while it was being perfused with maximal amounts of an alkylating agent. If vascular and lymphatic exclusion were complete systemic toxic effects should be eliminated while the specific activity of the agents would be brought to bear only upon the tumor and its immediate environment." Ionizing radiation was potentiated by high oxygen in the tissues, the chemotherapeutic agents had a radiomimetic effect, and he had therefore introduced a bubble oxygenator into their circuit in the hope of increasing the effectiveness of the mustard compounds employed. They undertook to treat with nitrogen mustard or phenylalanine mustard 24 patients with a variety of sarcomas and carcinomas, including six with melanoma. Appropriate limb artery and vein were cannulated,- and for pelvic tumors the aorta and inferior vena cava just above their bifurcation and pneumatic tourniquets applied to both limbs. One patient died of the toxic hematologic effects of the perfusate because of incomplete isolation of the lower limb. For lung perfusion, the therapeutic perfusion was left atrium-to-pump oxygenator-to-pulmonary artery, at the same time that a standard cardiopulmonary bypass supported the systemic circulation. In a number of patients there was a striking regression of palpable masses or radiologically visible masses, or of cutaneous metastases.

Discussion

Warren H. Cole, of Chicago, thought this ". . . a very clever idea" because the toxicity of most of the agents was so high "It's been a bit discouraging during the past 10 or 12 years to realize that perhaps as many as 50,000 chemicals have been screened for effect against cancer, yet none of them seems to be any more effective than the original one, nitrogen mustard . . . I believe we must give serious thought to methods of this sort, hoping to utilize them as the primary agent in destroying local tumors until we get better drugs." John Schilling, of Oklahoma City, asked whether they had microscopic observations on the effects on normal structures from the regional perfusion and whether they had perfused the liver, and what had been the results upon it. Denton A. Cooley, of Houston, said that in dogs they had been using an extracorporeal circuit with the aim of irradiating the blood as it passed through the circuit, using a 2 million volt Van de Graaff electrostatic generator, hoping to use the technique in leukemia. Oscar Creech, Jr., in closing, said that they had not

perfused the liver and that normal tissue had shown no more than edema.

* * *

Claude E. Welch, of Boston, Clinical Associate in Surgery, Harvard Medical School, and by invitation, Earle W. Wilkins, Jr., *Carcinoma of the Stomach,* brought up to date the experience at the Massachusetts General Hospital with cancer of the stomach, last reported in 1948, announcing ". . . a striking improvement in the survival rate." In the previous decade they had had admitted 637 patients with carcinoma of the stomach, and followed 99% of the patients to recurrence or death. Subtotal gastrectomy with negative nodes gave 63% five-year survival, and with positive nodes, 24% five-year survival. Total gastrectomy with negative nodes gave a 21% five-year survival, and, with positive nodes, a 6% five-year survival. Extended gastrectomy gave a 29% five-year survival with negative nodes, and a 7% five-year survival with positive nodes. The overall was, therefore, 51% five-year survival with nodes negative and 17% five-year survival with nodes positive. Patients were not coming into the hospital any sooner than they had in the 1927 to 1936 period. Mortality of exploration alone was 7.5%,- for palliative operations other than resection, 10.2%,- for palliative resections, 24%,- and for resection for cure, 8.7%. Extended gastrectomy, involving removal of portions of the transverse colon, pancreas, liver and spleen together with the primary tumor was done in 36 potentially curable cases, with a five-year survival in six. On the other hand, "Mortality has gradually risen with the inclusion of more viscera in the resection." The mortality was "subtotal distal resection, 8.2 per cent; of subtotal proximal resection, 7.0 per cent; of total gastrectomy, 14.5 per cent, and of extended total gastrectomy, 15.4 per cent . . . cancers of the distal stomach are treated adequately by subtotal distal resection, since 47 per cent of those surviving such resections for cure were living five years later . . . if nodes were negative, the survival rate was 63 per cent . . . For large cancers of the cardia or entire stomach, the preferable operation appears to be total gastrectomy with splenectomy and hemipancreatectomy . . . mortality rises with the extent of the procedure."

Discussion

Henry King Ransom, of Ann Arbor, Michigan, said that of 105 patients who died after total gastrectomy only six had lived for more than two years. One of them was alive 20 years later. Ralph F. Bowers, of Memphis, Tennessee, mentioned the hazard in failing to operate on tumors of the stomach because of their huge size, citing a lymphosarcoma and a leiomyosarcoma, which responded to irradiation and resection, respectively. Jonathan Rhoads, of Philadelphia, said that on the Surgical Service of the Hospital of the University of Pennsylvania, the gross five-year survival in 233 cases of carcinoma of the stomach was 15.5% ". . . and a 5 year salvage of 35.5% among the resections undertaken for cure." He had attributed this to ". . . greater emphasis on restricting test periods of medical treatment for supposed ulcer to 2 or 3 weeks. This view is supported in the literature in 2 studies of gastric carcinomas discovered at operation for ulcer, with 5 year survival rates of about 40%, and is also supported by the fact that more than 50% of those cases which were resected for cure in the Ravdin and Darrow series had negative lymph nodes." Earle W. Wilkins, closing, emphasized the fact that some of the total gastrectomy patients who survived operation had ". . . major functional problems."

* * *

Edward S. Stafford, of Baltimore, Associate Professor of Surgery, Johns Hopkins University, and by invitation, G. Rainey Williams, Jr., *Radical Transthoracic Forequarter Amputation,* presented the reports of two patients one with fibrosarcoma at the outer end of the clavicle and one with axillary metastases from carcinoma of the breast involving the brachial plexus. They performed in each a forequarter amputation, together with a resection of the first and second ribs and the associated chest wall. Both patients did well (see p. 1086).

Discussion

Discussers reported three additional cases. David W. Robinson, of Kansas City, mentioned two patients, one operated upon by C. A. Hardin, and one by Stanley Friesen. Dr. Hardin's patient operated upon for fibrosarcoma was alive and well after five years. Ralph F. Bowers, of Memphis, said by a similar operation he had obtained striking palliation and relief of pain for nine and a half months in a patient with recurrent melanoma in the axilla and chest wall. G. Rainey Williams, closing, said no prosthetic materials had been required to close the thorax under the flap.

The Business Meetings

The 1958 meeting took place on April 16, 17, and 18, at the Waldorf-Astoria Hotel, New York, President John H. Mulholland presiding.

The cost of printing the *Transactions* had been the subject of comment for several years and at this meeting J. Englebert Dunphy, the Recorder, said "During the year, we have received considerable correspondence pro and con relative to abandoning the practice of publishing the scientific papers in the Transactions. It is argued that inasmuch as this material is available to both members and libraries in *Annals of Surgery,* it would be unnecessary to print them in the Transactions. This would save considerable cost. On the other hand, many members feel very strongly that this step would change the traditional character of the Transactions. The matter was given careful consideration by the Council and it is recommended that the present form of the Transactions be continued."

H. W. Scott of the Program Committee said the number of abstracts this year was 110 from which 34 papers were selected.

Louis M. Rousselot, Chairman of the Committee on Arrangements, among other things said, "There will be five separate tickets for the total period of the meetings including three luncheon tickets at $6 each, the reception ticket Thursday afternoon at $6, and the banquet ticket for Thursday night at $18. The total package comes to $42.00." [At this point, a murmur of outrage arose through the room. The subsequent protestations to the Council over these, at the time truly exorbitant, rates led to the reassuring rumor that the Council had agreed that the Association would never again meet in New York!]

Dr. Coller reported once more for the Committee on Unnecessary Surgery, and expressed concern about a number of things that were going on. Five general practitioners in a city in Michigan were suing the hospital because they were not given full surgical privileges. Osteopaths had been taken into five Michigan hospitals built by Federal money. ". . . an infinite number of operations are done in this country by men who have no training. While our efforts are excellent and powerful, and I hope eventually successful, there is this group who still are opposed to higher standards because they interfere with their income."

Dr. William F. MacFee, the Chairman of the committee to study the problems of nursing, said that there was a serious shortage of trained nurses

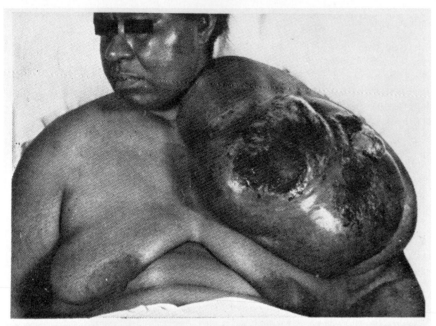

FIG. 4. Case 1. Preoperative.

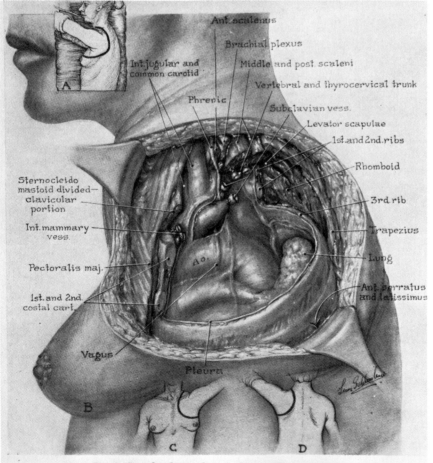

FIG. 2. Completed transthoracic forequarter amputation.

Stafford and Williams reported two forequarter amputations combined with a resection of the chest wall and the first and second ribs. The first, a patient with a fibrosarcoma (Figure 4), and the second, a patient with carcinoma of the breast, recurrent in the axilla after five years and invading the brachial plexus. Forequarter and humeral amputations of the arm for "cure" of advanced cancer of the breast, some with chest wall resection, had been discussed in the 1907 symposium on cancer of the breast [see pages 373 and 374] by J. B. Roberts, A. H. Ferguson, T. W. Huntington.

Edward S. Stafford, G. Rainey Williams, Jr., *Radical Transthoracic Forequarter Amputation*. Volume LXXVI, 1958.

"particularly of those who are interested in bedside nursing" despite a steady increase in their numbers. They concluded that the shortage of nurses ". . . trained and willing to do general duty and bedside nursing . . ." was serious, that the greatest source for such nurses was in the hospital schools of nursing, "currently designated as diploma schools". Here such training was obtainable by girls who could not afford a collegiate program. The college-trained faculty required for accreditation by the nursing boards was difficult for many hospital schools to maintain and such hospital schools should be accredited without college diploma teachers. Training and utilization of practical nurses was helping "but restrictions imposed by lack of education and the law place limitations on their usefulness."

At the Second Executive Meeting, the report of the Nursing Committee was presented as a resolution expressing ". . . approbation of measures that have been taken to increase the numbers of general duty and bedside nurses, as exemplified by the establishment of two-year registered nurse (Junior College) programs of training, and by sponsorship of practical nurse training programs . . . That the Association urge greater utilization and support of the hospital schools of nursing which currently are the principal source of general duty and bedside nurses . . . That the Association recommend top priority for the education of nurses for general and bedside duty, at least until the current shortage is over."

Among those elected to Membership were Marshall K. Bartlett, Charles Eckert, Ben Eiseman, George A. Hallenbeck, and William V. McDermott.

I. S. Ravdin, of Philadelphia, was elected President. [It is of some interest that until Ravdin was elected President of the Association in this year, no incumbent of the John Rhea Barton Chair of the University of Pennsylvania since D. Hayes Agnew had held that position. John Rhea Barton, a Pennsylvania alumnus, died in 1871 and the chair was endowed in 1877 by his widow. The successive incumbents were D. Hayes Agnew, 1877-1889; John Ashhurst, Jr. 1889-1900; J. William White, 1900-1910; Edward Martin, 1910-1918; J. B. Deaver, 1918-1822; Eldridge Eliason, 1936-1945; I. S. Ravdin, 1945-1959, now President of the Association, as his successor in the Professorial Chair, Jonathan Rhoads, was also to be. However, Presidents DeForest Willard, Richard H. Harte, and John B. Roberts listed University of Pennsylvania affiliations. Philadelphia, of course, had been the home of the Association in many ways. The College of Physicians of Philadelphia is the repository of the Association's Charter. Samuel D. Gross had long been in Philadelphia when he conceived of and organized the Association, but his school was Jefferson, and the Philadelphians who succeeded in the presidency of the Association were for the most part Jefferson men.]

John D. Stewart, of Buffalo, and Frederick C. Kergin, of Toronto, were elected Vice-President; and William Altemeier, of Cincinnati, Secretary.

LXXVII

1959

The 1959 meeting was held in San Francisco at the Fairmont Hotel, April 15, 16, and 17, President I. S. Ravdin, John Rhea Barton Professor of Surgery, Medical School, University of Pennsylvania; Surgeon-in-Chief, Hospital, University of Pennsylvania, in the Chair. Among those who died in the preceding year had been Daniel C. Elkin, of Atlanta, who was President in 1952, and Lord Alfred Webb-Johnson, the distinguished President of the Royal College of Surgeons, who had been present at the 1958 meeting.

* * *

In early years, Honorary Fellows,- v. Mikulicz, Sir Berkeley Moynihan,- had not rarely spoken before the Association, but none had done so for many years. Now, Sir James Paterson Ross, K.C.V.O., M.S., Professor of Surgery, University of London; Surgeon and Director of Surgical Clinical Unit, St. Bartholomew's Hospital, *The Vascular Complications of Cervical Rib,* emphasized his thoughts about the diagnostic and etiologic factors. Pain in the forearm was common, sometimes spreading proximally, felt on exercise and relieved by rest. It was produced more rapidly if the limb was elevated while being used, ". . . it indicates relative ischemia in active muscles, being strictly comparable with intermittent claudication in the leg." He spoke of coldness and sudden color changes or mottling, "Paresthesia, in the fingers, and numbness of the fingertips are frequent complaints, often erroneously attributed to compression of nerves." Small indolent ulcers were

common, gangrene was rare. It was often impossible to feel a pulse beyond the middle or even the proximal end of the brachial artery and occasionally even the axillary was pulseless. There was no discernible neurological sensory loss. "It is most important to recognize these symptoms and signs as indicating occlusion of the main arteries of the limb; and the sudden onset points to embolism as the cause of the arterial obstruction . . . the clinical histories . . . include several acute episodes indicating the more proximal lodgement of emboli . . ." There was always a systolic bruit over the subclavian artery and frequently a pulsating swelling. At operation, when the scalenus anterior muscle was divided, the second part of the artery was "seen to be greatly narrowed by a bony projection behind it . . . even after the muscle has been cut across the artery is still compressed, apparently as badly as ever. It is essential, therefore, to remove the bone to free the artery." In several patients, the artery, apart from being constricted, felt perfectly normal without suggestion of arteriosclerosis, and yet these patients had had emboli. He discussed the post stenotic dilatation of the artery "very comprehensively explored and clearly expounded by Emile Holman." Clots, he thought, probably formed in the eddies in the post stenotic dilated area. Relief required excision of the cervical rib. The dilated area, even if it was large enough to suggest an aneurysm, should be ignored. Upper thoracic sympathectomy was "essential if the maximal improvement in the circulation to the forearm and hand is to be obtained", particularly if there had

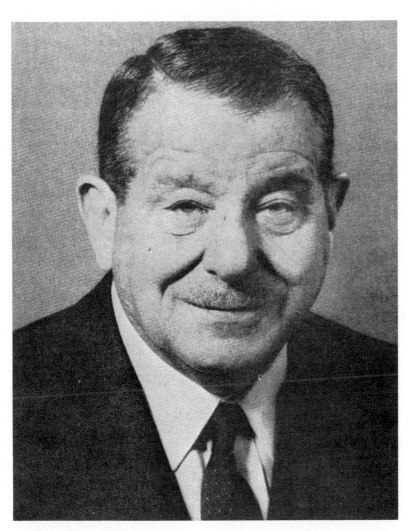

I. S. Ravdin, 1894-1972, President 1959 and of the American College of Surgeons 1960-1961. M.D., University of Pennsylvania 1918, where he spent his entire professional life. An ardent proponent and supporter of the importance of the physiologic and biochemical approach to surgery, he was early placed in charge of the laboratories for surgical research, became Professor of Surgical Research 1928 and Harrison Professor of Surgery in 1935. His early emphasis on the nutrition of the surgical patient led directly, through Rhoads and Dudrick, to total parenteral alimentation. He became John Rhea Barton Professor of Surgery and Chairman of the Department in 1945 when, a Brigadier General, he returned from his legendary service in India. A man of indefatigable energy, he conducted a major surgical practice, closely supervised his large and expanding department, was the strongest voice in the medical school. He was a stimulator of younger men. A short man with a rasping voice he was perceptive, an absolutist and an autocrat in most of his activities, a talented fund raiser, a wise and extraordinarily effective mover in medical affairs, and a major force in American surgery for more than three decades.

been embolic occlusion of the principal vessels. "When the cervical rib is a short pointed structure and there is a fibrous band joining it to the first rib, the lower trunk of the brachial plexus is compressed thereby, and the well known clinical picture of segmental sensory loss and wasting of the small muscles of the hand is the result. But when the cervical rib is a complete one articulating with the first thoracic rib, the brachial plexus comes off one segment higher up and there is no compression of the nerve roots . . . the complete rib presents a bony obstruction to the artery as it curves over the thoracic outlet to reach the neck and axilla . . . vascular and nervous complications of cervical rib do not appear together." Even though the fingers might be ulcerated, the digital vessels were usually intact, the emboli lodging in the radial, ulnar, or brachial arteries.

* * *

Owen H. Wangensteen, of Minneapolis, Professor of Surgery and Surgeon-in-Chief, University of Minnesota Hospitals, and by invitation, Peter A. Salmon, Ward O. Griffen, Jr., James R. S. Paterson, and Farouk Fattah, *Studies of Local Gastric Cooling as Related to Peptic Ulcer,* demonstrated that at the temperature reached with local gastric hypothermia ". . . gastric digestion is virtually suspended . . ." Frogs fed nasal oxygen, while lying in the chilled stomach of a dog for 20 to 36 hours, emerged apparently unharmed and ". . . digestion in all species studied so far, save for fish, suggests quite definitely that, gastric digestion virtually comes to a standstill when the temperature of the gastric mucosa is kept at or below 10° to 14°C." A sharp decrease in gastric blood flow corresponded with decrease in the temperature of the intragastric balloon which was used to produce hypothermia. Since motility of the stomach ceased at temperatures of 29.5°C, it seemed that it might be possible to cool the stomach by irrigating it with cooling fluid without a balloon. In any case, Wangensteen suggested that "direct perfusion of the gastric wall with a cold solution may prove to be an effective agency in the control of gastric hemorrhage. Whether this simpler variant of the balloon-perfusion technic will prove as effective in the control of massive gastric hemorrhage under a variety of conditions remains to be seen . . ." The antrum of a dog brought down to 14° or 15°C. still stimulated secretion in a Heidenhain pouch. With these moderate temperatures gastric secretion of acid and pepsin resumed as soon as the stomach was rewarmed, with what appeared to be a rebound phenomenon. They applied the balloon cooling system to 11 patients

with bleeding duodenal ulcer, three-quarters of whom were in shock, two patients with benign gastric ulcer and five patients with bleeding esophageal varices, two patients with hemorrhagic gastritis and five patients with postoperative bleeding during a complicated postoperative course, shock, sepsis, etc. They controlled the bleeding in all the duodenal ulcers,- one patient died. They had been 100% successful in gastric ulcers. They controlled the bleeding in four of the five patients with esophageal varices although two of them died; controlled the bleeding in both of the patients with gastritis, although one of them died; controlled the bleeding in four of the patients with postoperative stress ulcers, but two of them had died. Some bleeding recurred in those ulcers "ascribed to stress or steroid therapy."

Discussion

The Discussion was opened by Arthur H. Blakemore, of New York, who said that with balloon tamponade they had occasionally saved even profound cirrhotics with jaundice, ascites and massive hemorrhage. Wangensteen had said that balloon tamponade had not worked in his hands and Blakemore's comment was "we have never been able to get the doctors to read the directions in using this nasogastric double-balloon tube." John D. Stewart, of Buffalo, rose to applaud Wangensteen, "His studies show beyond doubt that by local cooling the motility of the stomach can be reduced, the volume flow of blood to the stomach can be lowered, and the rate of digestion of protein substances as well as the rate of secretion of acid pepsin can be slowed." Stewart still thought perhaps the best use of this technique "will be in the preparation of patients who are bleeding rapidly; preparation for more definitive surgical treatment . . ."

* * *

H. William Clatworthy, Jr., and E. Thomas Boles, Jr., by invitation, *Extrahepatic Portal Bed Block in Children: Pathogenesis and Treatment,* presented 11 children with extrahepatic portal obstruction. Four of them were infants presenting with troublesome ascites. The natural progress of the disease was for disappearance of the ascites in a year or two and then the appearance of varices after the passage of another year or two. Hemorrhage then became a risk, but in their experience had never been fatal, and caused relatively little morbidity even when it was large. A variety of procedures were available to buy time before the vessels were large

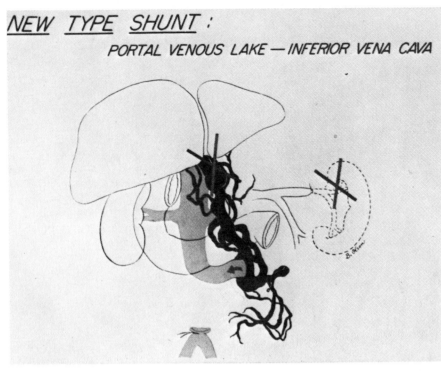

NEW TYPE SHUNT :

PORTAL VENOUS LAKE — INFERIOR VENA CAVA

FIG. 5. Side-to-end superior mesenteric vein-inferior vena cava anastomosis.

The illustration shows ligation of the vena cava and implantation of its cardiac end into the side of the superior mesenteric vein, an operation which Clatworthy had performed four times with success, once in a 10-month-old infant, all of the patients having had unsatisfactory splenic veins so that his preferred, portal end of the splenic vein-to-renal vein shunt which he called central splenorenal shunt, could not be performed.

H. William Clatworthy, Jr., and E. Thomas Boles, Jr., *Extrahepatic Portal Bed Block in Children: Pathogenesis and Treatment,* Volume LXXVII, 1959.

enough to permit a satisfactory portal systemic shunting procedure,- transesophageal ligation of the varices; esophagogastrectomy with jejunal interposition [Merendino, Volume LXXIII, 1955]. Hypersplenism and dangerous hemorrhage rarely occurred before the age of four. Splenorenal shunts, because of the size of the vessels, were rarely successful before the age of 10 or 11. They pointed out the disadvantage of using a long mobilized segment of splenic vein, and the great advantage of using a short stump of vein close to the confluence with the inferior mesenteric vein,- central splenorenal shunt. They had done three such central splenorenal anastomoses in children 11, eight, and four years of age. All lived from 12 to seven months with no further hemorrhage, and with good drops in portal pressure at the time of operation. An eight-year-old boy had had a satisfactory conventional splenorenal shunt and had not bled for three-and-a-half years. In four patients without a satisfactory splenic vein, they had performed a side-to-end superior mesenteric vein to inferior vena cava anastomosis. [Clatworthy 1955]

Two of these children had had previous splenectomies. One of the children was only ten months old at the time of the shunt, the second child was six years old, the third, 15 and the fourth, 13 years old. None of the children had bled since operation although in the 13-year-old child, thrombi were found in the superior mesenteric vein so that it was doubtful that the anastomosis remained open. In sum,- they recommended no operation for ascites, temporizing management for bleeding from varices in early childhood, transesophageal ligation if one was forced, after which proximal gastrectomy and jejunal or colonic interposition. Central splenorenal shunt was the preferred anastomosis and in the absence of an available splenic vein, they resorted to side-to-end superior mesenteric vein to inferior vena cava anastomosis. [No mention was made of Marion's 1954 publication in France, nor of Blakemore's statement, (Volume LXVI, 1948) that he had twice employed mesenteric-caval anastomosis.]

* * *

PORTAL DIVERSION THROUGH LARGE CONNECTING CHANNELS BETWEEN THE PORTAL AND SYSTEMIC CIRCULATIONS

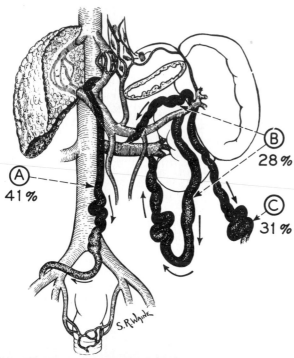

FIG. 2. Diagrammatic presentation of the main types of large channels connecting the portal and systemic circulations. A. Connections between the left intrahepatic branch of the portal vein and the iliac veins. These connections were usually mediated through the paraumbilical and deep epigastric veins. B. Channels emptying into the left renal vein. C. Channels in which the final site of communication with the systemic circulation could not be determined.

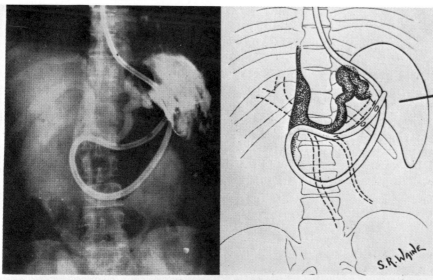

FIG. 8F.

FIG. 8. A group of splenic portograms with accompanying diagrammatic interpretations demonstrating large embryonic channels arising from the portal venous circulation and emptying directly into the systemic circulation via the left renal vein. These are representative films selected from percutaneous serial multiple-exposure splenoportograms of six different patients.

The most startling portion of Rousselot's presentation was the demonstration of numerous splenoportograms graphically showing very large spontaneous variceal anastomoses into systemic vessels, such as these spontaneous anastomoses with the renal vein, without any effect upon portal pressure because, he thought, of the slow flow in collaterals.

Louis M. Rousselot, Augusto H. Moreno, and William F. Panke, *Studies on Portal Hypertension*. IV. The Clinical and Physiopathologic Significance of Self-Established (Nonsurgical) Portal Systemic Venous Shunts, Volume LXXVII, 1959.

The mini-symposium was continued by Louis M. Rousselot, of New York, Professor of Clinical Surgery, New York University College of Medicine; Director of Surgery, St. Vincent's Hospital, and by invitation, Augusto H. Moreno, and William F. Panke, *Studies on Portal Hypertension.* IV. The Clinical and Physiopathologic Significance of Self-Established (Nonsurgical) Portal Systemic Venous Shunts. In 203 patients with portal hypertension, 135 with cirrhosis and 15 with a variety of types of extrahepatic obstruction of the portal system, the remainder without "evidence of pathology in the portal system", Rousselot and his colleagues determined splenic pulp pressures, portal vein pressures, before and after operation. Splenoportograms were made in every case and repeated after operation, often several times. They had demonstrated the wide variety and impressive size of spontaneous portal systemic shunts emphasizing the fact that "Spontaneous diversion of portal blood, either by reversed flow into branches of the portal system or through reopened embryonic channels, was not associated with alleviation of portal hypertension in this series." Although the appearance of esophagogastric varices was accompanied by a decrease in hepatic blood flow, diversion of blood through the varices "did not generally reduce the values of portal tension." Operative shunts produced a decrease in the hepatic blood flow of patients with varices, sharply reduced portal pressure, and abolished backflow into esophagogastric varices or other collaterals, and hemorrhage from varices was prevented.

Discussion

Discussion of the two papers was opened by Edgar J. Poth, of Galveston, who said that on a number of occasions, he had successfully divided the distal esophagus and then reimplanted it into the stomach, for bleeding esophageal varices or "better still, the interposition of a segment of jejunum, and doing a Heineke-Mikulicz pyloroplasty". Roy Cohn, of Palo Alto, California, said that Dr. Rousselot had shown venous anastomoses and "there has been a considerable amount of physiologic evidence for a long time that there are veno-arterial anastomoses in the presence of cirrhosis of the liver." Hearts were larger in cirrhotic patients, without evidence of heart disease, and there was an increased cardiac output. Arterial oxygen saturations were in the eighties. He then demonstrated a splenoportogram, "The injection into the portal bed shows the collateral veins going up and actually filling the pulmonary venous tree, so that because of the unique anatomy in this situation venous blood is able to pour directly into the arterial system, and therefore increase the cardiac output and desaturate the arterial blood." Arthur H. Blakemore, of New York, said that he and Rousselot had puzzled many times over the ineffectiveness of these huge collaterals and "Hunt's speed of blood flow measurements of such portal-systemic venous shunts suggest that it is the slow flow that makes this group of so-called collaterals very inadequate." Of Clatworthy's presentation, he commented that he had been in correspondence with Dr. P. Marion, of Lyons, France, in 1953, who was performing the mesenteric-caval shunts at the time, and that "Dr. Auvert of the Children's Hospital in Paris visited us recently and he brought along for us a beautiful colored movie showing the technic of Dr. Marion and we have started using it." They had done only two. In the first one thrombosis developed in the distal vena cava which had been ligated. In the second one, they sutured over the end of the distal vena cava. He was impressed by the "great efficiency of this type of shunt, considering the wide width of the vena cava in proportion to the superior mesenteric and, as you [Clatworthy] have mentioned, the decompression from both the areas above and below." [He made no mention of his own two pre-1948 cases.] Charles Eckert, of Albany, referred to his St. Louis experience, from 1946 to 1956, with 22 instances of bleeding varices in children. They performed splenorenal anastomosis in six, a superior mesenteric to vena cava shunt in five, splenectomy alone in seven, esophagogastrectomy in three, and no operation in six. There had been no further bleeding in three of the six splenorenal anastomoses, one had bled seriously but had not been reoperated upon and two had been reoperated upon. Of the five patients with mesocaval shunts, four had had no further bleeding, one had to have an esophagogastrectomy for major bleeding. David V. Habif, of New York, advised for those children who might require a partial esophagectomy "that it include at a minimum the lower third of the esophagus." In a group of seven patients with extrahepatic block, who had undergone almost total gastrectomy, five had rebled. He preferred the resection of the lower third of the esophagus, and a jejunal interposition. This had been done in 17 patients, the varices disappearing in all except three, two of whom had rebled and required a more extensive esophagectomy. Clatworthy, closing, said that he, too, had had a child with a jejunal interposition procedure who had bled massively within a year and now understood that further esophagectomy would be required. Rousselot re-emphasized what Blakemore had said, that the varices were under high pressure, but had a very slow flow "one of the reasons for their inability to control hemorrhage."

* * *

W. Dean Warren, by invitation, and William H. Muller, Jr., of Charlottesville, Stephen H. Watts Professor of Surgery, Chairman, Department of Surgery; Surgeon-in-Chief, University of Virginia Hospital, *A Clarification of Some Hemodynamic Changes in Cirrhosis and Their Surgical Significance,* presented the first in a long series of papers which were to come from Warren on portal hypertension [the hemodynamic changes in which have not yet been altogether "clarified"]. In eight cirrhotic patients, they performed extensive hemodynamic studies before, and immediately after side-to-side portacaval shunting, and subsequently. Pressures were measured in the unobstructed portal vein,- free portal vein pressure,- the wedged portal vein pressure, and, on either side of the occluded portal vein,- hepatic occluded portal pressure and peripheral occluded pressure. In all patients, they performed side-to-side portacaval shunts. They concluded that "The overall hemodynamic effect in cirrhosis is a post-sinusoidal outflow obstruction which leads to an elevation in the hepatic sinusoidal pressure. With increasing severity of the obstruction, the sinusoidal pressure may exceed the free portal vein pressure and lead to spontaneous conversion of the portal vein to the outflow tract from the liver. This reversal of flow in the portal vein was found in three of the patients." Six patients studied postoperatively showed normal portal vein pressures, disputing "the theory of significant perfusion of the hepatic sinusoids with portal blood following an adequate decompression of the portal system." Oxygen saturation studies suggested that "The blood leaving the liver via the portal vein has been venous in nature, not excessively saturated" and the hepatic vein oxygen content was normal "indicating sufficient perfusion of that portion of the liver drained by the hepatic venous system." Their own results and those from the literature indicated that a side-to-side shunt was as effective as an end-to-end shunt in lowering pressures, and Warren felt "The beneficial effects of side-to-side shunts are in maintaining this vessel as an outflow conduit and at the same time, increasing the effective pressure across the resistance in the portal bed." The "double-shunt" technique recommended by McDermott, they thought had no advantage. The splenorenal shunt was "similar hemodynamically to the side-to-side portacaval

anastomosis but involves working with a vessel that is often less than optimal size . . . predisposes to thrombosis and may not be large enough to decompress the portal system even though it remains open."

* * *

The symposium was continued by C. Stuart Welch, of Albany, Professor of Surgery, Albany Medical College, and by invitation, Harold F. Welch and John H. Carter, *The Treatment of Ascites by Side to Side Portacaval Shunt.* Welch based his "rationale for using side to side portacaval shunt for the relief of ascites . . . on the peculiar anatomical situation that prevails in the cirrhotic liver . . . It was shown by Herrick in 1907 . . . that there was an increased number of arteriovenous communications in the liver . . . the perfusate of the hepatic artery could be recovered from the portal vein in surprisingly high amounts indicating that retrograde flow could occur through the portal vein. Longmire has subsequently confirmed these findings *in vivo* . . . We have attempted to utilize this retrograde flow in a contrived surgical operation which would permanently decompress the liver. The side to side portacaval shunt allows splanchnic flow to enter the vena cava, diverting this volume flow from the liver. By decompression of the splanchnic system, the chance of esophageal bleeding is also reduced . . . in relation to ascites formation, it allows the arterial pressure to dissipate itself into the low pressure caval system via the naturally occurring intrahepatic arteriovenous shunts and the artificially fashioned portacaval anastomosis . . . the side to side shunt accomplishes arterial pressure reduction within the liver without the disadvantages of hepatic artery ligation." Welch was reporting 14 patients; it was known that 13 of the patients had not reaccumulated ascites. Three of the 14 died immediately after operation and four others had died since from hepatic failure, in each case without reaccumulation of the ascites. Welch pointed out that there were four possible shunts which might be used to take advantage of the physiologic principles as he understood them, all of them leaving the portal vein intact,- side-to-side portacaval shunt, double end-to-side portacaval shunt, the superior mesenteric vein-vena cava shunt of Marion [1954] and an H-portacaval shunt made with a graft, which he thought "should be avoided since closure by thrombosis is a hazard when vein grafts are used." He concluded that the mechanism for the formation of ascites was principally an outflow block and that

"Outflow block can be corrected by establishing a side to side portacaval shunt which provides a new egress from the congested liver via the portal vein to the inferior vena cava . . . Results of the operation have been consistently good."

Discussion

H. W. Scott, Jr., of Nashville, spoke of the work of "Dr. Carl Ekman, of the Department of Surgery of the University of Lund in Sweden, who has been working with us this year at Vanderbilt" and had demonstrated by splenoportogram the existence of reverse portal flow, in six of 85 cases of cirrhosis. Scott showed a splenoportogram with side-to-side anastomosis which he interpreted as showing that all of the injected material bypassed the liver. W. V. McDermott, Jr., of Boston, reported the use of his double shunt procedure [division of the portal vein and implantation of each end into the vena cava]. He had performed the operation 12 times with two immediate deaths. In the ten survivors "the ascites has been totally dissipated in all . . . without recourse to any salt restriction or adjuvant medical therapy of any kind . . ." Charles G. Johnston, of Detroit, had for years believed that the side-to-side shunt was superior and said that as done by Dr. Alfred Large it was actually the easier shunt. He had years before given up operating for ascites alone, and now operated only for bleeding, although "a rather large shunt" would relieve ascites. Robert R. Linton, of Boston, described a young woman who died of liver failure, five weeks after side-to-side anastomosis, with what looked like acute yellow atrophy, which he interpreted as the result of "shunting of not only her portal venous blood, but also her hepatic arterial blood into the inferior vena cava, thereby depriving the liver parenchyma of both its venous and arterial blood supply." He preferred the end-to-side portacaval shunt, "thus instead of permitting reversal of the blood flow in the portal vein, the arterial blood must traverse the liver and go out the hepatic veins." In any case, 80% of his patients could be cleared of ascites by nonoperative measures, others had either end-to-side portacaval shunts or splenorenal shunts with control of their ascites. John L. Madden, of New York, had performed side-to-side shunts in four patients for ascites, all four bled postoperatively, having never bled before, and three of them died of liver failure. Warren, closing, commented on Dr. Eckman's work, indicating that the frequent interpretation by others on splenoportography of thrombosis of the portal vein in cirrhosis might be "simply failure of the dye to get into the portal vein because of reversal of flow in this vessel." With regard to McDermott, Warren had "found no theoretical basis for the superiority of two shunts to decompress this vein, since we have measured the pressure and shown it to be normal after the creation of the side-to-side shunt." Dr. Linton's patient who had what "appeared" to be acute yellow atrophy might in fact actually have had that. Hemodynamically, Warren thought "the splenorenal shunt is very similar . . . to the side-to-side portacaval shunt", but the portacaval shunt provided better decompression of the portal system in the treatment of hemorrhage. He thought the side-to-side shunt would, in fact, relieve ascites in many cases. [This is one of the many times the expurgated, amended and "corrected" discussions are emasculations of the original. The very junior Dean Warren, not yet a Fellow, had begun his discussion by saying with charming effrontery to the much senior Linton, that he had never expected Dr. Linton to have a good word for direct portacaval shunt and Warren was glad that Linton was now beginning to see the light. Linton turned a fiery red, and given his total allopecia, this had a startling effect.] C. Stuart Welch pointed up the interesting fact that a few years ago ascites was considered a contraindication to portacaval shunt and now discussion centered on the technique of the shunt for ascites. As far as patients who had bled were concerned, the results with side-to-side shunt in his hands were as good as with end-to-side shunt. The loss to the liver of hepatic effluent blood in the side-to-side anastomosis did not seem to be harmful clinically in his patients. He had not seen bleeding come on for the first time after side-to-side shunt as Dr. Madden had, and "I don't see why bleeding should occur unless something has happened to the shunt, which, of course, could happen . . ." Welch dismissed the double end-to-side shunt by saying, "I am most pleased to find that Dr. McDermott's results in 10 cases of ascites with double shunts have corroborated our work."

* * *

Blood Transfusions and Serum Hepatitis: Use of Monochloroacetate as an Antibacterial Agent in Plasma, J. Garrott Allen, Professor and Executive, Department of Surgery, Stanford University School of Medicine, and others by invitation, despite the subtitle, centered on the problem of serum hepatitis, the study all having been done at the University of Chicago in the ten years, 1946 through 1956. A statistical sampling technique was employed in the follow-up of 11,382 patients who received blood in the period. Approximately one patient in every 500 receiving transfusion of whole blood and no plasma died of serum hepatitis. The overall mortality for serum hepatitis in their series was 13.9%. The hepatitis attack rate for all patients receiving blood, but not plasma, was 2.31%, but for those receiving blood only from family donors the attack rate was 0.69%, and for those receiving blood from professional donors, the attack rate was 4.13%. If patients received only a single unit of blood, the attack rate for blood from family donors was 0.3% and for blood from professional donors was 3.2%, the overall attack rate being 1.06%. The attack rate increased with the number of units of blood given, up to five units,- after which the mortality of the underlying condition affected the opportunity for the appearance of hepatitis. Thirty-six established cases of serum hepatitis occurred in their randomized 2,388 patient sample, and eight other patients developed jaundice, not certainly due to serum hepatitis. Five of the 36 and two of the eight died. Allen indicated, without emphasizing, that 36.5% of the patients in the sample study had received only a single unit of blood.

Discussion

Paul Hoxworth, of Cincinnati, interpreted Allen's figures as showing that one unit of blood in 127 transmitted hepatitis, whereas in Cincinnati one unit of blood in 386 transmitted hepatitis,- "Allen's attack rate is 2.3% and ours is 0.56." There were no paid donors in the Cincinnati study and the incidence of hepatitis from Allen's family donors was essentially that of Hoxworth's series. "The higher incidence rate, as Dr. Allen has shown, is apparently due to the use of the paid donor. The purchase of blood at low rates attracts many alcoholics or other unfortunates who return every eight to ten weeks and who know that they will not get the money if they answer 'Yes' to questions not only about jaundice but malaria and other infectious diseases. Blood banks should pay donors only after exhausting other methods of recruitment, and only then from controlled groups whose medical history is known before they volunteer . . . Another way for reducing disease transmitted in transfusions is by avoiding unnecessary transfusions . . . as in Allen's series, in our institution thirty to forty per cent of the total volume of transfusions is now being given in single-unit transfusions, most of which are probably unnecessary." Frank B. Berry, Assistant Secretary of Defense, commented from the national defense standpoint on the need for preparation of plasma by long-time storage or by heat treatment, "The objection we have heard to the long-term storage at room temperature of plasma is that it takes so long. Well, of course it will take long unless one starts it. Once started, the supply will increase. The heat-treated plasma is probably not as good . . . both have been accepted now by the National Research Council." He referred to the preservation of blood "by Dr. Merriman, assisted by the Linde Corporation, in which whole blood is drawn and promptly sprayed into liquid nitrogen and can be preserved indefinitely . . . preserved by storage in liquid nitrogen", and referred also to "The Cohn method of fractionation . . . now in routine use at the Naval Hospital at Chelsea . . .", in which program the practice was that "only the preserved red cells would be used for transfusions unless fresh blood were absolutely required", the plasma being used separately. "From the military standpoint, we are trying to encourage the formation of blood centers, four or five throughout the country, in the different services, but so far we have found that inertia is a very powerful force." Lieutenant Colonel H. F. Hamit, U.S.M.C., commented that the Navy's blood preservation program entailed "deep-freezing and a lot of heavy equipment and, taken in terms of mobility and field operations, we sometimes question the practicality of this method for our particular service." The army was trying to find a chemical additive for blood which would increase its usefulness beyond 21 days and emphasized the use of plasma to avoid the one-unit blood transfusion.

* * *

J. Englebert Dunphy, of Portland, Mackenzie Professor of Surgery and Head of the Department, University of Oregon Medical School, and by invitation, W. B. Patterson and M. A. Legg, *Etiologic Factors in Polyposis and Carcinoma of the Colon,* returned to the subject introduced by Ian Todd at the meeting in 1956 in the Discussion of Ravitch's comments about polyposis, that there might be "some agent, completely unknown that tends to make the polyps grow in the rectum and in the colon, and that having removed the greater part of this organ in some people, they will lose the tendency to form polyps." Dunphy commented on the occasional experience that, at the second operation of the two-stage procedure for carcinoma of the colon, the tumor mass was found to have been sharply diminished, usually attributed to "inflammation", but asked whether this might not, in fact, have been "a temporary regression in growth." He cited a remarkable example of that kind in which, two months after colostomy, the previously histologically confirmed carcinoma of the rectum had so regressed that no identifiable cancer was found on microscopic examination and the patient did well for years. Dunphy found two similar cases in the literature. In polyposis, he found reported cases of disappearance of the polyps distal to the anastomosis after subtotal colectomy and showed a decrease in the number of polyps in a patient of his own. Dunphy asked whether there might not "be a factor which leads to polyposis and carcinogenesis . . . either produced by the mucosa of the colon or activated by it, and . . . removed or deactivated by diversion of the fecal stream and partial or subtotal colectomy?" If so, diversion of the fecal stream by colostomy might have a specific value in preparing the patient for operation. He raised the question, "Is the greater frequency of carcinomatous implantation at the suture line in recent years attributable in part to the fact that, with improved methods of preparing the bowel, preliminary colostomy is seldom used today?"

Discussion

Jay L. Ankeney, of Cleveland, "on behalf of Drs. William Holden and Jack Cole, of the Western Reserve Department of Surgery" mentioned their "two interesting cases of disappearing polyps following subtotal colectomy with ileoproctostomy". Their proposal was that "Perhaps the ileum and the ileal contents play some part in preventing the formation of polyps, since the ascending colon in these patients contained very few polyps. Perhaps the ileal contents bathing the rectum after colectomy account for the disappearance of these tumors . . . perhaps the colon stimulates the formation of polyps in the rectum and the removal of this organ . . . removes this stimulus and therefore polyps disappear." James D. Hardy, of Jackson, Mississippi, mentioned a case of disappearance of residual polyps following ileoproctostomy. President Ravdin commented that he had had two patients whose polyps had disappeared after ileoproctostomy. William A. Altemeier, of Cincinnati, cited four patients with carcinoma of the rectum who had survived for long periods of time in the face of incomplete removal of the tumor, in all of whom, there had been massive infection and high fever. Dunphy, in closing, said that infection had been a feature in other of the cases of regression.

* * *

In the Discussion the year before, H. William Scott had referred to the Vanderbilt series of patients with vagotomy and antrectomy for duodenal ulcer, and now J. Lynwood Herrington, Jr., L. W. Edwards, Kenneth L. Classen, Robert I. Carlson, and William H. Edwards, all by invitation, and H. William Scott, Jr., of Nashville, Professor of Surgery and Head of Department of Surgery, Vanderbilt University School of Medicine; Surgeon-in-Chief, Vanderbilt University Hospital, *Vagotomy and Antral Resection in the Treatment of Duodenal Ulcer:* Results in 514 Patients, reported their experience in detail. Vagotomy, Dragstedt had shown, abolished the fasting continuous secretion of gastric juice. The original postulate of Edkins [1906] "that a gastric secretory hormone is liberated from the mucosa of the gastric antrum in response to the presence of food" had been amply confirmed and reinforced. Removal of the antrum seemed to remove the source of gastrin, the gastric secretory hormone, "thus making it unnecessary to sacrifice a portion of the body or fundus of the stomach". In animal experiments the combination of vagotomy and antral resection gave maximal protection against ulcerogenic procedures. The Vanderbilt group had performed vagotomy and antral resection for duodenal ulcer in 680 patients from January of 1947 through December of 1958 and were now analyzing the 565 patients operated through December of 1957. There were 18 deaths, for a mortality of 3.1%, and if the patients operated upon for massive hemorrhage were excluded, the mortality otherwise was 1.7%. None of the 18 patients who died subsequently had symptoms of ulcer at the time of death. 514 patients, 97% of the total survivors, were available for follow-up. Pain was the major indication for operation, 53%; hemorrhage, 30%; obstruction, 15%; and perforation, 1.4%. The 3.1% mortality included poor-risk patients with obstruction, massive bleeding, or coexistent systemic disease and the mortality was no different on the ward service than on the private services. Eight of the 18 deaths were in patients operated upon for control of massive hemorrhage, six dying of cardiac or pulmonary complications, one of pancreatitis and one of bleeding diathesis. Five deaths were in elderly patients operated upon for obstruction, three of these died of pre-existing cardiorenal disease, one of pulmonary embolism and one of stomal obstruction with electrolyte imbalance. A leaking duodenal stump was responsible for a single death, and another patient died with a subdiaphragmatic abscess. Six percent of the Billroth I patients and 4% of the Billroth II patients had delayed gastric emptying and six of the 11 such Billroth I patients required reoperation, whereas only two of 13 Billroth II patients required reoperation. There were two nonfatal leaks, one from a gastrojejunostomy and one from a gastroduodenostomy. The overall results were excellent in 62%, good in 30%. There was one recurrent ulcer in the Billroth I patients and one among the Billroth II patients,- a total recurrence rate of 0.38%. The overall good results were about the same with Billroth I and Billroth II, but not a single patient with a Billroth I reconstruction had severe dumping. Excessive weight loss was rare in both groups, presumably because of the limited gastrectomy. Billroth I patients lost somewhat less weight than Billroth II patients.

Discussion

Keith S. Grimson, of Durham, North Carolina, commented on his series of 276 patients operated upon for duodenal ulcer by vagotomy and gastroenterostomy since 1944, with one death, a one-half of one percent mortality. There had been recurrent ulcers in 4%. Stanley O. Hoerr, of Cleveland, in 100 patients with vagotomy and hemigastrectomy followed one to six years, had had a single marginal ulcer. His mortality was 2% for vagotomy and hemigastrectomy; when he did vagotomy with a drainage procedure, it was less than one-half of one percent. A survey in the state of Ohio showed "Mortality for procedures involving resection was 4.9%; for procedures involving drainage procedures without resection, 1.7%, a threefold difference." In 100 personal patients with vagotomy and posterior gastroenterostomy, he had 90% good clinical results, the same as in his 100 patients with vagotomy and hemigastrectomy. The 12 patients who had not been controlled by vagotomy and gastroenterostomy had been reoperated upon, "These twelve patients are just as happy as if they had had a primary gastric resection, and several of them are living that might be dead if I had performed gastric resection for every one of this group." He asked "should the mortality of elective operations for chronic duodenal ulcer exceed that of elective cholecystectomy for gall stones? . . . should we hesitate to advise a safe operation which may require secondary gastric resection in 5% or less of patients?" Jack M. Farris, of Los Angeles, who had been performing vagotomy with one or another gastric operation since 1945, said that vagotomy with gastrectomy and a Billroth I or Billroth II reconstruction, or with gastroenterostomy, or pyloroplasty gave essentially the same results from the

standpoint of recurrence. Since the recurrent ulceration with vagotomy and drainage procedure was only 2%, he could not feel that antrectomy was "necessary in the vast majority of patients . . . at the present time our operation of choice is vagotomy combined with pyloroplasty, reserving more formidable operations for the occasional patient in which this operation has failed." He reported the results of Dr. Joseph Weinberg from the Veterans Hospital, in Long Beach, 850 cases of pyloroplasty and vagotomy, mortality 0.3% ". . . I am sure that most of us agree that it is better to be dyspeptic and alive than to submit to a formidable operation which in the light of present knowledge has no greater (and perhaps lesser) chance of curing one's ulcer diathesis. The incidence of recurrence in Dr. Weinberg's cases is 5% . . ." Farris emphasized the necessity for a careful and complete vagotomy and a nonobstructing pyloroplasty. Robert M. Zollinger, of Columbus, Ohio, rose "to support the operation of vagotomy-antrectomy, combined with the Billroth I type of anastomosis." In 100 patients carefully followed, 95% considered the results excellent, but only 55% had reached ideal weight. J. E. Strode, of Honolulu, said that hemigastrectomy and vagotomy had given good results and he intended to continue doing it. H. William Scott, Jr., closing, thought the effectiveness of vagotomy and antral resection in controlling the ulcer diathesis had been demonstrated although "the role of the antrum in the genesis of peptic ulceration and the role of the antrum in surgical treatment of duodenal ulcer" were still subjects of controversy. Drs. Dragstedt, Grimson, Hoerr, Wangensteen, and others preferred saving the antrum, and Scott and those of like mind tended to resect it. He agreed that their mortality was too high, as pointed out in the Discusion, but reminded the Fellows that 30% of the patients in the Vanderbilt series had been operated upon for bleeding. He concluded by emphasizing the fact that all of the operations involved "either bypass or deliberate obliteration of the functional integrity of the pylorus. Once this is done, then our work and that of Dr. Randall and others indicate that all such individuals are potential dumpers and should follow an anti-dumping dietary regimen".

* * *

The age of organ transplantation had obviously been entered and Richard C. Lillehei, Bernard Goott, and Fletcher A. Miller, all by invitation, *The Physiological Response of the Small Bowel of the Dog to Ischemia Including Prolonged In Vitro Preserva-*

tion of the Bowel with Successful Replacement and Survival, demonstrated that in the process of excision and replantation "The majority of adult mongrel dogs tolerated up to 3.5 hours of superior mesenteric arterial occlusion if the collateral circulation to the small bowel was not disturbed", but died if the collateral circulation was occluded as well, for that period. The bowel tolerated occlusion of all circulation for two hours at 25° to 28° C. and for five hours at 5° C. If the bowel was resected and held *in vitro,* it could be kept for two hours at room temperature and successfully replaced, and if cooled to 5° C. would survive if replaced after up to five hours. The animals appeared to do well indefinitely. The divided lymphatics apparently were rapidly reconstituted, the stools were normal within 10 days and there was no evidence of impaired fat absorption. Eight dogs received homograft bowel either stored for two hours at room temperature or four to five hours at 5° C. Edema of the reanastomosed bowel was much more striking than in the autograft experiments. "Yet, the bowel was viable and functioned for periods up to seven days . . . at autopsy the homografted bowel appeared grossly and microscopically normal. The cause of death in each case could be attributed to other causes . . . we do not think that we have yet reached the true rejection . . ."

Discussion

Owen H. Wangensteen, of Minneapolis, commented "It occurs to me that Dr. Lillehei and his associates will presently address themselves to employment of shorter segments of bowel, establishing the vascular connections, making the intestinal anastomoses at a later date. There may be less risk of loss of the homograft for the recipient if the homograft transplant is done in this manner." J. Englebert Dunphy, said that "There is no doubt that cooling permits one to leave an organ, even a whole organ, a heart or a kidney, outside the body for an appreciably longer period of time than would otherwise be possible. We have brought hearts by a combination of dehydration and cooling to a -8° C. and find that when they are rewarmed and transplanted they resume a normal beat."

* * *

V. L. Willman, by invitation, and C. Rollins Hanlon, of St. Louis, Professor of Surgery and Director, Department of Surgery, St. Louis University; Surgeon-in-Chief, St. Louis University Hospitals, *Safer Operation in Aortic Saddle Embolism:* Four Consecutive Successful Embolectomies via the Femoral Arteries under Local Anesthesia, reported successful use of the technique which Ravdin had presented before the Association in 1941, although most reports emphasized the importance of a transabdominal or at least a retroperitoneal abdominal approach to the aorta. They recommended bilateral groin incisions, distal injection of heparin and application of vascular clamps distally to the femoral arteries, inserting a large thin-walled catheter proximally with a glass T-arm to allow inspection of the return and to permit venting of the artery without suction. It was sometimes necessary to aspirate first on one side and then on the other.

Discussion

James Alastair Key, of Toronto, said they had been using this technique for a number of years with instruments made by Dr. [Ray] Heimbecker, who had used that method in 15 patients, 14 of them under local anesthesia. The operation was immediately successful in all 15, one died of cardiac failure, four ultimately died of systemic emboli. A possible problem was arteriosclerosis constricting the common or external iliac vessels. Elliott S. Hurwitt, of New York, said his last three saddle embolectomies, done transabdominally, had all been successful, two of them occurring following the closure of the chest after mitral commissurotomy. The third patient entered the hospital with mitral stenosis and fibrillation, had a successful embolectomy, a week later had another embolectomy and on this occasion had a mitral commissurotomy followed by successful embolectomy. Harris B. Shumacker, Jr., of Indianapolis, had successfully operated upon seven saddle emboli, transabdominally, in the last ten years; in two of his patients, the embolism occurred during mitral valvotomy, and in two patients, mitral valvotomy was done in the presence of saddle embolism and the embolectomy performed immediately afterward. President Ravdin said only that "I personally am delighted to hear this paper. The patient I reported was a patient who had coronary infarction." V. L. Willman, closing, said that in many patients whose mitral lesions were not amenable to operable correction, prevention of the reformation of the clot and repeated embolism required heparin which he would prefer not to administer after transabdominal or retroperitoneal operation. Obviously, many patients could indeed tolerate general anesthesia and laparotomy for embolectomy, but there was no need to test them.

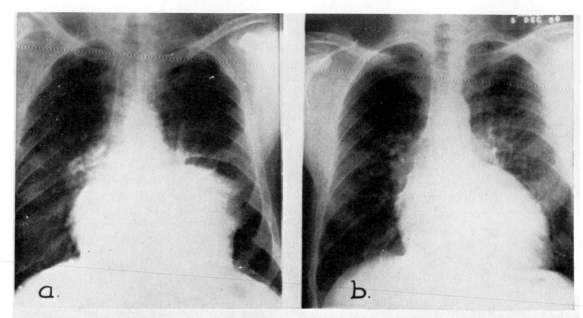

FIG. 2. Roentgenograms of chest in Case 2 made before operation (a) and five months after operation (b) showing improved cardiac contour and reduction in cardiac size. Patient had excellent improvement in cardiac function demonstrated clinically and by cardiac catheterization.

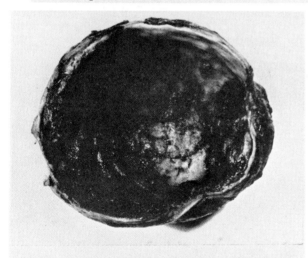

FIG. 3. Specimen of aneurysm of left ventricle removed intact in Case 2. Sac is composed predominantly of fibrous tissue and is partly lined by organizing and laminated thrombus. Note size of aneurysm in relation to 1.0 centimeter scale.

* * *

Denton A. Cooley, of Houston, Associate Professor of Surgery, Baylor University College of Medicine, and by invitation, Walter S. Henly, Kamel H. Amad, and Don W. Chapman, *Ventricular Aneurysm following Myocardial Infarction:* Results of Surgical Treatment, presented a series of six such opera-

As Cooley said, Gordon Murray in 1947 (Vol. LXV, p. ▲ 902) had shown in dogs the effectiveness of resection of infarcted myocardium, and Charles Bailey, by 1958, had five survivors out of six, in patients with left ventricular aneurysm, simply sutured and excised—Murray's original proposal. Cooley, under cardiopulmonary bypass, now had resected six left ventricular aneurysms, with survival and improvement in all, and in a footnote he added two more successes and two deaths. He favored operation some months after infarction when the scarred myocardium could be expected to hold sutures. In the Discussion, K. A. Merendino, of Seattle and J. Y. Templeton, III, of Philadelphia, mentioned their own successes with ventricular aneurysm resection under cardiopulmonary bypass.

Denton A. Cooley, Walter S. Henly, Kamel H. Amad, Don W. Chapman, *Ventricular Aneurysm following Myocardial Infarction:* Results of Surgical Treatment, Volume LXXVII, 1959. (Figure continues on facing page.)

tions using a pump oxygenator and cardiopulmonary bypass. The six patients were operated upon two-and-a-half months to ten years after their original infarction, were aged 45 to 57, all survived, four were working and two were listed as retired but active, although, with one exception, "all patients were severely handicapped and completely incapacitated

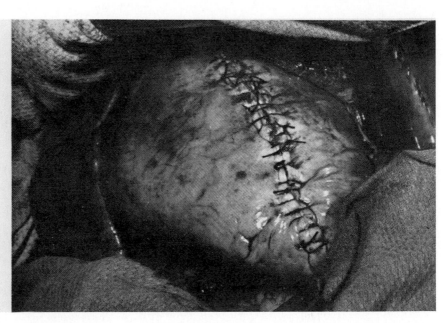

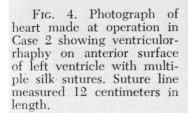

FIG. 4. Photograph of heart made at operation in Case 2 showing ventriculorrhaphy on anterior surface of left ventricle with multiple silk sutures. Suture line measured 12 centimeters in length.

from work prior to operation". They reviewed the literature of the knowledge of ventricular aneurysms, most of which followed myocardial infarction and most of which involved the left ventricle. In a collected series of cases, 73% of patients with cardiac aneurysms died within three years and 88% died within five years. The cause of death was usually congestive heart failure and not rupture of the aneurysm. Beck, in 1944, had attempted to reinforce an aneurysm with pericardium and a fascia lata graft, unsuccessfully, and Murray, three years later [Volume LXV, 1947] had reported the creation and resection of experimental myocardial infarcts with resultant improvement in cardiac output. Bailey, in 1958, had reported surgical excision of ventricular aneurysms without bypass in six patients, with five survivors. De Camp, in 1956, had similarly operated without cardiopulmonary bypass in a patient who died of hemorrhage eight days after operation. Cooley's first patient had been reported in the *JAMA* the year before and he reported verbal communication from C. W. Lillehei of a successful case also operated upon with cardiopulmonary bypass. Whereas Gordon Murray had advocated immediate resection of the infarction, Cooley said that resection "may be feasible after a delay of approximately three months. During this period sufficient scarring and fibrosis occurred with possible recovery of function of the surrounding myocardium to make the procedure feasible. [Gordon Murray was not present at the meeting.] Whether or not a similar operation would be possible on patients less than one month following the acute episode is somewhat doubtful." An addendum indicates that four more operations had been performed, between the time of the meeting and the time the galleys were received, with two deaths, in patients, both 63 years of age who had severe right and left coronary disease.

Discussion

K. Alvin Merendino, of Seattle, in his first 100 pump oxygenator cases had resected aneurysms in two patients, both of whom did very well and were very stable after operation, one patient, six weeks after his infarction, one long after. Cooley had shown a motion picture and Merendino commented that opening and separating the pericardium from the heart was inadvisable, since any collateral circulation to these hearts might be useful, so that, "the incision is made directly into the aneurysm without freeing the pericardium. Thus the pericardium is excised with the ventricular aneurysm; one has not devascularized the edges, and you also have the pericardium available for suture." John Y. Templeton, III, of Philadelphia, said they had operated upon three patients with post-infarctional left ventricular aneurysm under cardiopulmonary bypass. All three did well and were much more fit than before operation. Frank Gerbode, of San Francisco, agreed "that operating upon the relaxed heart, under extracorporeal circulation, is much better from the point of view of suturing than when it is full." Cooley and Merendino had emphasized the importance of preventing systemic embolism from the aneurysm and Gerbode agreed. Cooley, closing, thought that

Merendino's suggestion of using the pericardium in closure, which was somewhat analogous to Claude Beck's operation, might restrict the motion of the left ventricle. He agreed that intermittent occlusion of the ascending aorta was important to minimize the danger of embolism. His final casual sentence was that, "Our experience with pump oxygenator bypass numbers more than 600 cases, and we now recognize no lesions in which potassium arrest or other cardioplegics are needed."

* * *

Arthur D. Boyd, Richard E. Tremblay, and Frank C. Spencer, all by invitation, and Henry T. Bahnson, of Baltimore, Associate Professor of Surgery, Johns Hopkins University, *Estimation of Cardiac Output Soon after Intracardiac Surgery with Cardiopulmonary Bypass,* stated that among the problems which they had seen after intracardiac surgery with cardiopulmonary bypass were "metabolic acidosis, unexplained hypotension or tachycardia, cardiac failure, respiratory insufficiency, and even 'sudden death.'" A variety of explanations had been given for these states "including low flow during bypass, oxygen poisoning, pyrogens, air embolism, and pulmonary engorgement . . ." To see whether it might be the "activity of the heart as a pump in the critical period of several days after bypass" which was at fault, they reported "arterial and mixed venous oxygen saturation, oxygen consumption, cardiac output, and intracardiac and vascular pressures after bypass" in 34 patients, among the 65 undergoing intracardiac surgery between July, 1958 and March, 1959, tending to conduct the study on the sicker patients. They found a close correlation "between the volume of cardiac output and the clinical course of patients . . . In addition, measurement of cardiac output, or, more frequently, measurement of the oxygen saturation of mixed venous blood . . . often gave a clue to an inadequate circulatory status which was not evident by other signs." Postoperative pressures and sampling were through fine polyvinyl catheters placed in the pulmonary artery, left atrium, and femoral artery, at operation and simply withdrawn one to four days after operation. No complications resulted from the use of the catheters. Patients, who had a cardiac index above 2.4 liters and a venous oxygen saturation above 60%, had no cardiovascular complications in the first nine days. Of 15 patients with cardiac index of less than 2 liters per minute per M^2, ten died. In four of the 15 patients, there was an anatomic explanation for the low cardiac output. The so-called "sudden death" or "postperfusion" syndrome described in the literature was only seen in the patients with low cardiac outputs, and "Although the terminal event may have occurred abruptly and prior to this the usual clinical signs may have shown little change, a low cardiac output was always present for many hours before death." Five of the patients had a significant arterial unsaturation and in them "there were no clinical signs of anoxia . . . if blood oxygen studies had not been done routinely the arterial unsaturation would not have been recognized." In one such patient, tracheotomy and inhalation by respirator gave relief. "Measurement and replacement of blood volume, correction of acidosis with sodium bicarbonate, of respiratory insufficiency with tracheotomy and a respirator, digitalization, restriction of fluid intake, diuretics, control of fever—all have been used when indicated." They concluded that ". . . measurement of cardiac output, or its most important denominator, the mixed venous oxygen content, showed a decrease some hours before the low output was evident by clinical signs alone . . . The so-called 'sudden death syndrome' reported after cardiopulmonary bypass was seen in this series to be invariably preceded by a period of low cardiac output."

Discussion

John H. Gibbon, Jr., of Philadelphia, opened the Discussion, congratulating the authors,- "I believe this represents the first study of cardiac output in such patients postoperatively". He wondered whether the dye dilution technique, which he had used intraoperatively, might not be simpler. C. Rollins Hanlon, of St. Louis, had thought "some deaths after operations done under cardiopulmonary bypass are due to myocardial insufficiency brought about by prolonged cardiac arrest. We have used potassium cardioplegia, as have others, and we have gradually minimized its use on the basis of experimental observations which have been made by Dr. [Theodore] Cooper and by Dr. [Vallee] Willman in our laboratory." Reducing the temperature of a dog's heart to 28° C. permitted him to tolerate cardiac arrest for 30 minutes with less effect than from the same period of arrest in the normothermic animal. Prophylactic digitalization mitigated but did not avoid "the deleterious effects of 30 minutes of cardiac arrest in the dog". They now avoided cardiac arrest as far as possible, minimized the duration when they did have to employ it, and digitalized the patient in advance if they suspected cardioplegia might be necessary. Frank C. Spencer, in closing, said to Gibbon that they had considered using the dye dilution technique for determining cardiac output "although at the present time measuring the oxygen saturation from the pulmonary artery seems to be about as good an indicator as the cardiac output itself." As far as the harmful effect of arrest was concerned, they had wondered whether it might actually be due to the potassium but there had been no correlation between cardiac output and the use or non-use of potassium in their studies. "Nevertheless, like most workers in the field, we have gradually worked away from potassium and now almost never use it, using instead intermittent occlusion of the aorta from three to five minutes . . ." They felt digitalis was important and had been concerned about how much of it might be "bled into the pump". They usually digitalized the patients immediately after the operation.

* * *

Will C. Sealy, of Durham, Professor of Thoracic Surgery, Duke University; Ivan W. Brown, Jr., Associate Professor of Surgery, Duke University School of Medicine, and by invitation, W. Glenn Young, W. W. Smith, and A. M. Lesage, *Hypothermia and Extracorporeal Circulation for Open Heart Surgery:* Its Simplification with a Heat Exchanger for Rapid Cooling and Rewarming, described the clinical use of the in-line blood heat exchanger which Brown, Emmons, and Smith had described from Duke in 1957. The cylindrical heat exchangers were in the perfusion line, with jackets in which hot or cold or ice water could be circulated, and for extremely low temperatures two heat exchangers could be placed in series. They reported 95 cardiac operations under hypothermia with the heat exchanger with 16 deaths,- none in 23 atrial septal defects, three in 19 ventricular defects, four in 19 cases of tetralogy of Fallot, none in four cases of pulmonic stenosis, etc. Ventricular fibrillation occurred in 15 cases, with spontaneous reversion in eight and successful electrical reversion in the remaining seven. In patients cooled to below 20°, all electrical activity in the brain disappeared. With hypothermia at 28°-31° venous oxygen saturation remained at normal levels even with low perfusion rates, and metabolic acidosis was prevented. In seven patients, they had carried hypothermia down to profound levels, from 9° to 20° C. Three of these patients died and "the cause of death was obvious in all three and did not result from the hypothermia". There were no complications from the hypothermia in the surviving patients and they suggested the use of profound hypothermia for the more complex defects.

Discussion

Henry Swan, of Denver, also had been using hypothermia by perfusion. He said that under hypothermia, it was difficult to know exactly at what level the venous oxygen should be kept. He monitored arterial PO_2 and venous PO_2 constantly and thought the venous PO_2 should be at 70 to 75 and the A-V oxygen difference 4 to 6. Sealy, in closing, said they aimed to keep the venous oxygen saturations above 70% and rarely saw it between 60 and 70.

* * *

Bernard Zimmermann, of St. Paul, Associate Professor of Surgery, University of Minnesota, and by invitation, Walter H. Moran, Jr., J. C. Rosenberg, B. J. Kennedy, and Richard J. Frey, *Physiologic and Surgical Problems in the Management of Primary Aldosteronism,* presented five patients with the syndrome described by Conn in 1955 of "hypertension, hypokalemia, and metabolic alkalosis associated with excessive production of a mineral-regulating steroid of adrenal origin." Reichstein had identified aldosterone in 1953. In most of the reported cases, there had been a benign cortical adenoma, "non-neoplastic hyperfunction with or without gross or microscopic evidence of hyperplasia" accounted for other cases, and there were a few cases of adrenal carcinoma. They operated on four of their patients, the first of whom died of cardiac arrest on the day after operation, two patients survived operation for an adenoma, one survived operation for hyperplasia and all three were well. One patient had refused operation. Two of the patients had benign tumors and one had a carcinoma. ACTH in two of their patients caused a striking elevation of aldosterone excretion and one of these was the patient with a malignant tumor, so that ACTH could not be used to differentiate hyperplasia from tumor. In two out of three patients, addition of potassium to the diet caused an increase in aldosterone output. Nevertheless, it was "possible to produce positive potassium balance in these patients with quite rapid reversal of alkalosis, hypokalemia and electrocardiographic changes." Since the tumors might be quite small, transabdominal exploration was advised, and "Because of the possibility of incompletely restored potassium balance, curare-like drugs should not be used in conjunction with anesthesia."

Discussion

Victor Richards, of San Francisco, had operated on three of the four patients he had seen, each of whom had an adenoma. Dr. [John] Luetscher, in the Department of Medicine, had incubated slices of the tumors and these produced aldosterone in large quantities. Oliver Cope, of Boston, said that the tumors ought to respond to physiologic stimulation, ". . . these tumors are well differentiated, otherwise they wouldn't be hypersecreting. That being so they ought to respond", and he warned against loading with "chosen electrolytes. These patients, as I see them, have low serum potassiums because they have too much hormone, not too little electrolytes." Zimmermann, closing, said they had done some incubation of tumor slices with variable results. To Cope, he said "The matter of autonomy of these tumors and of hyperfunctioning adrenal states is, of course . . . variable and I am sure no generalizations can be made . . . In the matter of loading—I simply feel it is hazardous and unnecessary to operate on patients with hypokalemic alkalosis . . . The metabolic status can be restored in a relatively gradual way, and we feel that this should be done."

The Business Meetings

The 1959 meeting was held April 15, 16, and 17, at the Fairmont Hotel, San Francisco, I. S. Ravdin presiding.

The Treasurer announced that there would be a deficit of $3500 to $4500 owing to the fact that the banquet and luncheons at the Waldorf, at the New York meeting the previous year, had cost more than $3000 in excess of receipts.

Richard Varco reported for the Program Committee that in response to several dozen personal calls from himself and from Dr. Ravdin, a total of 98 abstracts had been received, only 22 of them having been received by the date of the deadline. Once more the Chairman of the Committee on Arrangements, Carleton Mathewson, Jr., said "Arrangements have been made for a cocktail party for members and their wives in the Nob Hill Room at 6:30 p.m. on Thursday, April 16. The By-Laws of this organization provide that this cocktail party is to be held exclusively for the members and wives . . . Immediately following the cocktail party on Thursday, April 16, the men's dinner will be held in the Gold Room, which is adjacent to the Nob Hill Room. The men's dinner is restricted to members of the Association . . ."

Frederick A. Coller was now getting a good deal more information from the various Blue Shield organizations and could say that "In the Atlantic Seaboard States the majority of the operations were performed by trained surgeons. The greater the magnitude of the operation, the greater the percentage performed by trained surgeons. In the predominantly rural population of the plains states having few cities and many small communities with small hospitals, a lesser per cent of operations were performed by trained surgeons, although, here too, we find that operations of greater magnitude are performed largely by this group. California, Pennsylvania and Michigan have the largest number of osteopaths so the information on their surgical activities is not available, but in Michigan and to a lesser extent in Pennsylvania, they perform an astonishingly large number, usually in their own hospitals which are small and not well equipped. In many states they cannot practice and in others they cannot perform operations; therefore, they are not generally a surgical problem. That they practice surgery at all is the responsibility of the legislators who write laws and the people who elect the legislators." As before it was Coller's feeling that such unnecessary operations as were done were being done in hospitals where there were no provisions for checking, inspection, medical audit and tissue committees, etc.

Among the recommendations of the Council was one that henceforth a registration fee be charged to all active and senior members at each annual meeting, which was accepted. An additional item proposed by Council was placed on the ballot for the election of new members so that there would be a written vote, which was ". . . whether or not wives, and distinguished invited guests and their wives, be permitted to attend future banquets. This is a matter which has been passed on to you", Dr. Ravdin said, "by Council without any recommendation. Numerous individuals have brought this to the attention of Council and a special ballot form has been provided for you to indicate your preference. Perhaps . . . one or another of the Fellows might wish to discuss this recommendation." Dr. Naffziger, was the first, and was recorded as saying that he thought ". . . there are many ladies who have felt embarrassment over being required to leave the cocktail party and not being able to attend the banquet. I think they have good reasons for such comments. I am not in favor of changing our tradition, however. This scheme has been in existence for a long time. Perhaps this is not enough reason to continue it, but there are no other social occasions in which the men get together. The opportunities for them to get together at tables and talk amongst themselves are infrequent, and I think it would be unwise to change our tradition. I do think that some provisions ought to be made for the ladies. We ought to see to it that some provisions for dinner and entertainment be made for them after the cocktail party other than inviting them to the annual banquet." Dr. Edward D. Churchill was recorded as saying "Knowing that it cannot possibly influence any vote, as they have already been cast, I feel very free to comment. One of the first duties ever given me by the American Surgical Association was to serve as a junior member on a Committee, of which Dr. Eugene Pool of New York was Chairman, whose obligation it was to reset the course of the American Surgical Association. The older members at that time felt that this Association had become entirely too social; in fact, it was so social that the first local caucus I ever attended in Boston was discussing whether the wives of candidates would fit in properly to the social milieu of the American Surgical Association. I just bring up those two historical points, hoping that the membership considers those aspects in casting their votes."

[The Fellows recall the discussion clearly, but not all identically.]

Owen H. Wangensteen, February 28, 1979. "Churchill, as I recall it, was one of the members of the committee who insisted that the Association was not to be a Club; that a Dinner should be delimited to men and that scientific papers and business should be the sole concern of the membership and the *Transactions*.

"In subsequent years I saw both Mary and Pete Churchill at such gatherings but I was never bold enough to ask him concerning the whyfore of his prior position of totally excluding wives from the sessions of the Association.

"On this score, Mark, I believe women have been discriminated against. Sally tells me that when she began attending sessions she frequently saw at the hotel or meeting place many a young lady, whose husband had just been elected to membership, neglected and crying in a corner. It is a problem for young wives, yet I do believe they should be encouraged to come, a view that Sally too strongly supports. Actually, a few years ago, she wrote Jim Maloney during his term as Secretary in the matter of the neglect of young wives. He took Sally's plea to the Council and they did finally establish a coffee hour. There is still much room for improvement on this score."

Loyal Davis, March 3, 1978. "The annual dinners were stag affairs until, I believe, during Bert Dunphy's presidency at the meeting in Washington, D.C., when the wives came in after dinner to hear General Eisenhower. Several couples gathered in Bert and Nancy's suite for a drink with the former President. We were about to go down to dinner when he received a telephone call. We waited there for over an hour and the members had to mill around waiting. It developed later that President Kennedy had him on the telephone discussing whether or not to send the first 15,000 troops into Vietnam. Bert Dunphy can give you the exact details.

"I believe it was the following year which wives were invited to attend the annual banquet. I always agreed that they should be present but there was considerable opposition."

Claude E. Welch, August 2, 1979. "One of the most important events in the history of the ASA occurred when Bert Dunphy was in charge and he invited his good friend President Eisenhower for the after dinner speech. It was this gesture of the President [see Minutes 1962] that led immediately to the inclusion of wives at the time of the annual banquet. Some of the footdraggers against this phenomenal change in the course of the organization included Bert himself. You may remember that he was very eloquent about this matter. He spoke against having the women present. He stated that as soon as they came, you would sit down next to a woman and her first question would be, 'and how are your grandchildren?' However, despite all of his objections he was voted down and women were invited to be present at the time of the next banquet. At that time I sat down next to Bob Linton's wife Emma and the first words that came out of her mouth were, 'And how are *your* grandchildren?' Obviously, despite grandchildren, however, this change has been very important and good for the Association."

One remembers that Dr. Churchill spoke at much greater length than is recorded, that he spoke of the fact that this was a scientific and professional association and not a social association, that its purposes would not be well served by inviting the wives however charming they might be, and moreover one recalls that he spoke with considerable heat. One also remembers Bert Dunphy spoke with his usual wit and pungency and that one spoke oneself. One has no recollection of anyone having spoken *for* the motion.] President Ravdin then said "I take it that your having been notified that this would come up for a vote today, every one has considered this; and that perhaps the wives, having heard that this vote would come up, have indicated to each of you their own feelings in the matter. This is a matter which has come up perennially. There was a great deal of discussion of this in the Council but no decision. It was for this reason that Council passed the question on to you." The Tellers reported that "The vote on the special ballot concerning invitations to wives and guests to dinner is as follows: 'Yes' 89, 'No' 49, and a large number of blank ballots were received."

Among the new members elected were Donald B. Effler, John W. Kirklin, Robert S. Sparkman, and as Honorary Member, Professor Philip R. Allison, of Oxford. The elected President was Warren H. Cole, of Chicago; as Vice-Presidents, Richard H. Sweet, of Boston, and Carleton Mathewson, of San Francisco; and as Secretary again, William Altemeier, of Cincinnati.

Dr. Ravdin announced that although the matter of the wives attending the annual dinner was not in the Constitution or By-Laws ". . . this is a matter of such importance that if I have your consent, I shall refer it back to the Council with the action taken, for them to make such recommendations to you as they believe should be carried out within the framework of this action. This is for you to decide. The vote was 89 and 49. I am sure that the question of whether or not this was a majority or not is beside the point, and I shall do whatever you wish about it, but I think perhaps this would be the best way of finally solving this question. There was a division within the Council concerning this." There was a good deal of discussion at this point. Dr. Moyer moved that the rules applying to modification of the By-Laws be applied to this vote, and that

was seconded. Dr. Altemeier, Secretary, said that there was nothing in the Constitution really about attendance at the banquet. There had been major opposition to the move in the Council and obviously in the Association, and perhaps the Council should establish what majority was necessary to pass such a proposal. Dr. James D. Hardy suggested that if it were referred back to the Council that it be limited to the wives with no added guests. Julian Johnson said that he had voted against the proposal "because it has been the tradition, and so far as I know it is the only Association to which I belong in which this distinction occurs. I thought it was a very nice arrangement and liked it." On the other hand he said there had been a vote and perhaps it ought to be left up to Council. Dr. Blalock, with regard to Dr. Hardy's statement, said that the mention of guests meant only those who appeared on the program as authors of papers. Dr. Naffziger rose again "I hesitate to speak again about this, because my feelings are not strong, but I believe many of the members who come without wives will say, 'Well, this is a big crowd; I think we will go to the theatre,' or something of the sort. We will lose out the one opportunity, the one time, when there is any social gathering of the membership." It was finally voted and agreed that Dr. Moyer's motion, which was passed, meant that the proposal would lie over for a year.

1960s

1960s

THE NEW YORK TIMES-MONDAY APRIL 4,1960-THE FIRST DAY OF THE MEETING OF THE AMERICAN SURGICAL ASSOCIATION IN WHITE SULPHUR SPRINGS, WEST VIRGINIA

Senators Kennedy and Humphrey were campaigning in the Wisconsin primaries [which Kennedy won], the Civil Rights Act of 1960 was close to passing, overt evidences of racial unrest were prominent in South Africa, the Dominican dictator was "imperilled"; the Russians were having economic problems; in this country, people were still going to Florida by train, candidate John Kennedy pledged to support a ban on atomic bomb testing and General Douglas MacArthur had had a prostatectomy.

"All the News
That's Fit to Print"

The New York Times.

LATE CITY EDITION

U.S. Weather Bureau Report [Page 36] forecasts
Cloudy, mild, rain today; fair
tonight. Fair, mild tomorrow.
Temp. range: 53-42; yesterday: 47-37.8

VOL. CIX . No. 37,326.

© 1960, by The New York Times Company.
Times Square, New York 36, N. Y.

NEW YORK, MONDAY, APRIL 4, 1960.

FIVE CENTS

SOVIET REPORTED WARNING ITS BLOC OF A CUT IN TRADE

Said to Foresee Move in '65 to Meet Home Needs and Commitments in Aid

RAW MATERIALS A KEY

Communist Lands Now Rely on Russia for Major Flow of Iron Ore and Grain

By M. S. HANDLER
Special to The New York Times

WARSAW, April 3—Moscow is reported to have informed members of the Soviet bloc that heavy economic commitments at home and outside Europe may result in fundamental revisions of trading policy toward Eastern Europe in 1965.

This was said to have been conveyed to the bloc at the February meeting in Moscow of Eastern European ministers and during recent bilateral negotiations for trade agreements covering the period 1961-65.

These trade agreements emphasized once again the magnitude of Soviet economic assistance to Eastern Europe. This assistance falls into three categories: industrial raw materials, ranging from iron ore and petroleum to almost the entire field of nonferrous metals, heavy industrial equipment and cereals.

Dependent on Soviet Ore

The role soviet raw materials play in the growth of heavy industry in Eastern Europe may be judged from the fact that all the great steel mills constructed or expanded in the last ten years in Poland, Rumania, East Germany, Hungary and Bulgaria are largely dependent on Soviet ore from the Krivoi Rog region in the Ukraine.

At the February ministerial meeting and in the trade negotiations the Soviet Government indicated that it would no longer be economically feasible to ship the ore because of the burden on the transportation system and the cost.

The Soviet Government was said to have suggested that it would be more economical for the mills to take deliveries of pig iron.

The meaning of this to the Eastern European steel mills is clear, considering that the entire industrialization program in Eastern Europe was based on the establishment of a great steel industry and that the mills are integrated, that is, they are set up to carry out the entire process from ore to finished steel.

The nature of the problem may also be judged from the fact that the trade agreements

Continued on Page 3, Column 5

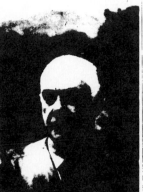

RESISTS GROWING OPPOSITION: Generalissimo Rafael Leonidas Trujillo Molina of the Dominican Republic.

The Dominican Struggle: Change Imperils Trujillo

Following is the first of three articles on the Dominican Republic by a correspondent who recently visited there.

By EDWARD C. BURKS

The pressure within the Dominican Republic is near the bursting point. But Generalissimo Rafael Leonidas Trujillo Molina turns on his bland smile, radiates confidence and goes on ruling like an ancient oriental potentate.

Behind that bland smile are a strong mind and an iron will. At 68 he has been master of his mountainous, tropical realm for thirty years.

Since breaking up a nationwide plot of the professional classes last January he has tightened his repression of parties. He even resigned from the dominant Dominican party, ostensibly so that others would feel free to form new parties.

But in fact the country remains a tightly run police state. Furthermore, General Trujillo demands ever greater evidence of support and solidarity, especially from those he knows to be his enemies.

Political Decisions Awaited

Should the calm continue, it is expected that leaders of the governing National party will turn their attention to whatever political decisions they feel must be made as a consequence of the rioting and unrest of the last two weeks, which have thrust South Africa to the center of the international stage.

But thus far the Government headed by Prime Minister Hendrik F. Verwoerd, has given no indication of making any basic change in its policy of racial separation, known as apartheid.

As a result of this attitude, there is much talk that political forces are at work that will dislodge the Verwoerd regime and replace it with one less

Continued on Page 4, Column 4

JAPAN AND KOREA TO RESUME TRADE

Rhee Regime Also to Reopen Talk Aimed at Establishing Normal Diplomatic Ties

By ROBERT TRUMBULL
Special to The New York Times

TOKYO, Monday, April 4—Japan and South Korea agreed today to reopen trade relations and to resume suspended diplomatic talks.

The Republic of Korea halted commerce with Japan last June 15, in retaliation against the Tokyo Government's agreement to the voluntary return of Korean citizens in Japan to Communist North Korea.

Meanwhile, protracted negotiations on property exchanges, return of Korean art treasures and numerous other issues between Japan and their former colony were halted. These discussions will be resumed April 15, it was agreed today.

Ambassador Yiu Tai Ha, head of the South Korean diplomatic mission here, and Hisanari Yamada, Japan's Deputy Foreign Minister, announced the new accord after a forty-five-minute conference this morning.

In return for the removal of restrictions on imports from Japan by President Syngman Rhee's Government, Tokyo agreed to buy 20,000 tons of swift-arrival and lost of property surplus from South Korea this year.

The negotiations to be resumed April 15 have as their objective the establishment of full diplomatic relations between the two countries. The beautiful, modern and clean, United States has been pressing

Continued on Page 11, Column 3

20 ON TRAIN HURT AT PENN STATION

19 Cars Here From Florida Jolted by Locomotive

Twenty persons aboard a passenger train that had just arrived in Pennsylvania Station from Florida were injured yesterday when the train was jolted severely as it was being coupled to a locomotive.

Nine of the injured were treated at St. Vincent's Hospital.

The train, an extra section of the Seaboard Railroad's Silver Meteor, arrived at 1:13 P. M. on Track 12. The jolt occurred five minutes later.

There was a loud crash and passengers who were in the aisles screamed as they were thrown to the floor. Washroom mirrors cracked.

Emergency calls brought policemen, and ambulances from St. Clare's and St. Vincent's Hospitals. The injured who were not taken to St. Vincent's were treated outside the station master's office at the north end of the main departure level.

The train is operated by Pennsylvania Railroad locomotives between here and Washington. The extra section's nineteen cars included some from Miami and some from St. Petersburg. The locomotive, a 4,600-horsepower model, was supposed to haul the empty section back to Washington.

Arthur W. Chapman was at

Continued on Page 16, Column 5

Police Jokes by Lt. Gov. Wilson And Sheen Rile Commissioner

About 6,000 city policemen laughed yesterday when Bishop heard a way to endure an Fulton J. Sheen and Lieut. Gov. prohibiting woman Malcolm Wilson told jokes from being served in bar. All about policemen who are quick, and their way, no trouble with their nightsticks and the backslaps after one of the others who take graft. offenders moved his nightstick

But Police Commissioner along one row of bodies, then Stephen P. Kennedy was not along another and another amused. The sermon roared. Mr.

"We are not children playing Kennedy at the noon table did a game," he said when he turn-

came to address the group "This The next speaker was Mr. is a serious business. There can Wilson. He told about his 'Uncle be no substitute for integrity Pat,' a police patrolman whose and fidelity and for moral and duties he described as 'getting spiritual courage' things rung out of court'

The occasion was the Police- when he stopped speeding men's Holy Name Society's forty- Holy Name Society's forty-second He lived 'frugally,'

second annual communion Mr. Wilson said and managed breakfast in the Waldorf to retire with $66,000 at a time Astoria Hotel. when the city gave no pensions.

Bishop Sheen, national direc- Then Mr. Kennedy spoke. He tor of the Society for the did not mention Bishop Sheen Propagation of the Faith, re-

called a joke the late Gov. Al-

fred E. Smith had told him Continued on Page 37, Column 6

"When 'Al' was Sheriff of New

Continued on Page 16, Column 5

TENSION DECLINES IN SOUTH AFRICA; POLICE ON ALERT

Only Minor Incidents Occur —Nation Is Awaiting Next Move by Government

By LEONARD INGALLS
Special to The New York Times

JOHANNESBURG, South Africa, April 3—Tension appeared today to be easing after two weeks of extreme racial strife in South Africa.

Only isolated incidents of petty violence, such as stoning of buses, were reported from such major trouble spots as Capetown, Durban and the African townships southwest of Johannesburg. Thousands of policemen and troops still maintained emergency patrols at African dwelling areas.

Johannesburg was enjoying its usual Sunday quiet. Workmen were busy completing the decoration of department stores and public buildings for the Union Festival that is being held this year to mark the fiftieth anniversary of the formation of the Union of South Africa.

Exposition to Open

The Union Exposition, organized as part of the observance will open on schedule tomorrow.

Hotels here are packed with visitors from many parts of South Africa and from abroad. The declaration of a state of emergency appears to have had no effect on the tourist trade. Communications and air, rail and bus services are functioning normally.

Both African and white window-shoppers strolled peacefully through downtown Johannesburg today. Yesterday thousands of persons attended a full program of sports events including racing, rugby football matches and tennis as on a normal Saturday.

Meanwhile the country was anxiously awaiting the next move from Capetown, the center of government when Parliament is in session.

Political Decisions Awaited

Wisconsin Voters Watch TV War

Humphrey Steps Up Attack — Kennedy Retains His Calm

By JAMES RESTON
Special to The New York Times

MILWAUKEE, April 3—The voters of Wisconsin have been sitting in this week-end on the noisiest TV war of the Presidential campaign.

Spin the dial and what do you get:

¶Senator Hubert H. Humphrey at a bean feed, scalding the Republicans as the party of "waste and neglect."

¶Vice President Nixon on film being introduced as "the man the nation needs and the world respects * * * The man who stood up to Khrushchev while the whole world thrilled"

¶Senator Kennedy with his wife, Senator Kennedy with his child, Senator Kennedy with his sisters and his in-laws, and his buddies in the war.

The campaign for Tuesday's Presidential preference primary vote is picking up speed and losing altitude. On the national television shows, Senators Humphrey and Kennedy have been elaborately generous to one another, but on the local level, here, Humphrey has been increasingly the attacker and Kennedy the defender.

It is Humphrey who is making the claims of victory and launching the charges. He has driven himself to the point of

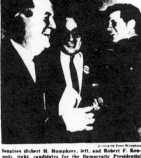

Senators Hubert H. Humphrey, left, and Robert F. Kennedy, right, candidates for the Democratic Presidential nomination, exchanging greetings yesterday during meeting in narrow corridor of television studio in Milwaukee.

exhaustion, crossing and recrossing the state in his way. Even then while the Minnesotan had recovered his voice by noon today he was speechless at noon today, his composure. He was pressed hard by the reporters on the question of campaign expenditures and hit back hard at

Continued on Page 21, Column 1

GEROSA IS WILLING TO FORGO PAY RISE

Says He Will Give Up Added Pension Payment if Other Elected Officials Do

By PAUL CROWELL

Controller Lawrence E. Gerosa declared yesterday that he did not believe elected city officials should be given increases in take-home pay by having the city assume part of their contributions to pension systems. He indicated willingness to forgo such an increase himself if his elected associates would do so too.

Mayor Wagner's $2,338,857,- 517 executive budget for fiscal 1960-61 provides take-home-pay raises for 105,000 city employes belonging to the New York City Employes Retirement System and the retirement systems for teachers in city schools and colleges.

Under permissive legislation voted in Albany last week, the city would pay in 1960-61 and 1961-62, in addition to the regular contribution to these employes pension funds, an additional amount equal to 2½ per cent of the employe's gross annual salary. This sum would otherwise be deducted from the

Continued on Page 23, Column 5

Kennedy Gives President A Pledge on Test-Ban Pact

Wrote to Eisenhower

By AUSTIN C. WEHRWEIN
Special to The New York Times

MILWAUKEE, April 3—Senator John F. Kennedy said today that he had pledged to support political observers to the conference.

President Eisenhower's efforts to end nuclear testing by negotiations with the Soviet Union.

He said he had informed the President and had also stated his belief that the United States should continue in the conference now going on at Geneva and should not resume nuclear testing.

"Dear Mr. President:

"I have been greatly disturbed by the possibility that our current nuclear test negotiations might be jeopardized by the approach of a Presidential election.

"You have consistently indicated your own belief that the present Geneva negotiations may be bringing us close to a final agreement to end testing. I share this belief with you. At the same time you may be running

Humphrey Is Confident

By DONALD JANSON

MILWAUKEE, April 3—Despite the unanimous opinion of political observers to the contrary, Senator Hubert H. Humphrey of Minnesota asserted today that he would win a decisive victory in Wisconsin's Presidential primary Tuesday.

He said on a nationally televised panel program that he forecast a solid Roman Catholic vote for his rival, Senator John F. Kennedy of Massachusetts.

Senator Kennedy, said in a letter to the President dated last Wednesday.

"I resent the fact that people vote on religious lines without proof," Senator Humphrey asserted.

He said Minnesota voters had not divided on religious lines in electing Eugene J. McCarthy, a Catholic, to the Senate in 1958 and he did not expect Wisconsin voters to do it in this primary.

Senator Kennedy is a Catholic. Senator Humphrey is a Protestant.

Senator Humphrey predicted yesterday that he would win six of Wisconsin's ten Congressional districts in Tuesday's primary. This would give him fifteen of the state's thirty contested votes. He would not name the districts he expected to win or forecast his chances in the popular vote, which will decide the four delegate-at-large votes.

The Minnesotan is given little chance to win the state-wide popular vote because his rival's strength is greater in the

Continued on Page 21, Column 3

Seen Proof Lacking

"I have been greatly disturbed by the possibility that our current nuclear test negotiations might be jeopardized by the approach of a Presidential election.

Continued on Page 21, Column 5

General MacArthur Returns Home From Hospital

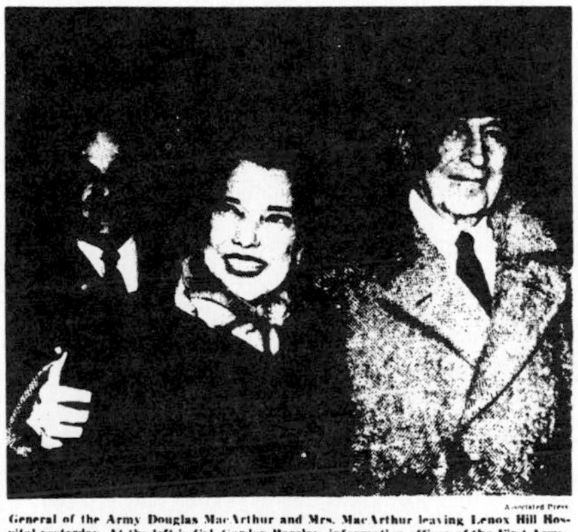

General of the Army examination and was operated on Douglas MacArthur left Lenox for removal of his Hill Hospital yesterday and prostate gland on March 19. returned to his Waldorf Towers apartment. The 80-year- The General issued a stateold former Far Eastern commander had entered the hospital Jan. 29 for a urological most striking stories in the examination and was op-

dead. I feel very much like a modern Lazarus whose resurrection is due to the extraordinary skill and efficiency of Dr. (George W.) Slaughter and his aides. A baseball telecast occupied his afternoon.

[Photo caption:] General of the Army Douglas MacArthur and Mrs. MacArthur leaving Lenox Hill Hospital yesterday. At the left is Col. Gordon Barclay, information officer of the First Army.

SENATE SEEKING VOTE THIS WEEK FOR RIGHTS BILL

Southern Resistance Easing —Both Sides Grow Weary of Prolonged Debate

FILIBUSTER IS UNLIKELY

Some Hope Is Seen for Quick Approval in House—Few Changes Are Expected

By ANTHONY LEWIS
Special to The New York Times

WASHINGTON, April 3—A weary United States Senate may finish its work this week on the Civil Rights bill.

The Senate has been debating civil rights since Feb. 15, and a conclusion this week would make just about every member happy.

Despite public protestations of continued ardor for or against the legislation, all sides are tired of the talk and of the issue.

The Southerners had threatened to filibuster in earnest to prevent a vote on final passage. But it appears now that they will be satisfied with fairly brief denunciations for the record. If so, the Senate vote could come soon.

South's Resistance Easing

Southern resistance has cooled as it has become more and more apparent that the final legislation will be limited primarily to voting rights. The only really significant provision of the bill as it stands permits appointment of voting referees by the Federal courts to enroll Negro voters where state officials will not do so.

There will undoubtedly be further attempts by Northern liberals to broaden the bill by amendment. But they cannot take much hope from last Friday's 48-to-38 vote to table, or kill, an amendment to set up a statutory commission against job discrimination by Government contractors.

Some Senators who had endorsed the commission idea in principle voted to table it, on the ground that broadening of the civil rights bill now would lead to all-out Southern resistance and prevent its passage. Among these voters was the Republican leader, Everett McKinley Dirksen, of Illinois.

Amendments likely to be

Continued on Page 19, Column 1

INTEGRATION AIDS CAPITAL'S SCHOOLS

Standards Found to Improve Steadily in Five Years

Special to The New York Times

WASHINGTON, April 2—Five years of desegregation are reported to have brought a marked rise in the educational level of District of Columbia public schools.

Dr. Carl F. Hansen, superintendent of schools, told in a report today of steady improvement in academic standards, teacher efficiency and school services, accompanied by a decline in delinquency.

The capital's schools were among the first to accept complete integration under the 1954 ruling of the Supreme Court.

"The nation's capital ought to symbolize a national dedication to the principle of superior education for every child," Dr. Hansen said. "There are many miles to go before we reach this goal."

The rise in academic standards, coinciding with a rise in the number of Negroes enrolled, is testimony to "the capacity of the Negro pupil to respond to educational opportunity," he declared.

His report was distributed by the Anti-Defamation League of

Continued on Page 20, Column 5

Mrs. Roosevelt Hurt By Car, Carries On

By ROBERT CONLEY

Mrs. Franklin D. Roosevelt suffered a sprained ankle yesterday morning when an auto backed into her and knocked her down as she stepped off a curb near her home on the East Side.

Her ankle was taped and bandaged by her physician and she had to use a crutch to walk. But Mrs. Roosevelt, indefatigable at the age of 75 was too busy to think much about the injury. She did not know the name of the motorist, she said, nor did she notify the police.

Instead, she had three speaking engagements in the city, a modern Lazarus whose and she kept every one of them. She finished the day about 10 P. M. by addressing a dinner for the Women's Coat and Suit Industry for Brandeis Univer-

Continued on Page 21, Column 5

LXXVIII

1960

The 1960 meeting was held at The Greenbrier, White Sulphur Springs, West Virginia, April 4, 5, and 6, with President Warren H. Cole, of Chicago, Professor and Head of the Department of Surgery, University of Illinois, College of Medicine, in the Chair. Among those who had died in the preceding year was William Edward Gallie, of Toronto, who had been President in 1948.

The Presidential Address, *Potentialities of Surgery,* dealt with the impact on surgery of the "Important medical discoveries . . . being made so rapidly these days . . ." Typhoid fever and diphtheria no longer concerned surgeons. Actinomycosis and lymphogranuloma venereum were rarely seen and surgical lesions of tuberculosis had decreased sharply in incidence. The incidence of cancer in the stomach, appendicitis, and diffuse toxic goiter had also decreased sharply ". . . during the past few decades but we are woefully ignorant of the actual reason." Would ". . . the pathogenesis of gallstones and peptic ulcer . . . be developed to the point where these two conditions can be eliminated?. . . I personally believe this, but I doubt that anyone in this room will see the day when cholecystectomy and subtotal gastrectomy for peptic ulcer will be erased completely from the operating room schedule . . . are we getting appreciably nearer the day when the surgeon's work will be limited to the repair of congenital defects and accidental injury to the body? I suspect we are, although, again I believe no one in

this room will see that day." Something was already known of the causation of congenital defects and even of their prevention. Cardiovascular surgery would be sharply decreased in volume ". . . if the problem of atherosclerosis was solved and a majority of the congenital defects prevented . . . rheumatic fever . . . will probably be erased . . . before atherosclerosis. Again, I suspect we are safe in saying no one in this room will see that day." "It requires no imagination to deduce that the successful transplantation of homologous tissue with persistent survival of the transplant would perhaps be surgery's greatest accomplishment of all time", and if any homologous tissue could be successfully transplanted, then almost any organ could be ". . . because the immunologic discovery resulting in the successful transplantation of one organ should permit other organs to survive . . ." The availability of cadaver organs he thought would remain a limiting factor in the wholesale application of organ transplantation. He suggested that the progress of medical science would so decrease the death rate from disease as to provide an inadequate number of donors so that thoughts would turn to the use of heterologous organs. He commented on Medawar's establishment of graft rejection as an antigen antibody reaction, the demonstration that cortisone was ". . . a powerful agent in preventing the development of immunologic reactions" [Wells and Kendall, 1940; Stoerk, 1950]. He made the cautious statement that

1110

"Consideration of the data known to date suggests that the decrease or prevention of resistance to homografts by cortisone, body radiation and other factors is sufficient to justify great optimism in homotransplantation . . . we cannot hope that the complete solution to homografting will be achieved within the next few years or even decades, but the progress already made makes the solution appear certain, at least to a limited degree." In the field of anticancer drugs, since Goodman and Gilman's 1946 presentation of the effect of nitrogen mustard on experimental tumors, and Farber's 1948 work on aminopterin in leukemia, more than 100,000 drugs had been tested, most of them inferior to the original ones, "with the possible exception of methotrexate for chorioepithelioma". The use of these agents as adjuvants to operations, for perfusion of tumor-containing areas, for irrigation of wounds, ". . . will probably improve results appreciably but they cannot change the results in any pronounced fashion until better drugs are made available." There was some evidence that tumor resistance to chemical agents ". . . was best explained by a failure or decreased activity of the enzyme systems", and there was some hope that this offered an avenue for specific therapy. It did not appear impossible to synthesize a specific DNA which would enter the cancer cell and accomplish this destruction. He was obviously fascinated by the work which suggested that many cancers were viral in etiology. He felt there was convincing evidence that a part of the human cancer problem was one of resistance "possibly immunologic in character", which might vary with a number of influences. He thought that ". . . the scientific world is waiting anxiously for the development of a test which will apply to all cancers and be specific." The test might ". . . detect susceptibility to cancer . . . detect the initial development of cancer . . . detect the time when the patient's resistance of his tumor decreases sufficiently to allow development of metastases." [He made no mention of the immense problem which would result if a sensitive test could show the presence of cancer in an asymptomatic individual with no localizable tumor.] He concluded that while scientific advances would make many operations obsolete, other advances would ". . . lead to the development of operations not yet conceived" and the ". . . greatest of these future discoveries, perhaps the most profound in all surgical history" would be transplantation of tissues and organs.

* * *

Quite appropriately, the President's paper was followed by *The Homotransplantation of Kidneys and of Fetal Liver and Spleen after Total Body Irradiation,* David M. Hume, of Richmond, Professor of Surgery, Chairman of the Department, Medical College of Virginia; and by invitation, Benjamin T. Jackson, Charles F. Zukoski, H. M. Lee, H. Myron Kauffman, and Richard H. Egdahl. It was known that in mice a sufficiently large dose of total body irradiation would prevent antibody formation and hematopoiesis, that bone marrow homotransplants from another mouse strain would take successfully, and that such mice could then accept skin homografts from mice of the donor strain. The use of adult bone marrow transplants led to a graft versus host reaction and the "runt syndrome", whereas transplant of fetal bone marrow did not produce this syndrome. The lymphocytes seen in dogs who rejected homografted kidneys were thought by some to be of donor origin and to represent a donor reaction against the host. Hume's group set out to determine ". . . whether infusions of homologous fetal liver and spleen cells would permit indefinite survival after lethal doses of total body irradiation . . . in the dog", whether prior irradiation of the host would prevent homograft rejection, and whether the lymphocytes and plasma cells seen in the rejected kidney were of host or donor origin. They demonstrated that 28 splenectomized dogs given 600r Total Body Radiation died within seven to 17 days, but four of the 16 dogs also given infusions of fetal liver and spleen cells, were surviving 12, 16, 18, and 22 months later, and a male host given female cells was shown to have female leukocytes for up to eight months but not at 12 months. In the case of renal homotransplantation in the dog, irradiation of the donor up to 1500r "did not prevent the appearance of the usual homotransplant rejection phenomena in the usual time", and irradiation of the host at doses of 600 or 1000r failed to prevent rejection. Irradiation at 1200r prevented rejection in half the cases, and irradiation at 1500r prevented rejection in all cases. "Irradiation of both host and donor prevented rejection at doses of 1,000r or greater in all cases, but not at doses of 600r." Long-term survival studies were not undertaken in this series of experiments. "The greater the degree of destruction of the lymphoid follicles of the host lymph nodes by irradiation, the greater was the likelihood that the renal transplant would persist without rejection." Prolonged survival of "fetal blood-forming cells can occur in hosts receiving a dose of irradiation which is lethal to the unprotected animal, but still too small to permit successful renal homografting." They found no evidence that a sublethal dose of irradiation ". . . would exempt a resident homografted kidney from ultimate rejection." Their evidence was that the lymphocytes and plasma cells in their rejected kidney were of host origin and represented "a reaction of the host against the graft."

Discussion

J. Englebert Dunphy, of Portland, Oregon, said that in their experiments, irradiation at 600r had ". . . no demonstrable effect upon the regeneration of autologous marrow", and that autologous marrow would regenerate after 2000r. Francis D. Moore, of Boston, said that in one patient given 650r ". . . at 28 days there was no histologic evidence of kidney rejection. The patient died essentially of the radiation injury." He asked Dr. Hume whether there were any long-term survivors in dogs receiving over 1000r. Herbert Conway, of New York, complained that research funds were not available to surgeons for immunologic work and that immunologists were not as aggressive in research as surgeons and were disinclined to accommodate surgeons in their laboratories. He urged that surgeons ". . . master the technics of immunology sufficiently to meet the criteria for successful scientific investigation" [and sufficiently to pass muster before granting agencies]. Hume, in closing, said that in fact there was convincing evidence from some experiments that bone marrow could be completely destroyed by irradiation and repopulated with foreign cells, and that in his dogs ". . . biopsies of the bone marrow . . . show complete absence of cells unless they've been given bone marrow . . ." Hume was interested that bone marrow cells injected intravenously ". . . gravitate to the host's bone marrow and multiply there . . ." and that spleen cells given intravenously migrated to the host's lymph nodes ". . . and will grow and produce foreign lymphocytes." As for Dr. Moore's patient with a normal appearing kidney at 28 days, Hume said that ". . . in some instances just by chance, even in unrelated humans, the kidney will function for a period as long as six months . . . in the experiments reported here, only those doses which destroyed the bone marrow and the lymph germinal centers were capable of producing a tolerance to a foreign graft, and this may also possibly be true in the human."

* * *

The discussion of transplantation continued with *Experimental Whole-Organ Transplantation of*

the Liver and of the Spleen, Francis D. Moore, of Boston, Surgeon-in-Chief, Peter Bent Brigham Hospital; Moseley Professor of Surgery, Harvard Medical School, and seven others, by invitation. The studies of transplantation, up to then, had been mainly of skin, bone marrow, and kidney, and it was important to study other organs and tissues, particularly ". . . organs involved either with a large antigenic mass, or those containing immunologically competent cells. Examples of such are to be found in the liver and in the spleen." For hepatic transplantation, the recipient's venous blood was shunted from the inferior vena cava to the jugular vein through flexible plastic tubing. In suturing the transplant in place, the suprahepatic cava was sutured first, then the portal vein after which blood was allowed to flow from the portal vein into the liver and into the heart. The infrahepatic vena cava was then anastomosed, and finally the hepatic arteries. The most satisfactory biliary anastomosis proved to be a cholecystoduodenostomy. No heparin was required. From their 31 homotransplants, 15 animals had lived over 24 hours, and eight had lived four to 12 days. However, in 27 autotransplantations, the liver being removed, cooled and perfused with refrigerated blood, and then replaced, ten survived 24 hours or more and seven four days or more, up to 14 days. They were not sure that any of the homotransplant animals had died of rejection. Some of the dogs succumbed to technical operative problems, hemorrhage, perforated ulcer, etc. Splenic homotransplants were carried out in 29 dogs, in ten of whom the anastomoses were thought to be satisfactory. If the blood supply to the spleen remained intact, the animals showed no symptoms. Histologic study of the spleens showed the evidence of a rejection process. For the liver transplant, they thought further experiments were required ". . . to view the unmodified rejection response more clearly", and then other studies with treatment of the recipient ". . . with radiation, radiomimetic drugs, with or without bone marrow or splenic transplant, to achieve a state of tolerance in which prolonged hepatic survival might be achieved." From the clinical standpoint, it appeared that ". . . the liver of a recently deceased animal appears to maintain viability so long as either the entire body, the liver perfusate, or the liver itself is rapidly cooled and maintained in the cool state . . . The treatment of cirrhosis or other liver disease by hepatic transplantation offers promise clinically only where there is a comparative lack of conjoint pathology in other organs. The treatment of metastatic carcinoma by liver transplantation would offer salvage only in those rare patients where the liver was the only site of metastasis." Chemical studies showed no change in blood urea nitrogen, usually a normal or elevated blood sugar, a progressive rise in alkaline phosphatase which often preceded the rise in the serum bilirubin, the one beginning on the third day, the other on the fourth or fifth day. A fall in serum albumin was characteristic. They found no abnormalities in coagulation studies. Histologically, the liver showed infiltration of the portal areas with mononuclear cells, lymphocytes and plasma cells, and dilatation of the lymphatics, and evidence of injury to the bile duct epithelium, but apparently not of the parenchymal cells. Again, experiments were required to see whether the spleen would be accepted after whole body irradiation or the use of radiomimetic drugs in the recipient. If the spleen could be accepted this would be ". . . an ideal situation for subsequent acceptance of other organs because such donor would then be available for transplantation studies of skin, kidney, liver, or other organs." It was necessary to establish the techniques of surgical transplantation and to understand the events that followed, and this they felt they had done for the liver and spleen.

Discussion

Thomas Starzl, of Denver [not yet a Member], said that he and Dr. Harry A. Kaupp had "been working on the problem of liver transplantation for the past 18 months. We have had experience with about 80 hepatic transplants, but we were not able to obtain survival for longer than three or four days until we were encouraged by Dr. Moore's results in Atlantic City last fall. Since then, our survivals have been longer." The arterial anastomosis had been usually made by taking a segment of donor aorta with the hepatic artery. They had done a variety of venous anastomoses including a reverse Eck fistula ". . . in which all of the blood from the inferior vena cava and the splanchnic system is deviated through the liver", a procedure with a very high immediate mortality. They had also done an anatomic reconstruction, and a small portacaval shunt to decompress the liver if that was required. This permitted a small dog's liver to be placed into a large animal. With either of these two methods, the survival time had been nine days. With a totally normal anatomic reconstruction, the maximum survival had been 20-1/2 days. The bilirubin started rising on about the fifth day. Many of the dogs died of hypoglycemia. W. V. McDermott, of Boston, said that they had been perfusing isolated livers at the same time that the donor animal was perfused, later reim-

planting the liver, and had been successful in three of five attempts after perfusion periods of up to two-and-a-half hours "In all three survivors liver functions, ammonium clearance and all standard parameters were entirely normal, and the longest survivor is now over three months." The liver of one dog, deliberately sacrificed, appeared entirely normal, supporting "Dr. Moore's observations that replant and transplant of the liver are technically and physiologically feasible and that the abnormalities described, particularly in the excretory functions of the liver, are a part of the rejection phenomenon and not due to any metabolic disorders attendant upon the operative procedure." Moore, in closing said that they had conducted some studies on ". . . hypothermic preservation of the postmortem liver . . . if the liver is cooled fast enough, it maintains excellent metabolic functional capacity up to 12 hours after death."

* * *

E. M. Bricker, of St. Louis, Associate Professor of Clinical Surgery, Washington University School of Medicine, and by invitation, H. R. Butcher, Jr., W. H. Lawler, Jr., and C. A. McAfee, *Surgical Treatment of Advanced and Recurrent Cancer of the Pelvic Viscera*: An Evaluation of Ten Years Experience, were reporting "Two hundred eighteen exenterations of the pelvic organs . . . for advanced pelvic cancer or for complications resulting from irradiation (9 patients) in the last ten years." Their total operative mortality was 11%,- 25 patients, and the initial mortality of 25% had dropped to 7% in the exenteration for carcinoma of the cervix, an operation which now took them four hours, and required 2500 ml. of blood. There were numerous and severe complications, wound infection, thrombophlebitis, hemorrhage, intestinal obstruction, postoperative psychosis, mechanical and bacterial urinary problems, fecal fistula, etc. "The most clearly defined indication for exenteration of the pelvic organs is cervical carcinoma persistent or recurrent after irradiation." All but three of their 150 operated women had been irradiated. Inoperability was demonstrated by the finding of tumor outside the pelvis,- the lungs, the cervical and inguinal lymph nodes, or by the signs of hopeless local extension such as ". . . sciatic nerve pain and swelling of the leg on the same side . . . Ipsilateral ureteral obstruction at the pelvic brim . . ." At laparotomy inoperability was indicated by ". . . metastases to the liver, periaortic lymph nodes or extrapelvic peritoneum . . ." or hopeless intrapelvic spread. Radiation fibrosis

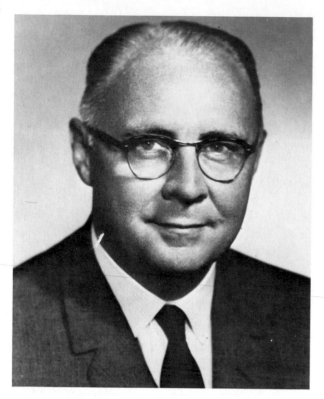

Eugene M. Bricker (c. 1962) 1908—. Vice-President 1967. M.D. Washington University, St. Louis, 1934. Trained, and entire professional life at Washington University, St. Louis and Barnes Hospital. Professor of Clinical Surgery, 1961-1975. By a lifetime of devotion to the problem demonstrated that the exenteration for pelvic cancer, pioneered by Alexander Brunschwig, could be performed with acceptably low morbidity and mortality and worthwhile long-term results, - establishing the indications and techniques, and contributing his method (Bricker's ileal loop) of urinary diversion.

was sometimes difficult to differentiate from cancer. The operation was not undertaken unless it was thought that all gross cancer could be removed, and only if recurrent cancer had been demonstrated histologically, although occasionally operation was justified even though no cancer was found in the operative specimen, if after radiation ". . . the lesion is associated with extensive pain, sloughing and fistula formation." As controls, they had 118 women who had either refused operation or whose physicans had refused to recommend operation. Taking 69 matched pairs of patients with or without pelvic exenteration, at the end of five years, 13 patients with exenteration were alive and only one without. For carcinoma of the rectum in women, total exenteration was rarely necessary since the uterus and the vagina protected

the bladder and ureters from direct extension. Bricker's statements here were somewhat contradictory, "Pelvic exenteration should be employed only rarely when there is no chance of complete excision of the cancer. However, we believe there is more frequent justification for a deliberate palliative resection for this lesion than for carcinoma of the cervix . . . Experience with the operation, and particularly with the results of ileal segment urinary diversion, has led us to employ exenteration more frequently in the treatment of advanced carcinoma of the rectum, especially in elderly men. So many of these patients have dysfunction of the lower urinary tract following abdominoperineal resection that we have been encouraged to proceed with the radical operation in questionable cases rather than to court a local recurrence of cancer with bladder dysfunction as the result of extensive dissection in the area between the rectum and the urinary tract." Five of 16 patients so operated upon five years ago or more were alive and free of evidence of tumor. On the other hand, reoperation by pelvic exenteration for recurrent carcinoma of the rectum had been disappointing. The urinary diversion was by ileal loop. In 150 women who had undergone pelvic exenteration, there were only 11 who had postoperative complications,- five instances of pyelonephritis, three of separation of the ileal stoma, and three of revision for ureteral obstruction or necrosis. Eleven patients subsequently had pyelonephritis, 12 subsequently required revision of the ileal stoma, and three required revision of the uretero-ileal anastomosis. In all, 15 postoperative deaths in the 150 women were attributable to the urinary diversion.

Discussion

Alexander Brunschwig, of New York, opened the Discussion. He was in complete agreement with everything that had been said. He had done 640 pelvic exenterations including both anterior exenterations,- leaving the rectum,- and total exenterations, over a period of 13 years. The operative mortality, within 30 days, was 19% in total exenterations. Bricker had said that "palliative" total exenterations for carcinoma of the cervix were unjustified and Brunschwig agreed. Earlier they had ". . . attempted not a few palliative resections, that is, taking out cancer where we know we left some behind, because the patient's symptoms were quite distressing . . . we have given this up . . . we do not do the operation unless all the macroscopic tumor can be removed." The anterior exenterations, 248, had a lower mortality,- 12%,- than the total exenterations.

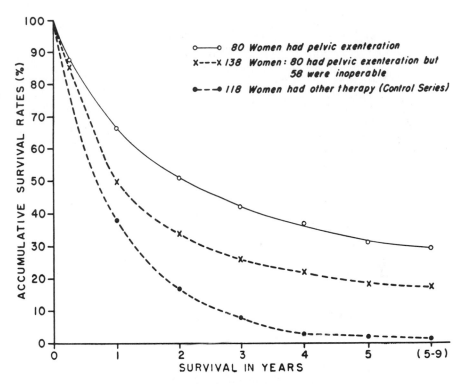

Fig. 2. Accumulative survival rates of women treated for postirradiational cancer of the cervix in the Barnes Hospital— 1950 to 1957.

○——○ *80 Women had pelvic exenteration*

×---× *138 Women: 80 had pelvic exenteration but 58 were inoperable*

●--● *118 Women had other therapy (Control Series)*

Graph showing the survival rate of patients with pelvic exenteration (open circles) to be much more favorable, five- to nineteen-year survival, 30%, than the survival of women refusing operation (closed circles) five- to nine-year survival, 2%.

E. M. Bricker, H. R. Butcher, Jr., W. H. Lawler, Jr., and C. A. McAfee, *Surgical Treatment of Advanced and Recurrent Cancer of the Pelvic Viscera:* An Evaluation of Ten Years Experience. Volume LXXVIII, 1960.

Brunschwig performed urinary diversion in a variety of ways, occasionally performed cutaneous ureterostomy when the operation had to be terminated rapidly. His usual operation was a "wet colostomy". Not infrequently he implanted the ureters into the rectum and performed a proximal colostomy, the rectal ampulla functioning as a bladder. Of the group of 448 done five years ago or more, there were 83 who had survived four-and-a-half years or more. He had 36 patients with total exenterations who were alive and well five to 13 years, and 30 patients with anterior exenteration alive and well five to 13 years. Bricker, closing, gave credit to Brunschwig ". . . for having pointed out the possibility of extended surgery in the treatment of cancer of the cervix". He commented on the sequence of papers arranged by the Program Committee, "The first two papers we hope are opening the doors for future surgery, while my paper represents a type of surgery that we hope will not have to be done for long . . . the needs of today require it, such as it is, and I think the procedure is justified by the results."

* * *

Jack Matthews Farris, of Los Angeles, Associate Professor of Surgery, University of California, and by invitation, Gordon Knight Smith, *Vagotomy and Pyloroplasty:* A Solution to the Management of Bleeding Duodenal Ulcer, suggested that direct suture occlusion of a bleeding vessel in the floor of a duodenal ulcer might be successful if vagotomy and pyloroplasty prevented ". . . recurrent peptic digestion of the suture site . . .", thus allowing a lesser operation than subtotal gastrectomy. They had begun with a few poor-risk bleeding patients in 1952 and reported an initial pilot study in 1957; of 21 patients with major hemorrhage, seven still bleeding at the time of operation, there were no deaths, and no recurrences of hemorrhage during the postoperative period. They now had data on 48 patients, 18 who had had major bleeding but were not bleeding at the time of the operation, and 30, who were bleeding at the time of the operation or within the previous seven days, had an average hemoglobin of eight grams or less and required four units of blood (2000 ml.) or more. In the emergency situation, a 10 cm. gastroduodenotomy was performed. The bleeding in

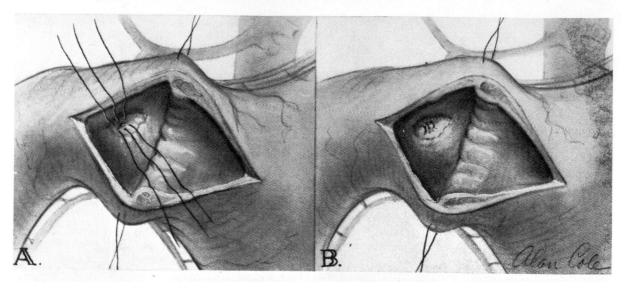

Fig. 2. (A & B) Transfixion sutures through base of ulcer securing vessel.

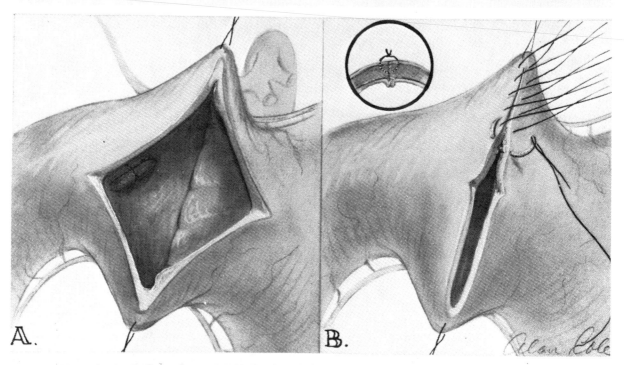

Fig. 4. A. Pyloroplasty. B. Sero-muscular sutures. Inset—illustrating avoidance of mucous membrane.

In 48 patients who had bleeding from a duodenal ulcer, 30 of whom conformed to Stewart's definition of massive bleeders, bleeding had been controlled by placing nonabsorbable sutures deep in the floor of the ulcer and tying them over the bleeding vessel, gaining access through a 10 cm. gastroduodenotomy which was closed transversely by one layer of sutures not penetrating the mucosa. In some cases, a plug of muscle was tied down over the ulcer bed. No patient rebled in the postoperative course. Of three patients who had subsequent melena, one subsequently required a gastrectomy, his recurrent ulcer problems being attributed to obstruction at the pyloroplasty. There were two operative deaths, both in elderly massive bleeders, neither from hemorrhage. [Joseph Weinberg, of Long Beach, had been advocating the technique for 12 years.]

Jack Matthews Farris and Gordon Knight Smith, *Vagotomy and Pyloroplasty:* A Solution to the Management of Bleeding Duodenal Ulcer. Volume LXXVIII, 1960.

the ulcer crater ". . . is secured by means of several stout nonabsorbable fine caliber sutures introduced deeply through the calloused base", occasionally tying a bit of skeletal muscle down into the ulcer with the sutures. Pyloroplasty was by the Heineke-Mikulicz technique, not penetrating the mucosa, and with only a single layer of sutures. "Almost without exception, all duodenums are now considered suitable for pyloroplasty, whereas those with edema, induration and obstruction were previously rejected in favor of gastroenterostomy or subtotal gastrectomy. An acutely perforated ulcer also lends itself particularly well to this operation." He performed a decompression gastrostomy in all patients. There were only two deaths, there were three patients who rebled months or years later, but only one who required reoperation. The first death was in an 86-year-old man who required seven units of blood, developed cardiac arrest at the conclusion of the pyloroplasty and vagotomy, and died six days later. His pressure was maintained throughout that time, and he did not rebleed. The second death was in a 69-year-old man who required eight units of blood and had had a recent stroke with hemiparesis. Restoration from shock was prompt. The operation controlled the bleeding satisfactorily but the cerebral thrombosis progressed. He died without further bleeding. Of the three patients who rebled, two had merely recurrent melena and one had melena and hematemesis, and required a gastrectomy for a duodenal ulcer. Outlet obstruction and gastric retention after the first operation were considered responsible. Farris asked, now that gastric acidity could be controlled so that the suturing of the bleeding point was secure, why one should treat hemorrhage from an accessible vessel in the duodenum differently than one would treat an accessible bleeding vessel elsewhere. He thought the initial hemorrhage was more dangerous than generally thought. Twenty-two of the 30 patients with massive hemorrhage were operated upon in their initial episode. The age of the patient was less important than had been said, "The risk of second hemorrhage is the same in all ages —approximately one-half will die, have other hemorrhages or operations within five years . . . even if one successfully combats an episode of bleeding in a patient . . . by nonoperative methods, little or nothing has been accomplished in the patient's life as a whole . . . he returns to his ulcerogenic environment with overwhelming odds that his symptoms will continue."

Discussion

Frederick A. Coller, of Ann Arbor, Michigan, opened the Discussion, stating he had been communicating with Doctors Farris and Smith over the ten years that they had been interested in this problem. He commented on the long history of papers before the Association on duodenal ulcer, with unsatisfactory results, and the change that had come about since the experimental work of Wangensteen and Dragstedt, and that ". . . Lester Dragstedt's work was not accepted widely because there were so many surgeons who still remembered the evils of the gastroenterostomy alone; they had forgotten or did not admit that something new had been added . . . I think that Dr. Smith and Dr. Farris have given a beautiful presentation. I always thought it was so stupid to resect a fine, big, handsome, strong stomach for a little ulcer just because it was in the neighborhood . . . these gentlemen have taken advantage of the more recent experimental methods and researches and I myself will go to them when I have my ulcer, you see, because I want to keep my stomach." Stanley Hoerr, of the Cleveland Clinic, said that while they had ". . . been very interested in vagotomy, pyloroplasty and gastroenterostomy for chronic duodenal ulcer, we had a deep mistrust of using this procedure for active bleeding that the doctors here describe . . ." However, they had now undertaken it on three extremely bad-risk patients with success in all three. He concluded by saying, "if it works for the poor-risk patient, perhaps we should consider it for the better-risk patients." H. William Scott, Jr., of Nashville, said the antrectomy associated with vagotomy which he had reported the year before was ". . . not, Dr. Coller, a radical resection of the stomach, but involved a physiologic procedure . . . elimination of the cephalic phase of the gastric secretion by vagotomy and excision of the antrum which produces gastrin as well as the inhibitor hormone . . ." They had performed the operation in 765 patients, in the same period of time as the Farris and Smith study, with 21 hospital deaths,- 2.7%. 220 of the patients had hemorrhage as the primary indication of the procedure. He did not have the breakdown as to the kind of bleeding, and there were ten deaths in the 220 or ". . . 4.5 per cent, essentially identical with that which we have heard tonight." He emphasized ". . . both vagotomy with antral resection and vagotomy with pyloroplasty attempt to solve the problem of gastric hypersecretion by essentially the same basic fundamental physiologic principle. The problem is: Is it safer from the pathologic standpoint to resect the bleeding ulcer, or is it safer to suture it and leave it *in situ*?" Mark Ravitch, of Baltimore, said that "Stimulated by Dr. Farris' comments at the last meeting anent the number of patients throughout the country who must be succumbing every year to more or less complicated operations . . . and his mention of the enormous series with a spectacularly low mortality and good results reported by Dr. Joseph Weinberg of Long Beach, California [1956], we got Dr. Weinberg on an eastern trip to give a staff conference at Hopkins." Encouraged by this, his resident, Dr. [F. M.] Steichen, at the Baltimore City Hospitals, ". . . and we specialize there in poor-risk patients", had performed the operation six times for actively bleeding ulcers, all of the patients doing very well. In relation to Scott's "beautiful" figures, he commented that the studies of Dennis and of Stewart had ". . . shown the extreme difficulty in assessing the mortality of the operations for hemorrhage unless every patient is treated in the same way and all are included in the study whatever method is under investigation." Ravitch said that they had also treated a patient with an acute perforation by pyloroplasty and vagotomy with equally good results, and concluded ". . . if there is a very sharp difference in the initial mortality . . . it may not be important if the recurrence rate is somewhat higher, although the reported evidence would not indicate that it will be." Clarence Dennis, of Brooklyn, reminding the Fellows of his paper at the 1958 meeting, said that ". . . the figures we are accumulating at Kings County Hospital now are not yet statistically significant, but begin to favor Dr. Stewart." Farris, closing, said that Scott's study ". . . represents one of the most carefully studied series of hemigastrectomy and vagotomy reported . . . Our belief at the moment is that pyloroplasty will just as successfully accomplish nullification of the antral phase as extirpation of the antrum." He objected to the Billroth I, principally because it required excision of ". . . a difficult duodenal ulcer under conditions much less than ideal . . ." He responded to Dr. Ravitch that "We, too, have been stimulated by our association with Dr. Weinberg over a period in excess of 10 years, and it is through this association that we were given the impetus to begin this small series approximately seven years ago." [Weinberg's first paper was published in 1948.]

* * *

The Use of Jejunal Interposition with Total Gastrectomy, George N. Cornell, Helena Gilder, Frank Moody, Charles K. McSherry, all by invitation, and John M. Beal, Associate Professor of Clinical Surgery, Cornell University Medical College, reported the results in 54 patients undergoing total gastrectomy and jejunal interposition at the New York Hospital over a six-and-a-half year period, an extension of studies which W. P. Longmire and Beal had reported from U.C.L.A. in 1952. Two of the patients undergoing total gastrectomy for cancer had had partial gastrectomies three years earlier for benign gastric ulcers of the lesser curvature. In 15 patients the entire operation had been done transabdominally. In 39 the incision had been carried across the costal margin into the left thorax. The spleen was regularly removed with the specimen, the pancreas transected at its neck and closed over with silk sutures. If the gastric cardia was involved, a portion of the diaphragm surrounding the esophagus was taken with the specimen. The jejunum was divided some 20 to 25 cm. beyond the ligament of Treitz and a 25 cm. segment of jejunum, with its mesentery intact, isolated, brought through the transverse mesocolon, and interpolated between the esophagus proximally and duodenum distally, using two layers of interrupted silk sutures, the jejunal continuity being restored by an end-to-end anastomosis. If the pancreas was transected, the area was drained. The spleen had been removed in 22 cases, part of the pancreas in 27, part of the liver in two, and the transverse colon in two. Their immediate operative mortality, three patients, was 5.6%. One patient operated upon three days after an exploratory laparotomy for biopsy of a gastric lesion at first reported, incorrectly, as benign, died six days after total gastrectomy with fibropurulent pleuritis and peritonitis with multiple organisms. "Anastomoses were intact" and it was thought that operation ". . . had been performed too soon after the first laparotomy." The other two patients died abruptly on the second and third postoperative days with what were presumed to be myocardial infarctions. There were four nonfatal esophagojejunal leaks, with subphrenic abscess in two, and one nonfatal jejunoduodenal leak. The fistulas all closed with expectant treatment, or drainage of the abscess cavity. Forty-six of the operations were done for carcinoma, six for lymphoma, one for benign gastric ulcer, and one for varices. Thirty-one patients survived a year or more without evidence of recurrent cancer. Sixteen patients had obvious recurrent disease in less than a year. Three operations were done less than a year before, and a single patient "who moved to Brazil was lost to follow-up". Eight patients who appeared to be free of cancer underwent extensive absorption studies. The operation had been done with a reasonable mortality and was no more complicated than total gastrectomy and reconstruction by Roux-Y. The interposed isoperistaltic jejunum prevented regurgitation into the esophagus, which was often troublesome with end-to-side esophagojejunostomy. The postprandial symptoms decreased quite sharply between six to 18 months after operation either because the patients could accommodate to hypertonic foodstuffs or because they

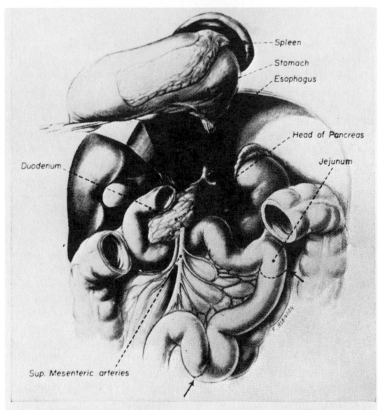

FIG. 2. The completion of specimen mobilization.

The arrows in Figure 2 indicate the sites of transection of the jejunum. In 54 patients, they had three operative deaths,- 5.6%. Gastrointestinal symptoms were common for six months. Thirty-one were N.E.D. at one year. They thought balance studies demonstrated an advantage to retaining the duodenum in the alimentary stream. W. P. Longmire, of Los Angeles, from an experience of 19 cases agreed. W. E. Abbott, of Cleveland, said weight gain and absence of distressing symptoms were attained "not by the type of operation performed but by instructing the patients to eat small, frequent, low carbohydrate feedings, preferably while recumbent." Edgar Poth, of Galveston, with 30 cases, described his jejunal pouch interposed between the esophagus and duodenum, and H. W. Scott, of Nashville, stressed the importance of keeping the duodenum in the alimentary stream.

George N. Cornell, Helena Gilder, Frank Moody, Charles K. McSherry, John M. Beal, *The Use of Jejunal Interposition with Total Gastectomy,* Volume LXXVIII, 1960.

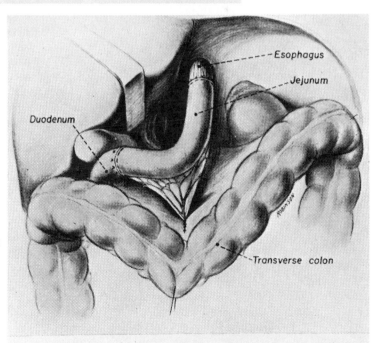

FIG. 4. The completion of jejunal interposition.

had learned by experience to avoid them. "Small capacity and immediate postprandial distention appear to be the most tenacious symptoms. However, the patients in this series who survived beyond 18 months have had good digestive function even though they had postprandial symptoms in the early postoperative period. Those who are under retirement age are employed gainfully, or do their own housework . . . the relationship of the patient's actual postoperative weight to ideal and preoperative weight reflects the incidence of digestive symptoms and adequacy of oral intake . . . some patients who have survived for more than two or three years have been found to lose weight without recurrent neoplasm. This has also been noted in patients who have survived three to five years after partial gastrectomy. Appetite may be reduced after gastrectomy, and it is probable that this late weight loss represents a reduced dietary intake." The metabolic studies demonstrated ". . . an absence of significant defects in protein absorption in seven. There was minimal malabsorption of fat in four patients and clinically significant malabsorption of fat in two of these patients . . . The interposition of the jejunal segment appears to be an effective method to restore gastrointestinal continuity, as it prevents regurgitation and facilitates digestion and absorption."

Discussion

William P. Longmire, of Los Angeles, initiated the Discussion, stating that F. A. Henley, in England, had undertaken jejunal interposition at the same time as Longmire and Beal had begun their studies in 1951. Longmire had 19 patients with total gastrectomy and jejunal interposition, apologizing that ". . . our results are much poorer than those that have been presented today . . ." They had had five deaths during the immediate postoperative period, three of them from suture line leaks, and only three of the 14 patients who survived the operation were alive, two at eight years and one at five years. The late deaths he believed were all due to recurrence. William E. Abbott, of Cleveland, said that to justify the jejunal interposition,- which he favored,- it was necessary to show ". . . that the patient has fewer troubles if ingested food passes through the duodenum rather than bypassing it", and he thought that "the important factor is the preservation of a segment of stomach or the creation of a pouch which acts as a reservoir rather than a conduit." Second, it was necessary to show that jejunal interposition had a favorable effect upon the patient's weight and nutrition. He agreed with H. T. Randall's previ-

ous studies ". . . if only protein and fat are fed to malnourished dumpers, essentially normal quantities of these nutrients will be recovered in the stool. If, on the other hand, high carbohydrate intakes are given with comparable amounts of fat and nitrogen, abnormal amounts of fat and nitrogen and even in some instances carbohydrate may be recovered from the stool." He made the important point that "A gain in weight, reduction or avoidance of distress or vasomotor symptoms and improved absorption of nutrients was obtained in the patients we studied who had interposed loops or direct esophageal duodenal anastomosis not by the type of operation performed but by instructing the patients to eat small, frequent, low carbohydrate feedings, preferably while recumbent. Before routinely advocating an interposed loop because of its nutritional advantages it should be demonstrated that it acts as a reservoir and permits the patient to eat a normal meal while sitting without abdominal distress, vasomotor symptoms, diarrhea and steatorrhea." Edgar J. Poth, of Galveston, responded to the challenge by showing a drawing of an interposition operation which ". . . illustrates the formation of a pouch from jejunum which, in addition to preventing regurgitation into the esophagus, serves as a functioning reservoir. The peristalsis of the reversed segment of jejunum which is the outlet of the pouch serves as a physiologic valve causing the pouch to empty piece-meal and over a period of two to four hours . . . Some 30 individuals have been so treated during the past five years." H. William Scott, Jr., of Nashville, said the studies of Shingleton at Duke and Gobbel at Vanderbilt had "demonstrated the importance of preserving the duodenum in alimentary continuity after doing a total gastric resection . . ." John M. Beal, closing, agreed with Abbott's analysis but said "We have been particularly impressed in our series that there are no patients who can be described as gastric cripples. Part of this we recognize as being due to the careful coaching and education that these patients have received in a special clinic that has been established to guide patients who have had operations upon their stomach . . . an interposed segment prevents regurgitation quite satisfactorily . . . our patients who have had the jejunal interposition have had a superior course to those who have a Roux Y anastomosis." He emphasized his low mortality.

* * *

L. Henry Edmunds, Jr., G. M. Williams, by invitation, and Claude E. Welch, of Boston, Visiting Surgeon, Massachusetts General Hospital; Clinical Associate in Surgery, Harvard Medical School, *Ex-*

ternal Fistulas Arising from the Gastro-Intestinal Tract, reviewed ". . . 157 patients with external gastric, intestinal, or colic fistulas . . . at the Massachusetts General Hospital . . . from 1946 to 1959 . . .", 113 of whom developed their fistulas at that hospital, the others having been transferred to the hospital with the fistulas in existence. There were 55 fistulas ". . . arising from the stomach or duodenum proximal to the ligament of Treitz." There were 46 patients with jejunal or ileal fistulas draining more than 100 cc. and frequently more than a 1000 cc. daily. Finally, the colonic fistulas and the few ileal fistulas, which drained less than 100 cc. a day, formed their third group. Since 1946, 37 gastrojejunal or duodenal stump fistulas had resulted from the 2,648 subtotal gastrectomies performed at the Massachusetts General Hospital, 1.4%. Most of the gastric and duodenal fistulas were preceded by operations for duodenal ulcer, and half of them were from emergency operations for hemorrhage. Eighty-two percent of the fistulas resulted from suture line failures, and in 22 of 26 duodenal stump fistulas ". . . the surgeon classified the stump turn-in as difficult." In eight of the 13 gastrojejunal leaks the probable cause was found. In three of the gastrojejunal leaks with palliative gastrectomy, the suture line contained cancer. In two cases splenectomy and high subtotal gastrectomy had been performed. The left gastric artery had been ligated at its origin "so that ischemia probably was a major contributing factor." In other patients, "Wound dehiscence, stomal obstruction, pancreatitis, tension on the suture line, and gross trauma to stomach or jejunum were obvious causes . . ." Three of their nine lateral duodenal fistulae ". . . followed duodenotomy for pancreatic sphincterectomy", two represented ". . . failure to close a perforated peptic ulcer successfully", and distal obstruction contributed to the formation of three of the lateral fistulae. In general, the gastric fistulae tended to close unless there was distal obstruction. Thirteen of the 17 patients with gastroduodenal fistulae and fluid and electrolyte disturbances died. Sepsis was always part of the problem and required prompt drainage for a suture line leak. Sump suction was the mainstay of care for gastroduodenal fistulae with "Quantitative control of fluid and electrolyte balance . . .", and either restriction of oral intake or a passage of an enteric tube beyond the fistula for distal feeding. ". . . devices to block the fistulous discharge, have proved uniformly unsuccessful in our hands." They used feeding jejunostomies relatively frequently,- 12 patients secondarily and 21 at the time of the original operation. Fifty percent of the patients with duodenal stump fistulae died, 67% of the patients with lateral duodenal fistulae died, 85% of the patients with gastrojejunal fistulae died, 50% of the patients with gastric fistulae died. The overall mortality for all of the patients in this group of fistulae was 62%. They emphasized that this was the mortality of established fistulas only. They made the obvious statement that "The incidence of blownout duodenal stumps is necessarily higher than that of stump fistulas . . . no patient recovers from a major leak or perforation without the formation of a fistula." To prevent stump leaks they suggested vagotomy and gastroenterostomy when a difficult duodenal dissection was anticipated, and prevention of afferent loop obstruction by an indwelling tube through the gastrojejunostomy. The record showed that in 26 patients with a stump fistula it was known whether the surgeon had used a drain or not, and of the 11 patients who had had a drain, four died,- 36%; of the 15 who did not have a drain, ten died,- 67%. "There is nothing to indicate that drainage *per se* increased the number of fistulas." As an operative technique to prevent fistula formation they had ". . . been interested particularly in catheter duodenostomy as an adjunct to gastrectomy . . . a planned fistula is established but is controlled completely by the indwelling catheter and replacement of the duodenal content through a jejunostomy tube. This method allows resection of the bleeding ulcer." Rodkey and Welch had recently reported 51 such cases of "planned duodenostomy", all with "difficult stumps", with a single death. When the catheter was removed, in only five cases had drainage lasted more than 48 hours. Drainage persisted for over two weeks in one patient. As for the established fistula, the "profuse use of antibiotics, blood, human albumin, and improved replacement of electrolytes . . ." had not lowered the mortality, in the last decade. While lateral duodenal fistulas were occasionally amenable to direct closure, fistulas from the duodenal stump were not.

Of their 46 small bowel fistulae, 33 were accounted for by anastomotic failure, surgical injury, or gross surgical error. Of their 56 large bowel fistulae, 25 were similarly attributed. With the small bowel fistulae it was notable that only one patient died of 17 treated by resection of the connecting bowel and anastomosis, whereas 80% of the patients treated less definitively died. Various attempts at bypassing and sidetracking the fistulae were in general unsuccessful, except for "The single patient with complete exclusion and end-to-end anastomosis . . ." who was cured. The high mortality in the patients with high fistulae was particularly notable. A long intestinal tube passed from above before operation helped at operation to identify the loop of bowel involved in the fistula. Inflammatory disease accounted for more large bowel fistulae than small bowel fistulae. Of the 55 patients with colonic or low output ileal fistulae, four had died of their fistulae, 7%. Twenty-two of the 55 closed their fistulae spontaneously. When definitive operation was undertaken,- either resection of the bowel or turn-in of the communication of the fistula,- it was successful 88% of the time. There were nine fistulae from appendicitis, four closed spontaneously, four were closed operatively and "one was not treated at the patient's request." The causes of persistence of colonic fistula, they listed as ". . . active disease at the internal fistulous opening, foreign bodies, fistulas of large diameter, (1 cm. or more) . . . distal intestinal obstruction . . . eversion of mucous membrane, and epithelialization of the fistulous tract." Since large bowel fistulae, once the infection was controlled, were not life-threatening, in the absence of distal obstruction general supportive therapy could be employed for six weeks to allow inflammation to subside, and decision for operation made then. With a fistula and peritonitis either immediate exteriorization or emergency resection was required, "Proximal defunctioning operations are inadequate since they do not stop the source of the contamination immediately . . . all four patients who succumbed because of their lower bowel fistulas died of peritonitis."

Discussion

Samuel P. Harbison, of Pittsburgh [whose paper from St. Louis on complete exclusion of the fistula segment and end-to-end restoration of continuity around it had been cited by Welch], said that he was ". . . a little surprised, as was Dr. Sweet, about the large number of fistulas . . ." [Dr. Sweet must have reconsidered his remarks, for his discussion is not published]. Harbison agreed that emergency gastrectomy for bleeding ulcer was demonstrably hazardous and that the procedure proposed by Smith and Farris at this meeting might be much safer for that reason. He agreed with Edmunds, Williams, and Welch that for the high output fistulae ". . . partial exclusion by bypass technics is to be condemned. Complete resection, or complete exclusion through a clean field is the obvious attack. In wounds complicated by infection and maceration, I still favor complete exclusion . . . Later removal of the isolated segment with its mucous fistula is very simple indeed." Francis D. Moore, of Boston, re-emphasized ". . . that the lesion should be adequately drained . . . many of these are an abscess

with a hole on both sides, a hole to the skin and a hole into the gut, and it must be adequately drained so a narrow cicatricial tract can form which then by contracture will close the fistula." The electrolyte disorder had to be rapidly and drastically corrected. Alexander Brunschwig, of New York, spoke of the special problem of the fistula in irradiated bowel ". . . if one encounters any type of fistula, small intestinal or colon, at any level where there has been radiation previously . . . immediate operation gives the patient the best chance . . . We have tried the conservative method and it has failed in most instances." Welch, in closing, re-emphasized ". . . that a controlled duodenal fistula is a far safer type than one which occurs after a blown-out duodenal stump . . . there are two types of catheter duodenostomy. In the first, the catheter is sewed into the open end of the duodenum, which is then closed tightly about it. In the second type the duodenal end is closed but the tube is put into the side of the duodenum a short distance below the closure . . . we have performed just over 50 of these catheter duodenostomies . . . there was one death, a mortality just below 2 per cent. In the 25 patients who had the duodenal stump blow-out after an apparently successful closure, 13 died, with a mortality of 52 per cent." [He failed to cite the relevant figure, the stump leak-rate and mortality in closures without catheter duodenostomy.]

* * *

John W. Kirklin, of Rochester, Minnesota, Surgeon, Mayo Clinic and Associated Hospitals; Associate Professor of Surgery, The Mayo Foundation Graduate School, University of Rochester, and by invitation, W. S. Payne, Richard A. Theye, and James W. DuShane, *Factors Affecting Survival after Open Operation for Tetralogy of Fallot,* had carried out 110 open intracardiac repairs for tetralogy of Fallot during 1958 and 1959. All patients who died within two months of operation were classified as surgical deaths. They used the Gibbon-Mayo pump oxygenator, primed with heparinized blood drawn the day of operation, normothermic perfusion at flow rates of 2.2 liters per minute per square meter of body surface for adults, and 2.4 for children. "Occasionally hypothermia was intentionally induced during the perfusion, and low flows or, more rarely, circulatory arrest was used . . . while simple valvotomy and excision of infundibular stenosis were sufficient occasionally, it was frequently necessary to carry out plastic reconstruction of the outflow tract and pulmonary valve ring, and, on occasions, of the pulmonary artery in order to relieve adequately the obstruction to outflow from the right ventricle." The ventricular septal defect was usually closed by direct suture, a teflon intracardiac patch being employed in only six patients. Cardiac asystole, originally produced with potassium citrate, was now produced by cross clamping the aorta, and in November, 1958, median sternotomy had replaced the bilateral transverse anterior thoracotomy. They had an 83% overall survival in their 110 patients. If there had been no cyanosis, the survival was 100%; with a mild or moderate cyanosis, 86%; and in severely cyanotic patients, 77%. ". . .the probability of survival after open operation for tetralogy of Fallot is high and is inversely related to the degree of cyanosis present prior to operation." Twenty-seven patients had had a prior anastomotic operation and only two of them died, which had surprised them because ". . .of the great increase in technical difficulties encountered in patients with previous anastomotic operations." In 22 of these 27 patients an outflow tract prosthesis had been employed, and the two deaths fell among these 22. They had only operated on two patients under two years of age, and both had died. Nine patients of the 104 developed heart block, and six of them died in the hospital. Kirklin recognized the problem of avoiding heart block in closure of the ventricular septal defect and yet insuring complete repair. Since March 1955, and through the period of the present study, ". . . all patients seen by us with tetralogy of Fallot, whose disability was sufficient to warrant operation, have been treated by operation save three . . . the only contraindication to open operation for tetralogy of Fallot at present is small size of the patient. An anastomotic operation is performed on disabled patients two years of age or less, and is followed in about three years by open operation." While the mortality of 39% in cyanotic patients three to four years of age was high, in the last ten patients only two had died and the last five represented consecutive successes. "In nine of the 19 patients who died after operation . . . severe hypotension began within an hour after termination of the perfusion and continued until death. These patients had clinical evidence of low cardiac output and died within five to 36 hours after operation . . . no deaths of this type have occurred since the vigorous application of knowledge concerning proper management of blood volume and of metabolic acidosis." Use of an outflow tract prosthesis was to be avoided whenever ". . . adequate reduction of right ventricular pressure can be obtained by valvotomy and infundibular resection", in which case they had 20 survivals in 20 cyanotic patients. In the majority of cases, some plastic reconstruction was required,

using ". . . a flexible prosthesis of woven Teflon . . . the latter part of this series." There had been only one heart block in the last 44 patients. While there was great argument over the danger of asystole, their clinic experience made it ". . . difficult to believe that under the circumstances in which it has been used, cardiac asystole induced by ischemia for periods up to 30 minutes has imposed more than a slight additional risk . . . compensated for by the favorable effect on risk afforded by the facility, accuracy, and gentleness with which the intracardiac operative procedure can be accomplished."

Discussion

Egbert H. Fell, of Chicago, initiating the Discussion, discussed two patients who had had the corrective operation and then developed loud murmurs and cardiac failure. The first was found to have a sinus of Valsalva—right ventricle fistula which was successfully closed, the second had had an injury to an aortic cusp which was successfully resutured. Denton A. Cooley, of Houston, was impressed by the better results in patients who had had previous systemic-pulmonary anastomoses. "If this can be confirmed by others, it may provide the solution to a problem which confronts us in selecting an operation for infants and for extremely cyanotic and polycythemic children." The shunt operation might ". . . increase the capacity of both the pulmonary circulation and left side of the heart." In the previous four years, he had performed anastomotic procedures in 45 infants under a year of age with a total mortality of 20%, and no deaths in the last 17. "Several years ago we had poor results in tetralogy of Fallot in attempts at open repair. Our own mortality in 86 cases has decreased progressively, and in the past 37 patients there was only one death." Two technical factors stood out in relation to the improvement. One was the use of Teflon outflow patches which were "used frequently over the pulmonary annulus and on the main pulmonary artery, but the portion which extends over the ventricle must be limited", and the second was employing ". . . a sump-type suction in the left ventricle inserted trans-septally . . . through a stab wound in the anterior muscular part of the septum", to keep the field dry. Richard L. Varco, of Minneapolis, said that his personal results were not as good as those of Kirklin. With respect to the question of a preliminary shunt procedure, he said, ". . . it seems to me, having gone from shunt procedures to the no-shunt procedures and now back to the shunt procedure for the tiniest tots, that for those infants and neonates, this temporizing approach is the treatment of choice for the child desperately ill from the tetralogy of Fallot defects at that early age." The excellence of Dr. Kirklin's results presented a challenge to them all. Henry Bahnson, of Baltimore, cited an additional technical problem. In three cases, sudden ventricular fibrillation had been caused by the transection of an aberrant coronary artery coursing across the right ventricle. Kirklin, closing, paid tribute to Gibbon's contribution and reminded the Fellows that ". . . it was before this Association that Dr. Lillehei, Dr. Varco and their associates presented the original report on what I think perhaps we should all call the Lillehei-Varco operation for the tetralogy." He agreed with Fell that the area around the aortic leaflets was a difficult one, and his answer to Bahnson indicated some experience with the problem of the aberrant coronary artery. ". . . there are a few patients with a tetralogy of Fallot in whom the left anterior descending artery as such appears to be absent. Large branches of the right coronary artery coming across the outflow tract of the right ventricle then supply blood to the left ventricle . . . that is probably an indication for an anastomotic operation, since, if these branches are the sole supply to this area of the left ventricle, it has been in our experience fatal to cut them." Of Cooley's comments, he said, ". . . I think his excellent results with the anastomotic operation in these little patients are even more encouragement to us for the time being, at least, to do this procedure in the sick, small infant rather than primary open repair."

* * *

Henry T. Bahnson, of Baltimore, Associate Professor of Surgery, Johns Hopkins University; Frank C. Spencer, Associate Professor of Surgery, Johns Hopkins University; and by invitation, E. F. G. Busse, and F. W. Davis, Jr., *Cusp Replacement and Coronary Artery Perfusion in Open Operations on the Aortic Valve,* had devised and fabricated individual Teflon cusps for the aortic valves, and in each of four patients they had implanted a single cusp for replacement of a diseased aortic cusp, but they always attempted valvuloplasty if possible ". . . since most stenotic valves can be treated by simple excision of the calcified scar. If this is not feasible or if large perforations are made in attempted valvuloplasty the prosthesis is then used." While the most involved cusp might have to be removed, if there was a choice, "The noncoronary cusp is most accessible and most easily replaced; replacement of the right coronary cusp is more difficult than replacement of the left." The operative field was continu-

ously flooded with carbon dioxide, the coronary arteries were cannulated and perfused, the flow being monitored by an electromagnetic flowmeter. They had performed the operation in four patients, three of whom, one with aortic stenosis and two with aortic insufficiency, were strikingly relieved of symptoms, and the fourth patient ". . . with aortic and mitral stenosis and insufficiency . . . treated with aortic valvuloplasty including replacement of the left coronary cusp, mitral commissurotomy, and removal of clots from the left atrium", had died of a myocardial infarction on the seventh day. They had made attempts in two patients to replace more than one cusp, both of these failed, and they had discovered that they needed smaller cusps and a greater range of sizes. The ultimate fate of the Teflon cusps was unknown, and one patient, at least, had gone four months without any change in the satisfactory function of the cusp. Their high flow coronary perfusion they thought, prevented the arrhythmia and myocardial damage they had previously seen with ischemic arrest.

Discussion

William H. Muller, Jr., of Charlottesville, Virginia, agreed that oftentimes normal function could not be restored except by partial or total valve replacement. He had used a compressed Ivalon sponge initially and now was using Teflon cusp prostheses, and had implanted them in nine patients including one patient, who had a total replacement and was now normally active at 15 months. Muller had developed a total prosthesis consisting of a solid Teflon ring covered with Teflon netting and made of leaflets like Bahnson's. It had been tried in two patients, both of whom had died soon after operation of uncertain causes. Charles A. Hufnagel, of Washington, demonstrated the somewhat similar cusp he had evolved, the movable portion of which was ". . . impregnated with silicone but that portion which is in contact with the aortic wall is of the cloth itself",- either Dacron or Teflon. He had a total replacement prosthesis and had made single, multiple cusp or total valve replacements in 40 patients using cold arrest, and not employing coronary perfusion. Cold arrest was originally achieved by perfusion with cold Ringer's lactate but now by external cooling of the heart, "With this we have held patients in arrest for as long as 100 minutes with only one patient with any difficulty with resuscitation of the heart and that one ultimately resuscitated successfully." He thought that with pure insufficiency ". . . a single cusp replacement is frequently

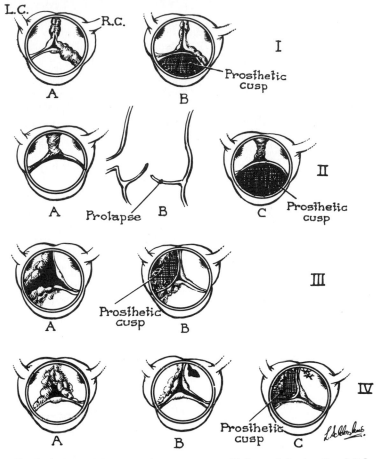

Fig. 5. Condition of the aortic valve in cases reported before and after insertion of Teflon cusp.

I. Case 1: Incision of the two fused commissures failed to relieve the stenosis; the noncoronary cusp was replaced.

II. Case 2. The noncoronary cusp was pliable but contracted so that prolapse and insufficiency occurred; this was relieved by the prosthesis.

III. Case 3: The left and noncoronary cusps were scarred, contracted, and the adjacent portions destroyed; the deficient portion of the noncoronary cusp was sutured to the prosthesis.

IV. Case 4: Right and left coronary cusps were fused, calcified, and contracted; valvuloplasty on the right cusp failed to relieve the insufficiency from contraction and resulted in a tear which could not be closed because of calcium in the adjacent cusp; excision of the left cusp allowed repair of the right and further correction of the deformity.

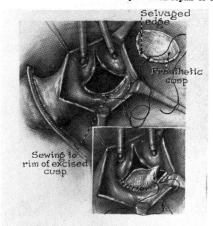

Fig. 4. Noncoronary cusp being replaced with Teflon fabric. The suture is begun at the bottom of the cusp and carried up on each side.

Under cardiopulmonary bypass, high flow coronary perfusion, flooding the field with carbon dioxide, Bahnson and Spencer replaced a single aortic cusp with Bahnson's Teflon valve. Three patients were much improved, one died. Attempts to insert more than one cusp, in two patients, had failed. Valvuloplasty was preferred when possible "since most stenotic valves can be treated by simple excision of the calcified scar."

Henry T. Bahnson, Frank C. Spencer, Edward F. G. Busse, and Frank W. Davis, Jr., *Cusp Replacement and Coronary Artery Perfusion in Open Operations on the Aortic Valve.* Volume LXXVIII, 1960.

adequate but there are certain groups, particularly those with endocarditis, in which it is highly desirable for total valve replacement." His "longest total valve replacement was not quite as long in time as Dr. Muller's." He gave no figures. Donald B. Effler, of Cleveland, had abandoned the sternal split incision and was now using the right anterolateral approach, transecting the sternum but not entering the left pleural cavity. He made sure of left ventricular decompression by a catheter placed from the left atrium venting into the venous reservoir. He had become a convert to Bailey's ". . . decortication of the calcific valves . . . It is incredible to me how well horribly calcified valves can be sculptured or decorticated and returned to a useful state . . . At present we have followed the policy of not using a foreign body, unless forced to do so at the time of operation." He employed cardiac arrest ". . . with regional hypothermia, perfusing the root of the aorta with cold blood and on occasion employing small amounts of potassium citrate." The majority of the patients fibrillated during rewarming. D. W. Gordon Murray, of Toronto, obviously appreciating his own singularity, said that his "only comment is to introduce a note of discord, as usual, on the application of these artificial valves. Despite all the terrific evidence yesterday against homotransplantation of tissue, I have put homo-aortic valves into the aorta in patients in the same position that Hufnagel has put his valves [referring to Hufnagel's old lucite valves inserted into the descending aorta]. Recently we have had one studied now four and a half years after transplantation of the valve and it is in good condition; it is working well with dye and catheter studies; it is intact. My thesis is that if it has to be rejected by the host, the host is a bit slow in getting on with it. I have done four in humans and they are all working well. So I am in favor of transplanting the normal aortic valves. All these beautiful valves produced as we have seen today do not approach the perfection of normal tissues." Bahnson, closing, suggested that perhaps hypothermia might be combined with coronary perfusion. Of hypothermia, "We will admit to its simplicity but not necessarily to its superiority over perfusion." Once one undertook perfusion it was remarkably simple. He agreed with Effler's emphasis on left ventricular decompression and the attempted "simple valvuloplasty". Bahnson said, very aptly, "Dr. Murray has raised a valid question and also described a valuable contribution. I suspect that some of Dr. Murray's contributions will be very much like Dr. Carrel's which were not appreciated at the time but to which we continually return." Bahnson put the current state of valve re-

placement in perspective ". . . almost any of the cusps shown make a much better valve than that which the patient had prior to operation. I suspect that we may have to re-operate upon some of these patients in the future but I do not believe that there will be a second set rejection phenomenon."

* * *

William H. Muller, Jr., of Charlottesville, Stephen H. Watts Professor of Surgery, Chairman, Department of Surgery; Surgeon-in-Chief, University of Virginia Hospital, and by invitation, J. Francis Dammann, Jr., and W. Dean Warren, *Surgical Correction of Cardiovascular Deformities in Marfan's Syndrome,* presented brilliant results in three stunning patients with Marfan's disease affecting the ascending aorta and the aortic valves. "In two, the large aneurysm was excised and a bicuspid aortic valve was created [by excising a cusp and a wedge of aortic wall]. The defect remaining in the aorta was bridged with a Teflon prosthesis. In a third patient who had only marked dilatation of the ascending aorta and a bicuspid valve with a large cleft in it, the aortic ring was narrowed at the cleft commissure to relieve the aortic insufficiency and a segment of the circumference of the aortic wall was excised. The ascending aorta was wrapped with a Dacron fabric band."

Discussion

Denton A. Cooley, of Houston, said that at Baylor, although they had operated on some 50 aneurysms of the ascending aorta, they had only recently had a patient with Marfan's disease ". . . a successful case of annulo-aortic ectasia". The aneurysm was excised along with the noncoronary cusp, the bicuspid valve ". . . repaired by annuloplasty", and the aorta closed. The patient did well. Charles A. Hufnagel, of Washington, D.C., said that in Marfan's disease one could have aortic insufficiency with or without a dissecting aneurysm, and that occasionally with enormous dilatation of the aortic root, aortic insufficiency arose in patients, without Marfan's stigmata. In four patients with dissecting aneurysm, three of them with Marfan's disease, ". . . a repair has been possible using the same methods which Dr. Muller has already described . . . obliteration and resection of the noncoronary cusp and either resection of the ascending aortic root or a plastic procedure . . ." Hufnagel further said that bleeding from the "friable aorta" in Marfan's patients was a problem and that ". . . the closure of the [aortic] root has been markedly facilitated by the use of small strips of Teflon felt through which each suture is placed on each side of the suture line. With this method, which we now routinely employ for all aortic closures in the ascending aorta, even in the heparinized patient leakage is insignificant . . ."

* * *

Benjamin A. Barnes, by invitation; Oliver Cope, of Boston, Associate Professor of Surgery, Harvard Medical School; and by invitation, Esther B. Gordon, *Magnesium Requirements and Deficits:* An Evaluation in Two Surgical Patients, for the first time directed the attention of the Association to the clinical significance of this electrolyte, There were endogenous supplies of magnesium in the soft tissues and in the bone, and it was ". . . a reasonable assumption that, as with calcium and phosphorus, the skeleton represents a reservoir to supplement the needs of the body when on a deficient intake." Studies of the mobilization of magesium and calcium had not been made to see whether either could be mobilized independently of the other, and they asked "Can a normal individual subsist on a diet deficit only in magnesium for more than a week without developing symptoms? How much magnesium is lost in a patient developing a deficit severe enough to produce symptoms?" The first patient was one with a tracheo-esophageal fistula who had been fed by gastrostomy with only glucose and water for 14 days. He was thereafter maintained on a special liquid diet with no magnesium intake, "The serum magnesium values were repeatedly checked and always found normal. The patient never developed any symptoms related to the magnesium-free diet and renal function was normal throughout the study." The second was a patient who had had a total colectomy and resection of 85 cm. of terminal ileum [the case report identifies the lesion of the small bowel as "regional ileitis" and the lesion of the large bowel as "chronic ulcerative colitis", without any comment]. In subsequent operations she had had several small areas of small bowel removed although it was thought much of the retained small bowel was diseased. She had tetany with only modest depressions of her serum calcium and was finally found to have a substantial depression in her serum magnesium ". . . 0.4 mEq. per liter (normal range at this hospital 1.5 to 2.5 mEq. per liter)." The patient's clinical condition responded strikingly to the administration of calcium and magnesium intravenously. Their final conclusions were that "The human body with normal bowel and renal function can tolerate magnesium-deficient diets for at least 38 days . . . There is no significant obligatory loss of magnesium by normal kidneys or gastro-intestinal tract in this period of time . . . Calcium deficient and magnesium deficient states are easily confused clinically and are each relieved in part by salts of either ion." In the magnesium-deficient patient with a short bowel, "Treatment with magnesium intramuscularly at the rate of 27 mEq. per week has prevented symptoms of deficiency developing in the same patient . . . the most common surgical situation where a magnesium deficit will develop is in those patients with abnormal gastro-intestinal drainage, extending over many weeks."

Discussion

William E. Abbott, of Cleveland, said that in 1956 his group had reported magnesium balance studies ". . . in four patients who were losing up to 4,000 ml. of gastric or intestinal fluid daily." With large amounts of fluid loss, magnesium was lost. They had several years earlier seen a patient ". . . with symptoms of magnesium deficiency similar to the one reported by Drs. Barnes and Cope", due to a low small intestinal fistula. Francis D. Moore, of Boston, reminded the Fellows that ". . . in the middle 1940's potassium entered the I.V. flask and surgical fluid therapy entered the cell . . . many patients who we care for now in a routine way without thinking about it would not get along nearly as well without their potassium supplements. The search for other intracellular electrolytes which might help us in surgical care has not been very rewarding. Phosphate and calcium are both found in the skeleton in huge amounts. Iron remains very important, but we easily provide it intravenously in blood transfusions. Magnesium remains the next one to look at." He interpreted Abbott's data as showing that ". . . skeletal mobilization is not particularly important in this particular form of electrolyte deficiency . . ." His group had seen magnesium abnormalities in alcoholics with cirrhosis, in the short bowel syndrome, and in patients with prolonged I.V. therapy who received no whole blood. Alkalosis made the symptoms of magnesium deficiency worse. Barnes, closing, re-emphasized the fact that ". . . under normal circumstances . . . an obligatory loss essentially does not exist. There is no requirement, except a very minimal one, of half a milliequivalent or so of magnesium per day."

* * *

The presentation by Angus D. McLachlin, of London, Ontario, Professor and Head of the Department of Surgery, University of Western Ontario, and

1128

by invitation, John A. McLachlin, Thomas A. Jory, and E. G. Rawling, *Venous Stasis in the Lower Extremities,* was one of those remarkably simple and clear demonstrations of a clinically practical principle. Lower extremity venous angiography in volunteers showed that, in the horizontal position, contrast material might remain behind the valve cusps for long periods of time, up to an hour, whereas if the whole table was tilted so that the legs were elevated 15°, there were only a few individuals in whom the dye could still be seen after brief periods of time. This elevation was more efficient than vigorous contraction of the thigh and calf muscles with the patient horizontal.

Discussion

Rocke Robertson, of Montreal, said McLachlin's technique was ". . . a most ingenious way of demonstrating the factor of stasis which everybody agrees is important in the induction of thrombosis but which I think everybody has found very difficult to demonstrate in the clinical case and even to test experimentally . . . It may well be too, that if he persists in operating in patients in a 15-degree head-down position that his incidence of thrombosis in his patient will be less than it has been before." Alton Ochsner, of New Orleans, said that there were two types of venous thrombosis, the one which McLachlin had shown, the coagulation thrombosis ". . . as a result of stasis, a precipitating factor and a predisposing factor increased coagulability of the blood, usually with the result of tissue injury", and that the second type was associated with thrombophlebitis ". . . the so-called phlegmasia alba dolens . . . an entirely different lesion . . ." The lesion of which McLachlin was speaking was ". . . the bland thrombus or the phlebothrombosis . . ." which predisposed to pulmonary embolism. Joel Baker, of Seattle, asked whether Dr. McLachlin had tested the effect of compression bandages or stockings. Robert R. Linton, of Boston, agreed with the importance of elevating the foot of the operating table and of the bed in the recovery room, and after operation making patients exercise their legs in bed pushing against the footboard with their toes ". . . which causes contraction of the gastrocnemius and soleus muscles where these thrombi so often begin. They are told that they must do this at least *one thousand times* a day . . ." McLachlin, closing, said addition of elastic bandaging to the 15° elevation improved the results not at all, "The elevation leaves very little blood in the superficial veins, and it is probable that pressure bandages are effective by directing the su-

perficial flow into the deep veins and so speeding its return from the legs." McLachlin reminded them that ". . . Dr. Ochsner has long advocated elevation of the foot of the bed in postoperative patients. We hope that elevation of the foot of the operating room table and recovery room bed will lessen the chance of venous stasis initiating thrombosis in the period of enforced inactivity."

* * *

The Business Meetings

The 1960 meeting was held at The Greenbrier, White Sulphur Springs, West Virginia, April 4, 5, and 6, Dr. Warren H. Cole presiding.

The Treasurer, H. W. Scott, Jr., after reviewing the financial status of the Association, said "It is clear that the traditional publication of the Transactions is the Association's major financial burden. If the Association is to continue to publish the Transactions, it must arrange to increase its annual income."

At the Second Executive Session, dues were raised to $40. The Acting Secretary [Altemeier was absent] reported the Council's recommendation "That, in accordance with the traditions of the Society and after the most careful consideration of all factors involved, the strongest recommendation be made to the effect that the attendance at the annual banquet be restricted to members only."

There was no discussion and this item passed, along with all the other recommendations of Council read to the Membership by the Acting Secretary. [The heated discussion *against* having the ladies at the Annual Dinner had prevailed over the majority vote *for* having the ladies at dinner.]

Walter Maddock moved "that the Council of the American Surgical Association consider the establishment of a standing committee to consider and report on various problems of American Surgery. It is hoped that such a committee would be composed of enough members of diverse interest to be able, through subcommittees, to evaluate problems in many fields."

Among the new Members elected were Curtis P. Artz, Gilbert S. Campbell, David C. Sabiston, Frank C. Spencer, and an Honorary Member listed as Professor John P. Sandblom, of Lund, Sweden. Elected as officers were President, John D. Stewart, of Buffalo; Vice-Presidents, Harris B. Shumacker, Jr., of Indianapolis, and Joel W. Baker, of Seattle; and Secretary, William A. Altemeier, of Cincinnati.

LXXIX

1961

The 1961 meeting was held at the Boca Raton Hotel, Boca Raton, Florida, March 21, 22, and 23, President John D. Stewart, of Buffalo, Professor of Surgery, University of Buffalo; Head of the Department of Surgery, Edward J. Meyer Memorial Hospital, in the Chair. Among those who had died in the preceding year were Gordon Gordon-Taylor, the distinguished British Honorary member, and Howard C. Naffziger who had been President in 1954.

* * *

James R. Jude, W. B. Kouwenhoven, and G. Guy Knickerbocker, all by invitation, *A New Approach to Cardiac Resuscitation,* from the Department of Surgery, The Johns Hopkins Hospital and Johns Hopkins University School of Medicine, presented the work, which from the moment of its first publication in the *JAMA* the year before, had achieved acceptance of its extraordinarily simple and effective way of restoring to life patients with cardiac arrest or ventricular fibrillation. They were now reporting 22 patients with a variety of surgical procedures who sustained cardiac arrest in either the operating room or the recovery room, and 18 other patients who had cardiac arrest in the postoperative phase after a cardiac surgical procedure. The "method of external cardiac massage consisted of compressing the heart between the sternum and thoracic vertebral column . . . The operator placed the heel of one hand on the patient's lower sternum just above the xiphoid . . . The other hand was placed on top of the first, and using some of his body weight the operator pressed the sternum vertically downward with a thrusting motion. Pressure was transmitted through the heel of the hand only—none with the fingers." They advised compression some 60 to 80 times per minute, and simultaneous artificial respiration by face mask or intratracheal tube. Electrocardiograms were obtained as soon as possible, and ventricular fibrillation treated by electric shock through electrodes applied externally. Epinephrine as a vasopressor, by the intracardiac or intravenous route was almost always used, and calcium chloride by the intracardiac route "to strengthen weak heartbeats." If there was any delay in restoring good cardiac action, sodium bicarbonate was given "to reverse the acidosis secondary to the low flow of artificial circulation." Quinidine or procaine amide was given at times when defibrillation was difficult or when the heart was irritable. After resuscitation, they employed "hypothermia and intravenous urea for cerebral edema as necessary." The 22 patients, with a variety of operations, underwent a total of 25 arrests, three of them with fibrillation. After 24 out of 25 of the arrests,- 96%,- the patients were "resuscitated to their pre-arrest central nervous system status" and 17 of the 22 patients survived to leave the hospital,- 77%. In 18 postoperative cardiac patients, there were 24 arrests and after 17 of these, the patient was resuscitated to the pre-arrest central nervous system status. Eight of the 24 cardiac arrests were associated with ventricular fibrillation. Resuscitation was successful in 13 of the

1129

24 [only one patient was discharged from the hospital]. "The other 12 patients survived in a condition as before the arrest for periods of a few hours to a week before succumbing to their primary cardiac disease." In all, they had attempted resuscitation in 11 episodes of ventricular fibrillation. All of the patients were defibrillated and in seven of the 11 episodes, resuscitation was to the pre-arrest central nervous system status. They noted that the first reported successful direct cardiac massage was by Igelsbrud, in 1901, that Crile, 1906, had demonstrated the value of epinephrine, and Beck, in 1947, had reported the first defibrillation of the human heart. Kay and Blalock in 1951 [Volume LXIX] had demonstrated the value of calcium chloride in cardiac resuscitation and Elam and others in 1954 had, ". . . reintroduced . . . expired air ventilation . . . a major step towards effective pulmonary ventilation." Although their present report concerned patients in the operating room or recovery room, "External cardiac massage has also been extended to the medical and surgical wards, the cardiac catheterization laboratory, the diagnostic radiology laboratory, the emergency room and even outside of the confines of the hospital itself." Success in resuscitation under such circumstances was 46%, expectedly, not as good as in the operating room. Complications of external cardiac compression were probably not as numerous as those from direct heart massage in which actual rupture and laceration of the heart had been reported. Within the operating room, the Hopkins group had seen "an occasional fractured rib." Rib fractures were more common in patients resuscitated outside of the operating room, and the liver had been known to be lacerated. The great advantage of the method was that it could be instituted at once, on mere suspicion, eliminating the delay that frequently occurred when people hesitated before making a thoracotomy in a patient who was suspected of having cardiac arrest.

Discussion

Alfred Blalock, of Baltimore [who had certainly been responsible for the appearance of this paper on the program], said that Kouwenhoven had been interested in the effects of electricity upon the heart for years, had studied fibrillation and defibrillation and "A few years ago, Dr. Kouwenhoven told me that he was about to retire as Professor of Electrical Engineering and Dean of the School of Engineering in the Johns Hopkins University. He did not wish to stop work, and inquired if he could work in the surgical laboratories? The immediate answer was yes.

He was interested in developing a better method of defibrillating the heart by external means . . . In the course of observations on dogs, in which they were monitoring the blood pressure, and putting the two heavy electrodes on the chest, they observed that pressure on the electrodes caused a slight elevation in blood pressure in these fibrillated hearts. This led them to use vigorous [external] manual massage . . . As he said, this has been used not only in the hospital, but outside the hospital. I think one of the most dramatic instances was that of a 68-year-old man who had had a previous myocardial infarction. Last May, he collapsed at home and had gasping respirations. The ambulance was called, and it so happened that these drivers had been given instruction a week before by Dr. Kouwenhoven and his group. They started positive pressure ventilation and external massage. They took the man to the hospital, which required 15 or 20 minutes. He arrived in the accident room about 23 minutes after he collapsed . . . he was in ventricular fibrillation. The massage was continued. He was defibrillated . . . This man made a total recovery without any neurological deficit, and he is alive today, almost a year following this episode." Blalock said that there were two conclusions worth drawing from this work, "One is that most important discoveries are simple in concept and design, and the second conclusion is that an occasional person past three score and ten makes an important discovery, and it could not happen to a better fellow than Dr. Kouwenhoven." Robert D. Dripps, of Philadelphia, Professor and Chairman, Department of Anesthesiology, School of Medicine, University of Pennsylvania, called it "a tremendous contribution" and emphasized the necessity for providing a return flow of blood for the heart to work on, suggesting the elevation of the lower extremities, perhaps "a rapidly flowing intravenous", and the use of a pressor drug, which Kouwenhoven had mentioned. Henry K. Beecher, Chief, Department of Anesthesia, Massachusetts General Hospital, Professor of Research and Anesthesia, Harvard University, [after Francis D. Moore's vigorous condemnation in 1954 of the rejection of anesthesiologist candidates for Fellowship, Adriani, of New Orleans, Beecher, of Boston, and Dripps, of Philadelphia, had been elected in 1955], said that they had had a good many fractured ribs perhaps because in their experience, fatal cardiac standstill had occurred particularly in elderly people, and that "To our minds, this discovery—this observation which has been made—ranks not too far behind that of the tourniquet in its life-saving potentialities when there is an occasion for its use. We use it with success and satisfaction."

Properly, Claude S. Beck, of Cleveland, who had made so many contributions in this area, concluded the Discussion. "This contribution speaks for itself. Death has been reversed without opening the chest. This had been done when the victim died outside the hospital, even by nonmedical personnel, by the rescue workers." He emphasized the fact that the heart, which had undergone sudden arrest was sometimes a healthy heart, and with restoration of the heartbeat the patient might essentially be quite well. [He referred to his own work without mentioning the fact that it was his own work] "I should like to refer to several historical accomplishments. The possibility of shocking the human heart out of fibrillation was presented to the American Surgical Association in 1937 [Volume LV]. At that time fibrillation and defibrillation was a laboratory curiosity without practical application. The first successful case of shocking the human heart out of fibrillation was in 1947. This occurred in the operating room. This patient is alive. The first patient dressed in street clothes who fell over dead from a heart attack was successfully defibrillated in 1955. This patient, a doctor, is alive . . . Death has been reversed and these heart victims are alive years later."

* * *

W. G. Bigelow, of Toronto, Assistant Professor of Surgery, University of Toronto Medical School and by invitation, P. J. Kuypers, R. O. Heimbecker, and R. W. Gunton, *Clinical Assessment of the Efficiency and Durability of Direct Vision Annuloplasty,* reported the first 20 consecutive patients in whom, under cardiopulmonary bypass with a bubble oxygenator, they had opened the left atrium and attempted to correct mitral insufficiency by placing sutures in one or other commissure, usually the medial one. The sutures were of 0 silk passed through Ivalon or Teflon buttons. There were three deaths in the first six cases and two in the next 14. The heart size decreased radically after operation. Patients who had all been Grade III or IV, New York Heart Association, were now, all but one of them, Grade I or II. The left atrial pressure dropped in all patients but one. They were encouraged "that plication of a valve ring carried out in this manner has a good chance of becoming efficient and durable", and recurrence of the insufficiency as time went on had not been a problem. There were four late deaths, five to 18 months after operation.

Discussion

Denton A. Cooley, of Houston, stressed the hazard of air embolism in these operations. He had now learned to control that with a Teflon vent inserted into the apex of the left ventricle. Donald B. Effler, of Cleveland, said that annuloplasty alone had not given them as good results as Bigelow here reported. Like Bigelow, he operated through a right thoracotomy. George H. A. Clowes, Jr., of Cleveland, said that his group had been operating from the left side and he wished "to state that there is no view obtainable of the mitral valve comparable to that which one can get from the left side of the chest, if the patient is rotated slightly forward . . ." W. G. Bigelow, closing, said that they had handled the prevention of air embolism by introducing a sucker through the mitral valve "once you have made it competent".

* * *

[Bigelow in 1950 (Volume LXVIII) had suggested the possibility, at the close of an intracardiac operation, of leaving a wire electrode attached to the heart, brought out percutaneously for pacemaker stimulation if need be.] Now Paul M. Zoll, by invitation, Howard A. Frank, of Boston, Chief of Thoracic Surgical Clinic, Associate Director of Surgical Service, Beth Israel Hospital; Assistant Professor of Surgery, Harvard Medical School; and by invitation, Leona R. N. Zarsky, Arthur J. Linenthal, and Alan H. Belgard, *Long-Term Electric Stimulation of the Heart for Stokes-Adams Disease,* whose work had already excited the medical world, discussed the possibilities of their pacemaker studies, and the clinical application. They had experimented with a considerable variety of metal wires and of insulating materials, the bare ends of the wire inserted into the myocardium, with "Sutures used to hold the wires or plates in place". The principal problem in the clinical application was the progressive "rise in the electrical threshold for myocardial stimulation . . . The rise in threshold appears to result from a reaction of the cardiac tissue to the implanted foreign body [the wire]." Platinum was the most successful wire for the electrode. They found no difference between bipolar and unipolar thresholds and thought that "Two electrodes in the heart do provide a safety factor . . ." They accepted "the need for thoracotomy for myocardial implantation of the electrodes in order to achieve their optimal placement and fixation." The passage of wire through the skin was avoided ". . . by the use of an induction circuit or radiowave transmission across the skin." They had developed a "transistorized, battery powered pulse generator and radio frequency transmitter that transmitted a signal through the skin to a small subcutaneous receiver (diode detector) from which wires delivered the stimulus to the heart." The buried receiver could be very small and the external power source was easily replaced. However, the necessity for and problems involved in maintaining close apposition of the external apparatus to the skin overlying the diode had led them to prefer the buried pacemaker with long-lived batteries. They proposed to drive the heart at a fixed and predetermined rate. Chardack had set at about 50 per minute the pacemaker he had developed. Zoll and his associates preferred a rate of 70 to 80 per minute, assuming that that would give a maximal cardiac output. They had applied their pacemaker in 14 patients with Stokes-Adams attacks and the apparatus had been successful in preventing further Stokes-Adams attacks in all the patients for up to 12 months.

Discussion

Elliott S. Hurwitt, of New York, discussed the experience at the Montefiore Hospital, in New York, with the intracardiac catheter pacemaker, a report of which had been published a few months earlier. "The catheter is threaded through the external jugular vein and the tip positioned in the outflow track of the right ventricle, as in a conventional right-heart catheterization." The patients were all ambulatory and some had returned to work. If pacing was no longer required, as in some of the patients, the catheter could simply be removed. Howard A. Frank, closing, said they, too, had used the intracardiac catheter electrode successfully but liked the implantation wire electrode, ". . . because the patients are free of external wires and equipment and, as time goes by, begin to forget their pulse rates and hearts."

* * *

Experimental Studies of Factors Influencing Hepatic Metastases: IX. The Pituitary Gland, by invitation, Bernard Fisher [not a Fellow until 1963], and Edwin R. Fisher, from the University of Pittsburgh, was another in the continuing meticulous and sophisticated studies of experimental cancer by the Fisher brothers, surgeon and pathologist [one of which presented before the Association in 1959 (Volume LXXVII), had demonstrated that surgical trauma to the rat liver enormously encouraged the development of hepatic metastases from innoculated cells]. They had previously demonstrated that "tumor cell dosage, partial hepatectomy, liver injury, cirrhosis, nutrition, liver blood flow, alteration of

the reticulo-endothelial system all affect the establishment of liver metastases, whereas adrenalectomy and cortisone do not . . ." In their present experiments, they demonstrated that hypophysectomized rats, pair-fed with normal controls, were far less susceptible to the development of hepatic metastases from tumor cells injected into the portal circulation, that injection of growth hormone, follicle-stimulating hormone, luteinizing hormone, adrenocorticotropic hormone, and thyroid-stimulating hormone in combination did not protect against the effect of hypophysectomy, but that injection of homogenized fresh anterior or whole pituitary glands did. It was true that the individual hormone preparations were bovine or ovine in origin, whereas the fresh homogenates were rat pituitary. While there was no question of the protective effect of hypophysectomy against the injection of even large numbers of tumor cells into the portal circulation, and the design of the experiments suggested that the pituitary effect was due to some substance other than the individual hormones studied, and that it represented a direct effect upon the liver, yet the manner in which the effect was produced was not established. They concluded that "it seems clear that the take and growth of experimental hepatic metastases, usually observed under the conditions of the experiments, requires an intact hypophysis."

Discussion

Bronson S. Ray, of New York, with his enormous experience with hypophysectomy for advanced mammary cancer, arose in Discussion, commenting on the need for imaginative studies of this kind to evaluate the effect of the pituitary on tumor growth. He pointed out that they had observed in hypophysectomized patients with breast cancer that those "known to have been benefited or worsened by the administration of estrogens or androgens before operation do not react to a repetition of the treatment after hypophysectomy", whereas "it is not an uncommon experience to find that patients may respond to estrogen or androgen therapy after combined oophorectomy or adrenalectomy, or after adrenalectomy alone in older women . . . there may be a factor of pituitary function which must be present for circulating estrogen or androgen to influence activity in breast cancer." Warren H. Cole, of Chicago, commenting that "others have shown that the removal of the hypophysis depressed the tendency for the growth of the liver metastases" asked whether this was "a hormonal reaction, or is the cause located in the liver itself?" He interpreted Dr. Fisher's feeling as leaning toward a direct hormonal effect, whereas he himself inclined to think it might be an effect upon the liver. Bernard Fisher, in closing, would only go so far as to state that "it would certainly seem that the pituitary is of major importance."

* * *

A series of papers on the significance of cancer cells recovered from the blood of patients had issued from the laboratories of the Department of Surgery at the University of Illinois and now Stuart Roberts, Olga Jonasson, LeRoy Long, Ruth McGrath, Elizabeth A. McGrew, all by invitation, and Warren H. Cole, of Chicago, Professor and Head of the Department of Surgery, University of Illinois, *Clinical Significance of Cancer Cells in the Circulating Blood:* Two- to Five-Year Survival, reported studies of the blood in 700 patients, 283 of them two to five years earlier, and 73 of the latter studied before and during operation. The emphasis of their observations was that "although there was no difference in the survival of the entire group of patients with positive or negative blood samples, a shower of circulating cancer cells during an operative procedure was associated with a survival rate only one-half that of patients with negative blood samples during operation." They appreciated that a 10 cc. sample of circulating blood was a minimal sample, that their patients were all patients with relatively advanced cancers, and that these facts might have blunted the adverse prognostic significance of cancer cells recovered from the circulating blood. Nevertheless, "Twenty-five per cent of patients with cancer cells demonstrated in one or more blood samples survived, indicating again that 'tumor embolism is not metastases' . . . a concept which is as germane today as it was in 1897 when first stated by Paget." Engell [1959] had previously reported "no difference in the survival of patients with and without circulating cancer cells" and had concluded that "in the majority of patients surviving five to nine years, tumor cells disseminated before and during operation must have perished in the blood stream", whereas the study by Watne, Sandberg, and George Moore [1960] had found a substantial decrease in survival rate in patients in whom demonstrated circulating cancer cells had been found. In general, Cole and his colleagues found "a prompt disappearance of cancer cells from the blood stream following removal of the tumor or clamping of the venous drainage . . . persistence or the appearance of cancer cells in the blood stream following a 'curative' type of resection

. . . may constitute an indication for additional therapy such as x-ray or chemical agents."

Discussion

Warren Cole, the only discusser of the paper, which Roberts had presented, stated that thus far they had demonstrated only a trend toward lower survival in patients with cancer cells recovered from the blood. He thought the evidence was "that the great majority of these cells found in the blood stream die. They are probably killed, of course, by the host resistance . . . with few exceptions, the vascular spread is what kills the patient . . . There is a close relationship of the survival of these cancer cells to the survival of bacteria in the body . . . a small number of bacteria are tolerated in a wound without production of an infection whereas a large number of bacteria will result in an infection . . . cancer cells in the circulating blood might behave in a similar way . . . a small number of cells lodging in a certain spot might not live, whereas a large number would . . . It appears that host resistance is the important factor in determining whether these cells will die or survive . . . It seems possible that cancers are developing in a person's body numerous times throughout his lifetime, but that these cells are being killed off, or suppressed (perhaps 'suppressed' is a better word)."

* * *

Harvey R. Butcher, Jr., of St. Louis, Associate Professor of Surgery, Washington University School of Medicine, *Effectiveness of Radical Mastectomy for Mammary Cancer:* An Analysis of Mortalities by the Method of Probits, analyzed ". . . the different cellular growth patterns . . . the frequency of axillary nodal metastases . . . sizes of the primary tumors . . . and . . . the relationship of postoperative survival to these characteristics." The growth patterns were what they called "I. Nonmetastasizing (not invasive)" cancers,- intraductal or comedo cancer, and Paget's disease, "II. Rarely Metastasizing (always invasive)" cancers, including mucinous or colloid cancer, medullary cancer with lymphocytic infiltration, and well differentiated adenocarcinoma, "III. Moderately Metastasizing (always invasive)" cancers or advanced adenocarcinomas, intraductal carcinoma with stromal invasion and infiltrating adenocarcinomas, and "IV. Highly Metastasizing (always invasive)", including "undifferentiated carcinomas having cells without ductal or tubular arrangement and without cellular inflammatory response about them *and all types of tumors*

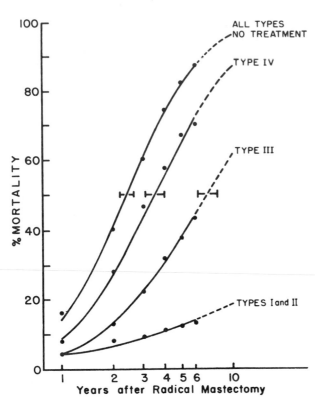

ALL TYPES
NO TREATMENT

TYPE IV

TYPE III

TYPES I and II

% MORTALITY

Years after Radical Mastectomy

FIG. 3. This graph compares the mortality expectancy of the different types of mammary cancer treated by radical mastectomy with the untreated series of Greenwood. The lines are calculated from the corresponding fitted probit transformation (Fig. 4). The dots about the lines are data points. The confidence limits (95%) for the time of median lethality are represented by the bars to the left and right of the point of 50% mortality.

Butcher's figure demonstrating the extraordinary difference in survival depending upon the histologic character of the tumor led him to say that "Women treated by radical mastectomy for Types I and II mammary cancers died at rates which hardly exceeded those expected among women of similar ages without mammary cancer (only 2 of 101 actually died of cancer during five postoperative years) . . . the inclusion of the individuals having Types I and II mammary cancers in any sample of breast cancer to be used for the assessment of the relative merits of radical mastectomy or any other manner of treatment would be almost as illogical as including fibromas of the breast in the sample."

Harvey R. Butcher, Jr., *Effectiveness of Radical Mastectomy for Mammary Cancer: An Analysis of Mortalities by the Method of Probits.* Volume LXXIX, 1961.

indisputably invading blood vessels." Analysis of 425 cases from the Barnes Hospital and 364 from the Ellis Fischel Cancer Hospital demonstrated that the mortality expectancy differed sharply according to the biological type of mammary cancer. Patients with Type III and IV tumors, with axillary nodal metastases died more rapidly than those without. An important result of Butcher's statistical analysis was that taking all cancers of the breast, without classification, the attrition rate beyond six years after operation was no different than it was for women without cancer of the breast. Butcher made the graphic statement that "The statistical analysis of the treatment of breast cancer as it has been generally practiced is somewhat analogous to attempting the collective assessment of the poisonous propensity of a pen full of varied kinds and sizes of snakes—including small, medium sized and larger garter snakes, water moccasins, rattle snakes, and king cobras—without any knowledge of the numbers of the various kinds of snakes within the pen. Obviously, without knowledge of the proportions of the various kinds of snakes that exist in the pen no real quantitative determination of the effects of pulling the fangs can be made." The variation in survival in association with size of tumors appeared to be actually dependent upon the histologic character of the tumors. A theoretical analysis of his data suggested to him that "the proportion of women with mammary cancer in a consecutive series who might survive as well after simple mastectomy as after radical mastectomy is rather high (75%)", those women being those who had no axillary metastases at the time of operation, and those who died before the point in the probit line for their particular tumor which he designated as "the point of truncation", but he indicated that obviously, this would have to be proved by the clinical test of the controlled trial of simple versus radical mastectomy in Types III and IV mammary cancers in whom axillary nodal metastases had been proved to exist.

* * *

Ira S. Goldenberg and John C. Bailar, III, both by invitation, and Mark A. Hayes, of New Haven, Associate Professor of Surgery, Yale Medical School, and Ruth Lowry, by invitation, *Female Breast Cancer: A Re-evaluation,* analyzed "the records of 1,458 women with histologically-proven breast adenocarcinoma diagnosed and treated at the Yale-New Haven Medical Center from 1921 through 1957." They concluded that survival was lower in younger patients and increased up to the time of menopause, after which there was a decline in survival associated, at least in part, with death from other causes. Survival was better [a little more than 50%] in the later years of the study and "Such an improvement in survival may reflect improved surgical methodology, i.e., adjuvant therapy, since radical mastectomy itself has changed little." Decreasing mortality from other causes, and earlier diagnosis, they thought, might have played some part. As in most previous studies, the lowest survival was with tumors in the lower and inner quadrant, the best survival in tumors in the lower and outer quadrant. Patients with the smallest tumors had the best survival, regardless of age. They were astonished to find that, despite the fact that "simple mastectomy is usually reserved for those patients in whom radical mastectomy is deemed too major an operation or for those with advanced disease", the five-year survival rate after simple mastectomy was "as good as that of patients treated by radical mastectomy" and the difference in ten-year survival could be explained by the greater average age of the patients undergoing simple mastectomy.

Discussion

David V. Habif, reporting from Presbyterian Hospital, where Cushman Haagensen had so continuously studied breast cancer, discussed the gross appearance of a whole section of the cancer, studied under low power, separating the tumors with well-delimited contour from those with less rounded, less well-delimited contour. The former had 41% axillary metastases and a smaller number of involved nodes, the latter 65%. The ten-year cure rate for those with the sharply circumscribed tumors was 80%, as opposed to 38% for the others. He suggested "we should try to do a radical mastectomy on those patients who may be cured, and relegate those with extensive or nonresectable disease to simple mastectomy and radiotherapy." Claude E. Welch, of Boston, said that 25 years before, he and Nathanson had analyzed their results with breast cancer and found at that time in the State of Massachusetts a relatively small effect in survival, compared to no treatment at all. He commented on "the importance of the two papers brought out tonight". [Particularly when the meeting was held at a resort, as in this case at Boca Raton, it was usually the practice to have one "free" afternoon to be followed by an evening session of papers. Some years, the evening papers seemed to be those devoted to a special or narrow phase of surgery, and small attendance might result. In other years, outstanding or strong

papers and new aspects of surgery were presented in the evening session, in the hope of encouraging the Fellows to leave the festive board in time for the session. Over the years, the Program Committee has demonstrated the same kind of ambivalence with respect to the nature of the program in the session on the last afternoon.] Welch continued, ". . . the two papers brought out tonight—both of them prepared some 25 years later than our study—. . . indicate the present marked spread between the life expectancy of untreated and treated cancer of the breast, now much greater than anything we were able to show 25 years ago. I believe these data indicate that those who adopt a laissez-faire attitude toward treatment of cancer of the breast are in error and that we must pursue treatment actively." Grantley W. Taylor, of Boston, was interested in Butcher's histologic classification and was concerned that other pathologists would group individual tumors in different Butcher types. He commented, with an overtly pejorative tone, on Habif's report from Presbyterian, where "he is using Dr. Haagensen's criteria of operability and deciding beforehand which ones are operable; and by sharpening these criteria, he is operating on fewer and fewer people, I gather. He has got his operability down to about 50 per cent. I think if he sharpens his criteria, he could bring his operability even lower than that, and get even better results on those which are subjected to operation." He was obviously describing the philosophical and emotional dilemma of the surgeon of the 60's dealing with breast cancer, knowing that radical mastectomy for all women subjected many of them to "futile operations", while at the same time, fearing that an occasional woman might be cured by a radical mastectomy who would not be cured by something less, so that "it seems to me we are under obligation to offer the benefit of the doubt to those patients who may be salvageable, if we carry out a properly planned, properly executed radical operation." Rudolph Noer, of Louisville, Kentucky, was persuaded by Butcher's presentation of the pathological classifications of Tornberg and Ackerman at Barnes, and said that at Louisville they were reviewing the material from the cooperative adjuvant breast chemotherapy group to see what influence the histological classification might have. Carl A. Moyer, of St. Louis, further emphasized the importance of the "Butcher-Ackerman classification". Simple mastectomy was all that was required for Type I breast cancer, radical mastectomy was unnecessary for Type II and Type III cancers without axillary metastases, and would not be required once "methods have been developed to determine with surety the absence of metastasis to the axillary lymph nodes, without having first to remove them. Whenever we shall be able to do this, simple mastectomy shall be sufficient for those types of cancers, whenever the axillary lymph nodes do not contain metastases." Hilger P. Jenkins, of Chicago, carrying to a logical conclusion the suggestion that radical mastectomy had a smaller place in the treatment of cancer of the breast than had been thought, said that "In view of some rather exuberant enthusiasm about a super-radical mastectomy involving the removal of mediastinal nodes, which has been popularized in some areas [Urban at the Memorial Hospital in New York, and Wangensteen at the University of Minnesota], I would like to provoke one or both authors into a statement pertaining to the so-called mediastinal node dissection of the supraradical mastectomy." Goldenberg had apparently not mentioned the significance of the quadrantal location of the tumor in his spoken presentation and Samuel J. Stabins, of Rochester, New York, pointed out that at Rochester they had demonstrated that "when the axillary nodes are involved in the inner tumor quadrant, only 8.0 per cent would be alive five years later." Butcher, closing, said that in fact the Haagensen criteria of operability had been applied to practically all of the patients with radical mastectomy in their series, agreed "that the prognosis is excellent among patients with well-delimited mammary cancers", but added that "A second factor which also appears to be of some importance is the degree of cellular differentiation in these cancers." As for Grantley Taylor's concern that pathologists would "start splitting hairs", he thought that the resultant intellectual turmoil might lead to better care for patients. Ira S. Goldenberg, closing, must have disappointed Jenkins by saying only that their experience with the super-radical operation had been too limited for them to draw any definite conclusions as to the advisability of the procedure. He agreed with Stabins that the lower inner quadrant lesions had the poorest prognosis whether the axillary nodes were involved or not.

* * *

Robert R. Linton, of Boston, Visiting Surgeon, Massachusetts General Hospital; Assistant Clinical Professor of Surgery, Harvard Medical School, and by invitation, Daniel S. Ellis and Joseph E. Geary, *Critical Comparative Analysis of Early and Late Results of Splenorenal and Direct Portacaval Shunts Performed in 169 Patients with Portal Cirrhosis,* were reporting the Massachusetts General Hospital experience from 1946 through 1958. Their earliest experience with portacaval shunts had been unhappy,- 15

patients, with two post-operative deaths from liver failure, one with a thrombosed shunt, and three other deaths in the subsequent months, two certainly from liver failure, leaving one third of the patients dead within a year or less after operation. In the same early two-year period, 1953 and 1954, 19 splenorenal shunts yielded two operative deaths, one in the immediate postoperative period, from failure to control esophageal bleeding, one later death from liver failure and one death from liver failure six months later. They then restricted portacaval shunts to those patients in whom "a satisfactory splenorenal shunt had failed to control the esophageal bleeding." The results had been increasingly clear "that the splenorenal group have done better on the whole than the direct portacaval ones . . ." All patients considered had an intrahepatic portal bed block. The review covered only Dr. Linton's own operative cases, 122 splenorenal shunts and 47 portacaval shunts. Although the mortality had decreased in recent years, all patients from 1946 on were included in the study. There were 13 operative deaths from splenorenal shunts,- 11%,- and seven operative deaths after portacaval shunts,- 15%. Seventy-two percent of the deaths after portacaval shunts were due to hepatic failure, and 15% of the deaths in the splenorenal group. On the other hand, one patient after splenorenal shunt died of esophageal hemorrhage from varices. There were more failures, more instances of postoperative bleeding, etc., after splenorenal shunts, indicating that it was a more difficult procedure. With increasing experience and better preparation of patients, they no longer lost patients with splenorenal shunts from postoperative hemorrhage. Jaundice, ascites, and premonitory signs of coma were commoner after portacaval shunt, whereas sepsis and pneumonia were commoner after splenorenal shunt. The portacaval shunt showed a moderate advantage in terms of late esophageal bleeding. Eight percent of the splenorenal patients and 4% of the portacaval patients died of esophageal hemorrhage. Duodenal ulcer developed in both groups with the same frequency. Twenty-five late deaths were attributable to liver failure,- 43% of the splenorenal shunt patients and 71% of those who had had portacaval shunts. A total of 10% of the patients died of cerebrovascular hemorrhage which Linton thought curious and perhaps attributable to clotting difficulties. Splenorenal patients had a 57% five-year survival and the portacaval shunt patients had a 36% five-year survival.

Discussion

John P. West, of the New York Hospital, demonstrated that of 97 patients with esophageal varices, who were thought inoperable, 40 died of the first hemorrhage, 10 more died in less than a year. They had offered operation to 42 during the same period, and operation had been rejected for 21 of them by the medical consultants. At the end of two years, 12 of the 21,- 57%,- who had had shunts were alive. Of the 21 patients for whom operation had been refused, six were alive,- 28%. "We think that this is in support of the operative treatment of esophageal and gastric varices." George A. Hallenbeck, of Rochester, Minnesota, said that they had similarly experimented with portacaval end-to-side, and splenorenal shunts, and came down on the side of the former "because it seemed much easier to do and because it accomplished better decompression of the portal system." The operative mortality of splenorenal shunt in their hands was only 5 or 6% and of portacaval shunt between 10 and 15%. Encephalopathy was much commoner after portacaval shunt and subsequent esophageal bleeding was pretty much the same with either operation,- about 20%. Remarkably enough, they found 73 patients who had had splenectomy alone and these had the same survival rate as those who had had shunts, "It looked as though survival rate was measuring something besides prevention of bleeding, because the people who had splenectomy bled in over 66 per cent of instances, where those who had shunts bled in only about 20 per cent of instances." When it appeared that the survival rate was better with splenorenal shunts than with end-to-side portacaval shunts, they switched to performing splenorenal shunts "whenever the splenic vein was large enough". However, as time had gone on, there seemed to be progressively less difference in survival between the patients having the two kinds of shunts. Hemorrhage from massive acute duodenal ulcers had occurred with both kinds of shunts. David M. Hume, of Richmond, came down, unequivocally, on the side of portacaval shunt as decreasing portal pressure much more dependably. He was "rather surprised at the mortality series in the two groups" since, in the 47 shunts he had done in the previous four years, he had had an operative mortality of 5.5%, operating on patients whose figures suggested they were worse risks than Dr. Linton's patients. No mention had been made by Linton of side-to-side portacaval shunts which Hume thought should be done from time to time. After shunting, he had had no bleeding from varices in the 47 patients. C. Stuart Welch, of Albany, said that initially, the splenorenal operation had seemed easier, but subsequent technical developments had eliminated that differential.

He was convinced of the superiority of the portacaval shunt in decreasing the incidence of hemorrhage,- from 20 to 25% after splenorenal shunt, to 1 to 2% after portacaval shunt [although admitting that some of his splenorenal shunts were done for extrahepatic portal blocks]. He favored the side-to-side shunt as "universal" both for the prevention of bleeding and for the treatment of ascites. The mortality, he thought, with any of the operations, was more directly related to the state of the liver than to the kind of operation performed. Linton, closing, said that they were dealing with cirrhosis,- chronic disease,- and he doubted "that any of these procedures that we have discussed benefit the liver in any way, other than to prevent esophageal hemorrhage and the troubles that accrue from repeated blood loss." He supposed most surgeons preferred the direct portacaval shunt because it was easier. He was particularly interested in the long-term outcome and survival and, in his series, that was best with splenorenal shunt. As to side-to-side shunts, he had done three, and those three patients were all dead. He thought a large drop in portal venous pressure was unsatisfactory and that if one insisted on performing a direct portacaval shunt, perhaps the anastomosis might be made a very small one.

* * *

P. S. Conner, in 1895 [see page 164, Volume XIII] had discussed carcinoma of the tongue, and more recently, J. C. Bloodgood in 1914 [see page 488, Volume XXXII]. Now from Philadelphia, Henry P. Royster, Professor of Surgery, School of Medicine, University of Pennsylvania; Assistant Surgeon, Hospital of the University of Pennsylvania; Consultant in Surgery, Skin and Cancer Hospital of Philadelphia, and by invitation, H. B. Lehr, A. Raventos, and W. E. Demuth, *Management of Patients with Squamous Cell Carcinoma of the Tongue*, discussed their experience with 146 patients seen in the 30 years between 1925 and 1955. The nature of their clinical material and their feeling about it is indicated by the statement that "The available data on these patients are devoid of controls; the treatment was at no time randomized or subjected to any other principle of experimental design which would make possible valid comparisons of the results among the several types of therapy employed. All of the treatments failed more often than they succeeded, and all were attended by morbidity and/or permanent disability of some degree." In the first 20 years, all patients were irradiated. The radical surgery of the earlier years had been abandoned by

1922 after which until about 1946, the operation was relatively conservative, limited to excision of the lesion and an occasional hemiglossectomy. The first modern radical neck dissection had been done in 1946. In the last ten years of the study the surgical treatment had been radical, with en bloc resection of the portion of the tongue involved, and a radical neck dissection performed in most patients with palpable nodes, and some without palpable nodes. Their accrued overall five-year survival rate was 24%, similar to that of other published series. They did not separately analyze the results in the three decades of essentially different treatment. Their current preference was for interstitial implantation in small lesions of the posterior third of the tongue or in the anterior two-thirds when resection would impair speech. The functional result was then essentially normal, although there was a risk, after radiation, of radionecrosis of the mandible. For lesions of the anterior two-thirds of the tongue, which could be resected without serious impairment of speech or deglutition, resection was preferred and particularly if there was extensive involvement of adjacent structures. A radical neck dissection was performed for resectable nodes whether the primary treatment was operation or irradiation.

Discussion

Arnold J. Kremen, of Minneapolis, referred to the early experiences of Billroth and Kocher, with cancer of the tongue, and the abandonment of operative therapy in favor of radiation until after the Second World War, since which ". . . there has been a renaissance of interest in surgical management of these diseases, and I think the results, as suggested by Dr. Royster, and others, bear out the assertion that this is a favorable cancer . . . a surgeon today . . . well versed in the technics and management of head and neck problems has more cures to show at the end of five years than surgeons concerned with most visceral cancer." The anatomical situation favored the attempt at a classical cancer operation. For exposure, Kremen preferred to split the cheek and divide the mandible, retracting it laterally, ". . . then one had the kind of exposure that every surgeon likes to have when he is doing surgery." Of thirty-eight of his own patients with operable cancer of the tongue, 26 had clinically negative neck nodes. All patients had resection of the tongue, floor of the mouth, and a radical neck dissection in continuity and there proved to be cervical node metastasis in 12 of the 26 clinically negative cases. John W. Baker, of Boston, cited 175 patients from the Massachusetts

General Hospital, 1946 to 1955, all with cancer of the anterior two-thirds of the tongue and a series of about the same number in the posterior third of the tongue. They found "at least a suggestive association between cancer of the oral mucous membranes and cirrhosis of the liver, or possibly the high alcohol intake and the vitamin and other nutritional deficiencies associated with cirrhosis." Their crude five-year survival thus far was 45%, all patients having been treated first by combined radiation and operation. Considering only the size of the primary tumor, if this was 1.0 cm. in greatest diameter or less, the five-year survival was 92%, between 1 and 4 cm., the five-year survival was 51%, and tumors larger than 4 cm. were associated with a crude five-year survival rate of 17%. He assumed that this was because the smaller tumors had not yet metastasized by the time the patients presented themselves for treatment. Frederick A. Bothe, of Philadelphia, having lost a patient from respiratory obstruction due to edema of the glottis after a radical tongue operation, now always performed a prophylactic tracheotomy. Grantley W. Taylor, of Boston, [responding to much of the program in the way that purely "clinical" surgeons so frequently have] said "It is very gratifying for us to find a clinical paper which we can react to and understand what we are talking about." Referring again to the Massachusetts General Hospital series, he said that it had been their experience that the very small early lesions did not require prophylactic neck dissections and even in the more moderately advanced lesions he was less radical than Kremen. Taylor thought that failure to cure with mouth cancer was "very often failure to control the primary disease, rather than because of uncontrollable metastatic disease." Royster, closing, agreed with Kremen, and opposed Taylor's stand, although admitting that for very small local cancer or cancer *in situ,* only a local operation was required. At Pennsylvania, they, too, had noticed an association between cirrhosis and cancer of the throat ". . . we are finding that a history of alcoholism is very common in most of these patients." While he had certainly seen edema of the glottis, Royster said that he did not routinely perform tracheostomy, reserving it for those with "previous radiation, previous surgery in the area, those who have had severe infections, and on those patients who have operations in the posterior part of the tongue . . . where the tongue has been dislodged, and the anterior mandible has been removed, the tongue may drop back and cause the epiglottis to close."

* * *

Benjamin A. Barnes, Glenn E. Behringer, Frank C. Wheelock, and Earle W. Wilkins, all by invitation, *Postoperative Sepsis:* Trends and Factors Influencing Sepsis over a 20-Year Period Reviewed in 20,000 Cases, were responding to, "The unanswered criticism of rampant hospital sepsis casually asserted by the lay press as well as by some doctors, the ill-defined impression of the limitations of antibiotics in the prevention and treatment of certain types of surgical sepsis, the avalanche of clinical reports without any statistical control purporting to show trends in sepsis rates, and the convincing reports of certain pediatric and maternity units of epidemic staphylococcal sepsis . . ." This was obviously a retrospective study, at the Massachusetts General Hospital. They studied abdominal hysterectomies and inguinal herniorrhaphies as being done usually in healthy adults, subtotal gastrectomy as representing a more severe operative stress and appendectomy for acute appendicitis "as an example of surgery applied to the treatment of a grossly septic process." The annual rate of sepsis for the 3,340 herniorrhaphies was 5.2%. Infection rate for removal of the normal appendix was 2%, for an acutely inflamed but not gangrenous appendix was just under 4%, for gangrenous appendices, almost 15%, and for hysterectomy, it was 4%. All of these figures were essentially constant over the 20-year period of the study. Gastrectomy in the pre-blood bank era,- 1932 to 1940,- was accompanied by a sepsis rate of 16%, which dropped sharply to 4.1% in the period of 1941 to 1953, and had risen to over 9% in the period 1954 to 1958, coincident with the change in hospital policy toward accepting more patients with massive duodenal ulcer hemorrhage for emergency operation. There was an increased rate of infection in the later periods in patients with ruptured appendices and appendiceal abscess, which was attributed to simultaneous lowering in mortality which provided a greater number of survivors at risk of developing infection. As far as they could tell, the " 'prophylactic' use of antibiotics prescribed in conventional ways did not influence the rate of postoperative sepsis." The single benefit of antibiotics they could demonstrate was in the lowering of the mortality in cases of advanced appendicitis. They were unable to demonstrate that wound infections, in these studies, were due increasingly to staphylococci.

* * *

From the laboratory of W. A. Altemeier at the Cincinnati General Hospital, W. R. Culbertson, by invitation, W. A. Altemeier, Christian R. Holmes

Professor of Surgery, University of Cincinnati, and Director of Surgery, Cincinnati General Hospital, and by invitation, Luis L. Gonzalez, and E. O. Hill, was now presented *Studies on the Epidemiology of Postoperative Infection of Clean Operative Wounds,* another of their detailed and meticulous studies of operating room infections. In *clean* wounds ["when the procedure had been performed under aseptic circumstances without a major break in technic, and was an operation which did not transect the gastro-enteric, genito-urinary or tracheal-bronchial systems and was not performed in the vicinity of any apparent inflammatory reaction"], the infection rate was 0.7%. [It was to be repeatedly commented on in national surveys of wound infections that the lowest rates were in the obsessively precise Cincinnati General Hospital operating rooms with their longstanding tradition of hostility to practices inviting infection.] Altemeier and his group noted "a striking lack of correlation between infecting bacteria and those recovered from the nasal flora of the operating personnel or the environmental air. It is interesting to note that the bacteria recovered from the wound at the end of the operation in two instances were the same as those recovered from the subsequent wound infection. Unfortunately, cultures were not obtained from the hands or gloves of the operating personnel or from the patients' skin or excised tissues such as gallbladder or lymph nodes." In *clean-contaminated* wounds [like clean wounds "except that opening or transection of viscera known to contain bacteria occurred"], there was a 5.1 incidence of infection. Of the 17 infections this represented, two were staphylococcal infections due to bacteriophage type 80/81, a hospital organism which again was not found in the naso-pharynx of the operative personnel or in the air of the operating room, and thus suggested no evidence of significant bacterial infection from aerial spread.

Discussion

Deryl Hart, of Durham, North Carolina, rose to initiate the Discussion, stating that the staphylococcus problem was much less severe than it had been from 1930 to 1943 when he had worked on the problem so intensively. In the winter of 1933–34, "we had within 72 days, six deaths; all patients had septicemia or meningitis. There was a concomitant high level of air contamination, with hemolytic staphylococcus aureus with over 80 per cent of our hospital personnel and of the general population carrying the staphylococcus aureus in their nose and throat." Hart's discussion mentions also streptococcal infection in the Boston Hospitals, and further infections in clusters at Duke, without stating the organisms responsible,- "over a five-year period the deaths from unexplained infections always occurred in groups, usually two or three, but on one occasion six, at which time we quit operating. In 1935, we had three such deaths in 32 days. We stopped operating except for emergencies. Since the installation of ultraviolet radiation in 1936, we had two deaths where we did not use it. I know of no death from an unexplained infection in a clean wound in the Duke Hospital since 1936, when ultraviolet radiation was used." William R. Sandusky, of Charlottesville, commented that phage group 80/81 could be "recovered from the nose and the skin of healthy individuals" and that staphylococci of other phage types could be equally virulent and invasive. He emphasized that in addition to the presence of bacteria, factors such as the presence of suture material, debilitation, malnutrition, cortico-steroid therapy, and of greatest importance "the presence in the wound of such factors as blood clots, tissue tension, dead space, devitalized tissue, and an inadequate local blood supply . . . the state in which the surgeon leaves the wound is of tremendous importance in determining whether or not wound infection will ensue." Frank L. Meleney, now retired to Miami, said that from 1945 to 1955 with the coming of antibiotics ". . . surgeons in many places began to let down the standards of strict aseptic technic, and at the same time the ubiquitous staphylococcus demonstrated its ability to develop resistance to the antibiotics . . ." He reviewed all the sources of organisms, all the factors responsible for infection. Curtis Artz, in a preceding paper on the problem of staphylococcal infection, had advocated instillation of a bactericidal ointment into the nares of staphylococcus carriers. Meleney thought a spray to the nasopharynx might be better. He urged further study of bacitracin [which he had introduced]. He disagreed with Barnes' findings that prophylactic antibiotics were not useful. "The time to use antibiotics is at the time of operation, applying them in bactericidal concentrations to the surface of the wound, where the organisms are, thus surrounding the bacteria with lethal effect before they have invaded the body, and thus rendering them impotent to produce infection . . . Antibiotics given systemically, prophylactically, may never reach this area . . ." Ultraviolet light would sterilize the air, but would not have any effect on surface contamination. Champ Lyons, of Birmingham, Alabama, spoke a little more clearly than some of his predecessors stating that there had been reports of increased hospital infections and that

many studies had "demonstrated a pollution of the air in the operating room by itinerant organisms derived from the environmental air of other parts of the hospital . . . The more generally accepted concept of the genesis of wound infection is that of direct contamination from pathogenic organisms harbored by the patient and referred to as endogenous bacteria, or from exogenous organisms derived from the secretions or excretions of the surgical attendants or immediately precedent patients." He agreed that Barnes' study indicated no increase of wound infections during the antibiotic age and that direct contamination was the likely source. Jonathan Rhoads, of Philadelphia, rose to comment on the joint study of ultraviolet light in the operating room, undertaken by five university hospitals. The study was not yet complete,- "the study has made clear to the participants in it that the clinic at which Dr. Altemeier is Chairman has achieved the lowest rate of infection in clean and clean-contaminated wounds among the participants in the study." Rhoads reiterated the necessity for careful operative technique, commented that "The study of wound infections per hour of operating time shows a definite rise in frequency as the length of the procedure increases." He tended to play down the significance of cultures of the nares of the operating room personnel, "No one in our own operating room personnel whose nares have been frequently cultured has consistently failed to show staphylococci." Altemeier responded, "The endogenous origin of wound infections is generally overlooked, and in the work presented by Dr. Culbertson [who had given the Cincinnati paper] there is evidence that the incidence of infection in clean wounds increased seven-fold whenever some area of the alimentary tract, including the gallbladder, was transected or resected . . . contact spread either by endogenous or exogenous sources are the most important means of significant bacterial contamination and infection of operative wounds." He stressed the importance, in addition, of obvious elements of technique, keeping the drapes dry, lest the passage of bacteria through them be facilitated. He now said quite bluntly "There is little or no evidence in our data to substantiate the importance of aerial spread and contamination of wounds. The evidence is more in favor of either exogenous or endogenous contact spread." Ivan W. Brown, Jr., of Durham, said that they had undertaken a retrospective study at Duke almost identical to that of Dr. Barnes. From 1930 through 1959 they had performed 2,956 herniorrhaphies under ultraviolet light irradiation with an infection rate of 0.12%. "This is to be compared with an infection rate of around 5.2 per cent for other reported series of herniorrhaphies covering essentially the same years." The infection rate at Duke for the ten years before the use of ultraviolet irradiation had been 8.3% in herniorrhaphies. Between 1930 and 1959 there had been 2,495 clean operations on the neurosurgical service performed under ultraviolet irradiation with an infection rate of 0.18% compared to a preceding infection rate of 8.9%. "We believe these figures speak for themselves with conclusive evidence that ultraviolet irradiation of the operating room is extremely effective in preventing the 'unexplained infections' in clean operative wounds." Curtis P. Artz, of Jackson, Mississippi, said there was "little doubt about the value of ultraviolet light." Benjamin Barnes, in closing, very gently pointed out that whereas Meleney had assumed that Barnes' comments about the increase of wound infections with increased transfusions was impugning the blood transfusions as the causative factor, he was, of course, impugning the insult of the condition for which correction by blood transfusion was required! He re-emphasized what Sandusky had said about the wound itself as a culture medium for bacteria. W. R. Culbertson, responding to Rhoads' allusion to the superiority of the Cincinnati results, said that it was due to "first and basically, an attitude of mind; second, meticulous maintenance of all the understood principles of aseptic and antiseptic technic; and above all, a continuous check of the technics by every individual involved in the operative team during the course of all procedures."

* * *

The Association had been hearing that some malignant experimental tumors were sensitive to chemotherapeutic agents and they had been hearing that tumor cells were recognizable in the blood of cancer patients at the time of operation. Now a large-scale attempt was underway, with 24 university departments of surgery cooperating, *Breast Adjuvant Chemotherapy:* Effectiveness of Thio-Tepa (Triethylenethiophosphoramide) as Adjuvant to Radical Mastectomy for Breast Cancer. The paper was presented by Rudolph J. Noer, Chairman, Surgical Adjuvant Chemotherapy Breast Group. The National Institutes of Health, Cancer Chemotherapy Center had set up a Clinical Studies Panel chaired by I. S. Ravdin, with George E. Moore as Chairman of the Surgical Adjuvant Chemotherapy Projects. The hope was "that chemotherapeutic agents given in association with excisional 'curative' cancer operations might diminish the recurrence rate and increase survival of patients suffering from cancer."

The chemotherapy projects had been set up to "test this thesis in cancer of the lung, stomach, colon, and rectum, ovary and breast." The initial Thio-Tepa dosage schedule, 0.8 milligram per kilogram of body weight, total dosage 0.4 mgm. at the time of operation and 0.2 mgm. on the first and second postoperative days, proved to be associated with too many side reactions and after the first 108 cases, the total dose was dropped 0.6 mgm. per kilogram body weight divided into 0.2 mgm. the day of operation and each of the next two days. There were 610 patients in the second series. The follow-ups were a little more than of two years' duration. While Noer emphasized the fact that the results were still preliminary he could not resist stating, "Although the confidence limits overlap, the absolute size of the difference between the curves is heartening and gives us cause to believe . . . that perhaps Thio-Tepa has demonstrable effectiveness as an adjuvant to radical mastectomy in the treatment of cancer of the breast." [It is remarkable how regularly, and up to the present day, sophisticated investigators employing complicated statistical analyses, report that the apparent differences in their data "are not statistically significant but clearly show an important trend". Noer and his group were obviously succumbing to the same temptation.] He concluded that "The data so far accumulated indicate a statistically significant decrease in the early recurrence rate among patients who received Thio-Tepa as adjuvant to operation in comparison with the control groups who received only radical mastectomy. It appears that the higher dosage was somewhat more effective." Noer said quite clearly that one would have to wait for the five-year results before an adequate evaluation could be performed.

Discussion

Arnold M. Seligman, of Baltimore, rose to dampen any enthusiasm which might have resulted from the presentation. Seligman did say that "the cooperative group method, involving many hospitals, a rigid protocol and independent statisticians, is probably the only way to obtain the kind of information needed today for evaluating a number of currently controversial surgical procedures." He challenged the wisdom of this study because "The experiments upon which Dr. Cole's hypothesis was based were performed in rats with the Walker tumor and nitrogen mustard. The Walker tumor is sensitive to this alkylating agent. Human breast cancer is not particularly sensitive to either nitrogen mustard or thiotepa, especially in the 'safe' dose level made nec-

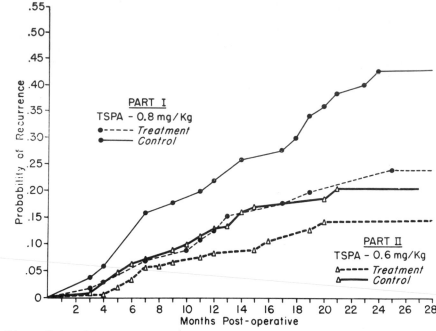

Fig. 8. Probability of recurrence in treatment and control groups, Part I and II compared.

In spite of the fact that the confidence limits of the control and treatment (thiotepa) lines for both Part I and Part II overlapped, hopeful inferences were drawn from the data and indeed, the lines as drawn might give reason for optimism.

Surgical Adjuvant Chemotherapy Breast Group, *Breast Adjuvant Chemotherapy:* Effectiveness of Thio-Tepa (Triethylenethiophosphoramide) as Adjuvant to Radical Mastectomy for Breast Cancer. Volume LXXIX, 1961.

essary by concomitant radical surgery." He indicated that many of those involved in the original decision doubted that "the drugs available at that time were good enough to test Dr. Cole's hypothesis, and we were concerned that the hypothesis might be discredited by premature trial with inadequate drugs. This is what has happened with the lung, gastric and colonic cancer groups." In any case, he said, "there was no evidence to support the idea that cells dislodged during radical mastectomy were more responsible for poor results than metastases already established prior to surgery." While it was inviting to believe that the danger was chiefly in the circulating cells at the time of operation and, "all that remained was to damage these circulating cells by adjuvant therapy and the survival results would be improved", he reminded the Association that Dr. Cole had commented on "the apparent lack of difference in survival of patients with and without circulating cancer cells". Seligman emphasized that these observations threw "some doubt on the validity of the hypothesis that short term adjuvant chemotherapy, no matter how good, can alter the survival rates." He urged that the data be considered preliminary and not the basis for clinical practice, when all that were available were two-year survival

data. William P. Longmire, of Los Angeles, thought the value of the gastric cancer chemotherapy study had been to set up a mechanism and familiarize surgeons and institutions with the technique of multi-institutional studies. Longmire made the interesting comment, without remarking upon it, that "in more than 20 university centers that were participating in our study, the mortality rates for gastric resection alone were somewhat higher than those that one would anticipate from a review of the operative mortality rate reported in the literature." Carl A. Moyer, of St. Louis, commented that multi-institutional cooperative studies had been under way at the Veterans Administration for 15 years, evaluating the therapy of tuberculosis, and had proved their value. He seemed to question whether the individual tumors in the present breast cancer study had been matched for size, specific characteristics, etc. If this were not done, the value of the chemotherapeutic program which might be useful to some tumors would be obscured by the combined results. Noer, closing, assured Dr. Seligman that "we are well aware of the fact that Dr. Cole's work was on nitrogen mustard and the Walker tumor, a very different situation than breast cancer and thiotepa." As for the significance of the study, Noer reminded Seligman that they had already said that the five-year survival rates would be more significant than the two-year recurrence rates, and concluded by affirming that this was, in fact, a preliminary report.

* * *

The last three papers had probably been adjudged by the Program Committee to be sufficiently exciting to keep the membership in attendance until the gavel came down after the discussion of the third paper on this last afternoon of the meeting. Frank C. Spencer, of Louisville, Professor of Surgery, School of Medicine, University of Kentucky Medical Center; Thomas A. Stamey, by invitation, [from the Department of Urology, the Johns Hopkins Hospital]; Henry T. Bahnson, of Baltimore, Associate Professor of Surgery, Johns Hopkins University; and Arthur Cohen, M.C. USA [from Walter Reed], *Diagnosis and Treatment of Hypertension Due to Occlusive Disease of the Renal Artery*, operated upon 27 patients, ages five to 69 in the previous three years "for hypertension caused by obstruction of a renal artery." They stressed, as much as the operative technique, the split renal function test of urea and inulin excretion [the Stamey test] which had proved to be the best test in their hands. They were already separating arteriosclerotic obstructions in 12 patients from fibromuscular hyperplasia causing obstruction in 11 [there were accessory renal arteries in two and an aneurysm of the renal artery in two]. They performed every variety of operation,- endarterectomy and patch graft, splenorenal arterial anastomosis, excision of stenosis and end-to-end anastomosis, endarterectomy, and bypass graft, and, in 12 patients, nephrectomy. Twelve of the patients had normal pressures after operation, and ten had a small degree of systolic hypertension. There was a single operative death.

Discussion

Stanley Crawford, of Houston, said that their experience was that results continued to improve with time in some patients. They had operated on 90 patients, relieved the hypertension in 84% and gotten significant improvement in 9% more. The incidence of arteriosclerotic disease was higher in their patients, and bilateral disease occurred in 40%. Split renal functions were not dependable in their hands and they insisted on aortography as "the only reliable method of screening at the present time." In the small shrunken kidneys, they attempted arterial reconstruction "and in most of the latter cases, the kidneys have returned to normal size and have as-

sumed normal excretory function." Edwin J. Wylie, of San Francisco, had also had difficulty with split function studies and had decided that "renal arteriogram is the more valid diagnostic procedure." They had had increasing interest in fibromuscular hyperplasia, in which the arteriogram showed "the distinctive pattern of 'accordion pleating' in the middle or distal third of the renal artery that appears characteristic of this disorder; this occurred in 19 women patients between the ages of 17 and 45 and a one-year-old boy." A resection and end-to-end anastomosis was performed in 11 patients and relief of hypertension was obtained in 10 of the 11, "a success rate almost double that obtained from renal artery reconstruction with a slightly larger group of patients with arteriosclerotic renal artery stenosis." He commented of the histologic appearance ". . . a uniform pattern of concentric rings of fibromuscular hyperplasia involving the media without significant changes in the intima." Spencer, closing, showed the histologic picture of fibromuscular hyperplasia, and said the intima and adventitia were involved as well as the media and that they had seen it in male patients. Spencer said [without indicating that it was Stamey's careful performance of his own split-function test that made it reliable in their hands] that they found it dependable and that "the rate of urine flow from the two kidneys does not vary in consecutive collection periods over 5.0 to 6.0 per cent." Of Crawford's revascularization efforts for shrunken kidneys, he said, ". . . they are defining one of the unknown limits in reconstructive renal surgery . . . how seriously can a kidney be injured from ischemia and yet recover after revascularization. We have revascularized all kidneys when it was technically possible, no matter how poor the preoperative renal function was . . . At the present we would revascularize any kidney unless gross anatomical abnormalities were present."

* * *

Michael E. DeBakey, of Houston, Professor of Surgery and Chairman of the Department of Surgery, Baylor University College of Medicine; Surgeon-in-Chief, Jefferson Davis Hospital; Surgeon-in-Chief, Methodist Hospital; E. Stanley Crawford and George C. Morris, Jr., by invitation; and Denton A. Cooley, Associate Professor of Surgery, Baylor University College of Medicine, *Surgical Considerations of Occlusive Disease of the Innominate, Carotid, Subclavian, and Vertebral Arteries*, demonstrated the exponential increase in the vascular surgery operating activity of the Houston group. "During the period of

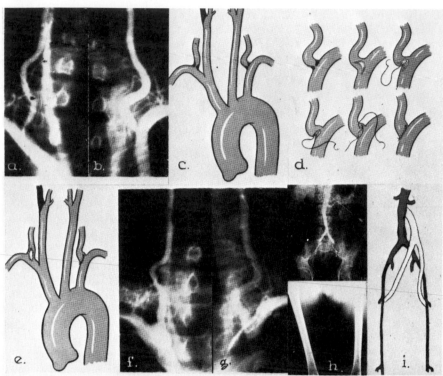

Fig. 13. Illustrations of patient with severe manifestations of cerebrovascular insufficiency resulting from multiple occlusive disease, including complete occlusion of right internal carotid artery and bilateral incomplete occlusive lesions of vertebral arteries, associated with complete occlusive lesion of both external iliac arteries and both superficial femoral arteries producing severe manifestations of arterial insufficiency of lower extremitus. Preoperative arteriograms of (a) right subclavian artery, and (b) left subclavian artery, and (c) drawing showing well localized severe stenotic lesions of both vertebral arteries at their origin from subclavian arteries and complete occlusion of right internal carotid artery of long duration and thus inoperable. (e) Drawings showing operative procedure consisting of endarterectomy with patch graft repair on right side and (d) technic of angioplasty on left side. (f) Arteriogram of right subclavian artery, and (g) left subclavian artery made 2 years after operation showing restoration of normal lumens and circulation. (h) Preoperative aortogram showing segmental complete occlusive lesions of both external iliac and superficial femoral arteries. (i) Drawing showing bypass graft procedure used to improve circulation in lower extremities. Patient has remained asymptomatic.

Complicated, multi-image, illustration characteristic of the DeBakey Group. In the lantern slides, C, D, E, and I would be shown in bright color. X-rays often had superimposed over them in color the specimen of the aneurysm, or whatever had been removed. They were now reporting 372 patients operated upon for occlusive disease of the carotid vertebral and subclavian arterial systems and in the 372 patients had, in fact, explored 521 occluding lesions and reconstructed 498 of them, "The remaining lesions, completely obstructing the internal carotid and vertebral arteries, were of long duration and inoperable."

Michael E. DeBakey, E. Stanley Crawford, George C. Morris, Jr., and Denton A. Cooley, *Surgical Considerations of Occlusive Disease of the Innominate, Carotid, Subclavian, and Vertebral Arteries.* Volume LXXIX, 1961.

a little over seven and one-half years following our first successful application of surgical treatment in a patient with occlusion of the left carotid artery, on August 7, 1953, we have employed this form of therapy in 372 patients with this type of extracranial segmental occlusive disease, involving the innominate, carotid, subclavian, and vertebral arteries." They frequently operated on multiple stenoses in the same patient, using variously endarterectomy, patch grafts, and Dacron prosthesis bypass of the lumbar aorta or the ileofemoral system. They had operated on 372 patients with a total of 498 individual lesions that were corrected operatively. Their patients ranged from 24 to 83 years in age, males predominated by the ratio of 2 to 1 and additional arteriosclerotic vascular disease was common, "Thus, some form of heart disease, usually coronary artery occlu-

sive disease, was present in 40 per cent of the patients, hypertension in 47 per cent, associated atherosclerotic occlusive disease of the terminal abdominal aorta, iliac, femoral, popliteal and renal arteries in 19 per cent, and aneurysms of the aorta in 3 per cent." The "great majority" of the patients with aortic aneurysms and disease of the ileofemoral system had their lesions in those areas corrected. For the internal carotid and vertebral arteries, short lesions were treated by endarterectomy and patch angioplasty. Extensive lesions of the branches arising from the aortic arch were treated by end-to-side bypass grafts. They were enthusiastic about their results, with success in restoring normal circulation in all obstructions arising from the aortic arch, and in 96% of the incomplete lesions of the carotids and vertebrals. In the carotid and vertebral lesions, of the 329 patients with neurologic disturbances, 93% survived, 85% of those with transient cerebral ischemia were relieved or improved, 80% of those with progressing strokes "and 50 per cent of those with completed strokes." The long-term results, likewise, were good. Operative mortality overall was 6.7% in these predominantly aged arteriosclerotic patients, "only about one-third" of the late deaths were due to arterial insufficiency and then, usually in patients who had originally presented a completed stroke.

Discussion

S. W. Moore, of New York, the only discussant, emphasized the importance in these patients of angiography "to have a complete survey of the body". DeBakey agreed on the "importance of a complete visualization, mostly because of the fact that multiple involvement is so often present, as exemplified by the fact that this was true in over 50 per cent of our cases . . . other lesions which may be present but can be missed at the time can produce subsequent disturbances . . ."

* * *

The pièce de résistance of the 1961 meeting was certainly the presentation by Albert Starr, of Portland, Oregon, and M. Lowell Edwards, B.S., both by invitation, *Mitral Replacement:* Clinical Experience with a Ball-Valve Prosthesis, from the Department of Surgery and Division of Thoracic Surgery, University of Oregon. Starr described previous reports of "flap valves . . . ball valves . . . sleeve valves without chordae . . . flexible sleeve or leaflet valve with chordae, homologous aortic valve and autogenous pulmonary valves . . . Human mitral resection and replacement has been reported by Kay [E.B., 1960], Braunwald [N. S. with T. Cooper and A. G. Morrow, 1960], Lillehei [C. W., 1960], Ellis [F. H. Jr., 1960]. While early satisfactory results were obtained in some patients, survival beyond three months has not been reported to now." Starr and Edwards had devised a ball valve with a ball at first of lucite, and a cage of lucite [used in their first two patients], the cage of the prosthesis consisting of four rods leading down from the ring of the prosthesis to join together sufficiently far beyond it to encase the lucite poppet when the valve was in the open position. The ring of the valve was covered with knitted Teflon cloth by which it was sutured to the mitral annulus. In some of their experimental studies, "Some of the valves . . . have radio-opaque

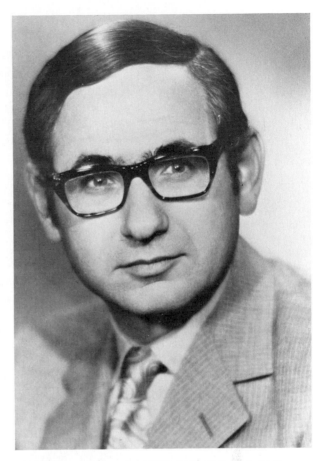

Albert Starr, 1926— (c. 1970). M.D. Columbia College of Physicians and Surgeons 1949. Intern, Johns Hopkins; residency, Bellevue-Presbyterian; University of Oregon, Instructor to Professor since 1957. The Starr-Edwards aortic ball valve immediately replaced the prosthetic leaflets which had brought some success, and was followed by a similar mitral prosthesis. With progressive changes in configuration of the cage, in the cloth covering of the ring, experimentation with cloth covering of the cage, change in the materials used for the ball, the Starr-Edwards ball valves in both positions remain in wide use. Starr's publications have been marked by careful and candid reporting of long-term follow-up, detailed analyses and persistent efforts to evaluate and improve the prosthesis, operative techniques and after-care in what is a prolonged clinical experiment.

balls or steel pins inserted into the balls so that valve function and ball spin have been observed with fluoroscopy." Stainless steel or "Stellite 21" had now replaced lucite for the cage, and the ball was made of silastic. They stressed the "mirror finish [of the metal]. . . produced by buffing and electropolishing. The surface is then silicone coated . . .

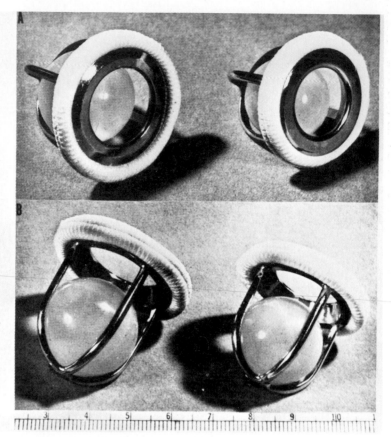

FIG. 4. The mitral ball valve prosthesis for human implantation. A. View of inlet side; B. View of outlet side.

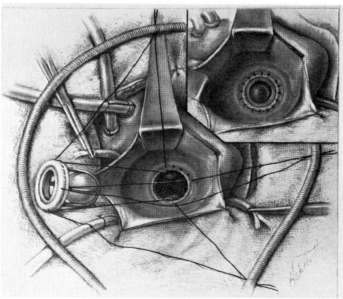

FIG. 9. Method of placement of silk sutures. Insert shows valve in place.

Unless flawless with regard to minor imperfections or irregularities of surface, the valve is rejected . . . the ball is of Dow-Corning medical grade heat-cured silastic." The change to metal decreased the external dimensions of the valve with no loss of strength. From July, 1960 to February, 1961, they had replaced the mitral valve of eight patients with rheumatic mitral disease. The first died of air embolism in ten hours, the second and third were well and at work, the fourth died of renal shutdown on the eleventh day. The fifth, sixth, and eighth were recently discharged well. The seventh was under treatment for staphylococcus endocarditis. [An Addendum to the paper, obviously inserted at the time of correction of the galleys, said that four more patients had been operated upon with no operative deaths, but one late death from staphylococcal endocarditis. Patients seven and eight of the original group had also now died of endocarditis, having been "operated upon during an epidemic of staphylococcal infections involving other cardiac surgical patients and requiring temporary closure of the operating suite. All seven survivors continue to maintain dramatic initial functional response."]

Discussion

Michael E. DeBakey, of Houston, rose to admit "that this paper persuades me to re-evaluate my attitude toward ball valves. I have been somewhat prejudiced against them because of my very early experience with their use in changing the directional flow in blood pumps. Our most recent experience with the use of such ball valves, as in the Hufnagel valve in aortic insufficiency [a lucite ball in a cylindrical lucite chamber made for insertion in the descending thoracic aorta], also tended to make me somewhat prejudiced." He supposed that newer materials and techniques might have been responsible for this "very impressive work on the part of Drs. Starr and Edwards." George H. A. Clowes, Jr., of Cleveland,

was equally impressed, "This is a most remarkable piece of work, to have had six out of eight patients survive." The previous problem had always been that the valves developed thrombi and the animals died of cerebral embolism. Starr, closing, said that they too had been "prejudiced against the ball valve for use as an intracardiac prosthesis, and it was difficult to state in the short presentation the various steps that led to the choice of this 'repugnant' intracardiac appliance." The ball valve proved to be the only one in dogs in which thrombosis did not occur without anticoagulant treatment. Starr believed that "the reason for this is that the valvular mechanism is not attached to the body of the prosthesis itself. The clot in the dog grows by direct extension like an infiltrating tumor rather than by multicentric origin, so that the clot which forms on the margin of the valve at its point of attachment is less likely to interfere with valve function with the ball valve as compared with other types of prostheses in which leaflets are anchored to the mitral annulus itself. I think this explains our ability to obtain long-term survival with the dog with the ball valve." Some dogs had developed embolic problems and "For this reason, the patients in this series are receiving anticoagulant therapy. All had atrial fibrillation. Many of them have had anticoagulants before operation. The price we pay for adequate hydraulic function in terms of anticoagulant treatment is really not great."

The Business Meetings

The 1961 meeting was held at the Boca Raton Hotel and Club, Boca Raton, Florida, March 21, 22, and 23, John D. Stewart in the Chair.

As the Second Executive Meeting convened President Stewart said that word had been received of the death of Howard Naffziger.

At this meeting the Report of Council read by the Secretary contained the recommendation "That

◄ The valve, at first made of lucite, was now made of either stainless steel or "Stellite 21", cast, then ground, buffed, electro-polished and finally silicon coated. The Teflon cloth fixation ring was held in place by a Teflon spreader and Teflon sutures. The poppet, at first of lucite, was of Dow-Corning silastic. With cardiopulmonary bypass, under mild hypothermia,- 32° C,- the left atrium was opened from the right chest, the mitral valve held open "so that foam is not expelled into the aorta" and the field flooded with carbon dioxide. Excision *in toto* was preferable, leaving three to four millimeters of valve in place for suturing the prosthesis, "without too deep a bite into the myocardium." The chordae could be divided individually, or the papillary muscles themselves divided. The valve was sutured in place with 0 silk, 16 to 20 sutures, preplaced as shown in Starr's figure 9, then all tied.

Albert Starr and M. Lowell Edwards, *Mitral Replacement:* Clinical Experience with a Ball-Valve Prosthesis. Volume LXXIX, 1961.

the original membership registration roster, the book in which all of the original signatures of the members of this organization since its inception in 1882 have been collected, be reproduced by the most practical and attractive method for distribution to the membership, the number of copies ordered to exceed that of the membership . . . That since the Association has no permanent archives of its own, the original registration book for the membership be thereafter permanently displayed in a safe and appropriate place, such as the Library of Congress, or some other National Scientific Library."

The Council recommended against the proposal of Dr. Walter Maddock for establishing a Standing Committee on "Various Problems of American Surgery." The report of Council was accepted.

A motion approved by Council was presented, dealing with vivisection and anticipating regulatory moves by the Federal Government, which stated among other things ". . . that the American Surgical Association believes that first things should be put first and that the progress of knowledge which will promote human welfare and relieve the great suffering still experienced by mankind is of paramount importance. Efforts in this direction should not be impeded with additional restrictions and time consuming recordkeeping. Rather we should trust to the proper motivation of the Universities, the responsible attitudes of University and Hospital administration, and existing local and state laws which protect animals against cruelty. Rather should the Federal Government assist institutions conducting medical research with funds for sanitary and safe animal quarters, and for employing competent personnel to care for them." In the discussion, Lester R. Dragstedt said "I am persuaded that the proposed Federal regulation for medical research represents the most serious threat to medical research in many years. Ostensibly, the bills that are introduced into Congress are designed for the humane treatment of experimental animals, but actually they represent antivivisection bills. The antivivisectionists have recognized that it is not possible for them to stop animal experimentation, and so now they have embarked on a program of harassment of investigators, and in an attempt to shackle the experimenter with red tape and regulations, so that they can reduce the amount of work that is done." He warned of the loss of time to the younger investigator, in making applications, receiving approvals, etc., when he was trying to get started. The motion was passed.

Fred Coller was ill at home [with carcinoma of the prostate] and Philip D. Wilson moved a message of good will and good wishes of the Association be sent for his recovery and that was done.

Among the new Members elected were Harvey R. Butcher, Jr., of St. Louis; Willard E. Goodwin, of Los Angeles; Joseph E. Murray, of Boston; and as Honorary Fellows, Professor John Bruce, of Edinburgh; and Professor René Fontaine, of Strasbourg. Elected President was J. Englebert Dunphy, of Portland, Oregon; Vice-Presidents, Nathan Womack, of Chapel Hill, North Carolina, and J. D. Martin, Jr., of Atlanta; Secretary, William Altemeier, of Cincinnati.

LXXX

1962

The 1962 meeting was held in Washington, D.C., at the Sheraton-Park Hotel, May 9, 10, and 11, President J. Englebert Dunphy, Mackenzie Professor of Surgery and Head of the Department, University of Oregon Medical School, in the Chair. In that year had died Bradley L. Coley, Willis D. Gatch, and Richard H. Sweet.

In his Presidential Address, Dunphy, more successfully than any of his predecessors attempting the same feat, discussed the nature of the Association's history and its contributions, in lucid and attractive prose. He made several suggestions pointing out that when Halsted had been admitted to the Association he had been 40 years age and had published ". . . about 24 papers at that time including his studies on local anesthesia, the radical cure of hernia, cancer of the breast, intestinal suture, and some observations on wound healing. The ideas were his own. Not only was he the principal author, he was the sole author. Today, the number of papers in a candidate's bibliography may vary from as few as 10 to over 200 and there is no easy way of comparing them." He suggested that "If, in addition to a bibliography on the candidate, the sponsors were required to submit reprints of what they regard as his three most important papers, it might be clear that a man with a total of 10 had made more fundamental contributions than a man with 150" [a suggestion implemented later at this meeting]. He suggested also that it would strengthen the Association to admit, as Senior Fellows, surgeons ". . . who publish comparatively little early in life but because they are accomplished surgeons and natural leaders attain great distinction in later life. These men wield enormous influence for good in all echelons of surgery but especially in their local communities . . . They become presidents of our great regional societies . . . They may become a regent of our College, but they are not admitted to the American Surgical Association. Why? Because when they were young, they had published too little to establish themselves and later when they have attained just recognition, we say they are too old. This is a mistake." [A suggestion implemented in 1964.] Finally, he proposed enlargement of the Association without specifying a number "The American Surgical Association cannot fulfill its purposes with a membership of 250 in a country of 200 million people. The American Surgical Association was never intended to be a surgical club. It is not a fraternity . . . The jet age makes acquaintances of us all, and means of communication have been so improved by better halls, better acoustics, and public address systems that 1,000 men can understand each other more effectively today than 100 did in 1880." [The active membership limit was raised to 300 in 1964.]

* * *

In an interdisciplinary presentation which impressively demonstrated the complex nature of the new field, Joseph E. Murray, of Boston, Clinical Associate in Surgery, Harvard Medical School; Associate in Surgery, Peter Bent Brigham Hospital [Plas-

1149

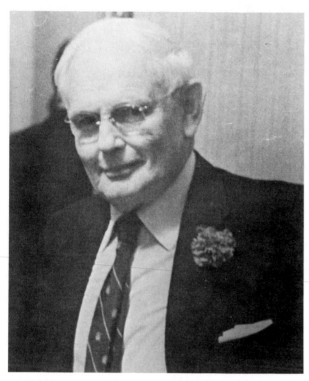

J. Englebert Dunphy (c. 1966), 1908—. (Recorder 1957-61, President 1962, President of American College of Surgeons 1964) M.D. Harvard 1937, trained at the Peter Bent Brigham. In 1955, Professor of Surgery, Harvard Medical School, left the Brigham to direct the Fifth Surgical Service and the Sears Surgical Laboratory at the Boston City Hospital. In 1959, accepted the Chair at the University of Oregon and in 1964 the Chair at the University of California, San Francisco. Broadly interested in general, and particularly abdominal, surgery and, in his investigative work, in the chemistry of wound healing. A man of great charm, puckish wit, and extraordinary capacity for persuasion, he has played a major role in American surgery and in national and international surgical societies.

(Photograph courtesy of C. R. Hanlon, M.D., Chicago, Illinois.)

tic], (and by invitation, John P. Merrill, of the Department of Medicine; Gustave J. Dammin, Professor of Pathology, Pathologist-in-Chief, Peter Bent Brigham Hospital; Guy W. Alexandre, Department of Surgery) and J. Hartwell Harrison, Clinical Professor of Genitourinary Surgery, Harvard Medical School; Urologic Surgeon, Peter Bent Brigham Hospital, initiated the meeting with *Kidney Transplantation in Modified Recipients*. At the 1958 meeting, they had presented the results of kidney transplantation between seven pairs of identical twins. They

now knew of at least 23 such transplants, 16 by their group, and others about the country and in Edinburgh, Scotland. They had undertaken to transplant kidneys in 18 patients, for the most part from living family donors but increasingly from cadaver kidneys or kidneys removed during an arachnoid-ureteral shunt for hydrocephalus,- "free kidneys". Total body irradiation followed by a bone marrow transfusion before grafting had not lived up to its early promise. Two of the 12 patients died before transplantation could be undertaken, and only a single patient was alive and surviving on the transplanted kidney, most of the failures having come from early massive rejection. They, therefore, shifted in their laboratory and clinical efforts to "Chemical suppression of the immune response . . ." With this they had performed six transplants and were able to say that "Five of six patients conditioned with thiopurine with or without Actinomycin C have had measurable renal function; one recipient still survives over 120 days. In others, death was due to drug toxicity." Earlier they had done over 300 kidney transplants in nephrectomized dogs under 14 different protocols, employing singly or in combination 6-mercaptopurine, dinitrophenolthiopurine, Imuran, nitrogen mustard, actinomycin C and actinomycin D, trypan blue, methotrexate, and azaserine. "The most encouraging are those using a combination of Imuran and Actinomycin C and Imuran plus azaserine. The longest survivors are over nine months and still on drug therapy. Stopping the drug even at eight months may lead to rapid rejection of the kidney . . . Striking reversibility of the rejection process by the use of the drug was noted in many animals". While they could say that "Chemical suppression of the immune response in both the experimental animal and in the human seems promising", and all of their recipients had been terminally ill, their results, one survivor out of six, were such that they thought that "In our present state of knowledge, it seems unwise to pursue further the use of living healthy donors for any type of human kidney transplantation except between twins."

Discussion

Francis D. Moore, of Boston, compared the action of irradiation, which ". . . has to do its whole job in one sledge-hammer blow. Each cell is hit hard—how hard, we never know—and recovery is slow or may never occur" with the action of the antimetabolites which ". . . can be used gently and with sequential discrimination, altering the dosage required by the sharply opposing needs of the graft (for immune suppression) on the one hand and the host (for survival) on the other." The fact that rejection had been shown to be reversible, permitted one to use border-line doses of the immuno-paretic agents. Richard L. Varco's (of Minneapolis) discussion, published after the succeeding paper, appears directed entirely to Murray's presentation. He said that he and Dr. James Pierce had had long-time survivals in dogs with a 6-mercaptopurine alone without any actinomycin D, and unlike Dr. Murray's experience, they had three animals who after 150 days on the drug had continued to have good renal function when the drug had been withdrawn. He made the entertaining suggestion that ". . . this suggests . . . that the *memory* of the host animal cells for this *foreign protein* has been lost . . . that group of multipotential cells participating in the immune response, having been replicated and differentiated a sufficient number of times, the newest (current) population eventually fails to distinguish these donated cells as *foreigners,* because the entire *lifetime* of these latter-day immuno-potential cells has taken place in an environment containing donor protein." He offered this as only a theory that "If one can keep the individual donor graft alive for a long enough period of time, protected against the rejection response by a drug such as this, it will then be possible to discontinue the drug with reasonable assurance that the individual recipient will continue to tolerate indefinitely that homovital graft" [would that it had been true].

* * *

Starting with the thesis that "Since immune responsiveness is a function of cell metabolism which in turn is determined by the nucleic acids of the cell genome, one possible method of altering immunologic reactivity would appear to be the introduction of new genetic information into potentially reactive cells", by invitation, John A. Mannick and Richard H. Egdahl, both from the Department of Surgery, Medical College of Virginia, Richmond, Virginia, *Transformation of Nonimmune Lymph Node Cells to State of Transplantation Immunity by RNA,* A Preliminary Report, introduced the Association to the exciting world of the manipulation of information systems in the cell. When skin from rabbit A was placed on the thigh of rabbit B and lymph node cells from rabbit A were injected into the foot pads of the same extremity of rabbit B, and eight days later the popliteal lymph nodes of rabbit B were injected into the skin of rabbit A, a *transfer reaction* was recog-

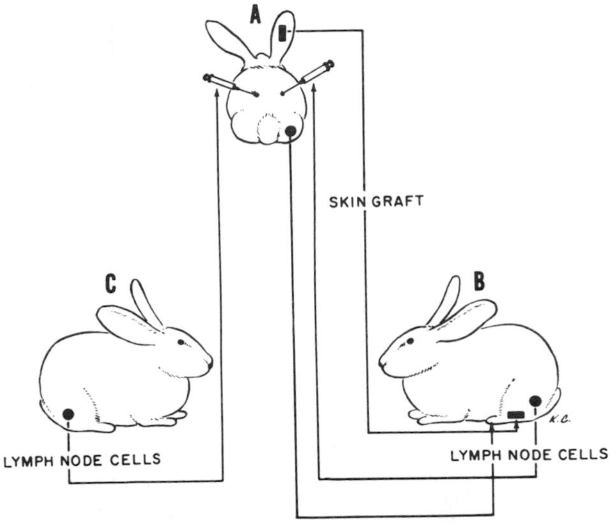

FIG. 2. Experimental design of the *transfer reaction* using immune cells.

Placing skin graft from Rabbit A to the left thigh of Rabbit B and lymph node cell suspension from A to the foot pad of B, and eight days later injecting into A's skin a cell suspension from the left popliteal nodes of B, produced in the skin the *transfer reaction.* Rabbit A did not react to cells from neutral Rabbit C, unless these cells were first exposed to lymph node RNA from Rabbit B. Exposing the lymph node RNA preparation to RNase prevented the reaction.

John A. Mannick and Richard H. Egdahl, *Transformation of Nonimmune Lymph Node Cells to State of Transplantation Immunity by RNA.* A Preliminary Report, Volume LXXX, 1962.

nized, as originally demonstrated by Brent, Brown and Medawar [1958]. Cells from a third rabbit, mixed with the lymph node RNA of rabbit B, produced the transfer reaction in rabbit A, suggesting that the RNA transformed the lymphocytes of a neutral rabbit into immune lymphocytes. Exposing the RNA to RNase prevented the reaction.

Discussion

The audience was obviously excited by the question which the young authors raised, "Whether or not lymphoid cells can be transformed to a state of tolerance as well as immunity, by incubation with RNA from an appropriate source, is a question of the highest significance which remains unanswered by the experiments reported here. An investigation of this possibility is currently in progress." Twenty-seven years later that question has unfortunately not been answered positively. Mannick writes, May 15, 1979,

> I did try to make rabbit lymphoid cells specifically nonresponsive to transplantation antigens. This work was subsequently published in the Journal of Clinical Investigation. What I found was that the RNA treatment did reduce the reactivity of the cells to transplantation antigens but the effect was nonspecific. We, therefore, abandoned this line of approach but went on to suggest that the RNA transfer of cellular immunity might be useful in transferring tumor immunity. (Journal of Clinical Investigation, 1964.)

The latter idea has subsequently borne some fruit. Ramming and Pilch in 1968 succeeded in demonstrating the successful transfer of tumor immunity by immune RNA. We and others have subsequently confirmed this, and have recently embarked on a clinical trial of 'immune' RNA therapy in patients with advanced renal cell carcinoma with a few encouraging results. There are other trials of immune RNA therapy underway in California as I am sure you are aware. I suspect, however, that the clinical value of immune RNA therapy, if any, will be in patients with minimal residual disease who have a high expectation of metastatic recurrence. Our recent animal experiments suggest that this is so in that RNA therapy after excision of a primary mouse melanoma effectively prevents death from pulmonary metastases which will kill 80-100% of control animals. (Science, 1978.)

The idea of specific nonreactivity transferable by immune RNA, which we abandoned years ago, may not be totally dead. We have recently reinstituted experiments to look at the possibility of transferring suppressor cell activity with immune RNA. We do not yet have any results to report, however.

* * *

The philosophy which Varco had expressed in his discussion of Murray's paper, also influenced Somers H. Sturgis, of Boston, Clinical Professor of Gynecology, Harvard Medical School; Surgeon (Gynecological), Peter Bent Brigham Hospital, and by invitation, Hector Castellanos, *Ovarian Homografts in Organic Filter Chambers.* Woodruff in 1959 had suggested the possibility of adaptation of the graft to the host as the result of experimental thyroid transplants in the anterior chamber of the eye. Sturgis and Castellanos in previously castrated rabbits and monkeys enclosed a bit of ovarian tissue in a sac of homologous corneal tissue and although the corneal envelope eventually became infiltrated with lymphocytes and slowly resorbed, and the imbedded graft became vascularized some ". . . recognizable ovarian elements . . ." persisted. At that point, exci-

sion of the implanted corneal chamber still resulted in changes characteristic of castration. They suggested that their results supported Woodruff's statement that ". . . it would be unwise to deny without further investigation the possibility of a fundamental change in the antigenic structure of the grafted cells."

Discussion

Herbert Conway, of New York, indicated as the authors had, that these experiments were comparable to those with millipore chambers becoming nonporous. Conway was apparently not convinced by the histological pictures of the grafts at a late stage, but correctly described the current state of transplantation research ". . . this problem is one which is being attacked by two arms of a pincher: the one is the strong arm of the investigative surgeon; the other, more academic and less furtive, that which is being carried on by the immunologists, immunogeneticists and immunochemists." Bradford Cannon, of Boston, pointed out that ". . . Dr. Sturgis possibly has answered the question or the speculation of Dr. Varco. If the homograft is protected for a sufficient period of time, there will be a loss of memory on the part of the host cells of the foreign protein." Joseph E. Murray, of Boston, commented "It seems to me that this paper of Dr. Sturgis fits in very well with that of Drs. Mannick and Egdahl. Dr. Mannick has demonstrated that you can transfer immunity or *sensitization,* whatever term you wish, by prior contact with RNA, by means of incubation. Dr. Sturgis allowed the host RNA to be perfused into the graft gradually over a period of time. It seems that the mechanism of the two effects might be exactly the same and that both are potentially useful for clinical application."

* * *

Russel H. Patterson, Jr., by invitation, and Bronson S. Ray, of New York, Professor of Clinical Surgery, Cornell University Medical College, *Profound Hypothermia for Intracranial Surgery:* Laboratory and Clinical Experiences with Extracorporeal Circulation by Peripheral Cannulation, stated that external body cooling and moderate hypothermia were providing no more than ten minutes of safe occlusion of the blood supply to the brain. Unwilling to add a thoracotomy to the operative insult, they had modified the suggestion of Woodhall and others two years before for cooling by partial bypass. Venous cannulation for the extracorporeal circulation was through the femoral vein and the jugular vein and the arterial return was into the femoral artery. Temperatures with the heat exchangers were brought down to between 5° and 7° and the brain temperature between 14° and 17°. Five of the seven patients fibrillated during cooling or rewarming, one reverted spontaneously and the other four were successfully defibrillated. Periods of circulatory arrest ranged from nine to 42-1/2 minutes. All of the operations were for cranial aneurysms. One patient ultimately died from what might have been clipping of the anterior cerebral artery. There was no autopsy. One patient, who, during induction, had a fresh hemorrhage from his aneurysm, died several days after operation. Five patients survived and were considered to have done well.

Discussion

Barnes Woodhall, of Durham, North Carolina, whose paper had initiated Bronson Ray's interest, said ". . . we have a good deal of basic confidence in this method . . ." They were restricting its use to patients with "aneurysms at the bifurcation of the basilar artery . . . we believe that these particular patients represent a very good proving ground." John W. Kirklin, of Rochester, Minnesota, said his neurosurgical colleagues at the Mayo Clinic had ". . . performed definitive intracranial surgery on 18 patients during total circulatory arrest in which the profound hypothermia was produced by the Drew technic of right and left heart bypass using the patient's own lungs as the oxygenator. This, of course, necessitates a thoractomy as well as a craniotomy", but in 12 subsequent patients, having heard of the work of Patterson and Ray, they had employed the closed chest technique. Woodhall, who had suggested that a catheter in the jugular vein would be in the way, and Kirklin also, employed two femoral venous catheters. Will C. Sealy, of Durham, who had been the cardiac surgical collaborator with Woodhall, said they had been employing this technique for deep hypothermia and cardiac arrest in dogs for several years. Flow rates had to be reduced, ". . . when the heart's temperature dropped below 25° C", to prevent an elevation in the left atrial pressure. In one patient the venous cannulation was into the superior vena cava through ". . . a small right anterior chest incision through the 4th interspace." Russel H. Patterson, closing, said that intracranial bleeding often occurred until the decannulation and the reversal of the heparin effect.

* * *

Watts and Freeman in Washington, D.C., [1946] created a wave of excitement with the use of prefrontal lobotomy for certain patients with psychotic disorders, and for the relief of pain. The procedures had fallen into disuse because of the unpredictable, and severe, personality disturbances which resulted. Now James C. White, of Boston, Professor of Surgery, Harvard Medical School; Chief of the Neurosurgical Service, Massachusetts General Hospital, *Modifications of Frontal Leukotomy for Relief of Pain and Suffering in Terminal Malignant Disease,* said of the earlier lobotomies that "Except as a procedure of last resort, bilateral extensive lobotomies have never been popular. The ensuing deterioration in personality and mentation can be appalling, much more so than in the psychotic who has undergone a similar procedure. Van Wagenen, who I believe first tried this, relieved the pain of phantom limb but was so dismayed by the ensuing mental changes that he never reported the case. Watts also has told me that the individuals whom he has submitted to bilateral transection of frontal matter for pain have never been able to return to work, although a gratifying number operated upon by him and Freeman for psychoses have subsequently become self-supporting." E. G. Grantham, beginning in 1951, had been employing the technique ". . . of inserting electrodes into the lower medial quadrants of frontal white matter and coagulating with the Bovie electrodesiccating current . . . increasing the extent of frontal leukotomy in stages." W. H. Sweet and White had for seven years been using ". . . the radio-frequency lesion-maker devised for this purpose by Aronow." Through small bilateral frontal trephines, needles were passed under X-ray control ". . . 1.0 cm. in front of the anterior horns of the lateral ventricles, which have been outlined by injecting 10 cc. of air." The electrodes were inserted through the needles, and the needles withdrawn. The electrodes being connected to the radiofrequency unit, "Tissue is coagulated by heating with a current of 30 to 40 watts for a period of five to 10 seconds. When bubbles of steam are heard the current is cut off. Single lesions are made at intervals of several days as the electrodes are withdrawn a centimeter at a time." The treatment could be repeated until the patient's concern for pain and need for narcotics ceased. The electrodes could be left for several weeks longer to be sure that the effect was permanent. They had employed the technique in 22 cases of malignant disease with effective relief in 18,- ". . . no spontaneous complaints or need for narcotics",- two patients with partial benefit, one death from pneumonia, and three patients with ". . . worth-while relief, narcotic intake greatly reduced". Some patients were mildly confused and had some memory loss and listlessness for a week or two. Some apathy and decrease in spontaneous speech persisted.

Discussion

James Watts, of Washington, D.C., the pioneer in psychosurgery, said that the technique represented a considerable advance and cited some background, "I thought I would take about one minute to tell you how some of this came about. In 1937, Walter Freeman and I had a patient who had been confined to bed for two years. She had severe arthritis of the spine, arthritis of the knees, and a diagnosis of conversion hysteria was made. A lobotomy was done because of the emotional symptoms. She walked on the fourth day, sprained her ankle, continued to walk, and she came back to the clinic and complained of pain. It appeared to be a relapse but it took us several years to realize that although the pain was still present, the fear was gone. This woman worked as a bookbinder for 20 years and died in 1959. The first patient with organic disease whom we operated on was in 1943: a man with carcinoma of the rectum with metastasis to the liver and lungs. The thing that led to operation was his statement, 'When the effect of this morphine wears off, you won't let me suffer, will you? you will give me another hypodermic, won't you?' It seemed then that the fear of pain was the chief cause of his suffering, rather than a disagreeable sensation. He lived for three months and was relieved." Watts was disturbed at White's condemnation of Watts' procedure ". . . Dr. White has done what everybody else who devises a new technic does. He says, 'All other technics cause deterioration of the personality or psychological crippling.' I think that is unfortunate. We have got some good ones and some bad ones, but those of us who are interested in using lobotomy as a method of treatment face the thing that every other author says every other method is bad except his own. I think Dr. White's work represents a real advance, but I do not think it is the only one." Dr. White, in closing, wanted ". . . to assure Dr. Watts I meant to imply that the deterioration that we saw from using his more radical method was from our own experience, and that is why we shifted." While he thought his technique was the most practical of all currently available, he was ". . . hoping in the future some of the new physical devices, such as ultrasound radiation or the proton beam, will make it possible to increase the extent of frontal leukotomy

just as effectively without any need for operating directly on the brain."

* * *

Kent W. Barber, Jr., by invitation, John M. Waugh, of Rochester, Minnesota, Professor of Surgery, Mayo Foundation, University of Minnesota; General Surgeon, Mayo Clinic; Oliver H. Beahrs, and William G. Sauer both by invitation, *Indications for and the Results of the Surgical Treatment of Regional Enteritis,* presented their experience with 257 patients operated upon from 1945 to 1955. Eighty-six percent of the patients underwent resections, 184 resections of the terminal ileum and right colon, 20 resections of the ileum, 13 of the jejunum, and four of the jejunum and ileum. Thirty-three bypass operations were performed,- 12.8%. Patients had laparotomy only for extensive disease, and one patient had gastroenterostomy for duodenal involvement. In the entire group of 257 patients, ". . . 49 patients ultimately required a total of 57 resections and 11 bypass procedures for complications of recurrent disease. The average time interval from initial operation at the clinic to the first recurrent surgery was 5.1 years. The over-all mortality rate for the 325 procedures was 2.4 per cent. Of the total of 49 patients requiring an operative procedure for recurrence, only 15 (30.6%) underwent a third procedure, and only four of the 15 patients (26.6%) needed still a fourth procedure. Of these 49 patients treated by one or more operations for recurrent disease, 77.6 per cent are in good health and symptom-free. Our initial surgical recurrence rate was 19.1 per cent." They concluded from their experience that "The treatment of choice is conservative resection of the involved bowel with primary end-to-end anastomosis. Removal of all the high-lying skip lesions or radical excision of the grossly involved bowel does not seem necessary in a certain percentage of these left-behind areas, for the disease will subside with postoperative medical treatment and sometimes even spontaneously."

Discussion

Bentley P. Colcock, of the Lahey Clinic, discussing, reported similar results in a similar series. They had had 304 patients, 20% of whom had required a second operation in a follow-up of at least five years, and averaging up to ten years ". . . over 50 per cent of our patients who required a second operation were cured by that second procedure. Furthermore, over 50 per cent of our patients who required a third operative procedure were permanently relieved of their symptoms by that third operation. The situation often is frustrating, but it is rarely hopeless." Like the Mayo group, the Lahey group preferred resection to bypass, ". . . removal of infected, indurated bowel, frequently associated with small abscesses, not only will help that patient to recover more quickly but should help him to resist a recurrence of his disease." [The figures which he gave, not altogether clearly, were] ". . . the mortality rate for these 273 resected cases was 2.4 per cent. Our mortality rate for 304 resected cases was 1.7 per cent." John Prohaska, of Chicago, said that in 50 patients operated on in the last five years, he had a 20% recurrence rate, no mortality, and also favored resection rather than bypass. E. S. Stafford, of Baltimore, asked why the right colon was removed when it was not involved in disease, and whether the 2.5% mortality was the mortality by procedure, and did that not bring the mortality per patient up to 10%. I. S. Ravdin, of Philadelphia, rose to ask "Dr. Waugh . . . with all the material at hand . . . whether the present study reconfirms the original study of the clinic that the incidence of recurrence in the elderly patient was very much lower than the recurrence in those of younger age. John, as I remember it, from 60 years and above, you had practically no recurrences. I say this because after an operation performed at Walter Reed Hospital a few years ago, one of the distinguished professors at the Harvard Medical School published an article in *The Atlantic Monthly*. He said that the operation which was done on this individual was an irregular operation, and should never have been done. The incidence in my experience is less in the elderly patient who has a burned-out lesion." [The patient Ravdin was referring to was, of course, President Dwight Eisenhower upon whom Ravdin and General Leonard Heaton had operated in an emergency when he became obstructed from burned-out ileitis and performed a bypass in continuity]. The record of Ravdin's discussion and of the President's remarks illustrates one of the problems involved in this History. Ravdin, in fact, went into a good many clinical details to suggest mismanagement of the patient by his medical advisors before surgical consultation was obtained and indicated the depleted state of the President when operation was undertaken. None of this appears in the printed Discussion, nor does the marvelous comment of the irrepressible and irreverent Dunphy, presiding at the session, who, as the eminent Ravdin (President of the ASA in 1959) left the platform, explained apologetically to the Fellows "At every meeting there is some country doctor with straw in his hair and manure on his shoes who gets up to tell you about his one case." John M. Waugh, closing, said that the results had been a little better in the patients in whom they had operated upon primarily at the Mayo Clinic with a duration of disease of 3.2 years, than in patients, previously treated elsewhere, who had had their disease over five years [without pointing out that the latter were a selected group of people who had already demonstrated the capacity for recurrence]. In answer to Stafford, he indicated that ". . . all of us in recent years have tried to preserve as much of the right colon as possible and it is always a joy when we find the disease does not involve the ileocecal valve, and certainly we would not remove it under these circumstances." As to the mortality question, he agreed that the 2.4% was of 325 procedures [The Clinic seemed to have forgotten that W. J. Mayo had more than once emphasized before the Association that their figures included all patients, all deaths from whatever reason and that they always calculated *patient* mortality not *procedure* mortality. Thus, (1921 in discussion of Ross) "I always want to know whether the discussion concerns the number of operations or the number of patients. For instance, one patient may have five operations, if he dies the operative mortality is only 20%. Multiplying operations improves percentages but does not necessarily mean fewer deaths".] In the 91 patients operated on first at the Mayo Clinic, there had been two deaths,- 2.0%, and in the other 188 patients, six deaths,- 3.0% patient mortality. As for their present view of the timing of operation he said that "I believe now, as the result of recent publications, including Dr. Colcock's and the others, as the result of our study, we will, if the surgeons have their way, operate on these patients earlier. I do not think there is any question that we can do a better job if we see them before they perforate." He supported Ravdin's choice of operation on the President of the United States, "I would like to emphasize, too, that the patient Dr. Ravdin and General Heaton operated on was actually obstructed—at least as I read the newspapers—and I believe that it would have been poor judgment to have done any resection under those circumstances, or even an end-to-side anastomosis, because I doubt if any of us would have wanted to exteriorize the distal ileum under those circumstances; as nearly as I have been informed, I think that this particular patient had excellent treatment."

* * *

It was now seven years since the Philadelphia meeting at which Zollinger and Ellison had pre-

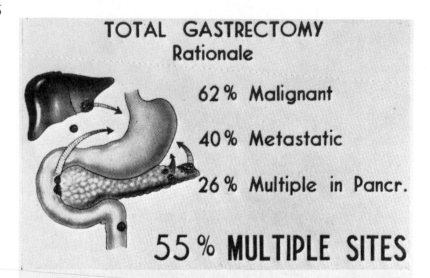

TOTAL GASTRECTOMY
Rationale

62% Malignant

40% Metastatic

26% Multiple in Pancr.

55% MULTIPLE SITES

FIG. 5. In 55 per cent of the cases reported, multiple sites for the potential production of the gastric secretagogue were found. This percentage corresponds closely to the incidence of recurrence following local excision of an obvious tumor of the pancreas. This finding constitutes the rationale for treatment with total gastrectomy.

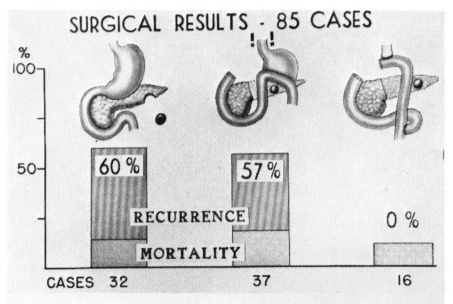

SURGICAL RESULTS - 85 CASES

%
100—

50—

60%   57%

RECURRENCE

MORTALITY   0%

CASES   32   37   16

FIG. 6. The surgical results of the three major operative approaches to the treatment of the ulcerogenic tumor of the pancreas are shown with the recurrence rate and mortality.

In the seven years since his original report, Zollinger had accumulated records of 132 cases,- ten of his own, 21 by "personal communication", and 101 published from other clinics. The illustrations demonstrate the rationale which led him to conclude that "Total gastrectomy remains the treatment of choice in the management of the ulcerogenic tumor of the pancreas."

Robert M. Zollinger, Dan W. Elliott, Gerald L. Endahl, George N. Grant, J. T. Goswitz, and D. A. Taft, *Origin of the Ulcerogenic Hormone in Endocrine Induced Ulcer*, Volume LXXX, 1962.

sented the evidence that established their new syndrome, and Robert M. Zollinger, of Columbus, Professor and Chairman, Department of Surgery, Ohio State University College of Medicine, and by invitation, Dan W. Elliott, Gerald L. Endahl, George N. Grant, John T. Goswitz, and David A. Taft, *Origin of the Ulcerogenic Hormone in Endocrine Induced Ulcer,* were able to report that they had records of 132 cases in which ". . . non-beta islet cell tumors of the pancreas are associated with intractable ulcer and/or enteritis . . ." Ten of the 132 cases were their own, 21 had been made known to them by correspondence, and 101 were found in published reports from other clinics. Priest and Alexander, only two years after Zollinger's original report, had described the occurrence of severe diarrhea and hypokalemia with non-beta cell islet tumors, a manifestation which Zollinger in this paper called "enteritis". This "enteritis" was found in association with ulcer in 30% of the patients and was the only symptom in 10%. In 36 cases, there was perforation of a primary jejunal ulcer just beyond the ligament of Treitz. Gregory, and Code had found a gastrin-like substance in these pancreatic tumors. Zollinger was able to say that employing Gregory's technique of extraction and a bio-assay on dogs with Pavlov pouches, ". . . a potent gastrin-like hormone was confirmed by bio-assay of the extracts of five islet cell tumors and two metastases." In a quarter of their cases ". . . one or more glands of internal secretion in addition to the non-beta islet cell tumor of the pancreas were involved. The most common of these was the parathyroid, 16; followed by the adrenal, 13; pituitary, nine; insulin-producing adenomas, nine; and thyroid, eight. There was a definite familial tendency in 15 of these cases." [No more was said about multiple endocrine adenomatosis.] As for the treatment, ". . . we continue to believe that total gastrectomy is the best way of controlling the fulminating ulcer diathesis associated with non-beta islet cell tumors of the pancreas . . . 62 per cent of these non-beta islet cell tumors are malignant and 40 per cent [of those] have metastases, which also produce the gastric secretagogue. In 26 per cent, the tumors are multiple throughout the pancreas . . . in 55 per cent of the cases there are multiple sites for the potential production of this potent gastric secretagogue. These statistics would predict recurrent ulceration in more than half of the cases if any acid-secreting surface of the stomach was allowed to remain." Local removal of the tumor had been followed by a recurrence rate of 60%, and ". . . radical gastric resection combined with partial removal of the pancreas with a recurrence rate of 57 per cent."

There had been no recurrences following total gastrectomy. The mortality was between 12.5 and 16% with each of the three approaches. Zollinger and his colleagues had, in addition, extracted by a similar technique, a pancreas from a patient with chronic pancreatitis in which there was ". . . tremendous hyperplasia and proliferation of islet tissue . . .", and the pancreas from dogs in whom the pancreatic duct had been ligated. The extracts showed an acid response in the same bio-assay.

Discussion

John H. Mulholland, of New York, was particularly interested in the demonstration of an acid stimulating substance from the pancreas of patients with chronic pancreatitis or from the dogs with experimentally atrophic acini, and asked "Dr. Zollinger, does he attribute the source of secretagogue to deteriorating acinar cells or to relatively well preserved islet cells?" Edgar J. Poth, of Galveston, commented that after total pancreatectomy, histamine in beeswax would produce fulminating peptic ulcer disease, as he had demonstrated in 1941, and wondered how that related to Dr. Zollinger's concepts. Edwin H. Ellison, now of Milwaukee [employing the eponym "Zollinger-Ellison Syndrome", which Zollinger had not], agreed ". . . that total gastrectomy with removal of the resectable tumor, but short of total pancreatectomy, continues to be the surgical treatment of choice, even when the presenting complaint is prolonged, persistent disabling diarrhea". He had performed such an operation four weeks before the meeting, with immediate relief of diarrhea, and rapid weight gain. Electron microscopic studies of the tumor cells grown in tissue culture showed what appears to be large secretory granules. Stanley R. Friesen, of Kansas City, appeared to challenge Zollinger on the chronic pancreatitis phase of the report ". . . he referred to a cycle in chronic pancreatitis in which secretin was mentioned as being stimulated by acid, this in turn stimulated islet cells . . . I really thought that secretion had to do with the stimulation of acinar cells." He was also concerned that in a recent patient on whom he had performed a total gastrectomy for the Zollinger-Ellison Syndrome, portions of the metastatic tumor in lymph nodes, liver and mediastinum were sent ". . . to both Gregory and to Code, both of whom failed to find this gastrin-like substance in this tumor. It is an islet cell tumor, not hypoglycemic, not beta cell. The only other thing about this particular patient is that five years prior to this time an adrenocortical adenoma was removed by Dr. Kittle; this patient had Cushing's syndrome at that time . . ." Charles B. Puestow, of Chicago, commented also on the pancreatitis, "We are not familiar with the possibility that an increase in islet cells might possibly cause the same kind of stimulation. If this is true, it might be an indication to perform more radical resections of the pancreas for pancreatitis . . . we have been trying to preserve as much of the pancreas as possible in order to allow a maximum amount of pancreatic regeneration or restoration of pancreatic function." So far as concerned the association of ulcer with pancreatitis, during a five-year period they had had 216 patients with pancreatitis, and ". . . only 13 (6.0%) had associated duodenal ulcers and no gastric ulcers were reported. I believe this percentage of peptic ulcer is lower than the average percentage found in all hospitalized patients. Might not the tremendous hyperplasia of islet tissue noted by Dr. Zollinger be more apparent than real and due to loss of parenchyma of the gland?" Lester Dragstedt, of Gainesville, Florida [he had "retired" to work at the University of Florida in the Department of his quondam resident, Woodward, and remained busily and productively engaged], said that "Many years ago . . . Dr. R. R. Bensley of Chicago claimed that ligation of the pancreatic ducts in animals caused hyperplasia of the islets, Drs. DeTakats and Wilder tried this operation in the treatment of human diabetes mellitus. It was a complete failure . . . we . . . learned in our laboratory that tying off the ducts of the pancreas caused not only atrophy of the parenchyma of the pancreas but also reduces the functional capacity of the islets by at least 50 per cent . . . It is difficult to show that in the dog any of the mechanisms of gastric secretion are dependent on the pancreas." He wanted to know ". . . how good is the evidence that these ulcero-genic tumors are of islet cell origin? My associates, Drs. Harry Oberhelman, Nelsen, Rigler and I have encountered nine of these tumors . . . Five of them were in the duodenum and five . . . were in the pancreas. One was in the duodenum beneath the mucosa about a centimeter distal to the pylorus. Is it not possible that these tumors arise from the cell, at present unknown, that manufactures gastrin? The isolation by Prof. Gregory and his associates, and now by Dr. Zollinger, of an agent which is indistinguishable in its physiologic action from gastrin, seems to support this theory. An objection, of course, is the fact that so far as I know, no one has found one of these tumors in the antrum of the stomach." Dan W. Elliott, closing, responded to Mulholland that all their evidence in pancreatitis, in their animal experiments, was that the secretagogue came from the islet and in response to Poth stated that since the histamine in Poth's animals ". . . acts directly on the parietal cells to produce acid, it is not surprising that it can produce an ulcer whether or not the pancreas is present." They, too, had been studying tumors by electronmicroscopy and said that Ellison's ". . . pictures are typical of islet alpha cells. In some of our material, there is evidence of alpha cell granules . . ." In response to Friesen, Elliott said they had ". . . postulated that if chronic pancreatitis is accompanied by islet hyperplasia, and the production of a gastric secretagogue, this substance will act directly upon the parietal cells to make excessive acid. If more acid is made, more secretin should be produced in the duodenum . . . this increased secretin stimulation of acinar cells against obstruction may be of definite importance in provoking further pancreatic inflammation." Friesen's tumor from which the gastric stimulant could not be isolated was "unique . . . However, we have noticed that if an ulcerogenic tumor also contains glucagon-like activity, it is more difficult to assay the gastric stimulant . . . It may be that glucagon present in his tumor extract inhibited the acid response that he otherwise might have obtained . . ." In response to Dragstedt, Elliott admitted "We do not really know for sure that ulcerogenic tumors actually arise from the pancreatic islets, but our best histologic evidence so far indicates this origin."

* * *

Owen H. Wangensteen, of Minneapolis, Professor of Surgery and Surgeon-in-Chief, University of Minnesota Hospital, and by invitation, E. T. Peter, E. F. Bernstein, A. I. Walder, Henry Sosin, and A. J. Madsen, *Can Physiological Gastrectomy Be Achieved by Gastric Freezing?*, gave the lie to the old aphorism that "If the title of a paper is phrased as a question the conclusion will be in the negative." Three years before, Wangensteen had presented to the Association the evidence that gastric cooling was effective in the treatment of bleeding ". . . in duodenal ulcer, gastric erosion, and in bleeding esophageal varices" with ". . . lesser levels of sustained effectiveness in gastric ulcer, steroid ulcer, and hemorrhagic gastritis." He had previously demonstrated that ". . . gastric secretion and digestion were depressed while local gastric cooling was in operation", the gastric mucosal temperature being lowered to 10° to 15° C. Experimenting with greater depressions of the temperature, as low as 0° to 3° C, and varying periods of exposure, they concluded that "Gastric cooling to near freezing temperatures

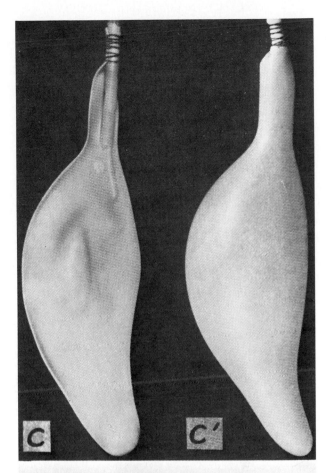

FIGURE 3 CC'

The stomach-shaped rubber balloon which Wangensteen finally came to for human gastric freezing, inserted through the mouth, and connected to an apparatus which delivered coolant at an inflow temperature of $-17°$ to $-20°$ C. Thirty-one of thirty-one patients with duodenal ulcer, originally referred for operation, had marked or complete relief of symptoms after a one hour gastric freeze, and thirty showed a significant reduction in HCl secretion. An addendum indicates that by the time the galleys were received the series had grown to 120 patients, "without serious complication".

Owen H. Wangensteen, E. T. Peter, E. F. Bernstein, A. I. Walder, Henry Sosin, and A. J. Madsen, *Can Physiological Gastrectomy Be Achieved by Gastric Freezing?*, Volume LXXX, 1962.

for two to four hours was attended by longer periods of depression of gastric secretion." A dog's stomach could tolerate freezing for varying periods of time so that ". . . in vivo gastric freezing was feasible and could be achieved within certain temperature and time relationships without injury to the dog or his stomach." The results seemed to be somewhat variable ". . . probably dependent, in large measure, upon the degree of gastric freeze. Intracellular ice crystal formation, with cell rupture and damage, is far more likely to be present in those instances in which the freeze of the gastric mucosa was accomplished quickly." Thereafter, some dogs remained unresponsive to attempts to stimulate acid production for as long as 35 weeks, and most of them for nine to ten months after a Heidenhain pouch was frozen. Gastric juice from previously frozen stomachs was not only achlorhydric but had ". . . little or no evidence of peptic activity . . .". Gastroscopy after freezing showed some reddening of the gastric mucosa which persisted for two or three days, and

some edema during the same period of time. "After the first week following gastric freezing, gastroscopic examination reveals a very normal gastric mucosa." Histologically, there was striking edema which lasted for three or four days, microthrombi in the submucosal vessels, and ". . . evidences of injury to Auerbach's plexuses within the gastric wall", but muscle seemed to be uninjured. Cooling was achieved by circulating a freezing solution through a "stomach shaped balloon" placed in the stomach. No histamine ulcers were produced in five dogs whose stomachs had been frozen, and after gastric freezing only one dog out of ten with an antral pouch in the transverse colon, developed an ulcer. "These studies suggest that gastric freezing does afford definite protection against ulcer provoking procedures." Since "No curative operation, which will preclude ulcer recurrence in 100 per cent of instances, having no undesirable side effects and without operative risk, has yet been found", and "X-ray irradiation for the purpose has not been followed by

1160

a high incidence of cure and the method is not without danger", they undertook to study gastric freezing in patients. "Thirty-one patients coming for elective operation for unobstructed duodenal ulcer were subjected to gastric freezing. All 31 of these patients received marked or complete relief of symptoms following an hour's gastric freeze. Thirty of the 31 exhibited a significant decrease in gastric HCL secretion . . . a significant decrease in the response to peptone and insulin stimulation also was noted. Seventeen of the 31 patients were achlorhydric on overnight gastric aspiration." Wangensteen's group had been progressively modifying the balloon, and the gastric-shaped balloon had been used in the last 19 patients all of whom ". . . were completely relieved of their symptoms and all exhibited a significant reduction in secretion of HCL. Fourteen of the 19 became achlorhydric judged by overnight gastric aspirations." Wangensteen concluded that "Gastric freezing appears to be a simple, effective and safe means of suppressing gastric secretion in the intact stomach without interfering with normal gastric motility." They had even conducted freezing as an outpatient procedure in one instance. In patients, the gastric inflow provided by the machine manufactured for the purpose was at -20° C. The patient was placed upon a warming blanket to prevent a downward drift in body temperature. "Gastric freezing is carried out for an hour, during which time the inflow temperatures range from -17° to -20° C." Sedatives were unnecessary. There might be a little initial pain, relieved by partial deflation of the balloon. "Strangely enough, no patient has complained of the cold tube in his mouth or throat nor have any evidences of frostbite of the tongue been observed." At the conclusion, the balloon was deflated and time permitted for the ice crystals between the balloon and the stomach to melt. There had been no complications in their 40 patients. They thought that the primary use would be ". . . in the management of the peptic ulcer diathesis . . . in patients with unobstructed duodenal ulcer . . ." They had seen improvement in patients with hiatal hernia, and in patients with stenosing esophagitis. An Addendum, written when the galleys were received, updated this series to 120 patients whose stomachs had been frozen ". . . without serious complication." Five of the last 96 had to be refrozen after three to six months for return of symptoms. Pyloric obstruction had proved to be an absolute contraindication to gastric freezing. Discomfort often persisted as long as a week after freezing. Eight patients of the 120 had had melena after the freezing period, and at the end of a year of experience, Wangensteen still thought

that it was ". . . a safe, simple, and effective way of managing patients with intractable unobstructed duodenal ulcer."

Discussion

A number of brief questions were answered by E. T. Peter in closing. The patient's temperature drifted no more than 1° C. and only if the warming blanket was not used. No anesthesia was employed except for spraying the throat with cyclaine. Laboratory experiments had been carried out under general anesthesia. Was the effect of the operation the result of "hypothermic vagotomy"? They believed it was to some degree. They had frozen the vagi in the chest and found depression of gastric secretory responses to insulin for six months when gradually it began to return to normal. There was histologic evidence of nerve injury in the gastric wall. The complication they had had was an anginal attack in an elderly patient. They did not know how long achlorhydria persisted, and one dog had been achlorhydric as long as 35 weeks. They had ". . . one patient who has gone almost eight months before return of secretion", but when secretion returned it was one-tenth or one-fifth of normal values. "We are fairly certain that it will last at least six months, and perhaps longer." Wangensteen had not been present for the Discussion, but Peter's final statement was that "Gastric freezing, embracing the concept of suppressing gastric secretion in the intact stomach, that is, physiological gastrectomy, offers promise of coming to occupy an important role in the treatment of peptic ulcer disease."

* * *

At the 1961 meeting, Spencer and Bahnson, in discussing renal vascular hypertension, had delineated a group of patients, female and younger, with fibromuscular hyperplasia of the renal arteries, and now Edwin J. Wylie, of San Francisco, Assistant Professor of Surgery, Vice-Chairman, Department of Surgery, University of California Medical Center, and by invitation, D. Perloff, and J. S. Wellington, *Fibromuscular Hyperplasia of the Renal Arteries,* [referring to no surgical publications but their own] reported an experience with 40 patients with hypertension and fibromuscular hyperplasia of the renal arteries, five seen in consultation, 35 evaluated, operated upon and subsequently followed at the University of California. Thirty of the 35 patients were female, and 63% of them had hypertension diagnosed in the third, fourth, and fifth decade of life. The five patients seen only in consultation were all females with onset in the same ages. Six patients had had the hypertension diagnosed before they were 20, and one at the age of six months. Drug therapy had been effective in no more than a third of the cases. Only five of the patients had arteriosclerosis and 83% of the 35 had a bruit at the epigastrium or flank. Urogram generally showed a decrease in size of the kidney, decrease in initial opacification, and increase in late opacification. In 13 of the patients, the lesion was unilateral. Arteriography made the diagnosis in all patients, showing ". . . closely grouped short zones of luminal constriction alternating with zones of normal or occasionally increased luminal diameter." The proximal artery was usually spared. The resected arterial segments showed ". . . irregularly spaced zones of concentric mural thickening with resultant narrowing of the lumen . . . which made the arterial wall appear corrugated when viewed from the intimal aspect." The thickening in the media ". . . consisted primarily of smooth muscle, similar in cellular organization to the smooth muscle in the medial coat of normal renal arteries." They operated upon 24 of the 35 patients,- nephrectomy in six, renal artery reconstruction in 18. In 17 of the 18, they performed segmental resection of the renal artery and end-to-end anastomosis, and in one early case, ". . . before the general feasibility of direct anastomosis was realized", performed a left splenorenal arterial anastomosis. In two of the patients, a venous patch graft was required in addition to the

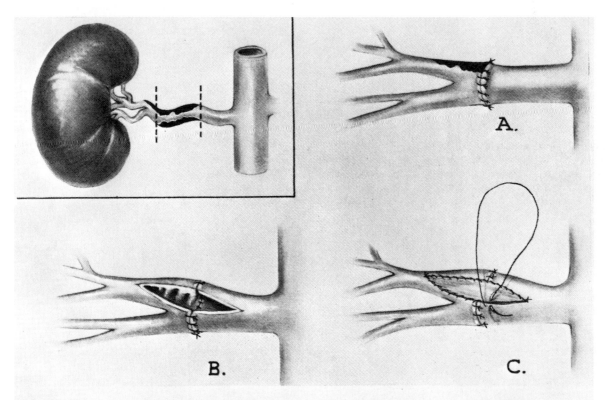

Fig. 12. Illustration of venous patch technic for lesions extending beyond the renal bifurcation.

Wylie performed the procedure indicated in 8A and B, a direct anastomosis, in 15 patients; in two he added the venous patch graft seen in his Figure 12; and in a single patient ". . .early in the series . . ." performed a splenorenal arterial anastomosis. There were no deaths. Six additional patients had had to have nephrectomy. Four of the patients with nephrectomy achieved normal blood pressure. The patient with the splenorenal arterial anastomosis had a normal blood pressure. Eight of the 16 patients with unilateral resection and anastomosis had normal blood pressure, and five had near normal blood pressure, one was improved, and two showed no change. One patient with a bilateral operation showed no change.

Edwin J. Wylie, D. Perloff, and J. S. Wellington, *Fibromuscular Hyperplasia of the Renal Arteries,* Volume LXXX, 1962. (Figure continues on overleaf.)

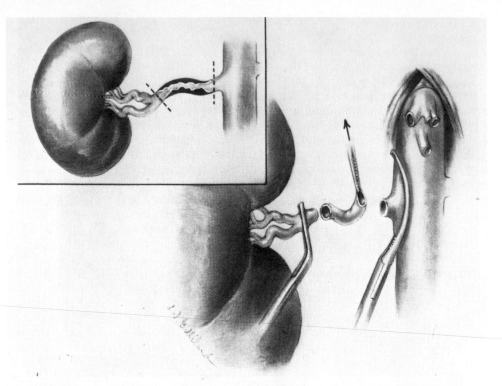

Fig. 8. A and B illustrate operative technics for segmental resection of renal artery. Note the ease with which the distal stump may be brought medially and the straightening of the distal branches. Gentle stretching of the opened arterial ends overcame local spasm (see insert in B).

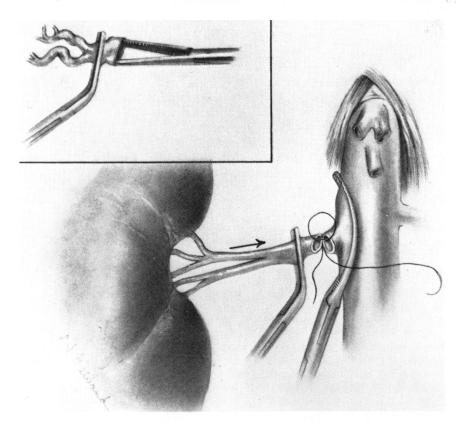

nd-to-end anastomosis. They had no deaths. Of the six patients who underwent nephrectomy, four now had a normal blood pressure. The patient with a splenorenal arterial anastomosis had a normal blood pressure. Eight of the 16 patients with unilateral resection and anastomosis had normal blood pressure, five near normal blood pressure, one was improved, and two showed no change. One patient, with a bilateral operation, showed no change. As for etiology, they speculated on the similarity of the lesion to the lesion in Marfan's syndrome, and the possibility that the occurrence largely in relatively young females, might suggest a ". . . possible endocrine factor". They suggested ". . . wider application of renal arteriography in hypertensive female patients."

Discussion

Frank C. Spencer, of Lexington, Kentucky, said ". . . the report represents one of the largest series reported thus far . . ." Spencer demonstrated the venous enlargement of the renal artery which he had been employing but commented that "With the good results of Dr. Wylie, I think I might be encouraged . . . to attempt to excise and perform a direct anastomosis." Watts R. Webb, of Jackson, Mississippi, commented that he and James Hardy had recently successfully operated upon a 14-year-old girl with fibromuscular renal artery hyperplasia who had an elevated aldosterone level in her adrenal vein blood at the time of operation, and high preoperative urinary aldosterone excretion which fell back to normal after operation, "Davis and Carpenter and others demonstrated that the renin angiotensin system can stimulate aldosterone. This is a clinical demonstration that this mechanism does pertain in the patient with the Goldblatt mechanism. If this can be confirmed with further patients, it will add to our understanding of the way the renin system can cause hypertension—not only by vasoconstriction but also by stimulation of aldosterone which with its salt-retaining properties adds to the vicious cycle of hypertension." J. Hartwell Harrison, of Boston, reported that in the 25 patients operated upon for renal hypertension from 1954 to 1961 at the Brigham, only one had shown fibromuscular hyperplasia. Wylie, closing, agreed that the venous patch graft technique demonstrated by Spencer had its uses. He preferred a patch of an autologous vein, rather than synthetic material. In general, he preferred direct anastomosis for fibromuscular hyperplasia, and "simple endarterectomy" for arteriosclerotic renal artery obstruction.

The Business Meetings

The 1962 meeting was held May 9, 10, and 11, at the Sheraton-Park Hotel, Washington, D.C., President J. Englebert Dunphy in the Chair.

H. B. Shumacker, Jr., for the Program Committee, reported that by the deadline for receipt of abstracts, they had received 112, and had selected a total of 33.

William S. McCune, for the Local Committee on Arrangements, announced the usual cocktail party for Members and their wives, "and a banquet for members only following the cocktail party. A dinner has also been arranged for the wives of the members following the Reception, in the Assembly Room directly across the hall." A tour of the White House had been arranged for the wives of members. [Dwight D. Eisenhower was President Dunphy's dinner speaker. Allegedly at Eisenhower's instance, the ladies were invited to cross the hall after dinner to hear the address.]

At the Second Executive Meeting, the report of Council included a suggestion for a special committee "to review, on a comprehensive basis, the interest of the American Surgical Association in surgical education in the Medical College Curriculum . . ." Council also proposed "That the application blanks for membership in the American Surgical Association by modified to include a listing by the sponsor (not by the candidate) of the applicant's three most significant published contributions."

The Secretary read a very strong resolution by Council condemning the creation of an American Board of Abdominal Surgery ". . . as an unnecessary and superfluous Board . . . and Whereas, those persons encouraging the creation of an American Board of Abdominal Surgery have persisted in their efforts despite the fact that numerous other established surgical societies have also rejected their request for sponsorship; these persons have also resorted to certain political moves to gain control of and the endorsement of the Section on General Surgery of the American Medical Association; therefore, be it *Resolved,* That the American Surgical Association reaffirms the previous statement of Council opposing the creation of separate Specialty Boards within the province of general surgery; and that the creation of an American Board of Abdominal Surgery is not in the best interests of the surgical patient, general surgical practice, or in the training of surgeons." [The American Board of Abdominal Surgery, self-ordained and self-established, apparently awarded certificates pretty much on payment of a fee. Its supporters had packed the meeting in the Section of Surgery of the American Medical Association and had taken over the meeting, elected new officers and voted to be an endorsing body of their "Board".] The report of Council and recommendations were accepted.

Among those elected as new Members were E. Stanley Crawford, of Houston; Milton Thomas Edgerton, Jr., of Baltimore; James Vincent Maloney, Jr., of Los Angeles; George L. Nardi, of Boston; Lloyd Milton Nyhus, of Chicago; and Kenneth Warren, of Boston. Officers elected were President, Oliver Cope, of Boston; Vice-Presidents, Frank Gerbode, of San Francisco, and William S. McCune, of Washington, D.C.; Secretary, William A. Altemeier, of Cincinnati.

LXXXI

1963

The 1963 meeting was held at the Hotel Westward Ho in Phoenix, Arizona, April 3, 4, and 5, President Oliver Cope, of Boston, Professor of Surgery, Harvard Medical School; Visiting Surgeon, Massachusetts General Hospital, in the Chair. Among those whose memoirs appear in this volume were Walter G. Maddock, whose early papers with Frederick Coller "marked the beginning of a new era which now embraces a vast literature concerning fluid and electrolyte balance . . . the related metabolic disorders", and Frank L. Meleney, who had made such significant contributions in surgical bacteriology.

* * *

Hiram T. Langston, of Chicago, Clinical Professor of Surgery, University of Illinois; Chief of Surgery, Chicago State Tuberculosis Sanitarium, and by invitation, George Milles and William Dallessandro, *Further Experiences with Autogenous Blood Transfusions*, had published a paper on the subject in 1962 and now reported in 113 patients the withdrawal of blood from a patient three days to a week before operation so that the patient could receive his own blood, eliminating the risks of serum hepatitis and mismatched blood transfusion. In their 113 patients, they had withdrawn 154 units of blood and had had to administer an additional 93 units of donor blood. They were unable to detect any deleterious effects of the preliminary venesection and said that ". . . within certain reasonable limits a patient can supply his own blood for transfusion to the extent of one,

two or more units. This decreases or obviates the problems of procurement and decreases, to the degree that transfusion requirements are met with autogenous blood, the hazards of incompatibility as well as serum hepatitis."

Discussion

H. W. Scott, of Nashville, asked about the interval before operation and the number of units that could safely be withdrawn. J. Garrott Allen, of Palo Alto, California, commented, as John A. Schilling, of Oklahoma City had, on autotransfusion of blood lost vaginally in obstetrical catastrophes, and the recent use by "obstetricians . . . faced with the problem of Rh negative incompatabilities in patients about to deliver", of a procedure similar to Langston's. He asked whether the preliminary venesection in Langston's patient had so "comprised" the patient's circulatory status as to make transfusion inevitable, led to the use of bank blood, and so increased the risk of hepatitis. Langston said that they had drawn blood as close as three days before operation, but thought four days to a week was "probably preferable". As to the amount, "We have on one occasion—at the time it was done it was by accident —removed four units in two separate bleedings for two separate operations from a single donor. He got only three of these units back, which will partially answer Dr. Allen's question." [Neither Langston, nor the discussers, seemed aware that C. H. Frazier in 1921 (Volume XL, 1922), twenty-four hours be-

1165

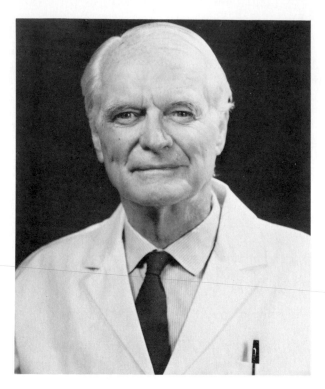

Oliver Cope, (c. 1965). 1902—, Vice-President 1957, President 1963. M.D. Harvard, 1928. Training and entire professional life at Massachusetts General Hospital, where he was acting Head of the Department of Surgery during World War II and again in 1964 and 1969, Professor of Surgery, Harvard Medical School. Precise, gentlemanly, early interested in surgical metabolism and in burns, major interest in hyperparathyroidism, contributed the concept and term of the "Delphic node" in thyroid cancer, deep interest in medical education, a penchant for philosophizing about surgery, education, and disease.

fore operation for suboccipital tumor, withdrew 500 cc of blood from the patient, citrated it, and successfully transfused it after the operation.]

* * *

Victor Richards, of San Francisco, Clinical Professor of Surgery, Stanford University School of Medicine; Chief of Surgery, Presbyterian Medical Center [who had relinquished the Stanford Chair when the Medical School moved to Palo Alto from San Francisco], and by invitation, Douglas Pinto and Paul Coombs, *Studies in Suspended Animation by Hypothermia Combined with Hyperbaric Oxygenation,* opened their paper with the imaginative statement that "The temporary suspension of life has been an intriguing concept to surgeons for years as a

method permitting singular and unmatched practices in the art of surgery." The needs of open heart surgery had stimulated intensive investigation of hypothermia to permit "regional cessation of circulation", surface cooling had been replaced by "core cooling" with the extracorporeal circulation and heat exchangers, and "Regional cooling of the ischemic heart can be produced safely by cross-clamping of the aorta, i.e., the application of a tourniquet to the heart, followed by packing of the pericardial cavity with iced saline . . ." with or without intermittent coronary perfusion. Their studies were based on the theory that "It should be possible to reduce the body needs for oxygen by lowering the body temperature, and to increase the body stores of oxygen available for tissue utilization by driving oxygen into the tissues under increased ambient pressures" and they had undertaken to study "the relationships and interconnections between hypothermia and hyperbaric oxygenation, particularly as they apply to suspended animation . . ." Boerema, of Holland, beginning in 1956, had begun applying hyperbaric oxygenation to the problems of cardiac surgery and had almost at once mentioned the combination of moderate hypothermia with hyperbaric oxygen, the "use of substances other than hemoglobin to carry physically dissolved oxygen to the tissues at 3 atmospheres of oxygen pressure", avoidance of fibrillation by deep hypothermia under hyperbaric oxygenation, the use of hyperbaric oxygenation for carbon monoxide poisoning and for the treatment of anaerobic infections. Illingworth, in England, in 1961, had reported clinical and experimental studies of hypothermia and found that dogs at 28° C could tolerate 35 minutes of complete circulatory occlusion under conditions of hyperbaric oxygenation, and others had studied the effect of hyperbaric oxygen therapy upon carbon monoxide poisoning, acute coronary occlusion, anaerobic infections. Boerema's experience with hyperbaric oxygenation in deeply cyanotic children was that "CO_2 transport is not interfered with . . . the condition of the patients is tremendously improved by saturating the polycythemic blood with oxygen under pressure. They performed aortico-pulmonary shunts in four patients under five years of age, the Potts' procedure, without difficulty, completely cross-clamping the aorta and pulmonary artery during the anastomosis. The ability to occlude the circulation completely simplifies the anastomotic procedure. Patients remained pink and well-oxygenated even during the periods of aortic and pulmonary occlusion." In their own studies, Richards and colleagues, employing cooling by immersion and then the refrigerated pressure chamber, in over 100 dogs monitoring EEG and EKG continuously and drawing repeated blood samples for study, found that dogs breathing 98% O_2 and 2% CO_2 at 3 atmospheres of pressure, withstood "apneic periods of 17 to 26 minutes with complete recovery. Adding circulatory arrest did not alter the results." Dogs cooled to 28° C to 30° C, withstood respiratory and circulatory arrest for 45 to 64 minutes with complete recovery. All animals cooled to 19° to 22° C with circulatory arrest for 75 to 80 minutes in the hyperbaric chamber fibrillated during arrest or rewarming, and all of those animals "had brain damage after resuscitation."

They concluded that "The combined effects of mild hypothermia and 98-2 at 3 atmospheres can allow total circulatory arrest up to one hour with no gross evidence of CNS or myocardial damage. Accompanying acid-base disturbances are transient and easily reversible." They mentioned no immediate intention to apply the technique clinically, planning to study "lower levels of hypothermia, defibrillate the heart electrically under CO_2 flooding to avoid explosive hazards . . . combine regional and total extracorporeal circulation to the study. Limited blood flows under these conditions may permit extended survival times."

Discussion

Ivan Brown, of Durham, North Carolina, said that at Duke they had been working in the hyperbaric chamber with dogs and monkeys for two or three years and agreed that "the tolerable and safe period for circulatory arrest . . . the safe period for severe circulatory collapse produced experimentally by a number of means can be extended by hyperbaric oxygenation." They were enthusiastic about the technique and had a pilot human chamber. He devoted a considerable portion of his long discussion to the hazards of the hyperbaric chamber in terms of oxygen toxicity and convulsions, the risk of fire, etc. Edwin H. Ellison, of Milwaukee, said that they had there a hyperbaric chamber which had been used since 1928 for decompression of divers for the relief of the bends, and like Brown, commented on the numerous problems associated with the use of hyperbaric chambers, stressing the hazard not only to the patients but to the surgical team in the hyperbaric chamber, ". . . surgical programs in the future might well include papers, panel discussions, *et cetera*, on compression air disease of surgeons, decompression sickness in surgical residents, or the influence of caisson disease on the fertility of operating room nurses."

* * *

Three papers on portal hypertension demonstrated the lack of agreement in almost every facet of the physiologic phenomena and operative treatment. R. C. Britton, C. H. Brown, and E. K. Shirey, of the Cleveland Clinic, all by invitation, *Intrahepatic Veno-occlusive Disease in Cirrhosis with Chronic Ascites:* Diagnosis by Hepatic Phlebography and Results of Surgical Treatment, had performed cine-fluorography by retrograde injection into the hepatic veins from the vena cava, as well as determining portal vein and vena cava pressures at operation. In patients with cirrhosis, their hepatic venograms showed "rigidity and loss of tapering contour of first, second, and third order vessels . . . reduction in the number of second, third, and fourth order branches visualized . . . reduction in caliber of all orders of branches . . . irregularity, tortuosity and segmental stenoses . . . ." If the force of the injection was sufficient to fill portal radicles, the subsequent flow was always "by drainage of medium in prograde direction towards the sinusoids and not into the portal trunk." The more severe the phlebographic changes the poorer the response of ascites to medical management, "All four of the patients with severe veno-occlusive disease had ascites which did not respond to prolonged and intensive treatment but they did not reform ascites from nine to 20 months after portacaval shunt." Their studies showed no support for reverse portal flow, even in the one patient in whom occluded portal pressures at operation showed an increase on the hepatic side, suggesting reverse flow. On the basis of their own experience and a less than lucid review of the literature, they concluded that "Chronic cirrhotic ascites associated with severe hepatic veno-occlusive disease may be relieved by portal-systemic shunts which preserve the portal vein intact."

* * *

Donald J. Ferguson, of Chicago, Professor of Surgery, University of Chicago, *Hemodynamics in Surgery for Portal Hypertension,* stating that "Whether it is preferable to make an end-to-side or a side-to-side portacaval shunt in cirrhotic patients may be decided primarily by the effect on portal flow", had measured portal pressures before and after occlusion in 48 patients. In the last seven he had measured the blood flows with a magnetic flow meter, repeating the flows after end-to-side or side-to-side portacaval anastomoses. "Measurements in the intact proximal and distal portal vein, after occlusion, invariably showed that pressure was higher proximally . . . In none of these patients, therefore, was there net flow away from the liver at the time of measurement." Both types of shunt produced a satisfactory fall in portal pressure which generally fell by 10% during the first day after operation. Portal flows approximately doubled after either type of shunt. After a side-to-side anastomosis, there was no measurable flow toward the liver in four of the five patients and a 200 ml./min. flow in one, a patient who had been overtransfused and whose vena cava pressure had been equal to portal pressure, so that this was interpreted as a temporary response to overtransfusion. "When proximal portal flow was shut off, portal pressure was lowered, and small retrograde flows were detected in two patients." Hepatic artery flow increased consistently when the portal vein was occluded. Ferguson considered that "It does not appear, if these cases are representative, that there is much to choose between the two types of operation so far as blood flow is concerned . . . The argument that side-to-side shunts are better for treatment of ascites can hardly be valid if there is not in fact appreciable retrograde flow through the distal limb. Moreover, ascites has been effectively treated by end-to-side shunts." He suggested that the potential retrograde flow in the side-to-side shunt was directed against the proximal flow and that the double end-to-side anastomosis of McDermott might actually facilitate retrograde flow.

* * *

In the third paper, W. Dean Warren, now of Miami, Professor and Chairman, Department of Surgery, University of Miami School of Medicine; J. E. Restrepo and J. C. Respess, by invitation; and William H. Muller, Jr. [the Recorder], of Charlottesville, Stephen H. Watts Professor, Chairman, Department of Surgery; Surgeon-in-Chief, University of Virginia Medical Center, *The Importance of Hemodynamic Studies in Management of Portal Hypertension,* sought to select patients who would benefit from portal decompression and to determine the stage in the disease process when operation would give the best results. Whereas Ferguson had measured portal and hepatic artery blood flow directly with the flow meter, Warren and his colleagues arrived at their Estimation of Hepatic Blood Flow [EHBF] by a radio-isotope technique utilizing colloidal radio-active gold with external monitoring of radioactivity. They made the flat assumption in their discussion that "with a side-to-side shunt, the portal vein is converted to an outflow tract" citing a 1959 paper of their own. From their studies they concluded that "Patients with less severe portal hyper-

tension (Stage I), usually maintained a normal, or near normal, estimated hepatic blood flow and showed less alteration in the portal venous perfusion of the liver . . . ascites was the commonest major complication of their disease . . . the response to portacaval shunt has generally been a significant reduction in the estimated hepatic blood flow, and an unsatisfactory clinical result . . . severe portal-systemic encephalopathy, persistent peripheral edema, marked weakness and inability to work . . . progressive liver deterioration with death from hepatic failure." Whereas, "Patients with a more fully developed portal hypertension (Stages II and III) . . . tolerated portacaval shunt quite well . . . continue full-time activity . . . The change in the estimated hepatic blood flow . . . is less marked in this group of patients . . . who exhibit bleeding esophageal varices." Warren and his colleagues suggested that an EHBF, "one-third or less of the normal mean, strongly suggests the possibility" that encephalopathy could appear after operation, and "Patients with markedly depressed liver blood flow appear to have an increased mortality from operation." The patients to be aware of, in consideration for operation were, "those with mild portal hypertension and those with markedly diminished preoperative hepatic blood flow."

Discussion

Warren opened the Discussion, insisting that "In our study of a large number of cirrhotics we have found that the basic hemodynamic change in all cirrhotics, exclusive of those who have portal vein thrombosis, is an outflow obstruction." The patients with ascites "appear to have a more acute form of hypertension . . . comparable elevations in pressure, but . . . a greater hepatic blood flow with less extrahepatic collateral . . . they will have less outflow obstruction than will the severe cirrhotic with bleeding varices without ascites." Louis M. Rousselot, of New York, was not convinced by Britton's Cleveland Clinic paper, "His conclusion that distortion of the hepatic vein vascular bed results in a functional Budd-Chiari syndrome reiterates the thesis of the numerous advocates of the outflow block theory in the genesis of cirrhotic ascites . . . the fact remains that passive venous congestion of the liver, as seen in Budd-Chiari syndrome, is not found in cirrhosis." Like Ferguson, Rousselot had been measuring portal flow with electromagnetic flow meters, but his findings were different. With end-to-side shunt, splanchnic flow increased substantially "in most cases in the range of 100 per cent" but after side-to-side shunt, in three patients, the "flow in the hepatic limb of the shunt was stagnant . . . In five patients . . . flow was toward the liver . . . in five patients there was definite retrograde flow", and he thought particularly significant the findings that "The eventual direction of flow in the hepatic limb of the shunt could not be predicted from the values of free or occluded portal pressure or the value of the preshunt flow." Their own attempt to use EHBF as an index of operability had been unsatisfactory, "We have had cases of patients with both large or small E.H.B.F. who did equally well or poorly after end-to-side shunt." In their experience, the incidence of hepatic encephalopathy was directly correlated with the age of the patients "and never occurred in patients under 40 years!" Donald G. Mulder, of Los Angeles, questioned Ferguson's findings that there was little or no retrograde flow. He had catheterized six patients under local anesthesia, six months to seven years after side-to-side shunt, "When a tracer substance is injected through the hepatic artery catheter, it can be detected both at the hepatic venous catheter and the portal venous catheter. If radiopaque material is . . . injected into the proximal portal vein catheter, placed well into its peripheral branches, there is immediate reflux back through the side-to-side shunt and into the inferior vena cava . . ." Charles Gardner Child, III, of Ann Arbor, said that after years of effort, "I have ended up moderately defeated in my efforts to relate validly phenomena of liver disease to pressure and flow in hepatic inflow and outflow tracts." George L. Nardi, of Boston, said that "I once belonged to the flow club, too", had measured "flows in all directions on a great many patients . . . we were unable to find a correlation between the preoperative flows we measured and the patients' post-operative results." His findings had been like Warren's in that "the patients who had the greatest reduction in blood flow were the patients who died or fared poorly." A flow reduced below 30% resulted in death, usually in coma. Richard C. Britton, in closing, said of Warren's technique, "The inaccuracies of indirect estimations of hepatic blood flow account, perhaps, for increasing interest in direct measurement using electromagnetic flowmeters . . . Drs. Ferguson, Schenk, and Rousselot have all shown . . . that there is usually a significant increase in hepatic arterial flow following occlusion of the portal vein or portacaval shunt." D. J. Ferguson, in closing, said that Mulder's retrograde [radio isotope] flow technique measured "smaller flows than one can measure with the magnetic meter and does not measure the volume of flow. The significance of such a flow depends on the volume."

* * *

The chemotherapeutic agents were being used systemically, had been injected into extremities isolated for regional perfusion, and now, Michael J. Brennan, R. W. Talley, E. H. Drake, V. K. Vaitkevicius, and A. K. Poznanski, all by invitation, and Brock E. Brush, of Detroit, Surgeon in Charge, First Surgical Section, Division of General Surgery, Henry Ford Hospital, *5-Fluorouracil Treatment of Liver Metastases by Continuous Hepatic Artery Infusion via Cournand Catheter:* Results and Suitability for Intensive Postsurgical Adjuvant Chemotherapy, in 13 patients, injected 5-Fluorouracil through a radial artery catheter passed into the hepatic artery at monthly intervals for continuous infusion of periods of five to 12 days. Nine of 13 patients with metastases from bowel carcinomas showed a decrease in size of the tumor as judged by Thorotrast injections.

Discussion

Warren H. Cole, of Chicago, who had been at the forefront of the move to employ chemotherapy prophylactically commented with gentle restraint, "The authors' figure of 60 per cent favorable results I think is splendid, although we realize that they are not cures." He urged continuation of the studies. F. W. Preston, of Chicago, had employed celiac artery instillation by radial artery catheter for carcinoma of the stomach in two patients who showed substantial clinical improvement, becoming able to eat and gain weight. E. T. Krementz, of New Orleans, had introduced small polyethylene catheters at operation into the right gastro-epiploic artery and threaded up into the hepatic artery for continuous intra-arterial infusions. Of 48 patients with continuous intra-arterial infusion, 28 had shown "definite objective responses, most of them of short duration." They believed that they had converted two patients with inoperable rectal cancer into operability. John M. Beal, of New York, said that they had found the technique safe but said nothing about effect. Brennan, who had presented the paper, now closed, and said that their hope had been to develop an effective method of prophylactic chemotherapy, "We believe, as Dr. Cole does, that the probability that one can destroy a tumor chemotherapeutically when it is very small is greater than the probability that one can destroy it when it is grossly visible."

* * *

The year before, Owen Wangensteen had presented his material on gastric freezing and now J. H.

Meredith and R. T. Myers, by invitation, and Howard H. Bradshaw, of Winston-Salem, Professor of Surgery and Director, Division of Surgery, Bowman Gray School of Medicine, reported their experimental studies, *Acid Secretion in Stomach Pouches Made after Freezing the Stomach.* They froze dogs' stomachs with the apparatus Wangensteen had invented, inflow temperature of the balloon, -17° C; outflow, -14° C, for an hour. A week later, Heidenhain pouches were made from the gastric fundus of these dogs and after a further week's delay, the gastric output of the pouch was measured. The acid production from these pouches was no different than that from normal dogs studied in the same laboratory. [Directly contradicting what Wangensteen had reported.]

Discussion

A vigorous Discussion followed. C. W. Lillehei, of Minneapolis, read Owen H. Wangensteen's discussion. They had had similar results with the same kind of experiment, the difficulty with which was that there was "no way of establishing a secretory base-line" since the pouch was not prepared until after the freezing. Since October, 1961, they had "frozen the stomachs of 350 patients with some manifestations of the peptic ulcer diathesis", most of them with "intractable duodenal ulcer", the second largest group being those with stomal ulcers. No deaths occurred, but after freezing they had had gross melena in 12 patients, and an acute gastric ulcer in eight patients. With respect to melena, "Our own experience . . . would indicate . . . there is no need for alarm." Gastric ulcer defects, they thought, would heal "with employment of a continuous Winkelstein drip of ice cold skim milk",- although they had one perforation. After a single freeze in man or dog, "gastric secretion has usually returned to pre-freeze levels within a period of six months", although half the patients remained asymptomatic and "For those having symptoms of any degree, we advise a refreeze." Their 350 patients had undergone 438 episodes of gastric freezing. It looked to them as if repeated freezing in dogs produced "what might be interpreted as an atrophic gastric mucosa" and such dogs' stomachs might remain achlorhydric to peptone or insulin but responded to histamine. Their clinical experience suggested "that gastric freezing is safe and that it is reasonably effective. Relief of pain is usual and dramatic. Ulcer craters heal quite consistently within two to six weeks (90%) . . . multiple freezes frequently will be necessary in order to cope effectively with some patients with the peptic ulcer

diathesis . . . multiple freezing can be done with impunity." Wangensteen's very long discussion concluded with the statement that he was "enthusiastic over the promise of gastric freezing in the management of several aspects of the peptic ulcer diathesis. However, we confess freely to being immersed still in the learning phases." Lloyd M. Nyhus, of Seattle, said that they had been studying freezing gastrectomy for six months and in their studies, they made the Heidenhain pouches before freezing [it was not indicated whether the pouch was separately frozen or simply assumed to be frozen because it was so close to the stomach]. Eight of 14 animals showed a "statistically significant reduction in acid secretion. There was in six, after the same type of procedure, no reduction in acid secretion." Nyhus proposed that this was like the effects of irradiation of the stomach for duodenal ulcer, "Reports in the literature indicate a reduction in acid in approximately 50 per cent of patients following gastric radiation. This figure approximates that reported from clinical studies of acid secretion following gastric freezing. Further, there is a tendency for acid secretion to return following radiation treatment, similarly many reports indicate that refreezing may be necessary as often as every six weeks to three months to maintain a state of achlorhydria. Will the high recurrent ulcer rate following gastric x-ray radiation be repeated following this new modality?" [It was obvious that many of the Fellows were evaluating the problem in the clinic and in the laboratory, and it was known that the apparatus for gastric freezing was being sold as fast as it could be manufactured. Nyhus' final recommendation was perhaps an allusion to this.] "We should restrict the study of the gastric freezing technic to three or four centers in the country until a more definite result can be predicted." Curtis Artz, of Jackson, Mississippi, said that he and Dr. John McFarland had studied 300 dogs and 59 patients. Ten of 37 patients with valid secretory studies showed no reduction in the overnight secretion. Nine patients had a 30 to 70% reduction, 18 had a 70 to 100% reduction, and eight of them were completely achlorhydric. "It is our conclusion from these few patients that diminution in acid secretion on the Hollander and peptone stimulation tests paralleled exactly the diminution in the eight-hour overnight secretion." Their animal studies showed that gastrotomy wounds made 24 hours after freezing were weaker than those made subsequently. He agreed that "Patients have an excellent symptomatic response after freezing. Ninety per cent of the patients are completely free of pain for a period of time." They had had two patients with melena requiring three units of blood. Both were completely achlorhydric and probably had too effective a freeze. They seemed to be enthusiastic, "It appears that this is an excellent technic for the treatment of duodenal ulcer and it merits further evaluation. Certainly we are not ready yet for every practitioner to change the treatment of duodenal ulcer to freezing in place of our currently accepted standards of management." Henry T. Randall's group in New York, had studied dogs with a gastric button inserted before the freezing. Within a week, the response to histamine stimulation was the same as it had been before and there was "no reduction in secretion following insulin or peptone stimulation." Their tritiated thymidine studies of the regeneration of the gastric epithelium had suggested that there was "virtually complete regeneration as judged histologically by light and electron microscopy and by the tritiated thymidine test . . ." In animals, therefore, there was a return to the control situation within three weeks of a freeze. Harold Barker, of New York, said that at the Presbyterian Hospital, Dr. Stephen Wangensteen had been employing the method clinically in some 50 patients, three of whom required operation, one for gastric perforation at 30 days, and two for persistent gastric ulcers, one of which was operated upon because it bled and the other because of persistent pain. In their patient operated upon at 30 days, there was still a good deal of edema of the gastric wall and he urged that operation, if possible, be delayed for at least three weeks after freezing. Meredith, in closing, admitted that "We have not been able to control freezing as well as we would like, and I believe that is the experience of most people who have frozen the stomach." [The gastric freezing apparatus was widely sold and employed throughout the country. Although in 1965 (Volume LXXXIII) Wangensteen still said "our group has shown that in interested and experienced hands gastric freezing can be done as an elective procedure with a low incidence of complications. There has been no hospital mortality in more than 1,000 episodes of elective clinical gastric freezing", the results with it were found to be inconstant and this fact, the necessity for repeated refreezing, the incidence of necrosis of the stomach and perforation from through-and-through destruction by the cold, all combined to retire gastric freezing from clinical use after a brief burst of frenetic excitement over its possibilities.]

* * *

Henry N. Harkins, of Seattle, Professor of Surgery and Executive Officer, Department of Surgery, University of Washington; Surgeon-in-Chief, Univer-

sity Hospital; Lloyd M. Nyhus, Associate Professor of Surgery, University of Washington, and, by invitation, Stanton Stavney, Charles A. Griffith, Lawrence E. Savage, and Tetsuo Kato, *Selective Gastric Vagotomy*, had been studying the preparation since 1955. Jackson, in 1947, had introduced it, and F. D. Moore in 1948 had reported upon it, stating "it might be possible to achieve the protection against ulcer which is apparently conferred by vagotomy, without denervating the upper abdominal organs. By such means the side effects of vagus resection might be reduced in number." Franksson, in 1948 had also employed the technique. None of them had employed a drainage procedure, which Harkins added to it in 1955. His group had now performed some 70 such selective gastric vagotomies and were reporting upon 52 patients with follow-up studies, and on animal experiments. In dogs and monkeys the hepatic and celiac branches of the vagus nerves could be effectively spared, and Harkins thought there was at least "a lessened incidence of diarrhea following selective gastric vagotomy as opposed to the classical truncal vagotomy." The important point was that "Assurance of completeness of vagotomy at the operating table is more certain by the selective technic because of the increased anatomic accuracy of the method." Initially, they had employed antrectomy with selective vagotomy, but more recently had simply used a Finney pyloroplasty as a drainage procedure with the selective vagotomy. Their recommendation was that "selective gastric vagotomy should be studied in a few centers on a trial basis as a refinement of the standard truncal vagotomy . . ."

Discussion

R. G. Jackson, now of Danville, Kentucky [his studies referred to by Harkins had been done at the University of Michigan], cited no numbers, but stressed, as Harkins had, the fact that to perform selective vagotomy, the operator had to identify the vagal anatomy accurately, ". . . selective vagus section can accomplish complete gastric denervation. The detailed dissection makes one less likely to do an incomplete gastric denervation. Preservation of the hepatic and celiac supply of the vagus is considered worthwhile." Joel Baker, of Seattle, said a visit to the University of Washington operating rooms had made him a converted skeptic, and he rose "to support the thesis that selective vagotomy is technically feasible . . . that in preserving the hepatic branch of the left vagus and the splanchnic branch of the right, one is forced to greater technical assurance of complete vagal denervation of the stomach.

This removes one of the chief objections to vagotomy, i.e., a 10 per cent failure to achieve complete vagotomy." Those who were "disenchanted with vagotomy" might perhaps now reassess it. He said that where the duodenum presents ". . . technical hazards . . . we substitute vagotomy with pyloroplasty . . ." Combining vagotomy with antrectomy, he considered ". . . too much, too early, exposing all patients to the hazards both of resection and vagotomy, and to the delayed morbidity of both sacrificing procedures, reduced capacity and total or near total achlorhydria—this in order that 5 per cent fewer will have recurrent ulcer. We reserve this greater combined sacrificial operation for the few patients *with* recurrent ulcer." Lester R. Dragstedt, of Gainesville, Florida, made a prescient statement, "I am indebted to Dr. Harkins and his associates for exploring the possibility of dividing the vagus nerves to the stomach in duodenal ulcer patients while sparing the vagus nerve supply to the other abdominal viscera. This is obviously just what we would like to do. In fact, if it were possible, I should like to divide the secretory fibers and spare the motor fibers in the vagus nerve supply to the stomach. Perhaps this too may be achieved sometime in the future." He had originally thought that a selective vagotomy might result in an incomplete vagotomy and in any case had believed that "the vagus nerves exerted only a minimal effect" on the pancreas and gallbladder, the chief stimulation of which was hormonal. Francis D. Moore, of Boston, emphasized that Harkins was talking about "*selective* vagotomy and not *incomplete* vagotomy". As far as diarrhea after vagotomy was concerned, he thought it was "gastric stasis with a foul colonic flora in the stomach that leads to diarrhea . . . and not the denervation of the colon." He sounded dubious that there would be confirmation of any physiological benefit of selective vagotomy from sparing of the nongastric fibers. H. W. Scott, Jr., of Nashville, said that their results with truncal vagotomy, whether with antral resection or pyloroplasty, were not "besmirched by a high incidence of post-vagotomy diarrhea", as Harkins said was frequently the case. The vagotomy-antrectomy series, begun at Vanderbilt in 1947 by Dr. Leonard Edwards, showed 68% of 1,073 patients with an excellent result, 94% with a good or excellent result. Only a small percentage had had diarrhea, 25% had had mild dumping. Like Moore, he thought that selective gastric vagotomy might be too difficult for wide application. Richard Kraft, of Seattle, reported 70 selective vagotomies with Finney pyloroplasty, and compared ten patients with truncal vagotomy and Finney pyloroplasty and ten with selective vagotomy and Finney pyloroplasty. There was no difference in the fecal fat in the two groups [Dragstedt, in his Discussion, had suggested this might be studied], nor was there any relation between the fecal fat content and post-vagotomy diarrhea. Similarly, there was no difference in the two groups in the fecal nitrogen content. Charles A. Griffith, closing, said that their post-vagotomy diarrhea had been "much much less" with selective vagotomy and did not know why.

* * *

There are repeated examples in the *Transactions* of surgeons who pioneered new methods with great success, and continued to adhere to the techniques which brought them success even after other developments and refinements had led other surgeons to abandon the techniques which once had meant so much. Robert E. Gross, at Children's Hospital in Boston, had produced the best results in this country, perhaps in the world, in many areas of pediatric surgery. In conditions requiring intestinal resection, particularly in the newborn, he had long espoused a Mikulicz double enterostomy and subsequent spur division and closure, and with this, had achieved truly enviable results. Perhaps in reaction to the increasingly frequent publications from other clinics favoring resection and primary anastomosis, J. G. Randolph and Robert M. Zollinger, Jr., by invitation, and Robert E. Gross, of Boston, Ladd Professor of Children's Surgery, Harvard Medical School; Surgeon-in-Chief, Children's Hospital, *Mikulicz Resection in Infants and Children: A 20-Year Survey of 196 Patients*, presented their results with this technique. Citing the publications of C. D. Benson, H. W. Clatworthy, C. W. Dennis, E. W. Gerrish, and Orvar Swenson, indicating the general trend toward resection and primary anastomosis "in even the smallest of subjects", they insisted that the Mikulicz double-barrelled enterostomy was the "sounder choice of operation" in meconium ileus with the great disparity in size proximal and distal to the resected segment, in congenital intestinal obstruction with similar disparity, in intra-abdominal catastrophes requiring intestinal resection in profoundly ill children in whom the duration of the procedure was important, and in instances of doubtful viability of the intestine. Gross' specially devised pediatric spur crushing clamps were applied on the fourth or fifth day, occasionally on the day of operation. The spur was usually cut through in four to five days and the stoma subsequently closed, usually extraperitoneally, with two rows of interrupted silk. Of their 196 patients, 147 came to closure, only nine of these requiring an intraperitoneal procedure. There were 40 patients treated in this way for meconium ileus and 27 survived, while 14 died months or years later from the pulmonary complications of cystic fibrosis, "This record for relief of meconium ileus obstruction is higher than other methods reported in the literature." Of the 39 babies with intestinal atresia, 28—71% recovered. For the most part, the paper makes no comparison of any experience of their own in comparing end-to-end anastomoses with double enterostomies but they did make the statement that "For the ileal atresias, we have had a distinctly higher rate of survivals following exteriorization when compared to treatment by primary anastomosis." They had had to perform resections in 30 patients with intussusception, had performed a Mikulicz double enterostomy in all, and 26 had recovered. In 32 patients, infants with some type of neonatal catastrophe, perforation and peritonitis,- 17, more than half, survived the Mikulicz procedure. In volvulus, when the viability of the bowel was in doubt, they at times resected only the bowel that was unequivocally necrotic, performing a double enterostomy and observed the exteriorized ends. There had been 25 survivors of 38 such babies. Complications in the 196 patients were not many. The stoma retracted in six, stenosed in two and the bowel prolapsed in one. There was skin breakdown in only four, there was an intra-abdominal perforation in seven, usually from an irrigating catheter, an abdominal abscess in three, and a wound dihiscence in one. Twenty-nine patients of the 147 who survived to have the enterostomy closed, developed an intracutaneous fistula after this closure, but only five required a second operation. One patient, years later, was found to have a jejuno-colic fistula which "probably occurred when the clamp extended beyond the depth of a short spur and crushed an interposed knuckle of colon." Four patients developed a "blind loop syndrome" which responded to resection of the involved segment.

Discussion

C. E. Koop, of Philadelphia, warm in his praise, listed himself among the critics of the Mikulicz procedure, ". . . the more experience I have with infant surgery the less often I do the Mikulicz procedure." He described the procedure which Bishop and he had reported for the treatment of meconium ileus, dividing the bowel, emptying it of its inspissated contents and performing a Roux-en-Y anastomosis, bringing only a single end out through the wound for instillation of pancreatic enzymes. H. W. Clat-

worthy, of Columbus, said that he favored primary anastomosis, "The Mikulicz procedure is distasteful to most of us because it is a multi-stage procedure." He was struck by the "exceptionally good" results with meconium ileus, and seemed not to agree with the use of the Mikulicz procedure for intussusception or for atresia of the jejunum and ileum for which he advocated "a more extensive resection, removing all of the abnormal dilated bowel and either performing an end-to-end jejunojejunostomy or an end-to-side ileocecostomy" which had yielded an 80% survival in their 25 cases. Faced with bowel of doubtful viability he preferred to replace it in the abdomen, undisturbed, then to reoperate 24 hours later. In the catastrophically ill newborn with perforation, he did perform the Mikulicz procedure. Clarence Dennis, of Brooklyn [not referring to his own outstanding results with primary anastomosis in intestinal resection in children] commented on "The excellent work of Edgar Poth and Isidore Cohn with regard to what happens when broad spectrum antibiotics are placed in the intestine . . . the technic that Isidore Cohn has suggested, of putting a very fine bore polyethylene tube into the intestine and dripping in the broad spectrum antibiotic at the time the anastomosis is made has seemed to me to be a very satisfactory solution to the problem of those patients who have bowel with marginal viability."

* * *

Arthur M. Vineberg, of Montreal, in 1946 had put forth his technique of implantation of the internal mammary artery in the ventricular myocardium to stimulate collateral circulation in the relief of myocardial ischemia. The matter had not been discussed before the Association. Now Donald B. Effler, of Cleveland, Chief Thoracic Surgeon, Cleveland Clinic Foundation, and by invitation, Laurence K. Groves, F. Mason Sones, Jr., and Earl K. Shirey, *Increased Myocardial Perfusion by Internal Mammary Artery Implant:* Vineberg's Operation, reported an experience with 46 patients operated upon at the Cleveland Clinic. Vineberg had proved in dogs that the internal mammary artery, carried through a myocardial tunnel, the side branches of the artery being left open, established communications with myocardial vessels. In 1962, two of Vineberg's patients with internal mammary artery implants of five and six years' duration were studied at the Cleveland Clinic by F. Mason Sones, Jr., who had been intensively developing selective coronary arteriography. In both cases, the implanted internal mammary artery was found patent and supplementing coronary blood flow. Effler's group had performed their first

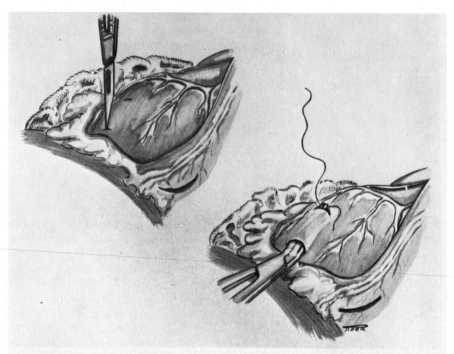

FIG. 6. Selection of the tunnel site is of utmost importance. As mentioned in the text, this will be determined by the position of the heart, the contour of the heart, and the distribution of the epicardial vessels. The tunnel is constructed in a plane that permits implantation of the artery with least chance for unfavorable angulation. The length and axis of the tunnel are designated by the two stab wounds that establish its position and limits. In the lower figure the dissecting instrument emerges from the proximal end of the tunnel to grasp the ligature affixed to the terminal *drag branch* of the artery.

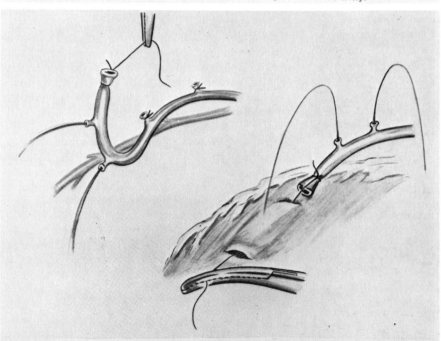

FIG. 7. The local application of papaverine upon the mobilized internal mammary artery may be impressive as the vessel is cut away from the chest wall; bleeding from the selective side branches can be forceful. The lower right-hand figure suggests the appearance of the mobilized artery and its bleeding branches as it is about to enter the proximal end of the prepared tunnel.

Effler and the group at the Cleveland Clinic had performed 46 Vineberg implants after Sones in 1962 had demonstrated in two of Vineberg's long-term patients that the mammary artery implant was patent and communicated with the coronary tree. They had had a single death. It was too soon for evaluation of the worth of the procedure. In seven patients, subsequent arteriography showed the implants patent, in two the implant was occluded.

Donald B. Effler, Laurence K. Groves, F. Mason Sones, Jr., and Earl K. Shirey, *Increased Myocardial Perfusion by Internal Mammary Artery Implant:* Vineberg's Operation, Volume LXXXI 1963.

Vineberg operation in May, 1962 and had now done 45 more such operations. All patients had preliminary coronary arteriography, were required to have clinically significant myocardial ischemia, arteriograms demonstrating predominant involvement of the anterior descending branch of the left coronary artery and not to have had a left anterior infarction. As for results, "the time factor does not permit clinical appraisal of this patient group".

Discussion

William P. Longmire, Jr., of Los Angeles, said that they had been skeptical about the operation, "not that it has not been demonstrated on a number of occasions that the vessel will remain open but skeptical in regard to the volume of blood that might be carried through this vessel and into the myocardium." He thought that the angiocardiographic demonstrations were encouraging. At UCLA, they had not employed the Vineberg procedure. In most of their 21 patients, they had performed coronary endarterectomy. In two cases, they had anastomosed the internal mammary end-to-end to the left anterior descending and in one to the right main coronary. In two instances, they had attempted to core out the coronary arteries through the root of the aorta. At the time of the meeting, 11 of the 21 patients had died, six of them at the time of operation, three postoperatively while still in the hospital, and two subsequently. Of the surviving patients, five were considered to have good results and four to be improved. Frank C. Spencer, of Lexington, Kentucky, commented on the 1957 studies of Sabiston and Blalock, that in the dog, a carotid artery implant in the wall of the left ventricle carried very little blood and was no more protective than the Beck procedure for producing pericardial adhesions. In 16 dogs, under cardiopulmonary bypass, operating upon a still heart with microsurgical techniques, he had anastomosed the internal mammary to the coronary artery. Fifteen of 16 dogs had patent anastomoses at five months, though to normal coronary arteries, true enough. Effler, closing, emphasized that this was a preliminary report "We are enthusiastic; we believe we have reason to be enthusiastic. But many of the things we say now may be obsolete or drastically changed a year from now." He stressed the importance of postoperative angiograms, and the unreliability of the relief of subjective symptoms such as angina.

* * *

The first discussion of a membrane oxygenator before the Association, *A New Method of Oxygena-* *tion:* A Study of Its Use in Respiratory Support and the Artificial Placenta, was by E. A. Maynes and J. C. Callaghan, both by invitation, from the University of Alberta, Edmonton, Canada. The presently employed oxygenators did not permit prolonged perfusion "due to blood damage and due to the possible toxicity of some of the plastics used in the circuitry . . . The more physiological approach seemed to be to attempt to utilize a blood-membrane-blood barrier similar to that found in the mammalian placenta . . . blood flowing on one side of a membrane could act as recipient or *fetal* blood, and that blood flowing on the opposite side of the membrane could act as vehicle or *maternal* blood." Of course, unlike the placenta, the membrane would be inert. In vitro tests with cellophane, polythene, Saran, Silastic, and Teflon demonstrated "Significant transmission of respiratory gases . . . only with 1/8 mil Teflon" testing it with out-of-date bank blood. They had tried both venovenous and arteriovenous perfusion of the dogs. They were able to carry out perfusions up to three-and-half hours using a single sheet of the membrane. In the first hour the plasma hemoglobin increased but not thereafter. There was no effect upon the thrombocytes or the white cells. Oxygenator blood flowed in a continuous stream on either side of a membrane sandwich and the recipient's blood flowed in the middle of the sandwich. They were able to increase the oxygen tension and decrease the carbon dioxide tension in the asphyxiated subject dog. Although ". . . a degree of respiratory support did occur", from subsequent experiments, "it was apparent that an impractical membrane area would be required to give appreciable respiratory support in this manner with existing membranes . . . Utilizing multiple membranes this form of oxygenation may ultimately permit the assumption of some of the other known functions of the placenta."

Discussion

Herbert Sloan, of Ann Arbor, emphasized the need for long-term oxygenation, "Every year there are thousands of infants delivered into this world who are just not ready to face life. They may be premature; they may have respiratory distress; they may have severe cardiac disease. If we can find some means of supporting these infants during these first hours after delivery we may be able to save a larger number of them. The artificial placenta technic which is being described today, or hyperbaric oxygenation, or a combination of these technics, may finally provide the solution to this problem. We heard yesterday that hyperbaric oxygenation is not without its difficulties."

* * *

J. Alex Haller, Jr., Assistant Professor of Surgery, and Berel L. Abrams, both by invitation, from the University of Louisville School of Medicine, Louisville, Kentucky, *Use of Thrombectomy in the Treatment of Acute Iliofemoral Venous Thrombosis in Forty-Five Patients,* referred to Howard Mahorner's presentation, at the 1957 meeting, of thrombectomy for acute and chronic venous occlusion of the lower extremities, a procedure which Haller said "had lain dormant since its initial trials by Leriche in 1928." Over a period of three years they performed thrombectomy in 45 patients with a diagnosis of acute ileofemoral venous occlusion. Diagnosis was suggested clinically by "massive edema of the leg from toe to groin, with tenderness along the femoral canal" and in 17 of the patients, confirmed preoperatively by phlebography. Operation was performed under local anesthesia with the venous tributaries isolated, taped, the patients heparinized once the clot was identified, clot cleared proximally and distally until there was free flow from both ends, the vessel and the wound carefully closed. Extraction of the clot was easiest in the patients with thrombosis of the shortest duration. Twenty-six of 34 patients with thrombosis of less than ten days duration had apparently normal veins and five had only slight to moderate disability. Poor flow was obtained after thrombectomy in three of the 34 patients and two of them had residual edema and moderate disability. Phlebograms in 13 of the 26 patients with clinically normal limbs showed a normal patency of the deep venous system in 11 and major venous obstruction with extensive collateral circulation in two. Venograms in three patients with residual edema and disability were normal. The procedure proved to be technically difficult in the patients with thrombosis of 14 to 21 days duration and in them the thrombosis could not be completely removed, and satisfactory bi-directional flow was reconstituted in none. Two of these patients died with thrombosis of the inferior vena cava, one required an above the knee amputation, one had a crippled postphlebitic limb, and one had only slight edema, no disability. The two patients who had fatal vena cava thrombosis had had true phlegmasia cerulea dolens,- the only examples in the entire series. Haller's optimistic conclusion was that "Our data strongly suggests that immediate thrombectomy in the acute stage of iliofemoral thrombosis can be expected to remove practically all of the occluding clot and to re-establish a normal deep venous circulation in the majority of patients."

Discussion

Robert R. Linton, of Boston, congratulating Haller on his results said however "I do not entirely agree with him on all counts." Linton was seeing less massive venous thrombosis than "25 years ago when we started doing femoral interruptions and thrombectomy for femoral iliac thrombosis. As you probably know, we surgeons at the Massachusetts General Hospital have performed this operative procedure on several thousands of extremities, a sizable experience. And yet I am glad to say that we have not witnessed the predicted postligation chronic ulcer of the lower extremity to be called 'the Massachusetts General Hospital type.'" His point was that "post-thrombotic ulcers develop because of canalization of a previously thrombosed femoral vein rather than because the femoral vein is occluded or interrupted." He was not sure that the restoration of venous continuity was the ideal method of therapy "because of the danger of recurrent thrombophlebitis and secondary pulmonary embolism". Linton insisted on the importance of wearing an elastic stocking for a prolonged period after venous interruption. He was "in whole-hearted agreement, however with Dr. Haller that thrombectomy is extremely important in the treatment of phlegmasia alba dolens and of utmost importance in the treatment of phlegmasia cerulea dolens, in order to open up the collateral venous channels, especially the large branches of the femoral vein in the femoral triangle, including the profunda femoris" which was easily done and left clean and smooth venous endothelium if undertaken within the first 48 hours after the leg had swollen to the groin. For venous thrombosis of the deep veins of the calf [a condition which Haller had not been discussing, of course] "I still believe the best treatment . . . is femoral vein interruption with anticoagulant therapy for a few days postligation; early ambulation; and later adequate elastic support. Once the venous interruption is accomplished, pulmonary embolism need not be feared in future years if venous thrombosis develops again in the leg." He was disturbed that there were so many cases for operation in Louisville, and feared that that meant that "both physicians and surgeons in his community need education in the prophylaxis and early diagnosis of deep venous thrombosis." Prevention was more important than treatment. Have the head of the bed elevated, the patient being provided with arm pulls to lift himself up and about, and a foot board at the foot of the bed so the patients push against it "at least a thousand times a day to contract the gastrocnemius and soleus muscles, and thereby prevent stagnation of blood in the deep veins in this area where deep venous thrombosis most commonly originates and from there extends up into the popliteal, femoral, and iliac veins." Harris B. Shumacker, Jr., of Indianapolis, had operated only upon patients with phlegmasia cerulea dolens, ". . . because in our hands the nonoperative management of acute iliofemoral phlegmasia alba dolens has been attended with very small risk and with very good ultimate functional results, and because we were not sure about the risks involved with thrombectomy." Patients with phlegmasia cerulea dolens, he operated upon under general anesthesia, exposed the iliac vein extraperitoneally and the femoral vein in the groin, always finding a residual clot in the iliac vein after a complete femoral thrombectomy. His patients [number not specified] "have survived and all have had excellent functional results." He was encouraged by Haller's results to think that he might consider operation now for phlegmasia alba dolens. Frank C. Spencer, of Lexington, Kentucky, had been interested in the procedure ever since Mahorner's presentation. He was impressed by Haller's excellent results but concerned about the danger of producing pulmonary emboli during the procedure, even though Haller had the patients strain during the embolectomy. Angus D. McLachlin, of London, Ontario, agreed with Haller and said that he believed that "the patients in Dr. Haller's series with no sequellae had essentially floating thrombi that were removed before there had been significant damage in the vein wall." In the thrombosed femoral vein of the dog, spontaneous fibrinolysis and recanalization occurred rapidly, leaving the vein open but the valves destroyed. They had been experimenting with transplantation of autogenous vein segments with normal valves. Howard Mahorner, of New Orleans, said that his results were much like Haller's,- ". . . 60 per cent of patients have a perfect or excellent result. Another 30 per cent will have great improvement, and 10 per cent will have failures, and these results will be correlated with the time from onset at which the patient is operated upon." The earlier after onset the operation was undertaken, the better the results. He thought one could still obtain dramatic improvement in the patients operated upon up to four to six weeks after the onset of thrombosis. He alluded, not very obliquely, to Linton's remarks, "It amazes me how surgeons who are really sincerely looking for the truth and trying to make the right decision as to what is the best to do for the patients, sometimes come to directly opposite conclusions. Our experience in the longstanding cases with post-thrombophlebitic edema is that if you ligate the vein you make them worse—always!" Haller, closing, said to Linton they had been primarily concerned with the prevention of the post-phlebitic state rather than with the possibility of later pulmonary embolism. He agreed with Mahorner, ". . . that interruption can not return the deep venous system to its normal function (although it certainly will prevent embolization). The thrombus material contained within the veins becomes organized, and if the vein reopens it is no longer a competent system because the valves are incorporated in this organized material and are no longer functional."

* * *

William A. Altemeier, [the Secretary], of Cincinnati, Christian R. Holmes Professor of Surgery, University of Cincinnati, and Joseph Todd, by invitation, *Studies on the Incidence of Infection following Open Chest Cardiac Massage for Cardiac Arrest*, reviewing the material in seven Cincinnati hospitals had found 43 patients who had survived open chest cardiac massage for at least 72 hours. So far as the overall results were concerned, 32 of the 43 patients, 74%, survived and were discharged from the hospital. Ten patients had died in the first two weeks, all of them with severe central nervous system damage and an additional patient died of pulmonary embolus on the eighth day. One patient died on the 21st postoperative day. There were only two wound infections in the entire group of 43 cases. "In both instances the wounds had been closed in layers with catgut, the four wounds closed with silk healing per primam." The current incidence around the country of postoperative infection in clean elective operations was considered to be 1 to 5% and in wounds associated with trauma, 8 to 26%. Altemeier considered that "The local circumstances for wound sepsis should have been unusually good . . . Since these wounds were made in the hospital environment, contamination by virulent and antibiotic resistant bacteria in the hospital reservoir was almost inevitable. Moreover, in some of the patients, bacteria were transferred to the thoracotomy wounds from areas of established and severe infections such as peritonitis." In addition to which, many of the patients had other profound diseases, diabetes, leukemia, far advanced malignancy, debility, etc. In the pre-Listerian era, "patients in civilian hospitals almost never recovered uneventfully from operations or open trauma. Surgeons in large hospitals seldom saw a wound heal by first intention and without inflammation or suppuration . . . The kindly healing of all but two of the 43 wounds in our series without cellulitis, suppuration, or even stitch abscesses, was thus considered to be most striking and intriguing." Most of the patients were receiving antibiotics, but one patient who received no antibiotic therapy healed his wound per primam and without inflammation. A review of the literature on cardiac arrest also suggested that post-operative wound infection was an infrequent complication. [Altemeier's published paper makes no suggestion as to his explanation.]

Discussion

William P. Longmire, of Los Angeles, commented that Stephenson's review of 1700 cases showed a very low incidence of infection. At UCLA, they had had ten open cardiac resuscitations, performed under unsterile conditions somewhere in the hospital, and surviving long enough to assess the outcome in the wound. Nine of the patients had primary healing; one patient, a severe diabetic under heavy steroid therapy, developed a staphylococcal wound infection. Longmire mentioned that the amount of devitalized tissue in the wound, the amount of foreign body, the duration of trauma might be the important factors. Jonathan E. Rhoads, of Philadelphia, indicated en passant, that he had not been quite persuaded of the virtues of closed chest cardiac compression,- "The surgeons caring for these patients are to be congratulated, I think, on the high percentage salvaged in the overall group. One wonders if it could have been fully achieved by the closed method", but offered no suggestion as to the cause for the low incidence of infections. Truman G. Blocker, Jr., of Galveston, thought that since most of the cases had been done in the operating room, there might have been a considerable degree of cleanliness, but like Rhoads, thought it was time to review every facet of what was now considered to be essential in sterile technique. Henry T. Bahnson, of Baltimore, said "Many of the thoughts I had used to explain the low incidence of infection in similar cases we have seen such as the fact that there is a lot of cutting and not much tying; that the operation is of short duration and there is not much trauma of lights and exposure, coexisting shock and so forth . . . have been carefully considered in the manuscript and in no instance did they seem to be of significant importance." William R. Sandusky, of Charlottesville, pointed out that in a study of 110 war wounds he had made, "24 per cent yielded pathogenic clostridia, yet only three cases of

gas gangrene ensued", emphasized the importance of even a sterile foreign body in a wound. He seemed to suggest that perhaps these patients had had less suture material implanted. J. E. Dunphy, of Portland, in agreement with Bahnson, quoted Mont Reid ". . . who was Dr. Altemeier's distinguished predecessor at Cincinnati . . . 'It is questionable if bacteria assume a role of greater importance in wound healing than do necrosis, debris and devitalized tissue . . .' " and went on to say that the infection rate in this group was, in fact, 5%, whereas, at the Cincinnati Clinic for clean operations it was 0.8% ". . . and if Dr. Altemeier were to have this rate in operations for hernia or thyroid he would be gravely concerned. The real feature here, and the best stimulus to normal repair and avoidance of infection, is what is called the clean sweep of a cold knife." David V. Habif, of New York, agreed that the infection rate at the Presbyterian Hospital in New York overall was between 1 or 2%, for thoracotomy wounds was 0.5%, and suggested that the infection rate in Altemeier's cardiac massage series was "10 times that which would be expected in a clean thoracotomy wound performed in the operating room". Altemeier, closing, said that, in fact, six of his patients were closed with silk so that foreign body seemed not to have been important. Dunphy had emphasized the atraumatic type of incision made and Altemeier agreed but still with hand massaging the heart sometimes for 45 minutes, he could not understand why infection did not occur more often.

* * *

David M. Hume, of Richmond, Professor of Surgery, Chairman of the Department, Medical College of Virginia, and by invitation, Joseph H. Magee, H. Myron Kauffman, Jr., Max S. Rittenbury, and George R. Prout, Jr., *Renal Hemotransplantation in Man in Modified Recipients,* presented his results in six patients receiving non-twin kidneys,- from a cadaver donor, three siblings, two parents. Two Rh— patients received kidneys from Rh+ donors and one group A recipient received a kidney from an O donor. The first four patients had been treated with total body irradiation, and subsequently with prednisone and Imuran "after the period of aplasia". The last two patients had been treated with a series of irradiation treatments to the transplanted kidney and with prednisone and Imuran. Hume performed bilateral nephrectomy before transplantation. In dogs, irradiation of the kidney could, alone, produce prolonged renal homograft survival. Rejection, marked by fever, swelling, and tenderness in the region of the transplant, decreased urinary output, rising BUN, leukocytosis and a positive needle biopsy, was reversed by treatment with actinomycin C and increasing the doses of Imuran and prednisone. Four of the six patients were alive at the time of the report and were still alive at the time Hume added an Addendum, when correcting the galleys. Hume's final sentence was that "Renal homotransplantation in man is showing signs of coming of age, but is still a highly experimental procedure with an uncertain ultimate outcome."

Discussion

Joseph E. Murray, of Boston, initiated the Discussion. They had now had over 60 human kidney transplants at the Peter Bent Brigham Hospital, 26 of them in modified recipients, 12 of those modified by total body irradiation and 14 by drug therapy alone. Four of the first 10 drug-treated patients had good renal function. William R. Waddell, of Denver, spoke of "the experience of the University of Colorado group, particularly that of Dr. Thomas Starzl." They had done seven renal transplant patients, six of them homotransplantations. Like Hume's patients, they had ignored blood groups and A kidneys had functioned well in O recipients, and B kidneys in A recipients, etc. He agreed that bilateral nephrectomy before transplantation was worthwhile. Five of the six patients had had a preliminary thymectomy and splenectomy. One of their patients had had a severe rejection crisis reversed by "Actinomycin C, heavy doses of Prednisone, Imuran . . ." One of their patients had had a "massive pulmonary embolus. It was necessary to resuscitate him by external cardiac massage and he underwent a Trendelenburg procedure on Wednesday afternoon with removal of a massive clot from his pulmonary artery. As of last reports by courtesy of the Bell Telephone system he has come through that satisfactorily and his kidney has continued to function . . ." Willard E. Goodwin, of Los Angeles, reported nine human renal homotransplantations from UCLA with a single long-term success in identical twins. J. Hartwell Harrison, of Boston, said he had worked with Hume, with Murray, and with Goodwin, on the problem. He emphasized the medico-legal problems involved with donors who were minors and for that matter with donors who were adults, since the only "benefit" to the donor would have to be considered to be psychologic. Among the purely urologic problems of the operation were several associated with suppuration. They had had to reimplant the ureter in five of their twin patients. Hume, closing, agreed with Murray that "the best modality we have at the moment

for the treatment of the patient undergoing renal homotransplantation is Imuran." On the other hand, survivals were not yet as numerous as they should be. It was a potent drug and that was why they were experimenting with irradiation of the kidney to kill the recipient cells bringing antibodies into the kidney to attack it. As for donors mismatched with respect to blood group, he knew of 18 thus far in the world, and six such kidneys had functioned.

The Business Meetings

The 1963 meeting was held April 3, 4, and 5, at the Hotel Westward Ho, Phoenix, Arizona, President Oliver Cope in the Chair.

Secretary Altemeier reported that "At the Council meeting on January 26 there was considerable discussion regarding the advisability of inviting wives of the members to the reception and the banquet. This is a recurrent discussion, as you all know, but after prolonged deliberation Council has recommended that the wives be included this year at the Annual Reception and Banquet. With your indulgence, the Committee on Local Arrangements was instructed to proceed with the arrangements on that basis, including the wives and the members for the Annual Reception and Banquet on Thursday evening. At the meeting on Friday this matter will come up for additional discussion in relation to any further continuation of the policy. Council also recommended at the meeting on January 26 that the membership of this organization be increased in the *Active* category from 250 to 300, yearly increments to be made at the rate of not more than 10 per year. A resolution will be necessary to activate this recommendation, and it will be held over for one year, at which time it will be voted upon." [Each previous increase in the membership has been preceded by years of resolutions and motions proposed, held over, and defeated, and it was obvious that on this occasion, the proponents of the increase were either working successfully through the Council or were members of the Council. The initiative this time had originated with Dunphy in his 1962 Presidential Address and he was now on the Council as the Presidents regularly were the year following incumbency.]

The subject of animal experimentation and Federal regulation was discussed at length once more.

Dunphy now formally introduced the motion to implement the recommendation of Council in respect to membership, increasing the Active membership to a maximum of 300 Fellows and not changing the Honorary membership limit of 25 Fellows.

Dr. Frederick Kergin, of Toronto, Chairman of the Advisory Committee on Membership, reported that they had that year considered 38 candidates for the first time, 20 for the second time, and 18 for the third time, "In relationship to the thousands of fully qualified representatives of the various surgical specialties in the United States and Canada, an active membership of 250 Fellows in the Association is very small."

At the Second Executive Session again there was a written ballot for the matter of the ladies' attendance at dinner, President Cope stating "Now, about the ladies. Dr. Sam Wilson Moore [never known to anyone, but apparently the President, as anything but Bill Moore] just came to the platform and reminded me that three years ago he was a Teller when a similar ballot to invite the ladies was voted upon favorably by the membership. By some parliamentary ruling, however, the motion was tabled. It was with this recurrent problem that Council had had to deal, and that is the reason that you have the vote before you again this morning. It was also, of course, stimulated by President Eisenhower's feelings last year." [Eisenhower had been President Dunphy's choice as the dinner speaker. He had insisted that the ladies be brought into the room for his talk.] Dr. Shumacker spoke in favor of the proposal "I think we have had a nice clinical experiment last night which proved without doubt that we lost nothing in the dignity of our annual banquet and gained a great deal in beauty." Dunphy spoke in his inimitable style "I hope I won't be misunderstood. I am terribly fond of women, and I love my wife, but I do think that there are occasions when it is extremely desirable to sit down at a banquet being able to talk with your colleagues in an association of this sort. My most cherished memories are of sitting at a round table in the presence of men like Fred Coller, Alfred Blalock, Bill Wilson, Mark Ravitch, etc. [Since there had *never* been a Bill Wilson in the Association, the group is perhaps not as illustrious as it sounds!] This is the way that I think we acquire something which we will miss if we bring the ladies to the annual banquet. It dilutes the intellectual exchange among men. I have nothing against the ladies. I had a delightful time talking about the number of children I had, where they go to school, and other interesting things. But there is a hard core of conversation that I think once, one day out of 365, the leading surgeons in the world today can give to each other. I am sure we will miss something if we don't continue. If we want to have the ladies, we can have them on Wednesday night. I think it is abominable to bring them to cocktails and send them out,

as we have in former years. We could leave Thursday night open for the ladies and let them do what they pleased to do. Most of them have a very good time when they are left to themselves. They just don't want to come to this cocktail party and be all dressed up and then sent away. On occasion, perhaps at the request of Council or the request of the President because of a particular speaker, I think they could be invited to attend the banquet, but I think if we make this a regular occurrence, we will lose something which we need." No other speakers were recorded. On this occasion there were 135 "Yes" votes and 55 "No" votes. President Cope said "I don't suppose we are going to come anywhere nearer. I can tell you that a great many people during the course of the year, stimulated by President Eisenhower, came to me individually about this matter, I don't know just how we can reconcile it differently than by the democratic process of abiding by the vote. At least next year I presume the ladies will again be invited, and I hope that in other ways, Dr. Dunphy, we can provide equally for those issues which you presented so well to us. For the moment this issue is closed."

A resolution was adopted calling upon the American Medical Association, the American Veterinary Association, the American Hospital Association, the American College of Surgeons, and other organizations to require that the inspection of animal laboratories be an integral part of the accreditation procedure, obviously an attempt to forestall Congressional action. At the same time, another strong resolution was sent to Congress decrying restrictive regulations on animal experimentation. Once more the proposal was made, this time by Dr. Donald Glover, that the American Surgical Association look into undergraduate surgical education. Secretary Altemeier said that there had been such a resolution on the books since 1958.

Among the new members were George Henry Clowes, Jr., Richard H. Egdahl, Keith Reemtsma, Paul S. Russell, and W. Dean Warren.

Dr. Dunphy proposed a motion for a change in the Constitution to add to the President, two Vice-Presidents, Secretary, Treasurer, and Recorder another officer, a President-Elect. This was to lie over for a year.

New Officers were, President, Warfield M. Firor, of Baltimore, who had been Vice-President in 1951; Vice-Presidents, Rudolph Noer, of Louisville, Kentucky, and Virgil S. Counseller, of Phoenix, Arizona, where he had retired from the Mayo Clinic; and Secretary, William A. Altemeier, of Cincinnati.

LXXXII

1964

The 1964 meeting was held at The Homestead, Hot Springs, Virginia, April 1, 2, and 3, Warfield M. Firor, of Baltimore, Professor Emeritus of Surgery, Johns Hopkins University, who had been Secretary from 1943 through 1948, and Vice-President in 1951, in the Chair. The preceding year had seen the deaths of three Fellows whose names had long been eponymically employed,—Harry H. Kerr, of Washington, of the Parker-Kerr stitch; Joe Vincent Meigs, of Boston, of the ovarian fibroma-ascites syndrome; and Allen O. Whipple, of the Whipple triad, and the Whipple operation for carcinoma of the pancreas, whose spleen clinic at Presbyterian Hospital in New York led the clinical thrust against the problem of portal hypertension. He had been President in 1940. Donald C. Balfour, Vice-President in 1923, had also died.

* * *

The scientific papers opened with two presentations on pacemakers, William W. L. Glenn, of New Haven, Professor of Surgery, Yale University School of Medicine, and by invitation, J. H. Hageman, A. Mauro, L. Eisenberg, S. Flanigan, and M. Harvard, *Electrical Stimulation of Excitable Tissue by Radio-Frequency Transmission,* discussed the cardiac pacemaker, phrenic nerve stimulation, and detrusor stimulation of the bladder. Verzeano and others in 1958 had reported radio-frequency stimulation of the dog heart, and in that year Glenn and Mauro had begun their studies of the problem. They had progressively developed the technique of implanting two electrodes of a cobalt-nickel alloy,- Elgiloy,- into the myocardium, connecting the Silastic rubber covered extracardiac portion of the wires to a receiving coil under the skin. The radio-frequency transmitter, glued to the skin over the receiving coil, connected to the power pack which the patient carried. Wire fatigue and breakage were a problem and the life of their antenna was three months "When the antenna fails, it is exchanged for a new one. A recent modification in antenna design may prolong the useful life, but as a practical matter it is wiser to have a second antenna on hand." The batteries for the pacemaker had originally had a life of only five to ten days, but with the newest model, a life of two months. They were anticipating a battery pack with a life of at least ten months. Their first application, in a patient with ". . . uncontrollable Stokes-Adams attacks . . ." was on January 27, 1958, and since then they had implanted pacemakers in 21 additional patients with complete heart block and Stokes-Adams attacks. In two of the patients ". . . both children, the heart block was surgically induced . . ." Eleven of the patients were alive, having been paced continuously for from four to 33 months. Ten patients were dead. One patient was alive and no longer required pacing. In three of the dead patients, ". . . the electrode wire broke, the patients refused reoperation and died in Stokes-Adams attacks." Four patients died suddenly with the pacemaker in place. Stimulation of the phrenic nerve for respiration had been initiated by Sarnoff in 1948, using both a percutaneous electrode and remote control by an induction

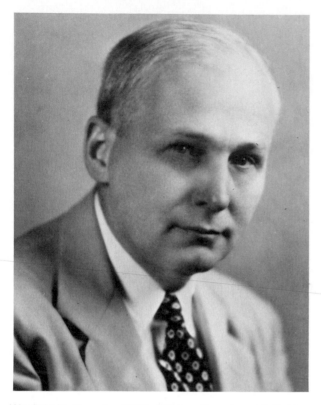

Warfield M. Firor, (c. 1950) 1896—, Secretary 1943-48, Vice-President 1951, President 1964. M.D. Johns Hopkins 1921. Began residency 1921 under Halsted, completed 1929 under Dean D. Lewis. Associate Professor of Surgery 1929-1960, Professor of Surgery 1960-1962. Acting Chairman, Department of Surgery 1939-1941. Inspiring teacher, imaginative investigator, in animals hypophysectomized by the technique he devised, he demonstrated the pituitary control of ovulation. Introduced intestinal antisepsis (sulfanilylguanidine) in bowel surgery. In the early days of the American Board of Surgery, instituted the residency review system. Upheld the Halstedian tradition at Hopkins and did much to restore the Department there during the 1938-1941 interregnum.

(Portrait courtesy of J. W. Humphreys, Jr., M.D., American Board of Surgery)

coil as well as a purely external stimulator. Glenn's group had developed a portable, transistorized, radio-frequency electrophrenic respirator, functioning on the same principle as the cardiac pacemaker but had not yet applied it clinically. In their laboratory, radio-frequency stimulation of the bladder of a paraplegic dog effectively emptied the bladder, as well when the electrode was applied to the bladder as when it was applied to the peripheral end of the divided sacral roots. They said no more of this than that further investigation was warranted.

* * *

Paul M. Zoll, by invitation, Howard A. Frank, of Boston, Assistant Professor of Surgery and Tutor in Surgery, Harvard Medical School; Chief of Thoracic Surgical Clinic, Beth Israel Hospital, and by invitation, Arthur J. Linenthal, *Four-Year Experience with an Implanted Cardiac Pacemaker,* referring to their publications beginning in 1961, the publication of Kantrowitz and others in 1962, and of Chardack and others in 1961, now reported their own experience of 77 patients with heart block and Stokes-Adams attacks since July 1960. Like Glenn they emphasized the initial difficulties with ". . . tissue reaction to the foreign body [the electrode], which in effect separates the electrode from excitable myocardium." A nonreactive platinum electrode surface had eliminated that problem. They had originally used platinum electrodes welded to multistrand stainless steel wire covered with Teflon, and now were using ". . . multistranded stainless steel wires . . . electroplated alternately with gold and platinum . . . then insulated with Teflon, except for a 1-cm. bare segment to form the active electrode." The pacemaker contained six mercury batteries, 1.4 volts each ". . . with an expected operating life span of 5 years." Since June 1961, with the most recent design, the pacemaker had functioned perfectly in 54 out of 55 patients, the longest for 30 months, "The methods of subcutaneous replacement of a pacemaker unit with attachment by crimp connectors to the orginal electrode wire have proved to be simple and effective." It was also possible to use batteries rechargeable percutaneously [as reported by Siddons and O'N. Humphries 1961]. The radio-frequency techniques required much smaller implanted components and battery replacement was effortless, but ". . . either the external source must be in close apposition to the subcutaneous unit or the external battery must be large. In either case, an ordinary bath or shower, for example, is difficult. Furthermore, preoccupation with the equipment creates a psychologic hindrance to normal activity." The patients of the Beth Israel groups ". . . with a fixed rate of 70 to 75 per minute can carry out normal activity, exercise, and other stresses without difficulty." The attempts of a number of investigators to conduct the atrial impulses by wires to the ventricle seemed to them to increase the complexity of the device unnecessarily. Implantation of the pacemaker was not problem-free, "Most of our patients have had ventricular standstill or fibrillation during the procedures. Adequate control requires continuous observation and readiness to stimulate, to countershock, to carry out cardiac massage, and to adminis-

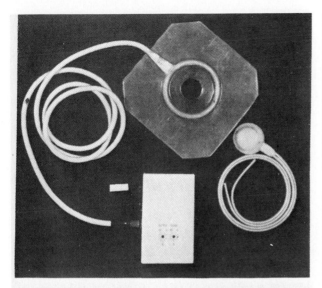

FIG. 3. The R-F cardiac pacemaker unit consisting of a transmitter which broadcasts a one millisecond impulse via the transmitting antenna coil. In use, the antenna patch is cemented to the patient's skin over the receiving coil, which is implanted subcutaneously. The attached electrode wires conduct the impulse to the heart.

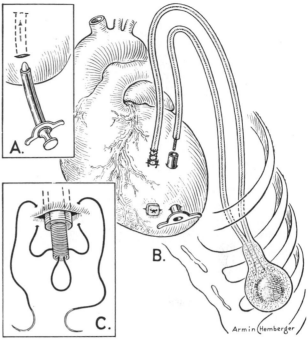

FIG. 4. Method of inserting electrodes into the myocardium.

Glenn's electrodes of a cobalt-nickel alloy were placed in a myocardial tunnel made with the aid of a tracheostomy tube used as a trocar and cannula. The Silastic-covered wires led to the Silastic-covered receiving coil which was implanted subcutaneously. The transmitting antenna coil was glued to the skin with cement and the patient carried the battery pack. They had employed the technique in 22 patients since January 1958. "Generally the antenna becomes loose after ten days to two weeks and must be removed completely from the skin with an appropriate solvent . . . An occasional patient develops asystole when the antenna is lifted off the skin."

W. W. L. Glenn, J. H. Hageman, A. Mauro, L. Eisenberg, S. Flanigan, and M. Harvard, *Electrical Stimulation of Excitable Tissue by Radio-Frequency Transmission.* Volume LXXXII, 1964.

ter dilute solutions of isoproterenol or epinephrine intravenously." They had used catheter electrodes in 13 patients ". . . to determine the usefulness of a pacemaker for the particular patient and its optimal rate, and to control cardiac action during necessary delays in surgery when drugs were unsatisfactory." They had perforated the heart in one patient, had intermittently ineffective stimulation in three—one of whom died—had staphylococcal septicemia in two, and clots on the catheter tips in two. The pacemaker unit, encased in Teflon mesh, was placed in "the retropectoral site". The left ventricle was broadly exposed, the wires passed through the myocardium with the attached needles, the needles cut away, the wires turned back, and sutured to the heart. Of their 77 patients, 71 had Stokes-Adams disease, five had congestive heart failure, one had angina pectoris, and all but one had an A-V block. None of the blocks had been surgically produced.

Twenty-nine of the 77 patients required more than one operation, and the entire system had been replaced 22 times in 17 patients, most of the secondary procedures being required by ". . . pacemaker failure, wire break, or sepsis, nearly all in the early phase of the program." The longest period of treatment thus far had been 40 months. One patient had died of respiratory failure in the postoperative period, and there had been 16 late deaths of which eight had been sudden and presumably were due to cardiac arrhythmia, only one due to broken wire and ineffective stimulation. They were able to say that "Our implanted, fixed-rate pacemaker has eliminated Stokes-Adams attacks due to ventricular standstill and has also largely prevented seizures due to ventricular tachycardia or fibrillation . . . improving congestive heart failure and other manifestations of diminished cardiac output in patients with heart block and slow ventricular rates." Even a sin-

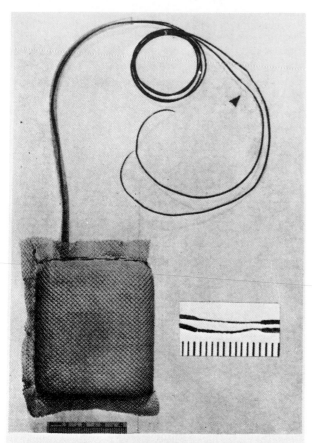

FIG. 1. The cardiac pacemaker-electrode system includes the pacemaker unit, the Teflon bag, 2 electrode wires, a length of Silastic tubing enclosing the proximal 6 inches of the wires, the bare electrode segments (*arrow* and *insert*), and needles at the ends of the wires.

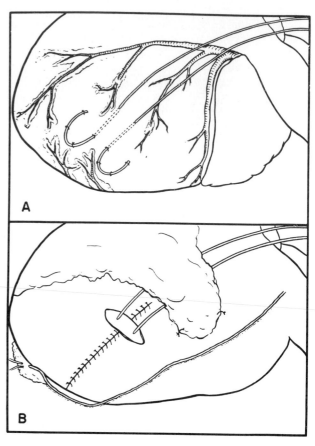

FIG. 3. Diagram of electrode implantation. A. The implantation tunnels are aligned toward the obtuse margin of the heart and the wires toward the base; the needles have been cut away and the distal wires turned back; all fixing sutures are distal to the tunnels. B. The pericardium is closed leaving an aperture about the wires; the wires are not sutured to the pericardium but are held in course by a flap of extrapericardial fat; the phrenic nerve has been displaced posteriorly.

Zoll's totally implantable cardiac pacemaker. The 77-strand steel wires were electroplated at the electrode end alternately with gold and platinum.

Paul M. Zoll, Howard A. Frank, and Arthur J. Linenthal, *Four-Year Experience with an Implanted Cardiac Pacemaker.* Volume LXXXII, 1964.

gle mild Stokes-Adams episode was an indication for insertion of a pacemaker. On the other hand, "we do not consider heart block alone in an asymptomatic patient to be an indication for treatment."

Discussion

Elliott S. Hurwitt, of New York, said that "Dr. Glenn's system has the unquestioned advantage of being adjustable to demand, including discontinua-

tion as indicated", and he agreed that application to the diaphragm, bladder, and bowel might well follow. Hurwitt mentioned the work in his department, "The first clinical application of the intravenously inserted intracardiac catheter pacemaker was carried out by Dr. Seymour Furman at the Montefiore Hospital in New York City on July 16, 1958. While still an assistant resident in surgery, he had the rewarding experience of developing a principle in the experimental laboratory and carrying it through to a successful clinical conclusion." Eighty-two patients with severe heart block had been managed in that way at the Montefiore Hospital of New York, and "While our group does not advocate the catheter for long-term stimulation, two patients have been managed this way for four years and three for three years . . . We believe the catheter pacemaker is the method of choice for initial treatment of the patient awaiting implantation of a permanent pacemaker, and for controlling the patient during anesthesia and operation." Frank C. Spencer, of Lexington, Kentucky, had used the pacemaker, which H. Frank had described, chiefly in ". . . elderly patients in refractory cardiac failure." He demonstrated the improvement in cardiac output in several patients with increased cardiac rate settings of the pacemaker up to a rate of 70 per minute, and endorsed ". . . what Dr. Hurwitt mentioned—that the catheter electrode is a superb method of preoperative management . . . preoperative pacing with a catheter electrode for two to three days may produce a diuresis of 2 to 4 L. of fluid . . . In addition, the risk of induction of anesthesia is greatly minimized by electrically controlling the cardiac rate." Sam E. Stephenson, Jr., of Nashville, had been experimenting with transmission of the atrial electrical impulse to the ventricle-, which Frank had decried-, and while ". . . this is a much more complicated gadget, it is still of the same relative size, and does function satisfactorily. We have had very little in the line of mechanical problems. We also have multiple problems with wire breakage." Benson B. Roe, of San Francisco, endorsed Frank's remarks on the basis of 35 clinical applications. He emphasized meticulous handling of the wires to avoid subsequent breakage. For the preoperative management of the patient ". . . we have introduced percutaneously through the chest wall a single myocardial electrode . . . a Teflon-coated stainless steel wire which is coiled in the form of a safety pin, to create a barb and is introduced through a No. 18 needle . . . does not interfere with the implantation of the permanent pacemaker and gives very satisfactory control during the investing period." Karl E. Karlson, of Brooklyn, also had found the endocardial pacemaker useful in the preoperative period before implantation of the permanent pacemaker, and had employed it in 54 patients. Patients with Stokes-Adams attacks ". . . uncontrolled with drugs or associated with myocardial infarction, shock, congestive heart failure, or azotemia . . ." had been treated with endocardial pacing first and had a 33% mortality in the first ten days. Subsequent permanent pacemaker implantation in the survivors carried a 15% mortality following implanta-

tion ". . . the same as that of pacemaker implantation in our group of patients who had endocardial pacemakers inserted only while they were being operated upon." He suggested that ". . . those patients who do not improve sufficiently with endocardial pacing to warrant intrathoracic pacemaker implantation might well be treated by continued endocardial pacemaking with subcutaneous implantation of the battery box." In dogs the best place for insertion of the electrodes was at the apex of the left ventricle, and the second best place at the apex of the right ventricle. W. W. L. Glenn, in closing, agreed with the value of temporary control of the heart with a catheter electrode. He repeated the advantages of the radio-frequency pacemaker, "It always controls the rate, duration, and amplitude of the impulse, and, of course, of the power source. This may prove to be of real advantage as time goes on." Electrolysis played an important part in failure in both systems. He questioned whether the complexity of Stephenson's apparatus was justified by the advantage of using the heart's own atrial impulse. Howard A. Frank, in closing, agreed with Spencer that there was an optimum cardiac rate, "We never set our rate below 70 . . ." They had used the intracardiac catheter ". . . but in our hands . . . less safe than Isuprel, given intravenously." There were obvious objections to placing the energy source inside, or outside, the body and time would have to tell which was best. The external source was subject to displacement and interruption and the patient never lost ". . . awareness of the fact that his heart is under artificial control." The capacity to vary the rate had ". . . certain desirable aspects, but it is not essential", and until the apparatus had been demonstrated to be completely reliable, the Beth Israel group did not believe ". . . that we have any right to add the complexity which is inherent in the variable rate systems."

* * *

Fifteen years before the technique was to be found useful clinically, [Starzl, Volume XCVII, 1979] Allan E. Dumont and Donald J. Mayer, both by invitation, and John H. Mulholland, of New York, David Stewart Professor of Surgery, Chairman of Department, New York Surgical Division, Bellevue Hospital; Attending Surgeon, University Hospital, *The Suppression of Immunologic Activity by Diversion of Thoracic Duct Lymph,* building on the work of Michael Woodruff, studied the results of thoracic duct diversion in patients and in rats. In 24 patients with a variety of disease not involving the lymphatics, one with rheumatoid arthritis, they cannulated the thoracic duct continuously for periods of one to

12 days. By the third to the fourth day, the serum gamma globulin fell "to less than one half the levels in control samples". Most serum iso-agglutinins fell two-to tenfold, peripheral blood lymphocyte counts did not change significantly. The 900 to 6,000 cells per cubic millimeter in the thoracic duct lymph were almost entirely small and large lymphocytes, but some eosinophils were always present. In all but two patients "The severity of skin reactions to bacterial antigens diminished". The "thoracic duct lymphocytes maintained in culture . . . synthesized and released several types of immune globulin into the culture fluid." In eight rats, the intra-abdominal portion of the thoracic duct was cannulated and the plastic tubing inserted into the jejunum. Rat skin homografts, placed into the kidney capsule, remained viable as long as three-and-a-half months in rats with thoracic duct diversion. They found it "tempting" to consider whether "in addition to temporary depletion of cellular or humoral antibody or both, antigens released from the graft may be transported to the gastro-intestinal tract where the materials are degraded and then absorbed in the form of haptenes. This process may render the animal nonresponsive when challenged with the complete antigen molecule."

Discussion

Alfred Ketcham, of Bethesda, said they had been experimenting with thoracic duct drainage in cancer patients at the Surgery Branch of the National Cancer Institute. The body response to antigen was depressed by thoracic duct drainage, and skin homografts "remained intact and grossly viable for up to 6 weeks after drainage. After 6 weeks, using small punch biopsy type of grafts, it becomes very difficult to determine continued viability of the graft . . ." He pointed up, more specifically than Dumont and Mulholland had been willing to do, the significance of the study, "As clinical transplantation programs continue to report their attempts at suppression of the rejection phenomena, this work of Dumont's becomes even more intriguing. It seems possible that the severe bone marrow depression and predisposition to infections which accompanies our present modes of suppression of the immune phenomena might be obviated through thoracic duct drainage. Obviously, technics will have to be refined which will establish prolonged drainage, allow adequate removal of the lymphocytes and subsequent reinfusion of the cellular depleted lymph." I. F. MacLaren, of Philadelphia, said that John M. Howard's group "has been interested for some time in

the possibility of prolonging homograft survival by means of thoracic duct lymph diversion." He had undertaken a thoracic duct cannulation, either prior to or at the time of renal homotransplantation in dogs, and had survivals up to 35 days, apparently without any other immunosuppressive measures. John H. Mulholland, closing, emphasized that the diversion of lymph into the gastro-intestinal tract in the rat was successful for only ten days or so ". . . and yet grafts persisted thereafter even though lymph was coursing in the normal manner. If this is so, then diversion of antigen or antibody contained in lymph (whichever is the case) is necessary for only the period during which the graft is being seated properly in its new bed, or for the time to bring about what is described as establishment."

* * *

Keith Reemtsma, of New Orleans, Associate Professor of Surgery, Tulane University School of Medicine; Oscar Creech, Jr., William Henderson Professor of Surgery, Chairman of the Department of Surgery, Tulane University School of Medicine, and eight others, *Renal Heterotransplantation in Man,* briefly discussed the reported experience with renal heterografts in humans, Jaboulay's 1906 goat and pig grafts anastomosed to the antecubital vessels, with failure; Unger's 1910 monkey transplant which failed because of thromboses and, Neuhof's 1923 lamb kidney transplant which survived for ten days. Immunosuppression now appeared to counter the rejection process. They had met ethical and legal problems in securing human kidneys in their renal homografting program, "Attempts to use cadaveric kidneys met with no prolonged success, and the supply of expended kidneys was inadequate. We were reluctant to press the use of volunteer humans for ethical, scientific and legal reasons", so that they undertook to study ". . . non-human sources for clinical renal transplantation." The six patients undergoing heterotransplantation were all terminally uremic patients for whom "no volunteer" [Reemtsma's quotation marks] donor was available, and when no cadaver kidney had become available in a stated period of time heterotransplantation was scheduled. Chimpanzees had blood types A and O ". . . offering the possibility of the *universal donor* from the standpoint of blood groups." The patients received pretransplantation treatment with azathioprine, actinomycin C and steroids. The transplanted tissue consisted of ". . . the entire renal complex, including both kidneys and ureters, aorta, and vena cava . . . removed *en bloc* after anticoagulation . . ." The aorta and vena cava of the graft were anastomosed to the recipient's external iliac artery and vein, and end-to-side. Postoperatively, all patients received azothioprine, actinomycin C, steroids, and x-radiation to the transplant. The patients died—at 63 days of sepsis, at seven weeks of sepsis, in eleven days of sepsis [a patient whose first chimpanzee kidneys did not function for two days and in whom a second transplant was performed], of sepsis at 18 days, and of sepsis at 27 days, the graft never having functioned. The third patient to receive a transplant was ". . . now asymptomatic and has normal renal function 6-1/2 months after transplantation." They thought the difficulties caused by infection had been greater than those from graft rejection, and felt that they had used excessive immunosuppression. The clinical behavior of the heterografted kidney, chimpanzee to man, seemed to be similar to that of the homografted kidney, man to man. They warned that their work was ". . . wholly experimental . . . historic experience shows that the field of heterotransplantation may be abused flagrantly. The use of non-human kidneys in man removes the problems of the human donor, but the consequence of this exchange is increased difficulty imposed by cross-species transplantation. Whether heterografted kidneys will function often enough, well enough and long enough to warrant their use remains unanswered, but the present study suggests to us that further work in this area is indicated."

Discussion

Joseph E. Murray, of Boston, opened the Discussion, stating that "None of us one year ago would have guessed that any primate graft would have survived for 12 weeks" [the length of survival of Case 3 at the time of the meeting; the patient was still alive at the time the Discussion went to press six-and-a-half months after transplant. "At the time of publication of the article, the patient had returned to full-time work, and was in good health with normal renal function. She was readmitted to the hospital in September, 1964, nine months following transplant. At the time of re-admission she showed slight deterioration of the renal function and marked electrolyte imbalance. She died within hours of admission. Post-mortem examination of the transplant showed well-preserved glomeruli and tubules, with mild cellular infiltration. There were mild to moderate vascular changes. The post-mortem did not establish the cause of death". Personal communication: Keith Reemtsma, June 11, 1979]. Murray would not go further than to say that "Primate grafts may in the future serve as a potential source

of donor organs, and this possibility alone warrants further laboratory study in their use." He mentioned, as Reemtsma had, the registry of human kidney homotransplants under the aegis of the National Research Council. David M. Hume, of Richmond, said that like Murray he had been ". . . among those who thought it was pretty foolish at the start . . .", that heterografts had not yet proved themselves but ". . . there are some types of grafts which will have to come from a source other than man himself, and the heterograft, if it works, may provide this source." He thought Reemtsma's group might well be encouraged to continue their experiments. Hume's group had done ". . . one chimpanzee transplant in man some time ago . . ." The two chimpanzee kidneys functioned at once and ". . . put out 54,000 cc. in the first 24 hours" in a patient who had been extremely edematous and ". . . lost all his ankle edema completely. He lost all of his ascites, and his face, which had been swollen, became sunken, and by the next morning he was dehydrated." The patient suffered a stroke, developed a coronary occlusion and died. T. E. Starzl, of Denver, reported for Dr. [William] Waddell on ". . . the six baboon heterografts which were done in Denver after considerable helpful guidance from the New Orleans group and in active collaboration with Dr. Claude Hitchcock of Minneapolis." Baboons were more plentiful and cheaper than chimpanzees. There was immediate good renal excretion from all six heterografts but ". . . cross-comparison with Dr. Reemtsma's data suggests that the baboon does not provide as good immediate or sustained function as the chimpanzee." The pathologic changes in the baboon kidney compared with those in the chimpanzee kidney, both reviewed by the same third party referee, suggested that ". . . the pathologic changes in the baboon [kidney] are also more severe than with the chimp." Four of their six patients were dead, two of them were still alive ". . . but only by virtue of a secondarily performed homotransplantation . . . the homografts functioned well despite the prior presence of the heterografts much like the experience which has been described with serial homografts." Starzl said that "Because of our experience with this group, it is our opinion that baboon heterografts cannot work on a long-term basis at the present time. The results we have obtained are less encouraging in terms of function and pathologic tissue injury than have been found in Dr. Reemtsma's chimpanzees. We have, therefore, abandoned the use of the baboon heterografts." Willard E. Goodwin, of Los Angeles, said that at UCLA they had thought kidney heterotransplantation was ". . . a study for the laboratory up till now." They had done dog to sheep, sheep to dog, dog to monkey, human to dog, human to monkey, and monkey to monkey—of different species—and human to chimpanzee "All of these have been rejected, usually with an accelerated pattern." In the dog to sheep and sheep to dog ". . . it happened while we were still watching it . . . The monkey to monkey of a different species was the most promising. This kidney survived for two months." The human to chimpanzee transplant lasted a week ". . . and the animal died probably not of rejection, but rejection was taking place in the kidney." Goodwin suggested the possibility that a primate kidney might be used as an artificial kidney for temporary situations. Francis D. Moore, of Boston, introduced a critical note "Intra-order heterografts, such as chimp (or baboon) to man are . . . susceptible to careful laboratory preparation and study. Now that this area has been invaded by assault, it would seem wise to slow down and entrench our position by careful laboratory study of the rejection immunology in intra-order primate heterografts involving the several available primate species *other than man,* in the hope of obtaining laboratory verification before pressing the human patient, *who has something to look forward to from a homograft.* The ethical problem . . . is that of science as a whole. Good science is ethical science . . . good biological science views the whole man and the whole problem with care and caution." Professor Michael Woodruff, of Edinburgh, Scotland, agreed with Moore that heterografts from primates needed more experimental work, and it had been assumed that heterografts were not worth investigating ". . . but if one looks at the behavior of skin grafts from rat to mouse one finds that it isn't much more difficult to make a rat-mouse skin graft than to make a mouse-to-mouse skin graft with a really unfavorable strain combination . . . if this were to apply with heterografts among primates, and could then be taken over to man, think of the problems it would solve!. . . After seeing Reemtsma's case [he had visited Reemtsma in New Orleans] I am convinced that one must investigate the whole problem with extreme thoroughness. I would also like to add that the achievement of making a heterograft of a kidney to a human being function, and continue to function after 12 weeks, is an absolutely astounding achievement. I am filled with admiration for Dr. Reemtsma and his colleagues." Reemtsma, closing, expressed his appreciation to the Association for having placed the paper on the program, "Historically the field of heterotransplantation has garnered a rather unsavory reputation because of outright abuses and extrava-

gant claims. The inclusion of the report on the program of the Association will aid immeasurably in restoring heterotransplantation to the position which we believe it deserves: an appropriate field for scientific investigation."

* * *

There had been a discussion of liver homotransplantation by Moore and his group from the Peter Bent Brigham, before the Association in 1960, and now T. E. Starzl, by invitation, T. L. Marchioro, by invitation, W. R. Waddell, of Denver, Professor and Chairman Department of Surgery, University of Colorado School of Medicine, and four associates, *Immunosuppression after Experimental and Clinical Homotransplantation of the Liver,* discussed the problem in 25 orthotopic transplantations in dogs, 15 auxiliary hepatic transplantations in dogs, and five human orthotopic liver transplantations. "From a histologic point of view, immunosuppression was most successful in the human cases despite the employment of badly ischematized cadaveric organs." Four of the patients had had primary liver tumors, the fifth a three-year-old child with congenital biliary atresia. The cadaver livers were perfused and cooled during removal, and transplantation was achieved in 164 to 420 minutes after death of the donor. Azathioprine and prednisone were used, in the patients, as well as actinomycin C. One patient received azaserine for two days. All of their dogs with orthotopic homografts died, 11 of them within three days, usually ". . . as a consequence of outflow block and/or hemorrhagic gastroenteritis." The remaining 14 died after three days to one month from a variety of obvious causes. It was difficult to tell the part that rejection might have played, and classic cellular rejection was not histologically apparent. Their first patient died of hemorrhage at operation, the next four at 22, 7.5, 6.5, and 23 days from pulmonary embolism, pulmonary embolism and gastrointestinal hemorrhage, pulmonary embolism and congestive heart failure, and from bile peritonitis due to common duct necrosis. The last patient was the only one in whom liver failure played a significant part, and that liver failure was heralded only by an attack of abdominal pain, indicating bile leakage. There was less evidence of rejection in the clinical cases than in the dog homografts, and substantially more evidence of rejection in the ". . . canine auxiliary livers which were placed in the right paravertebral gutter without removal of the recipient's own liver." [The data were presented objectively, describing techniques employed, observations made and results achieved. Neither in the paper nor in the Discussion did Starzl offer any comment on the prospects of solving the problem or of his reaction to his experience up to that time. An Addendum, submitted at the time the Discussion went to press, indicated that they had now achieved more than a month's survival in 11 of 20 dogs and up to four-and-a-quarter months in an animal which was still well, maintained on a regimen of ". . . daily azathioprine and intermittent intravenous doses of S^{35} methionine . . ."]

Discussion

Francis D. Moore, of Boston, said that with orthotopic liver transplantation in dogs, Starzl's results had been better than theirs, "We have never had a dog go longer than 14 days. He has had one at 30 days." However, no one had achieved a long-term laboratory survivor, ". . . we believe that the cause of this failure is vascular, probably a vasospastic or nonthrombotic vaso-occlusive feature of rejection. Our single human experience corroborated this interpretation." For that matter, long-term maintenance had not yet been possible with ". . . heart, lung, adrenal, or pancreas, to name but a few organs with which members of this society are laboring." He reminded the Fellows that the ". . . first successful long-term kidney transplantation in man between individuals related more remotely than fraternal twins was preceded by long-term survival in the laboratory using a protocol very similar, if not identical, to that later used in man." C. Stuart Welch, of Albany, had been working with liver transplantation in dogs, but as yet had not attempted it in humans, where he thought the greatest application would be in cirrhotics. He did not think the transplantation would have to be orthotopic. The large size of the liver made it difficult to transplant elsewhere in the abdomen but they had recently shown that a half-liver homotransplant ". . . will sustain life in hepatectomized dogs . . ." Joseph E. Murray, of Boston, asked "Is it a valid assumption that immune suppression is adequate because cellular infiltrate is lacking?" Starzl, closing, said that it had not been their ". . . assumption that the absence of immunocytes means that the rejection process has been controlled . . . it is our view that noncellular rejection is typical of the reaction which we are going to see with increasing frequency in livers, just as has been observed with kidneys." Like Dr. Welch, they had hoped that auxiliary liver transplants would avoid the necessity for a hepatectomy but they had been unable to control rejection in such animals. [An Addendum referred to the work of Dr. Thomas

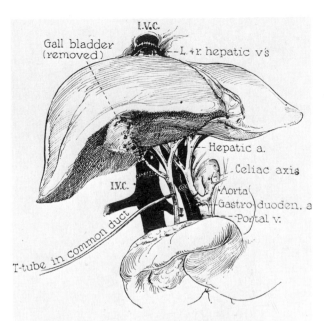

Fig. 2. Completed clinical homotransplantation. The reconstruction is anatomically normal. The T-tube is placed through a stab wound in the recipient common duct, rather than through the anastomosis as shown.

Technique of human orthotopic liver homotransplantation employed by Starzl in five cases. The first patient died of hemorrhage on the table, three others of pulmonary embolism, and one of bile peritonitis, perhaps associated with ascites [See Volume LXXXVI - 1968, for the technique in Starzl's successful human cases.] but the procedure was proved technically feasible in man.

T. E. Starzl, T. L. Marchioro, W. R. Waddell, and four associates, *Immunosuppression after Experimental and Clinical Homotransplantation of the Liver.* Volume LXXXII, 1964.

Marchioro which explained the previously observed shrinking of the heterotopic transplant, "When the homograft rather than the dog's own liver is vascularized with splanchnic venous flow, the auxiliary homograft retains its size and selective shrinkage of the autologous liver occurs."]

* * *

The pyrotechnics, and display of surgical virtuosity continued with *Transplantation of the Lung,* James D. Hardy, of Jackson, Professor and Chairman, Department of Surgery and Director of Surgical Research, University of Mississippi; Sadan Eraslan, and Watts R. Webb, both by invitation. They had studied lung replantation in the dog, finding that the pulmonary vein anastomoses were difficult

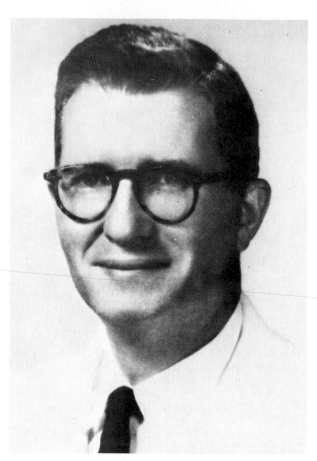

James D. Hardy (c. 1960) 1918—. President 1976, and of the American College of Surgeons 1980. M.D., University of Pennsylvania 1942; training University of Pennsylvania 1942-51; Assistant Professor to Associate Professor of Surgery and Director of Surgical Research, University of Tennessee, 1951-55; Professor and Chairman, Department of Surgery, University of Mississippi School of Medicine, 1955—. As multifaceted a clinician and investigator as the Association has had, with major contributions in vascular surgery, endocrinology and transplantation. Prolific author and editor.

and were best solved by taking a cuff of atrium with the veins. The gross mortality rate was 50%, but "Few deaths occurred after the fourth week . . ." Bronchospirometric studies showed a decrease in function to half normal values for the first few days, returning to ". . . low normal values . . ." by the 14th postoperative day. Subsequent contralateral pneumonectomy in three dogs was followed by progressive respiratory difficulty with death in two, 18 and 24 hours after the contralateral pneumonectomy, in the absence of any detectable anatomical defect. "Thus it appeared that the replanted lung

was not able to support the respiratory requirements of the animals after only approximately three months." When contralateral pneumonectomy was performed six months or more after replantation, the animal survived. Storage of the lung in cold solution at 4° for two hours, and sometimes as long as four after pneumonectomy and before replantation, was followed by successful function. Division of the pulmonary lymphatics, or of the bronchial arteries, or of the pulmonary branches of the vagus nerve, was studied, without conclusive results, "It was our impression that division of the bronchial arteries had relatively little effect, but that division of the nerve supply to the lung did apparently have an effect in reducing the functional capacity of the lung." The lymphatics appeared to regenerate within 12 days, and many lymphatic channels were established within two to three weeks, ". . . this regeneration of the lymphatics appeared to coincide with the reduction of congestion in the replanted lung and with the gradual improvement of the ventilatory and oxygen uptake capacity of the replanted lung." Homotransplantation in 108 dogs achieved a mean survival time of 7.4 days in untreated animals, and an average of 30.4 days in dogs treated with Imuran, including two permanent survivors, in whom ". . . at sacrifice many months later it was found that the homografted lung had been rejected at some time in the past and was encased in a fibrous envelope." Imuran proved to be more effective in lung homotransplantation in dogs than Imuran and hydrocortisone or Imuran and actinomycin C or Methotrexate, although Blumenstock, [at Cooperstown] three years before, had reported good results in dog homotransplantation employing Methotrexate. Hardy's group had undertaken a single human homotransplant in a 58-year-old man with ". . . a squamous cell carcinoma virtually occluding the left main stem bronchus with chronic purulent infection in this essentially destroyed lung. In addition, he had a chronic renal lesion bilaterally which had resulted in borderline renal insufficiency." [That patient had been reported in the J.A.M.A. the previous year.] The donor lung came from a patient who had died an hour before with a massive myocardial infarct and pulmonary edema. The nature of the problem in the recipient was suggested by the statement that "In this instance, venous anastomoses were employed rather than the atrial cuff, since the infection in the left hemithorax of the recipient rendered opening the pericardium of the recipient inadvisable." The patient's oxygen saturation improved immediately upon completion of the anastomoses, the lung remained expanded, and functioned for three weeks.

At autopsy "There was virtually no evidence of immunologic rejection." He was kept on a respirator and had "no particular problems referable to his lungs . . . throughout the period that he lived." Cancer had been left behind in the region of the aorta and esophagus. Immunoparalysis was with Imuran. The patient died of progressive renal failure on the 18th day after operation. At autopsy, "The gross appearance of the homotransplanted lung could not be distinguished from that of the patient's own lung, with the exception that once the vessels and bronchus were opened the anastomotic sites could be visualized." It was thought that a small bronchial dehiscence, closed over by adhesions, might have been produced by bronchoscopy two days earlier ". . . when the patient had become unable to remove his own secretions." Others had found lung transplantation in dogs practical and Magovern and Yates had just reported a human lung homotransplantation. Hardy thought that ". . . lung transplantation is technically feasible . . . the transplant supplies a considerable degree of respiratory activity until rejected, in the case of an homotransplant . . . not only acute and chronic respiratory insufficiency but also cor pulmonale could be improved by lung homotransplantation if immunologic rejection could be prevented."

* * *

An enormous amount of data in the *Analysis of Mechanism of Immunosuppressive Drugs in Renal Homotransplantation,* was presented by Joseph E. Murray, of Boston, Clinical Associate in Surgery, Harvard Medical School; Director of Surgical Research Laboratory, Harvard Medical School and Peter Bent Brigham Hospital; and by invitation, Gustave J. Dammin, Friedman Professor of Pathology, Harvard Medical School; Pathologist-in-Chief, Peter Bent Brigham Hospital, and four associates. As the result of studies in over 1000 animals with 24 different drug protocols, the most recent of which, employing Imuran and azaserine, produced 90%, 50-day survivors, and 50%, 100-day survivors, they had documented a number of observations. "All animals on prolonged drug therapy are immunologically competent; drug therapy can be stopped successfully in some but not all animals [vide Varco's suggestion at the Washington meeting in 1962, Volume LXXX], long surviving kidneys apparently are protected in some way in the new environment because a second kidney from the same donor can be rejected while the first survives; retransplantation of a long surviving kidney back to its original host did not lead to a decrease in renal function; long surviv-

ing kidneys successfully retransplanted back to their original donors are rejected when transplanted to third party, non-drug treated recipients; immune paralysis does not account for the prolonged survival because the second donor kidney which constitutes a double dose of antigen is rejected while the first continues to survive . . . all hosts are sensitized against the recipient and this sensitization continues even in those animals successfully weaned from drugs . . . skin homografts are universally rejected within 20 days by hosts treated with the drug regimen which protects kidney homografts sometimes permanently . . . drug treated animals, male and female, are fertile . . . multiple rejection processes can produce generalized immunological picture in the host similar to an autoimmune disease process."

Discussion

Paul S. Russell, of Boston, pointed out that Murray's long-term survivals were in animals "selected on the basis of genetic similiarity", and Russell suggested that ". . . it would appear that the use of drugs is only capable of controlling an immunologic reaction of a certain magnitude." And since the magnitude is determined by the genetic differences between the individuals, the long-term survivors will be selected on this basis." He agreed that there was ". . . a good deal of evidence that the immunologic deficit in the recipient is not a crippling one." The fact that a second kidney transplant would fail while a first transplant from the same donor continued to survive, suggested some change in the transplant itself despite the fact that it still would be rejected by a third dog, or accepted by the original donor. David M. Hume, of Richmond, felt there was, in fact, an adaptation of the graft ". . . not ruled out by the demonstration that retransplantation of the graft into the donor permits the graft to survive." T. E. Starzl, of Denver, agreed that adaptation occurred, demonstrating the data on a patient whose rejection was countered with Imuran and prednisone, the doses of which could subsequently be markedly reduced. They had five dogs in whom all immunosuppressive therapy had been stopped. Murray, in closing, said they were seeking 100% survivors, and were beginning to approach that. There was a difference among organs. He and most other investigators believed that suvival of the skin homograft was more difficult to achieve than survival of a kidney homograft. Finally, he spoke feelingly of the problem of the healthy living donor ". . . we must be clear and careful about our motiviation. When we take a healthy living donor and make him sick by subjecting him to a potentially fatal operation, we are reversing completely and qualitatively the very essence of our medical motivation . . . it must be done only after serious reflection and soul-searching. The motives of the donor are extremely important if we are to avoid what Lederberg has recently termed 'the potential dehumanizing abuses of a market in human flesh.' "

* * *

Robert P. Hummel, by invitation, William A. Altemeier, of Cincinnati, Christian R. Holmes Professor of Surgery, University of Cincinnati, and Director of Surgery, Cincinnati General Hospital, and by invitation E. O. Hill, *Iatrogenic Staphylococcal Enterocolitis*, continued to be concerned about what they conceived to be the effect of ". . . increased and widespread use of the broad spectrum antibiotics . . . in the development of clinical staphylococcal enterocolitis" concerning which they had written the year before. They had seen 155 cases of staphylococcal enterocolitis between 1958 and 1962, in which 58 of the patients had received broad spectrum antibiotic therapy alone or with penicillin, and 44 patients had been given ". . . neomycin alone or with sulfasuxidine prior to the development of the enterocolitis." Most of them had received a ". . . 24-hour gastro-intestinal preparation with a total of 8.0 to 10.0 Gm of neomycin." In the first group of patients, four had staphylococcus aureus in their stool prior to the administration of neomycin, and only one had not previously received antibiotics. At the time of the first postoperative bowel movement, staphylococci were cultured in the stools of 23 of the 30 patients. There appeared to be no correlation with the use of postoperative antibiotics. Eight patients had postoperative diarrhea, and all had stools positive for staphylococcus aureus. Six of the 30 patients died, two of them with wound infection, peritonitis, and pelvic abscesses, and in both of these staphylococcus aureus was recovered. One death was from severe enterocolitis. In a second group of patients, a third were treated with the neomycin sulfathalidine regimen, a third with sulfathalidine alone, and a third with paromomycin, 31 patients in all. Five of the neothalidine patients developed staphylococcus aureus in their postoperative stools, and three had moderate to severe enterocolitis, fatal in one. None of the patients with sulfathalidine alone had staphylococcus aureus in their postoperative stools or developed enterocolitis. Of the seven patients with paromomycin, one had staphylococcus aureus in the first postoperative bowel movement, and none developed enterocolitis. Hummel stated

that the evidence was that ". . . the oral administration of the various broad spectrum antibiotics including neomycin not only failed to *sterilize* the bowel but also seemed to predispose toward the colonization of the stool by virulent strains of *Staphylococcus aureus* that may be present in the environment and the development of staphylococcal enterocolitis." Their only recommendation was ". . . that if antibiotic agents including neomycin be used for the preoperative preparation of the bowel, they should be employed with caution and vigilance, the surgeon being particularly alert to the earliest signs and symptoms of staphylococcal enterocolitis . . ."

Discussion

Harold A. Zintel, of New York, enthusiastically applauded the findings. He quoted himself as having said two years before ". . . the intestinal antibacterial agents had probably killed more patients than they had saved from peritonitis." He maintained that the use of intestinal antibacterial agents had not decreased the mortality of colon surgery, and that sulfasuxidine and sulfathalidine were inadequate to reduce the bacterial content of the colon. Edgar J. Poth, of Galveston, said that 23 years of experience had shown that the value of intestinal antisepsis was "quite definite". Since 1941 he had performed over 250 open anastomoses following resection of carcinoma of the colon with his technique of intestinal antisepsis and ". . .there has not been a single breakdown of the suture line, there has not been a single localized abscess, there has not been a single instance of peritonitis, nor has there been a single operative death in the entire series." Since 1950 neomycin and sulfathalidine—not sulfasuxidine—had been the treatment of choice, "The proper dosage is 6 to 9 Gm. of neomycin and 9 to 12 Gm. of sulfathalidine on the short—20-hour—preparation schedule which is applicable if there is no contraindication to simultaneous purgation." He continued the neomycin and sulfathalidine postoperatively ". . . without development of pseudomembranous enterocolitis." The Air Force Hospital in Wiesbaden, Germany, had a large experience with neomycin and sulfathaladine in patients from all over the world "There has not been a single instance of pseudomembranous enterocolitis." John Prohaska, of Chicago, seconded Altemeier's comments. Isidore Cohn, Jr., of New Orleans, reported that his "experience with antibiotics is somewhat at variance with that reported by Dr. Hummel." Quantitative and qualitative stool cultures in 200 consecutive patients without bowel disease and not on antibiotics, had shown staphylococci to be present in about 30%, and very high counts in some. Kanamycin, which he had used in 800 patients with a single case of pseudomembranous enterocolitis, he considered better than neomycin and sulfathalidine. "We believe this is a low enough incidence so that we do not need to be afraid of enterocolitis if drug therapy is properly used for a period of three days." W. A. Altemeier, in closing, essentially repeated what had been said in the paper, that the neomycin-sulfonamide combination failed to sterilize the bowel, and seemed to predispose to colonization by virulent staphylococci. Once more he warned surgeons to be alert for the development of staphylococcal enterocolitis.

* * *

David C. Sabiston, Jr., Associate Professor of Surgery, Johns Hopkins University School of Medicine [Sabiston was actually Professor of Surgery at Hopkins when the abstract was submitted, and was now Professor of Surgery, and Chairman of the Department, at Duke, in Durham, North Carolina], and by invitation, Henry N. Wagner, Jr. *The Diagnosis of Pulmonary Embolism by Radioisotope Scanning,* had labeled macro-aggregated human serum albumin with I^{131} or Cr^{51}. The macro-aggregated isotope albumin had been shown to be "without significant effect on pulmonary hemodynamics in the amounts employed, and . . . without toxicity, radiation hazard, or antigenic effect." In dogs, Hypaque-filled rubber balloons tethered by a thread, were slipped into the jugular vein and allowed to occlude a pulmonary artery or branch at will. The scans clearly showed the nonperfused areas of the pulmonary parenchyma. In more than 100 patients with various forms of pulmonary disease, they had performed pulmonary scans. Sabiston presented a series of plain films, scans, and arteriograms demonstrating the accuracy of localization by their technique. The plain film could be relied upon principally if it showed radiolucency. Pulmonary arteriography was the most reliable and most diagnostic test, but somewhat laborious and time-consuming and presented some hazard of hypotension in an already ill patient. Others had suggested aggregates of radioactively-labeled human serum proteins as particulate matter which might be injected for a variety of purposes. Particles of appropriate size, Sabiston and Wagner said, could be injected intravenously ". . . with a majority of the particles becoming lodged in the lungs. This allows a scan to be performed which demonstrates the distribution of pulmonary blood flow and clearly delineates areas in which the pulmonary arterial flow is diminished or absent." The concentration of radioactivity provided the basis for quantitative determination of pulmonary blood flow. Initially they had employed pulmonary arteriography on the same patients but ". . . it is now believed pulmonary arteriography is not necessary, although it is of value in distinguishing massive embolism from multiple small emboli." Scanning established ". . . a firm diagnosis of pulmonary embolism and is especially useful in the selection of patients for direct pulmonary embolectomy employing extracorporeal circulation. In this group of patients it is particularly important to establish the diagnosis firmly and to thus exclude other serious causes producing similar clinical manifestations such as acute myocardial infarction." Their subsequent studies showed that arterial flow was restored after resorption of the emboli.

Discussion

C. Rollins Hanlon, of St. Louis, agreed that diagnostic accuracy was needed before proceeding to cardiopulmonary bypass and embolectomy. He reported the technique of his associate, V. L. Willman, passing a 21-gauge needle percutaneously under local anesthesia ". . . through the aorta and pulmonary artery into the left atrium securing pressure tracings in each area . . . The transfixion of these important structures is rather horrifying when one first sees the diagram, but the technic has been used safely in nearly 300 instances." A slide showing such pressure recordings from a dog which had been given ". . . a large embolus similar to that radiopaque oyster that you saw in Dr. Sabiston's presentation", showed elevated pulmonary artery pressure, decreased aortic pressure, diminished pulmonary arterial flow, and decreased left atrial pressure, as did another slide made of pressure tracings from a postoperative patient who had hitherto been incorrectly diagnosed as having ruptured chordae of the mitral valve. Peter V. Moulder, Jr., of Chicago, demonstrated a motion picture of pulmonary arteriography in a woman with pulmonary embolism in whom he had successfully performed pulmonary embolectomy, as he had also in another patient. He asked Dr. Sabiston whether the patient should also have the vena cava ligated and ". . . what are the scan findings when there is marked left atrial stasis?" Eric M. Nanson, Saskatoon, Canada, had been using I^{131} tagged fibrinogen ". . . with the idea of picking up deep venous thrombosis before the embolism has occurred . . .", and had found it effective in locating thrombosed veins both in animals and in patients

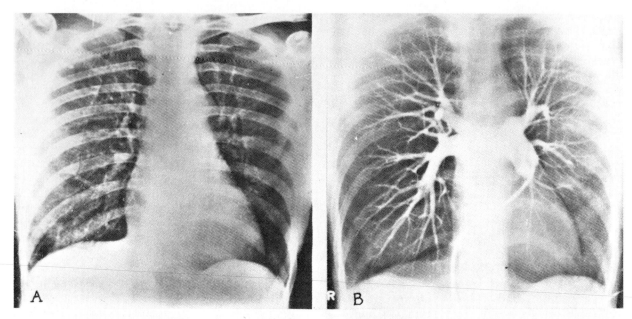

FIG. 12A. Plain chest film showing suggestive diminution of the vascular markings in this area. B. Pulmonary arteriogram clearly demonstrating an occlusion in the left lower lobe.

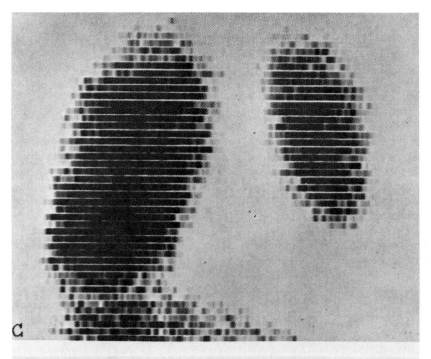

FIG. 12C. Pulmonary scan confirms findings in the arteriogram.

Macro-aggregated human serum albumin labeled with I^{131} regularly demonstrated the nonperfused pulmonary segments in patients with pulmonary emboli.

David C. Sabiston, Jr., and Henry N. Wagner, Jr., *The Diagnosis of Pulmonary Embolism by Radioisotope Scanning.* Volume LXXXII, 1964.

". . . we believe that this may be of some use—to use I^{131} tagged fibrinogen to seek out the oyster before it leaves the bed." Isidore Cohn, Jr., of New Orleans, showed studies of a patient of Dr. Bert Glass in whom pulmonary angiography demonstrated massive embolism which was successfully treated operatively. Sabiston, in closing, said that they had ". . . performed [vena cava] ligation or plication in each patient upon whom pulmonary embolectomy was done. In so far as left atrial stasis is concerned, this has not been encountered as a problem in the interpretation of pulmonary scans."

* * *

Albert Starr, of Portland, Oregon, Associate Professor of Surgery; Chief of Cardiac Surgery, University of Oregon Medical School, had, three years before, stimulated the Association with the presentation of his mitral ball valve, and now, with C. W. McCord, James Wood, Rodney Herr and M. L. Edwards, all by invitation, *Surgery for Multiple Valve Disease,* presented an experience with 27 patients who had had combined aortic and mitral valve replacements. The aortic prosthesis was very similar to the mitral ball valve prosthesis, and both had undergone steady improvement in design. "In June, 1962, the first patient in this series with known severe aortic and mitral disease underwent a double replacement procedure. Since then 27 such patients have been operated upon, 18 of whom had replacement of two or more valves. Seven patients had aortic replacement and repair of the mitral valve. Two patients had mitral replacement and repair of the aortic valve." Six of the patients had had previous cardiac procedures performed. All of the patients had rheumatic heart disease except for one with cystic medial necrosis of the aorta, aneurysm of the sinuses of Valsalva and aortic regurgitation, as well as mitral regurgitation from ruptured chordae tendinae. They operated through a midline sternotomy incision. The arterial return was through the left external iliac artery. They used a rotating disc oxygenator and roller pumps, and heparinized blood drawn 18 hours before operation, with added mannitol, but without hemodilution. Body temperature was brought down to 30°C. The mitral valve was approached through a long left atriotomy,- exposing the left atrium, by opening the posterior interatrial sulcus, retracting the right atrium and inferior vena cava sharply to the left. The aorta was clamped, intermittently ". . . if aortic regurgitation is not too severe." If continuous cross clamping of the aorta was necessary, the coronaries were perfused intermittently with cold blood from the oxygenating chamber. The mitral valve was replaced first because after the aortic prosthesis was in place it was difficult to explore the mitral valve. With the mitral and aortic prostheses in place the heart was closed, the aortic clamp removed, the heart defibrillated and the vent in the left ventricle withdrawn. If examination now showed tricuspid insufficiency, bypass was resumed, and a mitral prosthesis was inserted in the tricuspid position. The bypass in these patients varied from two hours and six minutes to five hours and eight minutes. Twenty of the 27 patients were still alive and in good condition at the time of the meeting, and in the last 24 patients there had been only four deaths, a 12% mortality. Patient 1 could not be resuscitated in the operating room and had a leak around the aortic prosthesis. Patient 2 died of acute yellow atrophy. Patient 6 died with shortness of breath on the second day, "In retrospect the earlier use of artificial ventilation in this patient may have changed the outcome." Three patients died of progressive low cardiac output, one of them despite a left atrial to iliac artery bypass 36 hours after operation. One patient died of supraventricular tachycardia, which he had had before operation. All of the patients who died were over 45 years of age, and all but one were in functional Class IV. One patient, eight months later, required re-exploration for a leaking tricuspid prosthesis. Two patients required reoperation for cardiac tamponade. Rhythm disturbances were common after operation. One patient on the 8th day developed ventricular fibrillation, was resuscitated and had done well since. Three-fourths of the patients had prophylactic tracheostomy and artificial ventilation for seven to ten days. More than half of the patients developed a psychosis some time after the third day, which cleared before discharge. Improvement in exercise tolerance was noted within a few months by nearly all, and "Those over four months postoperatively have had no cardiac symptoms despite full activity and normal diet." Six patients had been recatheterized. Those with pulmonary hypertension showed a fall in the pulmonary artery pressure, and all showed a "profound fall" in the mean left atrial pressure. Resting cardiac outputs were normal, and with exercise the patients could increase their cardiac output normally. All patients but one were on long-term anticoagulant medication. There had been no late emboli thus far, and only one during the period of hospitalization. [An Addendum to the paper states that there had been 13 additional multiple valve operations "including three triple replacements, eight combined mitral and aortic replacements, one aortic replacement with open mitral commissurotomy, and one mitral replacement with aortic commissurotomy, with no deaths." They thus, had no deaths in the last 18 patients.]

Discussion

John W. Kirklin, of Rochester, Minnesota, said that patients with severe aortic valve disease, and "clinical evidence of apparent moderate incompetence of the mitral valve in the form of some modest enlargement of the left atrium; an apical systolic murmur and on angiocardiography the passage of some dye from the left ventricle to the left atrium" might also have severe elevation of the left atrial pressure without in fact having any incompetence of the mitral valve even though to intraoperative palpation it seemed "modestly incompetent". In a number of such patients, the signs of mitral disease disappeared after aortic valve replacement. Kirklin and his colleagues had ". . . replaced simultaneously the mitral and aortic valves in 25 patients in the last 15 months. Twenty-one have left the hospital alive, and there have been no late deaths." Conrad R. Lam, of Detroit, said that they had some late trouble from leakage around the valve prosthesis ". . . three mitral replacements and one aortic with late leakage." The sutures appeared to have cut out and he now used ". . . a matress suture buttressed with Teflon . . . placing the prosthesis more or less as an onlay rather than trying to fit it tightly into the mitral valve annulus." W. H. Muller, Jr., of Charlottesville, Virginia, had had four multiple valve procedures with only one survivor. He announced ". . . we have discontinued using the tricuspid Teflon prosthesis, which had been used in our clinic during the past four years, because it does indeed have unfavorable fatigue characteristics. We are beginning to see some patients who had this prosthesis implanted return with stenosis or insufficiency and the valve has usually perforated because of wear at the base of one of the leaflets. Since September 1963, we have applied the Starr prosthesis in the aortic area." Muller asked whether the force of the ball moving back and forth could unseat the valve and cause fistulas. Starr, closing, said, in line with Kirklin's comments, that in 50% of all the aortic replacements the left atrial pressure was elevated, no mitral valve replacement was performed, and the left atrial hypertension disappeared after replacement only of the aortic valve. He congratulated Kirklin ". . . on the fantastic results of 21 surviving patients in 25 operations with multiple valve replacement. I think this is a tremendous accomplishment." [Starr's figures add up to 40 multiple valve operations with seven deaths, none in

the last 18 patients, and an overall mortality almost identical to that for which he was congratulating Kirklin.] Leaks could occur, and he had reoperated three times successfully for leaks around the mitral valve, "If a patient is not doing well after mitral replacement, they have a leak unless proved otherwise even if they have no murmur. The mitral valve prosthesis should function properly, and if it is not functioning properly, then re-operation should be performed." In the aortic valve, the techniques to prevent leakage consisted of ". . . proper selection of valve size, the use of a suture of plastic material rather than silk and proper preparation of the bed for the prosthesis." He had reoperated upon one aortic valve replacement for a leak, successfully.

* * *

Gilbert S. Campbell, of Oklahoma City, Professor of Surgery, University of Oklahoma Medical Center and Chief of Thoracic Surgery; Acting Chief, Department of Surgery, Veterans Administration Hospital, and by invitation, Robert H. Smiley, *Pneumatic Envelope to Avoid Hypotension following Removal of Aortic Clamps,* was concerned with the problem of "Catastrophic shock after aortic declamping . . . in elderly hypertensive individuals undergoing excision of aortic aneurysms." This did not happen in patients operated upon for chronic occlusive disease of the terminal aorta because there was already an arterial collateral circulation around the obstruction. To prevent the sudden pooling of blood in the extremities, they had devised a pneumatic counterpressure garment and in the laboratory had studied the use of one especially made for dogs. Blood pressure rose after aortic clamping whether the dogs had a pneumatic envelope on the hind leg or not, but after an hour of occlusion and sudden declamping the blood pressure in the animals wearing the pressure suit returned to normal levels whereas in the others there was a fall below the preocclusion level. Campbell discussed also the acidosis and the production of metabolites in the ischemic limbs with their adverse effect upon the body upon release of the occlusion. They had employed the suit in 31 elderly male patients undergoing aortic aneurysm excision. None of them developed hypotension after rapid aortic declamping and gradual reduction of pressure in the pressure suit over 15 to 30 minutes. Three patients died and with characteristic candor, Campbell commented "Obviously, the pneumatic envelope does nothing to alter blood loss through a faulty suture line or through an inadequately preclotted prosthetic graft." A fall in pressure after declamping the patient's aorta indicated that the patient was hypovolemic, the aorta was re-clamped, the hypovolemia corrected, and a second rapid declamping now produced no hypotension. Campbell commented that, of course, Crile had "first used an external counterpressure garment in surgical patients in the early 1900's, and later demonstrated his pneumatic rubber suit to the armed forces during the early development of G-suits for aviators. Counterpressure suits have been used in the treatment of postural hypotension [Sieker, et al, 1956] and during neurosurgical procedures in conjunction with hypotension anesthesia, [Gardner and Dohn, 1956]."

Discussion

William H. Moretz, of Augusta, said that Campbell's technique would correct the hypotension due to sudden pooling of blood in the lower extremities but not that due to the formation and accumulation of acid metabolites. They tried in patients to prevent the production of such acid metabolites by inserting a small arterial shunt around the occlusion clamp. "We found that this worked quite well in the animal, and that we did completely prevent the declamping form of hypotension. However, when we attempted to apply this to the clinical area, we found that the application of the shunt (inserting it into the aorta above the clamp and then suturing the holes after declamping, and removing the shunt) was quite inconvenient, and we thought that the amount of declamping hypotension that we observed did not justify this amount of inconvenience." Campbell's method, he thought more appealing, but he doubted that its routine use was justified. The insouciant Campbell responded "As far as the routine use of this suit is concerned, it is routine only with one group—us", but he thought that since it was impossible to predict in whom such pressure fall could occur, the use of the suit in all patients would prevent declamping hypotension and the subsequent necessity for overtransfusion, vasopressors, etc.

* * *

Michael E. DeBakey, of Houston, Professor of Surgery and Chairman of the Department of Surgery, Baylor University College of Medicine; E. Stanley Crawford, Associate Professor of Surgery, Baylor University; Denton A. Cooley, Associate Professor of Surgery, Baylor University, and by invitation, George C. Morris, Jr., Thomas S. Royster, and Walter P. Abbott, *Aneurysm of Abdominal Aorta*, Analysis of Results of Graft Replacement Therapy One to Eleven Years after Operation, pres-

ented another colossal series from Houston. Their total experience with aneurysms of the abdominal aorta from November 6, 1952 to January 1, 1964, was in 1,719 patients, of whom 1,449 treated before January 1, 1963, followed one to 11 years, were the basis of the present report, 98.8% of all of the patients having been followed. They used a simple tube replacement of the aorta, since 1957, always employing a Dacron graft. Nine percent of the patients died within 30 days, but 84% of the patients lived between one and two years and 63% of all the patients were still alive at the time of the report. Hypertension was associated with 89% of the early deaths and 74% of later deaths "A comparison of the long-term survival rates of patients treated surgically with those not treated surgically shows a significantly better life expectancy for the former group . . . these studies show that once the patient survives the immediate effects of the operation, his life expectancy closely approaches that of the normal population during the first five years, following which there is a gradual decrease in life expectancy. . . . Recent hemorrhage, indicating rupture of the aneurysm, was found at operation either in the tissues surrounding the aneurysm or in the peritoneal cavity, as well as in surrounding tissues, in 117 patients." In 1,332 unruptured aneurysms, the mortality was 7%, in 117 ruptured aneurysms the mortality was 34%.

Discussion

D. Emerick Szilagyi, of Detroit, compared 305 patients undergoing resection of abdominal aneurysm between 1952 and early 1963, with 200 cases not operated upon before and after 1952. The groups were otherwise identical, "It is evident that the survival rate of the surgically treated patients was consistently and considerably higher than that of the nonsurgical cases throughout a recorded period of eight years, at the end of which no patient without surgical treatment remained alive . . . The cause of death in 53 per cent of the nonsurgical cases was rupture of the aneurysm." David M. Hume, of Richmond, took particular note of DeBakey's 34% mortality in ruptured aneurysms ". . . in contrast to figures of 50 to 80 per cent given in the literature." At the Medical College of Virginia they had had 25 ruptured aneurysms in the past five years, 20 of them in the last three years with a 35% mortality for the five years and 26% for the past three years. Those were all patients with profound shock, ". . . no slow leaks were included in the series." He asked Crawford, who had presented the Houston paper, ". . . what he thinks about the use of mannitol . . .

this has contributed to the diminished mortality in our hands, together with getting the patient to the operating room as rapidly as possible and getting the aneurysm out as fast as possible, leaving a portion of the back wall of the aneurysm *in situ*." Crawford, said that he was not sure that mannitol was of value in the prevention of acute renal failure. He had "been dependent upon immediate expeditious surgery, adequate blood replacement, and conservative therapy for the renal problem, utilizing dialysis if necessary."

* * *

The first paper on the use of a new physical method for dividing or cutting tissues, *Surgical Applications of Laser,* Paul E. McGuff, by invitation, Ralph A. Deterling, Jr., of Boston, Professor and Chairman of the Department of Surgery, Tufts University School of Medicine; Surgeon-in-Chief, New England Center Hospital and Boston Dispensary; Director, First (Tufts) Surgical Service, Boston City Hospital; and L. S. Gottlieb, H. D. Fahimi, D. Bushnell, by invitation, was presented as a cooperative study from the Department of Surgery, Tufts New England Medical Center, Mallory Institute of Pathology, Boston City Hospital, and the Advanced Development Laboratory of the Raytheon Company, Wayland, Massachusetts. The laser, they defined, as "an acronym derived from Light Amplification by the Stimulated Emission of Radiation" which produced "a beam of light which is more coherent, more monochromatic and capable of greater intensity than any previous light source." Laser energy was "produced by controlled fluorescence in crystals and gases". Its essential characteristic was that its almost parallel beams of light afforded "extremely high radiation densities and may be focused on an area as small as a few microns." The synthetic ruby crystal laser was the earliest and still the commonest. Several hundred materials had been found which were excited to a high energy state and fluoresced upon the admission of photons when a high intensity lamp was flashed. Liquid gas, crystal, and semi-conductor lasers were all under study. The laser energy emission could be cut down to as little as ten to 50 nanoseconds and could be concentrated in an area as small as a few microns. In transplanted human tumors, including transplanted human melanoma, in hamster cheek pouches, the laser treatment was found to be completely curative. They had used laser in one patient with multiple melanoma metastases in the skin and had found the effect dependent upon the dose. Thus far, the major clinical use had been in the treatment of "retinal holes and tears".

Studying the temperature effect on experimental tumors, they were able to say that "temperatures within the Lased tumors most probably do not exceed 46° C. one second after the Laser burst" and thought the decay in temperature was much slower than that after the use of red hot cautery—one minute as opposed to five to ten seconds. They had had experience with the use of laser for hemostasis, and for the destruction of vascular skin lesions but were not reporting on that now.

Discussion

Captain Martin S. Litwin, of Washington, D.C., said that "The U.S. Army Medical Research and Development Command first became interested in the biological effects of laser radiation in 1961, shortly after its discovery", largely because of its uses in "ranging and communications". Laser presented a potential hazard to personnel. He pointed out the hazards of lasers to the skin, and stressed that the skin was not an effective protective barrier against deeper laser irradiation, showing instances of brain, liver, and intestinal injury. John P. Minton, of Bethesda, mentioned ruby and neodymium laser radiation effect upon a mouse meloma under study at the Surgery Branch at the National Cancer Institute stating that "both these sources of radiation are capable of permanently destroying this particular tumor system." Effect was immediate and if the tumor was "not completely and totally destroyed by the immediate effect of the laser radiation, it will eventually regrow and kill the animal", although McGuff had said that the effect of the laser lasted for some time. They had developed a theory which related tumor destruction "to the size of the tumor, the amount of laser radiation delivered to the tumor, the particular wave length of that laser, and the laser energy absorption capability of a particular tumor system." R. K. Gilchrist, of Chicago, said that as he understood it, the application of a 2 mm. beam made a much larger tumor disappear, "Now, these are straight beams. They do not diffuse at all. I do not know whether they diffuse after tissue is struck —or very much—but I would judge not. If this is so, some other thing than the direct, linear effect must be the cause of the death of this tissue." He asked whether the effect of the tumor was not an almost instantaneous thrombosis or vascular spasm. Had they more precisely measured the heat produced? McGuff, closing, said that with very fast thermocouples they had recorded "temperatures immediately upon laser impact of about 700° F." Microcirculation studies failed to show any interference with the blood flow in the tumor for two days after the laser burst exposure.

The Business Meetings

The 1964 meeting was held April 1, 2, and 3, at The Homestead, Hot Springs, Virginia, President Warfield M. Firor in the Chair. [The long and philosophical Presidential Address, in a tour de force of platform oratory, was faultlessly given entirely without manuscript or notes.]

Secretary Altemeier informed the Membership that at the winter Council meeting there had been discussion "regarding the advisability of inviting wives of the members and distinguished guests to the reception and banquet . . . after further deliberation, the Council has recommended that the wives be included again this year at the annual reception and banquet. With your indulgence, the Committee on Local Arrangements was instructed to proceed with the arrangements on this basis for the annual reception and banquet on Thursday evening." Secretary Altemeier informed the membership that the reproductions of the membership book had been distributed and the original deposited in the National Library of Medicine in accordance with Council action taken December 9, 1963.

Council did recommend the increase of membership from 250 to 300, yearly increments to be made at the rate of not more than ten per year, in accordance with the resolution made by Dr. Dunphy in the year before, and "held over for one year, and will be voted upon this morning in order to activate it if it is passed" [so that a larger slate of new members could be elected at the Second Executive Session].

John A. Schilling reported for the Program Committee that they had received 134 abstracts of which 33 had been accepted for the program.

Champ Lyons, reporting for the Advisory Membership Committee, said that J. E. Dunphy's Presidential Address "stimulated the nomination of several senior surgeons with great clinical competency and a few younger surgeons doing outstanding jobs in smaller community hospitals . . . A total of 28 candidates was favorably recommended and action was deferred on 12. Favorable action was recommended for one-half the candidates being consid-

ered for the first time, one-third of the candidates for the second time, and one-fourth the candidates for the third time. Another 20 candidates were believed to be alternatively acceptable for membership and only 10 were considered as unlikely to become important contributors to the annual meeting."

At the Second Executive Session, Dr. Oliver Cope rose "on behalf of your last five past Presidents to suggest and move a change in the By-Laws. The amendment is to include the Vice-Presidents as members of Council." That was moved and accepted and was to lie over for a year. [This obviously replaced the amendment proposed by Dunphy the previous year, and now conveniently ignored by Council, that there be a President-Elect, and had the effect in the interest of "continuity" of informing the Vice-President of the "functioning and actions of Council if he were called upon to assume the Presidency."]

Council recommended that an ad hoc committee be appointed each year "to advise Council regarding Honorary Members . . ." and finally the Council did recommend "That the President appoint an *ad hoc* Committee on medical education for a minimum of two or three years and, subject to annual continuing rotation, to study the present and future place of surgery in the medical curriculum." The recommendations of Councill were accepted.

Henry T. Bahnson was appointed Chairman of the ad hoc committee to advise the Council and Advisory Membership Committee on Honorary Members, and Oliver Cope, Chairman of the ad hoc Committee on Medical Education.

Among the new members elected were Wiley F. Barker, John Earle Connolly, Theodore Drapanas, Johann L. Ehrenhaft, Colin C. Ferguson, Albert Starr, and George D. Zuidema. Francis M. Massie, a distinguished and highly respected general surgeon of Lexington, Kentucky, and Walter P. Blount, of Milwaukee, known for his hip nailing technique, were elected directly to Senior Membership, the first "senior surgeons with great clinical competency" elected in accordannce with the Dunphy proposal. Elected to Honorary Membership were David H. Patey and Harold Clifford Edwards, of London.

Officers elected were Robert M. Zollinger, of Columbus, Ohio, President; Vice-Presidents, Clarence E. Gardner, Jr., of Durham, North Carolina, and Louis M. Rousselot, of New York; Secretary, Harris B. Shumacker, of Indianapolis.

LXXXIII

1965

The 1965 meeting was held at the Bellevue Stratford Hotel, Philadelphia, May 12, 13, and 14, Robert M. Zollinger, of Columbus, Professor and Chairman, Department of Surgery, Ohio State University College of Medicine, in the Chair. The previous year had seen the death, among others, of Alfred Blalock, who had been President in 1956, and whose contributions to shock and to cardiac surgery had been of such importance. Blalock's close friend, Frederick A. Coller, of Michigan, President in 1944, also died in that year.

The Presidential Address, *The Senior Surgeon's Responsibility,* emphasized the teaching of surgery in the medical schools at a time when there was a move among many to "think of surgery as a purely mechanical art and downgrade its importance in the medical school." He spoke of graduate training, of the changed role of the emergency room which had "assumed the role of general practitioners at night, on weekends and holidays", at considerable length about the training of operating room nurses. He noted the progressively infrequent appearance of contributions from the specialties to the program. Considering these and various other matters of the American Surgical Association, he proposed "that a permanent policy committee be established to press on with the task of translating our ideas into action. Assignment to this committee would imply qualifications of great merit. I would charge its members to bring important issues to this annual meeting for open discussion leading toward solutions." [This appears to have been the second suggestion for the formation of what ultimately (1974) came to be called the very important Committee on Issues, the first suggestion having been made as a motion from the floor by Walter Maddock in 1960.]

* * *

Ben Eiseman, of Lexington, Chairman and Professor, Department of Surgery, University of Kentucky, and by invitation, D. S. Liem and F. Raffucci, *Heterologous Liver Perfusion in Treatment of Hepatic Failure,* started with the argument that the "regenerative capacity of the liver provided the rationale for temporary support of the patient in reversible hepatic failure" and that the "metabolic complexity of the liver makes it unlikely that attempts to eradicate only a single 'toxic' product of liver failure would meet with much lasting clinical success. In all likelihood, only another normal liver can adequately substitute for one that has failed." In pigs they had demonstrated systematically that the excised pig liver, washed free of pig blood, functioned well infused with human blood whether through the hepatic artery and portal vein or the portal vein alone. Such an explanted liver cleared ammonia and bilirubin effectively even when exposed to high concentrations for long periods of time. Studies of BSP, Rose Bengal, and galactose excretion, and oxygen utilization, all showed physiologic function of the explanted liver. They now reported experience with eight patients with terminal liver failure treated by perfusion of their blood through an extracorporeal pig liver. The patients were all thought to have a hopeless prognosis and all but one were in terminal coma following esophageal bleeding and alcoholic cirrhosis. One patient had been comatose for 14 days with viral hepatitis. One patient was perfused twice, one patient perfused three times. A variety of perfusion techniques were employed with and without oxygenators, and with and without heat exchangers. Since the pig liver, emptied of blood, had a considerable capacity, the patients were given a transfusion of 500 cc. at the start. The use of systemic heparin created bleeding problems which were thought to be solved by the introduction of small amounts of heparin into the arterial blood as it emerged from the patient into the system. Pulsatile blood flow was thought to be associated with the best production of bile from the pig liver in the circuit. All of the patients showed some response in mental state. Five awakened sufficiently to respond to spoken commands. The patient with viral hepatitis, who had been totally unreactive for ten days, "began to respond within 15 minutes after the start of perfusion and was speaking coherently at the end of the 6-hour perfusion." The results lasted, at best, only a few days and in the most striking case, the patient with hepatitis was "coherent for 4 days after perfusion and then began a gradual deterioration that ended in death on the eighth post-perfusion day." None of the patients survived although "The seventh patient was eating and talking and appeared to be recovering from his liver failure 5 days after the first pig liver perfusion when he suddenly had a torrential hemorrhage from his esophageal varices" and ultimately died. Subsequent studies had shown that a calf liver would function as well as a pig liver when perfused with human blood, that a dog liver would not. The perfused liver did not synthesize gamma globulin but "Carbon tagged glycine and lysine both appeared in the albumin fraction of protein emerging from the perfused liver . . . it is assumed that such a protein carries the pig genetic code", raising the possibility that this might be antigenic and result in sensitization to pig protein. No sensitivity reaction occurred in either the original or subsequent perfusions although the patients were all profoundly ill and the longest interval between the first and last perfusion was no more than 10 days. Eiseman suggested the possibility that the technique might become useful in ". . . the cirrhotic with marginal liver reserve who has suffered an acute overpowering metabolic insult, but who might recover if he could survive the initial episode of coma . . . a patient comatose with acute viral hepatitis or acute toxic hepatitis with a potentially reversible hepatic lesion . . . a patient immediately prior to or following homograft replacement of an irreversibly damaged or diseased liver . . . the heter-ologous extracorporeal liver could function as a temporary support much as the artificial kidney or peritoneal dialysis supports patients undergoing kidney homotransplantation."

Discussion

Lloyd M. Nyhus, of Seattle, agreed "that these animal livers, used in perfusion technics, will clear by-products of metabolic processes . . ." They were interested in the nature of the protein produced by such livers and had perfused calf livers with human blood for six-and-a-half hours and showed by immuno-electrophoresis the production of new calf protein. The same was true of the circulation through a pig liver. In dogs perfused with bovine livers, very much as Eiseman had perfused patients with dog livers, they had challenged the animals days later with intravenous bovine plasma. One dog at 11 days died of anaphylactic reaction, one at 35 days had no reaction, one at 27 days recovered after an anaphylactic response, another had no reaction. One died of unknown causes 12 hours after challenge. Eiseman, closing, said that clinical trials were in progress and that "we are assisting four centers besides our own in Lexington to carry on these temporary heterologous liver perfusions."

* * *

Hermes C. Grillo, by invitation, from the Harvard Medical School, Department of Surgery at the Massachusetts General Hospital, Boston, *Circumferential Resection and Reconstruction of the Mediastinal and Cervical Trachea,* presented the successful results of resection and anastomosis of the intrathoracic trachea in four patients, and described a new technique for reconstruction of the cervical trachea. In the mediastinum it had been found by extensive cadaver dissections that "Over one half of the trachea (6.4 cm., 13 rings) was found to be removable." Full mobilization of the right hilum and division of the inferior pulmonary ligament could overcome a gap of 3 cm. If the left main bronchus were divided and brought above the aortic arch and implanted in the bronchus intermedius, another 2.7 cm. could be added. Dissection of the pulmonary vessels from the pericardium added 0.9 cm. One could thus overcome a gap of 5.7 to 10 cm.,- 11 to 18 rings. The measured tension produced was well below that required to disrupt the tracheal anastomoses in dogs. In their four patients, end-to-end anastomoses were done with success without the necessity for tracheostomy. His new technique for the cervical trachea developed in dogs and applied successfully in one patient is re-

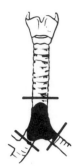 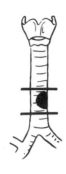 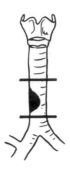 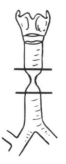

FIG. 2. Diagram of location of lesions and resection in Cases 1–4. See Table 1.

The four lesions treated by resection and anastomosis were from left to right cylindroma, squamous papilloma, squamous carcinoma, and cicatricial stenosis. All patients did well, no tracheostomies were required. The lengths of resected trachea, measured "from resected specimens, after shrinkage" were 4, 3, 3.5, and 2 cm.

Hermes C. Grillo, *Circumferential Resection and Reconstruction of the Mediastinal and Cervical Trachea*, Vol. LXXXIII, 1965.

markably reminiscent of the Wookey procedure for reconstruction of the cervical esophagus. The principal addition being the insertion of plastic rings to support the new trachea.

Discussion

James R. Cantrell, of Seattle, emphasized the increasing rigidity and loss of elasticity of the trachea with age and in his cadaver studies had found that "in individuals over 80 years of age, primary suture could not be accomplished after resection of even a single ring." Lyman A. Brewer, of Los Angeles, said that he had performed 21 tracheal resections, most of them involving only a ring or two, but six of them major, such as Grillo had described, employing moderate hypothermia "which tides the patients over those periods of hypoxia when the endotracheal tube is disconnected and the prosthesis is being sealed" and reinforcing the tracheal suture line with a pedicled pericardial fat graft. He reported a success with tracheal replacement with stainless steel mesh covered by fascia, and a failure with stainless steel mesh and Marlex. Grillo, closing, expressed appreciation of Cantrell's "experiments and measurements of tension in the experimental laboratory" and in mobilization of the trachea in the autopsy room. He indicated that patches of any kind tended to contract and to be replaced by scar. He had been pleased to find that the patient could clear his secre-

tions through the skin-lined reconstructed cervical trachea. "In the upper trachea the secretions are mobilized to that point by the usual mechanism and then cleared very easily with a cough."

* * *

Twenty-one years after Cameron Haight's discussion on atresia of the esophagus before the Association, C. Everett Koop, Surgeon-in-Chief, The Children's Hospital of Philadelphia; Professor of Pediatric Surgery, School of Medicine, University of Pennsylvania and by invitation, James P. Hamilton, *Atresia of the Esophagus:* Increased Survival with Staged Procedures in the Poor-Risk Infant, were able to say that "In the last 5 years, primary end-to-end anastomosis of the esophagus for atresia has resulted in a 92 per cent operative survival in a full-term baby, with no associated severe anomaly and without severe pneumonia. Yet the same procedure carried out in a premature or critically ill baby resulted in only a 38 per cent survival." The original approach to the problem before Haight's success, had, of course, always been staged and in 1962, Holder, McDonald, and Woolley had stimulated a new interest in staged procedures for the poor risk infants with esophageal atresia. Koop's earlier experiences with staging had all been with cervical esophagostomy which required reconstruction of the esophagus, usually with colon. The present staged

Grillo's experimentally elaborated technique for reconstruction of the cervical trachea, was successfully applied to ▶ one patient. The technique is remarkably reminiscent of Wookey's technique for reconstruction of the pharynx after cervical esophagectomy, the principal addition being the insertion of plastic rings to support the "trachea". Grillo's patient required resection of the trachea for involvement by carcinoma of the thyroid.

Hermes C. Grillo, *Circumferential Resection and Reconstruction of the Mediastinal and Cervical Trachea*, Vol. LXXXIII, 1965.

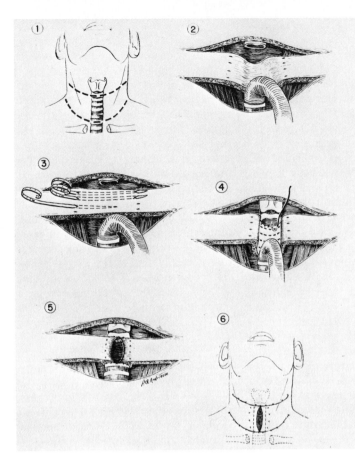

FIG. 8. Cervical tracheal reconstruction. Operative Technic. Stage I: (1) The incisions create a bilaterally pedicled flap of skin and platysma. (2) The trachea has been resected, the distal end intubated and the flap lies in the tracheal bed. (3) The ring-carrying needles are being inserted in the flap concurrently, through small lateral slits. (4) After placement of the rings between dermis and platysma, the outer layer of sutures has been inserted to form the posterior portion of the upper anastomosis and the posterior inner layer is being completed. The outer layer joins outer tracheal wall and platysma, the inner joins trachea and skin. (5) The upper and lower anastomoses have been completed, creating a longitudinal stoma. (6) Completion of the first stage by closure of the transverse incisions.

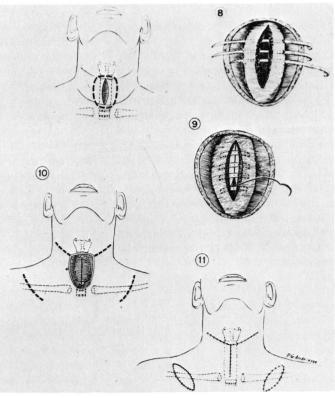

FIG. 8. Stage II. (7) The stoma is circumcised through skin and platysma. (8) The skin and platysma within the circular incision have been infolded. Additional segments of plastic rings are being added between dermis and platysma to supply more anterior support. (9) The internal skin tube is completed with a continuous subcuticular suture. (10) Platysma has been sutured over the rings. (11) Relaxation to permit midline closure of lateral platysma and skin over the reconstruction is permitted by incisions laterally over the clavicles. The resulting defects are surfaced with split thickness grafts. No tracheostomy tube is required.

1203

procedure involved a transpleural approach with division of the fistula, suturing the tracheal end closed, and tacking the closed esophageal end high onto the posterior chest wall. A gastrostomy was performed at the same time. The pharynx was kept empty by continuous suction with a sump catheter. There were now nine patients. One died of what was said to be an anaphylactic shock from penicillin, one died of respiratory compression of the trachea by a large pulmonary artery aneurysm, one, with a large ventricular septal defect, died from heart failure, one died of a recanalized fistula after esophageal anastomosis in the final stage. Four were living and well with end-to-end anastomosis of the esophagus, and one with intrathoracic colon transplant. Of 23 patients in their earlier group who had had a cervical esophagostomy and division of the tracheoesophageal fistula and gastrostomy in the first stage, 13 died before colon transplants could be carried out, nine of them of irremediable causes and four of them of preventable causes. All ten of the patients who had a colon transplant survived. Koop considered "staged procedures having much to offer those patients who have had such a low survival with a conventional approach." [It was not emphasized that these were consecutive and not simultaneous series, that the numbers involved were small, and smaller still when the deaths due to "other" causes were excluded.]

Discussion

Frank Allbritten, of Kansas City, reported for Holder, now at Kansas City, who had originated the staging method when in Boston. He thought there was general agreement that staging was indicated when there was atresia without a fistula, and in the premature infant. He performed immediate gastrostomy under local anesthesia, and 24 hours later retropleural division of the tracheo-esophageal fistula, under local anesthesia. The ultimate esophagoesophagostomy was transpleural, under general anesthesia. They now realized that lusty vigorous prematures could tolerate a primary repair. They had operated upon four infants four to five pounds in weight by primary repair with survival in all, had had five deaths in 15 treated by the staged approach at the same weight and lost two of four critically ill full-term infants who were staged, all as the result of associated anomalies. Harris B. Shumacker, of Indianapolis, said that since 1950, he and Battersby had had 178 consecutive patients with esophageal atresia. Patients over seven pounds in weight had had a survival rate of 88%, those from five to seven

pounds, 55 to 60%, and those from four to five pounds, 31%. W. H. Snyder, of Los Angeles, reiterated the importance of staging in ill or premature babies and in those with blind, widely separated esophageal segments. In the latter, they had twice applied the technique of Russell Howard, of Melbourne, Australia, of progressive stretching of the proximal segment by a mercury weighted catheter feeding the child by gastrostomy until, in both cases, it was possible to do a successful primary esophageal anastomosis. J. P. Hamilton, in closing, said that they had not used Howard's technique which they understood he had now used in eight cases. Hamilton now added in his recommendation for staging that not only should the fistula be divided but ". . . the aortic branches to the esophagus should be divided so that the collateral circulation to the distal esophagus can take over."

* * *

The problem which continues, in resolving the sometimes striking difference between results of treatment at the Veterans Administration Hospitals and those in other institutions was apparent from the presentation by Ralph F. Bowers, of Memphis, Chief of Surgery, Veterans Administration, Medical Teaching Group; Chief of Surgical Service, Kennedy VA Hospital, *Hyperthyroidism:* Comparative Results of Medical (I^{131}) and Surgical Therapy. [The paper also perhaps suggests the lament of the surgeon over the possible passage of another interesting lesion from the operative domain.] There were in all 102 patients treated by operation and 81 treated with the radioisotope. In the 102 operations, there were no deaths, there were two unilateral nerve injuries, one patient required re-exploration for hemorrhage. One patient developed transient hypoparathyroidism and two developed permanent hypoparathyroidism, in one resulting in death 11 years later. There were no infections and no hyperthyroid crises, and no permanent nerve injuries in the last 15 years. They administered dosages of I^{131} of one to 16 millicuries "to achieve euthyroidism without inducing a deep myxedemic state." The small dosages of I^{131} resulted in multiple admissions and delays in resolution of the hyperthyroidism, so that operated patients reached euthyroidism in 42 days, the I^{131} patients in 453 days with an even more dramatic picture in the thyrocardiacs. The surgical patients averaged 1.6 hospitalizations, the medical patients 5.0. There was recurrent hyperthyroidism in 5.8% of those operated upon and none in those treated with I^{131}. Myxedema occurred in ten patients after operation. Bowers anticipated that myxedema might occur after irradiation but with the small doses they had been employing they had apparently not yet seen myxedema. He concluded that "I^{131} therapy has proved to be exceedingly satisfactory in the mild hyperthyroid patient with diffuse toxic goiter", and superior to operation for malignant exophthalmos. "Operation appears to be more satisfactory in younger patients with moderate-to-severe toxicity in the diffuse toxic goiter." The rapid resolution of hyperthyroidism by operation was established, and this was preferable in the thyrocardiac patients. I^{131} therapy was probably preferable for the previously operated goiter with recurrence of hyperthyroidism. Bowers pointed up the problem that the decrease in frequency of thyroid operations was producing a generation of surgeons who had had relatively little experience in thyroid surgery and might have particular difficulty in operating for toxic goiter.

Discussion

George Crile, Jr. of Cleveland, commented that "everything that Dr. Bowers has said is true in the world that he lives in, but it bears absolutely no relationship to the world I live in." At Cleveland, the patients receiving I^{131} were treated as outpatients, so that there was no hospitalization at all and the average hospitalization for an operated patient in Cleveland was four days as opposed to Bowers' 52 [Bowers had said the patients became euthyroid in 42 days]. They used seven millicuries at a single dose, 70% of the patients were well within two months, most of the rest after a second treatment and the duration till cure averaged 89 days. He emphasized the gravity of even a low incidence of layrngeal nerve palsy or hypoparathyroidism. From operation, he said, "You can take your choice whether you want to have a high incidence of recurrent hyperthyroidism or a high incidence of hypothyroidism. You cannot get a perfect balance". They had now treated some 3,000 patients with radioactive iodine and apart from some patients with nodular goiter, he had not seen a patient "whose hyperthyroidism could not be controlled with radioactive iodine." Bentley P. Colcock, of Boston [the Lahey Clinic], supported Bowers and disagreed with Crile, ". . . we believe that for most of these patients—with the exception of those over 45 years of age and those with recurrent hyperthyroidism—thyroid surgery is the best treatment. In the last 8 years we have operated upon more than 500 patients with hyperthyroidism. There has been no mortality, no persistent tetany, and no persistent hoarseness. The incidence of myxedema is 8 per cent, which is about what Dr. Bowers found." The Massachusetts General experi-

ence, as Cope pointed out [Oliver Cope's discussion is referred to by other discussers but does not appear in the *Transactions*], indicated that the incidence of hypothyroidism or myxedema after radioactive iodine treatment was some 30%. Benjamin F. Byrd, Jr., of Nashville, supported the view that there were special indications for the use of operative therapy, referring to a series of 35 patients under 20 years of age treated operatively for hyperthyroidism, prepared for operation with iodine alone or iodine and one of the thiourea drugs. The complications "were negligible" and the children were "cured" in four days. Allen Boyden, of Portland, Oregon, quoted his series, indicating an 8% mortality for thyrocardiacs undergoing I^{131} therapy and was the only discusser to stress the progressive appearance of hypothyroidism and myxedema after I^{131} therapy,- 7.5% hypothyroidism during the first year and an increment of 3 to 5% in succeeding years, the expectation being that the ultimate incidence would be 50%. "This means that all patients treated with I^{131} must be followed regularly throughout their lifetime if the serious complication of myxedema is to be prevented." Bowers, closing, claimed that experience had shown that myxedema occurring after irradiation was more difficult to control than myxedema occurring after operation, and that irradiation myxedema was particularly dangerous to the thyrocardiacs. Of the deaths of thyrocardiacs under I^{131} therapy, which Boyden had referred to, Bowers said ". . . When a person dies from a surgical operation, that is obvious . . . when a medical man or any of us digitalize a patient and the digitalis goes wrong and the patient dies, they say he died of heart disease. They never say he died from the digitalis."

* * *

H. William Scott, Jr., of Nashville, Professor of Surgery and Head of the Department of Surgery, Vanderbilt University School of Medicine; John H. Foster, Associate Professor of Surgery, Vanderbilt University School of Medicine, and by invitation, Grant Liddle and Eugene T. Davidson, *Cushing's Syndrome Due to Adrenocortical Tumor:* 11-year Review of 15 patients, had in the same 11-year period seen "more than 50 patients with Cushing's disease due to overproduction of ACTH by the pituitary and bilateral adrenal hyperplasia . . ." The youngest of their 15 patients was nine months of age, the oldest 63, and three of the patients were males. One of the patients did not have central obesity, two of the patients did not have hypertension, two patients did not have impaired glucose tolerance and three patients showed no mental aberrations. Each of the other manifestations of the syndrome was absent in even more of the patients, so that "precise studies of adrenocortical function were often required to establish the diagnosis." They made the precise diagnosis of Cushing's syndrome, rather than Cushing's disease with bilateral adrenal hyperplasia, in every patient and accurately predicted that three of the tumors were carcinomas. Elevation of 17 hydroxy-corticosteroids in the urine and the ratio of 17-OHCS to the quantity of creatinine in the urine were the most practical indices of cortisol secretion. Dexamethasone in the normal individual suppressed ACTH secretion by the pituitary and caused a sharp drop in the urinary secretion of 17-OHCS. In patients with Cushing's syndrome due to an adreno-cortical tumor, dexamethasone in either small or large doses failed to cause suppression of urinary 17-OHCS output. In patients with adrenocortical hyperplasia, a large dose of dexamethasone decreased the urinary output of 17-OHCS. Metopirone, which blocked 11-beta hydroxylation in the adrenal cortex caused an increased output of urinary 17-OHCS in patients with pituitary-dependent adrenocortical hyperplasia, but not in those with adrenocortical tumor [nor in those with "the ectopic ACTH syndrome",- "bilateral adrenal cortical hyperplasia induced by a nonendocrine tumor (certain carcinomas of the lung, pancreas, etc.) "]. After trying the transabdominal approach, Scott had come to prefer the posterior retroperitoneal approach performed through the bed of the eleventh rib, bilaterally. In six cases, the intravenous pyelogram localized the tumor; in two cases, the tumor was large enough to be felt. In seven cases, a retroperitoneal pneumogram demonstrated the tumor. Aortography was applied successfully in one patient [its use not otherwise mentioned]. Of three patients, whose tumors could not be localized, one had bilateral tumors. The tumor was successfully removed in 14 of the 15 patients. An 11-year-old child died after an attempted removal of "a massive right adrenal carcinoma which involved the kidney, liver, inferior vena cava, aorta and retroperitoneal lymph nodes." Since the remaining adrenal had been suppressed because of the cortisol production by the autonomous tumor, the patients were treated with substitution therapy for periods of time ranging from a few days to one to two months and with a brief course of ACTH after operation. Twelve of the patients were very well after operation including two other patients with adrenal carcinoma. One patient died suddenly at home two-and-a-half months after operation, and one patient died of intestinal obstruction 17 months after operation. In general, the regression of the syndrome was rapid and complete.

Discussion

John W. Raker, of Boston, said that the dexamethasone suppression test had not been completely reliable in their experience at the Massachusetts General Hospital, neither had the Metopirone suppression test. They tended to rely on the ACTH stimulation test and the measurement of plasma cortisol, and the measurement of ACTH in plasma, "which Dr. Scott's colleague, Dr. Liddle, has developed so beautifully . . ." They preferred a transabdominal incision unless the evidence for unilateral tumor was good, in which case, they performed a lumbar incision, and for a large tumor, a transdiaphragmatic approach through the bed of the tenth rib. He stressed the danger, and the increased likelihood of, infection in the Cushing's syndrome patients. Frank Glenn, of New York, said that they had had 19 adenomas in a total of 66 patients with the Cushing's clinical picture. Four of the tumors were malignant, and they had one patient with bilateral tumors. He had observed that rapid advance of symptoms suggested either a large benign tumor or carcinoma. Four of their patients with adenomas also had tumors of the pituitary. James T. Priestley, of Rochester, Minnesota, said that they ordinarily employed the dexamethasone and Metopirone tests but not ACTH stimulation. After operation, they did not employ ACTH, giving only cortisone, in gradually decreasing doses. They had employed tomography but not retroperitoneal insufflation. Mark A. Hayes, of New Haven, said that of their patients, "One third has either unsuspected contralateral disease, or unlocalizable unilateral disease; and two-thirds have obvious bilateral disease . . . this makes the simultaneous exposure of both adrenals absolutely mandatory at the time of the operative procedure" and in the obese Cushing's patients this was more easily obtained from behind. Willard E. Goodwin, of Los Angeles, agreed that the posterior retroperitoneal approach was "by far the simplest, most direct, and most comfortable for both the patient and the surgeon." W. Eugene Stern, of Los Angeles, said that at UCLA they had had 15 patients with adenomas or carcinomas of the adrenal, none of whom had had an associated pituitary tumor. In 34 patients with adrenal hyperplasia, however, they had found three chromophobe adenomas, and two of these were secreting tumors. The dexamethasone test was not completely reliable and he cited several patients with pituitary tumors and adrenal hyperplasia in which it had failed. Could it be that in the small group of "adrenal adenomas or carcinomas which do not fulfill all the endocrinologic criteria of resistance to the ACTH suppression tests and so on . . . pituitary adenomas may be found and require therapy . . ." John H. Foster, closing, said that infection had not been a problem in their patients, that the dexamethasone suppression test and the ACTH stimulation test had given "rather consistent results" and the ability to determine plasma ACTH levels had improved their accuracy still further. None of their patients with Cushing's disease and hyperplasia of the adrenals had pituitary tumors. They used ACTH postoperatively for two to three months and were pleased with its effect. They did, indeed prefer the bilateral approach, employing two teams, operating simultaneously.

* * *

William J. Fry, by invitation, and Charles G. Child, III, of Ann Arbor, Professor of Surgery and Chairman of the Department, University of Michigan Medical Center, *Ninety-five Per Cent Distal Pancreatectomy for Chronic Pancreatitis,* reported their experience with 25 patients over the previous 10 years. They had been led to this approach because they had been "unable to reproduce the good results of sphincterotomy as reported by some investigators [Doubilet and Mulholland]", and because in intra-operative injections of the pancreatic duct, "Repeatedly pancreatic ductal obstruction was demonstrated within 2 to 3 cm. of the ampulla of Vater . . . we questioned the usefulness of sphincterotomy under these conditions and wondered how destruction of the sphincter of Oddi could be expected to promote pancreatic drainage in the presence of an obstructed duct." In 20 patients, they had performed 95% distal pancreatectomy with no operative deaths, 13 excellent results, five good results, and two poor results. They had in the same period performed five pancreaticoduodenectomies with one operative death from septicemia, one patient well at four years, two patients alive at four years, who had had a stricture of the common duct reoperated upon, and one patient alive at four years, but a hopeless narcotic addict. The magnitude of the operation of pancreato-duodenectomy and the complications suggested to them that 95% distal pancreatectomy was a superior procedure ". . . the spleen, the tail, the body and the uncinate process of the pancreas are removed completely. A small cuff of the head of the pancreas is preserved. This lines the lesser curvature of the duodenum and is estimated to be no more than 5 per cent of the entire gland. In addition to retaining some small portion of partially functioning pancreas, the cuff helps protect the superior and inferior pancreatico-duodenal arteries and the common duct from injury during the course of operation" and neither recurring attacks of pancreatitis nor pancreatic fistula had resulted. In their 95% pancreatectomies, they had not injured the common duct in any patient. The principal difficulty was "Irresponsibility in managing their diabetes and exocrine insufficiency . . . in only a very few patients." They had not found patients with obstruction of the pancreatic duct at a single point in whom distal pancreatectomy might drain the tail and sphincterotomy drain the head.

Discussion

Charles B. Puestow, of Chicago, said that in his studies, ". . .pancreatograms in chronic pancreatitis revealed a long proximal stricture of the main pancreatic duct, and intervening strictures throughout the balance of the duct, with dilated pockets between them. We found partial or complete ductal obstruction in nearly all of our patients. It has been our belief that all obstructive pockets would have to be drained into the gastrointestinal tract to relieve the patient's pain and pancreatic insufficiency . . . we split the pancreas longitudinally throughout almost its entire length and then anastomosed the pancreas to a defunctionalized limb of jejunum . . . in approximately 100 patients. In nearly 75 per cent, the results have been highly satisfactory." Fifteen percent of the patients showed an improvement and 10% had unsatisfactory results, continued to have pain, extensive calcification, were narcotic addicts, "I believe this group might be candidates for a 95 per cent pancreatectomy." He had had a single operative death. William S. McCune, of Washington, D.C., had had some successes with the operations of Puestow, DuVal, Bowers, and in four patients had performed total pancreatectomy, "All of our patients have been free from pain. We have had no problems of insulin coverage of their diabetes. We have had some problems with weight loss, but by the use of adequate pancreatic enzymes, these can usually be controlled." He thought that total pancreatectomy,- or 95% pancreatectomy would find increasing employment.

* * *

Two papers on gastric bleeding followed. Irving F. Enquist, by invitation, Karl E. Karlson, of Brooklyn, Professor of Surgery, Downstate Medical Center, Kings County Hospital; Clarence Dennis, Professor and Chairman of Department of Surgery, State University, New York College of Medicine at New York City, and by invitation, S. M. Fierst and

G. W. Shaftan, *Statistically Valid Ten-Year Comparative Evaluation of Three Methods of Management of Massive Gastroduodenal Hemorrhage,* reported the continuation of the studies which they had presented before the Association previously [1958, Vol. LXXVI], placing patients into three groups, *"Pattern I. The Nonoperative Pattern* . . . The method of A.F.R. Andresen and later adopted with slight modifications by Meulengracht . . . *Pattern II. The Immediately Operative Pattern* . . . The method of J. D. Stewart, consisting of rapid transfusion and prompt gastrectomy" and *"Pattern III. The Selectively Operative Pattern* . . . The method of Hoerr, Dunphy and Gray [1948], according to which operation was reserved for patients who failed to maintain stable vital signs during transfusion at a maximum arbitrary rate of one unit per 8-hour period [after restitution with a maximum of 1,500 ml. of blood]." Patients 50 years of age or older were all treated by Pattern III until June, 1958, when the factor of age was disregarded. Beginning in July, 1961, ". . . because of our medical colleagues' disillusionment with the Andresen nonoperative pattern, no patient was admitted to Pattern I. All were assigned in random manner to Patterns II and III." They had 121 patients in the nonoperative group, 133 in the immediate operation group, and 149 in the selective operation group, of whom 100 did not require operation. They found no differences in mortality rate among the three patterns of management, nor was there any when the age of the patients was taken into consideration. In all three patterns, advancing age was accompanied by increasing mortality rates. The mortality in the 1958 report had been 14%; the mortality now, 16.8%, was not significantly different. They had still been unable to conduct a satisfactory follow-up study, but knew "that several of the patients who were treated nonoperatively and ceased to bleed, died following the gastrectomy on subsequent admissions—a hazard not faced by patients treated by gastrectomy on the initial admission." The bleeding was from all of the usual conditions, but even "If consideration is focussed on patients with proved peptic ulcer disease, the mortality rates in the three patterns of therapy are statistically identical."

* * *

Raymond C. Read, H. C. Huebl, by invitation, and Alan P. Thal, of Detroit, Penberthy Professor of Surgery, and Chairman, Department of Surgery, Wayne State University College of Medicine, *Randomized Study of Massive Bleeding from Peptic Ulceration.* The patients were either operated upon immediately or an attempt was made to carry them

without operation. The operation was an anterior pylorotomy and gastrotomy, if necessary, the ulcer base obliterated with deep mattress sutures. In an occasional case, the major feeding vessel was ligated outside the stomach, and in most patients vagotomy and Heineke-Mikulicz pyloroplasty were performed. There were 41 patients in the immediate surgery group, 39 patients in the control group. An attempt had been made to eliminate patients with varices, gastritis or neoplasm and in fact, of the 41 immediately operated upon, 33 had ulcer disease and the four deaths were in patients with "chemical necrosis . . . gastric CA . . . hematobilia . . . varices . . ." In the 39 control patients, nonoperative management successfully controlled the bleeding in only 12 patients, only half of whom turned out to have ulcers, and delayed operation was required in 27 patients, 20 of whom proved to have ulcers. There were six deaths,- four patients with duodenal ulcer, a patient with a gastric ulcer and a patient with a marginal ulcer. The delayed operation was done on an average of 32 hours after admission, after an average transfusion of nine units of blood. They suggested that "if a patient bleeds into shock from peptic ulceration, he will usually require operative intervention to control the bleeding point. There is less morbidity and mortality when operation is performed as soon as possible, at which time local suture, drainage, and where possible, vagotomy have proved to be a satisfactory procedure."

Discussion

John D. Stewart, of Buffalo, opened the Discussion congratulating Dennis and his group on "clinical research of a very high order." His own series now included some 450 patients treated by "a standard two-thirds gastric resection with antecolic Hofmeister anastomosis". In patients under 50, the mortality was 3%, but two-thirds of the patients had been over 50 and the total mortality was 20%. He asked why Group I had been discontinued because of "medical disillusionment" when the results appeared to be as good as in Groups II and III. Mark Ravitch, of Baltimore, said "A surgeon would like to believe that it must be better to arrest bleeding as soon as possible, and that the patient who has bled as little as possible and been transfused as little as possible should offer the best possible operative risk. It has been a great source of disappointment that in the data collected for so many years it has not been possible to show this." He referred in the two reported studies to the "problem they have had in keeping to the protocol, and the numerous subgroups that gradually developed because of the exigencies of the clinical situation." It had been his policy for some years "whenever a complication of ulcer had been treated . . . to cure the ulcer diathesis at the same time" and in the bleeding patients, he had employed pyloroplasty and vagotomy. In 27 duodenal ulcers and an unspecified number of gastric ulcers, one duodenal ulcer rebled and five gastric ulcers rebled despite transfixion of the bleeding vessel at operation, but "none of these patients had to be operated upon for rebleeding; none of them died of hemorrhage." There were two deaths, one from hepatic coma and one from Zollinger-Ellison syndrome, recognized late. Despite a 5% mortality in patients referred late, he said "I think perhaps it still may be true that the quicker we operate on these patients and stop their bleeding, and the fewer transfusions we give them, the better they will do." J. Englebert Dunphy, of San Francisco, said that while Dennis' data showed no statistical difference in the three groups, "when no operation was done *11 patients died of exsanguination* . . . it is by moving these patients who would exsanguinate with no operation into the operative group that we raise the mortality on that side of the ledger . . ." He suggested that Stewart's approach and his own with Stanley Hoerr, were not far apart because the patients who fulfilled Stewart's criteria ". . . are indeed the ones who require large amounts of blood promptly. In our own experience we have been operating earlier and earlier on the patient we think is truly the massive bleeder, namely a patient who is losing a liter or more in a short period of time." They, too, to reduce the magnitude of the operation, had shifted from gastrectomy to pyloroplasty, vagotomy and suture ligation of the bleeding point. Their results with pyloroplasty and vagotomy were 11% mortality, all other operations 25%. In patients over 70 years of age, the figures were 14% and 46%. Jack M. Farris, of Los Angeles, had now treated 57 patients by vagotomy and pyloroplasty "occasionally with ligation or suture of the ulcer base" for duodenal hemorrhage. The 57 patients all conformed to Stewart's criteria. He had had three deaths, one cardiac, one from a stroke, and one from "a new, unrecognized gastric ulcer that could have been saved by operation." Five of their patients had ultimately required late operation for recurrent duodenal ulcer. It was their policy to restore rapidly the patients who came in bleeding and operate upon them promptly. Stanley O. Hoerr, of Cleveland, drew the lesson "from these two excellent studies . . . that patients who bleed seriously enough to be in shock when first seen should be operated upon promptly unless there is some cogent reason not to." Claude E. Welch, of Boston, discussed the safety of the operation and the subsequent course of the patients. So far as concerned safety, he referred to "a report by two of our residents, Drs. Austen and Baue", of 162 consecutive gastrectomies, a third for massive hemorrhage, with an overall mortality of 0.6%. He attributed "all of their success" to the "wide use of catheter duodenostomy, which was employed in almost 25% of these patients." As for the second factor, the ultimate course, a study made seven years after patients came into the hospital with massive hemorrhage showed that 29% of them bled again, three of them died. Fourteen percent of patients who had had the operation seven years before had bled again but none had died. Owen H. Wangensteen, of Minneapolis, whose long discussion ranged widely, agreed there did not seem to be much choice of treatment judging by the mortality, but he could not see how anyone well enough to take the Andresen diet could really be sick enough to be considered for an emergency operation. He mentioned the use of Pitressin in the control of bleeding from portal hypertension and for other causes, "We have come to administer Pitressin quite regularly to all patients with massive gastric hemorrhage as the first line of defense in the management of such problems. For many patients, administration of Pitressin alone appears to be quite adequate to cope with the problem." Wangensteen referred to his gastric cooling and gastric freezing, mentioning that "In all such endeavors there emerges the price of the learning process. In one's enthusiasm, it is easy to overextend use of a helpful device." They now carried cooling up to four hours and then operated if it was not effective in arresting bleeding. So far as general adoption of the technique was concerned, he said that "One of the problems is that many a young surgeon would rather operate than eat and assembling the apparatus and acquiring the skill to implement some time-consuming therapeutic endeavors often strikes him as a lot of unnecessary bother, like taking the patients' temperature or the blood pressure were at one time believed to be." Their mortality for massive gastric hemorrhage was now down to 18%, half what it had been before the use of gastric hypothermia. For bleeding from duodenal and gastric ulcer, their mortality was now 10%. He discussed his continued experience with gastric freezing as a treatment for ulcer, "Our group has shown that in interested and experienced hands gastric freezing can be done as an elective procedure with a low incidence of complications. There has been no hospital mortality in more than 1,000 episodes of elective clinical gastric freezing." Hilger P.

Jenkins, of Chicago, had studied the survival of catgut in gastric juice. Catgut knots would "untie within a period of 6 hours, or even 4 hours, when bathed and incubated in gastric juice . . ." so that if one were suturing an ulcer base, one should use silk. Clarence Dennis, closing, said in reply to Dr. Stewart that they had given up the Andresen regime, because as Dunphy pointed out, 11 patients had died of bleeding. In reply to Dr. Ravitch, he agreed that there had not been a comparison between the mortality rates of those ultimately operated upon in the Andresen group and those promptly operated upon and that should be undertaken. He agreed with Dunphy that pyloroplasty ulcer transfixion and vagotomy might be a better procedure but having begun the study with gastrectomy, they chose to continue the study with gastrectomy. Alan Thal, closing, agreed with Dr. Wangensteen's comments about patients well enough for the Andresen regimen not being patients with massive bleeding and described many of the patients in Dennis' group as "good-risk patients treated nonoperatively". He thought Dennis' reliance on blood volume and red cell mass determinations as criteria of massive hemorrhage not as good as his own cardiac output studies, which in the massive bleeders showed continuing shock and continued bleeding with a low cardiac output and high peripheral resistance, whereas in the patients with Dennis' low red cell mass, there was high cardiac output and low peripheral resistance. He re-emphasized his preference for vagotomy and pyloroplasty with suture of the vessel.

* * *

John W. Kirklin, of Rochester, Minnesota, Surgeon, Mayo Clinic; Associate Professor of Surgery, Mayo Foundation Graduate School; University of Minnesota; Robert B. Wallace, Dwight C. McGoon, and James W. DuShane, by invitation, *Early and Late Results after Intracardiac Repair of Tetralogy of Fallot,* 5-Year Review of 337 Patients, had undertaken open "intracardiac repair . . . for all patients over about 5 years of age. No case was deemed inoperable. A preliminary anastomotic operation was advised only for children less than about 5 years of age who were in urgent need of surgical help; intracardiac repair was then done when they reached the age of 5 to 6 years. Cardiac catheterization and angiocardiography were done only in selected cases." They employed ". . . a median sternotomy incision . . . Cardiopulmonary bypass . . . with a Mayo-Gibbon pump oxygenator, hypothermia to 26 to 30° C. . . . perfusion flow rates of 2.0 to 2.4 L./min./m². . . a single long period . . . of aortic

cross clamping profound cooling of the heart by the perfusate and by external cardiac cooling". Recently the right ventriculotomy had been transverse. If a septal patch was required, it was usually knitted Teflon, occasionally pericardium or Teflon felt. Pulmonary stenosis was relieved from within when possible, but occasionally "an inlay patch (usually of pericardium but sometimes of tightly woven Teflon) was used to widen the outflow tract of the right ventricle, pulmonary valve ring and first portion of the pulmonary artery." The hospital mortality had dropped progressively from 15% to 7% from 1960 through 1964,- as from 1955 through 1959 it had dropped from 50% to 16%. The improvement occurred despite the fact that more severe cases were seen and was attributable to "improvements in operative technic, reduced use of outflow patches, better preservation of myocardial function during the intracardiac procedure, improved hemostasis, use of hemodilution and some improvements in postoperative care." There was no difference in risk in a primary repair or after a previous Blalock anastomosis, but there was a higher risk after a previous Potts anastomosis. There had been no deaths from hemorrhage in the last three years, due "to a greater skill in establishing hemostasis surgically, to a policy of prompt re-exploration (within 6 to 10 hours postoperatively) in patients who bleed considerably through the drainage tubes, and, perhaps, to the use of hemodilution and maintenance of adequate heparin levels during long perfusions." For almost all patients over the age of five years, primary intracardiac repair was recommended and "Because of subtle inadequacies of cardiopulmonary bypass as now done and because of the technical problems of working inside the small heart of infants and small children with tetralogy", a palliative operation was recommended upon them, with open operation at five years, whether they were symptomatic or not. The greater risk of a secondary operation after a Potts operation suggested that the Potts operation be abandoned. The evidence was good that none of the children had pulmonary hypertension except those with a Potts anastomosis, and that pulmonary hypertension did not develop after complete repair of the tetralogy, so that "No evidence has been obtained that the lung is in any way unprepared to receive a full pulmonary blood flow." Permanent heart block had occurred in 1.5% of their cases and the clinical status was excellent in 93% of the patients at long-term follow up. There was no change in cardiothoracic ratio except in some patients with an outflow tract patch, when the ratio was somewhat increased after operation. "More than 90 per cent of patients gave evidence of essentially complete repair of the ventricular septal defect."

Discussion

David C. Sabiston, Jr., now of Durham, North Carolina, commented on 100 patients with tetralogy of Fallot corrected by open operation during the past two years, comparing those who had had a previous Blalock operation with those who had not. Although those patients who had had a previous shunt "had higher hematocrits, more intense cyanosis, and less exercise tolerance than those patients being operated upon for the tetralogy as a primary operation" and were shown by angiocardiography to have more severe malformations, ". . . those patients with a previous subclavian-pulmonary shunt had a *lower* mortality than did the patients who had not had a previous shunt procedure . . . a previous shunt operation does not increase the risk at the time of open correction and may offer certain protection." Frank C. Spencer, of Lexington, Kentucky, was impressed by Kirklin's operative mortality of 7% and the use of outflow patches in only 14% of the patients. He attributed the low mortality to precise operative techniques, to "adequate correction of the anatomic defect . . . avoiding any injury to a coronary artery . . . avoiding coronary air embolism." He interpreted Kirklin's data as meaning that a patch was not necessary if the right ventricular pressure had been reduced to below 60% of the left ventricular pressure. The incidence of heart block, he thought, might be smaller if the operation was performed upon the beating instead of upon the still, arrested heart. ". . . we have not had a permanent heart block in the last 3 years, but on the other hand, our mortality is much higher than Dr. Kirklin's . . ." Frank Gerbode, of San Francisco, commented also on the great improvement in the mortality. His own mortality in the "cyanotic tetralogy" was now 7%. They had gained a better understanding of the variations in the tetralogy. Good myocardial perfusion was important, circulatory arrest produced prolonged myocardial ischemia which damaged the myocardium. They used interrupted aortic occlusion for four-minute periods. Transverse ventriculotomy had practically eliminated right ventricular failure. The use of Dacron patch graft for the ventricular septal defect had eliminated residual shunts and their technique of application avoided the production of heart block. Physiologic monitoring made for more precise after care. Johann L. Ehrenhaft, of Iowa City, had between 140 and 150 operations for total correction of tetralogy of Fallot,

had used right ventricular outflow tract patches only four times, and emphasized "how much ventricular muscle can be resected from the right ventricular outflow tract, thus widening and reconstructing an adequate channel. If this is done rather aggressively but diligently, closure of the right ventricular incision without placing an outflow patch can be carried out without difficulty and with no serious obstruction to the right ventricular outflow tract." Kirklin, closing, agreed that patients with a *functioning* Blalock anastomosis could tolerate operation, but that it was important that the operation be undertaken while the anastomosis was still functioning. He agreed that "operative mortality in all centers has steadily reduced" and now emphasized the prevention of postoperative bleeding, the use of the median sternotomy incision as opposed to the transverse bipleural incision, and preserving myocardial function by whatever means, the use of the transverse ventriculotomy "which Dr. Gerbode and his associates first proposed" and the complete excision of the internal outflow obstruction. In their institution, the greatest improvement in postoperative care had been "the management of blood replacement on the basis of arterial and atrial pressures, rather than on the basis of blood loss . . ." He expressed the indebtedness of all to Dr. Ehrenhaft ". . . because he pointed out, I think, some 3 or 4 or 5 years ago that it was possible in most of these patients to make a complete repair without an outflow patch. Frankly, I did not believe it when he first wrote about it, but I am now in a position of having to support it."

* * *

Donald B. Effler, of Cleveland, Chief Thoracic Surgeon, Cleveland Clinic Foundation, and by invitation, F. Mason Sones, Jr., Rene Favaloro, and Laurence K. Groves, *Coronary Endarterotomy with Patch-Graft Reconstruction:* Clinical Experience with 34 Cases, said that Mason Sones' coronary arteriorgraphy at the Cleveland Clinic in more than 4,000 patients, had demonstrated "that few patients present occlusive disease that is sharply localized to a single segment of the main coronary artery." Nevertheless, occasionally there was a "remarkable localization of coronary atherosclerosis in proximal portions of main coronary arteries that otherwise are within normal, functional limits." They estimated that at that point only 200 patients had survived direct operative approaches to the coronary artery. They avoided endarterectomy and, to obviate dissection in the diseased vessel, dilated the stenotic artery with a small curved urethral sound until back flow occurred and then sutured the coronary artery incision open with a pericardial graft. The operation was performed under total body perfusion and cardiac arrest under regional hypothermia. Three of the 34 patients were also treated with transluminal dilatation of the proximal left coronary artery. There were 18 reconstructions of the right coronary artery, three with associated major cardiac procedures. Two patients died of ventricular arrhythmia and one was resuscitated but not rehabilitated after cardiac arrest from myocardial infarction. The nine operations on the left main coronary artery resulted in four deaths in the operating room and one late death from hepatitis. One of two patients, whose anterior descending branch of the left coronary was operated upon, died in the operating room and the other was not improved. An operation on the circumflex branch of the left coronary resulted in no improvement, and one patient died after an attempt to relieve proximal obstructions in both the right and left coronary arteries. Effler considered "the documented results . . . encouraging," despite the admittedly high mortality. He emphasized the importance of superb angiocardiography. He was enthusiastic about the advantage of transluminal dilatation and patch graft reconstruction. Late catheterizations had shown maintained patency and no aneurysms.

Discussion

Jack A. Cannon, of Los Angeles, rose to defend coronary endarterectomy against Effler's condemnation. His patients all had such extensive disease that it was obvious that if the operation did not help them, they would not survive the operation. [Effler in his presentation, but not in his published paper, had likened endarterectomy to the use of a snowplow which clears up the main thoroughfare but blocks up each of the side streets and driveways.] Cannon said that with gentle and careful endarterectomy dissection, the snowplowing simile did not hold. He showed motion pictures of the operation, and angiograms before and after operation showing extensive endarterectomy. He predicted "increasing numbers of such patients will be found to be surgical candidates if more coronary angiograms of this type are performed throughout the country." Effler, closing, pointed to the paucity of papers at this program and others on coronary surgery, the very small number of patients who had been operated upon and "the millions of people just in our country who have organic coronary atherosclerosis, who suffer from angina pectoris, and who will die of myocardial infarction." He emphasized the necessity to get cardi-

ologists to employ angiography more frequently. [By 1974, at the Colorado Springs meeting, Effler was able to say at the Cleveland Clinic they had done 4600 coronary bypasses in all, 1573 in 1973.]

* * *

John E. Connolly, Assistant Professor of Surgery, Stanford University School of Medicine, Palo Alto, and by invitation, A. Roy, J. M. Guernsey, and E. A. Stemmer, *Bloodless Surgery by Means of Profound Hypothermia and Circulatory Arrest,* Effect on Brain and Heart, declared that "Total circulatory arrest is one of the ultimate, but yet rarely employed, instruments of the surgeon." Dogs were cooled by whole body perfusion, with a heat exchanger in the circuit, brought down to temperatures of 2° to 5° C. Dogs' hearts usually went into arrest below 10° C. rectal. If fibrillation occurred during the rewarming period, the dogs could always be defibrillated with externally applied shock. Their dogs had undergone psychological training before operation. They concluded that "One hour and forty-five minutes of arrest was the maximum period tolerated without clinical brain damage. Results with long arrest periods were best with pure blood prime." Histologic brain changes, though subtle, "were noted only in animals surviving over 1 hour of arrest. Severe acute changes were presented in all animals subjected to arrest of 2 hours." They thought it possible that the brain injury reported clinically [Bjork and others] was not from "too low a temperature, we suggest that the clinical brain damage reported resulted from too high a temperature during circulatory arrest or during inadequate low perfusion . . . 1 hour of total circulatory rest and exsanguination can be effected safely with no detectable damage to the animal." Restoration of low flow bypass for short periods at the end of one hour would permit repetition of the total arrest of circulation. They experimented with a variety of major operations on the dogs, abdominal thoracic aortic replacement, hepatic lobectomy, organ transplantation, and found them greatly facilitated, but accompanied by severe and perhaps sometimes uncontrollable bleeding if arrest had been prolonged beyond one hour. They also experimented with a left heart bypass which eliminated the need for an oxygenator, employing the Dennis-Senning transarterial cannula and expressed some optimism for its possible application.

Discussion

Lars-Erik Gelin, of Göteborg, Sweden, commented that with hypothermia, there was an increase in vascular resistance because of an increase in the viscosity of the blood, and this implied a necessity to employ some form of hemodilution. Jonathan E. Rhoads, of Philadelphia, said that Sidney Wolfson, at his laboratory, had been infusing the carotids with ice-cold saline to protect the brain while the heart was stopped by electrically induced ventricular fibrillation. If the systemic temperature was lowered to about 25° and ice-cold saline run through the brain, "dogs withstood 60 minutes of anoxia fairly regularly and a number survived after 105 minutes." In green monkeys, survival was obtained "after periods of fibrillation lasting up to 60 minutes." Animals who had been psychologically trained before operation, "remembered what they had learned . . . they were taught a new trick and were able to learn it at the same rate as the trick they learned before they had had the experience with fibrillation and hypothermia." Connolly, closing, agreed with Gelin that hemodilution would probably be the best prime, but that it might be necessary to restrict the period of arrest to no more than an hour. He responded to Rhoads that he had thought about selective cooling of the brain, but thought it was "much more convenient and much easier to cool the entire patient and stop the total circulation, rather than just the cerebral circulation . . . the flaccid aorta that occurs under these conditions should be ideal for the type of thoraco-abdominal aneurysm case that Dr. DeBakey was talking about this morning, or for dissecting aneurysm or aneurysms of the arch of the aorta."

* * *

This is one of the occasions on which the Program Committee had placed one of the strongest papers as the last on the program, *Chronic Survival after Human Renal Homotransplantation.* Lymphocyte-Antigen Matching, Pathology and Influence of Thymectomy, T. E. Starzl, T. L. Marchioro, P. I. Terasaki, and six others, all by invitation, and W. R. Waddell, of Denver, Professor of Surgery and Chairman, Department of Surgery, University of Colorado. "From November 24, 1962 to March 30, 1964, 64 uremic patients were treated with renal homografts obtained from living volunteer donors other than identical twins. Thirty-seven of the original group lived for at least 1 year and 36 are still alive 13-1/2 to 30 months after operation." [see Vol. XCII, 1974] Twenty-three of the 27 deaths within the first year occurred within the first four months of operation. Of the remaining 37, only one died after the first year. No patient had yet had a late second graft. The patient who died after one year had

had a mild early rejection episode and a severe one at seven months "precipitated by discontinuance of prednisone". Rejection had been reversed by the use of cortisone, irradiation of the kidney, and administration of actinomycin C and the patient had been at work for months when he developed progressive jaundice and died with gram-negative septicemia. He was found to have a retroperitoneal abscess in the old left nephrectomy bed. "Thirty-one of the 46 who received kidneys from blood relatives are still alive (67%), contrasted to only 5 of 18 who had unrelated donors (28%)." Although the necessary dose of immunosuppressive agents declined with the passage of time, "nine patients in whom steroids were partially or completely withdrawn developed a late rejection . . . The function of the homografts after 13-1/2 to 30 months ranged from adequate to completely normal." A mild hypertension was common. All but one of the patients were at their normal activity,-either in school or employed. There had been more morbidity from steroids than from azathioprine. With respect to blood groups, the same precaution should be used as in transfusing blood, the risk otherwise being one of immediate failure, although successes had been achieved which violated the rules. If anything, the younger recipients did best. Late rejection, occurring in a total of nine patients because of reduction or discontinuance of doses of prednisone, had been reversed in all cases but one, "by resumption of or increased doses of prednisone with actinomycin C or local homograft irradiation or both." Four patients required late reconstructive urologic operations for ureteric strictures. The physical status of the patients and their rehabilitation depended to a considerable extent upon the pre-existing peripheral uropathy or hypertensive retinal disease. Three patients had an illness associated with jaundice, considered to be hepatitis. Whether this was drug-induced hepatic injury or the viral disease was not known. Comparing the antigen mismatches of the donor recipient pairs to control studies of a random population showed that the five surviving recipients thus studied "were clustered in the favorable half of a random distribution curve of antigenic compatibility . . . none fell into the unfavorable portion." There was some relationship between function of the graft and the degree of compatibility established by matching techniques, but there were some patients with a poor match and good function and vice versa. All four patients who had pre-transplant thymectomy were alive two to two-and-a-half years, with excellent stable renal function, none receiving steroids, none having had an episode of rejection, and all of them having proved easier to manage and having better histologic preservation of their homografts than that of most of the nonthymectomized patients, and all four of these patients had "exceptionally favorable" antigenic matches. Nine subsequent patients with thymectomy, long after transplantation, had no demonstrable benefit.

Discussion

The Discussion was begun by Dr. Wilhelm Brosig, of Berlin, who said that Starzl's results were "the best which have been reported." Willard Goodwin's address, in Berlin, in 1959, had stimulated their interest. In five attempts, they had only one survivor, alive, well, and with good kidney function. David Hume, of Richmond, had 40 transplants done more than a year before, with 21 patients alive. Thirty-one of the 40 were living donor, and nine cadaver kidneys. Five of the eight patients transplanted more than two years earlier were living, two of them having had cadaver kidneys and two having had second transplants. They had attempted no antigen matching. Twenty of the 21 patients surviving over a year, had "essentially normal kidney function". No patient had died after one year, although two patients had had chronic rejection and were doing well with retransplants. Ninety percent of the patients transplanted in the past year were alive and half of them had received cadaver kidneys. Of their total experience with 60 patients, 30 had had splenectomy, which they had given up "because of the increased complication rate, in splenectomized patients, of infection and thrombo-embolic phenomena, and because we could not demonstrate any immunologic benefit from this procedure." They had had no late ureter problems like Starzl's. They had seen similar late microscopic changes. Paul S. Russell, of Boston, said "The basic rules of immunogenetics are well substantiated in the results of the world experience of more than 500 kidney transplants . . . the more closely related the donor is to the recipient, the less will be the antigenic barrier between them. The method of matching now being developed by Dr. Terasaki of UCLA, with whom Dr. Starzl has collaborated, is an ingenious improvement over Dausset's original work, and appears to be quite promising from the retrospective studies so far done." He predicted "that full definition or typing of the operative antigens provoking transplantation immunity will eventually be possible." Russell's own experiments, with Anthony Monaco, had showed that "thymectomy in the adult mouse, quite distinguished from the newborn mouse, greatly delays the animal's ability to restore its lymphoid tissues following injections of the specific antilymphocyte serum. Splenectomy does not have this effect. These observations, therefore, suggest that thymectomy may prove to have a certain place in clinical transplantation in the future." Willard E. Goodwin, of Los Angeles, commented that better matching, better drugs, and possibly immunologic manipulations were future hopes and commented a little wryly of the burgeoning Denver program, that "We wish we could get Dr. Terasaki to do more of these matching tests for us at U.C.L.A.; but often he has been so busy working for Dr. Starzl that we could only get him to do it once in a while." He showed slides of a recipient, who received a kidney from a donor who died of carcinoma of the lung, and developed the carcinoma in the transplanted kidney. "We thought that when immuno-suppressive drugs were stopped the cancer would die. However, it did not work out that way . . . The transplanted tumor metastasized and killed the recipient." Nevertheless, he thought "we should not give up totally the idea of patients with cancer as prospective renal donors." Ralph Straffon, of Cleveland, reported 47 renal transplants in 40 patients, all cadaver kidneys, in 27 months. Twenty-three patients were alive, 21 with functioning kidneys. Some of the kidneys had been brought from other hospitals. All but five of their patients required postoperative dialysis for up to 24 days. Richard Wilson, of Boston, said they had added thoracic duct fistula and antigen competition, and thought their immediate incidence of acute rejection had been lowered. He compared splenectomized and nonsplenectomized patients and like Hume, had given up splenectomy. They had two thymectomized patients who had been doing well for over two years and were not on steroids. Roy Calne, of London, like most of the other speakers, lavish in his praise, commented that the paper "shows what can be achieved with technical excellence and attention to the minutiae of details in clinical care. Secondly, the collection and very careful documentation of comprehensive data on these cases will be of lasting importance." The Terasaki tests might be useful, but they did not establish tissue groups "that can be related from one case to another throughout the world in the same way as A.B.O. blood groups." In dogs, thymectomy was of "no value in prolonging survival of transplants when combined with a standard immunosuppressive therapy." Starzl, closing, said that they had only three cadaver transplants, all successful, which were not included in the report. He wanted to make it clear "that we have reached no conclusions about the effects of thymectomy in the human; the results are uninterpretable." Employing Terasaki's new matching techniques "Since last fall . . . the vigor of rejection in these later cases has seemed to be generally less than that observed in the original series. In fact, there have been no acute secondary anurias since Dr. Terasaki has selected our donors for us." He agreed with Calne that "The weakness of the method is, of course, the fact that one is measuring something unknown with a polyvalent antiserum, and as Dr. Calne has pointed out, it is a little bit like shooting buckshot in the air, hoping to strike an unspecified target."

The Business Meetings

The 1965 meeting was held at the Bellevue-Stratford Hotel, Philadelphia, May 12, 13, and 14, Robert M. Zollinger presiding.

Treasurer H. William Scott remarked once more upon the steadily increasing cost of the *Transactions* which was now about $5,000 a year. "If we wish to continue to publish the Transactions and to meet our financial obligations in the future, it seems clear that we must increase our annual income. An increase in dues to at least $50 per year seems mandatory."

The Amendment concerning the addition of the First and Second Vice-President to the Council, which had laid over a year, was now moved and carried.

Dr. Oliver Cope announced for the ad hoc Committee on Medical Education that they had been in touch with Professor Jerrold Zacharias, of Massachusetts Institute of Technology "the Professor of Physics who has spear-headed the new educational programs in mathematics and physics. He has developed a technic of getting people of various disciplines to work together toward a common end in education." [The national concern over the success of Russia's Sputnik, the first man-made satellite, had lead to a crash program for the acceleration and intensification of science courses, but curiously for the most part in primary and secondary schools.] A con-

ference had been organized for two weeks in July for some 30 scholars to meet at MIT under the leadership of Dr. Zacharias. "The participants will include distinguished representatives from biology, physics, pharmacology, pathology, microbiology, internal medicine, pediatrics, psychiatry, deans, provosts and presidents, and five from your Committee."

The meeting of the Association was held at the time of the 200th Anniversary of the University of Pennsylvania and at the Second Executive session the President read a telegram of congratulations from Lyndon B. Johnson, President of the United States.

The running battle with the American Society of Abdominal Surgeons, the sponsoring body for the Board of Abdominal Surgery, over the control of the Surgical Section of the AMA continued, and Charles G. Child, III, rose to urge as many members as possible "and as many surgical colleagues as they can gather together . . ." to come to the Business Meeting in New York in June. [They did, and won the hotly contested election, having lost when the "abominable surgeons" packed the meeting of the Surgical Section of the AMA in Chicago.]

The report of Council recommended that the dues be increased to $50. Council recommended, as well "That in line with President Zollinger's Address the President appoint a Committee to aid the Council in examining the policies and objectives of the Association, in making appropriate recommendations."

Among those elected to Fellowship were George W. Anlyan, of Durham, North Carolina; Franklin Henry Ellis, Jr., of Rochester, Minnesota; Lloyd Douglas MacLean, of Montreal; Marshall J. Orloff, of Torrance, California; Samuel R. Powers, Jr., of Albany; Seymour Ira Schwartz, of Rochester, New York; and G. Thomas Shires, of Dallas. The new officers elected were President, Leland McKittrick, of Boston; Vice-Presidents, Lawrence Chaffin, of Los Angeles, and David W. Robinson, of Kansas City; and Secretary, H. B. Shumacker, Jr., of Indianapolis.

LXXXIV

1966

The 1966 meeting was held at the Boca Raton Hotel and Club, Boca Raton, Florida, May 23, 24, and 25, President Leland S. McKittrick, of Boston, Clinical Professor Emeritus of Surgery, Harvard Medical School, in the Chair. Among those who had died in the previous year were Champ Lyons and Charles G. Mixter.

President McKittrick, *Leadership and Our New Alliance,* speaking of "leadership in medicine and the Government's increasing role in medical education and medical practice . . ." spoke from the vantage point of a man who had spent his life in clinical practice, albeit in a great medical center. He was concerned with the disappearance from activity in the affairs of the American Medical Association of major figures in American medicine, so that since World War II, ". . . the names of those most prominent in American medicine have rarely been related to organized medicine." He attributed this to ". . . the most significant contribution to medical education in the past half century, the full-time academic physician", the disregard of the academic physicians for organization work and their concentration on research and teaching. At the same time, he was fully aware that the American Medical Association was, in fact, controlled by the Board of Regents and not the Presidents, and that "Until the present policy, whereby election to the Board comes as a reward for conscientious service in the House of Delegates and/or as a stepping stone to the Presidency, is changed we cannot look to the American Medical Association for the quality of continuing leadership

we need so badly." He said that "The eventual disappearance of the nonpaying patient as a medium of surgical training has been clearly seen, but the abruptness with which it has come could not have been anticipated." He was particularly concerned that the young academic surgeon, precisely when he should have been sharpening the clinical skills and judgment which he was beginning to learn as resident, was relegated to the laboratory ". . . and must not permit clinical surgery to interfere with his research and teaching program . . . The patients on the teaching service are the responsibility of the resident", and the young academic surgeon had few private patients. He believed ". . . we should tell the young physician going into academic surgery that, as a future professor of surgery, he must be a surgeon in the true sense of the word and that in preparation for this his research and teaching activities must not jeopardize a continuing participation in clinical surgery . . . we have concentrated upon training at the resident level at the expense of the junior attending staff." He urged formalization of ". . . the mechanism by which those young men and women appointed to your junior attending staff may go into a well balanced program of research, teaching and clinical surgery, each contributing to his economic stability." Medicare, in fact, might be the very mechanism for achieving that and although the result might be to ". . . lessen the total number of patients operated upon by the resident . . . it should not lessen his educational opportunities."

* * *

TABLE 10. *MCV Series: All Transplants Performed Over 1 Year Ago (12–44 Months) (67 Transplants in 60 Patients) April 1966*

	Patients			Transplants		
	Total	Survival		Total	Success	
Sibling	18	12	67%	19	12	63%
Parent	21	13	62%	22	12	55%
Total related	39	25	64%	41	24	59%
Unrelated	3	0	0%	4	0	0%
Cadaver	18	8	44%	22	8	36%

TABLE 11. *MCV Series: Second and Third Transplants*

Patient	Duration of Function			Total Survival
	1st	2nd	3rd	
J. C. (#8)	2 mo.	32 mo.		36 mo.
C. S. (#15)	2 wk.	9 mo.		*Dead*
G. B. (#12)	16 mo.	24 mo.		42 mo.
K. E. (#34)	6 D	19 mo.		24 mo.
P. H. (#6)	15 mo.	3 mo.	12 mo.	36 mo.

Transplant survival was best in kidneys from living related donors, especially siblings. Although others feared second set reaction if a second kidney transplant replaced a non-functioning transplant, Hume "early adopted the policy of removing the transplant and performing a second one; and, if the second fails, of removing it and performing a third." The policy was successful and the single death in five second transplants was from an antibiotic reaction. When the second transplant failed, it nevertheless survived longer than had the first. There was no second set reaction.

David M. Hume, H. M. Lee, G. M. Williams, and nine associates, *Comparative Results of Cadaver and Related Donor Renal Homografts in Man, and Immunologic Implications of the Outcome of Second and Paired Transplants.* LXXXIV, 1966.

Organ transplantation and cardiac surgery dominated the first day of the meeting. David M. Hume, of Richmond, Professor of Surgery and Chairman of the Department of Surgery, Medical College of Virginia, and by invitation, H. M. Lee, G. M. Williams, and nine associates, *Comparative Results of Cadaver and Related Donor Renal Homografts in Man, and Immunologic Implications of the Outcome of Second and Paired Transplants,* reported their experience since August 1962. They had performed 89 non-twin renal homotransplants in 82 patients, 56 related donor transplants, and 29 cadaver transplants. The first four patients were given total body irradiation, two of them dying of radiation aplasia, the other two subsequently treated with Imuran and prednisone. All subsequent patients were placed on Imuran and prednisone on the day of the operation, and received radiation to the transplanted kidney on the first, third, fifth, and seventh days. Rejection was treated with increased doses of prednisone, actinomycin C, and additional doses of radiation. The spleen was removed in 31 patients and not in 51. Bilateral nephrectomy before, during, or after transplantation had become standard. The cadaver kidneys were perfused with cold Ringer's lactate solution with added albumin and heparin. The death-to-functioning-circulation time of the cadaver kidneys was 90 to 120 minutes. "Recipients with related donor transplants demonstrated somewhat better survival, function and immunologic acceptance of the graft than those with cadaver donor transplants." Rejection episodes were common in the cadaver donor group for up to a year and uncommon in the related donor group after eight months, and then common in both groups after one year. Over 60% of living donor kidneys were functioning at 36 months and little more than half that percentage of cadaver kidneys. In an unstated number of patients, a coil of Silastic tubing was connected to the patient's hemodialysis shunt and the coil surrounded by a Strontium[90] radiation source, to radiate the circulating blood in the treatment of rejection crises. If the renal homotransplant failed they "early adopted the policy of removing the transplant and performing a second one; and if the second fails, of removing it and performing a third. Despite the contrary arguments of others who anticipated a second-set reaction, the Table indicates that four of five patients with second transplants were alive from two to more than three years at the time of reporting. The patient who had died, had died of an antibiotic reaction. In the collection of data from "throughout the world . . . In 51 per cent of the second transplants, the second worked longer than the first, while the second transplant failed sooner than the first in only 16 per cent . . . surprising in view of the fact that the second transplant is often done under circumstances . . . less favorable than those of the first, and the patients undergoing a second transplant have already demonstrated their capabilities to reject a graft. These results suggest that second and third transplants may enjoy a privileged existence not conferred upon the first." He interpreted this as meaning that "Imuran thus prevents immunization to the antigens of the first transplant." In the eight times that the two kidneys from a cadaver were transplanted into two recipients,- "double-header",- both kidneys succeeded in seven, and both kidneys failed in one. In the world experience, in 12 such pairs both kidneys survived, in five pairs there was a mixed response, and in 12 pairs both transplants failed. Hume reasoned that "If one assumes that the alleles occur at equal frequencies and that there is a single major locus of histocompatibility in man, then results can be explained by the existence of three strong and five weak alleles at a single locus of histocompatibility." This suggested to him the possibility there might be a universal tissue donor susceptible of identification by simple serologic tests. One male patient on Imuran had fathered a normal child and one female patient on Imuran had given birth to a normal child. Urologic problems had been minimal. Four patients had developed temporary urinary fistulae, one patient had a mild hydronephrosis, and one patient with hyperparathyroidism developed a staghorn calculus and had now had a parathyroidectomy. Two patients had a urine leak from the bladder with retroperitoneal infection and death. They had successfully performed a transplant in one diabetic patient. Their overall patient survival was 66% up to three-and-a-half years. Patient survival had improved year after year.

Discussion

Lloyd D. MacLean, of Montreal, agreed with "Dr. Hume's thesis . . . that there are a limited number of strong transplantation antigens in man." Their experience with cadaver double transplants paralleled Hume's, and when rejections did occur they seemed to occur almost at the same time, "The chances that reactions such as these are governed by a wide variety of antigens seem quite unlikely . . ." They had also analyzed the relation of rejection to number of pretransplant dialyses and ". . . There are no patients with major rejection who have had over 50 hemodialyses", and in the group of 38 patients with very few dialyses there had been a large number of major rejections. W. R. Waddell, of Denver, reported Starzl"s experience to date. Patient survival was 65% with a follow-up of 12 to 40 months. The related living donor group had a better survival than the unrelated living donor group. After the first three fatal attempts with cadaver transplants, they had performed six more with four survivors and good function in all four kidneys. The kidney registry survivals showed ". . . the stability of the group that reaches into the 1-, 2- and 3-year periods." Hume, closing, said in relation to hemodialysis that "We have the general impression that multiple hemodialyses certainly do not prejudice the outcome, and may in fact be of some help. This may be related to the better results seen with second transplants. In other words, the more antigens the patient is exposed to, the more confused his antibody system gets . . ."

* * *

Albert Starr, of Oregon, had presented his results with cardiac valve replacements at the 1961 and 1964 meetings, and now Denton A. Cooley, of Houston, Professor of Surgery, Baylor University College of Medicine; Chief Cardiovascular Surgical Service, St. Luke's-Texas Children's Hospitals, and by invitation, R. D. Bloodwell, A. C. Beall, Jr., S. Gill, and Grady L. Hallman, *Total Cardiac Valve Replacement Using SCDK-Cutter Prosthesis:* Experience with 250 Consecutive Patients, presented their results with another type of ball valve prosthesis, differing in that the ball was seated partially behind the ring, contained by three prongs, and the three prongs of the cage, like the three prongs of the seat, did not meet. They used a disposable plastic bubble oxygenator primed with 5% dextrose in distilled water. Their perfusion time ". . . for single mitral or aortic valve replacement was 36 minutes; for double valve replacement, 73 minutes; and for triple valve replacement, 90 minutes." They had performed 101 mitral valve replacements with nine hospital deaths, 127 aortic valve replacements with ten hospital deaths and, adding the late deaths, had cumulative

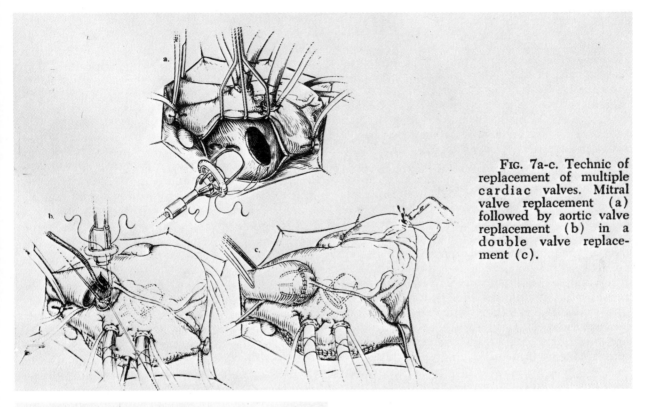

FIG. 7a-c. Technic of replacement of multiple cardiac valves. Mitral valve replacement (a) followed by aortic valve replacement (b) in a double valve replacement (c).

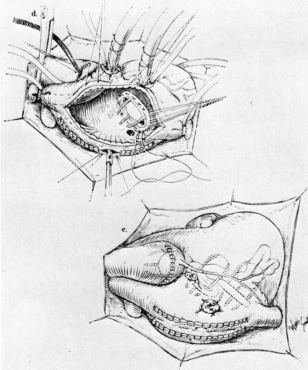

FIG. 7d-e. Tricuspid valve replacement (d) added to complete triple valve replacement (e).

In multiple valve replacement, the mitral valve was approached through the left atrium on the right, with the aorta cross clamped. The left coronary artery was perfused while the aortic prosthesis was inserted. There were nine hospital deaths in 101 mitral valve replacements, ten deaths in 127 aortic valve replacements, and eight deaths in 22 patients with multiple valve replacements. The outcome was not given for the two patients with replacement of three valves. By the time of the meeting, Cooley had given up coronary perfusion and had one death in 64 consecutive valve replacements.

Denton A. Cooley, R. D. Bloodwell, A. S. Beall, Jr., Sarjit S. Gill, and Grady L. Hallman, *Total Cardiac Valve Replacement Using SCDK-Cutter Prosthesis:* Experience with 250 Consecutive Patients. Volume LXXXIV, 1966.

mortalities of 14%, 16% and 41% respectively. For the mitral valve, they used a transverse sternotomy, exposing the left atrium from the right side. Their previous hospital mortality "using other prosthetic valves had been 16%." Ten patients of the 250 "demonstrated peripheral embolic phenomena or thrombosis about the valve prosthesis . . ." Patients were started on Coumadin from the third to the fifth day and maintained on it for three months after aortic valve replacement, and six months after mitral valve replacement. The drop in overall mortality from 16% to 11% with the new valve was encouraging as was the drop of thromboembolic problems from 17% to 4%. Since completing the series included in the present report, they had discontinued use of coronary perfusion during aortic valve replacement, and "Our current experience shows that the heart tolerates normothermic total ischemia, and cardiac function resumes promptly when normal coronary circulation is reestablished." In the previous two months they had performed 64 consecutive valve replacement procedures without coronary perfusion with only one death, and that after two weeks, from renal failure after massive hemorrhage.

Discussion

Albert Starr, of Portland, Oregon, suggested that Cooley's improving mortality might come from increasing experience and not from any change in valve, "For example, our initial mortality reported in 1960 with mitral replacement was 50%, and in 1965 our operative mortality with mitral replacement was zero." He went on to add that "In 1964 and 1965 the operative mortality of multiple valve replacement was 7%, with an over-all late mortality of 9%. This includes 25 triple valve replacements with two operative deaths." Nevertheless thromboembolism and the changes which occurred in the silicone rubber ball which might cause it to stick, as Cooley had mentioned, remained to be solved. Cooley's valve, which Starr had studied on the pulse duplicator had a built-in insufficiency. The regurgitant jet was unevenly distributed and not likely to reduce the risk of thrombosis. If the silicone rubber poppet swelled and the valve became completely competent, it could indeed stick in the closed position. Since the Starr-Edwards prosthesis was competent to begin with this could not occur, nor had the Starr-Edwards poppet ever changed as Cooley's had. They had continued to modify their cage to reduce the amount of material in the prosthesis. He questioned the wisdom of having a double cage. Herbert Sloan, of Ann Arbor, indicated that thrombo-embolism

was a major problem but there was a suspicious ring to his congratulations, "Dr. Cooley has just announced the millenium. If these valves show as low an incidence of thrombo-embolism as his early results suggest, most of our problems related to prosthetic mitral valve replacement will have been solved, and I hope devoutly, as all of you do that this is true." In mitral disease Sloan performed open valvuloplasty as frequently as possible and "In 115 survivors of mitral valvuloplasty there were only three instances of thrombo-embolism, while the incidence of thrombo-embolism in the Starr-Edwards valve replacements was considerably higher, and this figure is comparable to other reported series. It is also important to note that while none of the patients who had a valvuloplasty received anticoagulants, all of the patients with the Starr-Edwards prosthesis did receive anticoagulants." Atrial fibrillation had appeared to be the major selector of the patients who discharged systemic emboli and they now made vigorous efforts to accomplish cardioversion. They preferred heparin to Coumadin as an anticoagulant. Benson B. Roe, of San Francisco, had employed the Cutter prosthesis for six months but ". . . we cannot honestly and objectively distinguish its performance from that of the Starr-Edwards valve . . . I submit that it will take us a lot longer to separate the effect on results of a particular prosthesis from the improvement with experience, better methods of anticoagulation, more meticulous management of the patient and more rapid and effective operative technic. Thus I ask that we do not accept this nice series as evidence that this is a better gadget." Cooley, closing, felt it "important that we give each new prosthesis which is developed a clinical trial." He attributed to the discontinuance of coronary perfusion in January 1966, a fall in "mortality from the range of 10 to 15% to the range of 2%. We do not intend to use coronary perfusion in any valve replacement even where multiple replacements are done."

* * *

The National Heart Institute of the National Institutes of Health stimulated by Michael E. DeBakey and others had embarked on a heavily funded program to develop an implantable heart, and now Winton H. Burns, by invitation, Harris B. Shumacker, Jr., of Indianapolis, Professor of Surgery and Chairman of the Department of Surgery, Indiana University Medical School, and by invitation, Robert J. Loubier, *The Totally Implantable Mechanical Heart. An Appraisal of Feasibility,* presented the work which had engaged them for three years, say-

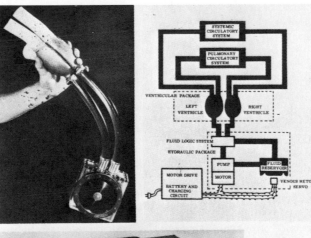

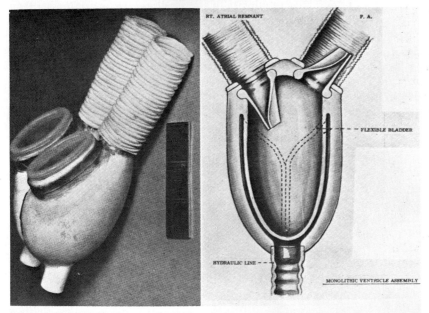

FIG. 2. Photographs of ventricular and electrohydraulic units (left upper) and external power supply-electronic control package (lower) and schematic drawing of the system.

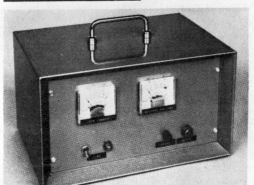

FIG. 3. Photograph of ventricular unit without atrial cuffs and schematic drawing.

Early model of Shumacker mechanical heart. Calves were maintained on it as long as 18 hours. The pump was powered by electricity, brought into the chest from an outside source. A newer model contained the motor between the two ventricles, was overall a little larger than the normal heart and could fit into the pericardium. It had not yet been used. The heat produced by the first model was not much more than that produced by the normal heart.

Winton H. Burns, Harris B. Shumacker, Jr., Robert J. Loubier, *The Totally Implantable Mechanical Heart.* An Appraisal of Feasibility. Volume LXXXIV, 1966.

ing that "Others, in clinics throughout the world, were studying the general problem of homologous organ replacement and some were specifically concerned with transplantation of the heart. We believed that a mechanical substitute would be much more widely applicable and were optimistic that a totally implantable mechanical heart could be developed." The technical developments which made such an approach possible were the introduction of prosthetic materials for aortic grafting by Blakemore and Voorhees in 1954, Gibbon's development of the heart-lung machine brought to clinical use in 1953, the development of satisfactorily functioning aortic and mitral valves, and the experience with implantable pumps of Kolff in 1959 and Hastings in 1961. While experimental models would require electric power from an external source, "It seemed possible that there might be developed atomic-powered batteries small enough for total implantation and of sufficient capacity to provide long-term function". It might also be possible ". . . by high-frequency radio transmission and reception, to transfer electrical energy through the intact chest wall in quantity . . . adequate for operating a mechanical heart." They had come to using leaflet valves molded of silicone rubber, and a two-chambered heart, each chamber with a "cuff of woven Dacron for connection with the atrial remnant." The collapsible Silastic ventricular chamber was separated from a rigid outer housing by a space for the hydraulic activating fluid of the pump. The miniaturized electrohydraulic package contained a pump ". . . about 1 inch in diameter, 0.7 inch long and capable of an approximate output of 12 liters per minute at 300 mm. Hg." With the earlier model, powered by an external electrical source, they had achieved survivals up to 18 hours in calves and very large dogs.

Discussion

Michael E. DeBakey, of Houston, said he had "had the pleasure to be associated with the support of activities in this field in a number of laboratories as well as in our own for some time. I, too, am convinced, like a number of others, and as Dr. Shumacker has just said, that this is a feasible objective." He had thought that the first step should be to develop a left ventricular pump bypass for temporary support of the left ventricle, and showed a motion picture of such a pump at work in a calf. He concluded optimistically [with what was in fact a declaration of intent] that "We believe that with this pump we are ready now to attempt its clinical use; that we have tested it sufficiently so that we can use

it for clinical purposes; and we are planning to do so within the immediate future." Shumacker, closing, was equally optimistic, "I do not think we are a long way from total human cardiac replacement. Indeed, I think it is just around the corner. If we have enough support, I am convinced that this development is not far off."

* * *

[In the previous year the Discussion of coronary sclerosis and angina pectoris concentrated on endarterectomy and direct plastic procedures on the coronaries. Arthur Vineberg, of Montreal, had been claiming for 20 years that the internal mammary artery, with its side branches opened, implanted in the myocardium, remained patent and established effective anastomoses with the coronary arteries. Bigelow had reported in 1963 that indeed one such long-term patient of Vineberg's had been demonstrated to have a patent internal mammary with intramyocardial coronary anastomoses. Mason Sones' selective coronary angiographies had made it possible to select appropriate patients for operation and to document the patency of an implanted internal mammary artery. Effler's 1963 report before the Association had been enthusiastic, but in 1965, discussing coronary arterioplasties, Effler had made no comments about his experience with the Vineberg operation and he did not now rise to comment on Bigelow's paper.] Strong support for Vineberg now came from W. G. Bigelow, of Toronto, Associate Professor of Surgery, University of Toronto Medical School; Head, Division of Cardiovascular Surgery, Toronto General Hospital, and by invitation, H. E. Aldridge, and D. D. MacGregor, *Internal Mammary Implantation (Vineberg Operation) for Coronary Heart Disease:* Cineangiography and Long-term Follow Up. Between 1953 and 1966, they operated upon a total of 65 patients, with a total of 11 deaths, seven in patients with decubitus angina. There had been no deaths in the 22 patients with exertional angina pectoris operated upon from 1963 to 1966. They had studied 26 of the patients by cineangiography. All 26 showed the internal mammary patent, and in 20 of them dye was demonstrated to enter the heart, with good to excellent branches in eight, fair branches in ten, and no branches, but a myocardial blush in two. Eighty-three percent of the patients showed improvement, most of them good to excellent, and 67% showed good to excellent treadmill performance after operation. There were ten late deaths in 54 patients available for study, eight of them two to four years after operation, none later than four years, and all from myocardial infarction. It was their "clinical impression that this operation may increase life expectancy . . ."

Discussion

Michael E. DeBakey, of Houston, arose in support having been ". . . converted to the procedure . . ." after seeing a patient that Dr. Vineberg had operated upon ten years before in whom a Houston angiogram showed the internal mammary artery implant functioning. They had modified the procedure "By utilizing a new graft attached by end-to-side anastomosis in the descending thoracic aorta . . . to use this approach for both the anterior and posterior areas of the left ventricle." They were enthusiastic about their experience with 100 patients in three years. They thought a vein graft might function in the same way.

* * *

In the Discussion of Zoll, Frank, and Linenthal's paper at the 1964 meeting, Elliott Hurwitt had spoken of the transvenous pacemaker developed in his department by Seymour Furman, and now by invitation, S. Furman, D. J. W. Escher, N. Solomon, and J. B. Schwedel, *Implanted Transvenous Pacemakers:* Equipment, Technic and Clinical Experience, described their permanently implanted transvenous pacemaker. The patients all had previously implanted temporary transvenous pacemakers, usually inserted through the femoral vein. The permanent pacemaker catheter was generally inserted through the cephalic vein. The catheter was advanced into the apex of the right ventricle, the position and function of the catheter tested, the catheter then tied into the vein, and attached to the pacemaker which was implanted "over the ribs at the anterior axillary line . . ." In the last nine months they had implanted 38 such transvenous pacemakers. They had noted the following complications, inadequate positioning of catheter tip, loosening of fixation ligatures, skin erosion over the pulse generator, electrical malfunction, threshold increase, and return of the catheter to the right atrium. One patient expired at home from gastrointestinal hemorrhage a month-and-a-half after implant, and one patient died of uremia 27 days after the implant. Electrode fracture and electrolysis of the leads had not occurred.

Discussion

W. W. L. Glenn, of New Haven, working with Furman and his group, had applied his own radio-frequency system to the transvenous intra-cardiac electrode connected to a radio receiver buried under the skin of the chest. This made it possible ". . . to change the battery or the rate of pacing or the intensity of the pacemaker stimulus externally. It is also possible to discontinue electrical pacemaking should it be no longer required by the patient."

* * *

S. H. Nadler, by invitation, and George E. Moore, of Buffalo, Director and Chief of Surgery, Roswell Park Memorial Institute, *Clinical Immunologic Study of Malignant Disease:* Response to Tumor Transplants and Transfer of Leukocytes, had performed an extremely simple experience on patients with ". . . histologically similar incurable tumors . . ." Bits of tumor from pairs of patients were cross implanted subcutaneously. Two weeks later "when homograft rejection is thought to have taken place", leukocytes were harvested and cross transfused daily for three weeks. At the same time "white blood cells sensitized to tumor during culture *in vitro* are injected intraperitoneally in the original patients" after ten days either daily or every other day. There had been abundant animal experimentation of this kind which indicated that lymphocytes could indeed be sensitized against tumors. Of their own work, they were able to say, "In seven patients with objective response to therapy there have been two complete responses, in one a complete remission of disease for about 2 years . . . Whether antibodies are being formed against tumors or whether some other 'anticancer' agent is being developed is not now clear but it is obvious that some mechanism has been enhanced by this method and is causing regression of tumor in a certain percentage of patients treated." Forty patients had been enrolled in the study and observations were considered adequate in 26, of whom seven had objective response.

Discussion

Warren H. Cole, of Chicago, said the principal point was whether a virus was involved in the etiology of the tumor being treated. He suspected that some of the spontaneous regressions of cancer, which he had recently reported, were evidence of immunological factors at work. Herbert Conway, of New York, considered this a classic presentation. He pointed out the close relationship between work on transplantation and work on cancer, and said that the National Research Council had recently at-

'EXCHANGE' OF TUMORS BRINGS REMISSION

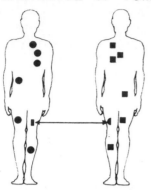

1. Tumor grafts are interchanged between two patients with histologically similar neoplasms.

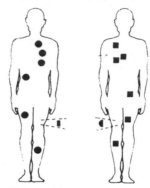

2. After 10 to 14 days, when graft rejection occurs, each patient is sensitized to tumor of the other.

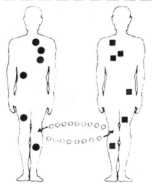

3. White cells from each sensitized patient are transfused into the other daily for 3 weeks.

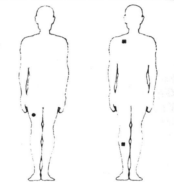

4. Sensitized to their own tumors by transfusions, patients have partial or total remission.

Fig. 1.

Pairs of patients with extensive cancer were cross implanted with their tumors and subsequently transfused with the new host leucocytes. The tumor did not "take" in any of the recipients. Seven patients with malignant melanoma had "objective response to therapy", two of them "complete response", and one patient had, at the time, a complete remission of disease for two years.

S. H. Nadler, George E. Moore, *Clinical Immunologic Study of Malignant Disease:* Response to Tumor Transplants and Transfer of Leukocytes. Volume LXXXIV, 1966.

tempted to bring together the members of the Tissue Transplantation Committee and members of the committees working upon cancer "hoping to prevent reduplication of extensive experimentation." As a note of caution he said there was a record of a human volunteer, the mother of a patient with malignant melanoma, the subject of an experiment like Moore's, in whom the melanoma killed the recipient in 308 days.

* * *

L. F. Urdaneta, D. Duffell, C. D. Creevy, all by invitation, and J. Bradley Aust, of San Antonio,

Professor and Chairman, Department of Surgery, South Texas Medical School, *Late Development of Primary Carcinoma of the Colon following Ureterosigmoidostomy:* Report of Three Cases and Literature Review, reported that of 23 patients at the University of Minnesota surviving more than ten years after ureterosigmoid implant, three had developed carcinoma of the bowel near the ureteral implantation. They were able to find 13 similar cases in the literature going back to 1929. Despite the relatively infrequent use of uretero-sigmoid implantations since the development by Bricker of the ileal loop in 1952, there were a large number of patients at risk who had been operated upon prior to that time.

Discussion

Victor F. Marshall, of New York, had reviewed 160 consecutive uretero-sigmoid implants at the New York Hospital, performed more than nine years earlier, and had found no carcinomas of the colon, although several patients had had carcinoma of the colon prior to ureteral implantation. Eugene M. Bricker, of St. Louis, said that as far as he knew ". . . there have been no cases of primary carcinoma of the ileum in association with diversion of the urine through an ileal segment. This operation has been done in significant numbers since 1950. I suppose at our place, between the General Surgery Service and the Urological Service of Dr. Justin Cordonnier, there must be close to 1,000 uretero-ileal urinary diversions that have been done." J. Hartwell Harrison, of Boston, said that Edwin Davis, of Omaha, 20 years earlier had "reported on the spontaneous regression of carcinoma of the bladder after urinary diversion" and that in 1947 they had made the same observation and in both cases the tumor had disappeared so far as cystoscopic observation was concerned, but was still present on histologic section. "This suggests some possibility, perhaps, of a carcinogen in the urine or some change which is beneficial after urinary diversion affecting the bladder and conferring an undesirable effect upon the bowel." They had had one case like those of Aust's "an adenocarcinoma of the rectum between the two uretero-sigmoidostomy implants 2 years after total cystectomy . . ." Willard Goodwin, of Los Angeles, said his personal preference continued to be for ureterosigmoidostomy. L. K. Ferguson, of Philadelphia, cited a case in support of Aust. [The general tenor of the discussions, by Prohaska and others not quoted, had been that the urine contained a carcinogen.] Aust, closing, said "A carcinogenic agent in the urine, capable of causing both a primary bladder cancer and bowel cancer hardly seems tenable when one reviews the literature, because most of these occurred in patients who had benign disease, and the crucial factor seemed to be time . . . The average latent period of 17 years is certainly suggestive of a carcinogenic stimulus." He thought, in fact, that it must be the urine, and suggested yearly sigmoidoscopy.

* * *

T. R. Miller, A. R. Mackenzie, both by invitation, and Henry T. Randall, of New York, Professor of Surgery, Cornell University and Surgeon, Memorial Center, *Translumbar Amputation for Advanced Cancer:* Indications and Physiologic Alterations in Four Cases, had in four patients with otherwise inextirpable but localized pelvic cancer, divided the vena cava, the common iliac arteries, the lumbar spine, the dura and cauda equina, removing the pelvis, with its contained viscera, and the lower extremities. Colostomy and urinary diversion had been accomplished in prior operations. None of the patients died. They demonstrated a patient walking with a prosthesis. All four patients had had excruciating pain which was immediately relieved by operation. Three of the patients had already developed metastases, and one had died of metastatic disease. Their final comment was "It is interesting to note that in 35 per cent of all women who die of cervix cancer, the disease is still limited to the pelvis and could be removed by this type of procedure."

Discussion

J. Bradley Aust, of San Antonio, who had four-and-a-half years earlier at the University of Minnesota, successfully performed the first operation of this type, was impressed by the degree of rehabilitation achieved in the patients at Memorial Hospital. Eugene M. Bricker, of St. Louis, told the Fellows of an episode of 15 years before, which a number of them remembered keenly, "Back in 1950 we were rounding a period in surgery in this country during which radical surgery had been re-introduced with the added benefits of increased knowledge of anesthesiology, blood banking, physiology of shock, et cetera. I was interested in pelvic exenteration, and Dr. John Modlin and I presented a paper in Durham, North Carolina, in 1950—I think it was—[Society of University of Surgeons] at which time we talked about the 'Role of Pelvic Exenteration in Surgery.' This subject and some others were being rather widely criticized in the editorials of the time as being an extension of surgery beyond justifiable limits. In the discussion of my paper, Dr. Fred Kredel took the floor and showed a picture of a cadaver that had been amputated through the middle, and he talked about this as being a possible extension of surgery for cancer limited to the lower half of the body. My reaction was that Dr. Kredel was criticizing me and had gone to great lengths to prepare a means of very strongly indicating his disapproval of the radical surgery that was being undertaken then. I later learned that I had misinterpreted Dr. Kredel's remarks and that he was indeed seriously, or semi-seriously, proposing such an operation. The possibility had already occurred to us, but we had not been disposed to consider it seriously. Now the operation is here for our serious consideration. I

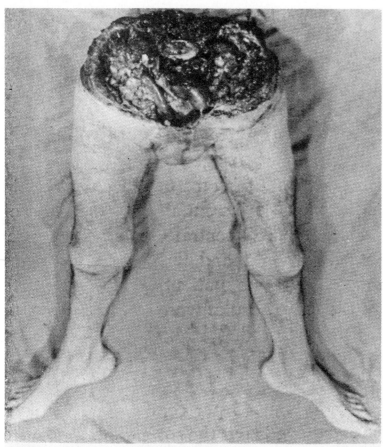

FIG. 2. Gross specimen from translumbar amputation.

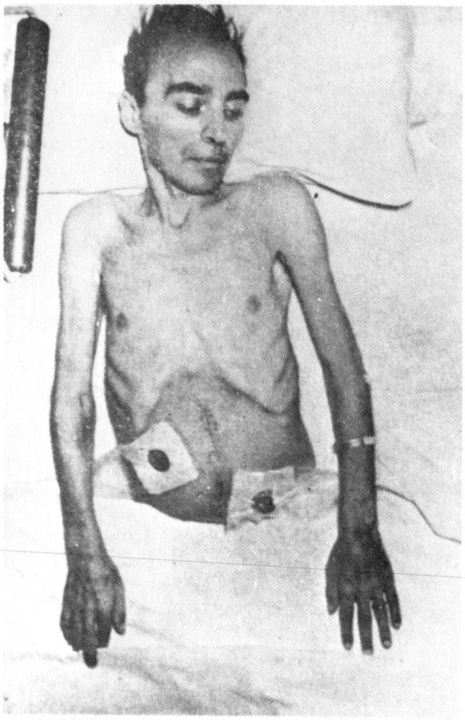

FIG. 6. Patient ten days postoperative.

In four patients, Miller and his associates at Memorial Hospital had transected the body, dividing the spine at the second, third, or fourth lumbar interspace. It is difficult to realize, perhaps to believe, that what is seen of the patient in Figure 6, ten days after operation, is all that there is of the patient. The four patients all survived operation, and one had already been rehabilitated to the point of being able to walk. At the time of this report, three of the patients had developed metastases and one had died.

Theodore R. Miller, A. Ranald MacKenzie, Henry T. Randall, *Translumbar Amputation for Advanced Cancer: Indications and Physiologic Alterations in Four Cases.* Volume LXXXIV, 1966.

wonder, considering today's possibility of organ preservation and perfusion, at what level of the body such efforts should cease. This consideration is a logical extension of the gruesome possibilities. I am skeptical of the advisability of offering such a procedure to a patient, and I wonder at the patient who is willing to accept the procedure in order to prolong life . . . let me urge that if such salvage surgery is to be investigated, that the study be limited to a few—a very few—centers with the willingness and the facilities to carry on extensive rehabilitation of the patient, which not only will involve the early postoperative period but will have to continue on through the remainder of the patient's life." Donald D. Matson, of Boston, asked whether their patients had phantom symptoms. "This is an unusual type of amputation, of course, in which not only the lower motor neurons are involved, but there is transection at the next proximal synapse, and I would be very interested in hearing the authors' comment as to whether they have had any phantom phenomena in these patients . . ." Henry T. Randall, closing, said that they had indeed employed a full panoply of social and rehabilitative services and that "All four patients, questioned some time after the procedure had been done, and by individuals other than our team, stated freely that they were glad they had done it and would go through it again." The patients had had phantom pain but that had not been a major problem. Randall thought they might continue to operate on a few patients of the kind.

* * *

Hiram T. Langston, of Chicago, Clinical Professor of Surgery, University of Illinois; Chief of Surgery, Chicago State Tuberculosis Sanitarium, and by invitation, W. L. Barker, and M. M. Pyle, *Surgery in Pulmonary Tuberculosis:* 11-year Review of Indications and Results, emphasized the shift in surgery for tuberculosis brought about by the anti-tuberculosis drugs. Hospital stays were shortened from years or months, to months or weeks, doubling or tripling the available beds, "Waiting lists for admission to sanatoria have disappeared and empty beds became so numerous that many small sanatoria have closed." He thought this was due as much to epidemiologic control and public health measures as it was to chemotherapy. The age of patients with tuberculosis had risen and patients now were more frequently males than females. At the beginning of the study, thoracoplasty was being performed in 9% of the cases, and at the end of this study period in 1%. Lobectomies had risen from 34% to 45%, segmentectomy had dropped from 14% to 7%, pneumonectomy, 10% at the beginning, had risen to 16% in 1960, and was now down to 8.7%. Wedge enucleations, not performed at all in the first five years, were now performed in 2% of the patients. The overall mortality for 879 resections was 3%; for 432 lobectomies, 1.4%; segmentectomy, 0.72%; for pneumonectomy, 5.9%; and for pleuropneumonectomy, 6.2%. In general, operation had been found necessary in 25% of the patients who had not responded completely to chemotherapy, and operation was increasingly more often resection, rather than collapse. Late residual advanced disease, and patients with advanced disease, were brought to operability by drug therapy, and were operated upon as "salvage" cases.

Discussion

Herbert Sloan, of Ann Arbor, congratulated Dr. Langston on his paper and his superb results but said ". . . I think this is a *swan song*. Surgery has a decreasing part to play in the treatment of tuberculosis, and I would not be surprised if this were the last paper to appear before the Association on the subject of pulmonary tuberculosis." [No other appeared in the remainder of the Association's first

century.] He suggested that in their area at least the sanatoria which were closed were needed by the teaching services for general, medical, and surgical beds. Edward F. Parker, of Charleston, S.C., said that in their part of the country, particularly among the Negroes, active tuberculosis was still a serious problem, and that the bronchiectatic residuum of tuberculosis was a particular operative indication. Frank B. Berry, of New York, said that "In 1945, Dr. [Edward] Churchill and I called upon Ferdinand Sauerbruch in Berlin, who, or course, was the father of the modern type of thoracoplasty. When Dr. Churchill mentioned resection for tuberculosis, Dr. Sauerbruch said: 'You don't mean to say that you are resecting lungs for tuberculosis?' And when we assured him that we were, and with success, all he did was to shake his head and say: 'But little foreign literature has come into this country for the past 15 years.' "

* * *

William Silen, of Boston, Professor of Surgery, Harvard Medical School; Surgeon-in-Chief, Beth Israel Hospital, and by invitation, E. G. Biglieri, P. Slaton, and Maurice Galante, from the University of California, San Francisco, *Management of Primary Aldosteronism:* Evaluation of Potassium and Sodium Balance, Technic of Adrenalectomy and Operative Results in 24 Cases, emphasized the need for preoperative correction of potassium depletion by combining sodium restriction with supplemental potassium intake in the conditions which Conn had described a little more than a decade earlier. All but one of their patients had hypokalemia, and all had hypertension, hypervolemia and increased aldosterone secretion. Spironolactone had not proved to be needed in correcting the potassium deficit. There was no correlation between the size of the lesion and severity of the clinical manifestations, nor between the severity of the hypertension and the amount of urinary excretion of aldosterone. They suggested, but did not employ, selective adrenal vein catheterization, and aldosterone determinations of that venous blood to determine the site of the lesion. Of their 24 patients, 15 had a unilateral adenoma, one had hyperplasia on one side; adenomata on the other, three had bilateral hyperplasia and one had "several 2-3 mm. nodules". There was "no correlation between the size of the lesion and the severity of aldosteronism as measured by the urinary execretion of aldosterone." There was a single death ". . . after uncontrollable renal hemorrhage from a needle biopsy of the kidney performed under direct vision at operation . . . nephrectomy was performed too late to save the patient." They would not take issue with those who preferred bilateral posterior incisions, particularly in obese patients. The urinary aldosterone fell in the first week or two after operation to abnormally low levels. Serum electrolytes returned to normal or remained normal. One patient became normotensive after a year, the others about the fourth or sixth week.

Discussion

Bernard Zimmerman, of Morgantown, West Virginia, had reported five cases to the Association in 1959, and had had eight more, including "six adenomas, two cases of hyperplasia, two instances of adenomatous hyperplasia, one carcinoma, and one undetermined." The urinary steroids other than aldosterone were usually not affected except in one patient with carcinoma, whose 17-ketosteroid excretion was high. They did pretreat their patients with both spironolactone and potassium chloride. Like Silen, they preferred the transabdominal approach. Their patients all had return of blood pressure to normal within two weeks. J. Hartwell Harrison, of Boston, had had 15 cases, two of them carcinomas. Dr. Thorn, at the Brigham, he said, would approve of Silen's performing total adrenalectomy for bilateral hyperplasia, whereas he himself would like to leave a little of the left gland behind and face the possibility of a second operation.

* * *

William B. Kiesewetter, of Pittsburgh, Professor of Pediatric Surgery, University of Pittsburgh School of Medicine; Surgeon-in-Chief, Children's Hospital of Pittsburgh, *Imperforate Anus:* The Role and Results of the Sacro-abdominoperineal Operation, presented the Fellows with the kind of sophisticated analysis of the modern understanding of a classical pediatric surgical problem which was beginning to be beyond most of them. Kiesewetter had adopted the principle of Douglas Stephens [Melbourne, Australia], modifying his sacroperineal operation to make it an abdominosacral perineal operation for bringing the proximal segment through the levator sling mechanism, close to the urethra. Like Stephens, he emphasized the important role the levator sling played in continence, adding to Stephens' explanation of its muscular action, his own observation that there was a sensory perception of pressure apparently received by the levator. In order to avoid the necessity for an extensive pelvic dissection which might interfere with this sensory perception, he added, for the distal rectal pouch, the mucosal denu-

dation technique of Romualdi, ignoring the urethral fistula, and bringing the proximal bowel down through the tube of undisturbed rectal musculature, within the levator sling, and through the perineum. He recommended a colostomy at birth and the definitive operation at six months of age. He had 22 of the primary pull-throughs and in 11 other patients, incontinent after a conventional operation, had reoperated to bring the bowel down through the levator ring. Thirteen of the patients with primary abdominosacroperineal operations had now been evaluated with six poor results, four of them in patients with lumbosacral vertebral anomalies. The other two were four and five years old and the reason for incontinence was not clear. He had thus far been able to evaluate only eight patients in the reoperated group. There were four poor results, two of them in children with mental or emotional problems. The other four, old enough to be evaluated, had been transformed from incontinence to complete continence or infrequent soiling only under stress.

Discussion

Orvar Swenson, of Chicago, agreed that "we are in need of better methods to improve our results." He agreed with "Dr. Kiesewetter's insistence that the surgeon conserve all possible neuromuscular structures . . . preservation of the feeble but intact external sphincter, and most important, the puborectalis portion of the levator . . ." He indicated some caution in accepting Kiesewetter's technique for accomplishing this, "This dissection sacrally and the utilization of a cored out rectum as described by the author is ingenious and elaborate. However, providing functional improvements are accomplished, this objection is overruled. It would seem that these patients with severe colonic inertia—that encasement of the distal colon in the additional rectal muscular walls may prove detrimental." Kiesewetter responded to the last comment, "as to whether the sleeve through which we do this pull-through proves inhibitory in any way to the evacuation of the stool", that this had not been his experience thus far, nor had it been in five patients of Soave's with Hirschsprung's disease whom Kiesewetter had examined [in whom the bowel was similarly brought down through a tube of rectum denuded of its mucosa].

* * *

D. Emerick Szilagyi, of Detroit, Chairman, Department of Surgery, Henry Ford Hospital, and by invitation, R. F. Smith, F. J. DeRusso, J. P. Elliott,

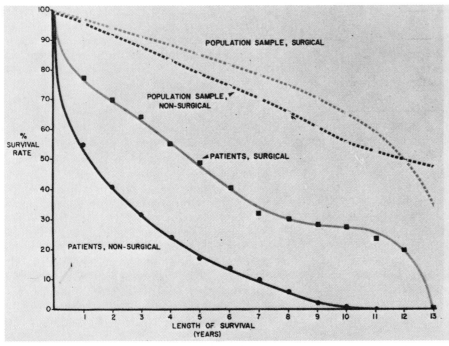

FIG. 4. Observed cumulative 13-year-survival experience of 434 surgically and 223 nonsurgically treated cases of abdominal aortic aneurysm and calculated survival experience of general-population samples compiled for corresponding sex and age distribution. (Source of data: Table 5.)

Comparing 223 non-operated patients with aortic aneurysm seen from January 1, 1944 to December 31, 1965, with 480 operated patients, Szilagyi and colleagues found that the overall survival was better for the operated patients, although poorer than in the population as a whole, that small aneurysms unoperated upon were accompanied by a much better survival than large aneurysms unoperated upon, and that small aneurysms operated upon were associated with a better survival than small aneurysms not operated upon.

D. Emerick Szilagyi, Roger F. Smith, Franklin J. DeRusso, Joseph P. Elliott, and Frederick W. Sherrin, *Contribution of Abdominal Aortic Aneurysmectomy to Prolongation of Life.* Volume LXXXIV, 1966.

and F. W. Sherrin, *Contribution of Abdominal Aortic Aneurysmectomy to Prolongation of Life,* compared the abdominal aortic aneurysms seen at the Henry Ford Hospital and not operated upon between January 1, 1944 and December 31, 1965, and the operated cases beginning in 1952. The survival for the 480 operated patients was substantially better than for the 223 nonoperated patients, although poorer in both groups than for the population as a whole or for a population matched by age and sex. When size of the aneurysms was taken into consideration, small aneurysms not operated upon were accompanied by much better survival than large aneurysms not operated upon, and small aneurysms operated upon yielded a survival superior to that of small aneurysms not operated upon. The operative mortality for ruptured, for expanding, as well as for asymptomatic aneurysms had been dropping steadily. For asymptomatic aneurysms, it had dropped from 21% to 7%, for expanding aneurysms, the mortality had dropped from 43% to zero, and for ruptured aneurysms, it had dropped from 75% to 55%. Of the patients whose aneurysms were not operated upon,

34.6% died of rupture of the aneurysm, and 17% of coronary heart disease. Aneurysms smaller than 6 cm. had a rupture rate of over 19% "and a survival expectancy that was about half that of treated small aneurysms."

Discussion

Harvey R. Butcher, Jr., of St. Louis, confirmed the validity of Szilagyi's statistical methods and said, "It would appear that the one question which has needed an unequivocal answer, namely, is the operative mortality less than the liklihood of rupture, has been, at least in part, answered. Late rupture of the aneurysm occurred in some 15% of the control series, the operative mortality, while 13% over-all in the operatively treated group, was only 6% in the more recent years." Szilagyi, in closing, said, "The problem of small aneurysms, because of the changing clinical picture of aneurysms of the abdominal aorta, has assumed increased importance. There is no doubt that in judging the operability of small lesions a greater degree of conservatism is justified than in the assessment of aneurysms of larger size. In any case of abdominal aortic aneurysm there is a race between the rupture of the aneurysm and coronary heart disease as the cause of ultimate death; when the aneurysm is small and the patient has clinically significant coronary atherosclerosis, the latter is more likely to win."

The Business Meetings

The 1966 meeting was held at the Boca Raton Hotel and Club, Boca Raton, Florida, on May 23, 24, and 25, Leland S. McKittrick in the Chair.

Dr. Frederick L. Stone, of the National Institute of General Medical Sciences, was introduced by Dr. McKittrick. He said that "With Dr. Ravdin's help, and with the help of others, about four or five years ago we began to provide support in a limited and restricted way for young, aspiring surgeons who wanted to be trained for a research career. It was decided that we would seriously attempt to provide the kind of training support that surgeons need who wish to prepare themselves for an investigative career in academic medical centers . . . our Institute was given a mandate in three clinical fields: anesthesiology, diagnostic radiology, and surgery . . . It is our intention to provide long-term training support for young men interested in an investigative career in surgery. By *long term* I mean somewhere in the neighborhood of seven years." In the marvelously encouraging spirit of support by the government for medical research and education in that day, Stone said, "You do not get good research training in a department which is not active in research. Therefore, we believe that our research grant funds should be used to affect in a beneficial way the environment in which research training will go on . . . we would like to use our funds to supply the needs that are not readily supplied by other sources of support. Therefore, our research grant program will be one in which the support will be made available rather on a custom-tailored than on a mass production basis." [This was the beginning of the Academic Surgery Training program begun in 1965, supported by the NIH, which successfully sponsored promising candidates selected by department chairmen early in their residency careers, for development as academic surgeons. The program, which had been initially proposed by W. P. Longmire when he was Chairman of the Surgery Study Section of the NIH, was finally approved and implemented through the efforts of Champ Lyons and Jonathan Rhoads. At what was generally perceived to be White House insistence

during the Nixon administration, fellowship programs and training grants were sharply curtailed, and the Academic Surgery Program was phased out. Some programs closed out as late as June 30, 1979.]

The question of registration fees at meetings had been discussed many times and Treasurer, William D. Holden, informed the Fellows that it was the Council's feeling "that the American Surgical Association should not follow a policy of charging a registration fee nor leveling an assessment to help defray the cost of its annual meetings, but should, instead, cover such costs from the income from dues of members and should, at the same time, continue its policy of charging those attending for the annual reception and banquet . . . the Council thought that the membership of this organization should support through its dues the cost of the Annual Meeting, and that this should not be supported solely by the members who attend the meeting."

At this First Executive Session, Dr. Cope's Committee on Education reported briefly. The membership already had the report which had been published by Lippincott as "the Endicott House Summer Study to Reconsider Medical Education.". The major conclusions were: "Physicians *are at present in short supply* and plans for increasing the number are inadequate . . . *There is an urgent need . . . for new medical schools* . . . beyond those presently planned . . . *Specialization is inevitable, desirable and here to stay* . . . *Adventurous experimentation in medical education is the order of the day* . . . *Teaching attitudes and teaching methods are to be sharply overhauled* . . . *The present traditional curriculum is obsolete.* Departmental autonomy obstructs thoughtful collaborative teaching and promotes bad habits of learning . . . *New schools with innovative curriculums should be launched* as quickly as possible . . . *Four experimental curricular plans were suggested* . . . All of them are based on the concept of an 8- to 10-year program, three years of college including a Leventhal type of program in biology, three years of medical school starting with the Bennett approach to pathology and 2 to 4 years of graduate education . . . the shortened curriculum is feasible because the students now in colleges are better at understanding and can learn faster." Psychiatry and the behavorial sciences apparently had aroused considerable discussions and disagreement and were left for a separate summer study. [The simultaneous creation of new medical schools and expansion of enrollment in established medical schools was to result in little more than a decade, in what was appearing to be an overproduction of physicians. For better or for worse, radical changes in curriculum did not occur except for the widespread acceptance of the 4th year of medical school as entirely a time for "elective courses",- a development which has not proved to an unmixed blessing.]

At the Second Executive Session, among the recommendations of Council was "That, in the future, the practice prevail of having no officer or member of the Council serve as a sponsor of a candidate for Fellowship during his period of service on the Council."

Among those elected to Fellowship, were Dwight C. McGoon, Henry G. Schwartz, William Silen, Thomas E. Starzl, and as Honorary Fellows, Mr. Hedley Atkins, Sir Charles Illingworth and Russell, Lord Brock.

Elected as President was Oscar Creech, Jr., of New Orleans; as Vice-Presidents, Eugene M. Bricker, of St. Louis, and Angus D. McLachlin, of London, Ontario; Secretary, Harris B. Shumacker, Jr., of Indianapolis.

LXXXV

1967

The 1967 meeting was held at The Broadmoor, Colorado Springs, Colorado, May 11, 12, and 13, President Oscar Creech, Jr., of New Orleans, William Henderson Professor of Surgery and Chairman, Department of Surgery, Tulane University School of Medicine, in the Chair. Among those who had died in that year were William E. Ladd, who had achieved in his lifetime recognition as the Father of Pediatric Surgery in the United States; Robert M. Janes, of Toronto; Francis Chandler Newton, of Boston; Grantley W. Taylor, of Boston; and John deJ. Pemberton, of the Mayo Clinic, of whom, reminiscing in his Presidential Address in 1977, Claude Welch said "who could forget a demonstration of flawless technique by Pemberton as he easily performed 19 thyroidectomies in the Mayo Clinic in a single morning?"

For the second time, the Association had elected as President a man whose days were more surely to be numbered than those of the other Fellows. When Elliott Cutler was elected in March, 1947, he was known to have osseous metastases from a prostatic cancer, and in fact, died the August after that meeting. Oscar Creech, known at the time of his election to be suffering from lymphoma which had escaped from control, died seven months after the 1967 meeting, over which he presided.

The Presidential Address, *The Surgical Residency Revisited,* reviewed the growth of the residency system beginning with Halsted at the John Hopkins Hospital in 1889. In the clearest fashion, Creech said that the residency training program as it

existed had served its purpose, that surgery had become more and more a postgraduate discipline, that to a considerable extent less productive service activities had replaced training and educational activities, and that the *education* of surgeons had been neglected for the *training* of surgeons. He proposed "that graduate surgical programs be divided into primary and secondary phases. Primary surgical education, consisting of three years including internship, should focus exclusively on development of clinical skills. It should begin with three to four months in the animal laboratory, where operative technic and applied physiology are learned. Instruction in technic should be given by expert surgeons who require proficiency for advancement of the student. Next should come training in surgical pathology, with emphasis on gross appearance of normal and diseased organs, as seen at operation and necropsy. Again, demonstration of competence should be required. The remaining time, perhaps as much as 24 to 27 months, should be spent on the surgical wards, including the specialties, and in emergency rooms, working under the close supervision of members of the attending staff. If the student were freed from the laborious, time-consuming, and largely unrewarding ancillary duties he now performs as an apprentice, he could, under close tutorial supervision, make each case an exciting learning experience. Responsibility for patient care would not necessarily be graded nor determined by months in training, but by the level of proficiency to which a student had advanced . . . On completion of the primary phase, examinations would determine whether or not a student were prepared to move to the secondary level . . . the student would be required to demonstrate his competence in diagnosis, in performance of the operation, in after-care, and in general knowledge, in much the same way as was required by the American Board of Surgery in its early years. If this preparation were considered inadequate, he would have an opportunity to remedy the deficiencies. All surgical students, irrespective of eventual subspecialty interest, would complete primary graduate education . . . *any* surgical subspecialty can be mastered within two years and some within one year, if the student is properly prepared. The secondary part of a surgeon's education should be in preparation for a specific career." Those who were going into academic careers would undertake a period of research training "either within or outside of graduate-degree programs. Upon completion of research training, the student would return to the hospital for clinical training in a specialty. Students planning a career in surgical practice would need only one or two years to acquire the special skills needed in a specialty. At the end of this period, the educational institution would examine its students to determine their proficiency as specialists. Those qualifying would be recommended to the certifying boards for final examination and certification. The important difference from the present system is that surgeons would be examined *first* by the institution in which they trained, before being recommended for examination by certifying boards." Such a system obviously meant that a good deal of what was done now by house officers would have to be done by "a new category of medical personnel, which I shall call medical or surgical *adjuncts.*" Such a man would have a special four-year baccalaureate program and a year of apprenticeship in a specialty, "The surgical adjunct would be a member of the surgical team. He would work in admitting departments and emergency rooms of hospitals and clinics, screening surgical patients and treating self-limited infections and injuries. He would assist at operations and would perform primary care of patients after operation. His work would be that of a bona fide professional member of the surgical team . . . for the most part, the surgical adjunct would have certain duties and responsibilities now assumed by surgical interns and residents, not nurses." The certifying boards in surgery, Creech indicated, had served their purpose splendidly up to this point, "Today, however, the primary purpose of some of the certifying boards appears to be the expansion of the anatomic and pathologic limits of the respective specialties, while

encroachment by another specialty is vigorously resisted . . . consider how much the practice of medicine has changed during the last thirty years. And consider how the specialties have responded, not by reconstituting themselves, but by accessions to insure their continued existence." Whereas ". . . a certifying board may decide arbitrarily that candidates for examination must be trained to do an operation which traditionally has been done by a specialist in another field, the opportunities for residents to do this operation are limited . . . In the process of enlarging the specialty while constricting the educational base on which it rests, the prime considerations of competence and welfare of the patient may be overlooked." [Although there were "trade union" jurisdictional disagreements among a number of specialties as to what "turf" belonged to whom, Creech's reference was generally understood to be applied to the problem presented by the otolaryngologists. Their board was increasingly "requiring" applicants for certification to have training in plastic and reconstructive surgery and in radical head and neck surgery, ignoring, as Creech indicated, the fact that the clinical material was limited and, as traditional general surgeons insisted, refusing at the same time to prepare their candidates in the techniques and principles of general surgery to the degree that was required for this extension of their interest. It was generally assumed that the virtual eradication of suppurative disease of the mastoids and paranasal air sinuses, and the resultant loss of these fields of operative surgery to the specialty, had been the driving force for this re-orientation.] Creech challenged "The legitimacy of the union of obstetrics and gynecology . . . Child-bearing and problems of fertility are more closely allied to medicine and endocrinology than to surgery. On the other hand, gynecology, which is concerned with surgical diseases of the female pelvis, is a narrow field indeed. Would it not be natural to classify obstetrics, or reproductive physiology, as a medical specialty and then to develop [other] specialists whose interests are in surgical diseases of women? One year of intensive training in gynecology after primary surgical education would adequately prepare the surgeon for practice in such a specialty." At the same time, he suggested ". . . another category of specialist . . . a systems specialist, trained to render all medical care within an organ system. The evolution of subspecialties in medicine and surgery has often resulted in needless duplication of facilities and personnel as well as fragmented patient care and teaching . . . gastroenterology and gastrointestinal surgery are concerned with the same organs, these fields overlap widely in teaching, prac-

TABLE 1. *The Clinical Spectrum of the Medullary Thyroid Carcinoma–Pheochromocytoma Syndrome*

1. Familial medullary thyroid carcinoma
   a. Usually bilateral
   b. Metastases to cervical nodes in about 2/3
   c. Distant metastases in about 1/3

2. Familial pheochromocytomas
   a. Frequently bilateral
   b. Rarely malignant

3. Familial medullary thyroid carcinoma associated with pheochromocytoma

4. Non-familial medullary thyroid carcinoma associated with pheochromocytoma

Parathyroid tumors, neurofibromas, diabetes mellitus, malignancy in other organs occur in a few patients in any of above categories

Melvin A. Block, Robert C. Horn, Jr., J. Martin Miller, John L. Barrett, and Brock E. Brush, *Familial Medullary Carcinoma of the Thyroid.* Volume LXXXV, 1967.

tice, and research. The same is true for cardiology and cardiovascular surgery, nephrology and genito-urinary surgery, and neurology and neurologic surgery. We should consider, at least on an experimental basis, the reorganization of departments by organ systems rather than by disciplines." And finally, for once the President chose not to blame the government or social changes, or educational theorists, "If blame is to be placed, however, for failure to anticipate disappearance of ward patients for teaching, fragmentation of surgery into isolated subspecialties, and evolution of certifying boards as policy makers in surgical education, the American Surgical Association must accept a large part of it. Nor may we shift responsibility to the boards, for they have been forced to extend their responsibilities far beyond the purpose for which they were created because their constituent organizations have not always furnished proper counsel . . . An era in medicine is drawing to a close, and although it has been a golden period,

highlighted by monumental developments in surgery, it *is* almost over . . . when maintenance of health will equal treatment of disease in importance and attention, when the role of the medical specialist will be that of consultant, when diagnosis will be a function of machines, not men, the surgeon may remain as the only physician closely and personally involved in the life of his patient."

* * *

Medullary carcinoma of the thyroid had been mentioned before [the term medullary carcinoma of the thyroid had been introduced by Hazard, Hawk and Crile, in 1959; and the distinctive tumor was described in seven cases by Horn in 1951, and by Wollner and others from the Mayo Clinic in 1961], but Melvin A. Block, R. C. Horn, Jr., J. M. Miller, and J. L. Barrett, all by invitation, and Brock E. Brush, of Detroit, Surgeon in Charge, First Surgical

Section, Division of General Surgery, Henry Ford Hospital, *Familial Medullary Carcinoma of the Thyroid,* now emphasized a special aspect, "Although thyroid carcinoma in general is not known to be hereditable, the medullary variety of carcinoma of the thyroid does occur in some families with a dominant autosomal inheritance." They had found two such families, the carcinoma affecting females more often than males. There were no pheochromocytomas in either family, but one patient had a parathyroid adenoma. The carcinoma was recognized histologically by its characteristic cells and by the appearance,- in eight of their nine cases,- of amyloid in it. They recognized the four clinical patterns of medullary thyroid carcinoma [as shown in the table]. They referred to the various syndromes of multiple endocrine tumors and were particularly insistent on separating the medullary carcinoma of the thyroid pheochromocytoma syndrome from the Zollinger-Ellison syndrome. The treatment of medullary carcinoma of the thyroid was "Total or near total thyroidectomy and lateral neck dissection, on one or both sides and modified depending on operative findings . . . if distant metastases are not evident." Parathyroid tumors occurred sufficiently often to ". . . justify obtaining a serum calcium determination prior to all operations for thyroid nodules." They went so far as to ask "Whether near total thyroidectomy is justified for healthy adult members of those families in which medullary thyroid carcinoma has occurred in approximately 50 per cent of previous generations . . ." and suggested ". . . periodic examinations of their thyroids, including the use of scintigrams."

Discussion

Samuel R. Powers, of Albany, reported on a family under study with ten proven and 15 probable pheochromocytomas, five medullary carcinomas of the thyroid, and two parathyroid tumors. "Four patients in this family have died from unsuspected pheochromocytoma during or immediately after surgical procedures on the thyroid gland. The pheochromocytomas in this syndrome tend to be multicentric and bilateral so that bilateral total adrenalectomy appears to be the treatment of choice. The high incidence of associated medullary carcinoma and parathyroid tumors . . . often bilateral, required careful investigation." Stanley R. Friesen, of Kansas City, pointed out that patients had to be followed for long periods of time since the pheochromocytoma ". . . may not occur at the same time."

* * *

John L. Madden, of New York, Director, Department of Surgery, St. Clare's Hospital, and by invitation, Souhel Kandalaft, *Electrocoagulation. A Primary and Preferred Method of Treatment for Cancer of the Rectum,* [acknowledgedly resurrecting a technique championed by A. A. Strauss, of Chicago, in 1935] aroused much more impassioned discussion in the corridors that day and in the succeeding years than is evident from the record of the *Transactions.* Between 1954 and 1956, Madden had treated primarily by electrocoagulation 28 cancers of the rectum. The lesions were located on the posterior wall in 12 patients, on the anterior wall in nine, on the lateral wall in two, and were circumferential in four. The level was at the anus in two, between 2 and 6 cm. in 17, and at 7 to 10 cm. in eight. The number of fulguration sessions required varied from one to 12. The tumor size was 1 to 4 cm. in 13, and 5 to 7 cm. in eight. Bleeding, which required electrocoagulation for control, occurred in a quarter of the patients, and two required blood transfusions. In two of the patients with circumferential lesions, the resultant stricture yielded satisfactorily to finger dilation. A perforation during fulguration occurred in one patient, requiring a temporary colostomy. One patient with a squamous cell carcinoma of the anus, involving the buttock and vagina,- considered inoperable,- developed a rectovaginal fistula. All patients were hospitalized, spinal anesthesia was employed, the surface of the tumor was first fulgurated, and the necrotic coagulum curetted away. Bleeding points were coagulated. "It has been observed repeatedly that the active bleeding ceases when all of the tumor tissue is removed . . . The fulguration and scraping are repeated until a soft pliable base is noted by palpation. A final fulguration is then done . . . In each fulguration session, three to six fulgurations and scraping are usually done. Ideally the tumor should be eradicated in one session. This goal was achieved in approximately one of every four patients treated." Early inspection, at ten to 14 days, was under spinal anesthesia, biopsies for frozen section were taken, and the fulguration procedure repeated if indicated. Re-examination at close intervals was required. Seventeen patients were alive and well an average of 50 months; two patients were alive with disease at 37 months; three patients were dead of disease at 24 months; and two were dead of other causes. In Madden's three original patients, who had refused abdominoperineal operation for resectable tumors, the result had been excellent and he had been encouraged to pursue the technique. Strauss had stated that even with incomplete fulguration the remainder of the tumor might disappear. Madden had not observed that. Strauss, in 1965, and Wassink, in the Netherlands, in 1956, had postulated an antigen-antibody reaction produced by the absorption of tumor destruction products which might not only result in destruction of cells in the regional lymphatics, but perhaps be aided by the persistence of the immunologic apparatus in the regional lymphatics.

Discussion

Alton Ochsner, of New Orleans, said ". . . the older surgeons of this organization . . . recall vividly how actual cautery was used 50 years ago, and used very effectively. Actual cautery is a modality of surgical therapy which is at times still worthwhile. I remember Vilray Blair, the father of plastic surgery . . . in the United States, using it extensively when I was a student at Washington U, and my mentor, Dr. A. J. Ochsner, used it very extensively. Alfred Strauss has called attention to the value of this, not only as a destructive agent, but he has observed, as some of us have, that individuals whose primary lesion is treated with cauterization and the primary lesion destroyed—that metastatic lesions have decreased; not always, but enough to be worthwhile. Dr. Strauss' idea about this, based upon his clinical and experimental investigations, is that as a result of the destruction of the tumor *in situ,* immune bodies are elaborated from this tumor which in turn have a beneficial effect upon the metastatic lesions." J. Englebert Dunphy, of San Francisco, said "I have only done this twice, in 1955, and probably didn't do it properly, because both patients developed a retrorectal recurrence and required an abdominal perineal resection. So I would hesitate to accept the suggestion that it become the routine therapy for all patients with carcinoma of the rectum." Madden, closing, hoped "that the members of this Association would try this procedure, using the same basic technic, so that we can obtain data which will be statistically valid. I do believe this is an excellent procedure, not only for the inoperable or for the elderly patient, but for the individual who has a resectable primary carcinoma of the rectum, because in our experience, the smaller the lesion, the better are the results that are obtained."

* * *

Rupert B. Turnbull, Jr., member of the Staff of the Cleveland Clinic Foundation, and by invitation, Kenneth Kyle, Frank R. Watson, and John Spratt [the latter two from the Ellis Fischel State Cancer Hospital and Cancer Research Center, Columbia, Missouri], *Cancer of the Colon: The Influence of the No-Touch Isolation Technic on Survival Rates,* presented the results of an analysis of 896 patients with cancer of the colon treated at the Cleveland Clinic Hospital from 1950 to 1964. [The collaborators from Missouri had performed the statistical analyses of the material.] Fisher and Turnbull, in 1955, "reported cancer cells in the portal venous blood of 8 to 25 resected segments . . . and suggested that the cells had been scattered by operative manipulation", [but prior to the report] Turnbull in late 1953 ". . . adopted a technic of colon resection for cancer wherein the cancer-bearing segment was not manipulated or handled in any manner until after the lymphovascular pedicles were divided and ligated and the colon was divided at the elected sites for resection . . . the name *no-touch isolation* was adopted." Turnbull had employed that technique in every colon cancer operated by him since then, at the same time that five other surgeons at the Cleveland Clinic Hospital had employed the conventional technique ". . . characterized by ligation and division of the lymphovascular pedicles *after* mobilization of the cancer-bearing segment." Turnbull's patients had an overall, age-adjusted five-year survival of 81.6% when resection was done for cure. Life table of stage A, B, and C cancers taken together, life table for A, B, C cancers resected for cure, and a life table for C stage cancers all showed substantially better survivals for the no-touch technique. There was not any difference in the A and B stages combined. Turnbull's conclusion was ". . . the greatly improved survival rates are due to the use of the *no-touch isolation* resection method and that the heretofore conventional manipulative resection technics for cancer of the colon should be abandoned."

Discussion

J. Englebert Dunphy, of San Francisco, said that this might be ". . . the most important advance in the surgical treatment in carcinoma of the colon in the last thirty years." The survival after operation for carcinoma of the colon and rectum had improved dramatically from 1920 to 1940 due ". . . to major advances in technic, wider resections, better resections, and lower surgical mortality", but there had not been much improvement since, ". . . this paper that we have heard today represents an almost 100% improvement in the treatment of carcinoma of the rectum with metastases to lymph nodes. I think

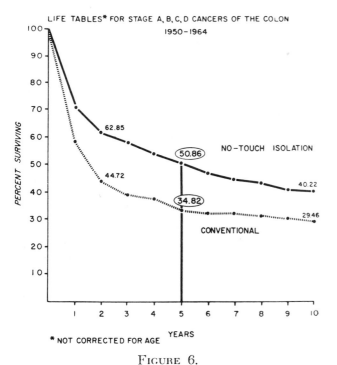

LIFE TABLES* FOR STAGE A, B, C, D CANCERS OF THE COLON
1950–1964

FIGURE 6.

* NOT CORRECTED FOR AGE

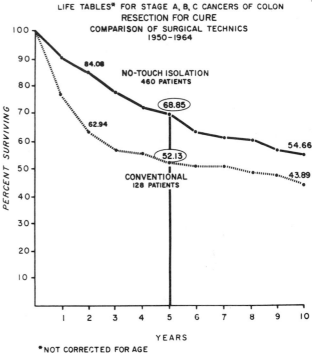

LIFE TABLES* FOR STAGE A, B, C CANCERS OF COLON
RESECTION FOR CURE
COMPARISON OF SURGICAL TECHNICS
1950–1964

FIGURE 7.

*NOT CORRECTED FOR AGE

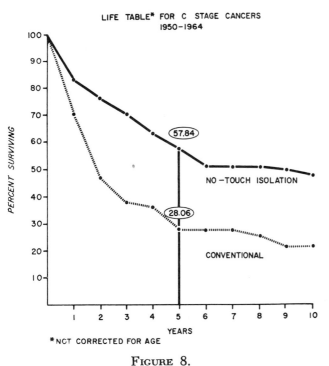

LIFE TABLE* FOR C STAGE CANCERS
1950–1964

FIGURE 8.

*NOT CORRECTED FOR AGE

Turnbull compared his own results at the Cleveland Clinic, in his technique of division of the vascular pedicle and division of the bowel at the points of resection before manipulation of the tumor, with results of the "conventional technic" of five colleagues at the Cleveland Clinic Hospital during the same time. There was no difference in the stage A and B tumors taken together, and the improvement, in Turnbull's patients, came in patients with stage C tumors.

R. B. Turnbull, Jr., K. Kyle, F. R. Watson, and J. Spratt, *Cancer of The Colon:* The Influence of the No-Touch Isolation Technic on Survival Rates. Volume LXXXV, 1967.

we must reserve final judgment, but I would agree 100% with the conclusions of Dr. Turnbull that the no-touch technic must be adopted by all of us at once. I don't think there is any need for a randomized study, because this advance is so significant, it's like trying to randomize whether ligation of the patent ductus will be beneficial or not. There just won't be any doubt about it, if it's going to be as good as he says." On the other hand, Dunphy did indicate that there might be a factor of selection of patients at the Cleveland Clinic and the fact that different surgeons used the two techniques might invalidate some elements of the study. Philip Schofield, of Manchester, England, agreed that the figures, particularly for the C cases were highly significant. J. Peyton Barnes, of Houston, demonstrated his use of the technique, saying that he had started applying the same technique to the right colon in 1951 and published it in 1952. Stanley R. Friesen, of Kansas City, said he had been practicing such a no-touch no-coagulation technique since 1952, and reported it in 1957, and that his results were ". . . comparable to those reported today by Dr. Turnbull", but then raised the question, "Is it really the avoidance of manipulation or is it the wider excision of the left colon mesentery that gives the better results?" Spratt closed Turnbull's paper stating that "Dr. Turnbull's paper could be retitled *The Importance of Ligating the Lymph-Vascular Bundle as a First Step in Resecting Colonic Carcinomas.*" He thought the figures were valid in representing a doubling of the survival rate for group C carcinomas. [At the 1979 meeting at The Homestead, Hot Springs, Virginia, (q.v.) Goligher, of Leeds, brutally dismissed Turnbull's work, in an almost parenthetical remark, expunged from the published Discussion, "Dr. Turnbull's trial was totally uncontrolled, and I think, of very dubious value".]

* * *

M. Kiselow, by invitation; H. R. Butcher, Jr., of St. Louis, Professor of Surgery, Washington University School of Medicine; and E. M. Bricker, Professor of Clinical Surgery, Washington University School of Medicine, *Results of the Radical Surgical Treatment of Advanced Pelvic Cancer:* A Fifteen-Year Study, presented their experience now that "Seventeen years have passed since initial reports by Brunschwig and Appleby indicated the possible benefit of exenteration of the pelvic organs in patients with advanced pelvic cancer." They had performed the operation in 312 patients, two-thirds of them with "Persistent postirradiational carcinoma of the cervix . . ." In the last five years the mortality of exenteration was 7%, but the morbidity remained high both in the hospital and with complications of operation manifested after the patient returned home. The only postoperative complications accounting for more than one death were intestinal obstruction, six deaths, and hemorrhage, three deaths. The absolute survival, two years after opera-

tion was 56%, and five years after operation was 35%. The operation was not to be undertaken except ". . . under rare circumstances . . ." and "unless the nature and extent of the lesion seem to offer a chance for cure." Clear indications for operation in patients generally suitable were ". . . postirradiational carcinoma of the cervix, confined to the central pelvis . . . Carcinoma of the rectum, involving the lower urinary tract in a man . . .", sometimes "recurrent carcinoma of the cervix or endometrium following simple hysterectomy . . .", but not recurrent carcinoma of the rectum following abdominal perineal resection, nor recurrent carcinoma of the cervix following a Wertheim type hysterectomy. The patient, treated for carcinoma of the cervix and presenting with rectovaginal or vesico-vaginal fistula, had a pelvis which often contained ". . . a sloughing dirty cavity from which a positive diagnosis of carcinoma cannot be obtained by biopsy. The peripheral pelvic tissues are solidly indurated and fixed to the lateral pelvic walls, and it is practically impossible to determine whether or not the patient has active cancer." Even if this represented only radio-necrosis, the patient would be "greatly benefited by pelvic exenteration." Admittedly "When uniformly early diagnosis of cervical cancer is attained and excellent primary treatment is universal, the number of patients for whom this type of surgery might be beneficial should be very few." Since that was not true, many more patients might be benefited than were being offered the operation, "Of less than 1,000 cases reported from other institutions in the past 10 years, over half are those of Brunschwig." The operation was to be undertaken in institutions and by surgeons with the resources, the skills, and the clinical volume to provide the necessary skill and care and long-term follow up. The paper, as published, contains an explicit plea for the training of individuals for surgery of this kind "Although there are a few notable exceptions, the majority of gynecologic training services in this country do not provide adequate training for the performance of the type of surgery under discussion . . . the requirements of the Board of Obstetrics and Gynecology are inadequate for this purpose, or for that matter, for the handling of many of the surgical conditions in the pelvis which may be encountered in the course of gynecologic surgery . . . In all fairness, it also must be stated that the average general surgical training program provides an inadequate exposure to gynecologic pathology, and to the technical problems attendant upon operations in the female pelvis. There is little assurance that an individual who has become a 'qualified' surgeon is in any way competent to operate on the female pelvis . . . what can the surgeons who direct American surgery do to insure the proper application of exenterative pelvic surgery to the patients who would be benefited by it?"

Discussion

Somers H. Sturgis, of Boston, agreed that "These patients are first seen by gynecologists, who, as the authors point out, are almost without exception unprepared for such surgery. Yet a 5-year salvage rate of 35%, presented by Dr. Bricker's group, surely must be considered a worthwhile goal for stimulating more responsible general surgeons to undertake these procedures." He believed that the operative skills and the postoperative expertise for managing the patients could come only from a large experience and that the operation should be performed only in special centers. However, ". . . gynecologists in general still follow the traditional pattern of referring their Stage 3 and 4 cancers of the cervix for radiation . . . Radiologists . . . are . . . not always quick to send their recurrent cases back to a surgeon." Alexander Brunschwig, of New York, congratulated ". . . Dr. Bricker and his group on . . . the best figures yet." When Brunschwig had begun pelvic exenteration ". . . it was not to achieve a 5-year cure; it was simply to explore the possibilities of alternatives to chordotomy . . . The fact that a 5-year cure could be achieved was totally unimaginable at that time." In patients with advanced cervical cancer previously untreated by any means, they had 38% five-year survivors in those with no lymph node metastases, 11% five-year survivors in those with lymph node metastases. In 393 radiation failures, they had 72 five-year survivors,- 18%. "Between 1947 and 1952—15 years ago—196 cases were performed among whom 14 are living and well 15 to 20 years later. All had cancer except one, who had massive radiation necrosis." His mortality had steadily dropped, and for 1958 to 1962 was ". . . for anterior exenteration, 8% surgical mortality; for total exenteration, 14%, for the whole group, 11%—still not quite as good as Dr. Bricker's group." Their total experience to 1960 was 699 cases with 19.4% five-year survival ". . . this operation, at first thought to be for palliation only, can afford an appreciable incidence of 5-year cures, or longer, in a group of patients ordinarily considered hopeless." He agreed that there was a need for "action to improve the situation regarding abdominal surgical training in depth for at least some of those going into gynecology." [Gynecological oncology is now a recognized subspecialty of gynecology.]

* * *

At the 1963 meeting there had been vigorous disagreement concerning the physiology of portal hypertension and the proper techniques of diversion, and now W. Dean Warren, of Miami, Professor and Chairman, Department of Surgery, University of Miami School of Medicine; Robert Zeppa, and John J. Fomon, both by invitation, *Selective Trans-Splenic Decompression of Gastroesophageal Varices by Distal Splenorenal Shunt*, pointed out that "Recent reports by Callow, *et al.* [1965], Conn and Lindenmuth [1965], and Jackson, *et al.* [1965]. . . in spite of a low operating mortality . . . have not demonstrated the superiority of the surgical group" in terms of survival. "Following portacaval shunt, the death rate from hepatic failure is greatly increased and completely offsets the undeniable protection afforded against fatal hemorrhage . . . portacaval shunt initiates or accelerates hepatic deterioration in some patients and the anticipated death rate from hepatic failure is substantially increased." Delayed death from hepatic failure did not appear to result from operative trauma unassociated with portal shunting. Nonshunting procedures,- gastric devascularization, splenectomy, etc.,- had given good results in some situations, particularly bilharzial cirrhosis, but continued and recurrent bleeding were common in alcoholic cirrhotics. Encephalopathy did not result from non-shunting procedures. Complete relief of splanchnic hypertension was probably not as important as it had seemed, because "resistant ascites" was now rarely seen, hypersplenism was uncommonly a problem and could be treated by splenic artery ligation. He implied that it might be an advantage not to achieve complete splanchnic decompression [which in 1959 and 1963 he had recommended accomplishing with a side-to-side portacaval shunt], "Ideally, an operation should allow continued perfusion of hepatic parenchyma by portal flow from the intestine and yet decompress the venous system in the gastroesophageal area. Gastrosplenic isolation with distal splenorenal shunt seems to meet these requirements." The procedure he had devised involved approaching the lower border of the pancreas through the root of the transverse mesocolon, elevating the pancreas to expose the splenic vein close to its junction with the inferior mesenteric vein. The splenic vein was divided, and dissected back toward the spleen securing the numerous small tributaries from the pancreas until the splenic vein had been sufficiently mobilized for an end-to-side anastomosis of its splenic end to the left renal vein. In addition, the coronary vein was "obliterated with

THE LIVER, PORTAL HYPERTENSION GROUP

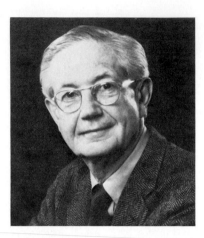

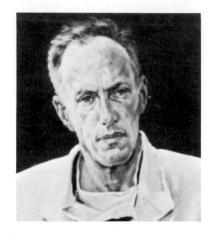

C. Gardner Child, III, (c. 1955-60) 1908—, M.D. Cornell 1934, Internship and residency New York Hospital 1934-42, Instructor and Associate Professor 1940-53, Professor and Chairman, Tufts 1953-58, Professor and Chairman, University of Michigan 1959-74, Professor, Emory University Department of Surgery 1977- . Diseases of liver and pancreas his lifetime work, devised the Child's system of gradation of the gravity of cirrhosis, published a basic monograph on portal hypertension. For a time spear-headed the move to resectional therapy for chronic pancreatitis advising near total pancreatectomy, safer than total pancreatectomy and not requiring duodenectomy. Tall, "professorial," thoughtful, he enraged a good many by an address in which he stated he hoped to see the day when, in his university at least, surgery would no longer be taught to medical students but would be reserved for post-graduate students.

Ben Eiseman (c. 1965) 1917—, M.D. Harvard 1943; Intern, Massachusetts General Hospital; Residency, Barnes Hospital, St. Louis, remaining until 1953 as Assistant Professor in Surgery; to University of Colorado 1953-61, Associate Professor to Professor and Chief, Surgical Service, Veterans Administration Hospital; Professor and Chairman, University of Kentucky, Lexington 1961-67; Professor of Surgery, University of Colorado 1967- . Dynamic, provocative, willing to challenge any doctrine. Remarkable series of innovative clinical and laboratory contributions,- like use of coconut milk as a volume expander in jungle conditions, use of a valve controlled peritoneo-venous shunt, use of ATP in shocked animals. Undertook in animals a systematic study of extracorporeal circulation through a heterologous liver in the treatment of hepatic insufficiency and conducted a clinical trial—demonstrating effective function of the perfused organ and sometimes dramatic improvement without altering the ultimate result in those desperate cases. Rear Admiral, U.S.N.R., relentlessly competitive, skier and mountain climber.

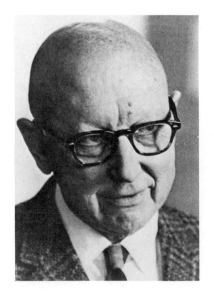

Robert R. Linton (c. 1955) 1900-1979, born in Scotland. M.D. Harvard 1925; Intern, Johns Hopkins; Intern-Resident, Massachusetts General Hospital and identified with it for his entire professional life, eventually Assistant Clinical Professor. A massive contributor to the development of peripheral vascular surgery,- the Linton procedure for post-phlebitic ulcers; the use of the saphenous vein for femoral artery replacement,- he had a major interest in and effect upon the surgery of portal hypertension. A meticulous and extraordinarily skillful surgeon, precise and thoughtful in his clinical analyses, he was characterized by blunt, direct, uncompromising presentation of his own views and equally forceful rejection of differing views. For the treatment of portal hypertension, he continued from first to last to espouse the operation of the original splenorenal shunt, achieving enviable results.

(Portrait courtesy of W. Gerald Austen, M.D., Boston)

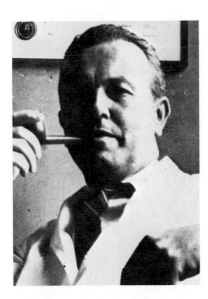

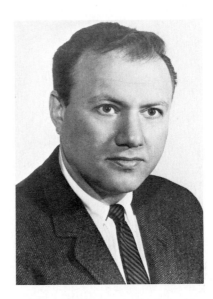

William V. McDermott (c. 1960) 1917—. M.D. Harvard 1942; Residency training at Massachusetts General Hospital; Instructor to Professor, Harvard 1951-63; Director, Fifth (Harvard) Surgical Service and Sears Surgical Laboratories at Boston City Hospital 1963-73; Director, Harvard Surgical Service, New England Deaconess Hospital 1973-   . In-depth studies of hepatic physiology and portal hypertension, particularly the nature, cause and prevention of ammonia intoxication. Developed his own double end-to-side portacaval shunt. Key element in the "Boston Liver Group".

Marshall J. Orloff, (c. 1960) 1927—. M.D. University Of Illinois 1951; Internship, University of California; Residency and Fellowship, University of Pennsylvania; Assistant Professor of Surgery, University of Colorado 1959-61; Professor of Surgery, UCLA and Chief, Harbor General Hospital 1961-67; Professor and Chairman, University of California, San Diego 1967- Wide interests in gastrointestinal physiology, with particular emphasis on liver disease and portal hypertension. Vigorously espoused immediate porto-systemic shunting for variceal bleeding, achieving results not matched elsewhere for emergency shunting.

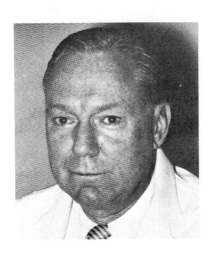

Louis M. Rousselot 1902-1974, Vice-President 1965. M.D. Columbia, 1927. Training, Columbia Presbyterian 1927-1933, remaining until 1948, then Associate in Surgery. 1948-67, as Director of Surgery, St. Vincent's Hospital, and Professor of Clinical Surgery, New York University School of Medicine, created a vigorous Department of Surgery. Genial, soft-spoken, suave and diplomatic, he spent the rest of his career in Washington in a variety of government posts, most important, Deputy Assistant Secretary of Defense for Health Affairs (succeeding another Fellow, Frank Berry) and Assistant Secretary of Defense for Health and Environment. In Washington, he played a major role in designing, modifying and pushing through to passage the legislation which resulted in the establishment of the Uniformed Services University of the Health Sciences, providing a medical school for the Armed Services,- something then and now not viewed with enthusiasm in all quarters. An early participant and principal actor in Allen Whipple's Spleen Clinic at Columbia, Rousselot contributed the first direct measures of portal pressure in patients with portal hypertension,- confirming the fact of its existence,- the concept of congestive splenomegaly and, in the United States, pioneered splenoportography, and demonstrated the presence of numerous porto-systemic shunts in cirrhotics, attributing to the low flow in them, their failure to decompress the portal venous bed.

(Portrait: *Surgery,* Volume 77, No. 2, February, 1975)

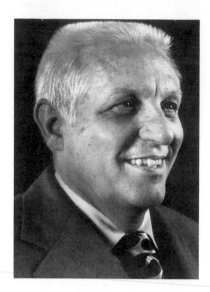

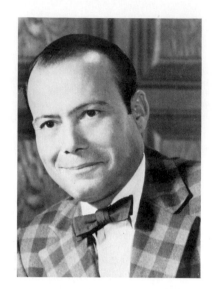

W. Dean Warren, (c. 1978) 1924—. M.D. Johns Hopkins 1950; Internship, Johns Hopkins; Residency, University of Michigan, and Barnes Hospital, St. Louis; Assistant Professor of Surgery, University of Virginia 1960-63; Professor and Chairman, University of Miami 1963-71; Professor and Chairman, Emory University 1971-   . Investigative and clinical activities largely involved with the physiology of portal hypertension and its operative correction, emphasizing the desirability of a "selective shunt" sufficient to prevent bleeding without inviting ammonia intoxication. Champions his eponymic distal splenal shunt, with verve, wit, and a massive laboratory and clinical experience.

Robert Zeppa (c. 1968) 1924—. M.D. Yale 1952; Intern, University of Pittsburgh; Residency, University of North Carolina 1953-58, leaving Chapel Hill in 1965 as Associate Professor of Surgery; Professor of Surgery, University of Miami 1965-, Chairman 1971-   . Closely associated with Warren in studies of portal hypertension and development and application of the distal splenorenal shunt.

a continuous suture." He considered that his operation succeeded in its specific objectives "selective reduction of pressure and volume of flow through gastro-esophageal veins . . . [Maintenance of] portal venous perfusion of the liver . . . [Maintenance of] continual venous hypertension in the intestinal bed." He had performed the operation in four patients with two deaths and two good results. The postoperative radiographic studies showed ". . . diversion of splenic flow through a distal splenorenal shunt while superior mesenteric flow continues to perfuse the liver. The proposed metabolic advantage has been confirmed by a markedly superior response to protein tolerance testing." Warren thought his procedure was indicated "in patients with high volume portal flow to the liver."

Discussion

Harold Laufman, of the Bronx, New York, said that a year-and-a-half ago ". . . two of our young men, Drs. Auguste Denize and Franklin Davidson . . ." had in dogs connected the end of the splenic vein which drained the spleen, into the vena cava rather than to the renal vein as Warren had. "They showed that it is unquestionably true that blood ammonia levels are kept remarkably low in the splenocaval, as compared to the portacaval shunt." They had attempted the operation in one patient, but had been unable to complete it because of extensive retroperitoneal varices. Robert R. Linton, of Boston, was not quite sure why Warren was ". . . dissatisfied with a splenectomy and a proximal end-to-side splenorenal shunt, and perhaps he will tell us why . . . I am a strong advocate of the latter type of shunt . . . because more patients have lived a longer and healthier life with this type of shunt than with any other . . . and with much lower incidence of post-shunt encephalopathy," He had performed 73 splenorenal shunts and 26 portacaval shunts. At five years, 58% of the spleno-renal shunt patients were alive, only 31% of the portacavals. At the end of ten years, the figures were 22 splenorenal shunt patients surviving,- 30%,- and four portacaval shunt patients surviving,- 15%. He thought of Warren's operation that it was ". . . an ingenious new variant, but I am

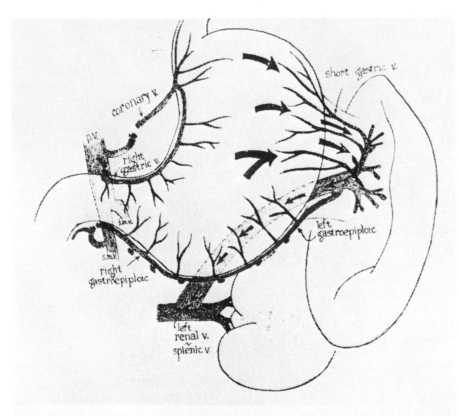

FIG. 9. The completed operation is depicted diagrammatically. Arrows indicate the direction of blood flow. The distal splenorenal anastomosis has been completed and the coronary vein has been ligated. The gastrocolic ligament has been divided and the right gastroepiploic vein ligated. At the time the gastro hepatic ligament is divided the right gastric vein is ligated. Blood from the inferior (i.m.v.) and superior (s.m.v.) mesenteric veins continues to perfuse the liver by way of the portal vein.

Warren conceived that his procedure would preferentially decompress the gastroesophageal venous circulation, at the same time that the superior mesenteric vein return would continue to nourish the liver. Two patients had good results, one ascitic died of peritonitis, one patient died in hepatic coma and was found to have extensive necrosis of the liver. Hepatic artery, portal vein and the shunt were patent, although there were thrombi in the renal and splenic veins.

W. D. Warren, R. Zeppa, and J. J. Fomon, *Selective Trans-Splenic Decompression of Gastroesophageal Varices by Distal Splenorenal Shunt.* Volume LXXXV, 1967.

afraid that for many surgeons it will be too difficult to accomplish . . .", and asked whether Warren had had technical difficulties, particularly in isolating the splenic vein, and what effect the operation had on hypersplenism. Was it possible to do Dr. Warren's operation as an emergency for massive bleeding? Warren, closing, said that in dogs, they too, had used the splenocaval anastomosis because it was simpler and physiologically similar to the splenorenal. The portal pressure did drop with his operation. In answer to Dr. Linton, Warren said that when there was a very large splenic vein, the conventional splenorenal anastomosis produced a marked fall in portal pressure and did not differ from the side-to-side shunt, and when there was a small splenic vein, most people reported a high incidence of thrombosis. Dr. Linton was right in suggesting Warren's procedure was difficult. Hypersplenism, he said, would be ameliorated as with any shunt. "The splenic pressure is lowered to normal, just as it is following a portacaval shunt." He indicated that this was not the procedure to choose in an emergency situation.

* * *

Marshall J. Orloff, of San Diego, Professor and Chairman, Department of Surgery, School of Medicine, University of California [but presenting work performed at the Harbor General Hospital, and the UCLA School of Medicine, Torrance, California, before he moved to San Diego], *Emergency Portacaval Shunt: A Comparative Study of Shunt, Varix Ligation and Nonsurgical Treatment of Bleeding Esophageal Varices in Unselected Patients with Cirrhosis,* presented the results of the challengingly simple program for treatment of massive bleeding from esophageal varices which he had instituted at the Harbor General Hospital in 1961. If it was determined that the patient had esophageal varices, no other lesions responsible for bleeding, and convincing evidence of cirrhosis, a portacaval shunt was performed "within 8 hours of admission to the hospital." Three patients were excluded because they had duodenal ulcers, eight because they had gastritis, and none of those had varices. Forty patients underwent emergency portacaval shunts. The patient received posterior pituitary extract, large transfusions of blood less than 12 hours old, iced saline lavage of the stomach, and magnesium sulfate and neomycin instillation in the stomach through a tube, as well as saline enemas with neomycin, and therapeutic doses of vitamins K, C, and B. "No patient was treated with esophageal balloon tamponade." Twenty-five patients received a side-to-side portacaval anastomosis and 15 an end-to-side shunt, the choice usually being left to the surgeon, "except when portal pressure determinations indicated reversal of portal flow and made a side-to-side shunt mandatory [five cases]." All their patients were chronic alcoholics and 26 had consumed large quantities of alcohol in the 24 hours prior to admission. Eight patients showed ". . . evidence of encephalopathy ranging from stupor to confusion, slurred speech and asterixis." The mean serum bilirubin was 3.5 mg./100 ml., the range 0.4-12.7 mg./100 ml. The serum albumin was 3.8 Gm/100 ml. in the range from 2.6 to 4.9. Twenty-one of the 40 patients survived for 30 days and left the hospital,- 53% early survival. Fifteen of the 19 who had died, died of liver failure, two from massive bleeding from gastric ulcer, one from perforated duodenal ulcer and peritonitis, and one was found to have had a thrombosis of an end-to-side shunt. All other shunts were patent at autopsy. Four of the 21 early survivors died, leaving 17 long-term survivals,- 43%, all but one for more than one year. One of the patients had died after an operation for a bleeding duodenal ulcer, when he seemed to be well otherwise. Three of six patients who continued drinking

vigorously died of liver failure in three, 14, and 25 months. Nine of the 40 had bled at sometime since operation,- seven from a peptic ulcer, one from a ". . . dyscrasia associated with liver failure . . ." and one from an undemonstrated cause. None were thought to have had varices. Clinical jaundice appeared after discharge in six of the 21 early survivors, in four instances in association with terminal liver failure. None of the 21 developed ascites. Five of the 21 had had encephalopathy at some time since discharge. In 1962 Orloff had reported a comparison between emergency varix ligation and modern nonoperative treatment and had studied a recent nonoperative group with "modern medical therapy". The groups were equivalent in terms of age, sex, the degree of hepatic insufficiency, etc. The early thirty-day survival in the nonoperative group was 17%, in the varix ligation group, 54%, and in the emergency portacaval shunt, 53%. The four-year survival of the nonoperative group was 3%, of the varix ligation group, 21%, and of the emergency portacaval shunt, "predicted", was 43%, so that ". . . both forms of operative therapy produced an early survival rate which was 3 times greater than that resulting from medical management. The four-year survival rate after emergency shunt was significantly greater than the survival rate with the other types of treatment . . . early and definitive operative control of varix hemorrhage provides the cirrhotic patient with the greatest chance of surviving. Although . . . larger numbers of patients are clearly necessary, it would appear that the emergency portacaval shunt is the therapy of choice for most cirrhotic patients who bleed from esophageal varices."

Discussion

Francis C. Jackson, of Pittsburgh, [who had headed a cooperative Veterans Administration study of portacaval shunting], said that in the Veterans Administration study there had been 55 emergency shunts, all end-to-side portacaval shunts. The mortality was much higher for the 34 patients who received truly emergency shunts than for 21 who had continued bleeding on nonoperative therapy and were finally operated upon,- 45% as against 33% thirty-day mortality. Life table analyses suggested that the two groups would have about the same survival at the end of 36 months. In two patients they had performed emergency shunts by an extracorporeal circuit from the umbilical vein to a systemic vein and wondered whether it was not ". . . possible to abort a massive hemorrhage by intermittent decompression of the portal system . . . to gain the lower operative mortality of an elective therapeutic shunt." In their studies, the life table analysis showed ". . . no significant difference in the probability of survival at the level of 42 months . . .", between controls and patients who had prophylactic, therapeutic or emergency shunts. Their impression was that ". . . death in the bleeding controls is offset by the operative mortality or complications occurring with greater frequency in the shunted groups following an operation." Robert R. Linton, of Boston, thought Orloff's 47% mortality was too high, although it was better than that of others utilizing the same method, "I have favored a two-stage procedure for the emergent treatment of the patient with massive esophageal bleeding, in order to avoid the construction of a direct portacaval shunt, because it is impossible, I believe, to construct a splenorenal one, either Dr. Warren's or the other type, as an emergency procedure." His two-stage method consisted of "an immediate transthoracic suture of the bleeding esophageal varices after temporarily controlling the bleeding by cardioesophageal tamponade using a 'Linton' single balloon tube." The splenectomy and splenorenal shunt were performed six weeks later. He had had a mortality of 34% in a group of 44 patients so treated. William P. Mikkelsen, of Los Angeles, thought Orloff's mortality ". . . horrendous . . . but when compared with nonoperative management it assumes a better perspective." [He seemed to be saying that the patient who was a good risk immediately before the hemorrhage would tolerate emergency shunt and that in the bad risk patient emergency operation might spare the patient and the staff the agony of continuing hematemesis and innumerable transfusions, though the outcome might be no different.] Orloff, closing, re-emphasized that there had been no patient selection, and despite the high mortality, he pointed out to Dr. Linton that ". . . the survival rate following emergency shunt was about 15 times [?sic] greater than the survival rate of comparable patients following medical management, and it was about twice as high as the survival rate of patients subjected to emergency varix ligation and then an elective shunt." All of Orloff's patients were alcoholics, many of Dr. Linton's patients had posthepatic or non-alcoholic cirrhoses; Linton's patients were mostly private, Orloff's were all indigent. Continued alcoholism was a grave problem in his patients. He suggested that in the Veterans Administration study, "several factors of selection have been introduced." He concluded by saying that "On the basis of the findings in our small study, plus the recent experience of several other groups . . . the treatment of large numbers of bleeding cirrhotic patients by emergency portacaval shunt is justified."

* * *

It had been obvious for some time that human cardiac transplantation was imminent. Shumway and Lower, in Palo Alto, then Lower, in Richmond, and Willman and Hanlon, in St. Louis, among others, had been studying the technique by autotransplantation over a period of five years, systematically studying the effect upon the heart. Now V. L. Willman, of St. Louis, Professor of Surgery, St. Louis University; J. P. Merjavy, and R. Pennell, by invitation; and C. R. Hanlon, Professor of Surgery and Chairman of the Department of Surgery, St. Louis University, *Response of the Autotransplanted Heart to Blood Volume Expansion,* continued their work upon the effect of the excision and reimplantation of the heart upon its function. With catheters in the femoral artery, right atrium, and left atrium,- passed transbronchially,- and an inlying urethral catheter, blood volumes, cardiac outputs, and urinary output were constantly measured before and after infusion of 50 ml./Kg. of homologous blood in 15 minutes and subsequently after the infusion of 110 cc./Kg. of Ringer's lactate in 60 minutes. Nine dogs were studied at three weeks and again six months after reimplantation of the heart, and compared with nine normal dogs. Animals whose hearts had been autotransplanted began with an increased blood volume and an increased left atrial pressure. Previous studies had shown that cardiac output was high in those animals and myocardial function normal. The differences in the two groups of animals after loading with whole blood and loading with electrolytes was not great. The autotransplant animals showed impairment of water execretion after loading with whole blood but responded normally to electrolyte loading. This was interpreted as meaning that ". . . an osmoreceptor mechanism can override the effects produced by denervation of pressure receptors and stretch receptors in the left atrium. The striking difference in urinary response to infusion of blood as contrasted with electrolyte infusion, although both increase left atrial pressure to comparable levels, suggests the importance of a mechanism other than atrial baroreceptors for fluid control in barbiturate anesthetized animals with a denervated heart." They considered that they had demonstrated ". . . that fluid retention presenting as 'cardiac failure' can be on the basis of decreased afferent stimuli from the heart and not impaired myocardial function."

Discussion

Richard Lower, of Richmond, was the only discusser. He attributed to the St. Louis group the introduction of ". . . the idea and the observation that reinnervation of the heart does seem to occur much earlier than we originally thought, and we have now made observations on more than 20 animals who are long-term after autotransplantation, and have found that we could demonstrate reinnervation of the heart in all of these animals as early as 3 months after operation . . . some 4-1/2 months after transplantation . . . a control heart rate of 135, with stimulation of the stellate ganglion . . . jumps to 225 beats per minute . . . 2-1/2 volts of stimulation to the vagus nerve at around 4 months produced complete asystole. These are essentially normal responses. . . . early return to the heart of autonomic control is probably important, and may provide the transplanted heart with certain advantages that the artificial heart will never have."

* * *

W. A. Altemeier, of Cincinnati, Christian R. Holmes Professor and Chairman, Department of Surgery, University of Cincinnati; and by invitation, Joseph C. Todd, and Wellford W. Inge, *Gram-Negative Septicemia: A Growing Threat,* discussed a phenomenon which had been concerning surgeons, "There is considerable evidence that Gram-negative sepsis has become a serious threat in modern surgical practice. The widespread use of a succession of newly developed and highly potent antibacterial agents during the past 24 years has not been followed by the anticipated reduction in incidence, severity, and mortality from septicemia . . . there has been a progressive increase in the number of cases and changes in their bacterial types with Gram-negative bacilli becoming more frequent than Gram-positive. Blood stream infections caused by *Pneumococcus* and beta-hemolytic *Streptococcus* have become infrequent, while those caused by *Staphylococcus aureus* are relatively more frequent, and those caused by the Gram-negative bacilli are much more frequent. The failure of antibiotic therapy to prevent and cure most cases of Gram-negative septicemia has become increasingly obvious . . . Gram-negative septicemias are playing prominent roles in hospital-acquired sepsis, usually associated with problems in diagnosis, difficulties in successful management, and high mortality rates, particularly in those patients who develop evidence of septic shock." They reviewed the experience at the University of Cincinnati Medical Center with septicemias from January 1955, to March 1967. During that period they had had 398 patients with Gram-negative sepsis and the incidence had been strikingly progressive and particularly rapid in the last two years. They thought that it had been "related to the rapid extension of new and

complex surgical procedures to elderly and other poor-risk patients whose resistance was diminished by extensive trauma, associated chronic diseases, and treatment with steroids, immunosuppressive agents and anticancer drugs." The more frequent organisms were E. coli, Aerobacter aerogenes, Proteus, and Pseudomonas aeruginosa. In over half the cases, the urinary tract was the source of the bacteria; the respiratory system, alimentary tract, and the skin being other important sources. The septicemia was acquired in the hospital by three-quarters of the patients and the prognosis was then particularly grave, ". . . prophylactic antibiotic therapy has been ineffective in preventing Gram-negative septicemia, particularly in poor-risk patients . . . our experience has suggested that antibiotic therapy, particularly with large and prolonged dosage, may have contributed to the development and increasing incidence of Gram-negative septicemia . . . Reduction of the incidence of septic shock during the past 2 years by earlier recognition of Gram-negative septicemia has been followed by a marked drop in mortality rate."

* * *

Lloyd D. MacLean, of Montreal, Surgeon-in-Chief, Royal Victoria Hospital; Professor of Surgery, McGill University, and by invitation, W. G. Mulligan, A. P. H. McLean, J. H. Duff, *Patterns of Septic Shock in Man—Detailed Study of 56 Patients.* At the Royal Victoria Hospital, MacLean had for years been establishing ". . . a hemodynamic diagnosis for all patients in shock. One of three possibilities is usually apparent after measuring cardiac output, central venous pressure, arterial blood pressure and urine output. Two abnormalities are frequently seen: 1) cardiogenic shock, in which state the cardiac output fails to meet the needs of the body despite an adequate filling pressure; and 2) hypovolemic shock, which is characterized by a low cardiac output and low filling pressure. The third possibility is peripheral pooling, which is also characterized by a low filling pressure and a low cardiac output but in contrast to hypovolemia, there is a failure of sustained response of the central venous pressure and cardiac output to volume replacement. As a guide to therapy and to ascertain the severity of the shock, we have found it useful to measure, in addition, arterial blood lactate, pO_2, pCO_2, pH and hematocrit." Of their last 120 studied patients in shock, 56 had sepsis as the clinical cause. Twenty-two patients died of shock and an additional 12 died from other causes before discharge from the hospital. "A syndrome of early septic shock was seen in 28 patients who were

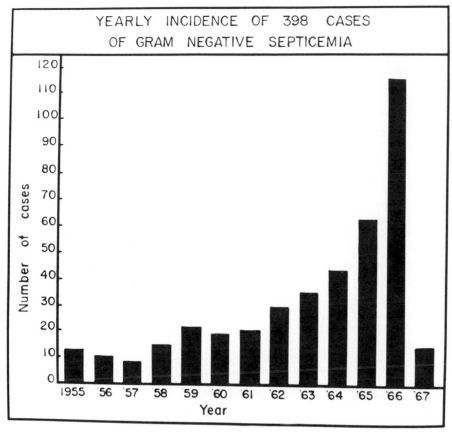

FIGURE 2.

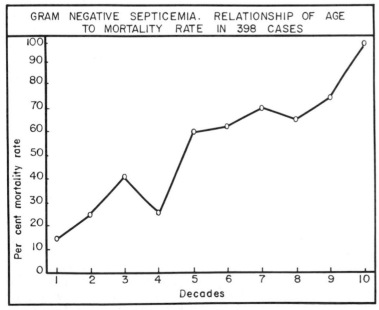

FIGURE 3.

The rapidly increasing incidence of Gram-negative septicemia and the rise in mortality from it with the age of the patient, show plainly. The most common organisms were E. Coli, Aerobacter aerogenes, Proteus, and Pseudomonas aeruginosa. Three-fourths of the patients acquired their septicemia in the hospital and the prognosis in them was particularly grave. The cause was thought to be the increasing gravity and complexity of surgical procedures applied to elderly and poor-risk patients with a multitude of invasive therapeutic and monitoring techniques.

W. A. Altemeier, J. C. Todd, and W. W. Inge, *Gram-Negative Septicemia:* A Growing Threat. Volume LXXXV, 1967.

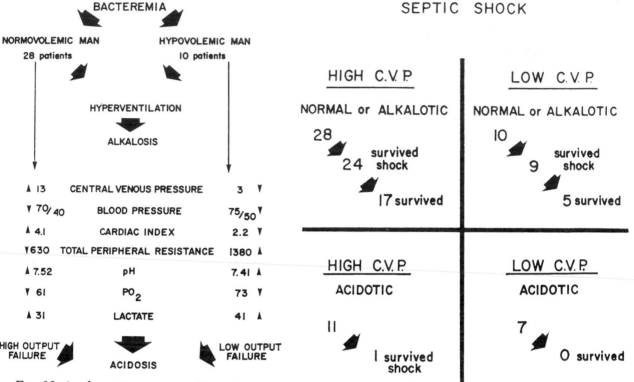

FIG. 13. A schematic summary of hemodynamic changes that occur with bacteremia in normovolemic man. In the former a high output state exists; in the latter, a low output. Both lead directly to metabolic acidosis which is extremely refractory to all forms of treatment. The early recognition of hyperventilation and respiratory alkalosis promotes early diagnosis.

FIG. 14. Mortality in 56 patients with septic shock. Only 6 of 38 patients died of shock if treatment was started before the onset of metabolic acidosis. Only 1 of 18 patients survived when treatment was started after the onset of metabolic acidosis.

MacLean's thesis was that "The natural history of septic shock . . . is from a state of respiratory alkalosis to metabolic acidosis." If the patient is normo-volemic at the onset of bacteremia, hyperdynamic circulation develops characterized by a high cardiac index, high central venous pressure, low peripheral resistance, hyperventilatory alkalosis, elevated blood volume, hypotension, warm dry extremities, lactate accumulation. If the patient, at onset of bacteremia has a low central venous pressure and low blood volume, as in patients with strangulated loops of bowel or peritonitis, "Cardiac index is low, central venous pressure is low, and peripheral resistance is high . . . the extremities are cool and cyanotic. Oliguria, hypotension, alkalosis and lactate accumulation also occur. While progression from alkalosis to acidosis has seldom been clearly documented in this group, we believe it does occur on the basis of clinical description of the acidotic patients prior to our period of observation."
Their Figure 14 demonstrated the importance of initiating therapy before the patient had become acidotic.

Lloyd D. MacLean, William G. Mulligan, A. P. H. McLean, and John H. Duff, *Patterns of Septic Shock in Man—A Detailed Study of 56 Patients.* Volume LXXXV, 1967.

normovolemic before the onset of the bacteremia or septic process and includes: 1) hyperventilation; 2) respiratory alkalosis; 3) a high cardiac index; 4) high central venous pressure; 5) low peripheral resistance; 6) elevated blood volume; 7) hypotension; 8) oliguria; 9) warm, dry extremities; and 10) arterial blood lactate accumulation. If recognized while still alkalotic, these patients responded to therapy designed to maintain cardiac output at an even higher level. There were only four deaths from shock among the 28 patients. If the patient was hypovolemic at the onset of sepsis, a quite different clinical picture was presented and consisted of: 1) low central venous pressure; 2) low cardiac output; 3) high peripheral resistance; and 4) cold, cyanotic extremities. Again, if found early, these patients were also alkalotic and responded to treatment which was primarily volume replacement and operation. If not seen until they were acidotic, a low fixed output persisted despite treatment, and a high mortality rate resulted. A classification based on central venous pressure and arterial pH was useful as a guide to treatment and prognosis. The four possibilities were: Group I—high CVP—alkalotic; Group II—high CVP—acidotic; Group III—low CVP—alkalotic; Group IV—low CVP—acidotic. Either high or low cardiac output failure characterized septic shock in man. Peripheral pooling, sufficient to prevent venous return to the heart, which occurs in the dog, did not appear in this series of patients. Gram-negative organisms were cultured from 42 of the 56 patients. Gram-positive organisms caused shock in 10 patients, of the hyperdynamic type in all but one. Candida albicans appeared to cause shock in four patients,- hyperdynamic in three and hypodynamic in one. Hyperbaric oxygen, used in five patients, did not lower arterial blood lactate in any, and all died. Patients who were able to raise their cardiac index over 1 L./min./M.^{2} in response to treatment had a much better prognosis than those who could not. Infections amenable to drainage and drained early were associated with improved survival. They identified as the most important predisposing factors in those 56 patients, "long-term treatment with cortisone; prophylactic antibiotic therapy including the preparation for colon surgery; cirrhosis of the liver; tracheostomy, urethral instrumentation; and chronic debilitating disease."

Discussion

Howard Frank, of Boston, said that they had not found "such well-defined patterns of cardiac output." In connection with MacLean's statement that some patients with septic shock were hypovolemic, Frank emphasized the importance of having both the blood volume determinations and central venous pressure determinations since "These parameters are not interchangeable. Our data show many instances of hypovolemia in the presence of a normal central venous pressure. There are also many moments, especially in elderly patients with peritonitis, when a normal blood volume cannot be tolerated by injured heart and lungs." John H. Siegel, of New York, agreed with MacLean's emphasis upon a continuum in patients in septic shock, the patient progressing from one stage to the next. He agreed with MacLean's observation that "*all* patients in septic shock, regardless of cause or bacterial etiology . . . have a significantly decreased vascular tone com-

pared to those with nonseptic shock." He was impressed by MacLean's demonstration of the effect of tissue anoxia, which correlated with their own studies "When patients in shock are evaluated with regard to the effectiveness of their oxygen transport, (milliliters of oxygen extracted per liter blood flow), the patients in nonseptic shock demonstrate one pattern, in that they have a direct relationship between decreases in the cardiac index and decreases in total oxygen consumption; whereas patients in septic shock show a variety of patterns which are output dependent. The patients whose septic shock has a low cardiac output basis are very similar to those in nonseptic shock in that their oxygen extraction ratio is greater than normal; whereas the hyperdynamic, or high output patients are different. They have a very inefficient oxygen extraction, so that to achieve any given oxygen consumption they require two or three or sometimes four times the cardiac index needed by the normal patient." He supported MacLean's emphasis on the importance of myocardial performance, "Both our data and those of Dr. MacLean demonstrate that patients in septic shock have a high incidence of myocardial failure which emphasizes, I think, the importance of using a cardiac inotropic agent to support the circulation of patients in septic shock." Francis D. Moore, of Boston, applauded MacLean's important studies ". . . using methods formerly confined to the physiology lab or the cardiac catheter lab . . . it's nothing but good. We must stoutly defend this sort of research in very critically ill patients against that increasing number of people who say that it is unjustified research using man as an experimental animal . . . Quite the contrary, it's those very patients who have had this sort of study and care *during* life who are most apt to stay alive; and then if they die, we know what they died of. We should realize the extreme shortcomings of the classical methods of pathology to tell us what these patients die of; the microscope is very unrevealing. It's the physiologic changes during life that really tell us what happened. We have been especially interested in the early alkalotic stage . . . early maintained spontaneous hyperventilation with hypocapnia is a harbinger of pulmonary trouble ahead. Those patients with long-standing hypocapnia will often be those who later have progressive pulmonary insufficiency. Hypocapnia decreases cerebral blood flow, and early coma can be seen in patients who are alkalotic. Early alkalosis, whether metabolic or respiratory, starts up a small lactate lead which may later become embarrassing; early cardiac arrest is favored in the alkalotic heart." John M. Howard, of Philadelphia, emphasized the enormous complexity, laboriousness, and costliness of studies such as MacLean's. An attempt had been made from Bethesda to encourage trauma centers, but most of the applications had been turned down. There was a lack of young career investigators interested in the acutely injured. Protocols were very expensive compared to those for the study of chronic disease, and were frequently scientifically substandard. George H. A. Clowes, Jr., of Boston, emphasized the pulmonary factors in death which MacLean had described. In dogs in septic shock but protected with penicillin, they had seen a pulmonary lesion which was not unlike that which was seen in patients and they thought that in patients this was sometimes reversible by the correction of the low flow state. Fraser N. Gurd, of Montreal said that in his laboratory there had been "defined a sequence of changes in the morbid anatomy of the lung, the stability of the alveoli and the metabolism of phospholipids in lung tissue. We believe that a definite series of intrinsic alterations in the lungs themselves can be related to that progressive respiratory failure which so often characterizes the patient's final hours. If we only knew better what was happening in those lungs, we might be better able to improve our treatment." MacLean, closing, showed "a slide of the pulmonary lesion to which Dr. Gurd and Dr. Clowes referred. A cardiologist studied this patient who had pulmonary edema within 12 hours of the time a transurethral resection was done, associated with septic shock due to E. coli septicemia . . . the pulmonary capillary wedge pressure was zero, indicating that left heart failure was not likely. Since the patient's albumin was over 3 Gm., the only other possibility to account for the edema was increased pulmonary capillary permeability, and I think this might be the basic pulmonary lesion in this syndrome." Perhaps responding to Moore's comments, he said, "I think there is a danger—and I hate to admit this—in studying shock rather than the patient, and there are some who have criticized intensive care, and they may have a point when the house staff knows the arterial blood gas of a patient, but not his name . . . This does not occur in well-run intensive care units that really provide intensive care by the doctors, rather than solely by the nurses . . . We have come to be able to select patients who required more aggressive surgery, because the prognosis is so bad in the presence of refractory acidosis and other unfavorable signs. In selected patients we have gone ahead with surgery that I think would have been debatable in the past, including total pancreatectomy for hemorrhagic pancreatitis associated with this syndrome, which I think might prove useful in the future. We are very fond of isoproterenol and we have received the support of our cardiologists on this recently, in that if the patient in shock with myocardial infarction doesn't respond to isoproterenol, they transfer that patient to us for counter pulsation or other extracorporeal support."

* * *

Jack M. Farris, of Los Angeles, Associate Professor of Surgery, University of California; and by invitation, Gordon K. Smith, *Appraisal of the Long-Term Results of Vagotomy and Pyloroplasty in 100 Patients with Bleeding Duodenal Ulcer,* 57 of them operated on for massive bleeding, and 43 operated on while they were bleeding, but not massively, had been able to follow 97 of the patients, for an average period of 7.4 years. The operative mortality was 6% in the group of massive bleeders, and zero in the others. Five patients subsequently required another operation for ulcer, and eight others rebled, "These postoperative difficulties are believed due to a poorly emptying pyloroplasty rather than to an incomplete vagotomy." The patients had retained good nutrition, eight had symptoms resembling dumping. The outstanding advantage they thought was the reduction of the initial mortality.

Discussion

Chester B. McVay, of Yankton, South Dakota, was in agreement ". . . there is certainly no quicker way to get to the point of bleeding than rapid incision through the abdominal wall and incision through the anterior wall of the duodenum and the pyloric antrum . . . When one ligates the bleeding ulcer base, it must be done deeply and thoroughly . . ." Stanley O. Hoerr, of Cleveland, agreed ". . . that direct ligation of the ulcer base in massive bleeding, coupled with vagotomy and pyloroplasty, is immediately effective and gives satisfactory long-term results . . . the ligation of the ulcer base may be difficult and awkward . . . I use silk with a small, thick needle to avoid breaking the needle." John R. Brooks, of Boston, had 38 patients with massive hemorrhage, most of them quite old. The mortality was 15%, which he thought acceptable. A series of comparable patients undergoing sub-total gastectomy had a 27% mortality. They had had no deaths in people under 65 with massive bleeding. They had had a 12% incidence of early rebleeding requiring reoperation and all of those patients had died. Claude E. Welch, of Boston, called Farris' paper ". . . the first long-term study of pyloroplasty and vagotomy, with an average follow-up of seven years." He still thought partial gastrectomy might be preferable, commenting on the low mortality of gastrectomy at the Massachusetts General Hospital, the incidence of rebleeding after suture of the ulcer, and of late bleeding after gastrectomy, admitting that "We found with partial gastrectomy without vagotomy that late bleeding occurred in 16% of our patients; this is certainly an argument to add a vagotomy to a resection whenever it can be done." J. E. Dunphy, of San Francisco, said that "Dr. Farris, Dr. Smith and Dr. Joseph Weinberg deserve the credit for having set the stage for the use of this operation in the patient with massive bleeding. I was very skeptical about this, but we tried the operation at the County Hospital in Oregon, in the belief that we would be able to prove in a short time that Dr. Farris was wrong. We adopted the same procedure in California, and we now have well over 150 patients with clear-cut criteria for massive exsanguinat-

ing hemorrhage, 50 of them over 70 years of age. The mortality in the over-all group is below 10%; in patients over 50 it is around 12 to 13%." They had had about a 7% incidence of immediate postoperative bleeding whether the patient was treated by vagotomy and suture or by pyloroplasty and suture, or by gastrectomy.

* * *

F. Henry Ellis, Jr., of Rochester, Professor of Surgery, Mayo Graduate School of Medicine, University of Minnesota; Chairman, Sub-Section Thoracic Surgery, Mayo Clinic, and five others by invitation, *Esophagomyotomy for Esophageal Achalasia:* Experimental, Clinical, and Manometric Aspects, presented their clinical and experimental observations with achalasia. Experimental esophagogastromyotomy in dogs demonstrated that esophageal reflux occurred after the original Heller double my-

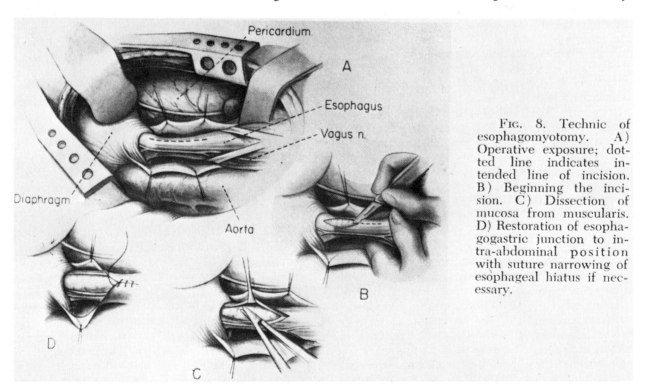

FIG. 8. Technic of esophagomyotomy. A) Operative exposure; dotted line indicates intended line of incision. B) Beginning the incision. C) Dissection of mucosa from muscularis. D) Restoration of esophagogastric junction to intra-abdominal position with suture narrowing of esophageal hiatus if necessary.

Ellis stressed a 6 cm. to 12 cm. incision in the esophagus, extending less than 1 cm. onto the stomach, and dissecting the muscle well back from the submucosa "so that approximately half to two-thirds of the circumference of the esophageal mucosa is freed and pouts freely through the incision." In 269 patients, he had had one death,- from hyperpyrexia,- excellent results in 46%, good in 36%, fair in 11%, poor in 7%. Ten of the 16 poor results were "almost surely caused by reflux esophagitis".

F. H. Ellis, Jr., J. C. Kiser, J. F. Schlegel, R. J. Earlam, B. Chir, John L. McVey, and A. M. Olsen, *Esophagomyotomy for Esophageal Achalasia:* Experimental, Clinical, and Manometric Aspects. Volume LXXXV, 1967.

otomy or after a long esophagogastromyotomy but not when the myotomy was restricted to the esophagus. However, after histamine stimulation, esophagitis developed in all animals ". . . suggesting that sphincteric function was impaired in all." Esophageal motility and pressure studies had disclosed impaired sphincter function after each of the operations and reduction of pressure at the inferior esophageal sphincter with each operation. They interpreted their experimental findings as meaning ". . . that a single longitudinal myotomy limited to the esophagus is preferable because longer and more radical incisions achieve no greater decrease in sphincteric pressure and yet may lead to greater disruption of the gastroesophageal sphincteric mechanism with the potential hazard of gastroesophageal reflux." They preferred to do the operation in patients transthoracically. They had performed the operation shown in the figure in 269 patients between January 1950, and January 1967, only seven of the operations being through the abdomen. The mucosa was opened 25 times and closed by suture. There was a single death, associated with hyperthermia of 43.3° C at the time of closure of the incision, and ventricular arrest. In five patients, a subphrenic abscess or empyema developed, obviously a result of a perforation, which had been recognized in only one. In 97 patients with postoperative roentgenography a year or more after operation, reflux was noted in only two patients, and reduction in the degree of esophageal dilatation in 70. No patient developed carcinoma of the esophagus. The clinical evaluation,- 95% follow-up,- showed excellent results in 46%, good in 36%, fair in 11%, and poor in 7%. The patients with fair results "although definitely better, continued to have episodes of dysphagia, regurgitation, or distress . . . despite only fair results, all these patients experienced significant symptomatic improvement and a gain in weight." In ten of the 16 patients with poor results, these were "almost surely caused by reflux esophagitis . . . Late postoperative manometric studies of esophageal motility demonstrated a decrease of sphincteric pressure and a shortening of the increased pressure zone between the stomach and esophagus at the expense of its suprahiatal portion. These changes persisted as long as 93 months postoperatively." Ellis emphasized esophagomyotomy as the operation of choice and recommended that it be done early in the course of the disease.

* * *

W. E. Ladd's 1938 report to the Association on the treatment of Wilms' tumor, reporting 14/45 survivals had shown a striking improvement over all previous results. Now Orvar Swenson, Professor of Surgery, Northwestern University School of Medicine; Surgeon-in-Chief, Children's Memorial Hospital, and by invitation, R. Brenner, *Aggressive Approach to the Treatment of Wilms' Tumor,* was able to say that whereas "In 1941 Ladd reported a mortality rate of 90-100% . . . recently Farber published an 89% 2-year survival rate. This change has resulted from more aggressive surgical treatment and a change from palliative therapy for pulmonary metastases to radiation therapy for cure. The contribution of dactinomycin to this improvement can not be fully evaluated at this time." In the preceding eight years, they had had 58 patients with Wilms' tumor at the Children's Memorial Hospital in Chicago, bilateral in five of them. Four of the five patients were living and well, usually after nephrectomy on the side of the larger tumor and partial nephrectomy on the side of the smaller tumor, some with irradiation and some with chemotherapy. Two patients had Wilms' tumor in a solitary kidney, both had a partial nephrectomy, one received dactinomycin as well, and both were alive and well. Their present treatment for pulmonary metastases was irradiation plus dactinomycin with operation if the tumor did not completely disappear. Five children under this regimen underwent operation, two upper lobectomies, one right pneumonectomy, one right upper and middle lobectomy and in one patient, a right upper lobectomy followed by a left upper lobectomy. All were well and free of disease two to five years after operation.

Discussion

C. E. Koop, of Philadelphia, said that in evaluating results, it was important to select out the two groups of high risk patients, those over a year of age and those in whom the tumor had grown beyond the kidney capsule. He showed slides of patients who had localized tumors and patients who had extensive tumors treated with and without actinomycin D, showing a benefit from actinomycin D. He had had six patients with bilateral Wilms' tumors, three of whom had survived. In one with very large tumors resection was not possible, ". . . and the only therapy has been 800r to the smaller tumor, 1,200r to the larger tumor; in conjunction with actinomycin D, which has been continued for several years . . . she is alive and well five years after her original diagnosis, with no evidence of disease and with normal kidney function. This makes us wonder whether the bilateral Wilms' tumor is a different entity from the unilateral tumor." Edward J. Beattie, Jr., of New York, said that at the Memorial Hospital, pulmonary metastases from Wilms' tumor were treated with actinomycin D, and for the drug resistant lesions, operation and/or radio-therapy. Nine of 26 patients with bilateral pulmonary metastases—30% —were free of disease five to 11 years later. W. E. Goodwin, of Los Angeles, recommended the operative placement of silver wire about the border of the Wilms' tumor in a solitary kidney, or on the second side, to permit precision radiation. In operating upon the solitary kidney, he urged isolation and clamping of the renal artery, and then securing the parenchymal vessels after amputation of the tumor. W. H. Snyder, Jr., of Los Angeles, said that at the Children's Hospital they had had three patients with bilateral Wilms' tumor in five years, all doing well thus far under the same type of therapy as Swenson's. Swenson, closing, said that there were still not enough data for definitive evaluation of actinomycin D and he had entered into a combined study of the matter with other Children's centers.

* * *

Mark M. Ravitch, of Chicago, Professor of Surgery and Chairman, Section of Pediatric Surgery, University of Chicago, and by invitation, F. Canalis, A. Weinshelbaum, and J. McCormick, *Studies in Intestinal Healing: III. Observations on Everting Intestinal Anastomoses*, had previously reported that with ". . . application of mechanical stapling devices to intestinal closure . . . healing was regularly achieved by the simple through-and-through closure of the cut end of the stomach, duodenum and large or small bowel with two staggered rows of wire staples. Healing occurred without abscess formation, localized peritonitis or excessive inflammation to suggest even a temporary leak . . . It seemed possible, therefore, that this method of closure might be applied to end-to-end, mucosa-to-mucosa, everting-anastomoses" in which the risk of constriction at the anastomosis was obviously less than with inverting anastomoses. Previous studies from their laboratory had shown that healing had occurred independent of formation of adhesions or coverage by omentum. End-to-end everting anastomoses made with a stapling machine or manually did indeed break down frequently when loosely surrounded with polyethylene, glove rubber or Silastic gauze but conventional inverting anastomoses similarly treated, broke down at almost the same rate. Travers, as far back as 1812, had pointed out that bowel would heal whether the anastomosis was inverting or everting.

All of this, of course, was contrary to the doctrines of Lembert and of Halsted and to generally accepted practice. Ravitch now reported the histologic appearance of anastomoses in the small bowel, inverted made with a single row of silk sutures, or everted made by mattress sutures, the bar of which was parallel to the circumference of the cut end. The present communication reported histologic studies of anastomoses harvested at intervals from six hours to six weeks. There was considerable edema, hemorrhage, and necrosis of the inverted portion of the conventional anastomosis and remarkably little reaction in the everting anastomosis, the serosal side of which was covered by mesothelial cells within six hours. India ink injected into arteries on one side at harvesting of the specimen, crossed over through the anastomosis at an earlier time in the everting anastomosis. It took a minimum of two weeks for inverting anastomoses to develop continuous mucosa on the luminal side, which was present from the moment of operation in the everting anastomosis. The everting anastomosis had the advantage that penetration of the submucosa, the importance of which Halsted had stressed, was obligatory. There did seem to be more adhesions with the everting than with the inverting anastomosis.

Discussion

William H. Moretz, of Augusta, cautioned against clinical application of the everting anastomosis. They had used the same everting horizontal mattress suture in the small intestine of dogs and found that if the pouting mucosa was excised, the dogs all survived, when it was not, two of nine dogs died of peritonitis. In another study, ten dogs with everting anastomosis with the mucosa excised all lived and five of ten with the pouting mucosa left undisturbed, died. Clarence Dennis, of Brooklyn, recalled his studies of some years earlier in end-to-end jejunal anastomoses in suckling pigs, slaughtered when they had increased in weight tenfold. Most types of anastomoses did not increase in size as the pig grew and the everting anastomosis, in fact, was "observed to decrease in absolute diameter while the rest of the animal grew". J. Englebert Dunphy, of San Francisco, commenting on the rapid healing powers of intestine made the inscrutable comment that "The question of inversion versus eversion is a biological variable that may be so inconsequential it cannot be measured. I think it's very important to continue studies of this type, and I congratulate Dr. Ravitch on his contribution." C. K. Holloway, of San Diego, [who with Getzen had introduced the so-called

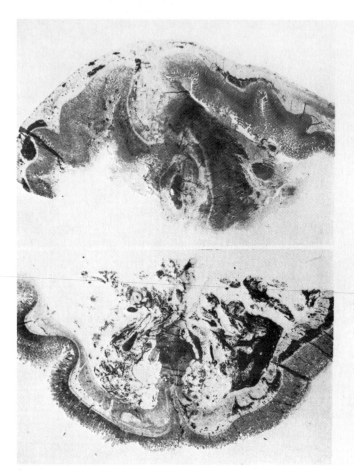

Fig. 2. Anastomoses at 12 hours. (Top) Inverting. The intraluminal protrusion of swollen hemorrhagic mucosa covered by hemorrhagic coagulum is more prominent than at 6 hours. The inverted flange seems firmly agglutinated at its base by the suture. (Bottom) Everting anastomosis. The mucosal surface continues smooth and unbroken, there may be a little crossover of India ink and the everted mucosa is not recognizable. There is remarkably little inflammation any where along the line of union or in the everted coagulum.

M. M. Ravitch, F. Canalis, A. Weinshelbaum, and J. McCormick, *Studies on Intestinal* ▶ *Healing:* III. Observations on Everting Intestinal Anastomoses. Volume LXXXV, 1967.

Navy stitch which, introduced as an everting stitch, actually produced a flush, end-to-end anastomosis] said that at the Naval hospital in the past several years, "We have performed 200 everting small intestinal anastomoses in dogs; and we came out with essentially the same findings that Dr. Ravitch has presented so well here." He described his differing suture and went on to say that "I don't recommend that we all do everting anastomoses in our patients, but as a result of this experiment I have gradually turned in less and less serosa in my own clinical work. I now prefer a single-layer end-to-end anastomosis in my clinical work, for both large and small bowel, and I have been very pleased with the results." Isidore Cohn, Jr., of New Orleans, said that in their earlier studies on the esophagus of a newborn pup, on the common duct of the dog, and in small bowel of dogs, "we have felt that the security

of the everting anastomosis was less than that of the inverting anastomosis, and that the long-term strength of the everting anastomosis was less than that of the inverting anastomosis." To determine the source of the bacteria which killed the dogs when any foreign wrap was applied about the anastomosis ". . . in consultation with Dr. Ravitch . . . We did both inverting and everting small bowel anastomoses in the dog, and after the anastomosis was completed we injected into the lumen of the bowel some *Serratia marcescens* which is not a normal inhabitant of the small bowel of dogs." The Serratia marcescens was never found on the surface of the bowel cultured at early intervals after the anastomosis. Bowel wrapped in solid plastic broke down as Dr. Ravitch had said but, [unlike Ravitch's findings with Silastic]". . . if the plastic is perforated, so that bacteria spilled at the time the anastomosis is made can get

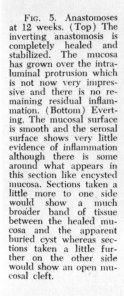

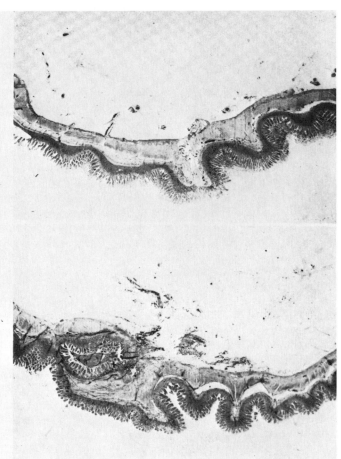

Fig. 5. Anastomoses at 12 weeks. (Top) The inverting anastomosis is completely healed and stabilized. The mucosa has grown over the intraluminal protrusion which is not now very impressive and there is no remaining residual inflammation. (Bottom) Everting. The mucosal surface is smooth and the serosal surface shows very little evidence of inflammation although there is some around what appears in this section like encysted mucosa. Sections taken a little more to one side would show a much broader band of tissue between the healed mucosa and the apparent buried cyst whereas sections taken a little further on the other side would show an open mucosal cleft.

out, or the peritoneal defenses can get to them, the animals survive . . . We believe that the spillage which occurs at the time of the anastomosis, not the leakage that occurs afterwards, determines whether the anastomosis will leak." Ravitch, closing, agreed with "Dr. Moretz's advice for clinical caution. We are not yet employing this ourselves. We have tried a number of dogs, a large series with excision of the omentum, and it made no difference. The everting anastomosis healed just as well." Others had studied the excision of the pouting mucosa which he thought a "messy and tedious" procedure. He was surprised at Dennis' findings in piglets that everting anastomoses failed to grow as the pigs grew.

The Business Meetings

The 1967 meeting took place May 11, 12, and 13, at The Broadmoor, Colorado Springs, Colorado, Oscar Creech in the Chair.

Edwin J. Wylie, for the Program Committee, reported that there were 139 abstracts submitted for the 33 places on the program.

Oliver Cope, reporting for the Committee on Education, said "The basic medical curriculum has seen almost no change since the founding of Hopkins in 1893. Western Reserve's new curriculum was the single exception when we began our work . . . The reorganization at Duke by Drs. Barnes Woodhall and William G. Anylan had already been planned but it was just that kind of experimentation which the Study felt was indicated. Since then, Dr. Child's curriculum [at Michigan] is, unfortunately, stalled and the effort of M.I.T. to enlist Harvard in a joint three-year curriculum has thus far been totally unsuccessful." A meeting of the Committee on Behavorial Science had been held and the report was to be published; the Interdisciplinary Study of the Graduate Phase of Medical Education had been held two weeks earlier. The Committee found "contemporary specialty education rigid, unimaginative, and unresponsive to growth of knowledge and needs of the community. It, therefore, recommended that universities assume responsibility for graduate medical education under interdisciplinary control . . . The Coggeshall and Millis Reports recommend it. The question is what do you do with it? How far out do you carry the recommendations? . . . how should the Universities relate to the Specialty Boards and Residency Review Committees?"

Once more a Fellow, Stanley O. Hoerr, of Cleveland, rose to implore the Fellows to pack the halls of the Section on Surgery at the convention meeting of the AMA, to prevent the Society of Abdominal Surgeons from taking over the Surgical Section. Hoerr said, "Dr. Blaise Alfano, the organizing genius and moving spirit behind the Society of Abdominal Surgeons, has notified the American Medical Association of his intent to file a slate of candidates challenging the current leadership of the section. This has been going on for some years. Last year, Dr. Alfano's slate was defeated by the frighteningly narrow margin of about 100 votes. He has greater strength, many followers and sympathizers along the Eastern seaboard."

At the Second Executive Session, among other items in the Council's report, was the recommendation "That in response to a request from an Ad Hoc Committee of the American Board of Surgery concerning a recommendation with respect to possible board certification in Pediatric Surgery, a reply be forwarded to its Chairman, Dr. John Kirklin, to the effect that the Council could not at the present time support a movement for a new certifying board in Pediatric Surgery." [At the 1966 meeting, Eugene M. Bricker reporting for the Board, said "At its annual business meeting on Monday the Board was asked to sponsor an affiliate Board of Pediatric Surgery. The request was presented by Drs. Mark Ra-

vitch and Clifford Benson and was discussed in detail before being referred to an *Ad-Hoc* Committee for further consideration." At the 1967 meeting, C. Rollins Hanlon reporting for the American Board, said "The important *ad hoc* committee, considering the revised application for a Board of Pediatric Surgery . . . received clear directives from the national surgical organizations which were generally opposed to the formulation of such a board. The *ad hoc* committee itself, while recognizing the importance of developing areas of special interest in surgery, did not feel that such developments required the establishment of a separate certifying board in each area. Therefore, in spite of the high regard and admiration for the accomplishments of pediatric surgeons and pediatric surgery, the *ad hoc* committee recommended disapproval of the application and in this recommendation the Board concurred. Dr. John Kirklin and his committee are highly commended for their objectivity and hard work in adjudicating this thorny problem." The Board ultimately agreed to a Certificate of Special Competency in Pediatric Surgery and the first examination was held in 1975.]

Among the new Fellows were Oliver H. Beahrs, of Rochester, Minnesota; John A. Mannick, of Boston; Norman E. Shumway, of Palo Alto, and William Gerald Austen, of Boston.

Officers elected were President, William P. Longmire, of Los Angeles; Vice-Presidents, Truman G. Blocker, of Galveston, and Richard L. Varco, of Minneapolis; Secretary, Harris B. Shumacker, Jr., of Indianapolis.

LXXXVI

1968

The 1968 meeting was held April 17, 18 and 19 at the Sheraton-Boston Hotel, President William P. Longmire, Jr., of Los Angeles, Professor and Chairman, Department of Surgery, University of California Los Angeles School of Medicine, in the Chair. Oscar Creech had died in the preceding year, not long after having served as President, and Willis J. Potts had died, who had contributed so much to the general and cardiac surgery of childhood.

President Longmire, *Some Wise Men in American Surgery,* chose to name "Halsted, Bevan, Archibald, the Mayos and Magnuson . . ." for their role in "shaping the manner in which surgery is actually practiced by the surgeon and specific surgical care is received by the patient." Halsted's was the credit for initiating the residency system of progressive surgical training although ". . . neither Halsted nor any other leader in surgery was more than vaguely concerned, at the time residency training was introduced, with the general level of surgical care in America". E. W. Archibald, in 1935 [Volume LIII] had argued the need for specialty certification in an address which was the immediate stimulus to the formation of the American Board of Surgery. Dudley P. Allen, of Cleveland, had made the same plea at his Presidential Address in 1907 [Volume XXV] and so had J. M. T. Finney in his address in 1922 [Volume XL]. Arthur Dean Bevan was cited by Longmire for the effect of his 24 years on the Council on Medical Education of the American Medical Association, from which Council as Chairman and member, he exerted an enormous effect, not least by his forthright statements, viz., "It is evident from a study of the medical schools of this country and their work that there are five especially rotten spots which are responsible for most of the bad medical instruction. They are Illinois with fifteen schools, Missouri with fourteen, Maryland with eight, Kentucky with seven, and Tennessee with ten, that is fifty-four medical schools in these five states and not more than six of these can be considered acceptable." It was the Council on Medical Education which, in 1908, held "an informal conference . . . with President Henry S. Pritchett and Mr. Abraham Flexner of the Carnegie Foundation", the result of which was to change the face of medical education in America. The brothers Mayo, Longmire cited for ". . . the world's first group practice . . . the inspiration for the formation of numerous such groups in this country and abroad." And finally, Longmire gave credit to Paul B. Magnuson for "the radical revamping of the Veterans' Administration medical service at the close of World War II . . ." Longmire suggested that for the future, problems of magnitude and importance comparable to those, the history of which he had discussed in his Address, would be those of continuing education of physicians and recertification, the nature of surgical training programs [in which he several times stressed "increase of latitude in the approval of training programs in university affiliated hospitals."] The problems of "day-to-day practice, including such concerns as methods to encourage the universal use of properly qualified surgical specialists, the place of the surgeon

1257

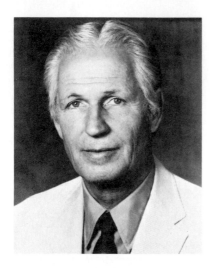

George Crile, Jr. 1907—. M.D. Harvard 1933; Interned at Barnes Hospital; Trained at Cleveland Clinic, eventually Head, Department of General Surgery. Shared with his father, G. W. Crile, a penchant for imaginative, incompletely supported, evangelistically preached, scientific hypotheses which he applied clinically, particularly in the areas of cancer of the thyroid and cancer of the breast. While his clinical recommendations, and his writings for the laity, were often vigorously condemned - viz., excision of the lump only, in breast cancer,- the germ of truth in his arguments left his audiences uncomfortable, hence, perhaps, their passion. Some of his proposals, specifically local excision of cancer of the breast, are still being evaluated.

in the nationwide expansion of health services with the suggestion that his role seems to fit most rationally into some type of expanded group practice arrangement, and a demonstration of our ingenuity and imagination in meeting the relicensing problem by a system that will continue to insure the rendition of informed, effective care by surgeons throughout their careers."

* * *

George Crile, Jr., Head, Department of General Surgery, Cleveland Clinic Foundation [with his father's gift for the provocative expression of new and iconoclastic approaches to old and important problems], *Results of Simple Mastectomy without Irradiation in the Treatment of Operative Stage I Cancer of the Breast* [a footnote to the title stated " 'Operative Stage I' means that no axillary involvement is palpable at operation"] compared 25 patients who underwent simple mastectomy without irradiation to 22 who underwent radical mastectomy with or without irradiation, none of them having palpable axillary nodes, but all of them ultimately proving to have positive lymph node involvement. In those undergo-

ing initial radical mastectomy, the involvement of the nodes was found by the pathologist, in the others it was demonstrated by the subsequent course of the patient, 22 of those 25 having secondary axillary dissection. The differences in treatment did not seem to affect the number of nodes involved at the time axillary dissection was done, nor did they affect survival. Sixty-eight percent of the simple mastectomy and irradiation patients with secondary axillary dissection, done on the average two years later, were living five or more years after operation and precisely the same five-year survival was achieved for those treated initially by radical mastectomy. During the same 1955 through 1962 period in which they had seen a total of 501 patients with carcinoma of the breast, 49 patients treated by radical mastectomy were found to have no axillary metastases and 110 treated by simple mastectomy without irradiation never showed evidence of axillary metastases "true stage I cancers". Of the total, 137 had tumors 1.5 cm. or more in diameter and they stated that there should be no irradiation in this group. "The patients treated by simple operation had a slightly higher 5-year survival rate than did those treated by radical ones, 82% compared to 65%." [As statistical methods and presentations before the Association have become more and more sophisticated, and their use essentially obligatory, the Fellows have more and more been plagued by the fact that their bald numbers favored one or another conclusion at the same time that statistical analysis insisted that the findings were "not significant". To this day, members seem to be unable to resist the temptation to say, "The figures are not statistically significant but they clearly show an important trend", and Crile succumbed to the same temptation, "Although the numbers are too small to be of much statistical significance, there is a higher rate of survival in the patients whose axillary nodes were left untreated either surgically or by irradiation."] If one lumped together all 119 patients with clinically negative axillae, there was again no statistical significance in survival between the radical mastectomy groups and the simple mastectomy plus irradiation groups, although the actual five-year survival rates, 66% and 79% favored simple mastectomy. He stated there should be no irradiation in this group, also. His final summary stated unequivocally that "The 5-year survival rate of patients whose axillae, at the time of operation, contained no palpably involved nodes, was 13% higher when the nodes were left in place and not irradiated than when they were removed with the breast." He further suggested ". . . that it is no longer necessary to inflict the morbidity of a radical operation on a patient with operative stage I cancer whose nodes, at the time of axillary exploration, are not palpably involved." He finally returned to the question of the immunological importance of the retained lymph node, to which he had made brief allusion in the body of the paper, "Although both clinical and laboratory evidence indicate that uninvolved regional nodes contribute to the host's immunological resistance to systemic metastasis, a large randomized study of patients with operative stage I breast cancer will have to be done before it can be stated with certainty that removal of uninvolved nodes promotes metastasis."

Discussion

Francis D. Moore, of Boston, expressed gratitude "to Dr. Crile for questioning orthodoxy, and attempting to base this question on familiar immunologic considerations." Moore indicated that "If a recommendation is made for simple mastectomy and irradiation without axillary node biopsy or dissection, then irradiation would be given without any need for it in 25 to 40 per cent of cases and given quite needlessly in *all* of those patients with small outer quadrant lesions without nodes." It was as necessary ". . . to avoid unnecessary radical irradiation . . . as to avoid unnecessary radical surgery . . . The nodal status is controlling in determining the biological balance between tumor and host, the prognosis, and further treatment . . . we have heard Dr. Crile recommend simple mastectomy *without* irradiation, in which case early nodal dissection becomes less critical in early management. His program is therefore consistent and his statistics are indeed impressive . . . We can still inquire of Dr. Crile a question about the patients he lost! What fraction would have been cured by radical mastectomy with irradiation amongst those in whom the nodes are involved, his so-called 'occult' group?" Data suggested that some of those patients might have been saved and Moore asked whether "the loss of the breast and some disfigurement of the axillary folds" was too high a price to pay for the increased survival. Nathan A. Womack, of Chapel Hill, called the subject "emotional" and Dr. Crile's views "provocative". Pointing out that cancer of the breast was a continuing process and a variable disease, he said that ". . . an unusually large population must be studied for the sampling to be valid. I doubt, therefore, if the number of patients observed by Dr. Crile in this paper is large enough from which to derive firm conclusions. This, I think he realizes for he so stated in his talk." Womack cited the experiments of

Dr. Colin Thomas in his department, "injecting a radioactive tag the day before operation in the region of the breast cancer". Thomas demonstrated that "all nodes in the axilla were involved with equal ease in this short length of time . . . no tendency for the material to extend from one node to another in consecutive fashion . . . when several nodes were involved with cancer, resistance to lymph flow was inserted and there was directional change of flow with a tendency for random distribution of the tag as a result." The lymph nodes "afford cells ready access to blood vessels." Womack's point was that "when the primary breast cancer is removed, only those metastases already present at the time of operation tend to be of significance . . . whether in the lymph node, or lung, or bones". The metastases might stay and grow for an uncertain period of time, and Womack appeared not to be surprised that "Dr. Crile finds that removal of uninvolved axillary lymph nodes at a later date does not alter his survival figures . . ." Womack felt that "ultimate improvement in results from operation for cancer of the breast resides in removal or destruction of the primary tumor before metastases occur. Because many times, this will necessarily be before the lesion is palpable, we need look for no startling improvement in our results from operation for cancer of the breast with our present diagnostic methods. Extensive and meticulous dissection of the axilla, I believe we now know is not the answer. Our attention . . . must be directed at means of recognizing breast cancer before it can be felt. We have spent some 50 years in this society, primarily talking about the value or the disadvantage of meticulous lymph node dissection. I think we must change our sense of direction if we want to alter the end results in the treatment of cancer of the breast." Bernard Fisher, of Pittsburgh, indicated that Crile had been voicing his challenge to conventional cancer surgery for some time, "He continues to pose the same questions as he has in the past. Does it make any difference if the lymph node is removed before or after it's clinically involved with the tumor? Do tumors spread from one node to another?" Crile answered "No" to both questions. Fisher, who had been studying the effect of lymph node metastases in experimental preparations, indicated that the "role of the lymph node in tumor biology" was just coming under consideration and accurately predicted of Crile's paper that "whether or not it answers to everybody's satisfaction the biologic questions posed, [it] will have an impact on surgical practice and will add to the disquiet concerning the proper treatment of breast cancer." He spoke of the National Surgical

Adjuvant Breast Project clinical trials and urged participation, "What is needed are more agnostics; those people who have not acquired the faith and do not know for sure what the best treatment for cancer of the breast is but would like to find out." John W. Cline, of San Francisco, said that the Commission on Cancer of the American College of Surgeons had proposed to the Board of Regents a randomized study of the relative value of simple and radical mastectomy in the treatment of stage I cancer, but "it has been extremely difficult to find people willing to undertake this study . . . Such a study is needed. Either we are overtreating patients with Stage I cancer of the breast and they should all have simple mastectomy, or we are undertreating patients with Stage I cancer of the breast by performing simple mastectomy." Crile, closing, responded to Francis Moore's plea for axillary dissection so that tumors could be staged and postoperative irradiation given if need be. He wished to remind Dr. Moore "of Dr. Paterson's huge randomized trial in England in which he found prophylactic radiation did no good if nodes were involved and perhaps did a little harm if they were not. It does not seem to me that we gain very much useful information by removing nodes when we are not going to use radiation anyway." Crile suggested to Cline that it might be possible to conduct a clinical study because one group of surgeons might be willing to compare radical mastectomy and modified radical mastectomy in which the pectoral muscles were left while another group of surgeons might be willing to compare modified radical mastectomy with simple mastectomy, both groups having in common the modified radical mastectomy patients.

* * *

"In 1957, under the auspices of the National Institutes of Health, Cancer Chemotherapy National Service Center, representatives of 23 institutions . . . adopted a common protocol which was to determine the efficacy of administering chemotherapy in conjunction with 'curative' cancer surgery to decrease recurrence and extend survival of patients with cancer of the breast." At the 1961 meeting [Volume LXXIX] R. J. Noer, who was then Chairman of the Surgical Adjuvant Chemotherapy Breast Group, had reported to the Association. The Executive Committee of the National Surgical Adjuvant Breast Project currently had as Co-chairmen, Bernard Fisher, of Pittsburgh, and George E. Moore, of the Roswell Park Institute in Buffalo. Now, Bernard Fisher, Professor of Surgery, University of Pittsburgh; Robert G. Ravdin, Associate Professor of Surgery, University of Pennsylvania; Robert K. Ausman and Nelson H. Slack, by invitation; George E. Moore, Director and Chief of Surgery, Roswell Park Memorial Institute; and Rudolf J. Noer, Professor and Chairman, Department of Surgery, Louisville School of Medicine, presented *Surgical Adjuvant Chemotherapy in Cancer of the Breast:* Results of a Decade of Cooperative Investigation. They were concerned with the evaluation of 826 patients who had been studied for five years in the Thio-TEPA study, considered the Phase I study, and the 1341 patients in the second study who had received either Thio-TEPA, placebo, or 5-FU and had been followed at least 18 months. The Phase I study had compared the Halsted radical mastectomy followed by either Thio-TEPA or a placebo. Dr. Fisher reported for the group that the five-year recurrence after Halsted radical mastectomy was 20% in patients with negative nodes and 70% in patients with positive nodes indicating "the inability of conventional radical surgery to eradicate all cancer cells because of their dissemination prior to or at the time of operation. More extensive regional dissection, carried to the limit of feasibility and sensibility, has not produced a substantial improvement in results. The advantage of irradiation, another form of regional therapy, as an adjunct to surgery remains to be proven", and that was to be included in future studies by their group. Their thesis was that ". . . until cancer of the breast can be prevented or a therapy becomes available which is capable by nonsurgical means of destroying both primary and secondary tumors, systemic therapy as an adjunct to surgery affords the most likely means for escape from the plateau on which the prognosis and salvage rate of this disease has been ensnared for the last 30 or more years . . . It was hoped that by the use of adjuvant chemotherapy, cells dislodged into the blood and lymph during surgical manipulation could be eliminated." The fact that they had failed to show benefit from TSPA or 5-FU, except, as they added, "in one sub-group", did not "repudiate the concept of systemic adjuvant therapy." The complexity of the cancer-host relationships was beginning to be appreciated and factors now realized to require consideration were that ". . . cells are drug sensitive during only part of their mitotic cycle . . . therapeutic success may be equally or more dependent upon destruction of occult metastases than upon 'free' cells in the circulation . . . the per cent reduction of neoplastic cells for a given treatment is constant regardless of the number of cells present . . . host immunologic factors may be involved . . ." It was now thought that prolonged adjuvant therapy was important and Phase III of their program would evaluate that aspect. "Only if many clinical trials cast in differing detail as a result of new knowledge prove unrewarding will a searching reappraisal of the concept of adjuvant chemotherapy be in order. These studies have demonstrated that it is possible to collect a substantial number of patients treated in a prescribed manner from a large number of institutions. Aside from providing patients more rapidly than could be acquired by a single investigator or multiple investigators working at one institution, they as Schneiderman has pointed out, have advantages over single institutional trials in that they contain within themselves a basis for internal verification. 'A diversity of trials in a diversity of places at different times . . . is possibly the strongest evidence one can see of the worth of a treatment before it is employed on the whole population.' " In sum, for patients in the Phase I study who received Thio-TEPA or placebo on the day of and for two days after, a radical mastectomy, there was no evidence of any increase in local complications and the only immediate death was in a patient receiving placebo. The recurrence rate at five years was 40% in the Thio-TEPA group and 42% in the placebo group. Twenty percent with negative nodes had a recurrence and 60% of those with positive nodes. Patients with one to three positive nodes had a recurrence rate of 47%. Those with four or more nodes had a 77% recurrence. Analyzing the patients into subgroups indicated "that TSPA had a beneficial effect in premenopausal patients with four or more positive nodes". Fifty percent of the placebo controls had tumor recurrence within 12 months, whereas recurrence did not occur in 50% of the Thio-TEPA group until the 44th month. By the 60th month, there was no difference in the two groups. In the three-armed Phase II study, comparison of 5-Fluorouracil, Thio-TEPA, and placebo, in addition to radical mastectomy, suggested still a benefit of Thio-TEPA for the premenopausal patients with four or more positive nodes, but "Whereas in Phase I at 18 months after operation there was a 38 per cent difference in recurrence rate, in Phase II this difference was less impressive, being only 21 per cent." This was still a sufficient advantage to justify the use of Thio-TEPA in premenopausal women with four or more positive lymph nodes, but "Its use in others is *not* justified." 5-FU had proven to be both immediately toxic and without sufficient demonstrated therapeutic effect to warrant its further use as an adjuvant to breast surgery in the manner employed.

The Discussion was brief and unilluminating.

* * *

Loren J. Humphrey and Paula M. Lincoln, by invitation, and Ward O. Griffen, Jr., of Lexington, Professor of Surgery and Physiology, Chairman, Department of Surgery, University of Kentucky, followed with *Immunologic Response in Patients with Disseminated Cancer.* In their study ". . . pairs of patients with disseminated malignancies were challenged with an acellular homogenate of each other's tumors as well as heterologous red cells as an immunologic marker. General immune responsiveness and immunity to tumor antigens were investigated and correlated with clinical response following the immunization and after exchange of plasma and white blood cells . . . no effect on tumor growth was noted in those patients who developed a low hemagglutinin titer or those patients whose titers failed to show the expected anamnestic response after injection of erythrocytes . . .", after the fourth "immunization", the patients underwent plasmapheresis, exchanging 500 ml. plasma transfusions a total of ten times with reimmunization in the middle of the series. The studies were conducted in 14 pairs of patients of the same major blood group and with tumors of the same type. "Three patients with disseminated malignant melanoma are alive and well 10, 7, and 5 months after treatment. Two patients with disseminated carcinoma of the colon responded to treatment: one gained weight, returned to full time employment for 3 months, and then died; the other is alive without evidence of tumor 8 months later."

Discussion

Erle E. Peacock, Jr., of Chapel Hill, said that the tumor which was used minced, homogenized and repeatedly frozen and thawed, might produce less specific antigenicity than "if an ultracentrifugation technic were used to isolate various components of the cell such as membranes, cell sap, mitochondria, etc." James T. Grace, Jr., of Buffalo, hoped that "Dr. George Moore, who is in the audience some place, will relate some of his and Dr. Sigmond Nadler's experience with similar studies." [No recorded response, see p. 1223, 1966.] Grace thought that "tumor immunology has finally arrived. In many animal tumor systems, there is no question that tumor specific antigens exist and these can produce an effective immunity against the tumor with appropriate manipulation. There is also good evidence that certain human tumors also contain antigens which appear to be tumor specific although the antigens of some tumors may be found in embryonic human tissues." [Grace then made the first mention before the Association of carcinoembryonic antigen.] "A recent report by Dr. Philip Gold of studies of a large number of colon carcinomas in the human demonstrated, using immunodiffusion, that there were antigens present in the tumors that were not present in the normal mucosa of the bowel and they appeared to be similar in all the tumors studied. The same antigens were also found in human embryonic bowel mucosa. The fact that human embryonic gut also contained these antigens suggests that they might represent enzymes which were repressed during the process of differentiation. Then during the process of dedifferentiation, involved with malignant change, they became derepressed and again expressed themselves . . . the important question about these antigens . . . is whether they can act as transplantation type antigens in the sense that immunization with them can provide protection against the tumors." Edward T. Krementz, of New Orleans, said that at Tulane, they had performed studies like those at Lexington on "ten pairs of patients, nine with melanoma and one with renal cell carcinoma . . . one patient had a complete regression of melanoma for one year including subcutaneous nodules, a four-centimeter cutaneous implant, and pulmonary nodules; two other patients had objective responses; and two patients had increased activity following the cross-transplantation and cross-transfusions of a subjective nature." They had used minced live tumor. Humphrey, in closing, answered Peacock by saying that obviously selection of the proper cell fraction containing the antigen would be important. He agreed with Grace "that the antigen very active in the carcinogenic process may be a derepressed antigen."

* * *

Transplantation of the liver had been discussed as a vastly complicated clinical project at the 1964 meeting [Volume LXXXII] and now Thomas E. Starzl, of Denver, Professor of Surgery, University of Colorado School of Medicine; Chief of Surgery, Denver Veterans Administration Hospital, and C. G. Groth, L. Brettschneider, Israel Penn, V. A. Fulginiti, J. B. Moon, H. Blanchard, A. J. Martin, Jr., and K. A. Porter, all by invitation, *Orthotopic Ho-*

motransplantation of the Human Liver, suggested that the clinical problems were beginning to be solved, "Until last year, the kidney was the only organ which had been transplanted with subsequent significant prolongation of life. There had been nine reported attempts at orthotopic liver transplantation; seven in Denver and one each in Boston and Paris. Two of these patients had succumbed within a few hours after operation, and none had lived for longer than 23 days. This dismal picture has changed within the last 9 months, inasmuch as seven consecutive patients treated with orthotopic liver transplantation from July 23, 1967 to March 17, 1968 all passed through this previously lethal operative and postoperative period. Three of the recipients are still alive after 9, 2-1/3, and 1 months; the others died after 2, 3-1/2, 4-1/3, and 6 months." Five of the recipients had biliary atresia and two of them had hepatoma. The donors were all people who previously had had "irreversible central nervous system injury, with no spontaneous respirations and with isoelectric electroencephalograms. In each, life had been maintained for days or weeks with mechanical ventilators and in all but one there had been repeated previous cardiac arrests." Ventilatory support and cardiac massage were continued after death in the first six cases, and the liver was cooled by immediate infusion of cold balanced electrolyte solution containing heparin, inserting the cannula into the superior mesenteric vein. In the seventh, cardiopulmonary bypass for perfusion and cooling of the liver was established immediately after death. Starzl was now willing to say that "the actual operative procedure can be done in man with relative safety . . . subsequent survival is possible for at least as long as 9 months." The early postoperative convalescence in these patients was very satisfactory, probably due to better organ preservation, better donor selection, and improved immunosuppression. The four patients who had died had all died with or because of a septic liver infarction. "The sequence of events seemed to be, first, infarction of portions of the homografts and, then, overgrowth of gram negative bacteria in the necrotic areas." Autopsies in all four of the patients had shown thrombosis of the right hepatic artery which had been found also in a patient transplanted by Fonkalsrud, at UCLA. Early putative immunologic explanations for this had now given way to the feeling "that mechanical factors predispose man (or at least small children) to a right lobar vascular accident, possibly because of the erect position used by humans." In the last two patients the homograft had been fixed in position and these two patients had shown no evidence of acute liver necrosis. Other complications had been relatively minor and the gastrointestinal hemorrhage and pulmonary embolism seen in the earlier patients had not occurred. The emboli had probably arisen from the sites of venotomy for the plastic tube temporary bypasses which had been used in those patients and now had been demonstrated to be unnecessary. They had kept the azothioprine doses below 1 mg./kg. per day, had reduced the initial large dose of prednisone as quickly as possible and had employed antilymphocyte globulin "which in many dogs can delay or prevent liver homograft rejection when used as the only therapy [Starzl, 1964]". Study of liver biopsies 60 days to six months after transplantation, showed "portal fibrosis, a slight infiltration by small lymphocytes around the portal vein branches, proliferation of small bile ductules and some central cholestasis. One of the two longer surviving homografts had progressed to cirrhosis and in both many of the small hepatic artery branches were narrowed by intimal thickening. These various changes are thought to be the result of rejections; they were least severe in the homograft which was shown by lymphocyte typing to be most compatible with its recipient." A dated addendum of three months later [the first time such an addendum appears with a dateline] says, "The 3 patients surviving at the time the manuscript was submitted are still alive. The first patient will be one year post-transplantation in 10 days. The other 2 have now been followed for 5 and 4 postoperative months respectively. Three other recipients treated 3 months, 6 weeks, and 3-1/2 weeks ago are well. There have been no septic hepatic infarctions in the last 5 cases."

Discussion

Francis D. Moore, of Boston, used terms like "absolutely outstanding . . . banner day . . . magnificent achievement . . . an entirely new look . . ." Now that suppression without hepatotoxicity was possible, that antilymphocyte globulin was available and that there were groups with "practical capability in transplant immunology and histocompatibility matching, as well as surgical experience with transplantation and the postoperative care of patients on immunosuppression, there is no need for consultant boards to declare the patient operable or a team from another institution to decide that the donor is dead." One knew the time and temperature relationships controlling the viability of the donor organ,

". . . the same for liver donation as for heart, with the heart somewhat less vulnerable to normothermic ischemia." Moore was actually aiming at the writers of "a statement issued by a committee in Washington that attempts to deal with these matters as applied to the heart . . . none of the authors . . . has busied himself with the transplant problem over these last 15 years; the document makes no reference whatsoever to the long work of many Departments in this country . . . the obvious fact that actual experience in immunogenetics, immunosuppression and surgical transplantation are the essential normal prerequisites to moving ahead with any newly transplantable organ. Nor . . . that the moral security of the next 25 years of American surgery, in exploring this new field, will rest secure just where it has in the past 20 years; and giving free and untrammelled opportunity for development to those Departments and individuals . . . willing to take the time and trouble to develop both the immunological and surgical aspects of organ transplantation, as Dr. Starzl has demonstrated today with a project that was held in abeyance until the fundamentally ethical nature of science itself indicated that it was time again to move ahead." Eric W. Fonkalsrud, of Los Angeles, in animals and in one patient with biliary atresia, had used chlorpromazine as a "hepatic cell stabilizing" drug. His patient was ambulatory and excreting bile well when he became septic on the fourth day and proved to have a "large area of necrosis in the dome of the right lobe of the liver . . ." and was subsequently found at autopsy to have "thrombosis of the small branches of the right hepatic artery . . . similar to those described in Dr. Starzl's paper today." The vascular anastomoses were all patent. Starzl, closing, commented that by first placing the liver in a perfusion chamber and testing it under perfusion, they had been able to evaluate it "before anything was done to the recipient."

* * *

Starzl's revolutionary paper on the apparent solution of the problems of hepatic transplantation was followed by a comprehensive review of five years' experience from the Peter Bent Brigham, where renal transplantation had begun. In *Five Years' Experience in Renal Transplantation with Immunosuppressive Drugs:* Survival, Function, Complications, and the Role of Lymphocyte Depletion by Thoracic Duct Fistula, Joseph E. Murray, Clinical Associate in Surgery, Harvard Medical School; Chief Plastic Surgeon, Peter Bent Brigham Hospital; Director of Surgical Research Laboratory, Harvard

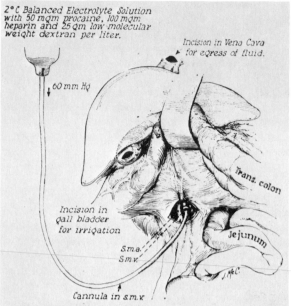

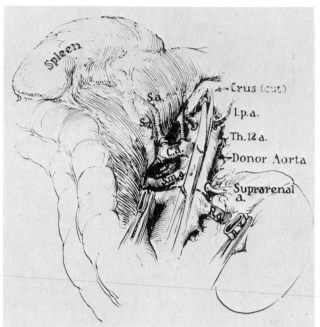

Fig. 2. Core cooling of cadaveric liver used for infant donors. Immediately after entering the abdomen, the cannula is placed into the readily accessible superior mesenteric vein. This vessel is far enough away from the portal triad so that the portal vein, which will ultimately be used for anastomosis, is not in danger of injury. Egress of the perfusion fluid is provided by the venotomy in the suprahepatic inferior vena cava. Bile is washed from the gallbladder through the cholecystotomy. For the adult donor (Case 7), the liver was cooled by total body extracorporeal perfusion, and the flushing carried out after completion of the hepatectomy.

Fig. 3. Mobilization of the aorta during donor hepatectomy. Rapid identification and ligation of the branches is facilitated if variable traction is applied to the distal aorta. During the initial dissection, all the aortic branches except the coeliac axis and superior mesenteric artery are ligated and divided; the latter vessel is cut only after it has been shown not to give rise to an anomalous hepatic arterial branch.

In six out of seven instances, Starzl cooled the donor liver by immediate postmortem introduction of cold saline into the superior mesenteric vein, allowed to escape through an incision in the vena cava. He had somewhat modified his original technique of donor arterial preservation, as indicated in the legend of figure 3. In six of the seven patients, the homograft was evaluated in a perfusion chamber. Excision of the recipient's liver was frequently the most difficult part of the procedure. Figure 4 (facing page) indicates changes in Starzl's original technique. Biliary drainage was now by cholecystoduodenostomy instead of choledochocholedochostomy, and bypasses "to decompress the splanchnic and systemic venous systems during the anhepatic phase" had been abandoned.

Thomas E. Starzl, C. G. Groth, L. Brettschneider, I. Penn, V. A. Fulginiti, J. B. Moon, H. Blanchard, A. J. Martin, Jr., and Ken Porter, *Orthotopic Homotransplantation of the Human Liver*, Volume LXXXVI, 1968.

Medical School and Peter Bent Brigham Hospital; Richard E. Wilson, by invitation; Gustave J. Dammin, by invitation [Friedman Professor of Pathology, Harvard Medical School; Pathologist-in-Chief, Peter Bent Brigham Hospital]; Hartwell Harrison, Elliott Carr Cutler Professor of Surgery, Harvard Medical School; Urologic Surgeon, Chief of Service, Peter Bent Brigham Hospital; and eight associates, reported their experience from the time of "first living volunteer donor for a drug-treated recipient" on

into the beginning of their experience with horse anti-human-lymphocyte globulin. In this paper, they eliminated from consideration their monozygotic twin transplants, their experience with total irradiation, and their "early introductory trials with drug therapy in cadaveric and unrelated living donors." They had done 110 kidney transplants, the 18 to 20 a year doubling in the last year to 37 ". . . primarily because of increased use of paired transplants from cadaveric donors." Pre-transplantation bilateral ne-

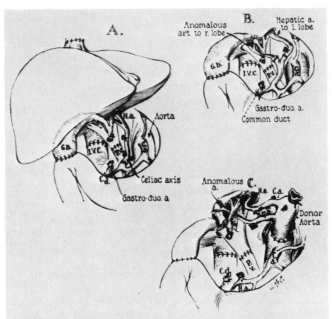

FIG. 4. Recipient operations. Cholecystoduodenostomy was performed in all 7 cases. A—The kind of arterial anastomosis used in Cases 1, 3, 4, 6, and 7. The homograft coeliac axis or common hepatic artery was attached to the proper or common hepatic artery. B—Arterial anastomoses in Case 2. The right hepatic originated from the superior mesenteric artery. C—Anastomosis of the homograft aorta to the recipient aorta (Case 5). This technic was used because of the double arterial supply.

phrectomy, and chronic hemodialysis were now standard. All donors underwent Terasaki leukocyte typing, but transplantation was done without regard to the result. They had developed an interest in the problem of secondary hyperparathyroidism. Immunosuppressive regimens had varied, azathioprine had been used in every patient. Discontinued in four after one-and-a-half to four years, rejection followed a variable period thereafter in all four patients. Almost all patients received corticosteroids either primarily or for treatment of rejection. Actinomycin C and azaserine had been used earlier, but azaserine because of its "questionable beneficial effect . . . increased morbidity . . ." had been abandoned and actinomycin C was now used only to treat rejection. Typhoid vaccine had been used in 12 recipients and given up. X-ray over the transplant had been used to treat rejection in living donor transplants and as part of the primary therapy in "all cadaveric and unrelated donor transplants since 1965". It had never been used as the sole treatment of rejection and they could not, therefore, attest to its value.

They had studied the benefit of splenectomy. It did not permit the use of larger doses of drugs, did not protect against drug induced leukopenia, platelet counts tended to be excessively high, there seemed to be an associated increase in major sepsis and in the number of rejection crises. They had abandoned splenectomy since 1965. Extracorporeal irradiation to achieve lymphocyte depletion had been employed in 12 patients and despite "one striking incidence of reversal of rejection" this method had been abandoned. They had begun thoracic duct cannulation as a means of lymphocyte depletion in March, 1965, and were still employing it beginning five to seven days before operation and continuing it after operation in those cases in which clotting at the time of operation or early postoperatively did not occur. Horse anti-human lymphocyte globulin, ALG, had been first used by them in 1967 in patients undergoing preoperative thoracic duct cannulation and pre- and postoperative ALG therapy. Azathioprine "started 2 days before transplantation and continued as the sole method of immunosuppression from

THE TRANSPLANTERS

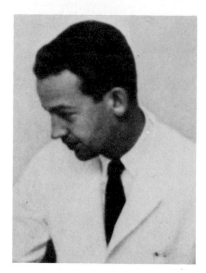

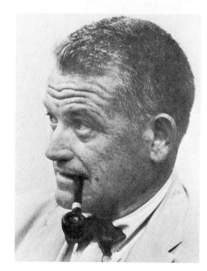

Folkert O. Belzer, (c. 1960), 1930 in Indonesia,- M.D. Boston University 1938; Intern and Assistant Residency Grace-New Haven Hospital 1958-62; Resident, University of Oregon 1962-63 and Instructor 1963-64; Senior Lecturer, Guy's Hospital, London 1964-66; Assistant Professor to Professor, U.C.S.F. 1966-74; Professor and Chairman, University of Wisconsin 1974—. Working at the University of California, San Francisco with Kountz, devised and applied a new preservation technique, involving pulsatile perfusion of a cooled kidney, with an oxygenated medium. Cadaver transfusion ceased to be an instant emergency. Remarkable impact on the practical problems of harvesting and transplanting, maintaining regional computerized networks of potential recipients, etc.

Willard E. Goodwin (c. 1958), 1915-. M.D. Johns Hopkins 1941, Residency Brady Urological Institute, Johns Hopkins, 1941-49, and Instructor to Assistant Professor 1948-51. Professor and Chief Division Urology, U.C.L.A. 1951-70 and Professor of Surgery, Pediatric Urology 1970-. Scholarly, ingenious, original talents combined with urologist's irreverence, and skier and mountain climber's derring do. Saw potentialities of transplantation, spent 1958-59 sabbatical year with Murray at Peter Bent Brigham and Woodruff in Edinburgh, returning to set up renal transplant program. Was both a gadfly stimulus and restraining influence during first years of clinical transplantation. His 1963 publications made the critical observations of the effectiveness of steroid therapy in reversing rejection. First also to employ cyclophosphamide, first "en bloc" transplantation of kidneys, aorta and vena cava, first ureteropyelostomy in transplanted kidney. In urology, made early use of trigone transplants into rectum, for vesical exstrophy.

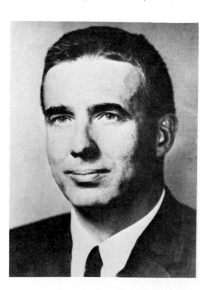

David M. Hume, 1917-1973. M.D. University of Chicago, 1943; Intern and Resident, Peter Bent Brigham Hospital 1943-51. Director, Laboratory for Surgical Research, Harvard Medical School, 1951-56; Stuart McGuire Professor of Surgery, Chairman, Department of Surgery, Medical College of Virginia Hospitals, 1956-73. Had been associated with Hufnagel and

Landsteiner in the 1947 attachment of a cadaver kidney to the antecubital vessels of a uremic patient, began laboratory renal transplantations in 1949, and shortly thereafter, human cadaver, renal transplants to unmodified recipients with encouraging temporary graft function. The work was interrupted by his call up for a second tour of duty, in the Navy, at the sudden outbreak of the Korean War. He was away when the opportunity arose at the Brigham for the performance of grafts between identical twins. At Richmond, established a major transplant center, a productive laboratory, evaluating step-by-step technical, immunological, and clinical features of renal transplantation. He was almost as deeply involved in surgical endocrinology,- (first quantitative bio-assay for serum ACTH), and led brilliantly in both fields. His analytic expositions of the problems in transplantation made him an international influence of first importance. His deep, and deeply analyzed laboratory and clinical experience, his cocky and aggressive good-naturedly belligerent manner enlivened meetings and chastened opponents. Died flying his plane from a medical visit to the West Coast.

(Portrait courtesy of Lazar Greenfield, M.D., Richmond, Virginia.)

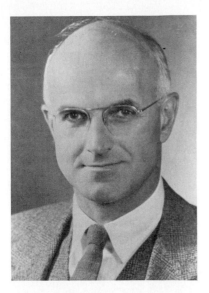

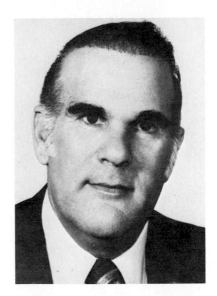

Joseph E. Murray, (c. 1963) 1919—, M.D. Harvard 1943; Vice-President 1979; Surgical House Officer, Peter Bent Brigham 1943-50; Plastic Surgery, New York Hospital 1951; Professor of Surgery, Harvard, Peter Bent Brigham and Children's Hospitals, 1970—; Chief of Division of Plastic Surgery, Children's Hospital 1974—. One of the authentic pioneers of transplantation, followed David Hume In the laboratory of Francis Moore, where successful renal transplantation had its genesis. Independently (of Küss in France) devised the still employed anatomical techniques of renal transplantation. Performed with Hartwell Harrison the first permanently successful transplantation, between identical twins, at the Peter Bent Brigham in 1954, the first transplant after total body irradiation in 1959, the first clinical use of azothioprine in 1961. Major role in founding the International Kidney Transplant Registry. Withdrew from the transplantation field to devote himself entirely to plastic surgery, making a major effort in the field of craniofacial reconstruction.

J. S. Najarian, 1927—. M.D. University of California, San Francisco 1952; Internship and Residency to 1960, devoted three years at the University of Pittsburgh and at Scripps Clinic, to immunopathology and transplantation immunology; Assistant Professor of Surgery to Professor, U.C. San Francisco 1963-67; Professor and Chairman, University of Minnesota, 1967-   . With Kountz initiated major renal transplant program at U.C. San Francisco, in the "second wave" and developed a second major program at University of Minnesota with particular emphasis on the effectiveness of renal transplantation in children and in patients with diabetic nephropathy. Vigorously pursued the use of A.L.G., adapting it to intravenous injection.

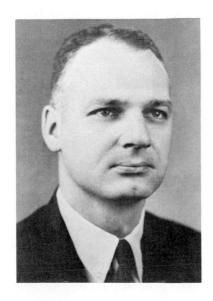

Keith Reemtsma (c. 1964), 1925—. M.D. University of Pennsylvania 1949; Residency, Presbyterian Hospital, New York 1949-57; Assistant Professor to Professor, Tulane University 1957-66; Professor and Head, University of Utah, 1966-71; Professor and Chairman, Columbia University College of Physicians and Surgeons 1971—. Undertook renal hetero-transplantation from non-human primates, with some success and an astonishing 6-month survival. Active in field of pancreatic and islet transplantation, developed procedure for parallel, auxiliary heart transplantation.

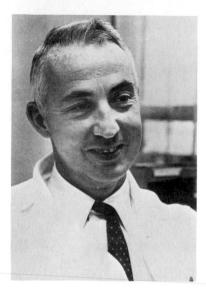

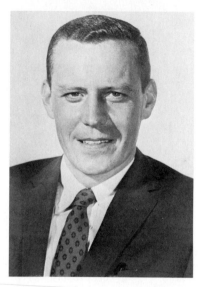

Norman E. Shumway (c. 1970) 1923—. M.D. Vanderbilt 1949; Cardiac Surgical Training University of Minnesota 1954-57; Stanford University, Instructor to Professor and Chairman, Department of Cardiovascular Surgery 1958—. Multiple contributions in surgery of acquired heart disease. With Lower, in a series of careful experiments, established feasibility and technqiue of cardiac transplantation and was in search of an appropriate first patient when the initial and successful cardiac transplantation was precipitately performed by Barnard in Capetown after a flying visit to the States. (Hardy had by then transplanted a chimpanzee heart to a human recipient who survived a few hours.) Most clinics have abandoned cardiac transplantation after their discouraging experience during the epidemic flurry of cardiac transplantations by cardiac surgeons in the first flush of the Capetown and Stanford successes. Shumway's was the second successful human cardiac transplantation and his large, systematic, carefully followed and continuing series of cardiac transplantations has long outdistanced all others in numbers, quality of results, and yield of scientific information and established the value of the procedure.

Thomas E. Starzl (c. 1963), 1926—. M.D. Northwestern University 1952; (Ph.D. in Neurophysiology), Internship, Fellowship, and Residency, Johns Hopkins 1952-56; Residency, University of Miami, 1956-58; Instructor to Assistant Professor of Surgery, Northwestern University 1958-62; Associate Professor, 1962, to Professor and Chairman, University of Colorado, 1972- Phenomenal and prodigious worker; intense, systematic, thoughtful, analytic,- superb scientist, audacious and skillful surgeon. His major renal transplantation effort begun in Denver in 1962, at the same time as Murray's in Boston and Woodruff's (Honorary Fellow) in Edinburgh, has been one of the major sources of technical, clinical, and immunological observations and advances,- the first trial with a significant number of long-term survivors, the first clinical use of histocompatibility testing, introduction of antilymphocyte globulin. He early recognized and documented the tumorogenic effect of immunosuppression, revived, studied and made practical, thoracic-duct drainage. Established the first,- and still the premier,- liver transplantation program (Roy Calne, Honorary Fellow, in Cambridge conducts the only other major liver transplantation program). Suggested and performed portacaval transposition for glycogen storage disease. A steady flow of fellows and long and short term visitors have gone forth from his laboratories and clinical program to establish programs of their own.

the day of transplantation onward" was part of the standard protocol and "Steroid therapy is reserved only to treat rejection." It was still too early to evaluate this experience of only six months. Their "Successive yearly survival rates . . . improved from 60% to 85%, a change which approaches but does not reach statistical significance . . . In the entire series of 110 transplants, five failed after 1 year, and eight more failed after 2 years". They now had two patients surviving for five years and six, between three and five years, all appearing well. The thoracic duct fistulae seemed to be associated with significantly better survival, not affected by the Terasaki match. There were six deaths, from sepsis or hemorrhage, as a result of ureteric anastomotic complications. Spon-

taneous rupture of the transplant occurred within 72 hours in three patients who had received kidneys from living, related donors with "complete recovery of function in all following re-exploration and tamponade of a bleeding surface." One cadaveric transplant kidney ruptured and was removed. Thus far, they had seen no new primary neoplasms develop in their immunosuppressed patients although "one cadaveric recipient developed the same epidermoid carcinoma that had caused the death of the donor. This transplanted tumor was rejected as was the kidney on discontinuation of the immunosuppressive therapy. The patient is now surviving on a secondary inter-familial transplant." They thought their improvement was due to better immunosuppression and better management of the patients and not due to better matching of donor recipients because they had not done prospective matching. Nevertheless, "There is no doubt that close tissue matching is desirable; in our series, as with others, *retrospective* analysis of leucocyte typing by Terasaki reveals that 90% of well matched recipients have continued good function whereas only 50% of poorly matched transplants continue to function. It is only coincidental that these are the same percentage survivals for the Group I [successful thoracic duct fistula] and Group II [failed thoracic fistula] in our thoracic duct fistula series." There was general agreement that after the first three months, immunosuppressive therapy could be reduced without danger to the graft. Murray postulated that "Thoracic duct cannulation may . . . exert its beneficial effect on kidney transplantation by the removal of the unsensitized small lymphocytes prior to their contact with the antigen . . . In some patients, more than ten times the total population of circulating small lymphocytes had been removed." In addition, sensitized cells might be removed as well. Eleven patients who had been recognized to have secondary hyperparathyroidism due to chief cell hyperplasia had undergone excision of three-and-a-half of the four parathyroids,- in seven of them before the transplant, and in one, four months afterwards and three more in preparation for transplantation which had not yet been performed. "Once good renal graft function has occurred, the need for calcium therapy ceases and serum calcium levels remain normal with healing of the bony lesions. Our preferred policy at present is to perform parathyroidectomy prior to the transplantation while the patient is on chronic dialysis."

Discussion

Paul S. Russell, of Boston [the Massachusetts General Hospital], discussing immunosuppression, stressed the "steady movement toward immunological specificity of action". Whole body irradiation had been abandoned, the "conglomerate treatment involving Imuran and steroids" produced numerous and often serious side effects. He mentioned, for steroids, "collapse of the femoral head, pancreatitis, bleeding ulcer, and intercurrent infection". Now "antilymphocyte serum and various serum fractions" were being evaluated with the hope that they would be "effective particularly against peripheral

lymphocytes leaving relatively intact humoral antibody responses", although even then defense against viruses might not be preserved intact. He was interested that the effect of thoracic duct fistula seemed to last for months so that "perhaps we cannot completely dismiss the possibility that thoracic duct fistula could favor a specific accommodation . . . between the host and the transplant." Thomas C. Moore, of Torrance, California, spoke for Dr. David Hume's Richmond, Virginia group [with whom he had worked] with "138 renal transplants in 117 patients, 116 first transplants, 13 second transplants, 3 third transplants and 1 fourth transplant." They had not employed thoracic duct fistula and in "42 consecutive related living donor transplants, we have had a 86% one year functioning survival of the transplant kidney." In 25 recent consecutive cadaver donor transplants, they had had a 76% one-year survival of the transplant kidney, but the two-year survival had fallen to 48%. Overall, they had six patients living more than five years after transplantation, with functioning kidneys, "three on the same kidney and three on second, third and fourth renal transplants." They had not seen rupture of a transplanted kidney. They always performed a capsulotomy, which Dr. Murray's group had not done. There was a "ten-fold greater fall-off in patient survival between one and 2 years in the cadaver donor group" than in the living donor group and it appeared to be due to thrombotic and embolic complications, gastrointestinal ulceration and bleeding, hepatitis, and sepsis. Thomas E. Starzl, of Denver, showed the survival curve in 64 patients treated from the fall of 1962 until March of 1964. Thirty-one were alive at from four to five-and-a-half years after transplantation. The results were better with living, related donors. From 1964 to 1966, they had not been able to improve their results and therefore added their own antilymphocyte globulin, "raised in horses and prepared and purified in our own laboratories", in addition to azathioprine and prednisone. "Since then the mortality has, for intra-familial transplantation, been almost eliminated. Of the first 20 patients, treated since this change was made in June of 1966, 19 or 95% have good function of their original homografts from 16 to 22 months later . . . only five deaths in the last 70 consanguineous renal homotransplantations . . . and there has not been a late loss of any of these kidneys. 80% of the recipients of cadaveric transplantations treated in this same interval are still alive . . . kidney transplantation has become a spectacularly successful way of treating terminal renal disease. No one has contributed more to this present state of affairs than Dr.

Joseph Murray. . ." The "role of host immune potential in curbing the growth of the malignant tumors, presumably by reacting to tumor-specific antigens" had already been commented upon at the meeting, and Starzl reported that "we have now seen three patients develop reticulum cell sarcoma from 8 months to 2-1/2 years after renal transplantation. Two similar cases have been seen in Minneapolis and another one in Edinburgh, Scotland. An increased incidence of mesenchymal cell malignancy may therefore prove to be one more complication of homotransplantation." J. Fish, of Galveston [to whom Murray, in closing, expressed appreciation for his having taught the group at the Peter Bent Brigham the technique and management of thoracic duct fistula], said they had treated five patients "with long-term lymph fistula, with lymph dialysis and destruction of lymphocytes in preparation for renal transplantation. These patients have had functioning thoracic duct fistulae present for 35 to 108 days with average lymph flows from five to ten liters a day and with destruction or removal of 100 to 330 billion lymphocytes prior to receiving the transplant." In two patients, as long as an open fistula was maintained, no Imuran or prednisone was employed and no rejection occurred. J. E. Dunphy, of San Francisco, [his name unfamiliarly written by the stenotypist, and recorded in the Discussion, as "Dr. John E. Dunphy"] presented the work of Drs. Najarian, Belzer, and Kountz at the University of California at San Francisco. Seventy-five percent of 87 recipients of January, 1964 were alive and all but one or two had functioning kidneys. In the last year, there had been no failures due to technical problems or rejection and a 93% survival, the patients who succumbed dying of their underlying disease. Murray, closing, said that Dr. Russell's thought that thoracic duct fistula might "give some specificity to immunosuppression" had not occurred to him. He had thought of the fistula as merely "bulk removal of uncommitted cells, thus decreasing the total numbers of attacking forces." Murray was impressed by Fish's two patients with successful transplants maintained 30 to 60 days solely with thoracic duct fistulae.

* * *

There had recently been a flurry of interest in the possibilities of pancreatic transplantation, and Keith Reemtsma, of Salt Lake City, Professor and Head, Department of Surgery, University of Utah, College of Medicine; and by invitation, Nelson Giraldo, D. A. Depp, and E. J. Eichwald, *Islet Cell Transplantation*, presented the results of their work

in dogs and rats preserving the arterial and portal venous attachments of all of the pancreas but the head, thus transplanting it solely by two vascular anastomoses, and tying off the pancreatic ducts. In some of the dogs and some of the rats, the pancreatic duct had been ligated some weeks before the grafting. The recipients had had a total pancreatectomy before grafting. In 40% of their pancreatectomized dogs, transplant of the pancreas achieved normal blood sugar levels and this rose to 80% if the donor pancreas had had a previous ligation of its duct. The maximum survival of islet function had been two weeks, significantly prolonged by immunosuppression. In inbred rats, the pancreas functioned at least 150 days. In general, they thought that "enzymatic factors may contribute to early graft failure but . . . long-term success of islet cell transplants is determined by immunologic factors."

Discussion

John R. Brooks, of Boston, whose work had been referred to by Reemtsma, said that in their dog experiments, they had done a combined pancreaticoduodenal graft, "we use the duodenal segment as a drain to allow pancreatic secretion to come out. This has been our way of avoiding serious pancreatitis. . ." They used Imuran suppression. Early death was due either to bleeding, or thrombosis of vessels, or to overwhelming pancreatitis. Most dogs eventually survived, getting over their pancreatitis. They had seen no late pancreatitis. Late death at 30 to 40 days was due to infection and inanition, occasionally to rejection. If the serum amylase rose after transplantation and if it remained high, the dog could be expected to succumb. Pancreatic exocrine function seemed to disappear by eight to 12 weeks. He thought that Reemtsma's pancreases showed more histologic reaction and that this might be due to ligation of the pancreatic duct. John M. Howard, of Philadelphia, suggested that pancreatic transplantation would be useful for the juvenile diabetic and for chronic pancreatitis and perhaps for cystic fibrosis. Their own dog experiments with pancreatic transplantation led them to think "that the necrosis which the homografted pancreas undergoes does not represent pancreatitis in the clinical sense. We consider it necrosis and autolysis."

* * *

Stanley R. Friesen, of Kansas City, Assistant Professor of Surgery, University of Kansas School of Medicine, *A Gastric Factor in the Pathogenesis of the Zollinger-Ellison Syndrome*, had been struck by the fact that these patients were not only cured of their ulcer symptoms after total gastrectomy, but that metastases did not progress and, in fact, regressed. It was already known that excision of the pancreatic islet cell adenoma rarely cured, presumably because there were already metastases, and that nothing short of total gastrectomy produced relief of symptoms. It seemed to Friesen that "That entire spectrum of islet cell growths from simple hyperplasia to multiple primaries with metastases in nine of the patients suggests that these abnormalities are manifestations secondary to another stimulus such as the stomach." The fact that the patients who had diarrhea were relieved by total gastrectomy suggested "that the cause of diarrhea or steatorrhea is related to gastric acid hypersecretion alone or to a gastric stimulation of islet cell gastrin or other islet cell hormone." Reports in the literature, similarly, described patients who, after total gastrectomy, had had either remissions or long periods without change in growth of metastases. In fact, Wilson and Ellison in 1966, reviewing 78 collected cases of total gastrectomy for ulcerogenic tumor of the pancreas "stated that there had been only four deaths attributable to tumor and cachexia." Friesen pondered the relationship of the Zollinger-Ellison syndrome to multiple endocrine adenomatosis usually with tumor in the parathyroid glands and occasionally in the pituitary as well. Friesen postulated ". . . a genetic neurohumoral basis", and suggested several mechanisms.

Discussion

Robert M. Zollinger, of Columbus, thought that Friesen's "stimulating concept . . . may give moral support to the surgeons who have been afraid to do a total gastrectomy or have been hesitant to do it." Zollinger supported Friesen's observation that metastases might remain static for years and asked "why do we sometimes find only microscopic evidence of metastasis in the adjacent lymph nodes without gross evidence of tumor in the pancreas? How do you explain this? I wonder why the pathologists can't give us an answer?" With his customary tongue-in-cheek outrageousness, Zollinger concluded by saying "I like this concept of Dr. Friesen. I don't know that I believe a word of it, but I'd like to thank him." Edwin H. Ellison, now of Milwaukee, said they now had "over 600 proven cases of the Zollinger-Ellison syndrome in the registry; 120 of these are living and well after total gastrectomy." Those who died of total gastrectomy usually died early, of technical mishaps, in what was frequently the patient's fourth or fifth gastric operation No

children had survived without total gastrectomy, ". . . this is a more serious disease in children but it responds better to total gastrectomy. These children continue to grow and some of them have had children . . . Stan Friesen may have a point, that removal of that end organ, although he is saying it in a different fashion, does have an influence on the growth of tumors. Certainly the ones I have seen personally and have done total gastrectomies for them are still living and the tumors have not grown."

* * *

Robert M. Zollinger, of Columbus, Professor and Chairman, Department of Surgery, Ohio State University College of Medicine; Ronald K. Tompkins and four other associates by invitation, *Identification of the Diarrheogenic Hormone Associated with Non-Beta Islet Cell Tumors of the Pancreas,* continued the discussion. Islet cell tumors had been demonstrated to produce insulin, gastrin, serotonin, and glucagon "singly or in combination with other hormones". Still another hormone had been postulated for patients whose chief symptom was diarrhea from a non-beta islet cell tumor of the pancreas. They described two patients with watery diarrhea, hypokalemia, and achlorhydria, one of whom had a very large islet cell adenoma, removal of which was curative; the other of whom was found to have extensive metastases to the liver. The pancreas was edematous but not certainly the source of the primary tumor. The second patient was irradiated but succumbed to multiple hepatic metastases. Neither tumor, on assay, proved to have any gastrin activity. In Patient 1, the duodenum refilled with secretion during the operation and the gallbladder was greatly enlarged, "The unexpected finding of high chloride and bicarbonate levels . . . in the otherwise very dilute bile led to the suspicion that an unusual choleretic agent was being liberated by the islet cell tumor." The second patient evidenced very similar chemical results in the bile. The fact that the achlorhydria in the first patient was gone within a week of resection of the large pancreatic tumor confirmed the suspicion that the tumor secreted a substance inhibiting gastric acid output. In fact, they had data that "five of the six patients with malignant islet cell tumors . . . in 12 proven cases of non-beta islet cell tumors with watery diarrhea, hypokalemia and achlorhydria collected to date . . . had histamine-fast achlorhydria. This suggests that such malignant tumors may be capable of more marked production of the responsible hormone." On a parallel tack, Greenough in 1965, had suggested that the diarrhea of cholera might be due to biliary or pancreatic juice hypersecretion and suggested at that time that "an excess of secretin, released from the duodenum by large numbers of cholera vibrios, might cause biliary and pancreatic hypersecretion in amounts as high as 8 liters per day." Wormsley had demonstrated that secretin injected in man could cause "attacks of explosive, painless diarrhea . . ." without cramping pain, although Zollinger had been unable to reproduce this effect of secretin in dogs. Both of Zollinger's patients had parathyroid hyperplasia and the first patient had hypercalcemia. Bioassay of the metastatic tumor from the second patient showed "the classic secretin-like pancreatic response of high volume of juice with an increased bicarbonate concentration and a decreased enzyme content as evidenced by total protein."

Discussion

Lester R. Dragstedt, of Gainesville, said that "There is no evidence that the normal pancreatic islets produce secretin and the evidence that they produce gastrin is scant and contradictory. It is, therefore, probable that the pancreatic tumors that produce gastrin and secretin arise from heterotopic or embryologically misplaced cells that occur normally in the stomach [gastrin] and duodenum [secretin], respectively." Dragstedt, alluding to the fact that the one tumor did not occur in the stomach and the other tumor did not occur in the duodenum, both of them occurring in the pancreas, made one "think of the suggestion of Cohnheim many years ago that heterotopic or embryologically misplaced tissue is more apt to undergo neoplastic transformation than is tissue in its normal location." Edgar J. Poth, of Galveston, said that while a Zollinger-Ellison tumor, and insulinoma, and carcinoids from the lung and the stomach might look alike under the light microscope, they were very different under the electron microscope, because of the different appearance of their specific granules. William Silen, of Boston, agreed with the technique employed for extraction of the secretin from the tumors. He was in the process of doing that in two such tumors in his own laboratory and as yet had no results to discuss. He asked Zollinger whether the hormone in question might be glucagon or a substance related to glucagon, "since glucagon has many of the properties of secretin and certainly has a choleretic effect as strong as, and perhaps more so, than secretin and it also depresses gastric secretion." Gerald W. Peskin, of Chicago, had studied a similar patient when he was at the University of Pennsylvania, and in a golden Syrian hamster ileum preparation, felt that he had demonstrated that the diarrheogenic activity "was due to a mucosal to serosal transport inhibition produced by the humoral agent within this tumor." When he had tested secretin, cholecystokinin, histamine, serotonin and other agents from gastrointestinal sources, he found "that only secretin and cholecystokinin produced a similar effect." The pattern on gel-electrophoresis of secretin was essentially the same as that of the extracts of the tumor, so that "With these three indirect bits of evidence, I think we can support further the hypothesis that a secretin-like substance or secretin itself is a part of the overall elaboration of this particular tumor." H. W. Scott, of Nashville, said that Longmire at UCLA had "reviewed the literature recently on the pancreatic cholera syndrome associated with a non-beta cell islet tumor . . ." had collected 15 cases and there were perhaps four more, representing perhaps 10% of all Z-E cases. They had had a patient at Vanderbilt with inoperable metastases from an islet cell tumor and massive explosive diarrhea, who, as the tumor progressed, developed hypercalcemia and then finally extreme hyperchlorhydria "producing as much as one liter of strongly acid gastric juice per hour during this 4 day period. He required as much as 20 to 25 liters of fluid per day, parenterally, to keep up with his losses." Scott raised the question as to whether the tumor, originally producing only a secretin-like substance, was now perhaps producing gastrin as well. Autopsy showed only "the massive pancreatic islet cancer with liver metastases and no other endocrine tumors." Edwin H. Ellison, of Milwaukee, was willing to "predict that a secretin antibody could be prepared and tagged with radioiodine in a fashion similar to that described by one of my surgical trainees, Dr. John Stremple, for a synthetic gastrin, thus permitting a highly sensitive radio immuno assay." He was attracted to the "concept Dr. Bill Scott spoke of, that there may be mixed tumors . . . because many of the patients in the collected series started out with diarrhea and then developed the ulcer syndrome later. We have no idea whether they made acid initially or not. They may not have, as gastrin is certainly a potent substance . . ." William P. Longmire, of Los Angeles, said that in one patient with diarrhea, they had failed to extract an active principle from a large beta cell tumor, but had noted that the gallbladder was very large, and that there was a large amount of free fluid and gas in the small intestine, the walls of which were slightly thickened and edematous. Their patient had normal gastric acidity both before and after operation. The reported diarrhea-producing tumors all seemed to have been large, whereas the gastrin-producing tumors were frequently small and sometimes difficult to find. R. K. Tompkins, closing, said the physiologic action of their tumor extract was different from that of glucagon. With respect to H. W. Scott's question about the possible production of gastrin by the tumor late in its life, he asked whether it was possible that the ulcer effect in Scott's patient occurred at the time that steroids had been exhibited.

* * *

There was a remarkable two-paper symposium on the use of computers for surgical patients, which brought into sharp focus the fact that computers were being widely used in surgical care but possibly not appropriately, that there was not yet full agreement as to what information it was desired to obtain from a computer, and that there were differences among the Fellows as to the actual purpose of the computers, whether they were to complement or replace the human brain. From the University of Alabama, Louis C. Sheppard, Nicholas T. Kouchoukos, Mary Alta Kurtts, all by invitation, and John W. Kirklin, of Birmingham, Professor and Chairman, Department of Surgery, University of Alabama College of Medicine; Surgeon-in-Chief, University Hospitals and Clinics, *Automated Treatment of Critically Ill Patients following Operation,* presented the details of studies they had been performing since July, 1967, in two beds of the surgical intensive care unit for postoperative cardiac patients, employing an IBM 1800 digital computer system "to facilitate the automatic measurements and to implement the rules and logic for treatment of the patients." In 124 patients, they monitored heart rate from the electrocardiogram, systemic arterial pressure from a Teflon catheter in the left brachial artery passed into the descending aorta, right and left atrial pressures through fine catheters placed during the operation, drainage from mediastinal or chest catheters collected "in a small reservoir which is automatically emptied by a metering pump when a limiting volume is reached" and urine output similarly. Central temperature was determined with a rectal thermistor. The amount of blood infused was measured with a metering pump and drugs administered intravenously similarly measured. Cardiac output was "estimated from the systolic arterial pressure, the pulse pressure and contour, the quality of the peripheral pulses, the rate of urine flow, and the temperature of the extremities." He indicated that methods for frequent determination of cardiac output and stroke volume had proved to be "time consuming and impractical". They were evaluating "A method of estimation of stroke volume from the central aortic pressure contour . . . from the detection of beat by beat changes in stroke volume and hence for frequent determinations of cardiac output." A good correlation was found between values obtained by this technique and values obtained by dilution methods. Current values were all displayed at the bedside and new measurements made automatically every five minutes or on request. Data were printed out every four hours and incorporated into the hospital record "This makes it unnecessary for the nurses to record anything but rate of respiration and progress notes." They had developed "clearly defined rules for the infusion of blood in patients after open intracardiac surgery . . . and blood is automatically infused by the system, using these rules." The mean atrial pressure being within a few millimeters of the ventricular end-diastolic pressure, "When cardiac output is judged to be less than optimal, consideration is given to increasing it by increasing atrial (ventricular end-diastolic) pressure with infusion of blood or crystalloid solutions. The tolerance of the individual to such augmentation is best judged by observation of the atrial pressures. The left atrial pressure, in particular, is the limiting factor in the ability of the organism to withstand continuing infusion of blood and fluid because of the deleterious effects upon the lungs of pulmonary venous (left atrial) hypertension . . . there is a level of atrial pressure above which infusion of blood or fluids is undesirable despite an apparently low cardiac output. There is also a level, as yet not clearly defined, above which further augmentation of blood volume does not result in increased cardiac output." The surgeon entered into the computer the desired value for systemic arterial pressure and for left atrial pressure,- usually between 12 and 25 mm. Hg. "When neither of the pressures exceeds its limit, 20 ml. of blood is automatically infused." They had written, but not yet employed a program for infusion of mannitol, which would be automatically administered if urine output was "less than 6 ml. in any one hour, or less than 15 ml./hour in any two successive hours . . ." Infusion would be stopped if atrial pressure exceeded the limit set. Observations of respirations, and the use of intermittent positive pressure through an endotracheal tube, were outside the system. Their emphasis was "on the performance by the system of real work of patient care, measurement and analysis of data, record preparation, and systematic treatment based upon a set of clearly defined rules. Close surveillance of these critically ill patients by the nursing and surgical staffs has not been eliminated by use of the system. Rather, the efficiency and effectiveness of the staff in caring for these patients has been enhanced by the work performed by the system." Refinements and additions to the system were necessary. The cuff pressure method for measuring arterial blood pressure was feasible except in patients with low cardiac output. They were working on a "convenient, semi-continuous method of measuring cardiac output . . ." and planning to incorporate measurements "for detecting and treating impaired pulmonary performance". Logic and rules for treatment had been determined on the basis of recent research and clinical experience, "Since the system applies them automatically and precisely as instructed, the logic and rules are not forgotten, neglected, or misinterpreted as can happen when they are applied by human beings." They estimated the cost, in a 14-bed intensive unit at 50% utilization, would be $77 per patient per day, and at 100% utilization would be $39 per patient per day.

* * *

James V. Maloney, Jr., of Los Angeles, Professor of Surgery, UCLA School of Medicine; Chief, Division of Thoracic Surgery, UCLA Medical Center Hospital, followed with, *The Trouble with Patient Monitoring,* a remarkably lucid analysis of the application of the computer to bedside problems. He was concerned that in many places, nurses watched computers instead of the patients and that actual contact with the patient was decreased by the use of computers. Much of the equipment was inappropriate for the needs. "The fault does not lie with the engineers, for they provided the equipment for which the physician asked. Rather, the fault is that the physician has only the most primitive understanding of what is meant by the term 'clinical acumen'. We do not understand the cognitive processes that permit critical judgment in the practice of medicine. Our inability to describe the process by which we make clinical decisions has resulted not only in fundamentally unsound monitoring equipment, but is at the root of the current turmoil in medical education. (If we cannot define in precise terms how clinical judgments are made, how can we build a machine to make them? How can we teach students to make them?)" He was concerned about the role of the nurse. The shortage of nurses has led to the employment of a team of nonprofessionals under the direction of the nurse, "The development of team nursing has, unfortunately, changed the nurse from a professional colleague of the physician to a data collector at the central nursing station, while non-professionals contact the patient. To counteract this trend, the surgeons invented the intensive care unit.

The confinement of two or three nurses in a small room with several critically ill patients restored the nurse to her appropriate position as a professional colleague of the physician in the care of the critically ill. Remote monitoring threatens again to remove the nurse from the bedside . . . A 24-hour a day digital display at the nursing station of a half dozen physiologic variables is inferior in information content to a 60-second confrontation between nurse and patient." An area in which computers were inferior to the human brain was in pattern recognition, " 'Clinical acumen' is pattern recognition in medicine. There are few areas in computer technology and psychology which are in such a primitive state as the understanding of the pattern recognition process . . . At some future time, when the nature of the cognitive process is understood, it will not only be possible to design meaningful monitoring systems, but a major advance will have been made in medical education." In the computers, improvements could be made in extracting information from the data already available as for instance from the electrocardiogram and the electroencephalogram, "There is no question that the electroencephalogram contains far more information than we have yet extracted from it. For example, Adey and associates at this institution have demonstrated that by autospectral analysis of the electroencephalogram of Gemini program astronauts and chimpanzees it is possible to anticipate errors in performance before they actually occur. Analytic devices tied to monitoring equipment might well establish valuable relationships between, for instance, venous pressure, pulse rate, and arterial pressure, ". . . a decrease in arterial blood pressure may have a different significance when it is associated with a decreased pulse rate and increased central venous pressure, than when it is associated with an increased pulse rate and a decreased venous pressure." He cited the need for "a whole new series of physiologic transducers", for instance for monitoring skin color by reflectance spectometry. An example of a new technique was the esophageal balloon technique of Lewis and of Peters which "together with the air flow from a pneumotachygraph, can be used to estimate pulmonary compliance, viscance, air flow resistance, work of breathing, and whole series of derived variables." Basic research in critically ill patients would establish the general principles which might obviate the need for routine complex studies just as was true of the work of "Moore [Francis] in studying body composition in the ill patient . . . The extremely complex multiple isotope dilution studies done in these patients produced a mass of data which were often not available for analysis until many months after the patient had died or recovered. Yet, the results of these studies have affected the care of tens of thousands of surgical patients." Maloney concluded "Contemporary technology has provided the physician with valuable tools for observing and studying the critically ill patient. Transducers, oscilloscopes, recorders and computers are providing multiple-patient remote monitoring systems in intensive care units. The inappropriate use of this combination technology may be detrimental to the patient's well being. The fundamental errors in the trend toward remote monitoring are: 1) *Failure to Employ the Man-machine System Concept:* This concept is concerned with achieving an objective (e.g., better patient care) by optimal use of the best features of both man and machine. Present trends in monitoring eliminate man from the detector-effector loop by replacing him with 4 or 5 relatively unimportant physiologic transducers. 2) *Overemphasis on the Importance of Temperature, Pulse, Respiration and Blood Pressure as Physiologic Variables:* Ninety-five per cent of useful information comes from talking with, seeing, smelling and feeling the patient. A monitoring system is inappropriate if it removes the professional, either doctor or nurse, from direct contact with the patient in exchange for a digital display of the respiratory rate. 3) *Failure to Understand the Importance of Low Probability Events in Medical Care:* Machines can be designed to perform more accurately and reliably than man certain repetitive tasks. They cannot be designed to respond appropriately to infrequently occurring, unanticipated events. The detection of, and response to low probability events requires a rationality which is unique to man. Most events of clinical significance which occur in postoperative patients are of the low probability type, e.g., pink fluid on the wound dressing, flaring of the nasal alae, the onset of pain, and abdominal distension. It is a common, and erroneous presumption that the nurse is required to feel the patient's wrist every 4 hours for a pulse count when the only purpose is to assure regular, direct nurse-patient contact. The valuable contributions of monitoring technics to patient care and to the understanding of the physiology of critical illness are too well recognized to need defense or justification. A critical evaluation of present trends in patient monitoring is necessitated by the evidence which suggests that neither physicians, nurses, nor engineers know what can reasonably be expected of patient monitoring at the present time. The major efforts in the monitoring field should be directed at fundamental research. The investigations should involve the analysis of information content of physiologic signals, the development of new transducers, and the nature of clinical pattern recognition."

Discussion

Francis D. Moore, of Boston, opened the Discussion of the two papers, emphasizing the frequency with which large amounts of unimportant data were produced and the need for "more research on what to measure" rather than data storage and retrieval. "Things in surgery are too unpredictable to be programmed and you have to simplify what you put in the machine and ask the machine to simplify what it gives back to you." Kirklin's contribution, he called outstanding and pointed out that Kirklin's group dealt with patients who had been intensively monitored in the operating room so that their basic condition was known before they came to the intensive care unit,- as opposed, for instance, to the situation of an automobile accident victim with multiple trauma, in whom, in addition, left atrial monitoring, for instance, was "almost out of the question". Richard M. Peters, of Chapel Hill, warned as others had, against the indiscriminate purchase of attractive hardware, "Computers are the glamor instruments of our age and computer salesmen have developed the art of 'huckstering' to its maximum limit. It is important for the members of this society to develop some immunity to these two antigens and give some adjuvant to our colleagues to reverse the immunosuppressive medication of the computer 'huckster'." He emphasized the disadvantage of large amounts of undigested data and the need for logic programs to analyze and use the data, "Together we must work out and analyze how we make judgments and from this work out algorithms for the computer programmers. Dr. Kirklin has clearly illustrated one step in this process. He is not using his system only to collect data but also to suggest changes in therapy." Roger D. Williams, of Galveston, had been using the computer to measure and record intake and urine output and gastrointestinal output. F. John Lewis, of Chicago, whom Maloney had cited, said that "I suppose we have all, as these comments have illustrated, been a little disappointed with the unfulfilled promise of digital computers in providing day to day patient care, yet work like that of Dr. Kirklin, Dr. Sheppard, Dr. Kouchoukos and associates suggests that computers are more likely to reach a day to day practical usefulness, first in intensive care units. It can be done already, as you have seen, if the computer is fed data from critically placed sensors, but most patients, as Dr. Maloney pointed out, who might be attached to such a machine provide less valuable numbers. As one retreats from clinical examination of the patients as carried out by a skilled physician to inspection of a few numbers, it is worthwhile noting that there may be a great reduction in the quality of information which can actually be quantitized." Like Maloney, Lewis emphasized the negative effect of the interposition of "a barrier of oscilloscopes between the patient and the attendant". In addition to which, a computer monitoring a patient displaying six three-digit numbers had, "in jargon of cybernetics . . . sixty bits of information in this data . . . In contrast, a lower bound estimate for the information transmitted by the optic nerve is 2,000 bits per minute, just one of the sensory organs the clinician uses. The computer, therefore, in addition to the other problems, has much less information to work with than the brain of the examining physician. There is a very important problem of inadequate transducers in this business." In addition, "The machine works in a rather simple, logical fashion with a binary type of logic and it simply cannot match the trained brain and the trained brain's ability to make subtle pattern recognitions, or pattern identifications rapidly from sensory information . . . Yet the machine is untiring and patient. It is accurate. It is amazingly fast at arithmetic. Its memory is infallible and it does not complain!" Frank Gerbode, of San Francisco, had been employing the computer for two years in some 300 cardiac surgical patients. The computer "provided constant accurate display and storage of parameters conventionally used in following seriously ill patients, but more important it has provided a method of observing parallel variables such as following blood pressure parallel to body temperature and a variety of respiratory parameters. This has brought out relationships not seen before. In the field of respiratory mechanics and respiratory physiology, we have learned a great deal by using computer technics with accurate and reliable sensing devices. I would say that this is a worthwhile effort. Certainly it is not economical at all . . . It does not save in personnel among nurses or others; it adds personnel." J. E. Dunphy, of San Francisco, complaining [tongue in cheek] that at the University of California, they had not had the funds to buy expensive computer hardware, had redesigned their wards "so that we now have ward managers and clerks at the desks and the nurses are at the bedside. This has been a remarkable revolution because the chief nurse makes rounds every morning with the chief resident. They are both fully informed as to what is going on . . . The most exciting thing of all is the tremendous increase in morale amongst students, nurses, residents—everyone wants to work on our ward . . . Now, I do not say that within this there is no place for some nice, small, modest hardware at the bedside and if we can get Mr. Reagan to relax a little bit, we will add that to our system, too." [Ronald Reagan, the conservative Republican Governor of California had slashed University budgets.] Kirklin, closing, said that their prime focus had been to counteract the nursing and resident shortage. "Those of you who have adequate numbers of skilled surgeons, those of you who have superb surgical residents who stay with you long enough to know exactly what you want done in these very low probability circumstances that come up only once in a blue moon, those of you who have large numbers of superior and well qualified nurses, need have no interest whatsoever in automated programs for the management of critically ill patients. We went into this purely and simply to reduce some of the mortality inherent in being critically ill in our hospitals today . . . I do not think there is anything magical about touching the patient or seeing him or using clinical judgment, and I have had reasonable experience in attempting these methods . . . as we gradually identify these rules and logic and teach a piece of equipment to use them—a piece of equipment that does not rotate off the service every 3 months—then I think we will have really better patient care. I think this is really particularly true in the low probability events that Dr. Maloney mentioned for it is these events that your resident sees for the first time, while you are away from the hospital and he sometimes does not know what to do." He disagreed with Moore's suggestion that "the arterial pulse contour has other features more significant to us as clinicians than those used for estimating cardiac output" and stressed the great importance of knowing the cardiac output. "The thing I, at least, would like to learn from the arterial pressure pulse contour is stroke volume and that plus heart rate would give us cardiac output and I think that is the central measurement that we need in dealing with the circulatory system in critically ill patients." It was possible to build into the system "something that tells about metabolic demand or oxygen consumption" but for the moment they had not chosen to do that. They did keep the displays at the bedside so the nurses were not separated from the patients, and as for using the massive data, surgeons would have to learn to use the computer just as they had learned to use hemostats and scalpels. He thought he had understood Lewis to say ". . . among other things that the clinical impression was better than the data that came out of the computer.

Again, I disagree! I do not think there is anything magical about clinical impressions. Many superb clinicians do very well treating patients but often they cannot tell us why they do well, or how they do well and if we are going to succeed in training people to reproduce the performance of these experts, if we are going to use all the technology available to us, we have got to go through that thought process and find out how we do it and once we do that, well, I think a machine can do it very well." Maloney, closing, agreed with Kirklin's summary "Anyone who disagrees with him is in the position of the pilots who said in 1929, when flight instruments first became available, 'I'd much rather fly by the seat of my pants!' Time proved those pilots wrong, as flight instruments are now generally accepted. I'm sure that when we look in retrospect at this discussion in print years from now, the analogy will be complete. Physicians will be making much greater use of automated equipment for patient care." The brain, he said, "is a computer having some marvelous attributes. An investigator once estimated on the basis of cerebral blood flow and oxygen saturation in the carotid artery and jugular vein that the brain does all its work on a tenth of a watt of power. An even more remarkable attribute of the human brain is that it's the only computer that can be mass produced by unskilled labor!"

* * *

The heavy concentration on the pancreas in the program continued with *Pancreatico-Duodenectomy* Forty-One Consecutive Whipple Resections without an Operative Mortality, John M. Howard, of Philadelphia, Professor of Surgery, Hahnemann Medical School. This was a personal series of 41 consecutive pancreatico-duodenectomies in 13 years without a death within 30 days of operation or resulting directly from the operation "under any circumstances". In fact, no patient died within six months of operation. He employed a bilateral subcostal incision. He was not insistent upon biopsy, feeling that "*Erroneously resecting a benign lesion is not considered as bad a mistake as that of leaving behind an early, resectable, malignant lesion on the basis of histologic evidence, on biopsy, of inflammation.*" None of the 41 resections was done mistakenly for a benign lesion, "A carcinoma, however, was resected in one patient after 8 biopsies had all been negative for malignancy" and in two others, a single biopsy and then the frozen section of the pancreas failed to find malignancy, which was finally confirmed only on the permanent sections. In two patients, failure to re-

sect, on the basis of pathological report, resulted in a delayed operation for gross tumor, "the early lesions of the head of the pancreas and of the distal common bile duct which offer the best prognosis are the most difficult in which to prove the diagnosis histologically." The common bile duct, portal vein, and hepatic artery were isolated, the pancreas mobilized from the vena cava, and the pancreas separated from the superior mesenteric vein with finger dissection. The distal third of the stomach was resected, the common bile duct divided, cholecystectomy performed, the pancreas transected to the left of the tumor and of the superior mesenteric vein in a V "to permit hemostatic suture of the inferior and craniad borders of the line of resection." The jejunum was divided beyond the ligament of Treitz, the entire duodenum mobilized and the specimen delivered. The jejunum was brought up through the transverse mesocolon and an end-to-end anastomosis accomplished with the transected end of the pancreas. A small rubber catheter "is allowed to sit loosely in the main pancreatic duct, bridging the pancreatico-jejunostomy . . . left in place to be . . . passed spontaneously." The choledochojejunostomy was performed 15 to 20 cm. distal to the pancreatico-jejunostomy and a long arm T-tube placed in the common duct with the long arm extending through the anastomosis and into the jejunum. A gastrojejunostomy was then performed 45 to 60 cm. distal to the biliary anastomosis. He had four subdiaphragmatic abscesses, four pancreatic fistulae, four biliary fistulae, and one gastric hemorrhage among the complications, none of them fatal. The paper did not address itself to the question of survival.

Discussion

George L. Jordan, of Houston, said that "mortality rate is lower in the hands of the senior, accomplished surgeon than in the hands of the occasional operator or of the surgical resident . . ." In the 50 most recent pancreatico-duodenectomies, by the senior staff, there had been five deaths for a mortality of 10%, ". . . not significantly different from that of operation for cancer in the other areas, particularly carcinoma of the lung with pneumonectomy, for example." In 300 patients with carcinoma of the pancreas in the Houston experience, "the only long-term survivals really occur in those patients who do have pancreatico-duodenectomy." Only one patient without a resection had lived as long as three years and a number of patients had lived that long after the Whipple procedure. Charles Eckert, of Albany, said that while Howard's results would be equaled by few, "the mortality rate for this procedure is declining over the country as a whole". At Albany, they had had 22 Whipple resections for carcinoma of the head of the pancreas since 1952 with three deaths none of them after 1957 "and this includes cases operated upon by the resident staff, practically always with the assistance of a senior surgeon." He thought the improvement was due simply to the fact that "we know how to do the operation better." Richard L. Varco, the Vice-President, presiding, said that "the Chair believes also that there is a real point that is raised in terms of the futility of the biopsy—often followed by a disregard of the biopsy diagnosis when it comes back pancreatitis." He asked Howard whether biopsy prejudiced survival. Kenneth W. Warren, of Boston, said Howard had demonstrated what they had "preached for many years, that this is a reasonable operation in certain hands." At the Lahey Clinic, they had done over 300 resections for periampullary carcinoma and he emphasized the distinction between the tumors arising in the ampulla of Vater, the distal common duct, and the duodenum around the papilla, on the one hand, and the carcinomas of the head of the pancreas on the other, taking opportunity for minor disagreement with Howard, because, as he said, "Some of the largest tumors are the most favorable." In 1966 and 1967, they had done 35 pancreatico-duodenectomies with a single death. He did not like to do biopsies and 80% of the patients had no biopsy. At one time they had done 56 consecutive Whipple operations without a death. He had also done 120 Whipple procedures for chronic pancreatitis [14 were actually total pancreatectomies] with three deaths and worthwhile results. As far as "salvage rate" [which he did not define] was concerned it was approximately 12% for carcinoma of the head of the pancreas, 35% for ampullary carcinoma, 36% for carcinoma of the common duct, 36% for carcinoma of the duodenum and 52% for carcinoma of the ampulla of Vater, if the Lahey clinic operation was the first procedure. Vice-President Varco asked another question of Howard, "Does the record of successes that he has achieved without mortality condition him to believe that more operations should be done of a palliative type, and if so, what results has he achieved by extending this procedure in that fashion?" Leon Goldman, of San Francisco, said the initial high mortality and brief survival after the Whipple operation led to a loss of enthusiasm for it, but that results had improved markedly. He had performed Whipple's operation in 12 patients in eight years with 11 survivals, the one death being in a Jehovah's Witness. He mentioned the use of curettage of the common duct or of the

tumor area for immediate cytologic study. Jonathan E. Rhoads, of Philadelphia, congratulated Howard saying, "I had not known that Dr. Cattell and Dr. Warren have run 53 cases [Warren had said 56] without a death. Prior to that, I thought that Mr. Rodney Smith of London had the record with 30 or 31." He mentioned the technique of Millbourn, of Stockholm, inserting the stump of the pancreas in the posterior gastric wall to minimize the risk in the pancreatic anastomosis. They had 15 such Whipple procedures done by seven different surgeons, with only a single death and that in a patient *not* operated by a resident. "Follow-up studies through a flexible gastroscope have shown that the stoma remains open, the mucosa seems to grow right down to the margin of the duct." The pancreas had been shown to respond to secretin after this procedure. Howard, closing, replying to Dr. Varco's question about biopsy, said "it is hard in a teaching institution to disregard an attempt to make a histologic diagnosis when you are training young surgeons. I think Dr. Varco should probably not biopsy, but it is hard to teach compromise." Unlike Warren, he had shifted away from the Whipple procedure for chronic pancreatitis toward "Puestow's operation, the short-term results have been impressive."

* * *

William R. Waddell, of Denver, Professor and Chairman, Department of Surgery, University of Colorado School of Medicine; and by invitation, W. R. Coppinger and R. W. Loughry, *Pancreaticoduodenectomy for Zollinger-Ellison Syndrome,* in four patients with Zollinger-Ellison syndrome, due to tumor in the head of the pancreas or in the duodenum or near the ampulla, had performed a Whipple resection. All of the patients had done well. He felt the operation for Zollinger's syndrome might be chosen to fit the patient, ". . . those patients with non-resectable malignant tumors of the pancreas and those with hepatic and extensive lymph node metastases should have total gastrectomy . . . the patients with localized disease in the duodenum and head of the pancreas, even with peripancreatic lymph node metastases, should have pancreaticoduodenectomy if total extirpation of the gross malignant disease can be achieved . . . In conjunction with extirpation of the tumor, subtotal gastrectomy with vagotomy should be carried out . . . A third group of patients comprised of those with resectable lesions of the tail and body of the pancreas should have partial distal pancreatectomy over the superior mesenteric vessels and total gastrectomy." In 1959, Waddell had sug-

TABLE 5. *Causes of Hospital Mortality*

63 Elective Side-To-Side Shunts
(1961–1967)

Cardiac-hepatic-renal failure	3
Shunt closure with ascites	2
Myocardial infarction	1
Bile peritonitis	1
Severe atelectasis	1
Total	8

TABLE 7. *Causes of Long-term Mortality*

55 Operative Survivors of 63 Elective
Side-To-Side Shunts

Liver failure (hepatoma-1)	12
Exsanguinating ulcer hemorrhage	1
Serum hepatitis	1
Epistaxis with aspiration	1
Brain abscesses with septicemia	1
Bizarre neurologic syndrome	1
Partial followup; considered dead from date of last followup	4
Total	21

The St. Vincent's Hospital experience with 63 side-to-side shunts for cirrhotic ascites was interpreted as providing a better overall survival than end-to-side shunts, at the cost of a slight increase in encephalopathy and in cardiac decompensation.

Albert R. Burchell, Louis M. Rousselot, and William F. Panke, *A Seven-Year Experience with Side-to-side Portacaval Shunt for Cirrhotic Ascites,* Volume LXXXVI, 1968.

gested a "unified concept" based on the known occurrence of associated lesions of the hypothalamus, "the known relationships existing between the hypothalamus and the pituitary gland and overlap of secretory function of the stomach in the Zollinger-Ellison patients . . . evidence . . . that endocrine end organ failure could result in hyperplasia and tumor formation of other glands and tissues under pituitary control." He thought the theory "almost as good now" as it was then, and suggested "A concept of the antrum, duodenum and pancreas as an endocrine organ of common embryologic origin . . ."

Discussion

Stanley R. Friesen, of Kansas City, agreed that Waddell's previous experiments and assay suggested pituitary involvement in the syndrome, and urged that the pituitary of any patient dying with the Z-E syndrome be sent to him or Dr. Waddell for analysis.

* * *

Albert R. Burchell, by invitation, Louis M. Rousselot, Assistant Secretary of Defense (Health and Medical), Washington, D.C., and by invitation, William F. Panke, *A Seven-Year Experience with Side-to-Side Portacaval Shunt for Cirrhotic Ascites,* reported the experience at St. Vincent's Hospital, in New York, from which Rousselot had recently gone to Washington. They had in seven years treated 63 patients with cirrhotic ascites by side-to-side portacaval shunt. Their previous experience with end-to-end shunt demonstrated its efficacy "but also a high incidence of an ever growing list of complications, and a disappointingly low, long-term survival rate." The side-to-side shunt had been subject to many of the same criticisms despite a much smaller experience with it. Their overall operating mortality was 12%—eight cases—in the 63 shunts, as low as 8% in some years. Their long-term survival rate was about 60% from the third to the seventh year, "more than twice as good as the survival rate for the end-to-side group which included a preponderance of good risk patients", among 210 elective end-to-side shunts with variceal hemorrhage. Post-shunt encephalopathy occurred in 17 patients and was severe only in nine. The causes of hospital mortality and of later mortality are as given in their Tables 5 and 7. The mortality was much like that they had experienced with end-to-side shunt. They were most impressed with the better survival of the patients with side-to-side shunt, despite the slightly increased frequency of encephalopathy and cardiac decompensation. Their plea was for "a pause in currect trends against shunts and a reassessment and further study of the value of the side-to-side portacaval shunt."

Discussion

Marshall J. Orloff, of San Diego, from an experience with use of the side-to-side shunt for intractable ascites in nine patients, supported the conclusions of Burchell and Rousselot. His metabolic studies showed dramatic reversal of abnormal patterns of sodium and aldosterone excretions, and improvement in nutrition. However, he thought the group of patients with intractable ascites was a small one. Jere W. Lord, Jr., of New York, said that at first, "following the lead of Dr. Gliedman and Dr. Dennis, we have employed the mesocaval shunt, end of the inferior vena cava to the side of the superior mesenteric vein as the procedure of choice for massive hemorrhage from varices due to cirrhosis of the liver." Ten months earlier, they had changed "to the use of a woven teflon prosthesis to join the side of the inferior vena cava to the side of the superior mesenteric vein . . . We used a woven teflon 18 to 20 mm. in diameter because of its tendency to maintain a circular shape." [For Drapanas' vigorous espousal of this technique with three-and-a-half year follow-up, see page 1363, Volume XC, 1972]. In a patient with bleeding and massive ascites, such a shunt was successful. William V. McDermott, Jr., of Boston, said that "when Nikolai Eck constructed the experimental vascular fistula which bears his name it was proposed for the treatment of ascites." The initial experience of Whipple, Linton, Rousselot and others had been that ascites was a contraindication to a shunt. With the development ten years before of the "concept of an out-flow-block as one of the predominant features in the development of cirrhotic ascites" shunt surgery was reintroduced specifically for ascites. He agreed with Burchell and Rousselot, with Orloff, and Lord that a side-to-side shunt was effective for "truly intractable ascites", however, occasionally end-to-side shunt would dissipate ascites. Louis M. Rousselot, closing, said that "whereas some fifteen years ago, I was personally guilty of stating that ascites was a total contraindication to shunt surgery, we have moved along a somewhat tortuous road and are able to begin to present some criteria that offer some hope for what was formerly a totally fatal and malignant disease."

Rousselot was dubious of Lord's use of a prosthetic H graft "in view of the experience of a number of surgeons with the 'H' graft using autogenous vein in portacaval shunts, in which there was an extremely high closure rate . . ."

* * *

The Business Meetings

The 1968 meeting took place at the Sheraton-Boston Hotel, Boston, Massachusetts, April 17, 18 and 19, President William P. Longmire, Jr. in the Chair.

The Secretary recorded that this was the last year since the *1964* change in the Constitution in which the total membership would be increased by ten, bringing it to a total of 300 Active Members. There were at the time of the meeting, 271 Active Members and thus potential places for 29 new Fellows.

There had been 120 papers submitted, and 33 selected.

William R. Waddell, Chairman of the Advisory Membership Committee, in his report very nicely encapsulated what he understood to be the requirements for entrance into fellowship,- "The American Surgical Association has been heavily oriented toward academic and scholarly attributes in selection of its members since the beginning. This is no less true now than at any time previously. Therefore, to rank high in the evaluation of the Advisory Membership Committee, the candidate must have not only shown promise and good intentions in his younger years, but to have actually contributed in a signficant way to the science and art of surgery. The majority of the committee's activity is a peer evaluation of this aspect of the candidate's qualifications. Bibliography and the so-called 'Zollinger Index' (the number of candidate's publications divided by his age) are taken into consideration, but content rather than actual numbers is obviously the only factor of importance. A career in teaching is considered an attribute and sometimes this is the most important contribution. The candidate must be an operating surgeon. Only in most exceptional instances have men been nominated to the Council whose entire reputations and careers have been based on their laboratory work. High public office, distinguished contributions to community, public and scientific life, prominence in politics and even tenure in a chair of surgery at an important university would not in themselves be sufficient to insure a candidate's nomination. As far as the writer can recognize, there has not been and there is not now any distinction between those in private practice and those in pure academic surgery . . . In summary, there are no ground-rules except as specified in the by-laws of the Association, but there are certain factors as outlined above that weigh heavily in the minds of the committeemen."

At the Second Executive Session among those accepted to membership were Paul C. Adkins, of Washington; Frank W. Blaisdell, of San Francisco; Ward O. Griffen, of Lexington; Harry H. Leveen, of Brooklyn; John S. Najarian, Minneapolis; and as Honorary Fellows, Fritz Linder, of Heidelberg, Germany; and Rudolf Zenker, of Munich, Germany.

Officers elected were: Owen Wangensteen, of Minneapolis, who had been Vice-President in 1952, President; Leon Goldman, of San Francisco, and Bentley Colcock, of Boston, Vice-Presidents; C. Rollins Hanlon, of St. Louis, Secretary.

LXXXVII

1969

The 1969 meeting, April 30, May 1 and 2, was held at the Netherland-Hilton Hotel in Cincinnati, President Owen H. Wangensteen, of Minneapolis, Regents' Professor and Chairman, Department of Surgery, University of Minnesota Medical Center; Surgeon-in-Chief, University of Minnesota Hospitals, in the Chair. Among those who had died in the year since the last meeting were Claude F. Dixon and Willis J. Potts, Jr.

President Wangensteen, *"We Cannot Escape History"*, neatly outlined and subdivided his address for easy reference. The familiar tenets of his philosophy emerge, ". . . the American Surgical should be a working organization and not an honor guard for surgery . . . Honor is not a hollow sound when accompanied by a full acceptance of the responsibilities which accompany honors. Whenever a small company of our Fellows come together, faint strains of that familiar refrain, 'Yes, we are the finest and fairest in the Land,' can almost invariably be heard. We need to hear less of honor and more of implied responsibilities." He was critical of the increasing rigidity and length of surgical training programs inspired by the requirements of the Boards so that ". . . a large proportion of future surgical academicians . . . are kept away from the experimental laboratories during their most impressionable and creative years." His opinion of Halsted and his trainees emerges, "The end effect is a virtual return to the training scheme of Halsted (1904), from which emerged the most talented and versatile group of clinical surgeons that this, or probably any, country

has produced. Surgery and the universities need surgeons with such unique talents, but especially for our discipline's continuing advance surgery needs future Teachers, anxious to create an atmosphere that will encourage research and creative scholarship, so vital in enabling those privileged to work in such an environment to grow to their full potential." Wangensteen's concentration was on the young men who stayed on with him after they had completed what he called "our somewhat unconventional surgical training program" rather than to the residents themselves and he was aware of that, but insisted that "Preservation of flexibility and latitude in our surgical training program, I feel, is not only desirable but essential." [His department for a generation was a continuing source of exciting contributions, particularly to gastrointestinal and cardiac surgery and transplantation contributed by these men.] Like a number of his predecessors he urged the wisdom of enlarging the membership roster. When W. T. Bull returned to New York in 1875, after training abroad, he was "the first American surgeon to delimit his professional activities solely to surgery . . . Today, 50% of Initiates admitted annually to membership in the American College of Surgeons are surgical specialists . . . If the American Surgical Association is to play the role of Sentinel in the overall picture of surgery, and do it effectively . . . it must identify itself more closely with the surgical specialists." Like a number of previous Presidents, Wangensteen proposed ". . . trials at our meetings of divided sessions determined by the Program Com-

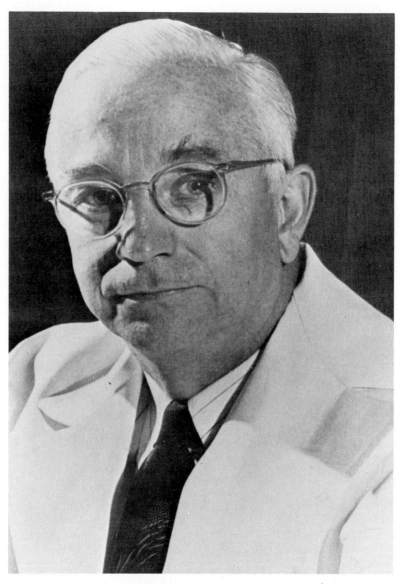

Owen H. Wangensteen (c. 1945), 1898 Vice-President 1952, President 1969. M.D. University of Minnesota 1922, training there and at Mayo Clinic, and after his European wanderjahr (de Quervain, at Berne), entire career at Minnesota, Professor and Chairman 1930-1967, where he built one of the major departments of surgery in the country. Massive contributions of his own, in intestinal obstruction (his book received the Samuel D. Gross Prize), its physiology, and treatment (continuous nasogastric suction); gastrointestinal physiology, particularly the physiology and treatment of duodenal ulcer, introducing a variety of experimental procedures and clinical operations and treatments successively put to the test; tumor surgery, (the "second look" concept); history of medicine. A voracious reader with awesome recall, and impatient curiosity, he put innumerable ideas to laboratory investigation and conducted his own large surgical practice and that of his clinic as a series of clinical investigations, stimulating other clinics and laboratories to verify or disprove his postulates. He chose aggressive, competitive young men, imbued them with his own agnosticism and daring in the laboratory and in the operating room, and provided the climate in which they in turn were at the front of surgical developments, particularly in cardiac surgery, and sent them forth to chairs of their own.

mittee . . .", indicating this would be along lines of special interest, but commented that "Many past the meridian of 50, well over the halfway mark of a long and active professional life, already begin to find it difficult to interpret or to evaluate the experimental data of their younger colleagues in a field not closely allied to their own interest . . . it is a foregone conclusion that such presentations have a Tower-of-Babel-like flavor." Like Evarts Graham before him, he urged election of men at a younger age "Our constitution permits election to membership at age 30, but the precept, as far as I know, has never been put to the test." The report of Council later in the meeting did not mention it, but the President in the Address which opened the meeting said, "Your Council has approved appointment of a Committee under Jonathan Rhoads to study the future directional course of our Association, a report which all will await with keen anticipation." [This led to the appointment of the important Committee on Issues which has played such a prime role in the Association ever since.] Wangensteen now voiced his pet project for an American Congress of Surgery referring back to the proposal of Claudius Mastin in 1886 which culminated in the Medical and Surgical Congress and Wangensteen urged that "Our Association, the most distinguished of American surgical societies, should take the lead in amalgamating and bridging interests and aspirations of the many existing surgical organizations into a coherent and cohesive whole that will benefit all."

* * *

M. M. Eisenberg, by invitation, E. R. Woodward, of Gainesville, Professor and Head, Department of Surgery, University of Florida, T. J. Carson, by invitation, and Lester R. Dragstedt, Research Professor of Surgery and Professor of Physiology, University of Florida [on retirement from the University of Chicago, Dragstedt had joined Woodward, his former Resident, in his Department at Gainesville], *Vagotomy and Drainage Procedure for Duodenal Ulcer:* The Results of Ten Years' Experience, presented the results of vagotomy and drainage in 455 patients. Some 95% of the patients had been operated upon by resident surgeons. The inclusion of patients from the Veterans Administration and state prison hospitals accounted for the 10:1 male/female ratio. Eighty-eight percent of the operations were elective. Only 46 patients were operated upon for acute hemorrhage and eight patients for perforation. There were only four deaths after elective operations, one in a patient who had a walled-off perforation and abscess at the time of operation, one in a

patient who had pyloric obstruction, one from an unrecognized injury to the esophagus, and one from a leaking pyloroplasty suture line. There was one death after emergency operation for massive hemorrhage in an 83-year-old woman, who died of cardiac arrhythmia without further bleeding. There were 13 proved and three suspected recurrent ulcers, an overall rate of 6.3%. Eleven of these 16 patients had had postoperative gastric secretory analyses, and in nine of them the basal gastric free acid secretory rate was in excess of 2 mEq./hr. and in five of seven patients so examined, the Hollander insulin test showed incomplete vagotomy. Sixty-five patients, 14%, had symptoms suggestive of dumping, but only one patient required operation. In 79% of the patients, weight after operation remained unchanged or increased. Basal or augmented histamine gastric acid analysis was more reliable they thought than the Hollander insulin test in determining the completeness of vagotomy. The maximal recurrence rate of 3.6%, the overall mortality of 1% for elective cases, and 1.85% for the emergency operations, the occurrence of only a single death in the 46 patients operated on for massive hemorrhage, a low postoperative morbidity, and the good postoperative weight status of the patients ". . . demonstrate that vagotomy and drainage is an effective, safe, and extremely well-tolerated operation, useful in the management of patients with duodenal ulcer."

Discussion

Ward O. Griffen, of Lexington, Kentucky, said that it had been "most disturbing to us that our results, particularly regarding recurrences, have not been anywhere near as good as the results reported today . . . the most recent recurrence rate in the 112 patients who originally underwent pyloroplasty and vagotomy at the University of Kentucky Medical Center is 28 per cent . . . with a 100 per cent follow-up for the four years." They had a 21% incidence of incomplete vagotomy ". . . no greater than that usually reported." [The Woodward-Dragstedt paper, in fact, did not give their incidence of incomplete vagotomy.] Griffen thought that it was due to the fact that, whereas in his own series only 11% of the patients were operated upon for intractability, that was the indication in 72% of the Florida patients, and wondered if ". . . since we have an admittedly-safe procedure in vagotomy and pyloroplasty . . . by operating on a high percentage of patients for intractable pain we may be operating on individuals who would not have been considered for surgery in the heyday of resection." Francis Moore, of Boston, said that ". . . with regard to pyloro-plasty and vagotomy . . . we are employing an operation that is less crippling, with a much lower mortality and morbidity than gastrectomy, but we still are plagued by the same old recurrence rate." He wondered whether postoperative testing could indicate the patients liable to recurrence, who could then be more carefully followed and dieted, "We feel very strongly that it is essential to measure the insulin secretory test after vagotomy", and he asked if ". . . Dr. Eisenberg in his discussion would tell us what his incidence of complete vagotomy by insulin test was . . ." E. R. Woodward, closing [Eisenberg had presented the paper], emphasized ". . . the extreme efficacy of vagotomy and pyloroplasty in the control of massive hemorrhage. Thirty-eight of our patients operated on as an emergency procedure for bleeding met all the criteria for massive hemorrhage laid down so well by Dr. John Stewart some years ago. There was only one postoperative death in these 38 critically ill patients." Most of their recurrences had occurred relatively early in the follow-up period, only a single one after more than three years. In reply to Dr. Moore, he said that they had found ". . . the comparison of the pre- and postoperative basal gastric secretory rate is considerably more effective than the insulin test in measuring the completeness of vagotomy. The patient who does not get a profound suppression of his basal gastric secretory rate is recurrence prone and the great majority of recurrences have occurred in this group." [He did not provide Dr. Moore with the figures for the incidence of incomplete vagotomy.] Dr. Dragstedt said that the data and the discussion this morning were "all in harmony with the view that duodenal ulcers are caused by a hypersecretion of gastric juice of vagus origin. I believe that the cause of the hypersecretion is an excessive tonus, secretory tonus in the vagus nerves . . . I am persuaded that gastric ulcers are caused by a hypersecretion of gastric juice of humoral origin, of hormonal origin . . . It is significant that one of the causes of failure after vagotomy for duodenal ulcer is stasis of food in the stomach which causes an excessive secretion of gastric juice of humoral origin."

* * *

Edward E. Mason and Chikashi Ito, from the Department of Surgery, University of Iowa, by invitation, *Gastric Bypass,* spoke of the mortality and morbidity of massive obesity, the appropriateness of operative treatment when other methods had failed, and the undesirable effects of intestinal sidetracking. They proposed a 90% gastric bypass operation, anas-

tomosing the jejunum to a small proximal pouch of divided stomach, reasoning that ". . . there is sufficient acid secreting mucosa excluded with the antrum so that after the stomach is stimulated to secrete acid, the antrum and first part of the duodenum should be bathed in acid gastric juice unbuffered by food. This should in turn inhibit release of gastrin and thereby tend to regulate gastric secretion at a relatively low level." In dogs a 70% gastric bypass "provided almost as much inhibition of secretion as 70% gastric resection." In the previous three years, he had performed 90% gastric bypass in 24 massively obese patients, two of them with proved duodenal ulcers, and a 70% bypass in eight normal weight patients with duodenal ulcer. Two of the obese patients died of the operation, one from peritonitis and pulmonary congestion although no leak was found at autopsy, the second from pulmonary embolus. A number of the patients had nausea and vomiting. The weight losses, large but inconsistent, seemed to be accounted for by decreased food intake. Half of the patients had a dumping syndrome. Two patients had maintained weights of 300 pounds "by physical inactivity and continuous slow eating." Only one of the duodenal ulcer patients and none of the obese patients had developed a jejunal ulcer. Mason was not recommending the operation for acid peptic disease, but the operation was recommended for the reduction of massive obesity provided the patients were ". . . physically active, young, or middle-aged people weighing in the range of 200% of estimated normal body weight."

Discussion

Lloyd M. Nyhus, of Chicago, said that "Antral exclusion for the treatment of duodenal ulcer has been of interest since von Eiselsberg's paper in 1895 . . . Dr. Woodward in 1956, and subsequently we, demonstrated, that an acid cuff left on the antrum will, indeed, prevent hypersecretion from a Heidenhain pouch. However, in the clinical setting, Kay of Glasgow performed the antral exclusion procedure with an acid cuff upon patients and an unacceptable number of stomal ulcers developed." Nyhus commented upon the similarly unsatisfactory experience of Devine, of Australia, and Ogilvie, of England, ". . . it would appear that the antral exclusion procedure for the treatment of ulcer disease should never be suggested again . . . As far as the matter of the antral exclusion procedure for obesity, in addition to possible development of a stomal ulcer, there are other undesirable side effects which will result from the high, gastric transection—dumping syn-

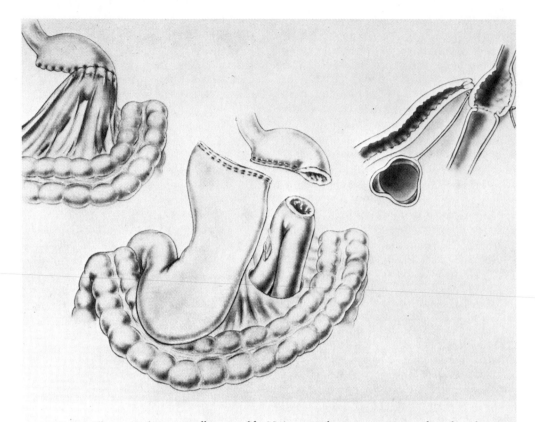

FIG. 1. Illustrates the potentially reversible 90% gastric bypass operation with a short loop, retrocolic gastroenterostomy. The ligament of Treitz is divided. The mesocolon is secured to the 10% stomach pouch and the closed distal 90% of excluded stomach is attached to the anterior wall of the fundic segment. These steps are important in preventing proximal loop stasis.

Mason's operation for massive obesity involved stapling and dividing the stomach, leaving an approximately 10% remnant which was anastomosed to the proximal jejunum by manual sutures. The distal stomach was anchored to the proximal pouch. Of 24 patients, two died of the operation, two "outate" the operation and others lost weight, for the most part, satisfactorily.

Edward E. Mason and Chikashi Ito, *Gastric Bypass,* Volume LXXXVII, 1969.

drome, et cetera. The two long suture closures will give increased morbidity and mortality rates. The procedure suggested today, devised for the treatment of a psychological metabolic problem probably should be extended cautiously to the human patient, if at all." Edgar J. Poth, of Galveston, supported Mason's physiologic reasoning and suggested that reflux of acid from the proximal gastric remnant into the duodenojejunal junction and into the distal duodenum would inhibit gastric secretion. Mason, closing, said that Kay, referred to by Nyhus, had done only a 50% exclusion and that Haberer in 1920 "called attention to the fact that stomal ulcers do not occur after antral exclusion procedures, except in patients who have previously had duodenal ulcers." Mason agreed with Poth that acidification of the duodenum and of the antrum was important. He

had studied, with the beeswax and histamine technique, dogs with varying degrees of exclusion, and found that ". . . with a small exclusion the dogs do develop stomal ulcers . . ." but with large exclusions they did not. He made it clear to President Wangensteen, who interposed the question, that he did not employ vagotomy with this operation.

* * *

Injury to healthy tissues in the course of irradiation of cancer had been recognized almost as soon as roentgen therapy had been undertaken [Volume XV, 1897, J. W. White, and XXV, 1907, Porter]. J. J. DeCosse, R. S. Rhodes, W. B. Wentz, J. W. Reagan, H. J. Dworken, all by invitation and W. D.

Holden, of Cleveland, Oliver H. Payne Professor of Surgery; Director, Department of Surgery, Western Reserve University School of Medicine, *The Natural History and Management of Radiation Induced Injury of the Gastrointestinal Tract,* reviewed 100 patients who had sustained significant injury to the gastrointestinal tract from irradiation between 1922 and 1968. The number of irradiated patients from whom these complications were derived was not known, but it was stated that "During the past 15 years at this institution, the frequency of gastrointestinal complications following radiation therapy for cervical cancer was 11.6 per cent, results comparable to that observed in the contemporary literature." In 75 of the patients, irradiation was for carcinoma of the cervix, in nine for carcinoma of the endometrium, in five for carcinoma of the vagina. Ninety-six of the patients were known to have died,- of these 28 died of cancer, 22 of radiation complications to the gastrointestinal tract, and three of other radiation complications. Calculating the possible influence of a variety of factors, it was found in a series of 34 consecutive injured patients treated for carcinoma of the cervix, that hypertension, arteriosclerosis or diabetes, and supracervical hysterectomy, were correlated with subsequent irradiation injury. "Radiation of the gastrointestinal tract produces an immediate and potentially reversible effect on the sensitive generative epithelium of the intestinal mucosa and a more prolonged and progressive obliterative vasculitis. Vascular damage includes endothelial proliferation, endarteritis, hyaline rings and subendothelial foam cell formation. It was the vascular occlusion induced by radiation that was critical in the pathogenesis of ulcers, strictures and necrosis, which developed months or years after primary therapy", histological effects which had long been known. Because of the malign correlation with hypertension, diabetes, and cardiovascular disease, DeCosse postulated "An inter-relationship between low splanchnic blood flow and radiation vasculitis . . . Those patients who sustained perforations of the intestine after intestinal resection for radiation injury all had varying degrees of cardiovascular disease." In 17 patients with hypertension and irradiation injury of the gastrointestinal tract ". . . radiation therapy appears by all standards to be within a tolerable range." Other patients had indeed received excessive internal or external radiotherapy. The increased risk of injury to the bowel after hysterectomy was attributed to fixation of the bowel to pelvic scar. Radiation induced rectal ulcers were usually noted 4 to 12 months after initiation of radiotherapy . . . on the anterior rectal wall at the level of the cervix . . .

Rectal stenoses were located higher than ulcers, usually 8 to 12 cm. from the anal verge." Proctitis, ulcers and stenosis tended to appear early and might all regress. Rectovaginal fistulas did not heal spontaneously. Proctitis persisting more than a month after completion of radiotherapy merited evaluation which included simultaneous assessment of the urinary tract. Rectovaginal fistulae did not yield to direct repair, and colostomy or exenteration were frequently necessary. The most complicated clinical problem was that of irradiation injury of the small bowel and the colon. Chronic abdominal pain was frequently the only symptom, often crampy, with or without diarrhea or obstructive symptoms. In the operative treatment of severe symptoms from radiation enteritis, ". . . a wide resection is preferable to a wide bypass; both are superior to limited procedures. A meaningless dissection of adhesions should be avoided and no attempt made to free intestine unless its removal is intended", for fear of a late perforation. Twenty-nine of their patients had rectovaginal fistulae in the absence of recurrence of the cancer, with onset three months to 12 years after irradiation. Twenty-seven of the 100 patients required a colostomy, and in 21 of these it was for a rectovaginal fistula. Of 17 patients with irradiation injury primarily to the small bowel, 14 presented with symptoms of ileitis or intestinal obstruction, eight with intestinal ischemia or necrosis, and three with enteric fistulae. "Sixteen patients had an intestinal resection; one had a lysis of adhesions which was followed by perforation and death . . . two had a bypass procedure . . . success in one and failure in the other . . . Adhesions . . . were not the cause of the obstruction . . . the cause of obstruction was a fibrotic, grey, stenotic segment of small bowel associated with diffuse thickening of the intestinal wall." Two patients of the 16 died and only six of the 16 were relieved of their symptoms. All of those six were dead, three of other radiation complications, two of recurrent cancer, one of myocardial infarction. The remaining eight were disasters, "seven developed a perforation of the intestine postoperatively, and one had an obstructed ileal anastomosis requiring an ileotransverse colostomy." The perforations in the seven patients occurring three weeks to six months after intestinal resection ". . . could not be attributed to a technical failure of surgery . . . the evidence supported continuing progression of vascular occlusion . . . three had evidence of heart failure or severe peripheral vascular disease at the time of perforation . . ." and four had documented hypertension. A single patient 31 years after irradiation developed an adenocarcinoma of the rectum.

Discussion

Bentley P. Colcock, of Boston, pointed out the seriousness of the problem,- ". . . almost as many patients died as a result of the radiation treatment as died from recurrent cancer. In the 41 patients of ours that I reported about 10 years ago, five patients died as a direct result of the radiation treatment, and in two of those patients there was no evidence of residual cancer." Correct clinical recognition was made difficult ". . . because the clinical effects of the radiation injury are delayed for many months and even years . . . in Dr. DeCosse's paper, the interval between radiation and surgery was 6-1/2 years for patients with small bowel injury, and 5-1/2 years for patients with colon injury . . . The key to a successful result is adequate surgery which includes resection of bowel, well beyond the obvious disease." J. Englebert Dunphy, of San Francisco, commented on ". . . the unexplained perforation which occurs after lysis of adhesions or sometimes after resection. The perforation often occurs in an area in which the surgeon realizes he could not possibly have inadvertently damaged the bowel during the operation." His laboratory had demonstrated that ". . . after a bowel resection, the normal, otherwise uninjured colon and small bowel undergoes a remarkable loss of collagen. There is a marked activation of collagenase in the small bowel . . . in the colon, and this can lead to loss of substance and then perforation of the normal, intact bowel. In radiation damaged bowel resynthesis of collagen is depressed. Therefore, the effects of lysis are increased . . . additional reasons why we should carry out not merely lysis of adhesions around the involved area, but resection and extensive resection if we are going to operate at all."

* * *

Wylie F. Barker, of Los Angeles, Professor of Surgery, University of California, Los Angeles School of Medicine; by invitation, L. Sperling, A. H. Dowdy, L. J. Zeldis; and W. P. Longmire, Jr., Professor and Chairman, Department of Surgery, University of California, Los Angeles School of Medicine, *Management of Nonpalpable Breast Carcinoma Discovered by Mammography,* discussed the management of the patient with a radiographic indication for operation. They were speaking from the perspective that cancer of the breast ". . . accounted for 2,626 of 19,232 new cases of cancer in Los Angeles County in 1967, a rate of 37.3 per 100,000. The death rate from breast cancer has not changed significantly since 1930 in spite of advances in selected

cases . . . the death rate from cancer of the uterus has declined sharply, probably largely because of early diagnosis. Although exception to his thesis has been reported [I. G. MacDonald 1951], diagnosis at an earlier period should reduce the ultimate death rate. Smaller cancers predispose fewer patients to lymph node metastases; the fewer the patients with nodal metastases, the better the survival rate." They ascribed the origin of clinical mammography to S. L. Warren, 1930, and its popularization and improvement to Egan, 1960. The U.C.L.A. technique was "Biopsy of the roentgenologically suspicious area, in the absence of a palpable mass . . . after consultation between surgeon and roentgenologist. A generous specimen was radiographed immediately to be sure the biopsy included the suspicious area after which the biopsy wound was closed. No attempt was made to confirm the diagnosis by frozen section or to proceed with definitive therapy on this date. (Because of a previous contralateral mastectomy, advanced age, or widely spaced suspicious lesions, several patients were subjected to an initial simple mastectomy, in which the entire breast became the biopsy specimen.) The biopsy specimen was cut into many thin slices, maintaining careful orientation, and again the 'bread-loafed' specimen was x-rayed . . . the pathologist is greatly dependent on the radiologist's study of the films of the bread-loafed specimen to select areas for histologic study . . . lacking guidance by the radiologist, an area harboring a small intraductal or lobular carcinoma may be no more distinctive grossly than areas of fibrosis or sclerosing adenosis in benign mammary dysplasia." A radiographic diagnosis of "benign" was correct 91% of the time, a suspicion of carcinoma was confirmed 22% of the time, a positive diagnosis of carcinoma was verified by section 95% of the time. Seventy-seven operations were performed in 1,543 patients examined. It was of interest that in 1,211 women in a cancer screening program, 1.1% were found to have carcinoma, but that of 332 women referred because of ". . . a mass, a previous history of cancer of one breast, or a strong family history of cancer of the breast", 4.8% were found to have carcinoma. Of the 29 carcinomas found ". . . 21 . . . were probably capable of being diagnosed without mammography, eight were nonpalpable . . . [and eight were Stage 1 lesions] The almost standard procedure was radical mastectomy unless age or advanced disease precluded it . . . On the basis of this initial experience we hope to design a prospective study to evaluate simple mastectomy in comparison with modified axillary dissection in patients with nonpalpable, stage 1 carcinomas of the breast."

Discussion

Walter J. Burdette, of Houston, emphasized the usefulness of thermography [which Barker had said had some virtue for screening, but was less accurate than mammography]. He preferred a circumareolar incision of the skin and a subcutaneous radical excision of the breast, being guided by a needle which the radiologist had inserted into the roentgenologically suspicious area. George Crile, Jr., of Cleveland, devoted his remarks to the question of lymphadenectomy and the possible immunizing effect of irradiation of the primary tumor. Bernard Fisher, of Pittsburgh, dismissed Crile's remarks "I personally feel it would be a great shame if the value of this paper became diverted by a polemic relative to the merits of the operative procedures employed; for who of us can be so sure of the correct procedure? " The situation with respect to the stage of diagnosis of breast cancer was illustrated by the fact that of ". . . 2,578 breast cancer patients entered into the National Breast Cancer Study during the past decade . . . almost two thirds of the tumors were greater than 3 centimeters, that only five per cent were smaller than 1 centimeter . . ." He was waiting to see whether mammography, Xeroradiography, and the like, resulted in smaller tumors being found. The National Study suggested ". . . that little progress has been made since about 1950 relative to the removal of smaller breast tumors." The U.C.L.A. paper suggested to Fisher that progress was now being made but "Will such accomplishment improve results? If . . . a six centimeter tumor had been removed when it was one centimeter or less, would the fate of the patient have been similar to that following the removal of a small tumor of similar size. While the popular hypothesis that removal of smaller tumors will cure more patients seems reasonable, only time will prove its validity . . . in this national breast cancer study series of patients, 22 per cent of those with tumors less than one centimeter had axillary node involvement . . . I think it fair to conclude that size alone is not as significant to the fate of the patient as are other factors relative to the tumor and/or host which determine the development of metastasis . . . if one has a group of patients with tumors 1 to 1.9 centimeters in size, the fate of the patient is not related to the size of the tumor, but . . . to whether or not there are nodes involved and how many nodes are involved . . . with large tumors the fate of the patient is . . . related, not so much to the size of the tumor, but to the nodal involvement." Joel W. Baker, of Seattle, had initially been skeptical of mammography but was now convinced of its value ". . . particularly in the large breast with borderline physical findings. In those with a family history of cancer, in those with cancer phobia, and in following the contralateral breast after mastectomy for cancer, and in search for the primary in unexplained metastatic disease, it has a definite value." William P. Longmire, Jr., closing, reassured Dr. Crile,- who had doubted it,- that "all of these carcinomas were invasive carcinomas." He agreed with Dr. Fisher that it remained to be seen "Whether the small size of these lesions and their early detection will make any significant difference in the ultimate results of treatment . . ." He reemphasized that they did not rely on frozen section examination but waited for the permanent section except in the occasional cases in which a simple mastectomy seemed to them indicated.

* * *

E. J. Wylie, of San Francisco, Professor of Surgery, Vice Chairman, Department of Surgery; Chief, Vascular Surgery Service, University of California, and by invitation, D. L. Perloff, and R. J. Stoney, *Autogenous Tissue Revascularization Technics in Surgery for Renovascular Hypertension,* depended upon renal arteriography for the operative decision, "A hypertensive patient was considered to be a candidate for renal revascularization if operable obstructive lesions judged to be sufficiently advanced to impair blood flow in one or more renal arteries were identified by arteriography and if the potential benefit from a successful operation was believed to outweigh the surgical risk." They made the diagnosis of *fibromuscular hyperplasia* in 136 hypertensive patients, 25 of them with minimal disease controllable without operation. Thirty-one had bilateral disease involving peripheral branches and were considered inoperable. Eighty patients were operated on, 14 with unilateral disease undergoing nephrectomy when their lesions proved uncorrectable. A secondary nephrectomy was performed in five patients after stricture of the reconstruction, or after a successful correction of the condition in the opposite kidney. Fourteen of the 19 nephrectomized patients were cured of hypertension, and four were improved. As in their 1962 report before the Association, for *fibromuscular disease,* "Resection of the diseased arterial segment and simple reanastomosis . . ." was the technique of arterial reconstruction, performed in 23 patients,- bilaterally in five of them,- hypertension cured in 19 and improved in five, and one death from rupture of an intracranial aneurysm ten days after operation, when the patient had been normotensive. Subsequent recurrence of hypertension in three patients was proved to be due to ". . . stenosis

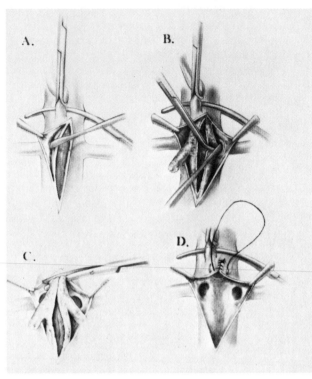

FIG. 6. Artist's drawing of the procedure for transaortic endarterectomy of the renal arteries in which the renal lesions are removed with a sleeve of aortic intima. This method is applicable when there is diffuse involvement of the aortic intima.

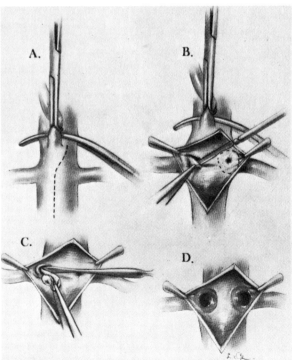

FIG. 8. Artist's drawings of the procedure for transaortic renal endarterectomy in which only a disc of aortic intima surrounding the renal artery orifice is removed. A tapered renal artery orifice is assured by cutting a disc with a diameter twice the external diameter of the renal artery.

For renal hypertension on the basis of an arteriosclerotic obstruction, even for unilateral disease, Wylie had come to favor the transaortic procedure shown. This required "Complete mobilization of the mid-abdominal aorta to the level between the celiac and superior mesenteric artery orifice . . . facilitated by division of the ligamentous surfaces of the crura of the diaphragm on each side of the aorta proximal to the origins of the renal artery. An 8-9 cm. longitudinal anterior aortotomy extending superiorly to a point adjacent to and to the left of the superior mesenteric artery provides excellent exposure of the renal orifices . . . extended inferiorly if exposure of more distal accessory renal arteries is required." In the last five years they had employed the transaortic approach in 37 patients, and transrenal in five selected patients with sharply localized disease and a normal aorta.

E. J. Wylie, D. L. Perloff, and R. J. Stoney, *Autogenous Tissue Revascularization Technics in Surgery for Renovascular Hypertension*, Volume LXXXVII, 1969.

of the main renal artery." The hypertension had been relieved in two by nephrectomy and in one by an autograft bypass. Splenorenal autograft was immediately successful in two patients, one of whom developed a suture line stenosis with hypertension, and was cured by nephrectomy. On-lay vein patch was employed in patients whose disease extended out beyond the main renal artery, with five cures, one improvement, and one death from a ruptured intracranial aneurysm. Their single saphenous vein bypass from the aorta stenosed and required nephrectomy. In 27 of the last 35 reconstructions, they had employed "Arterial autograft replacement for main renal artery lesions . . .", employing the hypogastric artery in 25 operations and the external iliac, which they replaced by a Dacron graft, in two. With an average follow-up of two-and-a-half years in the 25 patients, all beyond six months, hypertension was considered cured in 16, improved in eight, and with no late recurrences. One patient had a postoperative graft thrombosis and persistent hypertension. In their hands ". . . autograft bypass is less susceptible to technical failure than the other methods. The nature of the postoperative arterial stenotic lesions in the patients who developed this complication after partial renal artery resection and reanastomosis or a spleno-renal bypass operation suggests that abnormal tension on the foreshortened traumatized artery contributes to stenosis." Although Foster [of Nashville] had achieved good results with a saphenous vein bypass, Wylie thought the arterial autograft was more easily employed. In 110 patients with *arteriosclerotic* lesions, operated for hypertension, they had performed nephrectomy in 19, which cured the hypertension in eight and improved it in seven, spleno-renal anastomosis in four with a cure in two, Dacron bypass grafts in two with improvement in one, and death in the other, with a single kidney, whose graft thrombosed five months after operation. Arterial autografts in three patients resulted in death from hemorrhage in one, improvement in one, and no change in another, ". . . the most generally applicable surgical technic . . . has become . . . renal endarterectomy through a transaortic approach . . . Renal endarterectomy was performed in 83 patients. The obstructing lesions were unilateral in 47 patients and bilateral in 36. The approach was through a renal arteriotomy in 22 operations and a longitudinal aortotomy in 61." They had progressively favored transaortic endarterectomy, employing the direct approach through the renal artery ". . . for the removal of short proximal lesions in normal sized renal arteries when the aorta is free of intimal thickening or aneurysmal degeneration." They employed

the transaortic approach even for unilateral renal artery lesions. This required "Complete mobilization of the mid-abdominal aorta to the level between the celiac and superior mesenteric artery orifice . . . facilitated by division of the ligamentous surfaces of the crura of the diaphragm on each side of the aorta proximal to the origins of the renal artery." In the last five years, 74% of their atherosclerotic hypertensive patients were cured or improved and 26% of their patients were dead or unimproved, a significant improvement over the results of the previous seven years, 56% cured or improved and 44% dead or unimproved.

* * *

The limits of vascular reconstruction were being tested. DeBakey's group, the year before, had reported distal tibial bypass with autogenous vein grafts in 56 cases. R. Robert Tyson, and Frederick A. Reichle, both by invitation, from the Department of Surgery, Temple University Health Science Center, Philadelphia, *Femoro Tibial Bypass,* also had "more than 50 cases" in their five-and-a-half year experience. The Baylor two-year follow-up had shown a 70% rate of salvage. The Temple series employing a reverse saphenous vein graft to the anterior tibial, posterior tibial, peroneal, or tibioperoneal arteries in a total of 48 cases resulted in salvage of 33,- 69%. The operation was considered feasible if a catheter inserted distally could be easily and rapidly injected with saline-heparin solution. Tyson thought they had not "reached the distal limit as yet, but would not expect to go distal to the plantar arches." They used ". . . small instruments, magnification and seven '0' coated dacron sutures. A simple over and over suture . . .", for the distal anastomosis, and six "0" suture material for the proximal anastomosis which was usually at the level of the ". . . femoral bifurcation but . . . also . . . to the common femoral, superficial femoral and popliteal arteries."

Discussion

Anthony M. Imparato, of New York, said that at New York University Hospital they had operated on some 35 patients with arterial reconstruction below the knee, since late 1963, initially by endofemoral tibial endarterectomy, and more recently by "femoral to dorsalis pedis bypass grafts . . ." with or without an arterio-venous fistula. All patients were candidates for operation and almost all were diabetic. Immediate failures with resultant amputation occurred in about a quarter, and late failures,-

after six months,- in a third. [Tyson and Reichle had alluded to late failures.] Imparato's dorsalis pedis bypass grafts had not remained patent longer than eight months, but "This aggressive approach seems definitely to delay the need for amputation, and the longest such delay has been 6 years with a patient returning for a similar operative procedure on the other side." John E. Connolly, of Irvine, California, said his results had not been as good but ". . . even if you save only two or three legs out of 100 . . . it is worthwhile to consider this type of reconstructive surgery below the knee before you amputate." He thought that, particularly for distal anastomoses low in the leg, ". . . the nonreversed saphenous vein technic has many advantages." [If the saphenous vein was left in place, the valves were ruptured by an instrument passed down its lumen.] R. Tyson, closing, said that they had ". . . done very little endarterectomy, and we have used no distal fistulae . . . we have not used any veins with reversed [ruptured?] valves . . ."

* * *

Six years before, E. A. Maynes and J. C. Callaghan from Edmonton, Alberta, [Volume LXXXI, 1963, p. 1175] had introduced the Association to the concept of a membrane oxygenator for extracorporeal circulation, and now J. Donald Hill, M. L. Bramson, E. Rapaport, M. Scheinman, J. J. Osborn, all by invitation, and Frank Gerbode, of San Francisco, Clinical Professor of Surgery, Stanford University School of Medicine, and University of California School of Medicine; Chief, Department of Cardiovascular Surgery, Presbyterian Medical Center, *Experimental and Clinical Experiences with Prolonged Oxygenation and Assisted Circulation,* presented their experimental studies and their clinical experience in five patients. Three of the patients were in cardiogenic shock from massive coronary occlusions, one was a child with massive trauma and fat embolism, and one a woman with overwhelming pneumonia. The two latter patients had veno-venous perfusion from a catheter in the inferior vena cava to a catheter in the superior vena cava; in the patients with myocardial infarction, the blood was returned to the femoral artery. Experimental data had shown that the blood, and the experimental animal, would tolerate 36 hours of membrane oxygenation support. In four of their five patients ". . . definite improvement in the heart or lung function was attained . . . evident in . . . the clinical appearance of the patient and the measure of physiological parameters. In both instances of respiratory insufficiency the lungs improved sufficiently in 24 hours to enable the pa-

tients to maintain their own oxygenation . . . both . . . patients later died due to secondary complication of the disease." In cardiogenic shock, the subsequent failure after the initial response in two of the patients led them to recommend, ". . . that since the risk of the procedure is minimal and the prognosis is otherwise poor, assisted circulation should be instituted after 2-3 hours of aggressive treatment."

* * *

W. Dudley Johnson, Robert J. Flemma, Derward Lepley, Jr., all by invitation, and Edwin H. Ellison, of Milwaukee, Professor of Surgery and Chairman of Department of Surgery, Marquette U. Medical School; Director of Surgery, Milwaukee County General Hospital, *Extended Treatment of Severe Coronary Artery Disease:* A Total Surgical Approach, took an aggressive attitude toward coronary disease and the work of others in the field. ". . . left or right heart failure, massive aneurysms, dyskinetic or akinetic myocardium, or, left main coronary disease have all been listed as surgical contraindications . . . Our emphasis has been on the extensive revascularization and reconstruction of the end stage heart, rather than on the replacement of a sick heart with one soon likely to become even sicker. [Two papers on cardiac transplantation were given later in the same meeting.] . . . During the past 27 months, over 97 per cent of all patients presenting with significant disease have been accepted for surgery. In the past 11 months, no patient has been refused on the basis of the extent of the coronary disease. A total of 301 patients have undergone surgery since our initial efforts in February, 1967. Seventy-one per cent have had one to six previous infarcts . . . 33 per cent have had mild to severe degrees of left ventricular failure with end-diastolic pressures as high as 53 mm. Hg, and 12 per cent of patients have had ventricular aneurysms resected. The total mortality has been 12 per cent." They employed two techniques of coronary revascularization: (1) their modification of the Vineberg operation in which the side branches of the internal mammary were left long, the internal mammary lying on the surface of the heart, "the individual side arms . . . carefully positioned beneath all major coronary branches. From four to nine implants have been made into each heart." (2) ". . . a system of fine vessel anastomosis has been perfected in which free vein grafts can successfully be sutured [from the aorta] to any coronary artery 1-1/2 to 2 mm. or larger. Single or double vein grafts are inserted into any one or combination of arteries." In addition, all ventricular aneurysms were resected. "The day is

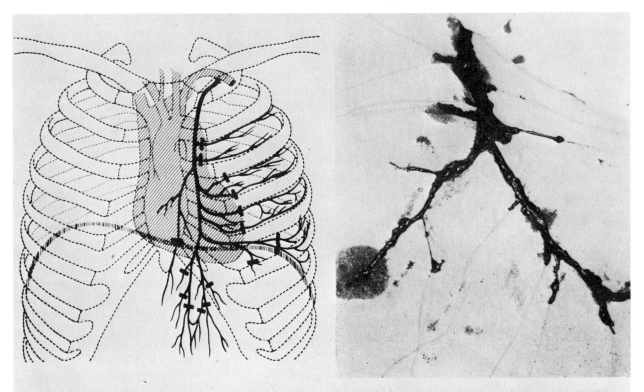

FIG. 1. The pedicle used for the multiple implant procedure is obtained through a sternal splitting incision. Intercostal, mediastinal and superior epigastric branches are left attached to the main mammary artery. As the pedicle is placed over the surface of the heart, the side branches are individually implanted beneath all major coronary arteries.

In addition to saphenous vein, aortocoronary grafts, double vein grafts in 40% of cases, Johnson and Lepley employed, in the same hearts, the modified Vineberg procedure pictured, implanting the multiple side branches, four to nine in a single case "into all areas of the left ventricle". All ventricular aneurysms were resected, no patient was refused operation and their total mortality was 12%. In the previous 12 months, no patient had received fewer than three coronary vein grafts.

W. Dudley Johnson, Robert J. Flemma, Derward Lepley, Jr., Edwin H. Ellison, *Extended Treatment of Severe Coronary Artery Disease:* A Total Surgical Approach, Volume LXXXVII, 1969.

gone when coronary surgery should be thought of in terms of one or two arterial implants. We have not done a single or double implant in over 12 months and consider this an outmoded procedure." The vein grafts ran from the aorta to the coronary arteries, "There is almost no limit of potential arteries to use. Veins can be sutured to the distal anterior descending or even to posterior marginal branches. Double vein grafts are now used in over 40 per cent of patients and can be used to any combination of arteries. We consider one or two vein grafts inadequate therapy for most patients with two or three vessel disease and, therefore, combined direct and indirect revascularization procedures in most patients." They considered it important not to limit grafts to the proximal portions of the large coronary vessels, to make the vein grafts as long as necessary to reach

distal normal arteries. The anastomoses were always end-to-side. It was important to "*Always work in a dry quiet field*", achieved by 15-minute intervals of aortic cross clamping. The hematocrit was kept above 32. "Coronary patients come off bypass poorly or not at all if the hematocrit is low. Hemodilution in the pump oxygenator should be minimal." As far as aneurysms were concerned, ". . . the larger the aneurysms the less the operative risk", and they had never seen a large aneurysm when all three arteries were over 75% occluded, and the risk in that group was 44% ". . . high . . . but considerably below that of transplantation." In 122 patients without aneurysms who had had direct reconstruction, there were 14 deaths, four from cardiac failure, three from stress ulcers, three considered technical. Only six survivors out of their entire group were not clinically improved and they had received implants only. They said flatly that "Direct reconstruction of coronary flow can be achieved in over 90 per cent of all coronary patients . . . End stage coronary disease can nearly always be managed without transplantation."

Discussion

Jack A. Cannon, of Los Angeles, opened the Discussion of this bravura presentation, commenting upon the experience at UCLA with endarterectomy for coronary artery obstruction. There had been nine long-term survivors in the original UCLA series [begun with Longmire] treated solely by endarterectomy, and one seven-year survivor who was completely asymptomatic. In a subsequent series of 58 operations on 52 patients, the mortality was 23% with a late failure rate of 9%. He made no overall comments except that "our problem with the implant is that we never do find really impressive distal perfusion and these patients never do, in our experience, show a negative treadmill test." Frank Spencer, of New York, reported studies by Dr. George Green, done in Spencer's department at the New York University [applying in patients the experimental technique Spencer had reported from Lexington, Volume LXXXI, 1963, p. 1175], "In the past year Dr. Green has electively anastomosed the internal mammary artery to the left anterior descending coronary artery in 23 patients, performing an end-to-side anastomosis . . . with a dissecting microscope, using 9-0 nylon." Flow meter studies showed a flow rate in the internal mammary artery "between 25 and 90 ml./min., an average flow of 50 ml./min. Saphenous vein grafts between the aorta and the right coronary artery had somewhat higher flow, a mean flow of 70 ml./min." There were no deaths on the operating table, four patients died in hospital after operation, and one died five months later from hepatitis. The grafts were patent in all the patients who succumbed. "In these 18 surviving patients, successful angiographic studies have been performed in seven, finding a patent vessel in each." The clinical results in all of them had been excellent, and "The low operative mortality has been most encouraging . . . We may have heard a milestone in cardiac surgery today, because for years pathologists, cardiologists, and many surgeons, [Szilagyi, Vol. LXXVI, 1958] have repeatedly stated that the pattern of coronary artery disease is so extensive that direct anastomosis can be done in only 5 to 7 per cent of patients. If the exciting data by Dr. Johnson remain valid, the grafts remain patent over a long period of

time, a total revision of thinking will be required regarding the feasibility of direct arterial surgery for coronary artery disease." He asked Johnson whether there was any disadvantage in using a vein as opposed to the internal mammary artery. How did Johnson find patent tributaries of the anterior descending artery, "how are the anastomoses performed?" By direct vision? With a microscope? Johnson, closing, said of Cannon's work with endarterectomy that ". . . one of the beauties of the vein is that you don't have to work with diseased arteries and you bypass into normal distal portions of an artery which almost invariably is present in one or more areas." To Spencer, he said, "We have never used the internal mammary-coronary anastomosis. With the pedicle system we have used, we can bring blood supply into any area of the heart with the mammary system and we are reluctant to sacrifice this for use in one coronary system only. Furthermore, with the veins we can attack a combination of vessels and do more than one bypass. We have used no magnification with the vein anastomosis which apparently is required for the internal mammary artery to coronary connection. The suture lines are all made with free hand suture using 6–0 and occasionally 7–0 sutures on the smallest arteries . . . All coronary anastomoses are made first and the veins are attached to the aorta secondarily." They had not yet seen vein aneurysm.

* * *

Robert Hodam, by invitation, Albert Starr, of Portland, Oregon; Professor of Surgery and Head, Cardiopulmonary Surgery, University of Oregon, and by invitation, Rodney Herr, and William R. Pierie, *Early Clinical Experience with Cloth-Covered Valvular Prostheses,* said that ". . . the problems of thromboembolism, long-term anticoagulant treatment, and lipid infiltration of silicone rubber prevent the earlier application of valve replacement at a more optimal time for complete restoration of normal circulatory dynamics." To eliminate thrombosis and embolism they had experimented with a totally cloth-covered prosthesis, and to eliminate the changes in the plastic poppet, had substituted a hollow metal ball. Experiments in dogs in 1966 with replacement of the aortic or mitral valves or both, which yielded them 48 surviving dogs, ". . . showed conclusively that a cloth-covered orifice either of dacron or of teflon implanted in the mitral or aortic position of dogs can heal perfectly without fibrous stenosis . . . Cloth-covered struts of teflon or dacron can heal completely in the mitral position of dogs." Thrombus deposits occurred on the ring but

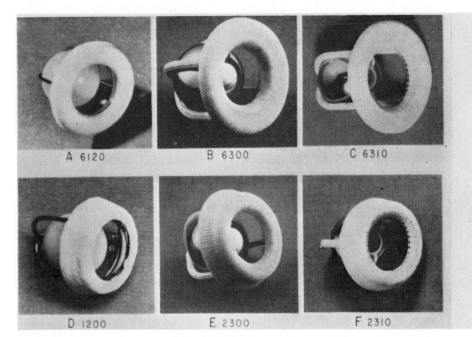

Fig. 1. Ball valve prostheses and modifications. Upper: Mitral prostheses. A. Model 6120—extended cloth model. B. Model 6300—early cloth-covered model. C. Model 6310—composite seat model. Lower: Aortic prostheses. D. Model 1200—extended cloth model. E. Model 2300—early cloth-covered model. F. Model 2310—composite seat model.

The object of covering the entire prosthesis with cloth was to prevent thrombosis and embolism and the need for anticoagulants. Thrombus might deposit on the ring but not on the struts. The substitution of the Silastic poppet by a metal ball was intended to prevent lipid infiltration of the Silastic ball and ball variance. They had 12 embolic complications in 126 patients and none after ten months.

R. Hodam, A. Starr, R. Herr, and W. Pierie, *Early Clinical Experience with Cloth-Covered Valvular Prostheses,* Volume LXXXVII, 1969.

not on the struts. From April, 1967 to January 1969, they had inserted 38 mitral valves with three operative deaths and four late deaths, 67 aortic valves with eight operative deaths and three late deaths, 21 multiple valves with six operative deaths and four late deaths. [In the same period of time other patients were being operated upon with the earlier valves and the present report excluded patients in whom multiple valves were implanted, any of which were not cloth covered.] There were 12 embolic complications in the 126 patients, six in the first four weeks after operation. Starr had discarded ". . . perfusion of the myocardium with ice-cold blood . . ." and now used intermittent coronary perfusion with blood at 34° and 35°. In the total group of 126 patients, 12 embolic complications had occurred, six in the first four weeks after operation and they had begun a double blind study with respect to the use of anticoagulants. Most patients began to take coumadin on the sixth postoperative day. As the valve design had changed,- including covering the struts with teflon cloth,- the incidence of late emboli in mitral replacement dropped from 48% to 3% and in aortic replacement from 28% to 6% without any change in the incidence of early embolism. Starr considered that "Ideal healing without thrombotic or fibrous stenosis has been demonstrated to occur both in the mitral and aortic position of dogs." He was obviously pleased with the early and late thrombo-embolic complications of 6% each, and the fact that no emboli had occurred beyond the ten-month mark.

* * *

B. G. Barratt-Boyes, and A. H. G. Roche, by invitation from the Cardiothoracic Surgical Unit, Green Lane Hospital, Auckland, New Zealand, *A Review of Aortic Valve Homografts over a Six and One-Half Year Period,* reported their massive and pioneer experience,- 590 homograft valve replacements from August 1962 to the end of 1968. It was ". . . the only form of aortic valve replacement used at Green Lane Hospital and the series therefore embraces all pathological variants of aortic valve disease and includes multivalvular operations." The overall hospital mortality was 9.8%. In the 66 patients with multiple valve replacements, the mortality had been 18.2%, but in the last 37 operations only 5.5%,- two deaths. The overall mortality for isolated aortic valve replacement was 6.8%, but re-

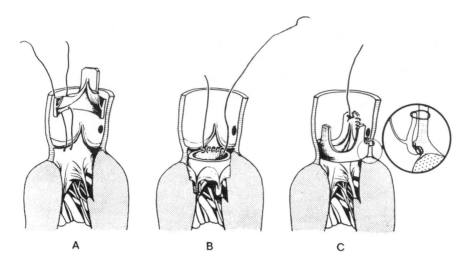

Fig. 4. Semi-diagrammatic drawing to show double suture line technic for homograft valve insertion. (Reproduced with permission from Brit. J. Surg., 52:847, 1965.)

A   B   C

Aortic valve homograft replacement was ". . . the only form of aortic valve replacement used at Green Lane Hospital" and had been employed in 590 patients from August 1962 to the end of 1968 with an overall hospital mortality of 9.8%. The mortality for multi-valve replacement had dropped from 18% to 5.5%. The mortality for isolated aortic valve replacement had risen from 6.8% to double that ". . . attributable largely to the referral of increasing numbers of elderly patients with associated severe coronary artery disease . . ." Of the 532 patients leaving the hospital alive, 4.9% died of aortic valve incompetence, the total incidence of valve failure was 10.7%. Fifty-six patients underwent second operations and 38 of those survived, ". . . no patient has died from embolism despite the fact that anticoagulants have not been used.

B. G. Barratt-Boyes and A. H. G. Roche, *A Review of Aortic Valve Homografts over a Six and One-Half Year Period*, Volume LXXXVII, 1969.

cently had doubled because of ". . . the referral of increasing numbers of elderly patients with associated severe coronary artery diseases in whom the risk of valve replacement is increased." Seventy-five deaths,- 14% of the patients who left the hospital,- were accounted for, half of them by progressive arteriosclerotic myocardial disease, a number to unrelated causes, and 26, 4.9% of the total cases leaving the hospital, to valve failure,- ". . . in each instance due to incompetence. The causes of incompetence were, peripheral suture line leak, malplacement of the valve at operation with a central leak, cusp rupture and endocarditis, both producing central leak . . . no patient has died from embolism despite the fact that anticoagulants have not been used." Incompetence, Barratt-Boyes thought, was purely a technical matter depending upon the method of placement and the surgeon's experience, but often due to an over large aortic root, so that he had begun excising the ellipse of aorta from behind the noncoronary cusp to narrow the aortic root. The valve was competent in 83% of patients, there was unimportant incompetence in 12%, an important leak in only 5%, and ". . . the most experienced surgeon in the group . . ." achieved a competence of 95%. Rupture occurred from six to 18 months after operation, rarely after two years and was ". . .

higher with chemical sterilization and freeze-drying . . . than with chemical sterilization and wet cold storage in Hanks solution. Valves collected sterile and stored for short periods in Hanks solution, of which 16 have now been followed from 5 to 6-1/2 years, have never ruptured, nor has rupture so far occurred with valves sterilized and stored in antibiotic Hanks solution . . ." Calcification of the leaflets was rare and also had not occurred in valves collected sterile and stored in Hanks solution. Barratt-Boyes concluded that his hospital mortality was comparable to that with use of other prosthetic devices, that "Emboli do not originate from a homograft valve and anticoagulants are not required." Incompetence "In experienced hands . . . would appear to be no more common than with a Starr-Edwards aortic prosthesis and possibly less so, although regrettably, there is not a recent serial angiographic study of the Starr-Edwards aortic prosthesis available for comparison with the homograft valve." Late valve failure was an uncommon cause of death and sudden death had never occurred so that "Reoperation is always technically feasible and usually successful." The method of storage was important "Histological study of human material indicates that host tissues never penetrate a leaflet which has been chemically sterilized . . . while such a leaf-

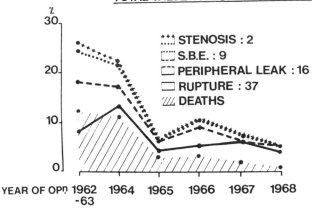

ALL PATIENTS (590)
TOTAL VALVE FAILURE INCIDENCE

STENOSIS : 2
S.B.E. : 9
PERIPHERAL LEAK : 16
RUPTURE : 37
DEATHS

YEAR OF OPⁿ 1962 1964 1965 1966 1967 1968
-63

FIG. 7. Total valve failure incidence. In this graph incompetence due to malplacement is included in the peripheral leak group. The two late valve failure deaths listed as "uncertain" in Table 1 have been divided between the peripheral leak and rupture groups.

The late performance of aortic valve homografts was very satisfactory. Rupture was related to the method of preservation and did not occur with preservation in Hanks solution with added antibiotics.

B. G. Barratt-Boyes and A. H. G. Roche, *A Review of Aortic Valve Homografts Over a Six and One-Half Year Period,* Volume LXXXVII, 1969.

let can function well for at least 6-1/2 years, it remains inert and can be expected finally to deteriorate and calcify . . . untreated leaflets, examined at intervals from 4 months up to 5-1/2 years after insertion, contain an increased amount of acid mucopolysaccharide ground substance and fibroblasts." He hoped that the Hanks penicillin, streptomycin, kanamycin, amphotericin B storage solution would not damage "the acid mucopolysaccharides, collagen and elastin which make up the leaflet . . . and provide an ideal valve transplant."

Discussion

Arthur C. Beall, Jr., of Houston, speaking of ". . . the Portland presentation regarding the cloth covered valves" thought that ". . . most thromboembolic complications result from thrombi beginning at the cloth sewing ring to metal cage interface, and to eliminate this problem we have attempted to develop a prosthesis with complete cloth coverage of the base." They had thought it better to avoid covering the cage legs with cloth. In May of 1968, they had presented 202 patients with isolated mitral replacement with a 9.5% mortality and had now followed those patients, so that the shortest follow-up was one year with a total of four late deaths,- ". . . one, I believe, we can consider unrelated. He was shot twice in the head." The incidence of emboli was less than 2% in these patients followed one to two-and-half years, "Dr. Jack Greenberg at Mt. Sinai Hospital in Miami has used more than 100 of these prostheses and has had only one embolus. Dr. Byron Dooley at Lackland Air Force Base has now used in excess of 50 of these valves. He has used no anticoagulants of any kind and has had no emboli . . . I think the cloth covered principle, as presented this morning, has gone a long way toward lowering the incidence [of embolism] to a very low and acceptable level." Frank Spencer, of New York, who had implanted 147 cloth-covered [Starr] prostheses in 113 patients, said there had been only four emboli, the single fatal one occurring 14 days after operation. No embolus had occurred more than six months after operation "All of these patients had received anticoagulants continually, starting with heparin 4 days after operation." He considered that the embolism problem was close to being solved, but "The major problem with the present cloth-covered prostheses is the fact that the small models are hemodynamically too small. Changes in valve design are required to make the small prostheses hemodynamically satisfactory." Raymond O. Heimbecker, of Toronto, endorsed Barratt-Boyes' ". . . preference for the homograft valve not abused by the rigors of chemical sterilization and freeze drying", and said that "I had the pleasure of assisting Dr. Gordon Murray at the implantation of fresh homograft valves in two patients, 11 and 14 years ago respectively, in the thoracic aorta as shown here. [See Volume LXXVIII, page 1126, 1960] These patients have continued to do beautifully clinically . . . These valves are totally free of calcium, are functioning beautifully with no stenosis, only a whiff of insufficiency which has undoubtedly been present since surgery." John W. Kirklin, of Birmingham, Alabama, spoke of the presentations by ". . . the two brilliant innovators so far as valve surgery is concerned . . ." He had been operating with homografts for about four years and now had 139 patients of whom 89 corresponded to the time frame of Starr's report. The hospital mortality was 4%. During the same period of time they had implanted, in a fifth of their patients, the Starr valve for patients older than 65 or with a very large aortic root, and the mortality was 3%. There had been no late deaths with homografts, no reoperations, no infections, no patients who had had anticoagulants, and there had been no thromboembolic complications. Angiocardiography, undertaken in some, had shown some incompetence in 13%, significant in only a single patient. There had been no cusp rupture. Kirklin asked whether irradiation, freezing and preserving the valve at -72° C would not be acceptable. Starr, closing, thought the operative and late mortality was remarkably parallel in his series and in Barratt-Boyes' . He and Dr. Beall were in agreement upon ". . . reduction of thromboembolic complications with extension of the cloth to the orifice for more complete healing of the prosthesis." Spencer's early initiation of anticoagulant therapy was probably good, Starr's group had "been interested in the development of a prosthesis which would require no anticoagulants at any time, and for this reason have put it to the test in our double-blind series." His late mortality was higher than Kirklin's but not related to the nature of the valve. No one had alluded to ". . . the problem of lipid infiltration of silicone rubber which has resulted in a very high incidence of valve failure with the use of the earlier type of aortic prosthesis and is one of the main forces driving us to the use of cloth-covered prostheses with metallic poppet." They had followed 40 patients from July 1963 to June 1964 and ". . . 28 have proven ball variance from lipid infiltration. Five of these patients died of this complication and all the others were reoperated." Barratt-Boyes, closing, said that ". . . the method of valve collection and sterilization is the most important single factor in the operation of aortic homograft valve replacement or the use of any homograft valve." Freeze-dried valves kept chemically sterilized with beta propiolactone or ethylene oxide never showed ingrowth of host tissue and were prone to rupture. In answer to Kirklin, he thought irradiation might be no better than chemical sterilization. Sterile harvesting of valves was impracticable in any large series, "Although we did this in our earliest cases, and have a long follow-up on these sterile valves, I think they behave extremely well as Dr. Heimbecker has said; this is not a practical solution to the problem. The solution is, I think, for the pathologist to collect the valves as cleanly as he can. They are then placed in Hanks solution containing antibiotics (penicillin, streptomycin, kanamycin and amphotericin B). Within 14 days 80 per cent of the valves are sterile and within 3 weeks, about 90 per cent."

* * *

The first mention of the diagnosis,- and treatment,- of gastrointestinal hemorrhage by selective angiographic techniques, *Clinical Experience with the Diagnosis and Management of Gastrointestinal Hemorrhage by Selective Mesenteric Catheterization,* Moreye Nusbaum, and Stanley Baum, by invitation, and William S. Blakemore, of Philadelphia, Professor and Chairman, Department of Surgery, The Graduate Hospital, University of Pennsylvania, presented their seven-year experience, four years after their first report on the method. In 45 of 60 patients they had localized the source of massive hemorrhage from the gastrointestinal tract. In 40 patients with previous massive bleeding or with occult bleeding at the time of the study, there were 12 who "were found to have a variety of vascular ectasias or arteriovenous malformations which were presumed to be the site of hemorrhage." In an additional 15 patients, there was on arteriography indirect evidence of a source of bleeding, so that the bleeding was localized in 72 of a total of 100 patients. Through an arterial catheter they had infused Pituitrin into the mesenteric circulation in eight patients. Bleeding was arrested in four of five patients bleeding from esophageal varices and the note was made that intra-arterial infusion of Pituitrin during the operation for a portacaval shunt, ". . . resulted in complete collapse of the collateral circulation, significantly decreased blood loss during operation and facilitated exposure of the portal vein." Infusion of Pituitrin into the left gastric artery in a patient bleeding from a gastric ulcer controlled the bleeding. The recommended dose of Pituitrin in patients with variceal bleeding was 0.2 of a pressor unit per cc. per minute, continued for 24 hours, then decreasing doses for ". . . anywhere from 5 days to 2 weeks . . ." They had no complications at the catheter site from infusions continued for as long as two weeks. Thus far they had noticed no antidiuretic effect from the doses of Pituitrin used.

Discussion

Philip Sandblom, of Lund, Sweden, demonstrated studies which showed bleeding from an aneurysm into the pancreatic duct. [A discussant, not identified, mentioned the fact that it was appropriate for the father of hematobilia to describe what might be called "hematopancreatia".] Blakemore said that it was Nusbaum who had started the work "in the laboratory and developed into the clinical work with Dr. Stanely Baum and others." They could catheterize "most of the branches from the aorta selectively . . ." and the addition of microangiography had been particularly useful. Moreye Nusbaum, closing, said that it was Sandblom's ". . . group in Lund, especially Dr. E. C. Boijsen, who have perfected selective arterial catheterization so that it is almost as accessible as venous catheterization for the infusion of solutions." The demonstration of vascular malformations by microangiography disclosed lesions which "were not recognizable on gross inspection by the pathologist. We have had to take the surgical specimens, have them injected by a special technic developed by Dr. Oscar V. Batson in our institution, in which he can dissolve away the extraneous fatty tissue and display the vasculature. The lesions are then identified and marked for histological examination by the pathologist . . . we now use mesenteric aorteriography as the initial study for the bleeding patient upon admission, reserving barium studies for later if they are then required."

* * *

[In 1968, in Brooklyn the widespread riots after the assassination of Martin Luther King had overwhelmed the King's County Hospital with stabbing victims. The observation that many of those without obvious signs of intra-abdominal catastrophe and therefore put aside while patients with more pressing injuries were operated upon, ultimately survived without any operation at all stimulated a series of reports by Shaftan and others supporting the policy of selecting for immediate operation only those with clinical evidence of intra-abdominal injury.] Now Francis C. Nance, by invitation, and Isidore Cohn, Jr., of New Orleans, Professor and Chairman, Department of Surgery, Louisiana State University School of Medicine, *Surgical Judgment in the Management of Stab Wounds of the Abdomen:* A Retrospective and Prospective Analysis Based on a Study of 600 Stabbed Patients, presented their results from the Charity Hospital in New Orleans of the "selective approach to the management of stabbed patients" since 1967. Their prior policy had been that "all patients were explored if they had a wound which possibly could have entered the peritoneal cavity." In the three-year period, preceding the study, of 480 patients, 8% refused operation, 50% were explored and found to have no injury, 9% explored and found to have injury usually the liver, requiring no repair, and 31% required repair. Of the 296 patients in whom nothing needed to be done within the abdomen, 29 developed wound infections, five developed an evisceration, in four the spleen was injured at operation, three developed an intra-abdominal abscess, in three the bowel was torn by the operator, two developed intestinal obstruction,

and one died. Under the new protocol, 1967 through 1969, operation was undertaken for evisceration, shock, or obvious, peritonitis, a positive peritoneal aspiration, or air under the diaphragm. Of 122 patients, 72 (60%) escaped operation. Among these there were no complications and the average hospital stay was 2.1 days. Three patients observed presently required operation, one after 13 hours for a lacerated mesenteric vein,- uneventful recovery,- one after 11 hours for a through-and-through laceration of the jejunum,- uneventful recovery,- and the third for what proved to be blood in the peritoneal cavity from the abdominal wall, not bleeding at the time. Twelve patients operated upon had negative explorations, two of them having presented with omentum in the wound. Cornell, at Johns Hopkins, had introduced the technique of forced injection of radiopaque material into the abdominal wound to demonstrate intraperitoneal penetration, but Nance and Cohn pointed out in their study ". . . a major concern was to evaluate the reliability of *clinical criteria* for diagnosis of intra-abdominal injury . . . the injection technic of Cornell can reduce the number of negative explorations, it does not identify the patients who have penetration of the peritoneum without serious injury. We sought to reduce to a minimum the number of unnecessary operations . . . it appears that clinical criteria *are* sufficient to differentiate seriously injured patients from those who can be managed non-operatively . . . More than 80% of patients with hollow viscus or other serious injury had unequivocal indications for surgery at the time of first examination. A period of observation for 48 hours identified the remainder without increasing morbidity or mortality. The overall complication rate in stabbed patients has been reduced from 27% to 12% and the average period of hospitalization reduced from 7.9 days to 5.4 days . . . Observation and selective management have a primary role in the care of patients with abdominal stab wounds."

Discussion

Clarence Dennis, of Brooklyn, spoke for G. W. Shaftan, of the Kings County Medical Center, stating that "After the original observations of Dr. Dwight Spreng, Jr., in 1955, at Kings County, a prospective study of penetrating abdominal wounds was reported by Shaftan in 1960, and by Shaftan, Herbsman, and Ryzoff in 1966." Their overall data indicated that 24% of 535 patients had criteria for immediate operation. Of the remaining 406 patients observed, only one was lost and that one had blood aspirated from the peritoneal cavity and should have been operated upon. Dennis emphasized the necessity of peritoneal aspiration. Their indications for operation were the same as those presented by Nance and held ". . . for penetrating wounds of all types including stab and gunshot wounds as well as for exploration in blunt abdominal trauma". He emphasized the need for repeated careful examination. The injection of radiopaque material into the wound showed peritoneal penetration, but "The true concern is in the first place, with intra-abdominal injuries, not with peritoneal invasion . . ." George D. Zuidema, of Baltimore [on whose service Cornell's study had been done], brought their studies up to date. Injection studies had been made in 192 patients, 124 of them negative, the other 68 patients having been explored, of whom 14 had peritoneal penetration, but no visceral injury requiring correction,- 22% of the positive studies, 7.3% of the total group. In the entire study, there was one false-positive study, and three false-negative studies. Zuidema stated specifically that the technique was recommended for patients with stab wounds of the abdomen and "It is not recommended in any way for patients with bullet wounds." Carleton Mathewson, Jr., of San Francisco, attempted by retrospective studies to show the danger of a policy of nonoperative observation of patients without mandatory indication for operation, concluding that ". . . we still believe that every penetrating wound should be explored in the operating room." Under some circumstances, local anesthesia sufficed to determine whether the peritoneum had been violated. President Wangensteen said that he would ask Isidore Cohn, in closing, to comment on bullet wounds. He had happened to see a patient in Dennis' clinic who had been observed with a bullet wound and passed the bullet in a stool three days later. What about pneumoperitoneum? Did Cohn explore patients with pneumoperitoneum? Cohn said that they had not extended their study to include gunshot wounds or bullet wounds but had it under consideration. As for the radio-contrast technique to which Zuidema had referred, Cohn said that ". . . with the use of x-ray in Dr. Zuidema's own hands he has explored 22 per cent of his patients that would not have been explored in our particular hands . . ." He made a final comment, "When the study was proposed by Dr. Nance—and I would assure everyone in the audience that the study was Dr. Nance's idea—when the study was proposed by Dr. Nance, almost everyone on the staff objected to it rather violently because it went against the grain of everything all of us had ever practiced at Charity, what most of us had been taught elsewhere, and what had been practiced in the service by all the members of our staff who had been on active duty during World War II or subsequently. As a result of a very prolonged, heated staff conference, in essence I challenged Dr. Nance to answer the question with our own material, with the one proviso that he personally see every patient, so that it could be his responsibility and not an error that we could lay at the feet of the residents. He accepted the challenge, and he has seen every one of these patients . . . . One other thing . . . When we started this technic, the residents resisted it very strenuously because the residents felt that they were being cheated out of some of the surgery that they really wanted to do. As the study has progressed, the residents have become convinced that we really are handling the situation better now than we were before. Any time you can convince your own residents that a nonoperative approach is a better one, you know you have accomplished something."

* * *

[Shumway and Lower at Stanford; Hanlon and Willman in St. Louis; Kantrowitz, in Brooklyn; and Webb, in Jackson, Mississippi, had been intensively studying the technique and consequences of cardiac replantation. Renal transplantation was becoming increasingly successful and it was obvious that human cardiac transplantation was imminent when Christian Barnard of South Africa, returning from a visit to the United States, performed the first human cardiac transplantation in Capetown, at the end of 1967.] E. B. Stinson, Eugene Dong, Jr., J. S. Schroeder, all by invitation, and Norman E. Shumway, of Palo Alto, Professor of Surgery, Stanford University School of Medicine, *Cardiac Transplantation in Man. IV. Early Results,* presented to the Association their experience in 13 human cardiac transplantations, eleven men and two women, ten with coronary artery disease and three with cardiomyopathy. "All patients suffered Class IV disability and three were moribund at the time of operation . . . Preoperative lymphocyte typing and cross-matching were performed in all patients and served as the basis for recipient selection in most. A compatible match was obtained in three instances; four patients were mismatched for one and six patients for two of the 11 antigens typed. In all instances ABO compatibility was observed." In the first five patients, femoral cannulation, which they had carried over from the laboratory, produced lymphatic fistulae in two and wound infection in one, so that thereafter they employed ". . . central cannulation of the inferior vena cava and aorta, and cannulation of the superior vena cava through the right internal jugular vein." The

Patient Survival

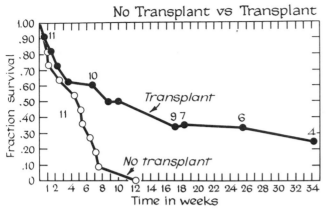

FIG. 1. Survival curves for transplanted versus non-transplanted cardiac recipients. Numbers indicate number of patients at risk.

In Shumway's first 13 patients, the three-month survival was 45% and six-month survival 29% of those at risk, obviously better than that of the patients who, having been accepted into the program, died while awaiting transplantation, after a maximum of 12 weeks.

E. B. Stinson, Eugene Dong, Jr., J. S. Schroeder, N. E. Shumway, *Cardiac Transplantation in Man.* IV. Early Results, Volume LXXXVII, 1969.

donor heart was immersed in cold saline at 4° to 6° C. immediately upon excision, "Myocardial anoxia time has averaged 55 minutes." Azathioprine, prednisone, and antilymphocyte globulin were employed in all but the first two patients. Eight patients were treated preoperatively with azathioprine for one to four weeks, but immunosuppression was now begun on the first postoperative day. Their current regimen was like Starzl's. Ten of the 13 patients had at least one episode of rejection, the diagnosis based ". . . primarily upon electrocardiographic changes, notably progressive decrease in voltage, atrial arhythmias, right axis deviation, and ischemic-type ST depression . . . by the development of an early diastolic gallop rhythm and significant changes in ultrasound cardiographic measurements of right ventricular diameter, left ventricular wall thickness, and total heart size." Immediate cardiac function was good in 12 of 13 hearts and in the 13th, the donor had had anoxic cardiac arrest and had been resuscitated. The recipient of that heart had a second transplant which functioned. Six of the 13 patients were alive two weeks to eight months after operation. The three-month survival was 45% and the six-month survival was 29%. "Comparison of these survival data with those for nontransplanted patients who died before surgery could be performed reveals maximum survival in the latter group of 12 weeks following acceptance into the program . . . Of the six currently surviving patients, three were treated for rejection on three separate occasions, two on two occasions, and one once postoperatively. Only one rejection episode was diagnosed and treated more than 3 months postoperatively." In this small series there was ". . . no apparent relationship of compatibility to survival, number of rejection episodes, or myocardial function." The survivals pointed out the difference between the maximum survival of 12

weeks of the nontransplanted potential recipients contrasting ". . . sharply with the generally accepted 10% annual mortality for patients maintained on chronic hemodialysis." They felt the transplanted hearts were particularly sensitive to pulmonary vascular disease and that there was as well ". . . an increased susceptibility to pulmonary sepsis in the presence of immunosuppressive drugs." A precise index of chronic rejection was not available, "The onset of intractable myocardial failure is a late manifestation of chronic rejection related to irreversible coronary insufficiency. The value of temporizing support and retransplantation in these instances remains unknown."

* * *

Grady L. Hallman, R. D. Leachman, Louis L. Leatherman, R. D. Bloodwell, J. J. Nora, John D. Milam, all by invitation, and Denton A. Cooley, of Houston, Professor of Surgery, Baylor University College of Medicine; Chief Cardiovascular Surgical Service, St. Luke's-Texas Children's Hospitals, *Factors Influencing Survival after Human Heart Transplantation,* had performed their first transplant on May 2, 1968, and were reporting 18 human transplantations. Over 100 human transplantations had already been reported [and they cited 13 of their own publications on the subject beginning in 1968]. They had performed 19 transplants in the 18 patients over a period of 11 months. Survival varied from 14 hours,- a two-month-old infant with a combined heart-lung transplant,- to nine months. Two patients were currently alive at two and five-and-a-half months. Their patients all had either C or D Terasaki lymphocyte matches and the duration and quality of survival correlated with the grade of the histocompatibility match. Eight of the hearts resumed activity and sinus rhythm spontaneously, ten fibrillated and required defibrillation. Survival seemed better in those that spontaneously resumed beating in sinus rhythm. Eleven of the 18 patients developed infections, pneumonia in five which caused death in three in them; two patients died two months after transplant with *serratia marcescens* septicemia, and one "long-term survivor" died of rejection and cytomegalovirus isolated from the lungs. Cooley suggested that "All donors over 50 years of age should have coronary arteriograms." Diabetes, hypogammaglobulinemia, and agranulocytosis from the immunosuppression predisposed to infection. The paper makes no statement as to their evaluation of the place of cardiac transplantation.

There was no pertinent Discussion of the two cardiac transplantation papers.

* * *

Anti-Serum to Cultured Human Lymphoblasts: Preparation, Purification and Immunosuppressive Properties in Man, John S. Najarian, of Minneapolis, Professor and Chairman, University of Minnesota; with R. L. Simmons, Henry Gewurz, A. Moberg, F. Merkel, all by invitation; and George E. Moore, of Buffalo, Director and Chief of Surgery, Roswell Park Memorial Institute; Clinical Professor of Surgery, University of Buffalo School of Medicine, documented ". . . the development of a high titer purified horse antiglobulin prepared against pure cultured human lymphoblasts. Such material can be given for prolonged periods of time because immunological tolerance to the administered globulin can be induced. The material is effective in prolonging human skin allografts and as an adjunctive agent with other immunosuppressive agents in the prolongation of renal allografts." The lymphocytes were grown constantly in culture at the Roswell Park Memorial Institute, shipped by air to the University of Minnesota, and injected at ten-day intervals into multiple sites in the neck and hind quarters of a horse. The horses were bled after the third and each succeeding injection, and were used for six months. The serum was purified by a chromatographic technique at first and more recently by an electrophoretic technique. Both the serum and the globulin would prolong the life of human skin homografts, and the serum had been used "as an adjunctive immunosuppressive agent in renal, hepatic and pancreatic transplantation. Of 19 related renal allografts performed in the past 15 months utilizing EAHLS, equine antihuman lymphocyte serum, none has been rejected." Intravenous administration was free from local reactions, sensitization to horse pro-

teins had occurred in only half of the recipients, and reactions were mild.

Discussion

Sir Michael Woodruff, of Edinburgh, said that he had published his first paper on an antilymphocyte serum in 1950 and produced an effective ALS by 1963, "Another six years have elapsed and, despite the example of Dr. Starzl and others, we have used anti-human serum in only a few patients." They had been concerned about painful local reactions at the site of intramuscular injection and about throbocytopenia. He confirmed ". . . what Dr. Najarian has said about the advantage and safety . . ." of intravenous administration. Thrombocytopenia had been a problem perhaps because they had used spleen cells. "Stimulated by Dr. Joseph Murray and his colleagues in Boston, and Dr. Traeger in Lyons, we are now raising horse-anti-human ALG with cells obtained by thoracic duct cannulation. Whether this will be as good as serum raised with the products of Dr. George Moore's spectacular lymphoblast factory remains to be seen. Certainly the apparent absence of anti-platelet activity in Dr. Najarian's serum is impressive . . ." He referred to ". . . one important complication of immunosuppression which Dr. Najarian did not mention; namely, the development of malignant tumors and, in particular, of reticulum cell sarcoma. Let me hasten to add firstly that ALG has been implicated in only about half the cases reported so far, and also that it may actually slow down the growth of some experimental tumors . . . the goal must be to avoid the present necessity for prolonged immunosuppression by making the donor specifically tolerant of the transplant in as short a time as possible. Monaco, Medawar and others have achieved this with ALG in animals, but so far it has not proved possible in man." David M. Hume, of Richmond, asked ". . . against what antigens of the lymphocyte ALG is made . . . how many of the HLA antigens Dr. Najarian feels it is important to immunize the horses with", what assay of ALG was useful. Since cytopenia was not produced in his patients whether ". . . the purified ALG is, in fact, as good an immunosuppressive agent as ALS . . ." how long should ALS be given,- it could not very well be given indefinitely intravenously,- how good was the evidence that his ALG "was, in fact, effective in producing immunosuppression of organ transplantation in man . . . which I am not convinced the paper actually demonstrates." Najarian, closing, said they had, in fact, been seeing "increasing numbers of tumors in these patients" and that this happened of course in patients receiving immunosuppression for lupus and other disease. "All of us are constantly throwing off a variety of cancer mutations in ourselves every day, and we have a surveillance system and immunosurveillance system which destroys these 'foreign' cells so that cancer won't flourish and survive. As we get better immunosuppression, we decrease this surveillance system, and there is no question that we are going to see increasing numbers of tumors, and, hopefully, this is going to shed some light in the general area of cancer immunology. This has not been a serious problem to date . . ." In answer to Hume, he said that they could identify seven or eight histocompatibility antigens in their stimulating cells and since they were "ubiquitous throughout the body . . . if you say you are making anti-human antibody, that is correct. This is exactly what we're making, and that is what we want." He thought their eight-day prolongation of skin-graft survival was very significant, "I think there are such things as kidney specific antigens, but histocompatibility antigens are ubiquitous and what can be achieved in a skin graft can be achieved very well and much better with a vascularly anastomosed organ graft." They did in fact get less lymphopenia than with the pure material and whether that was important or not was not known. As for the duration of administration of the ALG, they hoped to induce tolerance to it so that doses could be spaced farther apart and "In one patient, 2 months after receiving his last intravenous dose, he still had highly significant amounts of horse ALG in his circulation." Starzl had strongly supported the claim of benefit from ALG together with standard immunosuppression [No discussion by Starzl is recorded.], but Najarian said ". . . we have a series in San Francisco which Dr. Belzer and Dr. Sam Kountz are going to report . . . with an 80 to 85 per cent 4-year survival of kidney grafts without ALG and almost identical, if not better, survival statistics than have been shown by investigators using ALG." Their own results with ALG in cadaver transplants had shown an improvement over the 50% one-year survival, "It is hoped that we can use higher doses and more effective doses with our tolerant material, and that we will be able to significantly improve the survival of the cadaver grafts."

* * *

John L. Cameron, Robert K. Brawley, and Harvey W. Bender, by invitation, and George D. Zuidema, of Baltimore, Professor of Surgery, Director of the Department of Surgery, The John Hopkins Medical School; Surgeon-in-Chief of the Johns Hopkins Hospital, *The Treatment of Pancreatic Ascites,* discussed an experience with nine patients who presented with painless ascites, massive in eight of them, and in seven the reason medical help was sought. Six of the nine had a history of heavy alcoholic intake, two had documented episodes of acute pancreatitis,- one at seven months before the development of ascites. Ascites was straw-colored in eight and serosanguineous in one. The protein content of the ascitic fluid was always elevated, ranging from 2.2 to 5 grams per 100 ml. The ascitic fluid amylase was elevated in all, ranging from 360 mg./100 ml. to 16,800 mg./ml. The serum amylase was elevated in all but not quite to the same degree, the highest level being 1,970 mg./100 ml. Three of the patients were found to have pseudocysts, two had a leaking pancreatic duct and one had a duct stricture with no demonstrable leak at operative pancreatography. Three of the patients were not operated upon. Two of these were treated by repeated paracenteses, parenteral alimentation and diamox. The third was a child with pancreatitis and mild ascites which was not treated. One cyst was excised with Roux-en-Y drainage of the pancreatic stump and sphincterotomy, one cyst was simply excised. In one patient, a cystogastrostomy was performed with death two weeks later from pulmonary complications,- the only death in the series. One disrupted pancreatic duct was treated with a Roux-en-Y drainage and one leak from the posterior surface of the pancreas was treated by sump drainage and prolonged support with recovery. The patient in whom only a duct stricture was found had the Puestow type of Roux-Y pancreatojejunostomy. The patients had been originally thought to have, variously, cirrhosis with ascites, constrictive pericarditis, and carcinomatosis. The Hopkins group recommended a relatively brief trial of nonoperative treatment with nasogastric suction, parenteral alimentation and diamox and paracenteses. In the absence of rapid response, they recommended operation, transduodenal pancreatography, resection if cysts were present, or direct drainage from the pancreatic lesion to a Roux-Y loop. In several of their patients they had performed pancreatic sphincterotomy.

Discussion

George Jordan, of Houston, said that 6% of their patients with pseudocysts had had ascites but they had not demonstrated a leak in any of them at operation. Thomas T. White, of Seattle, preferred to make his pancreatograms by direct injection into the duct rather than through the ampulla. In his 172

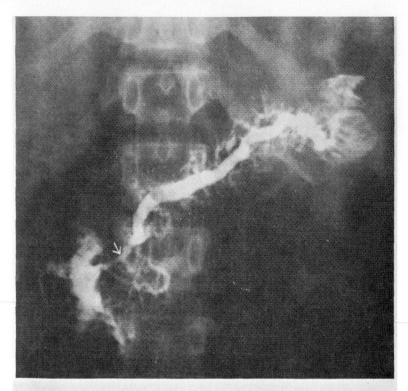

FIG. 2. Operative pancreatogram of Patient 1 showing proximal duct stricture (arrow) and distal pseudocyst filled with contrast media. Pancreatic duct is ectatic distal to the stricture.

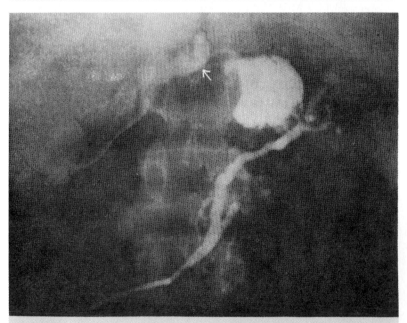

FIG. 4. Operative pancreatogram of Patient 2 demonstrating distal pseudocyst. Contrast media is seen extravasating free into the peritoneal cavity (arrow) from the cyst.

Six of nine patients were operated upon. Three were found to have pseudocysts and in one of these, extravasation was demonstrated from the cyst. Two were demonstrated to have extravasation from the pancreas in the absence of a cyst (see facing page). Five of the operated patients remained well, one died of pulmonary complications after operation. Two of the unoperated patients ultimately recovered after prolonged treatment,- nasogastric suction, parenteral alimentation, multiple paracenteses, thoracenteses, and diamox. For pancreatic ascites they recommended operation if a brief nonoperative trial gave no relief.

John L. Cameron, Robert K. Brawley, Harvey W. Bender, and George D. Zuidema, *The Treatment of Pancreatic Ascites,* Volume LXXXVII, 1969.

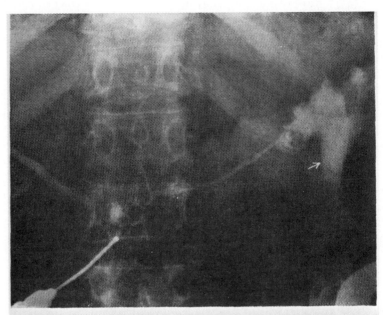

FIG. 6. Operative pancreatogram of Patient 4 showing free extravasation of contrast media through the hole in the pancreatic duct into the peritoneal cavity.

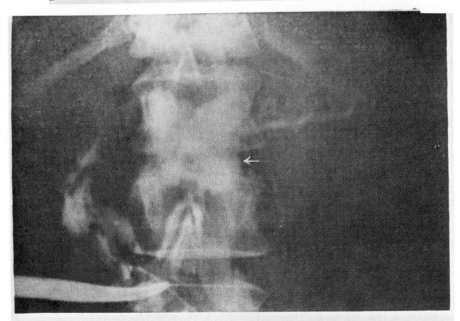

FIG. 7. Operative pancreatogram of Patient 6 showing retroperitoneal extravasation of contrast media (arrow) from the pancreatic duct.

operative cases of pancreatitis, 34 had pancreatic cysts and eight of those had ascites as the primary presenting symptom, five of them being alcoholics but two having gallstones and one, recent abdominal trauma. The Roux-Y pancreaticojejunostomy, he thought, was the appropriate operation in all cases. Zuidema, closing, said it was important in "all patients presenting with ascites, to study the serum amylase and the ascitic fluid amylase and protein in an effort to detect more of these patients and thereby offer them operative treatment." He performed whichever type of internal drainage was most convenient and preferred to perform the pancreatography through the ampulla of Vater "in an effort to pick up proximal duct damage or strictures, feeling that this is important in management as well."

The Business Meetings

The 1969 meeting, April 30, May 1 and 2, was held at the Netherland-Hilton Hotel in Cincinnati, President Owen H. Wangensteen, in the Chair.

Secretary C. Rollins Hanlon complained that in spite of the adoption in 1962 of the requirement for three copies of each of the three publications considered by a candidate's sponsors to be his best work ". . . one of the best kept secrets in American Surgery is the fact that one needs nine reprints to accompany the application. I assure you it is a rarity to get nine reprints. I have on occasion received 27, at other times, none, with many permutations in between. One member was so touched by my repeated entreaties that he sent me nine of his own reprints . . ."

[For some years the Treasurer had been indicating in his report the Council's concern for the expense of producing the *Transactions* and it now became obvious that the Council wished to take action. A long and spirited debate took place, essentially between the pragmatists and the traditionalists.] William D. Holden, the Treasurer, indicated that the Association's cash assets had fallen from $11,000+ in 1967 to $9,000+ in 1968 and $7,000+ in 1969. "The major item of expense for the Association each year is the cost of publishing the *Transactions*. Each year it amounts to more than 40% of the Association's income accruing from dues and initiation fees. In 1963 the cost of publication was $4,265.46. In 1968 it was $6,239.34." He was not recommending an increase in dues but indicated that ". . . added income or a reduction in expenses will be required in the foreseeable future . . ."

The Recorder, John Kirklin, announced that the *Transactions* of the previous year had only just been mailed out. "There seems to no way to overcome this clumsy and complex situation unless a mechanism is devised allowing the publication of the *Transactions* within a few months of the Annual Meeting. Your recorder urges strongly that the Association take appropriate action to allow this. This action might well recommend omission of inclusion of the scientific papers within the *Transactions*, since they are published also in the *Annals of Surgery*. Considerable cost reduction would also thereby be achieved." Kirklin presented a number of recommendations,- that the scientific papers not be published in the *Transactions* since they were being published in the *Annals*, that the Presidential Address be published in the *Transactions*, that the *Transactions* be published soon after the Annual Meeting together with the Minutes, that *Transactions* continue to include listings of officers, committees, etc., and ". . . memoirs with photographs of members recently deceased." Robert M. Zollinger moved to approve these proposals. Leo Eloesser, who had long since retired from Stanford to Tacambaro, Michoacan, Mexico, whence he came annually to this meeting and to the meeting of The American Association for Thoracic Surgery, and who had been inducted in the Association in 1936, rose to ask whether it would be "feasible to keep the *Transactions*, if you so desire, as they are, but to issue them as a volume that is to be paid for by the members who are interested? . . . As a suggestion, you might have a small volume containing the minutes of the meeting and the business that pertains to the Association separate from the scientific transactions. That would reduce the cost greatly" [precisely the suggestion that was ultimately adopted]. Dr. Kirklin said that Dr. Eloesser's comments in fact represented his proposal "That the *Transactions* continue to be published, but that they will be smaller to the extent allowed by omitting the scientific papers, but they would still be published annually and submitted to the membership." A dialogue disclosed that the saving would amount from $10 to $15 per member per year. Dr. Kirklin indicated that unless the Minutes, etc., were separated from the scientific papers, there was no way to get the publication to the members in less than a year. Claude E. Welch, of Boston, said he would "hate to see the *Transactions* go down, because this has been a wonderful publication. I personally refer to it very frequently, and I imagine many others do." He asked whether using the type from the *Annals* issue would save any significant sum of money. [This, of course, is what was done during World War II, but

THE MEDALLION OF THE AMERICAN SURGICAL ASSOCIATION FOR
DISTINGUISHED SERVICE TO SURGERY.

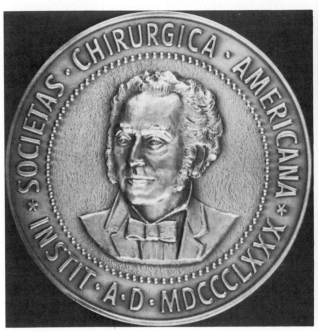 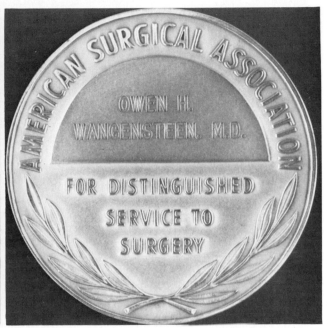

In awarding the Medallion to Dragstedt, its first recipient, Wangensteen said it was "an award for distinguished service to surgery", and that is the inscription on the Medallion. The Secretary's 1971 report of Council calls it a Medallion for Scientific Achievement. One would suppose the first awarding President and the inscription have the right of it. There have been five other awards since despite the original implication that the award would not be made frequently.

no one at the meeting seemed to remember that.] Dr. Hanlon said that they had anticipated this and nevertheless had been told that the saving would only be $1,000 or $1,500 [that is what is now done]. Warfield M. Firor, of Baltimore, who was President in 1964, suggested that the matter was too important to be rushed through after only brief discussion, and recommended that it be carried over to the Second Executive Session, and that at the very least, the *Transactions* should contain the titles of the papers with reference to the volume of the *Annals* in which they appeared. Loyal Davis, of Chicago, who was President in 1957, asked ". . . if this suggestion of Dr. Kirklin's has been considered by the Council, and is it a recommendation of the Council, or has the Council not considered this matter?" President Wangensteen said that it had indeed been discussed at Council the day before and at the January meeting and reminded the Association that "30-odd years ago, when Dr. Evarts Graham appointed a committee, a very knowledgeable committee consisting of Dr. Poole as chairman and Dr. Wilder Penfield, Dr. Churchill, Dr. Phemister and Dr. Harvey

Stone, they recommended that the *Transactions* be discontinued." Wangensteen indicated that there was a financial problem and that ". . . nothing really will be lost, and what we will preserve is vital in the *Transactions,* excluding the papers and the discussion." Joel W. Baker, of Seattle [who had been a Fellow since 1951; Loyal Davis had been a Fellow since 1933; W. L. Firor had been a Fellow since 1937; Claude E. Welch had been a Fellow since 1951], said "Mr. President, I was never so aware of the generation gap as I am now. I am old enough to honor tradition. I would hate to see this great surgical organization be the first to abandon the *Transactions.* I feel that having the *Transactions* at hand for reference and exploration and re-reading is very important. Therefore, despite opening myself to the criticism of being resistant to change, I would strongly urge you not to give up this tradition without further thought." "President Wangensteen: How much are you willing to contribute?" "Dr. Baker: I think that the organization looks pretty well fed to me, and this is just a mark of $20,000 a year of inflation. I don't think we can resist inflation, and I

THE RECIPIENTS OF THE MEDALLION FOR DISTINGUISHED SERVICE TO SURGERY.

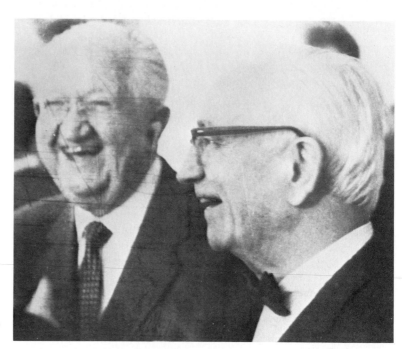

Lester R. Dragstedt, Medallion 1969, with Owen H. Wangensteen, Medallion 1970. (see also page 954, 1950 Dragstedt, and page 1283, 1969, Wangensteen).
   Photograph courtesy of H. T. Bahnson, M.D., Pittsburgh, Pa.)

Robert E. Gross, Medallion 1973. 1905—, M.D. Harvard 1931, training Peter Bent Brigham and Children's Hospital, where he spent his entire professional life ultimately becoming Ladd Professor of Children's Surgery and Surgeon-in-Chief of the Children's Hospital, 1945 until 1964 when he became Cardiovascular Surgeon-in-Chief, retiring in 1972. Made innumerable contributions to general pediatric surgery,- either solving problems previously hopeless,- Gross' operation for omphalocele,- or improving procedures and achieving the best results in the largest series to date in innumerable conditions. His world's first successful ligation of a patent ductus and second, after Crafoord, correction of coarctation of the aorta established interest in cardiac surgery. He developed the field and moved rapidly with it into open heart work, beginning with his atrial well technique for open but blind closure of atrial septal defects. His own work made a massive contribution to cardiac surgery and many profited by visits or training with him. A quiet, reserved man, intense in his work, he could demonstrate a coldness and aloofness which hurt and puzzled, but his trainees in Pediatric Surgery filled most of the positions available in the country for the young specialty, brought to respectability and prominence by his predecessor, Ladd and himself. The Ladd and Gross 1941 *Abdominal Surgery of Infancy and Childhood* and Gross' 1953 *Surgery of Infancy and Childhood* remain timeless classics.

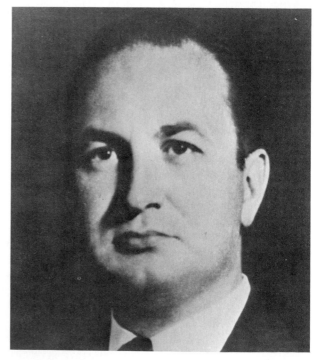

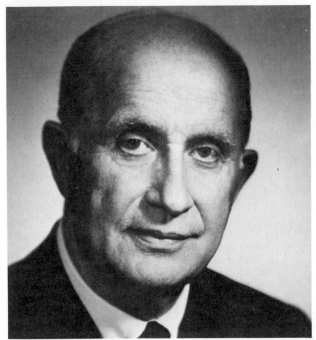

Robert M. Zollinger, Medallion 1977. 1903—, President 1965, and of the American College of Surgeons 1962, M.D. Ohio State University 1927. Intern, Peter Bent Brigham 1928-29; Assistant Resident and Resident, Lakeside Hospital, Cleveland 1929-32; Resident Surgeon, Peter Bent Brigham 1932-34; Instructor to Assistant Professor, Harvard University 1932-46; Professor and Chairman, Department of Surgery, Ohio State University 1946-74. Multiple contributions in general, particularly abdominal surgery, eponymically memorialized in the Zollinger-Ellison syndrome, his *Atlas of Surgery,-* originally Cutler and Zollinger,- a perennial classic. Distinguished by a quick, occasionally merciless, and often outrageous wit, he is one of those who has made a sweep not only of the presidencies of the major surgical organizations, but, as an acknowledged expert on roses, of horticultural organizations.

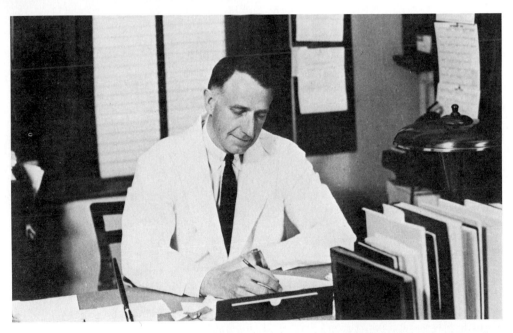

Francis D. Moore, 1913—, Medallion 1978. President 1972; M.D. Harvard 1939; Training, Massachusetts General Hospital 1939-1943; Instructor in Surgery to Assistant Professor 1943-48; Surgeon-in-Chief, Peter Bent Brigham and Moseley Professor 1948-76; Elliott Carr Cutler Professor 1976—. Established a biological laboratory at the Brigham from which have poured a steady stream of contributions to the understanding of body composition and the metabolic aspects of surgical care. His book, *The Metabolic Care of the Surgical Patient* is unique and a classic. Renal transplantation and hepatic transplantation had their beginnings in his department and renal transplantation took off there. With a wide range of scientific understanding, broad cultural interests, great articulateness, a powerful voice, and unfailing conviction, he has been an extraordinary force in American Surgery in its scientific, educational, and organizational life,- and as chairman of the Surgical Manpower Committee played a major role in SOSSUS.

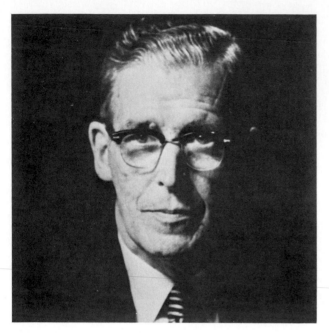

Jonathan E. Rhoads, (c. 1972) 1907—, Medallion 1979. President 1973 and of the American College of Surgeons 1971-72; M.D. Johns Hopkins 1932; House Officer Training 1932-39 and entire career at University of Pennsylvania; Professor in 1949, Provost 1956-59; John Rhea Barton Professor of Surgery and Chairman 1959-1974. Continued and deeply expanded Ravdin's interests in surgical nutrition ultimately culminating in the contribution of Dudrick and Rhoads to total parenteral nutrition. An extraordinary breadth of knowledge and interest in clinical and experimental surgery and science in general, with a talent for getting to the nub of issues. In institutional and organizational matters, thoughtful, perceptive, wise and remarkably effective,- and always expecting to be,- with an invaluable talent for seeing issues in their broadest light, while remaining intensely practical. He initiated, with Allen, Harkins, and Moyer, the first of the great, modern, multiauthor textbooks of Surgery,- *"Surgery–Principles and Practice"*

don't think the first cut in our overhead should be in our continuing education." Dr. Wangensteen attempted to close the discussion, "Thank you. We will bring up the matter again, then, on Friday morning", but the discussion continued and Leland S. McKittrick, of Boston, who had been President in 1966, rose to ". . . confess to you that I am a convert. I was one like Joel Baker, who has adamantly felt that the *Transactions* as now printed were a very intimate part of my professional life, and I didn't quite see how things would be the same without them. After having heard this discussed at length twice in the Council and having been opposed to any change a year ago, I now enthusiastically endorse the changes suggested by the Recorder . . . I really don't see any reason for printing the scientific papers a second time, when we all have them available in two volumes of the *Annals* . . . I think the *Transactions* will be more meaningful if, in addition to what they now contain, they contain the minutes of the meetings." [No further comments are recorded.]

W. Dean Warren, of Miami, for the Program Committee, announced that they had received 133 abstracts for the 33 program spots.

The report of William R. Waddell, of Denver, for the Chairman of the Advisory Membership Committee, indicated for the first time the fate of the records of applications. "As in the past with the candidates who were elected last year, and those who passed through three times without being elected, we have destroyed the records of these candidates . . .

Therefore, if a candidate is to be renominated after having been proposed previously; a completely new start must be made. A new application, new supporting letters and all other material is to be sent in as with a completely new entry."

At the Second Executive Session, the Recorder, John W. Kirklin, of Birmingham, Alabama, said that there were at least three alternatives with regard to the *Transactions,* to continue publishing them precisely as before in terms of paper and binding, but without the scientific papers except the Presidential Address, and adding the listing of the titles of the scientific papers. That would save the Association $3,500 to $4,500 annually. "A second possible course of action is a new one since Wednesday that has grown out of the suggestions of many of you, including Dr. Eloesser, Dr. Gilchrist, and others. This new proposal has the approval of your Council . . ." The *Transactions* would be published precisely as in the first proposal, but in addition the members would have the opportunity to purchase later in the year ". . . a bound volume containing all of the papers of the Annual Meeting . . ." The third alternative was to make no change. William P. Longmire, Jr., of Los Angeles, moved that the second proposal be accepted and the proposal carried.

Among the recommendations of Council was the revolutionary one that, ". . . in view of the increased size of the organization and the continuing difficulty in establishing an orderly procedure for registration and recording for attendance by Fellows and guests, consideration should be given by the Association to the advisability of wearing name badges at meetings to facilitate the conduct of the meeting." [It had, of course, long been apparent that the younger members did not know many of their seniors, and that each year the seniors knew by sight a progressively smaller number of the younger members. The polite fiction had been maintained that the Association was so small and select, of course all the Fellows knew each other. There was possibly also some feeling that the guests, who were numerous, should be marked as such. There had always been a separate Register for the Fellows. Many of the years show a signature crossed by a ruler-guided line, indicating that a visitor had inscribed his name in the Member's Register. For many years now, the Fellow's Register and the Guests' Register have been separated at the Registration desk, behind large signs, in addition to which the registration staff,- generally representing the office force of the Secretary of the Association,- have gently but clearly asked each advancing signatory whether he was a Fellow, and directed him to the appropriate book.]

For some years it had been necessary to schedule meetings long in advance, and at this 1969 meeting the dates, cities, and hotels were announced for all the meetings though 1977.

Fifty-one new candidates were proposed for consideration for the first time in 1970.

President Wangensteen announced that "The Council has asked me to make a very special announcement. They have decided to establish an award for distinguished service to surgery. In this select company there is one man very signally qualified for this recognition, Dr. Lester Reynold Dragstedt . . . A brillant investigator who has blazed trails . . . has illumined the ideology of peptic ulcer and its physiologic management. He is essentially a physiologic surgeon who has contributed richly to the development of his discipline . . . in a sense he has followed the Claude Bernard pattern of hypothesizing, and trying and establishing factual confirmation or 'disfirmation' of the theses which he has set

up." President Wangensteen asked the Fellows to approve by acclamation the recommendation of Council, which they enthusiastically did. Lester R. Dragstedt, coming forward, said only "I am overwhelmed by this gesture of friendship on your part. I cannot tell you how I appreciate it. I thank my good friend, Owen, for this tremendous statement that he has made. [And couldn't resist stating] I hope, gentlemen, that I will live long enough to see Owen do a vagotomy . . ."

Among the new Members elected were Moses Judah Folkman, of Boston; Richard R. Lower, of Richmond; John L. Ochsner, of New Orleans; Richard E. Wilson, of Boston; and Robert Zeppa, of Miami. The new officers elected were William A. Altemeier, of Cincinnati, President; Leonard D. Heaton, of Pinehurst, North Carolina [the former Surgeon General], and Robert T. Tidrick, of Iowa City, Vice-Presidents. C. R. Hanlon had accepted the post as Director of the American College of Surgeons, and was succeeded as Secretary by G. Thomas Shires, of Dallas.

[The 1969 *Transactions* are the first in which a slender separate volume contains the list of the Officers of the Association, the committees and representatives on boards, location of past meetings of the Association, Fellows of the Association, Honorary Fellows of the Association, Minutes of the meeting, the Presidential Address, and the list of papers presented, as well as the memoirs of the Fellows of the Association deceased in the previous year, and a list of all of the deceased Fellows of the Association with the dates of death. It is bound in the same brown cloth traditional with the old *Transactions,* with the Presidential seal on the front cover. The companion volume containing all of the papers presented at the meeting has imprinted on the spine, *Transactions of the American Surgical Association,* Scientific Papers. The Association was not above saving the $1,000 or $1,500 which came from using the type of the two issues of the *Annals of Surgery* in which papers appeared, using at first even the pagination of the September and October issues.]

1970s

THE NEW YORK TIMES - TUESDAY, APRIL 28, 1970 - THE SECOND DAY OF THE MEETING OF THE AMERICAN SURGICAL ASSOCIATION IN WHITE SULPHUR SPRINGS, WEST VIRGINIA

The war in Indochina continued and had been deliberately extended to Cambodia; the Supreme Court agreed to rule on an abortion case; John Lindsay was Mayor of New York and applying a job freeze, but excluded the Sanitation Department; the era of student revolts in colleges was nearing an end; Hunter College cracked down, and the Yale University Law School student body voted against a student strike in sympathy with the Black Panthers.

The New York Times

LATE CITY EDITION

Weather: Mostly sunny, warm today;
Cloudy tonight, Fair, warm tomorrow.
Temp. range: today 77-54; Monday
73-60. Full U.S. report on Page 82.

VOL. CXIX..No.41,002   © 1970 The New York Times Company   NEW YORK, TUESDAY, APRIL 28, 1970   10 CENTS

POLICE 'JOB ACTION' IS DUE TOMORROW IN WAGE DISPUTE

City Gets Injunction as the P.B.A. Asserts Sick Calls Will Keep 80% Off Job

PACT BREAKING CHARGED

Raise for Sergeants Without One for Patrolmen Called Ratio Clause Violation

By EMANUEL PERLMUTTER

The Patrolmen's Benevolent Association announced yesterday that beginning at 12:01 A.M. tomorrow four-fifths of the 25,000 patrolmen on the force would call in sick and refuse to report for duty.

The city obtained a court order last night banning the threatened mass sick call by patrolmen, but it was not immediately clear whether it would be obeyed. The order, returnable Thursday, was signed by State Supreme Court Justice George M. Carney at his home in Manhattan.

Edward J. Kiernan, president of the P.B.A., said the sick call was being started because the city had violated its contract with the patrolmen by giving police sergeants a raise without giving the patrolmen more money.

He said that he and other officers of the P.B.A. were prepared to go to jail because of the patrolmen's job action. The state's Taylor Law prohibits strikes, work stoppages and slow-downs by public employes.

4,000 to Stay Home

Mr. Kiernan said that of the approximately 6,000 patrolmen scheduled to report at 12:01 A.M. tomorrow 4,000 would stay home. He said the sick absence ratio would be maintained on the 8 A.M. to 4 P.M. tour and the 4 P.M. to midnight tour, he added.

The P.B.A. staged a similar job action in a contract dispute in 1968, but only 20 per cent of the patrolmen on each shift were asked to take part then.

Patrolmen also ignored that first sick-call then and showed their anger by going "by the rule book." They ended their work-rule actions after the city obtained a court order that forbade the tactic.

Mr. Kiernan said that he might be charged with a crime by his action to match pay of fire sergeants, patrolmen were entitled to $1,200 more a year, to $2,700 in their 27-month contract retroactive Oct. 1, 1968, for 25,000 patrolmen.

Continued on Page 36, Column 6

FREEZE EXEMPTS SANITATION FORCE

But All Other Jobs in City Are Affected by Embargo

By EDWARD RANZAL

The freeze quietly imposed on new jobs in February affects every agency except the Sanitation Department, a spokesman for Mayor Lindsay said yesterday.

The disclosure was made in a statement by Budget Director Frederick O.R. Hayes explaining that the job embargo affected "only the unfilled positions and the Sanitation Department."

Asked why Mr. Hayes had singled the Sanitation Department and had not mentioned it to other city departments, the Lindsay spokesman said:

"I guess Fred didn't get the message."

Mr. Hayes referred all questions to the Mayor's press aide, Tom Morgan.

Mr. Morgan explained that last February, when Mr. Hayes foresaw financial troubles ahead, he made several suggestions.

Continued on Page 37, Column 4

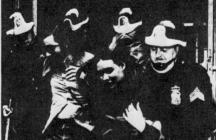

AT HUNTER COLLEGE: Police removing two of 13 persons, including a professor, arrested yesterday. Arrests followed the suspension of seven students for rest of the spring term.

11 Students, 2 Teachers Seized in Hunter Protests

By ALFONSO A. NARVAEZ

Thirteen persons, including two faculty members, were arrested at Hunter College yesterday during a day of hit-and-run disturbances by bands of dissident students. The arrests followed the announcement that seven students had been suspended for the rest of the spring term and that she would no longer tolerate "violence, force and bully tactics."

"I've drawn the line," she said at an 11 A.M. news conference at her office.

As she spoke, about 10 policemen were in the basement cafeteria of the school, at 69th Street and Lexington Avenue, quelling a disturbance by students who were helping themselves to food and who overturned a rack of dishes.

Other disturbances included the following: files in the office of the dean of students were overturned and sprayed with a fire extinguisher. Books and papers in the offices of the departments of sociology, history, English, German, political science and education were strewn across the floor.

Also, fire alarms were pulled and fire hoses were turned on, flooding the fire stairs and causing the second floor where Mrs. Wex-

Continued on Page 48, Column 1

CITY OPENS STUDY OF POLICE GRAFT

Rankin Rejects Investigation by State—Mayor Pledges Funds for Staff Inquiry

By MARTIN TOLCHIN

Corporation Counsel J. Lee Rankin yesterday rejected a call for a state investigation of charges of police corruption after presiding at the first meeting of a special committee, appointed by Mayor Lindsay to investigate the allegations.

A state investigation was urged on Sunday by Adam Walinsky, a Democratic candidate for Attorney General. Samuel S. Leibowitz, retired Supreme Court justice, said Supreme Court Justice, said that he favored investigation by a commission whose members "have no involvement with the operation of the [Police] Department or the courts or political offices."

Mr. Rankin told newsmen yesterday after the two-hour closed-door session in his 16th floor office in the Municipal Building:

"I don't think that an outside committee, having no familiarity [with the problem] could do the work with the same skill and effect required of us."

The committee was appointed by the Mayor last week after he had learned that

Continued on Page 36, Column 3

High Court to Hear Abortion Law Plea

By FRED P. GRAHAM

WASHINGTON, April 27 — The Supreme Court agreed today to consider the constitutionality of the District of Columbia's antiabortion statute, which is similar to the abortion laws in effect in most states.

By granting the Federal Government's request for a hearing, the Court entered the growing national controversy over whether abortion should be solely a matter between a woman and her physician.

The local statute, like the laws of most states, makes it a crime for a physician to perform an abortion except for therapeutic purposes that are narrowly restricted. Under the district's statute, doctors could perform abortions only when

Continued on Page 31, Column 3

STUDENTS REJECT YALE LAW STRIKE

But Many Voice 'Sympathy' for Panther Protest— Books Are Burned

By JOSEPH B. TREASTER

NEW HAVEN, April 27 — Students at the Yale University Law School voted today against suspending classes while the campus is engulfed in debate about the Black Panther trial here. In a second vote, however, the students approved giving professors and students a choice of whether to continue academic work now

Louis H. Pollak, dean of the Law School, said that it was the policy of the school to leave the choice of classroom attendance to professors and students and that the second vote had been tactical.

But many students said they wanted the votes to show that they were in "full sympathy" with an undergraduate student strike that began six days ago at Yale today.

A fire, which New Haven fire officials said had been set by an arsonist, destroyed $2,500 worth of books in the basement of the Law School Library.

President Kingman Brewster Jr. released the text of a

Continued on Page 44, Column 2

PRESIDENT WARNS U.S. COULD LOSE ARMS RACE LEAD

G.O.P. Aides in Congress Told Soviet Would Take Advantage of ABM Lag

By JOHN W. FINNEY

WASHINGTON, April 27 — President Nixon has moved to assume personal command of the fight to expand the Safeguard missile defense system by issuing a stern warning to Republican Congressional leaders that the United States is in danger of becoming militarily inferior to the Soviet Union.

The President also cautioned his Congressional lieutenants that it would be "destructive" for the United States unilaterally to halt expansion of the Safeguard antiballistic missile (ABM) system or to stop deployment of the Multiple Independently Targeted Re-entry Vehicle (MIRV) missile warheads.

Such a "unilateral moratorium," the President was reported to have argued, "would remove the incentive" for the Soviet Union to negotiate a strategic arms limitation in the arms control talks now under way in Vienna.

The President staked out his emphatic position in favor of expansion of the Safeguard system and a start on deployment of MIRV warheads on Minuteman missiles at a meeting last Thursday with Republican Congressional leaders.

Permission to Quote

It was the first time that the President had raised the ABM issue with the Congressional leaders since the proposed expansion of the ABM system in January.

That he was intending to convey the Administration line of attack on the Safeguard arms opposition in the Senate was evident from the fact that he gave the Congressional leaders permission to quote his statements.

From the President's statements as well as from recent speeches by Defense Secretary Melvin R. Laird and Dr. John S. Foster, Director of Defense Research and Engineering, it is becoming apparent that the thrust of the Administration's argument will be to emphasize the growing Soviet strategic threat and thus the necessity for the United States to act to protect its ability to deter or deal with nuclear attack.

The implication of the President's statements at the Congressional briefing was that if the Soviet strategic build-up continued, the United States

Continued on Page 8, Column 1

Indochina Leftists Pledge Mutual Help Against U.S.

Sihanouk and Representatives of Hanoi, Vietcong and Pathet Lao Confer— They Urge a Stepped-Up Fight

By TILLMAN DURDIN
Special to The New York Times

HONG KONG, April 27 — Prince Norodom Sihanouk, the deposed Chief of State of Cambodia, and Communist and other leftist leaders of North Vietnam, Laos and South Vietnam have pledged mutual support in their fight against the United States and other forces that oppose them in Indochina.

A Hanoi radio report received here today said that, on the initiative of Prince Sihanouk, the four groups met last Friday and Saturday "in a locality of the Lao-Vietnam-China area" for what was described as a summit conference of the Indochinese people.

The groups adopted a 2,000-word declaration that denounced the United States as an "imperialist aggressor" bent on prolonging and widening the war in Indochina and called on the peoples of Vietnam, Cambodia and Laos to "step up the fight against the common enemy — American imperialism and its lackeys in the three countries—until total victory."

Hsinhua, the Chinese Communist press agency, gave the text of the declaration this evening.

While the declaration affirmed the support of each delegation for the cause of the others, it notably did not report any decisions about common action or the establishment of a permanent agency for common action.

The conference followed

Continued on Page 4, Column 3

Profits of G.M. and Ford Down Sharply in Quarter

By JERRY M. FLINT
Special to The New York Times

DETROIT, April 27 — The nation's two largest automobile makers, the General Motors Corporation and the Ford Motor Company, announced today that their profits slumped sharply in the first three months of this year.

The profit drop is another sign of the sputtering in the nation's economy that has hurt the auto industry.

The reports of lower profits from the two—last week the

Stock Market Plunges

The stock market plunged yesterday to its lowest level since the assassination of President Kennedy on Nov. 22, 1963. Under the pressure of reduced corporate profits, economic uncertainty and tensions abroad, the Dow-Jones industrial average fell 12.14 points to 735.14. Details on Page 61

third biggest car maker, the Chrysler Corporation, said it lost $29.4-million in the first quarter — come as the United Automobile Workers is readying its new contract demands. The union's president, Walter P. Reuther, has said that the industry's troubles would not mean a softer tone toward Detroit, a sign of strike potential this fall.

The reports by the two companies also showed sharp employment reductions and lower weekly pay for those on the job, and even a drop in taxes to the Government.

G.M.'s net income fell 33 per

Continued on Page 58, Column 5

ALLEN TO STEP UP INTEGRATION FIGHT

Seems to Go Beyond Nixon's Stand on de Facto and de Jure School Practices

By DONALD JANSON
Special to The New York Times

WASHINGTON, April 27 — James E. Allen Jr., United States Commissioner of Education, took a stand today for desegregation that appeared to go substantially beyond that of President Nixon and his Secretary of Health, Education and Welfare.

The former Education Commissioner for the State of New York said in a statement: "In the position of national leadership which I occupy, I shall continue to emphasize the educational value of integration and the educational deprivation of segregation regardless of cause."

This appeared to put the Commissioner in opposition to all segregation, both de facto and de jure.

In a policy statement March 24, the President pledged to

Continued on Page 44, Column 1

KEY SENATE UNIT OPPOSES SENDING CAMBODIA ARMS

Decision Is Still Pending on the Request, Rogers Tells Fulbright Committee

ITS STAND IS BIPARTISAN

Soviet Opposes Indonesian Call for Parley on the New Crisis in Southeast Asia

Special to The New York Times

WASHINGTON, April 27 — The Nixon Administration encountered nearly unanimous bipartisan opposition in the Senate Foreign Relations Committee today to the extension of military aid to Cambodia.

Secretary of State William P. Rogers told the committee that the Administration had made no decision on the urgent request of the Government of Premier Lon Nol for military aid running into hundreds of millions of dollars. But he suggested that the executive branch had authority to send at least limited amounts of military equipment without seeking Congressional approval.

Mr. Rogers appeared before the committee in closed session for two hours and 15 minutes to discuss the crisis in Cambodia, where the Vietnamese Communists are on the attack, and to obtain the committee's advice on whether to provide military aid.

[The Soviet Union expressed opposition to the convening of an international conference to deal with the crisis in Cambodia. Authoritative articles in both Pravda, the Communist party newspaper, and Izvestia, the Government paper, criticized Indonesian efforts to organize an Asian regional meeting on the situation.]

Nixon Cancels Appointments

President Nixon, meanwhile, continued to ponder his decision on the aid—a decision widely regarded on Capitol Hill as a fateful one. A meeting of the National Security Council scheduled for today was postponed until tomorrow and the President canceled several appointments so he could confer on the Cambodian crisis.

In the Senate hearings, the advice to the Administration, not unexpectedly, was negative, but what was surprising to the committee members was the virtually unanimous and bipartisan nature of the opposition.

Senator J. W. Fulbright, committee chairman, told reporters after the meeting that the committee members were "virtually unanimous" and "very firmly" against "sending any military assistance under the present circumstances alluded to by the Secretary."

The opposition came not only from Democrats but also from such senior Republicans as Senator George D. Aiken of Vermont and Senator John J. Williams of Delaware, both of whom have refused to support

Continued on Page 5, Column 1

19 Youths Arrested With 40 Bombs Here

By FRANK J. PRIAL

The police raided a basement club at 517 West 134th Street last night and seized more than 40 homemade bombs. Nineteen teen-agers, who, the police said, were making the bombs in production-fashion for use in a gang war, were taken into custody.

Charged with possession of bombs at the West 126th Street police station were 15 boys and 4 girls, most of them under 16 years old. All were of Puerto Rican, Dominican or Cuban extraction, the police said, and were members of a gang called The Royal Aces.

The police said the bombs apparently were to be used in a fight with a rival gang called The Saints. The Saints were said to be situated uptown near West 163d

Continued on Page 38, Column 1

Kienast Quintuplets, Calm in Spite of Chaotic Atmosphere, Taken to Their Jersey Home

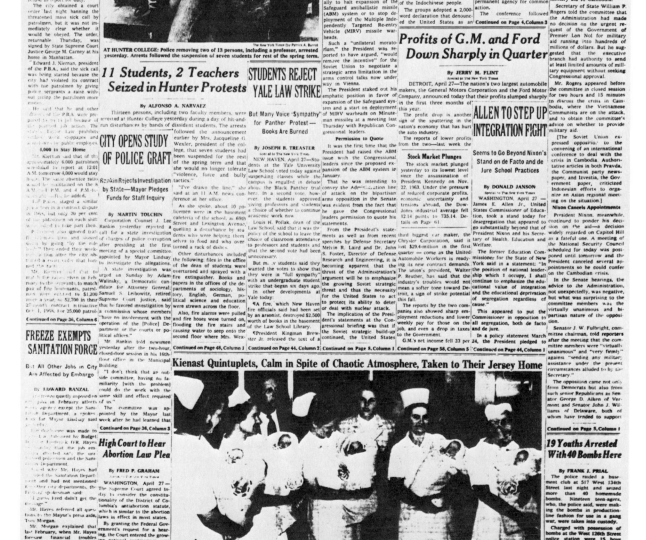

Mr. and Mrs. William G. Kienast at Babies Hospital with nurses holding the quintuplets, from the left: Edward, Abigail, William Gordon, Sarah, Amy

By DEIRDRE CARMODY
Special to The New York Times

LIBERTY CORNER, N. J., April 27 — Five healthy and remarkably composed quintuplets, wrapped in blankets and strapped into car seats, came home today by ambulance under police escort with their parents, Mr. and

Mrs. William G. Kienast.

The infants were given a send-off in the lobby of Babies Hospital at Broadway and 167th Street, Manhattan, at 11:30 A.M. by 40 newsmen who shoved, pushed and yelled to each other in confusion under the strong lights for television cameras.

An hour and a half later, the infants arrived at their 100-year-old farmhouse here. The not yet completed addition and were greeted by their 4-year-old sister, the 20-month-old brother and more newsmen, who marched all over the lawn.

The babies, who will be

nine weeks old tomorrow, never once uttered a cry. They slept, wrinkled their faces, stretched their fingers out of the blankets and yawned. Several times they opened their eyes and looked as if they were staring with great interest, if not understanding, at the performance.

It was as if they had inherited the calm that seemed to be shared by both their parents and even their sister, Meg, and their brother, John, who did not appear to be in the least perturbed by the commotion attending the ar-

Continued on Page 24, Column 4

LXXXVIII

1970

The 1970 meeting was held at The Greenbrier, White Sulphur Springs, West Virginia, April 27, 28, and 29, President William A. Altemeier, of Cincinnati, Christian R. Holmes Professor and Chairman, Department of Surgery, University of Cincinnati; Director of Surgical Service, Cincinnati General Hospital; Surgeon-in-Chief, Christian R. Holmes Hospital and Cincinnati Children's Hospital, in the Chair. Among those who had died in the preceding year were the salty Ralph F. Bowers, of Memphis, Herbert Conway, of New York, and Frederick L. Reichert, of San Francisco.

In his Address, *Crisis and Apathy,* the President identified ". . . many problems which are producing great confusion and seriously affecting our efforts . . . those which seem to be of the greatest significance include the following: 1. Student unrest and militancy. 2. Internal disruptions within universities which threaten academic independence and demand radical changes in teaching and faculty orientation. 3. General unrest of the public and its growing interest in the delivery of health services and the development of 'corrective' changes. 4. Growing political and economic pressures from Government. 5. Inflation and its effects on the hospital environment and the practice of surgery. 6. Critical shortages of professional and supporting personnel needed for the expanding demands of medical and surgical practice. 7. Rising incidence of malpractice claims and the spiraling cost of malpractice insurance." Altemeier

chose to concentrate on four of the problems: "Student Unrest and Militancy" [which had been at its height in the late 60's and involved "sit ins", takeovers of administrative offices, destruction of equipment, and a cult of dress and appearance which ran to oddments of old and tattered clothing, long hair, and beards, in which,- it seemed to the faculty at least,- soap and water had been rejected along with civility, neatness and conventional dress. One recalls the possibly apocryphal exchange between two deans, "How are your students?" "Revolting."] Altemeier appreciated that "urgent problems related to national defense and the continuing demands of World War II, the Korean War, and the Vietnam War, found their way to American universities for solution. This trend has seemed to lead progressively to growing student turmoil which appeared to be related primarily to concern over the war in Vietnam, its mortality and propriety in relation to University function, its threat to their future, and its cost in manpower and money needed for the solution of other demanding problems of society in the United States. In addition, many American students have professed to be worried by problems peculiar to our society such as the disruption of city life, racial problems, the persisting inequality of opportunity, the destruction of their natural heritage, the need for 'community medicine,' and the rapidity of growth of crime as a major industry." The "university students have frequently rioted in the streets and within our universities, and with considerable destructiveness." Equally, he deplored "Internal Disruptions Within Universities". Altemeier was concerned about the future of sponsored research which had been so magnificently productive. [President Lyndon Johnson had urged that research be "relevant" and there had been some resultant pressure for what university faculties perceived as "applied research". President Richard Nixon had been making a deliberate effort to cut the costs of medical research both by decreasing the funds available for research and by abandoning the system of training grants, the result of which was calculated to be a decrease in the number of scientists who would press for research support. Mark M. Ravitch reporting to the Association concerning the meeting of the National Society for Medical Research, had chosen not to tell the Association for publication, although Dr. Visscher's remarks had been made in what was essentially a public forum and to a large audience, that Maurice B. Visscher, of the University of Minnesota, President of the National Society for Medical Research had said that he had just returned from a meeting in Washington at which it was announced that the Administration, seeking to decrease expenditures for medical research, had concluded that the most effective way was to decrease the number of investigators and had adopted the calculated plan of eliminating training grants and thus the entry into medical research of scholars who would need and want the research funds. In fact, the government had implemented this policy, and training programs in the various fields of medicine were being phased out. At the First Executive Session at this 1970 meeting, William Holden representing the American Surgical Association at the Council of Academic Societies of the Association of American Medical Colleges, reported that the 1971 federal budget provided for training grants and fellowships ". . . amounts which are slightly below the fiscal year 1970 level, which in turn is about 10% below the fiscal year 1969 level. The reduction in intramural training programs for fiscal year 1970—a reduction of $18 million below the 1969 figure—necessitates looking at training objectives and goals realistically. The reductions in the 1970 budget will require a reduction in the number of trainees and programs. In order to protect the training environment during this period of fiscal constraints, the fellowships program necessarily must absorb a proportionately heavier share of the reduction." The general research support grants were also to be cut by 20%, 19 clinical research centers were being phased out. Dr. Holden concluded "The immediate future is dismal. A blue ribbon

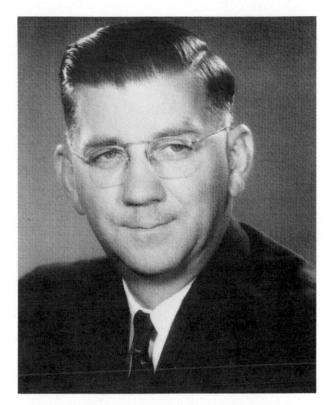

William A. Altemeier (c. 1956) 1910- . Secretary 1958-64, President 1970 [and of the American College of Surgeons 1978]. M.D. Cincinnati, Internship Cincinnati General Hospital, Residency, Ford Hospital. Returned to the University of Cincinnati in 1940 and succeeded Mont R. Reid as Christian R. Holmes Professor of Surgery and Chairman of the Department, in 1952. Major contributor to surgical bacteriology and the role of antibiotics. Maintained the discipline of the Heuer-Reid surgical school to the extent that in a multi-institutional wound infection study the infection rate at Cincinnati was the lowest, and the records adjudged the best.

committee has to be formed from within the membership of the Council of Academic Societies to study this matter in depth. Please note that surgery is represented by Dr. Gerald Austen."] Altemeier said "The recent withdrawal during the past 2 years of 30 to 50 percent of Federal research funds has created a crisis which, added to the demands of expanded health programs under Medicare, is producing chaos in our university hospitals and faculties. It would seem imperative that we find an adequate way of financing our universities and at the same time maintain their academic freedom. Otherwise, there is great risk of their being destroyed by inflation and the rising resentment against the Vietnam war." Shortness of faculty and staff might well result from "reorientation of clinical faculty members toward health service delivery in the hospital and in the community, with less emphasis on research and education . . ." The third problem Altemeier chose to concentrate upon was "Critical Shortages of Professional and Supporting Personnel." It was generally advertised "that a medical manpower shortage of 50,000 doctors currently exists in the United States . . ." However, the physician population ratio had increased steadily from 1940 to 1970 and the ratio of surgeons to population had increased even more. He felt, therefore, that the shortages ". . . are not related primarily to the number of licensed physicians and certified general surgeons . . . the shortages appear to be related more to the geographic location and function of physicians and surgeons in medicine . . . the concentration of physicians in metropolitan and suburban areas, their involvement in specialty practice, industry, or the Vietnam War, and their non-participation in clinical practice with involvement in medical administration, public health, or research activities not directly concerned with the personal delivery of patient care." As a number of Presidents before him had, Altemeier directed attention to the "critical nursing shortage which grips our hospitals today . . . probably one of our greatest problems facing the delivery of surgical care to society." This, he thought, required "that crash programs for educating sufficient numbers of nurses be undertaken with Federal financial support to meet the needs of society . . . I can see little hope of any change short of active governmental support on a major, comprehensively planned basis." The fourth problem, "Malpractice Claims and Spiraling Cost of Malpractice Insurance", he attributed to the public's having been "educated" to an exaggerated belief in the powers of medicine and of surgeons, to the system of contingency fees which encouraged lawyers to undertake malpractice suits, to outrageous jury verdicts, and to the doctrine that the surgeon was responsible for an unsatisfactory result whether negligence existed or not. President Altemeier seemed interested in the idea of the patient carrying his own insurance for untoward results of medical care. He recommended that these issues be "actively pursued by a special committee of the American Surgical Association on 'Issues in Surgery.'" [The Committee on Issues had, of course, already been recommended to the Fellowship by Jonathan E. Rhoads, in his ad hoc committee report at the First Executive Session just before the President gave his address, and obviously had been extensively discussed in Council. As so frequently happens by the time crises are finally officially recognized the answers to the crises are already being generated. Student unrest and militancy de-

creased sharply with the ending of the Vietnam War and with Watergate and Nixon's abdication, and while the academic world was not the same, by the time the Association's centennial year rolled around, a decade after Altemeier's address, student unrest and militancy, and much of their outward behavorial signs, were a thing of the past. The nursing shortage in hospitals persisted, but what had been perceived as a physician shortage had been "corrected" by increasing the output of American Medical Schools from 8,000 at the end of 1969 to 14,000 at the end of 1979, at the same time that the "population explosion" in the United States rather suddenly ceased. The statistical studies of SOSSUS, the direct result of the efforts of the Committee on Issues and of the American Surgical Association, as well as other studies, suggested that on the one hand there was possibly an overabundance of physicians by the centennial year, and that on the other hand, surgical needs were being adequately met. By the same token, for causes that were not exactly clear, "Malpractice Claims and Spiraling Cost of Malpractice Insurance" seemed not as threatening, perhaps, because of public outrage and professional indignation at the absurdity of awards and the cost of maintaining the system, causing many surgeons in California, for instance, to "go bare", carrying no insurance at all to remove the incentive for baseless suits. The assumption of insurance risks by hospitals, and societies of physicians themselves demonstrated that the premiums they had been paying had been grossly excessive. The "Internal Disruptions Within Universities" resulting from the decreased availability of research funds, the decreasing significance of endowments in view of the progressive inflation and the costs, and the increasing need for support of the medical schools by the clinical earnings of the faculty all contributed to increase the problems of the universities. Although with the ending of the Vietnam War, and the acceptance of the changed status of black Americans and of women, despite the nuisance of sometimes meaningless and burdensome regulations intended to further the resolution of the problems of race and sex, the *direction* of change was no longer challenged. The major problems within the university were those of finances, and the degree to which the university yielded to the pressures "toward health service delivery in the hospital and in the community, with less emphasis on research and education . . ."]

* * *

Robert P. Hummel and Bruce G. MacMillan, by invitation, and William A. Altemeier, the President, *Topical and Systemic Antibacterial Agents in the Treatment of Burns,* reviewed the experience at the University of Cincinnati and the Shriners Burns Unit, Cincinnati, for the previous five years. In earlier years, the incidence of staphylococcus aureus septicemia in burns had decreased with the use of antibiotics. There then emerged "a growing number of gram-negative septicemias in severely burned patients usually caused by *Pseudomonas aeruginosa",* for which a number of agents had been proposed,- silver nitrate, Sulfamylon, gentamicin, silver sulfadiazine. They had used each of these agents in some of the 354 patients included in the report. There appeared to be a lower mortality with gentamicin, "The overall mortality rate in the various groups studied ranged from 12.5% (gentamicin) to 27% (silver nitrate). When all of the variables (including age of the patient, per cent of total and third degree burns, etc.) are considered, however, the variation in mortality rate may be more apparent than real." Silver sulfadiazine allowed the earliest autogenous skin coverage,- 47-day mean, and silver nitrate the latest, 84-day mean. They had used systemic antibiotics in all of the patients, intravenous penicillin initially, then a variety of antibiotics chosen "on the basis of sensitivity studies of the patient's cultures." They concluded that "Infection continues to be the principal cause of death in patients suffering from extensive burns. Treatment of these patients with topical and systemic antibacterial agents is an important factor in the containment of burn sepsis." Their final conclusion was that "Although all of the agents were of value in containing invasive burn wound sepsis, the lowest mortality rate and the fewest complications were seen in the group treated with gentamicin ointment." Comparing their results to a previous group of patients treated with an occlusive Polysporin ointment dressing they found only that the ". . . overall mortality rate was not greatly changed but the length of time patients survived before developing fatal sepsis was much greater with the newer methods of topical therapy." Pseudomonas aeruginosa infections increased in frequency during the progress of treatment with all forms of local therapy, but perhaps least with Sulfamylon and silver sulfadiazine. Systemic gentamicin therapy had been effective in gram-negative septicemia "particularly if begun when the condition is first suspected because of positive verdo-globinuria or clinical signs and prior to obtaining positive blood cultures."

Discussion

Curtis Artz, of Charleston, South Carolina, said that indeed, ". . . tremendous advantages have been

made in the last 10 years." Sepsis was the major problem and "if you can minimize the sepsis then the body can withstand this insult and survive." He was still enthusiastic about Sulfamylon despite the pain which it caused. Although gentamicin was good, "The experience at the Grady Hospital is that almost all of the pseudomonas organisms during the past year have become resistant to gentamicin." Silver sulfadiazine, he thought, was promising but not yet established. He asked what the Cincinnati experience had been with gentamicin-resistant pseudomonas, and with vaccines. John A. Moncrief, of Charleston, [Artz and Moncrief had been successively Directors of the U.S. Army Burn Unit at Brooke General Hospital] said that at the Surgical Research Unit at Brooke, the overall incidence of sepsis had not decreased though burn wound sepsis had diminished rather markedly while pneumonia, septic phlebitis and other infections had increased. Staphylococcal infection could be controlled with systemic antibiotics. Gentamicin and Sulfamylon were the most effective agents controlling wound sepsis, because they had been "those which penetrate the wound actively in effective concentrations". He would expect that if therapy were begun late in the first week, silver nitrate would, therefore, not be effective "since the invasive sepsis is already beneath the surface of the wound and the silver nitrate does not affect those areas, whereas with gentamicin and Sulfamylon penetration in active concentration is effective and one could expect even at this late date some control of the therapy." Given the variation in the problem and the numbers of drug and treatment regimens employed by the Cincinnati group, Moncrief suggested the numbers were insufficient. He pointed out the discrepancy between the fact that, "in the Sulfamylon group the mortality rate over-all was not much less than some of the other agents, yet the incidence of burn wound sepsis with the Sulfamylon group was the smallest of any." Topical therapy had made the greatest difference in children where "prior to topical therapy . . . 35 of every 100 . . . who came in the front door of the hospital . . . died of burn wound sepsis", and asked what the Cincinnati data was with respect to age of the patients. Bruce G. MacMillan, closing, said the gentamicin resistance previously reported by Harlan Stone, from Emory, had been largely with organisms arising in their hydrotherapy unit and this had now been corrected. Their own gentamicin resistance study showed gentamicin resistance to be between 1 and 2%. He recommended the use of multiple antibiotic agents, rotated. Yeast infections, in patients surviving burns for more than a month, had recently become a problem in their unit. They had tried "a heptavalent vaccine developed by Dr. Wesley Alexander" and had lost only one of 76 patients from pseudomonas sepsis.

* * *

Folkert O. Belzer and Samuel L. Kountz, both by invitation from the Department of Surgery, University of California, San Francisco, *Preservation and Transplantation of Human Cadaver Kidneys:* A Two-Year Experience, described the use of the portable perfusion pump which Belzer had developed, employing human plasma with added mannitol and electrolytes as the perfusate in a sterile self-contained system providing pulsatile perfusion at temperatures of 8° to 10°C. The perfusion apparatus served not only to preserve the kidney but to assess its function. If the pump was set at 60 strokes per minute and the systolic pressure maintained at 60 mm., resultant venous outflow,- renal blood flow,- indicated the likelihood of success. "If the flow is 50 to 100 ml./min., the grafts can be transplanted, although postoperative tubular necrosis is possible. If renal blood flow is over 100 ml./min., the organ is satisfactory and renal function is usually excellent after transplantation." In the two-year period, they had transplanted cadaver kidneys into 63 patients with preservation periods of up to 50 hours. In the first 36 patients, graft survival was 34%. In the next 22 patients, followed more briefly, graft survival was 77%. They seemed to attribute this to their having added kidney-cell typing to their conventional tissue typing. They still thought that "renal transplantation from unrelated donors probably should still be considered a research effort." Their apparatus had permitted them to assess the value of and to employ some kidneys with warm ischemia time of up to an hour because of delayed harvesting. Tissue typing could be delayed until after the kidney had been harvested and found to be suitable for transplantation. "This allows salvage of organs from donors who have died shortly after arrival in the emergency room, before the results of typing can be obtained, or, more often, are even initiated. It eliminates unnecessary typing of potential donors from whom the organs are never obtained for various reasons . . .", and, of course, it permitted kidney-cell typing. While they were studying much longer term storage, they had not found it necessary to go beyond 50 hours and in most cases, the perfusion on the apparatus was 24 to 36 hours. They provided no detailed figures.

Discussion

T. C. Moore, of Los Angeles, had used one of Belzer's machines and been impressed by it. Willard E. Goodwin, of Los Angeles, said they had no such machine, but harvested "the kidney as quickly as possible . . . get it cold, perfused and transplanted into the patient." Belzer commented to Goodwin that "we all know that the kidney is a remarkably sturdy organ." He stressed that while a good kidney taken at the moment of death could be simply cooled for up to 10 hours, their apparatus permitted not only preservation but testing of function, "We received a kidney from Oregon some time ago. After it was put on the preservation unit it did not seem to perfuse very well, so it was not used for transplantation. We subsequently discovered that the other kidney which was transplanted immediately in Portland never worked sartisfactorily either." [Belzer had mentioned earlier, as others had during renal transplantation discussions of previous meetings, that to a considerable degree a cadaver donor's two kidneys either both failed or both functioned.]

* * *

Richard C. Lillehei, of Minneapolis, Professor of Surgery, University of Minnesota Medical School; Richard L. Simmons, by invitation; John S. Najarian, Professor and Chairman, Department of Surgery, University of Minnesota; and by invitation, R. Weil, H. Uchida, J. O. Ruiz, C. M. Kjellstrand, and F. C. Goetz, *Pancreatico-Duodenal Allo-Transplantation:* Experimental and Clinical Experience, pointed out that the interest in transplantation of the pancreas in relation to diabetes was that, despite insulin, generalized vascular disease frequently progressed, involving particularly the kidney and the retina. "As a result over three quarters of juvenile-onset diabetics have significant retinopathy or nephropathy by age 30 no matter how carefully they have been managed." In considering the available techniques, they reviewed the extensive literature with transplantation of minced or sliced pancreas, and finally of the entire pancreas with vascular anastomoses either to systemic vessels or intraabdominally and with provision of porto-venous drainage. In the dog, the technique was developed of re-establishing the arterial supply and anastomosing the portal vein of the graft to the host inferior vena cava. The duodenum was taken with the pancreatic graft, the proximal end of the duodenum closed, and the distal end anastomosed into the recipient jejunum. The recipient dog underwent pancreatico-duodenectomy. With azathioprine and steroids, they

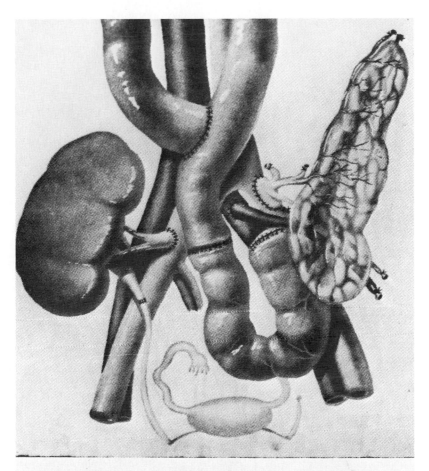

FIG. 22a. Technic used in G. M. and in
all subsequent patients.

This was the pancreatic transplantation technique employed in the last six patients, the first four having had the duodenum draining externally. The pancreas was taken together with "a cuff of donor aorta containing the celiac axis and superior mesenteric artery" and the donor portal vein was removed together with the pancreas. The graft was placed in the iliac fossa, the aortic button implanted in the iliac artery, the portal vein into the iliac vein, the proximal end of the duodenum closed and the distal end anastomosed to the host's jejunum. Nine of the ten patients had a simultaneous renal graft from the same donor. At the time of reporting, two of the patients were living five and 12 months after operation, others had survived as long as five, seven, and 12 months after operation, never requiring insulin. Rejections of the kidney graft were frequent. None were recognized in the pancreas.

Richard C. Lillehei, Richard L. Simmons, John S. Najarian, Richard Weil, Hisanori Uchida, Jose O. Ruiz, Carl M. Kjellstrand, and Frederick C. Goetz, *Pancreatico-Duodenal Allotransplantation:* Experimental and Clinical Experience. Volume LXXXVIII, 1970.

had gotten survivals up to six months, "results equal to that achieved with renal allografts in dogs". The pancreatico-duodenal grafts could be preserved "for 24 hours using combinations of hypothermia and hyperbaric oxygen" and the graft when perfused, discharged insulin from its vein, suggesting that a perfusion test might be applicable, much as employed by Belzer and Kountz for the kidney. At this point, Lillehei said, ". . . we now had a successful technique for the procedure; we could prevent rejection of the pancreatico-duodenal allograft at least as well as we could for other organs that are transplanted in the laboratory; and, finally, have dispelled the myth of the sensitivity of the pancreas to ischemia." Patients with juvenile-onset diabetes and terminal renal nephropathy appeared to justify a clinical trial of pancreatic transplantation. They had begun their clinical trials in December, 1966. After an initial failure of a partial pancreatic homograft, they had performed "pancreatico-duodenal allografts in 10 other patients and nine of these patients have simultaneously received a renal allograft from the same cadaver. Neither pancreatic fistulas nor pancreatitis has occurred in these patients." Two of the patients were still alive, one in the hospital and one out. Four were said to have died of "sepsis", the others of "acute hyperkalemia", "acute perforation graft, duodenum, with sepsis", "sepsis secondary to ATN—?? rejection", "acute necrosis" of the renal and duodenal grafts. One survivor was 12 months after operation, one five months after operation. The patients who had died had lived from one to seven months. "Almost without exception, the pancreas has functioned normally in all patients and insulin had not been required in the postoperative period. The principal problems have been associated with the cadaver kidney." They thought it "clear from these studies that the pancreas is far less antigenic than the kidney and possibly less than other organs as well. Pancreatico-duodenal allotransplantation alone is now planned for juvenile-onset diabetics who have significant but not terminal renal nephropathy. If the characteristic vascular disease of diabetes mellitus can be altered by a pancreatic allograft, then this will become one of the most commonly performed transplant procedures."

Discussion

John R. Brooks, of Boston, [to whose previous work Lillehei had referred] said they had tried pancreas fragment transplantation in patients and subsequently had "obtained long-term successful grafts of pancreatico-duodenal tissue in dogs such as seen in Dr. Lillehei's slides" but had not yet employed the technique in patients. The graft would have to survive for months or years to affect the vascular complications, it was not clear whether vascular disease was secondary or independent, and there was the interesting question whether the insulin pro-

duced by the transplant would, with time, prove to be antigenic. He mentioned that a suggestion had been made "that a small machine combining both a glucose monitoring system and insulin delivery system might be devised which a patient could carry with him, as a pacemaker or a chemotherapy infusion machine, to control accurately his blood sugar level from moment to moment during the day and particularly at night." John Connolly, at the University of California at Irvine, had six months before "placed a donor pancreas and kidney into a 32-year-old woman with juvenile diabetes, who was in terminal renal failure." In the succeeding six months, there had been three episodes of rejection of the kidney, but none of the pancreas and "Blood sugar, blood amylase and glucose tolerance tests have been repeatedly normal . . . No insulin has been given since operation and the patient has consumed unlimited amounts of sugar." They had had a large pancreatic fistula but the pancreas having been placed retroperitoneally, this ultimately closed. In the future, they planned to trim the "donor portion of duodenum down to just a tuft of bowel wall containing the ampulla of Vater and then placing a loop of jejunum alongside and using this tuft of donor duodenum as a side patch." Lillehei, closing, said that "It was John Brooks' summary of endocrine organ transplantation in 1959 which first aroused our interest in pancreatic transplantation." He did not know whether the insulin would be antigenic. They were working on the artificial pancreas idea. They had had no fistulae. He agreed with Connolly that it would be well to have as small a bulk of duodenum in the transplant as possible.

* * *

T. E. Starzl, of Denver, Professor of Surgery, University of Colorado School of Medicine; Chief of Surgery, Denver Veterans Administration Hospital, and 11 associates, *Long-Term Survival after Renal Transplantation in Humans:* (With Special Reference to Histocompatibility Matching, Thymectomy, Homograft Glomerulonephritis, Heterologous ALG, and Recipient Malignancy, presented their report on 189 patients "given kidney homografts at a remote enough time to permit relatively long follow-up in the event of continued survival." From the fall of 1962 to March, 1964, they employed azathioprine and prednisone and no tissue typing. From October, 1964 to 1966, they typed lymphocyte antigens (HL-A System) and selected the best donor. In Series 3, they added horse antilymphocyte globulin (ALG) and continued tissue typing, without accepting a poor match as a contraindication. "In all three eras of our experience, the majority of the recipients of related kidneys derived long lasting benefits with one-year survival rates in Series 1, 2, and 3 of 67%, 68%, and 92% . . . With follow-ups of 2 to 7-1/2 years in these familial cases, 91 of the 131 consecutive patients (69.5%) are living and 88 (67.2%) of the originally transplanted homografts are still functioning." Degree of consanguinity was not significant, but "With non-related donors (both volunteer and cadaveric) the salvage of life and the degree of social and vocational rehabilitation were less gratifying." There had been a striking improvement in the one-year results with unrelated kidneys. Two out of three died in their early group, whereas in their third group, only three out of 17 died in the first year. Late survival was much poorer than with familial kidneys, 33% at one to seven years, and three of those as a result of a second transplantation. After a year or more, renal biopsies showed glomerulonephritis in almost three-quarters of the kidneys, interpreted as a result of "slow rejection mediated primarily by humoral antibodies." This type of glomerulonephritis, seen in kidneys in which the original disease was not of autoimmune etiology, occurred less commonly with good histocompatibility matching. Thymectomy before transplantation, in 46 patients, had not proved to give superior results. Ten of the 189 patients,- 5.3%,- had developed carcinoma or mesenchymal malignancy and they had accumulated reports of 27 other cases from other institutions, so that "an increased risk of neoplasia is yet another penalty for chronic iatrogenic immuno-suppression . . ." Eight of the ten malignancies in their patients "were cured by conventional forms of treatment; the other two died of widespread reticulum cell sarcoma." It had been anticipated that this risk would be found to exist.

Discussion

T. C. Moore, of Los Angeles, as he had the previous year, commented on the Richmond review conducted by Hume and Moore, reporting that the 49 of the 75 related living donor recipients alive then had been reduced by eight, two of the deaths being from malignancy, one of leukemia, one of lymphoma. He mentioned also the long-term risk of hepatic failure as well as tumor, "Both of these late hazards probably are related to long-term azathioprine administration . . . we must raise the question of the feasibility and desirability of substantial, gradual reduction in azathioprine administration in long-term survivals." Richard E. Wilson, of Boston, said

that they had typed all their patients but never rejected a patient because of a poor match. Living donors with an A match resulted in very good results, but B matches did no better than C or D matches and he agreed with Starzl that "this probably represents a fault in the sophistication of typing . . . we must continue to type . . . become more sophisticated . . . certainly do not believe that at the moment we have all of the antigens properly matched, nor can we for any given patient predict the exact outcome of a given kidney." Two-and-a-half years earlier, they had begun alternating patients with and without ALG for both living and cadaver donors. Thus far, there had been no differences in survival at three months, or at one year and ". . . the only thing that appears to be better in the ALG treated patients is less severe and probably fewer rejections." He agreed "completely with Dr. Starzl's points about late rejection and failure to be able to really differentiate this from chronic glomerulonephritis. The changes in these late kidneys are certainly severe, vascular in nature and are the end result of immunologic damage, be it glomerulonephritis or transplant rejection." David M. Hume, of Richmond, was "willing" to accept Starzl's figures as indicating that ALG had improved his results in the unrelated donor groups. His own results during the same period had improved without the use of ALG, "The most recent group of related living donor transplants had a functional survival at 1 year of 92%, and a survival to 3-1/2 years of 80%. This is survival of functioning grafts, not just patient survival, which is, of course, better . . . In the cadaver donor group, the 1 year survival of 19 consecutive recent cadaver donor transplants was 95%, while the 2- to 4-year survival was 53%. These figures do not greatly differ from Dr. Starzl's with ALG and illustrate the difficulty in comparing recent results with past results as a consequence of the over-all improvement in the handling of the patient, apart from the addition of ALG." The incidence of recurring nephritis was much less in his experience than Starzl indicated. Starzl, closing, said that they had indeed found "a significant incidence of liver disorders at all times postoperatively" ranging from minor crises to death from hepatic failure, two deaths occurring 18 to 25 months after renal transplant. He agreed with Hume that they needed to try controlled clinical studies with and without ALG, but "Because we are convinced of the value of ALG, we cannot in good conscience perform such studies which will have to be left to those who are more skeptical."

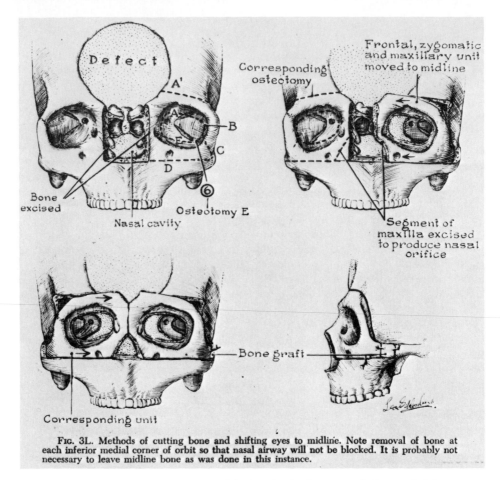

FIG. 3L. Methods of cutting bone and shifting eyes to midline. Note removal of bone at each inferior medial corner of orbit so that nasal airway will not be blocked. It is probably not necessary to leave midline bone as was done in this instance.

Drawings showing hypertelorism in a child who also had a congenital cranial defect. Portions of the maxillae were excised, the orbital assemblies isolated, and moved medially.

Milton T. Edgerton, George B. Udvarhelyi, and David L Knox, *The Surgical Correction of Ocular Hypertelorism.* Volume LXXXVIII, 1970.

* * *

A striking example of the capabilities of the combined efforts of plastic surgeons, neurosurgeons, and ophthalmic surgeons was presented by Milton P. Edgerton, Jr., of Charlottesville, Professor and Chairman, Department of Plastic Surgery, University of Virginia Medical Center; George B. Udvarhelyi [by invitation from the Division of Neurosurgery at the Johns Hopkins University], and David L. Knox, [by invitation from the Department of Ophthalmology at the Johns Hopkins University], *The Surgical Correction of Ocular Hypertelorism* [the work had been done at Hopkins before Edgerton's move to Charlottesville]. Tessier, in France, in 1967, had shown the possibilities of radical craniofacial osteotomies in re-arranging malformations and correcting hypertelorism, and Edgerton electrified the

audience at the night session with a succession of operative photographs and artist's drawings to indicate the kind of reconstructions which were possible. They had operated upon eight patients with hypertelorism and multiple and severe associated defects, all of them significantly improved "and in the four most recent instances, complete correction of the hypertelorism has resulted. There has been no operative mortality, no loss of vision, and no development of ocular palsies in these patients . . . We have had no meningitis, although spinal fluid leak has been observed at operation in several of the patients."

Discussion

Joseph E. Murray, of Boston, opened the Discussion, saying of the patients with these deformities "Previously considered beyond the possibility of

1322

therapy, these patients now have a chance for an improved outlook of living." [There seemed then, and now, not to be much justification for his hope that "Experimental intrauterine surgery is possible and neonatal surgery in the human may become feasible as a method by which these adverse growth influences may be altered following the production of these deformities".] They had been working on deformities of the same kind at the Boston Children's Hospital for a period of eight years and were enthusiastic about the results. W. Eugene Stern, of Los Angeles, suggested that, in those patients of Edgerton's who had nasal encephaloceles, a preliminary intracranial approach for that might make an appropriate first-stage. He asked what had been done about CSF leakage during the operation. He marveled at the ocular result, "You could not have done these procedures under local anesthesia and therefore, could not have asked the patient to cooperate in balancing his ocular visual axes. I am fascinated to know whether you have, in fact, been able to create patients who have binocular vision but without diplopia. Your operative procedure must bring you into the vicinity of the superior orbital fissure and once again I admire the fact that you have not caused any extra ocular palsies as a result of disturbing the function of extra ocular muscle innervation." Edgerton, closing, said to Dr. Stern that Tessier had in fact performed two-stage operations, and he, having had experience with massive reconstructions at the same stage as resections for malignant disease had been encouraged to attempt one-stage procedures. "We have had no fatal meningitis despite several postoperative spinal fluid leaks. Encouraged by these cancer resections, we have done all hypertelorism procedures as one-stage technics. Almost all patients showed spinal fluid leak in the operating room, but most of them had ceased two or three days to a week after operation. Before operation, the children developed "an alternating use of the eyes, depending on which side of the head the viewed object is located. Postoperatively, some of the children appear to fuse [their vision]—at least from a clinical standpoint . . . the eyes will track together, and we have observed this to occur as early as 5 to 6 days after operation—and without special training . . . The extra-ocular muscle unit is sometimes disturbed preoperatively and the amount of squint should be carefully measured in advance." By the same token, the children were frequently retarded and it was important to establish this before operation so that it was not attributed to the operative insult.

* * *

William H. ReMine, by invitation; James T. Priestley, of Rochester, Emeritus Staff, Mayo Clinic; Edward S. Judd, Professor of Surgery, Mayo Graduate School of Medicine; and John N. King, by invitation, *Total Pancreatectomy*, presented the results of 36 such operations performed between 1942 and 1968. Twenty-three of the operations were undertaken for carcinoma, five patients dying of the operation—21.7%. At the time of the report, four of the 18 survivors were alive and well and others had lived from two to five years. "One patient died 4-3/4 years after operation from insulin shock, and at postmortem examination, no evidence of recurrence of tumor could be found." Ten patients had a total pancreatectomy for islet-cell tumor, with one death, the second patient, of hypoglycemia and shock after operation. Two of the patients had multiple endocrine adenomas and one subsequently died of a total gastrectomy for his Zollinger-Ellison syndrome. The others were well of their symptoms. Eight of the ten patients with islet-cell tumors had had previous partial pancreatectomies without success and the eight survivors had lived five to 27-1/2 years after operation, six of them still alive and well. Three patients had had total pancreatectomy for chronic pancreatitis, all three surviving the operation. One died two-and-a-half months later from an overdose of insulin, one at home in diabetic coma and one requiring operation for a stomal ulcer ultimately died of massive gastrointestinal hemorrhage. Total pancreatectomy avoided the hazard of the pancreatico-jejunal anastomosis after the Whipple operation, "Although Howard reported 41 consecutive Whipple resections without mortality and Warren reported one death in 35 operations, such a remarkable accomplishment is far from being representative of general experience." They thought it possible that "most surgeons" might be able to perform a total pancreatectomy with a lower mortality than for the Whipple operation. They accepted the argument of Collins, Craighead and Brooks, 1966, that total pancreatectomy might be a better cancer operation, because with the Whipple operation, ". . . a new cancer may develop in the remaining portion of the pancreas . . . cancer may be left at the line of resection . . . implantation and growth of cancer cells . . . within the ductal system . . ." In addition, the surgeon could not determine by gross examination whether cancer remained at the line of resection in the Whipple procedure, "Most frequently, the so-called recurrence, which accounts for most deaths of those who survive a Whipple operation, probably is a 'persistence' of the neoplasm that was left at the line of pancreatic resection." Pancreatic insufficiency after total pancreatectomy, could be managed satisfactorily. They thought total pancreatectomy was the best operation for cancer and the results would improve when it was applied to smaller tumors than the rather large ones for which they had employed it. It was rarely indicated for hyperinsulinism, and never as a primary procedure. They were inclined to think that Child's 95% pancreatectomy should be evaluated further before any large series of total pancreatectomies for pancreatitis was undertaken. The requirement of insulin was usually "modest" but there might be "increased sensitivity to insulin. In order to avoid hypoglycemic episodes, it is probably better . . . not to be too assiduous in attempting to keep levels of blood sugar within normal range." The available substitutes for the external secretions of the pancreas were satisfactory.

Discussion

John R. Brooks, of Boston, said their 1965 review of the results with the Whipple procedure had indicated "that a new look at the treatment of cancer at the head of the pancreas was needed." Their Whipple operative mortality was 25%, a third of these due to pancreatic leakage. Forty percent of the patients had evidence of tumor left behind. The average survival was six months. They had begun then a planned program of total pancreatectomy which they had now performed 12 times with one postoperative death, two patients alive longer than two years and one patient alive four-and-a half years, seven of the 11 surviving patients outliving the Whipple operation patients. They had had no major problem with insulin replacement. George Jordan, of Houston, said that some years earlier he had collected the published reports of total pancreatectomy,- 147 patients, 113 of them for cancer and only two had survived for five years, one with a cyst adenocarcinoma, and one with a neuroblastoma. Only two patients with adenocarcinoma lived as long as two years and the mortality rate was 36%, higher than for the Whipple procedure. During the period of ReMine's low mortality for total pancreatectomy, the mortality for the Whipple procedure had dropped. Claude E. Welch, of Boston, said it was going to be hard with total pancreatectomy to reduce the mortality below that for the Whipple procedures in "the reports of Drs. Howard, Warren and others who presented long series of cases with zero mortality." It might well be that in some of the advanced cases represented in ReMine's group, total

pancreatectomy was indicated. They had not done any at the Massachusetts General Hospital.

* * *

Jesse E. Thompson, of Dallas, Clinical Professor of Surgery, University of Texas, Southwestern Medical School, and by invitation, D. J. Austin, and R. D. Patman, *Carotid Endarterectomy for Cerebrovascular Insufficiency:* Long-Term Results in 592 Patients Followed up to Thirteen Years, indicated that since the 1954 publication of Eastcott, Pickering, and Rob, it had been accepted "that 74% of patients with ischemic stroke syndromes have at least one significant stenotic lesion in the extracranial vasculature at a surgically accessible site . . . the intracranial vessels are surprisingly free of demonstrable disease . . ." and that it had become "feasible to restore cerebral blood flow by surgical means with an acceptable mortality and morbidity." In the 592 patients, they had performed 748 carotid endarterectomies with an overall operative procedure mortality of 2.7% and "In the last 6 years, using a shunt routinely and avoiding operation on acute strokes, mortality was 1.47%." In transient ischemia, the mortality was 0.77% and it was 0 for asymptomatic bruits. In patients with transient ischemia or asymptomatic bruit, operation produced transient weakness in 0.9% and permanent deficits in 2%. Of the 172 ultimate long-term deaths, only 23 were due to cerebral causes. Of the frank stroke survivors, 30% were normal and 59% improved, and of the transient ischemia survivors, 81% were normal and 16% improved. They had operated upon 65 patients for asymptomatic bruits with no mortality and subsequently two had had strokes, one mild and one severe. Twenty-four of thirty-seven "control" patients,- 65%, with asymptomatic bruit, some of whom had refused operation, "developed symptoms of transient ischemia or frank strokes." In 118 totally occluded carotid arteries, flow could be restored in 40%. They now advocated the use of an in-lying shunt when operating for incompletely occluded vessels.

Discussion

Edward A. Stemmer, of Long Beach, California, had performed 109 carotid endarterectomies, 15% of them for asymptomatic bruits. They had abandoned the use of vasopressors, as being detrimental, still used general anesthesia with hypercarbia, and preferred to use a shunt. Their single death was in a patient who died of myocardial infarction. Seventy-two percent of the patients with transient episodes were cured or markedly improved and "No patient who had undergone a so-called prophylactic endarterectomy suffered any adverse effects from operation." Charles G. Rob, of Rochester, New York [one of the originators of the procedure, when he had still been in London], asked about the asymptomatic bruit, "Operations on these patients are 'entirely prophylactic' . . . we are still worried about operating on the asymptomatic bruit, but essentially our definition of asymptomatic has changed. We have relaxed it considerably and we now feel that a symptomatic bruit is a patient with mild early forgetfulness, or early so-called senile mental changes and I believe that when you look carefully at these patients with so-called asymptomatic bruits as we do, extremely few of them are in fact asymptomatic." Jesse E. Thompson, closing, agreed with Stemmer that hypercarbia was satisfactory, but "all the published statistics to date show that it is not any better than the use of a shunt; in fact, a shunt is a bit more effective than hypercarbia alone." He repeated that 74% of the patients with cerebrovascular insufficiency syndromes had at least one operable extracranial vascular lesion and often intracranial vessels free of demonstrable disease. He emphasized "the recent work of Dr. Javid and his group in Chicago on the natural history of atheroma. They have studied patients serially with arteriograms who had lesions in the neck . . . only 38% of the lesions remain unchanged in size; 62% . . . changed as they followed them along . . . 34% of these increased in size at a rate greater than 25% per year . . . These studies . . . coincide with our own clinical observations . . . As Dr. Rob has pointed out, perhaps we are finding more of the patients with bruits who are not entirely asymptomatic and this gives us reassurance about operating on them."

The Business Meetings

The 1970 meeting was held at The Greenbrier, White Sulphur Springs, West Virginia, April 27, 28, and 29, President William A. Altemeier in the Chair.

At the First Executive Session, the Treasurer, William D. Holden said, "The savings anticipated by the reduction in the cost of publishing the *Transactions* will not be realized until next year since payments in the current year are made for the *Transactions* published in the previous year." The Association's cash assets had decreased from more than $11,000 in 1967 to less than $3,000 in 1970 and an appropriate recommendation would be made at

the Second Executive Session on the final day of the meeting. The recorder, John Kirklin, of Birmingham, said that the *Transactions* were now published in two parts, Part I containing the Minutes of the meeting, lists of Members, Fellows, Officers and the Presidential Address; Part II, "made available to the membership at $5 a copy, contains the scientific papers and their discussions presented at the 89th Meeting. The scientific papers continue to appear in the September and October issues of *Annals of Surgery.*"

W. H. Muller, of Charlottesville, Chairman of the Local Arrangements Committee, announced a very large attendance,- 565 reservations for members and wives and 94 for guests.

David C. Sabiston, of Durham, Chairman of the Advisory Membership Committee, reported that they had considered 97 candidates, 51 of them for the first time, 29 for the second time and 17 for the third time. There was a maximum of only 19 places and Sabiston commented that "These figures just presented indicate the clear need for increasing the active membership, such that at least a portion of those highly qualified candidates for whom there will not be a place this particular year, according to the Constitution and By-Laws, can be elected next year."

Jonathan E. Rhoads, Chairman of the ad hoc Committee appointed the previous year, "on the Purpose and Functions of the American Surgical Association", recommended "four innovations for the favorable consideration of the Council and the Fellows". Although the membership could not be rapidly increased in size, and should remain restricted, yet ". . . the number of academic surgeons in the United States and Canada has approximately doubled in the last 15 years". The Committee was "opposed to the multiple session type of meeting, although it would be willing for the Program Committee to have one half day for pilot programs, pilot formats and frank experimentation." Material from the specialties should be included in the program. The Committee agreed that "it is best that the Council transact most of the business of the Association. We believe the Council should feel free to hold a greater number of meetings if the business to be considered warrants it. It does not appear useful to occupy more of the time of the general sessions for business that is now allotted, nor would we recommend less for fear that this would dissociate the membership from the Association as an entity." They approved of the current system of recommendation of the names of new members to the Council for action [before the vote by the membership]. Rhoads transmitted four principal recommendations of his committee, "*I—A Committee on Issues*". There were many issues which more perfectly belonged before the American College of Surgeons and the Association of American Medical Colleges, however, examples of issues which could appropriately be "resolved or influenced" by the Association were "The fragmentation of surgery through specialization . . . The integration and coordination of undergraduate and graduate surgery . . . Core or basic surgical education prior to specialization . . . The effect of third party payments on graduate surgical education . . . The relationship of university departments of surgery to graduate educational programs in community, municipal and veterans' hospitals . . . Matching plans for the selection of residents . . . Recertification and relicensure of surgeons . . . Manpower requirements for academic surgery . . . Women and minority groups in surgery . . . The representation of academic surgery to the federal government and other organizations . . ." They anticipated that such a standing committee would require an appreciable amount of financial support which would require an increase in annual dues and perhaps special funding, "although the Association should avoid becoming beholden to the federal government or any agency." They suggested that the substance of deliberations and recommendations of the committee be presented at the annual meeting, one of the possibilities being, "A breakfast meeting of one-and-a-half to two hours, probably on the second day . . ." [the procedure which has been adopted]. Recommendation II was that as time was wanting for all the good papers proposed, the meeting could be extended to a fourth day or there could be two meetings a year and the committee recommended "that the present policy of holding one annual meeting be continued, but that consideration be given by the Council to extending this meeting whenever possible to four days" which would permit 24 additional presentations. The Committee believed "that some innovation and experimentation in developing the yearly program should be encouraged" and recommended that the Program Committee "be authorized to experiment with up to a half-day of the time assigned to the regular program and that, with approval of the Council, it be permitted to depart from the standard format", suggesting the possibility of "symposia on topics of unusual interest . . . inviting a guest speaker to deliver a lecture of particular relevance [both common in the Association's early years] . . . the presentation of a special

lecture reflecting an extraordinary accomplishment by a member of the Association." They rejected the possibility of multiple simultaneous sessions "each dealing with a topic of interest to only a portion of the membership . . . because . . . it would seriously undermine the very important object of unifying the various surgical specialty disciplines." They considered that "insufficient use has been made of honorary membership, which could bring us more closely in contact with surgery in other parts of the world", suggested exchange programs with comparable foreign organizations, and official representation of the Association at meetings of similar organizations abroad. Dr. Wangensteen had asked them to consider "the sponsorship of a triennial congress of surgical specialities." They thought that the Congress of the American College of Surgeons and the meetings of the Societé Internationale de Chirurgie and of the International Federation of Surgical Colleges made such a Congress unnecessary for the present. The report was accepted in principle and referred back to Council for implementation.

At the Second Executive Session, the recommendations of Council presented by Secretary Shires included, finally, the recommendation "That badges would be tried at this Annual Meeting. As you will note, three colors were used: white for Fellows, blue for new Members, and yellow for distinguished visitors." All past minutes of the Association were to be bound in three separate volumes [this suggestion had come from Dr. Robert Sparkman, of Dallas]. The Council recommended that "Dr. Robert Sparkman and the Secretary be given a year to attempt to enlist a sale of one hundred or more subscriptions from libraries and other agencies, thereby reducing the cost to about $135 per set [from $9,500 for six sets for the Association]." The Council did recommend the appointment of an ad hoc Committee on Issues to function for three years with a special assessment of the Fellows up to $20 per Fellow per year, the first two issues to be "the need for manpower availability and distribution including academic and community surgeons, nurses and paramedical personnel, and . . . Corrective measures for delivery of health services." The Program Committee was authorized to experiment with up to one-half day of the regular program. A registration fee of $20 was established for invited guests [others than interns and residents]. The Council recommended constitutional amendments [to lie over for action the following year], to increase the active membership from 300 to 350 Fellows, adding no more than 10 per year and limiting the Corresponding Fellows to

30 and the Honorary membership to 25. Corresponding members were to be foreign surgeons from abroad "whose scientific contributions to the discipline of surgery are comparable to those of Active Fellows of the Association." Honorary Fellows were to be "distinguished foreign surgeons whose contributions to surgery have been unusually noteworthy, of lasting value and worthy of the highest international recognition." Neither Corresponding nor Honorary Fellows would be required to pay fees or dues nor would they be privileged to vote or hold office. Council recommended the establishment of "The American Surgical Association Medallion for Scientific Achievement" to be awarded "to those individuals whose scientific contributions have been worthy of the highest recognition the Association can bestow. It is assumed that the Association will see fit to only make occasional awards of this distinction." [In fact, in 1969, at the Cincinnati meeting, President Wangensteen had announced the Council's award, and made the presentation of the Association's 'Award for Distinguished Service in Surgery' to Lester R. Dragstedt. This now proposed the regulation of the award and the creation of a medallion.] There was concern about the "federal retrenchment of research and research training grant funds" and the Council asked approval of a letter to the American Association of Medical Colleges supporting their plan to obtain information from the medical schools to present to the Federal Government, stating as well that the Association agreed with the Council of Academic Societies that an information effort with the laity and the legislators "about the problem of research support and the role of research and research training in schools of medicine" should be instituted. The Council believed "that several avenues of influence should be employed to accomplish this objective but that the single most important is direct communication with the President of the United States by individuals or agencies which have access to him." The Council also proposed informing the AAMC that "The As-

sociation believes that there can be physicians' assistants developed who can relate to the delivery of surgical care."

There was vigorous discussion of ways and means to impress the Government and the country with the needs of the medical schools and medical research, and discussion of the public image of American medicine. Francis D. Moore said the problem was "We just do not have the facts and this committee that we are discussing and this group is going to have to do much more than sit around and utter platitudes and gather bold phrases to tell the press. We do not know anything about the distribution of surgical care in this country. We do not know anything about the discontinuity of this distribution; places in which there are patients who need care and doctors who can give it, but these patients and doctors are not getting together and I believe this is a problem of our big cities, mostly, also in some rural areas. We do not know about surgical incomes which is so much faulted. We do not know what is happening in group practice and in prepayment; efforts have been made by Fellows of this Association to create an atmosphere in which the patient is not penalized financially for the nature of his disease process over which he has no control. We know practically nothing about so-called unnecessary surgery, despite the work of our beloved, former member, Dr. Coller. We all realize that public relations with the Madison Avenue approach is a terrible thing and that good public relations are only effective when they are based on facts. We must get those facts and I remember an old aphorism, 'It don't pay to advertise if you don't have the goods!. . . the 'goods' . . . are . . . the facts about the sociology of surgery and I hope the new committee will get those facts." The report of Council was approved.

The officers elected were William D. Holden, of Cleveland, President; Hartwell Harrison, of Boston, and E. S. Judd, of Rochester, Minnesota, Vice-Presidents; G. Tom Shires, of Dallas, Secretary.

LXXXIX

1971

The 1971 meeting was held at the Boca Raton Hotel and Club, Boca Raton, Florida, March 24, 25, and 26, President William D. Holden, of Cleveland, Oliver H. Payne Professor of Surgery and Director of Department of Surgery, Case Western Reserve University School of Medicine; Director of Surgery, University Hospital of Cleveland, in the Chair. Among those who had died in the preceding year were Arthur H. Blakemore, of New York, contributor in so many areas of vascular surgery and from whose laboratory had come prosthetic grafts; Edwin H. Ellison, already eponymically enshrined in history, though only 52; and Cameron Haight, who first had successfully repaired esophageal atresia and tracheoesophageal fistula in the newborn.

President Holden addressing himself to the *Dilemma of the 1970's* spoke about the "comfortable evolution in this country" of the health profession, "unencumbered by rigid non-professional controls and direction." The extraordinary development of medicine had been accompanied by a fragmentation of the profession so that "each segment of medicine has attained a degree of autonomy that encourages a disinterest, at times amounting to disdain, for what the other segments are doing, and especially for the total health care system." The profession had concentrated for the most part on the cure of disease rather than its prevention and was being "challenged by society and its governmental representatives to redefine its goals and to provide the human and material resources required to exercise as much influence upon the maintenance of health as it has upon remedial care, and to do so for all segments of soci-

ety." He spoke of the fact that ". . . the medical profession has considerable apprehension about socialistic programs for the delivery of medical care", and that the quality of professional services seemed not to be considered in such programs. He characterized "the current condition of the medical profession . . . now engaged in a conflict with society. The profession will continue to make a maximum effort to preserve its independence and capacity for self-determination. Society will make progressively greater demands for more prevention of disease, standardization of methods for delivering care, better distribution of care for all social and economic groups, and increased opportunity to participate in designing the structure of medicine." He thought it was possible in a democratic society to achieve both objectives. Whereas, ". . . observations of the incidence of malnutrition, neonatal mortality, lack of immunizations, and the advanced stages of many diseases unrecognized at a time when more effective medical care might have been provided" were taken to be the fault of the system of medical care, these were basically social and economic problems and not medical ones, ". . . Most of these problems are intrinsic to the environment in which medically indigent people reside and they will be resolved not by any dramatic change in the way medicine is practiced but by vastly improved opportunities for education, housing, and employment." Physicians could contribute to the correction of these problems as citizens no more than other citizens, and through their associations, but no more than could other associations within society. He recognized the problem of the disappearance of the guiding general practitioner, the resort to emergency departments of large hospitals because "primary physicians" were unavailable and "because of an increasing appreciation by people from all social levels of the capability of a general hospital to provide whatever professional and material resources are required to contend with an acute illness", but, apart from improvement in the organization of emergency services, made no recommendation. As for numbers, while not accepting the figure generally bandied about of a deficit of 50,000 physicians in the country, he suggested that even if that many new physicians were available, unless their distribution within the specialties met actual needs, the problems would not be solved and that therefore, the medical profession must obtain the needed facts "about the quality, quantity, and distribution of service now provided" and within the profession there needed to be developed "some mechanism . . . to exercise some form of incentive, guidance, or even control" to achieve a reasonable balance and distribution of professional capability. The medical profession needed to be vigorously involved in the planning of national health programs. It was unfortunate that the medical profession had been repeatedly put in the position of responding defensively to proposals by the government. He attributed this to the "lack of acceptance of a communal objective" by the various specialties and interests within the medical profession, citing as an example close to home the rivalries among the specialties of surgery within a medical school. He seemed to despair of the possibility of a united national effort by the medical profession short of its being dragooned into government service under "an arbitrary federal system of delivering health care", referring to "The events that have taken place in the Province of Quebec within the past year" [where the Provincial government had struck consternation into the medical profession by assuming great powers over the practice of medicine and the remuneration of physicians which had been met with what was in essence a strike of the physicians, and the departure of numbers of them for other provinces or other countries, particularly the United States, and with, of course, the eventual success of the Provincial government, imposing its will]. Since he saw no hope that the entire medical profession of the United States would move concertedly, in a way which would have "society's best interests in mind and which can act voluntarily and effectively for the entire health care system", he was pleased that the surgical profession, represented by the American Surgical Association

and American College of Surgeons in the SOSSUS, had undertaken to "evaluate the potential for improvement in the organization and delivery of surgical services to the people of the United States so as to assure that surgical needs will be met in an efficient and effective manner whereby all individuals will have these services available and accessible, and whereby the surgical profession will be able to maintain a high level of quality in the delivery of those services." He said quite rightly that the study "represents a new era in professionalism in that a large segment of the medical profession has acquired a social conscience, is mature and secure enough to subject itself to a probing self-analysis, is committed to examining the results of the study in the best interests of the public and is sufficiently responsible to make rational changes for improvement."

* * *

Eli Wayne, Robert E. Miller, both by invitation, and Ben Eiseman, of Denver, Professor of Surgery, University of Colorado Medical School, *Duodenal Obstruction by the Superior Mesenteric Artery in Bedridden Combat Casualties,* while subscribing to the general skepticism "as to the frequency with which an overlying superior mesenteric artery . . . causes symptomatic duodenal obstruction in an ambulatory patient" documented the syndrome in five soldiers injured in Vietnam, sustaining massive weight loss,- 55 to 80 pounds. They described in graphic terms the anatomical features involved, "The duodenum is immobilized by its retroperitoneal attachments and lies wedged within the mouth of an anatomic scissors. The hinge is the origin of the SMA from the aorta. The posterior jaw is the aorta and the vertebral bodies (L2, L3) . . . Normally, the jaws of this scissors are kept open by a generous fat pad providing a wide angle between the aorta and the SMA." With massive weight loss, such as in their combat casualty patients, the angle between the SMA and the aorta was sharply decreased. The effect of posture was to open the angle when the patient was erect, leaning forward, or prone, and to decrease the angle in a patient normally recumbent. By feeding the patients prone or in the left lateral position, they were able to overcome the obstruction, eliminate the vomiting and permit the patients to regain their weight. The first patient of the five had been treated, also successfully, simply by duodeno-jejunostomy, first suggested by Bloodgood in 1907. Eiseman and his colleagues studiously avoided any comment about the occurrence of arteriomesenteric ileus in other situations than that of massive weight loss in the patient confined to bed.

Discussion

Basil Pruitt, of the Brooke Hospital Army Burn Center, San Antonio, said that they had seen the syndrome in 17 patients with severe burns. Fluoroscopic studies suggested to them that in most patients, barium passed best "in the left lateral decubitus, rather than in the prone position." In some patients complicating features of the patient's illness, inability to maintain position required for relief, etc., had led to corrective operation. T. J. Whelan, Jr., of Washington, D.C., at Tripler General Hospital, in Hawaii, and in Okinawa, had seen the syndrome in wounded men "associated with extreme weight loss . . . the development of duodenal obstruction aggravates the symptoms". He was a little concerned about the explanation of the angle of the SMA with the aorta, ". . . this angle varies considerably from one individual to another. I would wonder whether or not there is any evidence that, after recovery from this syndrome, the angle is any wider or any greater than it was when it was measured by aortogram when the patient was symptomatic . . ." Eiseman, closing, answered that in fact they had "not performed lateral aortography after successful treatment to see whether restoration of body fat changed the aortic-SMA angle" and agreed that this ought to be done. Whether, as General Whelan had suggested, individuals with narrow SMA angles were particularly prone to the sequence of events that he had described, he did not know.

* * *

James A. DeWeese, of Rochester, New York, Professor of Surgery, University of Rochester, School of Medicine, and Charles G. Rob, Professor of Surgery, Chairman, Department of Surgery, University of Rochester, School of Medicine, *Autogenous Venous Bypass Grafts Five Years Later,* had come by 1957 to the use of autogenous veins as the preferred material for bypass grafts after the early disappointing experience with arterial homografts which tended to thrombose or to become aneurysmal, after the unsatisfactory results with synthetic grafts, the laboratory demonstration by themselves and others that autogenous vein grafts were superior to arterial grafts, and the clinical work of Kunlin, in France [1949], and of Linton, in the United States [1962], "that autogenous veins could be successfully used as long femoro-popliteal bypass grafts." They presented their analysis of "103 consecutive patients with 113 grafts who were operated on more than 5 years ago." Seventy-two percent of the patients were

between the ages of 50 and 70, 35 patients had known arteriosclerotic heart disease, 25 of the patients were diabetic, 30 of the patients had hypertension. The operations were undertaken for intermittent claudication in 46, rest pain 26, gangrene or non-healing ulcers in 41. The patient's own, excised, and reversed saphenous vein was employed with end-to-side anastomosis to the arteries. There were three hospital deaths, 31 deaths within two years of the operation, and at the end of five years, 54 of the patients,- 52%,- were alive. Two of the in-hospital deaths and 26 others, for a total of 26%, were from myocardial infarctions, seven patients died of other arteriosclerotic complications,—stroke, mesenteric artery occlusion, etc., and 14 of a variety of causes. If operation had been undertaken for claudication, the five-year mortality rate was reduced from the 48% overall to 26%. For rest pain, the five-year mortality was 42%; for patients in whom the operation was undertaken for gangrene the five-year mortality was 76%. The mortality in patients with arteriosclerotic heart disease was 71%, in the others it was 35%. Mortality in the diabetics was 80%; 37% in the non-diabetics. All of the 14 patients who had both diabetes and arteriosclerotic heart disease were dead within five years, nine of them within two years. Fifteen of the total developed symptoms requiring operation or amputation in the opposite limb. There were 54 patients alive five years after operation, 32 had a bypass graft patent in at least one extremity but in 22 the grafts were occluded. The patency rate was 76% at one month, 60% at the time of death or five years after operation. Percentage of patency varied with the indication for operation just as had the mortality, the indications of claudication, rest pain, and gangrene having been accompanied respectively by patency rates of 72%, 62%, and 46%. The patency rate was better for bypasses from the common femoral artery to the popliteal above the knee than from the superficial femoral to the popliteal below the knee and was substantially better if two or three of the major lower leg vessels were patent on the preoperative arteriogram. Forty-five of the grafts were known to have thrombosed,- eight times following infection. Three patients were shown by arteriography to have small aneurysms which did not progress and required no operation. They were particularly pleased at their clinical, arteriographic and histologic studies indicating "that veins are very satisfactory arterial replacements". They noted "thickening of all three layers of the vessel wall, primarily due to fibrous tissue, and the preservation of smooth muscle and most elastic fibers" with very little in the way of dilatation or aneurysm formation.

Discussion

George C. Morris, of Houston, introducing himself as "a 15-year veteran of the saphenous autograft procedure" made the surprising statement that "With practically no exceptions, the only long-term degenerative changes [aneurysmal dilatation] in these grafts have been seen in children . . . For this reason, in children, I believe the hypogastric artery is the autogenous reconstructive material of choice . . . to substitute for a right renal artery." Arteriographically, repeated studies showed what he called "the arterialization that typically takes place in these venous autografts." He predicted "that in 10 years in this Association we will be hearing reports of arteriosclerosis occurring in vein grafts in increasing numbers . . ." W. Andrew Dale, of Nashville [who had been associated with DeWeese in the 1959 report], emphasized the importance of placing the distal anastomosis to the usually better vessel below the knee. He demonstrated that with returning ischemic changes, in the face of a pulsating graft, arteriography could show a remediable thrombosis in the distal end of the graft. Emerick Szilagyi, of Detroit, said that "in all the carefully followed, larger series of reconstructive procedures on the femoropopliteal trunk utilizing autogenous vein grafts, the results are remarkably similar and relatively stable. The overall, immediate patency rate is about 70 to 80%, and the yearly postoperative attrition of patency is about 3%, giving a 5-year patency rate of about 65 to 70%." In his own 183 cases, followed five years or more, the late success rate was 68% which, given the advanced cases in his material, he considered satisfactory. "Homologous arteries have a patency rate at 5 years of about 20%, and the Dacron prostheses about 10%." Seventy percent of the failures were ultimately due to primary thrombosis of the graft and he thought that his routine follow-up arteriograms showed local lesions which it might be possible to correct before thrombosis occurred. D. W. Gordon Murray, of Toronto, reminded the Association that he had, in 1930 [in discussion of McCune and Blades, Volume LXIX, 1951], presented before the Association "the use of autogenous vein grafts to replace arteries" and he was interested to see, after a period of enthusiasm for plastic prostheses "a return to the autogenous vein . . . I have seen within the last year one man who had a vein graft in his popliteal artery, a young man with an injured artery. Thirty-eight years later it functions well. Another vein graft placed in the femoral artery of a young man, still functions well. He went through the Second World War, and his vessel withstood the stress

of military work . . . another vein graft in the brachial artery has survived 34 years . . . I am suggesting that the veins have the possibility of survival." James A. DeWeese, closing, agreed with Morris "that we are going to see some degenerative changes in venous grafts." He thought they had found "less evidence that arteriosclerosis progresses in the vein grafts than is seen in the rest of the body . . ."

* * *

B. T. Williams, S. Sancho-Fornos, D. B. Clarke, L. D. Abrams, all by invitation, and Worthington G. Schenk, Jr., of Buffalo, Professor and Acting Chairman, Department of Surgery, State University of New York, *Continuous, Long-Term Measurement of Cardiac Output after Open-Heart Surgery,* had developed an electromagnetic flowmeter which could be "positioned around the ascending aorta at operation, the cable emerging to the exterior through the second intercostal space" for continuous recording, and permitting ultimate removal "by gentle traction on the protruding cable." They stated that hitherto postoperative monitoring had been "restricted to pressure measurements or their derivatives" whereas the aortic root pulsatile flow signal permitted the derivation of cardiac work, of stroke work, and cardiac output. The electronic instrumentation with which it was combined permitted the display of Starling curves of the left ventricle. Flowmeter measurements were much more reliable and consistent than pressure measurements through catheters. In any case, arterial pressure measurements reflected both changes in peripheral resistance and in cardiac output. Dilution techniques for measurement of cardiac output were subject to errors, particularly in low-flow states and, at best, could be used only intermittently. "Conversely the electromagnetic flow meter not only provides a continuous display of the mean cardiac output, but also a pulsatile flow trace, from which many parameters of cardiac function may be derived using relatively simple electronic equipment." The extractable flow probe had been previously reported by B. T. Williams, C. Barefoot, and W. G. Schenk, Jr. [1969].

Discussion

Frank C. Spencer, of New York, opening the Discussion, said that "For over a decade we have used a technic of monitoring, originally developed at Johns Hopkins, in which a catheter is left in the pulmonary artery after operation and withdrawn 1–3 days later. Through this catheter blood can be sampled for periodic determinations of mixed venous

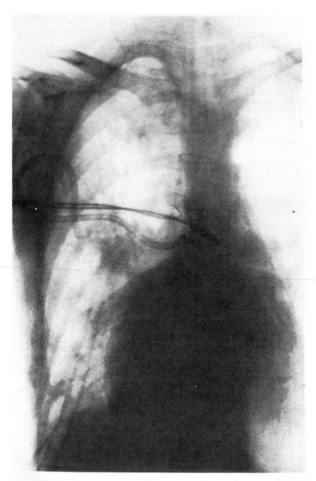

FIG. 2. Chest x-ray of patient shows position of probe around ascending aorta.

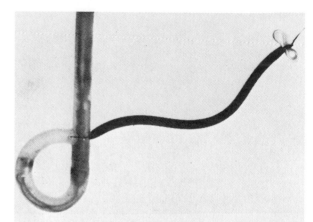

FIG. 3. Probe shows method of fixation around the aorta using a nylon snare.

Worthington G. Schenk, Jr., and his associates had employed the removable flowmeter in 20 patients for up to eight days of postoperative monitoring. The probe was bent to lie around the aorta and was removed by pulling upon the end emerging from the chest. There had been no complications.

Bryn T. Williams, S. Sancho-Fornos, D. B. Clarke, L. D. Abrams, and Worthington G. Schenk, Jr., *Continuous, Long-Term Measurement of Cardiac Output after Open-Heart Surgery.* Volume LXXXIX, 1971.

oxygen saturation, an index of efficacy of oxygen transport . . . the oxygen saturation is a valuable guide for indicating adequacy of oxygen transport, and has been a routine part of postoperative management of patients following open-heart surgery for several years." He agreed that the importance of knowing the cardiac output was so great that it would be good if there were a ready method for determining cardiac output continuously, but "My only question regards a potential complication which has not been reported to date. What does one do when repeated traction on the pacemaker does not remove it from the chest? Pull harder, and for how long?" Russell M. Nelson, of Salt Lake City, said that they had experience "with approximately 5,000 cases of continuous monitoring of cardiac output by an indwelling small Teflon catheter introduced percutaneously (retrograde) in the radial artery at the wrist. This catheter has a 1 mm. outside diameter and is 100 cm. in length; it is introduced up to the level of the origin of the subclavian artery from the aorta . . . we can withdraw blood gas samples when desired, and otherwise have it connected to a strain gauge transducer, measure the area under the pulse pressure curve, and heart rate and provide this information into the computer. This gives us a continuous monitoring of the cardiac output, as well as stroke volume and other parameters which we have indeed found very useful, as Dr. Williams has suggested." Williams, closing, said that thus far they had had no difficulty in extracting the probe and "the longer the probe remains in, the easier it is to extract, because it has become surrounded by a nice smooth tunnel." Spencer's oxygen saturations for estimation of cardiac output provided only isolated readings. Nelson's technique of arterial catheterization "may give results which one could question in low flow states, and certainly, as far as I know, there is no good way of accurately calibrating this technic in absolute terms." The flowmeter "represents a degree of monitoring precision hitherto unobtainable . . . by providing a pulsatile aortic flow trace, many sophisticated indices of cardiac function may be easily derived, and such a system may be very easily incorporated into a computerized postoperative management system, such as practiced by Dr. Kirklin, for example."

* * *

L. J. Humphrey, C. Barker, C. Bokesch, D. Fetter, J. R. Amerson, and O. R. Boehm, all by invitation, from the Department of Surgery, Emory University School of Medicine, *Immunologic Competence of Regional Lymph Nodes in Patients with Mammary Cancer,* noted that McWhirter had proposed leaving the lymph nodes after simple mastectomy and radiation therapy, that Crile's "plea has been to save the regional lymph nodes and remove only the mammary cancer" and that animal studies had suggested "that tumor memory resides in the regional lymph nodes . . . removal of these lymph nodes decreases host resistance and enchances recurrence and/or dissemination of cancer." In an inbred strain of mice, a methycholanthrene-produced sarcoma, transplanted into the hind leg which was subsequently amputated, rendered the mouse immune. They studied the effect of both spleen and lymph node cells from the immune mice upon growth of the tumor cells in tissue culture and upon the transmissability of the tumor into other mice after incubation with cells from lymph nodes and spleen. The spleen cells were much more effective in reducing transplantability of the tumor than were cells from regional and distal lymph nodes. In patients, Humphrey attempted to see whether tetanus toxoid injected in the triceps muscle, with a booster dose four weeks after operation,- radical mastectomy or simple mastectomy,- would show differential results in the production of antitoxoid titers in the serum. The patient studies indicated normal immune response to tetanus toxoid of patients who had only breast biopsies for benign tumors, but failure to respond in patients not only after radical mastectomy, but after simple mastectomy for cancer as well. Humphrey had some difficulty in interpreting the data of the studies with patients.

Discussion

George Crile, Jr., of Cleveland, jumped up to respond, "I think that this paper has been put forward as though it were a challenge to some things that I have said, but I don't believe that anybody in immunology believes for a moment that any one experiment in a certain set disproves any principle . . . immunological relationships depend too much upon time, dose, and other intricate factors." He claimed that in his own experiments, the mouse tumor had been isogeneic and that he got increased numbers of

metastases when the regional nodes were removed. He questioned whether the tetanus toxoid experiments had anything to do with the regional lymph nodes in human breast cancer. He had seen "a specific inter-reaction between cancer cells in the primary tumor and the lymphocytes from axillary nodes." He thought it was "too early to write off the role of the regional node." Bernard Fisher, of Pittsburgh, agreed that Humphrey's studies showed spleen cells more effective than lymph node cells against the tumor cells. He was concerned that the removal of the cells from the organ in which they resided altered things radically and in his own experiments with a naturally occurring tumor, "we have obtained data which have provided evidence that removal of the regional nodes is of great importance in the initiation of tumor immunity", decreasing it sharply. In his preparation, removal of the regional lymph nodes before, during, or after tumor transplantation resulted in some loss of immunity but removal of the spleen had no effect. He agreed with Humphrey that "failure of a response to tetanus toxoid may possibly reflect a systemic depression rather than a single inadequacy of regional nodes." In his characteristically vigorous style, Fisher said that "as far as I am concerned, the data relative to the role of the regional lymph nodes, both experimental and clinical, fail to provide a consensus which justifies the therapeutic adventurism which is becoming so commonplace in the treatment of breast cancer." He was happy to announce "that this May we shall begin the long-planned and long-awaited clinical trial to compare the results of operations which do or do not leave axillary nodes." William Hammond, of Bethesda, Maryland, said that worrying about the regional lymph node immunity might be irrelevant because of studies which had shown "that peripheral circulating lymphocytes are quite active against the autochthonous tumor." Humphrey, closing, responded spiritedly to Crile, "Dr. Crile's statements do need some housecleaning, I feel." He thought Crile's tumor, carried in many strains, its source unknown, was in fact allogeneic.

* * *

The Fellows were visibly disturbed by the paper presented by Leslie Wise, F.R.C.S., Aubrey York Mason, F.R.C.S., Lauren V. Ackerman, from the Department of Surgery, St. Helier Hospital, London, and the Departments of Surgery and Surgical Pathology, Washington University School of Medicine, all by invitation, *Local Excision and Irradiation:* An Alternative Method for the Treatment of

Early Mammary Cancer. The patients had all been operated upon in London and the pathological material all studied by the distinguished pathologist, Lauren V. Ackerman, of St. Louis. Ninety-six patients between 1950 and 1964 with Stage I and Stage II breast cancers were treated by local excision followed by irradiation to the tumor, supraclavicular, posterior axillary, and parasternal regions, to a total dose of 6,100 rads in nine weeks. During the same period of time, 207 patients were treated by radical mastectomy with or without radiotherapy depending upon the status of the nodes, and radiotherapy given only to those with involved nodes. A variety of sophisticated statistical methods was used to construct survival curves on the basis of the observed data, the result of which was that "there was no statistically significant difference between the ultimate survival times for the local excision and radical mastectomy series." The previous studies of Adair (1943), De Winter (1961), Porritt (1963), Crile (1965), Peters (1967), had all suggested "that the simple and non-deforming operation is at least as effective as the radical one", most of the studies having included irradiation as well. In the present study, "Apparently the mode of treatment did not alter the overall prognosis. There was, however, a significant difference between the histopathological pattern of the two groups; namely, there was a significantly higher percentage of tumors with infiltrating borders in the radical mastectomy group (74%), than in the simple exicision group (54%) . . . local excision with modern irradiation may be a suitable alternative to radical mastectomy for early breast cancer. Further prospective, controlled, clinical trials would be needed, however, before this method could be advocated for general use."

Discussion

Stanley O. Hoerr, from the Cleveland Clinic, said that "For some years in carefully selected instances I have been doing local excisions for clinical Stage I cancer of the breast." The lesion had to be small, the anticipated cosmetic result pleasing ["better than an absent breast with a scar"], and the excision had to be clear of the tumor. From 1955 through 1966, he and George Crile, Jr., had performed local excision without postoperative irradiation for Stage I cancer in 31 patients "less than 10% of all surgery for this stage of mammary cancer." The five-year survival had been over 80% and the local recurrence rate less than 5%. "This has suggested to us that local excision without irradiation also may well have a place in selected instances of

favorable cancer of the breast." Oliver Cope, of Boston, said of the report that "If one looks at this extraordinary series of nearly 100 patients treated by radiation, one can see that there is an alternative to surgery, and the alternative could be very important. Dr. Hoerr is suggesting that one patient should be treated this way, and another that way. Of course, there will be improvement, not applying a single therapy to all. That alternatives may now be offered to many women will have an enormous meaning to women psychologically." George Crile, Jr., of Cleveland, said that "For nearly a century women have feared the treatment of breast cancer almost as much as the disease, and I think that when they realize that there is, perhaps, going to be a reward for reporting a lump when it is small, and that in many cases the breast can be saved, it is possible that they will come earlier to the surgeon, and the cure rate of breast cancer will actually rise." He suggested that their very high five-year survival rate of 81% with simple excision alone and no irradiation "may be related in part to the fact that we did not irradiate. I have a feeling that irradiation may have an adverse effect . . ." He expressed his own philosophy, "The next great experiment must be in the favorable cases to see what wide local excision alone can do, because you can always irradiate; or you can always remove nodes later if they become palpably involved. We are firmly convinced, on the basis of a large experience, that if one waits until nodes become palpable and then removes them surgically, or irradiates them, the results are just as good, if not even better, than if one did it prophylactically." Francis D. Moore, of Boston, said, of the fact that the patients in both of the groups studied by Dr. Wise, in London, had been irradiated, "If *both* groups were irradiated, what evidence does he have that the local excision contributed anything to their care?" He attacked Cope's "emphasis on psychological impact to the woman of losing her breast . . . There is developing psychiatric evidence that the loss of the breast may be more meaningful to the male surgeon than, often, it is to the female patient. She has usually finished nursing her children and doesn't any more think of her breast as an immensely important cosmetic or sexual symbol. Most of our patients have said quite clearly that the loss of their breast is not as important to them as is cure of the disease. They would like us to tell them what is *best for them*." Claude E. Welch, of Boston [like Cope, from the Massachusetts General Hospital, obviously disturbed by the results in some of Cope's patients and visibly seething, undoubtedly in part because of the publicity given to Cope's views in a nationally distributed women's journal], commented that "what purports often to be a local excision turns out to be a partial excision of the carcinoma. This can be exceedingly dangerous. In the past few years we have had quite a number of local excisions of carcinoma of the breast followed by irradiation in our hospital. We have had several patients who I know of personally that have returned with extensive local disease in the chest wall, a situation that is absolutely hopeless, completely incurable by any other measures, because everything else has been exhausted . . . a careful follow-up of these patients will be done and should document this impression, which has been of more importance to me than 'controlled series' which usually consider only deaths." J. Montgomery Deaver, of Philadelphia, probably expressed the die-hard feeling of some of the Fellows, "And the paper, by Dr. Wise, on simple mastectomy—I don't understand it. I don't see what it proved. Radical mastectomy in properly selected areas I feel is still the procedure of choice." L. J. Humphrey, of Atlanta, emphasized that "Radiation therapy is immunosuppressive . . . the patient who has had radiation therapy has a significantly depressed total peripheral lymphocyte count for years . . . we surgeons should not accept radiation therapy lightly . . . we need to get on with studying these patients and finding improved treatment methods, instead of trying to condone or accept the inadequate ones we have." Leslie Wise, closing, agreed with Dr. Moore that "radiotherapy had a significant role in the therapeutic effect, but in some cases it could possibly have been harmful." Their retrospective study showed that "results of lump excision with radiotherapy compared very favorably with the classical treatment of radical mastectomy, with or without radiotherapy" and urged a well-controlled prospective study.

* * *

Two papers on carcinoma of the rectum followed. George E. Block, of Chicago, Professor of Surgery, Coordinator of Clinical Oncology, University of Chicago, and by invitation, Warren E. Enker, *Survival after Operation for Rectal Carcinoma in Patients over 70 Years of Age,* noted that the electrocoagulation of malignant tumors of the rectum, first proposed by Byrne in 1889 according to A. A. Strauss, of Chicago, who had reintroduced it and vigorously championed it in 1935, was once more being proposed [see page 1235, Volume LXXXV, 1967], particularly for the treatment of carcinoma of the rectum in the elderly. They had undertaken the review of their total of 111 patients over 70 years of age, of whom 64 underwent operation for cure, 41 of

the 64 had an anterior resection with a low anastomosis and 23 had an abdominoperineal resection. There were 10 postoperative deaths in the 64 cases, a 15.2% mortality. Absolute survival of the patients with resection was 56.6% at five years, and if operative deaths were excluded, it was 67.2%. Five-year survival, relative to the longevity of a similar population, was 84% including operative mortality, and 100% if that were excluded. Reviewing the published material on local cautery excision of cancer of the rectum, they found the five-year survivals of 40.7% and 46% "far short of the result of radical operation in the elderly population." They thought there might be a place for local electrocoagulative therapy in particularly fragile elderly patients or for palliation.

* * *

John L. Madden, of New York, Director, Department of Surgery, St. Clair's Hospital and by invitation, Souhel Kandalaft, *Electrocoagulation in the Treatment of Cancer of the Rectum:* A Continuing Study, presented their further experience with the method which Madden had discussed before the Association in 1967. They now had 77 patients, over half of them were alive and well for an average of four years. Four patients were alive with disease, 16 had died of disease and three more had died of other causes but with disease present. In patients whom they judged inoperable by conventional means, their failure rate was 60% as opposed to 23% in "operable" patients. Nevertheless, in the "inoperable" patients, five,- 20%,- were alive and well for an average of 49 months and five more had died of other causes without evidence of disease, one of them more than five years after fulguration. Madden had had no treatment deaths in his 77 patients, but had 22 complications in the 77 patients, 28.5%,- bleeding in 17, severe in seven. Four patients had had repeated episodes of bleeding. The peritoneal cavity had been perforated in two patients, a rectovaginal fistula had occurred in two. One patient had a nonfatal pulmonary embolism. He suggested that in the hands of highly skilled surgeons, the operative mortality for abdominoperineal resection varied from 2.4 to 8.5%, that in some hospitals it was as high as 17% and that "12.0% would be a fair estimate for the average mortality rate throughout the United States." His results with electrocoagulation in the patients with what he considered to be operable lesions,- 24 patients with a 66% cancer-free survival for four years or longer and 54% of the total number of the patients available for an absolute four-year survival,- persuaded him that "the results of electrocoagulation are at least equal to and in many respects superior to abdominoperineal resection in the treatment of cancer of the rectum."

Discussion

George Crile, Jr., of Cleveland, said that he had learned about rectal cancer from Tom Jones, who had performed electrocoagulation in selected patients and Crile had continued to employ the technique. In patients considered potentially operable, excluding cancers in polyps and villous tumors with cancerous changes in them, including only invasive carcinomas "The only selection was towards polypoid form", there was an 89% five-year survival in 19 patients and "None died of cancer in less than 5 years." Five patients required abdominoperineal resection for failure of coagulation and four of them "were cured by this procedure". He made the interesting statement that "Patients who did not undergo combined abdomino-perineal resection did not develop carcinomatosis, and none of the patients who died of cancer in the entire coagulated group ever had pelvic pain" [the implication being that palliation by electrocoagulation did not disseminate tumor as an operative resection did]. William Hammond, of Bethesda, said they had been led by the reports of electrocoagulation on rectal cancers to wonder whether "there is something different in the tumor-host relationship when a large mass of tumor has been killed promptly and left *in situ* . . ." They found destruction of tumor left *in situ,* whether by cryosurgery or by ligation of blood supply just as significant to subsequent immunity, whereas there was none when the tumor was sharply excised, "the killing of the tumor *in situ* by some mechanical means (whether it be infarction, hyper- or hypothermal insult) and leaving it *in situ* to be absorbed rather strikingly affects the immunologic component of the tumor-host relationship . . . it might be more productive to think and work in this area than to engage in a polemic between electrocoagulation and abdominal-perineal resection." J. Englebert Dunphy said that this was exactly what A. A. Strauss, of Chicago, had maintained. His own experience was smaller than Madden's and had been similar, "I think this is the ideal treatment for a superficial, exophytic lesion in the older patient." The lesion had to be at 10 cm. or less, which would restrict the number of patients to whom it was applicable. They had had no significant bleeding, "It may be that we have been picking rather favorable cases." R. K. Gilchrist, of Chicago, [with his long interest in carcinoma of the rectum and colon, lymph node studies, and his attachment to the traditional concept of cancer surgery] took vigorous issue with Madden "It is

very dangerous for this prestigious group to propose that this operation is now satisfactory as primary treatment, since in the punched-out lesions that are not polypoid at least 60% having involved nodes which will not be reached by cautery. This may be acceptable as an experiment; otherwise, I think we are setting a dangerous example . . . the large polypoid lesion is a very favorable lesion no matter what you do, because they seldom have early metastases to the nodes." He did not understand how Madden could have described some of the patients treated by electrocautery as inoperable since 20% of them were reported to have been cured by electrocautery. "This is remarkable . . . After the end of an operation for cancer it is said, 'This is incurable,' . . . the patient is alive after any kind of procedure, you are obviously going to have a cure rate much higher than is the true state." George Block, in closing, said "a patient should not be considered for less than a curative operation, just because that patient happens to be aged," but for the particularly poor risks, electrocoagulation might be acceptable. John L. Madden, closing, agreed that his results were identical with Crile's and that like Crile, he had found that "if electrocoagulation fails, you can always do an abdominoperineal resection . . . one should not persist in treating these patients by electrocoagulation beyond . . . 6 months. If the lesion does not respond during that time, abdominoperineal resection is advised." He responded to Dunphy that compared to the complication rate of abdominoperineal resection, his complication rate for electrocoagulation was low. He referred to "the recent study of Grinnel . . . that whenever the nodes about the inferior mesenteric artery are invaded, the disease has spread elsewhere and the patient is absolutely incurable. In his series of 19 patients who had metastases to the nodes about the inferior mesenteric artery, none were cured. All of them died of disease." Madden warned Hammond against "transferring the results in experimental models, the rat, to the human which is most dangerous. I have never seen clinically any evidence of an autoimmune response in the treatment of the rectal cancer by electrocoagulation" [without stating what evidence might have been seen].

* * *

John L. Sawyers, of Nashville, Professor of Surgery, Vanderbilt University; Chief of Surgery, Nashville Metropolitan General Hospital, and H. William Scott, Jr., Professor of Surgery and Head of Department of Surgery, Vanderbilt University School of Medicine, *Selective Gastric Vagotomy with Antrec-*

0

tomy or Pyloroplasty, impressed by the "enthusiastic reports" of Harkins,- 1963, Griffith,- 1966, Burge,- 1964 with the selective gastric vagotomy originally described by Jackson, 1948, and Franksson, 1948, had undertaken a prospective randomized clinical trial comparing truncal and selective vagotomy in 145 patients. Although ". . . the clinical results of truncal and selective gastric vagotomy in this group of patients indicated little significant difference",- 93% of good to excellent results with truncal vagotomy and 96% with selective gastric vagotomy,- ". . . there was a highly significant difference in the effectiveness of the two procedures in achieving vagal denervation of the stomach". The Hollander insulin test indicated incomplete vagotomy in 19% of the patients with truncal vagotomy, and in only one of 42 patients with selective vagotomy. They found the alleged metabolic and other advantages of the selective gastric vagotomy to be "much less impressive and in no way statistically significant." In 2,150 patients with truncal vagotomy and antrectomy, they had had good to excellent results in 94%, a 0.7% ulcer recurrence rate but in the difficult cases such as those with massive bleeding and operations in poor-risk elderly patients, there was a mortality of 2%. Weinberg, in his series of 1,129 patients with truncal vagotomy and pyloroplasty had had good to excellent results in 91.5% with a 0.5% mortality and a recurrence rate of 4.5%. Others had reported an even higher recurrence rate after truncal vagotomy and pyloroplasty and this Sawyers and Scott thought to be due in most cases to incomplete vagotomy and perhaps due to antral stasis and stimulation of gastrin production in others. The failure rate of truncal vagotomy could be decreased by selective vagotomy and the gastric retention following pyloroplasty could be eliminated by antrectomy. For four years, they had been comparing patients with selective gastric vagotomy who had had either an antral resection or a pyloroplasty by either the Finney or Jaboulay techniques. There were 79 patients in the study, followed 12 to 45 months. Evidence thus far was "that selective gastric vagotomy and pyloroplasty affords patients an equally good clinical result as selective gastric vagotomy and antrectomy. This is contrary to our past experience of superior clinical benefits from truncal vagotomy and antrectomy compared to truncal vagotomy and pyloroplasty in the surgical treatment of duodenal ulcer."

Discussion

Lloyd Nyhus, of Chicago, interpreted the results as meaning that "the margin of error is de-creased when selective vagotomy is performed; decreased, I believe, by the meticulous dissection of the vagal fibers. Thus antrectomy may not be necessary to obtain a low recurrent ulcer rate, as had previously been thought." Lester R. Dragstedt, of Gainesville, was "very pleased to have heard this paper. It is a good demonstration of the value of a prospective randomized study . . . if the vagotomy is complete in the duodenal ulcer patient and the drainage procedure adequate to prevent stasis of food in the gastric antrum, resection of the antrum makes no contribution to the operation . . . In my early experience with vagotomy incomplete nerve resection was the chief cause of failure. Later failures were usually due to an inadequate drainage procedure. Removal of the antrum will often make an incomplete vagotomy satisfactory because of the potentiation between the nervous and hormonal phases of secretion." Dragstedt [now 78 years of age] continued, "I am pleased that selective vagotomy has proved to be a practical operation in the hands of many surgeons. I am disappointed, however, that attempts to deprive the parietal cells of vagus innervation while preserving the vagus innervation of the antrum have so far not eliminated the need for a drainage operation [the first reference in the *Transactions* to parietal cell vagotomy]. Perhaps more work needs to be done in this area, as my son, Lester, II, has assured me that many of the duodenal ulcer patients upon whom I did a simple vagotomy in the early days have remained entirely well." Jack M. Farris, of Los Angeles, had performed some "Eighty-odd selective vagotomies" with pyloroplasty and had been unable to see any advantage. Paul H. Jordan, Jr., of Houston, was looking for something other than the paradoxical claim that "selective vagotomy with pyloroplasty is a more efficient operation in the prevention of recurrent ulcer than is truncal vagotomy and pyloroplasty . . . because . . . meticulous efforts required to perform selective vagotomy . . . more likely to result in an adequate vagotomy than truncal vagotomy." He was more inclined to believe that it might be that truncal vagotomy, affecting the duodenum, decreased the production of secretin, one of the functions of which was to inhibit the secretion of gastrin. Sawyers, closing, appeared willing to accept Jordan's suggestion as another reason for preferring selective gastric vagotomy although still believing that its chief virtue was the completeness of the gastric denervation.

* * *

The Question of Bile Regurgitation as a Cause of Gastric Ulcer, Lester R. Dragstedt, of Gainesville,

Research Professor of Surgery and Professor of Physiology, University of Florida; Edward R. Woodward, Professor and Head, Department of Surgery, University of Florida, and by invitation, T. Seito, J. Isaza, R. Rodriguez and R. Samiian, essayed to respond to the suggestions of DuPlessis, Capper, Schrager, that "regurgitation of bile and pancreatic juice into the stomach occurs in a large proportion of gastric ulcer patients . . . these patients regularly display varying degrees of gastritis in addition to the ulcer." When, in the modified McCann-Schmilinsky procedure, the duodenal, biliary, and pancreatic secretion was emptied into the corpus of the stomach rather than in the antrum, ulcers were not produced either in the stomach or at the gastroduodenostomy, whether vagotomy or an antral resection was done or not. If the duodenal loop into which the bile and pancreatic secretion emptied was anastomosed to the esophagus, ulcers developed and perforated,- if the preparation had transplanted all of the duodenum. If the distal duodenum was still anastomosed with the pylorus, no ulcers developed, presumably because the outpouring of gastric juices into this portion of the duodenum had inhibited the secretion of acid. They concluded that in the Schmilinsky-McCann operation, jejunal ulcers were produced in the efferent loop because of "Hypersecretion of gastric juice due to absence of the duodenal brake of gastric secretion" which normally cancelled out the neutralization of the gastric acid by the alkaline duodenal secretions. In other preparations, so long as there was access of gastric juice to duodenal mucosa, ulcers were not produced. In all of their experience, "The formation of ulcers at the efferent stoma where there is contact with the acid gastric contents and not in the esophagus or stomach where there is contact with bile and pancreatic juice suggest that the latter are relatively impotent as ulcerogenic agents."

Discussion

D. Walford Gillison, of Chicago, from the laboratories of Lloyd Nyhus, reported that they had consistently produced esophagitis in monkeys with chronic esophagogastric reflux, after an operation in which all of the bile was diverted into the stomach. William Silen, of Boston, disagreed with Dragstedt because "it has been clearly shown in our own laboratory and that of Dr. Horace Davenport and others that bile salts and pancreatic enzymes such as phospholipase A will disrupt the gastric mucosal barrier to hydrogen ion" and he suggested that in Dragstedt's experiment the gastric juice might have been

sufficiently alkaline so that ulceration would not have occurred despite the disruption of the mucosal barrier. Were measurements of gastric pH made throughout the experiments? Owen H. Wangensteen, of Minneapolis [one remembers that he walked into the room, as he went to the platform, commenting that he regretted not having heard the presentation], took the opportunity to remark that "What a great day it was for surgery when Dallas Phemister persuaded the budding young physiologist, Lester Dragstedt, to become a surgeon. I would like to express the hope and belief that some day there will be enough relaxation among surgical boards to provide the opportunity for academically minded surgical aspirants to spend considerable time in the laboratory . . . when that practice becomes the rule in University surgical clinics, we shall certainly continue to lead the world in the academic surgical area. Basic training in research must continue to be an important ingredient in the training of future surgical academicians." He did, in fact, quite directly say "Unfortunately, I did not have the opportunity to hear your paper, Lester, but I heard you say, finally, that acid peptic juice is much more important than bile, pancreatic juice, and succus entericus in the production of gastritis, with which suggestion, I agree completely. However, I did read your abstract." Wangensteen then went into details of the work of Schmilinsky and of Frank Mann and of McCann [which are discussed in detail in Dragstedt's published paper], discussed the experience which he and Richard Varco had had in performing the operation on three patients, after laboratory experiments in animals,- with disastrous results in two of the three patients, a neostomal ulcer in one and massive hemorrhagic gastritis in another. In 1951, Wangensteen and Fred Cross had anastomosed the proximal duodeno-jejunal loop into the dog esophagus, one of the procedures by Dragstedt and Woodward, and had produced esophageal erosion and substantial bleeding. René Menguy, too, Wangensteen said, had demonstrated that in "the canine antrum, even when completely isolated from the stomach . . . bile and pancreatic juice can corrode the antral mucosa." He concluded by saying that "while agreeing completely with Dr. Dragstedt over the importance of acid peptic juice in the genesis of manifestations of the peptic ulcer diathesis, I submit we must be mindful that bile and pancreatic juice *per se* also can erode the esophagus and produce neostomal ulcer and even diffuse hemorrhagic gastritis when refluxed into the stomach." J. Lynwood Herrington, Jr., of Nashville, discussed the clinical problem of gastric ulcer. Local excision with vagotomy, and pyloroplasty had shown strikingly disparate results, published recurrence rates running from 3 to 38%. He now employed distal gastric resection with added vagotomy because "we have noted recurrent ulceration following gastric resection alone, without vagotomy, for treatment of benign gastric ulcer." The recurrence rate after gastrectomy for benign gastric ulcer without vagotomy was 2.5%. Dragstedt, closing, said that gastroenterostomy for the treatment of peptic ulcer was abandoned because of the occurrence of gastrojejunal ulcers but it was not noticed at first that gastrojejunal ulcers did not occur after gastroenterostomy for gastric ulcers. He was pleased that Dr. Wangensteen had discussed his paper particularly because of his work in the field and his early recognition of Schmilinsky's work. Dragstedt appeared to agree that "The gastric ulcer that Wangensteen and Cross observed after diversion of bile and pancreatic juice into the stomach seemed to support the view of DuPlessis and Capper that regurgitated bile is the cause of gastric ulcer." For gastric ulcer "The beneficial effect of antrum resection (the Kelling-Madlener operation) on high-lying gastric ulcers left *in situ* is readily accounted for by the concept that these ulcers are of gastrin origin."

* * *

H. William Scott, Jr., of Nashville, Professor of Surgery and Head of the Department of Surgery, Vanderbilt University School of Medicine, and by invitation, H. H. Sandstead, A. B. Brill, H. Burko, and R. K. Younger, *Experience with a New Technic of Intestinal Bypass in the Treatment of Morbid Obesity,* had four years earlier begun to study the effect of the Payne-DeWind [1969] intestinal bypass implanting the proximal 14 inches of the jejunum into the terminal ileum four inches from the ileocecal valve. Metabolic studies indicated "that weight loss resulted chiefly from malabsorption of fat and carbohydrates; body fat appears to be the principal component of weight loss." Five of the patients had had unsatisfactory weight loss and this had been attributed to reflux into the bypassed bowel and they had since operated upon 12 patients anastomosing the proximal jejunum end-to-end to the terminal ileum, emptying the bypassed small bowel into either the sigmoid or transverse colon. They required of their patients a history of at least five years of massive obesity, weights two to three times ideal, with evidence of attempts at dietary control, absence of correctable endocrinopathy, an assurance of cooperation in the metabolic studies. "Pickwickian syndrome, hyperlipidemia, adult onset of diabetes, and

hypertension" were specific indications for operation. There were no deaths, weight losses had been impressive. The longest follow-up was 13 months. Diarrhea was controlled with diphenoxylate Hydrochloride—Lomotil—and had "gradually ceased to be a problem in the period of postoperative follow-up. No patient in the group has required regular medication for control of diarrhea after the first 1 to 3 months following operation." The patients showed a great increase in fecal fat excretion, a drop in serum carotene and serum cholesterol, a drop in serum triglyceride levels, and a reduction in carbohydrate absorption. The four patients with diabetic glucose tolerance curves now had normal curves. Fecal nitrogen excretion was excessive and exceeded the normal in four patients and four patients had hypoalbuminemia. Vitamin A serum levels tended to be reduced. "Despite the steatorrhea induced by the operation serum calcium, magnesium and potassium levels have remained in the normal range." Hematocrits had remained in the normal level, B_{12} and serum folate serum levels had not yet been followed long enough for any statement. All patients but one [with an 18 inch proximal segment] had satisfactory weight loss and "Further study of these patients over a longer period of time is obviously needed before this procedure can be recommended for wide clinical use."

Discussion

Richard L. Varco, of Minneapolis, rose to present his work and that of his associate, Dr. Buchwald. He agreed that the results of the "conventional jejuno-ileal 'bypass' ", the Payne operation with an end-to-side anastomosis were erratic, "due to proximal ileal loop reflux after end-to-side jejuno-ileostomy". He and Buchwald had come to the same conclusions as Scott although their interests had been chiefly in hyperlipidemic patients. The subset of arteriosclerotic lipidemic patients had elevations of cholesterol values into the 300 mg. per 100 ml. range, and were usually not obese. In them, they bypassed 200 cm. or one-third of the ileum. There was no weight loss, but a 40% reduction in the circulating cholesterol concentration because of "failure to absorb an average 60% of the exogenous and endogenous cholesterol. This shortened piece of bowel also dumps unabsorbed bile salts into the colon where they are degraded to a non-absorbable form. As a result of that breakdown in the normal enterohepatic bile salt recirculation, an excess daily loss of bile salts occurs. Since bile salts can only be synthesized from cholesterol, a second and indirect

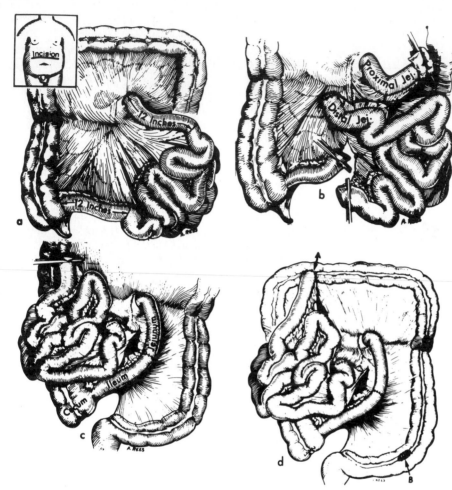

FIG. 2. Steps in a new technic of intestinal bypass for morbid obesity. Proximal end of jejunum is anastomosed to distal end of ileum. Distal jejunum is closed, sutured to mesentery. Bypassed jejunoileum is drained by anastomosis of proximal ileum to (A) transverse colon or (B) sigmoid.

Approximately 12 inches of jejunum was anastomosed end-to-end to the terminal 12 inches of ileum, the proximal end of the bypassed bowel was closed, and the distal end was implanted either into the transverse colon or to the sigmoid colon. After one year the results, in 12 patients, were satisfactory.

H. William Scott, Jr., H. H. Sandstead, A. B. Brill, H. Burko, and R. K. Younger, *Experience with a New Technic of Intestinal Bypass in the Treatment of Morbid Obesity.* Volume LXXXIX, 1971.

drain on the body cholesterol is created." There were also "catastrophically corpulent" patients with hyperlipidemia. In those they anastomosed the proximal 40 cm. of jejunum to the distal 3 or 4 cm. of ileum. It was the length of the segment of ileum retained which was significant. Edward R. Woodward, of Gainesville, had also had failures with end-to-side bypass, and subsequent good weight loss after conversion to end-to-end bypass which they had now done in six patients. Woodward asked whether Dr. Scott had had difficulty with fatty liver, "About half our patients have developed acutely fatty liver with not only hepatomegaly, but considerable temporary disturbance in liver function. This leads us to wonder a little bit about the long-term prognosis of their livers." He thought there had been less trouble with the diarrhea in the end-to-end bypass. He warned

"that this is certainly no panacea for morbid obesity. It should not be undertaken for cosmetic purposes . . . above all, don't let your enthusiastic resident staff sell this procedure to a reluctant fat person, because that patient will have intractable postoperative diarrhea." He concluded with a warning that ". . . I still have some reservations that we may be producing nutritional cirrhosis in some of these patients years later." H. William Scott, closing, said that like Varco, he was "more interested in the problem of hyperlipidemia and atherosclerosis than in the problem of obesity." In spite of the fact that he left 12 inches of terminal ileum in the alimentary stream, the cholesterol and triglycerides had fallen satisfactorily. As for the liver, biopsy before operation had shown fatty liver. Thus far they had detected no hepatomegaly after operation and had no evidence

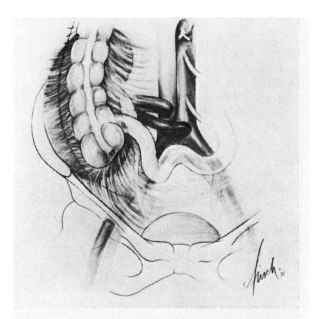

FIG. 1. Technic for transplantation of adult kidneys to infants or small children. A mid-line abdominal incision is made, both kidneys and spleen removed, the colon mobilized as shown and the anastomoses made to the aorta and vena cava or the ileac vessels. Appendectomy is performed and the colon is replaced as shown. The transplanted ureter must be placed in the retroperitoneal position.

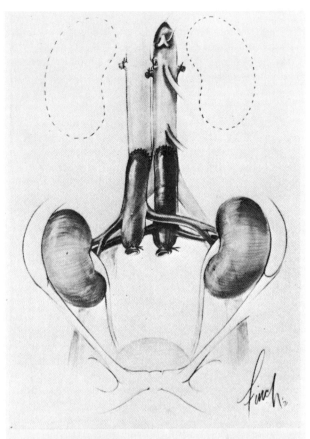

FIG. 8. Technic of transplantation of two newborn cadaver kidneys to newborn recipient. Aorta is anastomosed to aorta, and vena cava to vena cava. The kidneys are fixed by the sigmoid mesentery on the left, and the cecum on the right. The Ureters are implanted separately into the bladder by conventional tunneling technics.

In children weighing less than 20 kg., operating through a midline incision, Najarian performed splenectomy and bilateral nephrectomy at the time of transplantation. The arterial anastomosis was made to the aorta or iliac artery and the venous anastomosis to the vena cava or iliac vein. In two infants, as shown in Najarian's Figure 8, the two cadaver kidneys were removed en bloc together with segments of the vena cava and aorta, and anastomoses performed as shown [the technique reported to the Association by Reemtsma in 1964 (q.v.) for the transplantation of chimpanzee kidneys to man]. One 3 kg. infant had perfect initial renal function but died at four-and-a-half months, three months after operation, of uncontrollable rejection. The second infant, 3.9 kg. at four months, died abruptly during endotracheal suctioning on the second day after operation.

50% of the recipients of related kidneys transplanted before 1968 were well with their first transplant, and 15% with their second. Of 24 since 1968, only one had died and only one kidney had been lost. The results with cadaver kidneys were poorer.

John S. Najarian, R. L. Simmons, M. B. Tallent, C. M. Kjellstrand, T. J. Buselmeier, R. L. Verneir, and A. F. Michael, *Renal Transplantation in Infants and Children.* Volume LXXXIX, 1971.

of increasing hepatic damage. He agreed that the patients seemed to have less diarrhea than after the Payne operation. He wondered whether lipocaic, a great interest of Dr. Dragstedt's for years, might be used prophylactically "against nutritional fat accumulations in the liver of these patients."

* * *

John S. Najarian, of Minneapolis, Professor and Chairman, Department of Surgery, University of Minnesota, and by invitation, R. L. Simmons, M. B. Tallent, C. M. Kjellstrand, T. J. Buselmeier, R. L. Vernier, and A. F. Michael, *Renal Transplanta-*

tion in Infants and Children, reported their results with renal transplantation in 56 children, one to 16 years of age and two infants, in the previous eight years. In children under 20 kg., the vascular anastomoses were made to the vena cava or the common iliac vein and to the side of the aorta or the common iliac artery. They had given up peritoneal dialysis in favor of hemodialysis for all children. Most of the children in the last three years of the study had undergone bilateral nephrectomy and splenectomy, a week or two before transplantation. In the smaller children, one to 20 kg. the nephrectomy and splenectomy were carried out at the time of transplantation, except in the presence of active urinary tract infection. Prior to January, 1968, the immunosuppressive regimen "consisted of azathioprine, prednisone, Actinomycin D., and local irradiation. Since January 1968, almost all patients . . . received a 2 to 4 week course of intravenous antilymphoblast globulin (ALG)". Local irradiation of the kidney was employed only during rejection episodes. Azathioprine and prednisone were employed but not actimonycin D. The two smallest patients, weighing 3 and 3.9 kg., received transplantation of two newborn cadaver kidneys at once. The first died of uncontrollable rejection. The second died abruptly in the immediate postoperative period. He commented that Cerilli [at Ohio] had "reported a successful case of transplantation in an infant nine months who is well more than year later." Of the 24 patients transplanted before 1968, 50% of the recipients of related kidneys were well with their first transplant and 15% were well with their second transplant. Of the children receiving cadaver kidneys, 16% were well with their kidneys and 16% well with their second kidneys. "Of 24 children aged 1-16 transplanted with kidneys from related donors since 1968, only one has died, and only one has lost his kidney. Of six children aged 1-16 transplanted with cadaver donors since 1968 all are alive and five have good renal function." If the ureter was removed, patients with obstructive uropathy did as well as patients with nephritis. In four children, they had used ideal loop diversion. They thought the patients with steroid resistant nephrosis did poorly. Children grew normally after transplant but "catch up growth" was uncommon, and "Growth appears to stop several years earlier than normal in both girls and boys" irrespective of renal function or maintenance doses of steroids.

Discussion

Joseph E. Murray, of Boston, said that "It was Dr. Starzl, I believe, who first popularized the tech-

nics of kidney transplants in infants and children, and Dr. Hume who first presented a series of transplants before the Transplant Society a few years ago." He thought transplantation to children who had ileal loops was something which probably ought to be studied in a few major centers for the time being. He was concerned about the use of a young parent as the donor in families who frequently had other children. This sometimes required the parent to be away for a long period of time, and frequently presented serious family problems. Immunologically, Murray thought children should do no worse than adults and might have a better survival chance even if the cadaveric donors were used "because children have more resilient cardiovascular and pulmonary systems ." Thomas E. Starzl, of Denver, said that "For reasons that have never been very clear, the pediatric patient has been considered in many centers to be an unfavorable candidate for organ transplantation. In fact, we agree with Dr. Najarian that the pediatric patient is actually a favored recipient." Starzl had reported 20 renal transplantations in children in 1965 when 14 of the 20 patients were alive. "Today these same 14 patients are still alive, now 7 to 8 1/2 years post-transplantation, and in all but two of the 14 cases their original transplants are still functioning." He now had a total of "about 60 pediatric patients . . . all with minimum potential follow-ups at least 3 years." In their earlier experiences, particularly "in the pre-ALG days before 1966, there was often a real cessation of growth for the first year or two after transplantation or even longer. Then, as long as 4 and 5 years postoperatively, a surprising catch-up growth spurt occurred." They had seen catch up as late as 18 or 19 years of age "at which time growth of almost a foot has occurred over a year's time". He thought it was necessary to follow children at least five years or more before concluding there would not be such growth. In children, particularly, the use of ALG permitted the use of smaller doses of steroids, "an especially important factor in their social rehabilitation . . . At one time we were extremely wary of using cadaveric kidneys for pediatric patients, because of the predictable need for greater steroid doses, the consequent stunting of growth on these children, and the very real possibility that they could thereby be turned into iatrogenic pariahs." Najarian, closing, agreed with Murray about the social and economic problem involved with the use of a parent donor. The children, however, were rapidly rehabilitated, "all the children that we have done that are living and well (when you talk about survival of children, it is almost 95% survival) all but one in the school age group has returned to school . . ." He agreed with Starzl about the social effect of the Cushingoid appearance with prednisone and the beneficial effect that ALG had had in that regard. They had seen occasional catch up growth but thought it was rare even as long as seven years.

* * *

T. E. Starzl, of Denver, Professor of Surgery, University of Colorado School of Medicine, Chief of Surgery, Denver Veterans Administration Hospital, 10 others by invitation, *Immunosuppression, Liver Injury, and Hepatitis in Renal, Hepatic, and Cardiac Homograft Recipients:* With Particular Reference to the Australia Antigen, studied "the problem of hepatic damage with or without hepatitis in a large transplantation program." The question had been raised as to whether the liver malfunction which was seen was the result of a toxic reaction to the immunosuppressive agents, or of an actual hepatitis. They found "The hepatitis associated or Australia (Au) antigen . . . in the sera of almost one-fifth of a group of 89 chronic survivors after renal, hepatic, or cardiac transplantation", and two patients were found to possess anti-Au antibody. Ultimately, "28% of the studied patients had serologic evidence of having had or, more commonly, of having contact with the serum hepatitis virus . . . Once Au antigenemia developed in the immunosuppressed patient, it seldom disappeared and these organ recipients became infectious carriers." Before it had been possible to detect the Au antigen, "a number of Au positive patients were unknowingly entered into the transplantation program already infected from dialysis or blood transfusion. In turn, staff members treating these carriers frequently developed acute hepatitis and in one instance the consequence was the death of a research technician." The Au antigen was known to occur "with increased frequency in patients with a variety of natural immunologic deficiency states including Down's syndrome, leukemia, leprosy, and uremia." It had been suggested "that the virulence of hepatitis under conditions of immunosuppression is considerably less than in a normal person" because of "the coincidental prevention of autoimmune sequellae of hepatocellular injury", suggesting the possiblility of employing immunosuppressive treatment in patients with chronic aggressive hepatitis, and indeed whereas one technician had died of hepatitis none of the transplant patients had died of hepatitis itself. In a patient, dying of hepatic failure from chronic aggressive hepatitis, they had performed a hepatectomy and liver transplant and ". . .removal of the diseased organ was fol-

lowed within a few minutes by the complete disappearance of all serologic evidence of the Au antigen from the peripheral blood, indicating that the primary source feeding the antigenemia had been the liver." The hepatitis recurred "at about the same time as would have been expected with an initial exposure to virus at the time of transplantation." Thus far, the patient was surviving. A potential homograft recipient, who was Au positive, was not a prohibitive risk for transplantation but "a decision against the undertaking could be justified on the basis that the creation of a dangerous endemic hepatitis pool within the hospital is unwarranted." Starzl's unit had decided to accept such patients but to employ rigorous infectious precautions. In their unit, "The single most important identifiable source of hepatitis . . . has been pretransplantation renal hemodialysis. . ." Clearly, "Au antigen tests should also be performed on all prospective organ donors" including cadaveric donors.

Discussion

John S. Najarian, of Minneapolis, recounted the sudden increase in his unit of serum hepatitis "among hospital and laboratory personnel, transplant personnel, dialysis personnel" after performing a hepatic transplant on a patient who had "subacute hepatitis with decreasing hepatic function" after a renal transplant, and Najarian himself was one of those who developed hepatitis. In that outbreak, they recognized no increase of hepatitis in dialysis or transplant patients. He agreed with Starzl "that the ones not at risk are the dialysis patients and the transplant patients—the dialysis patients perhaps because they are immunosuppressed from their uremia, and the transplant patients, perhaps because they were immunosuppressed as well. All of us nonimmunosuppressed patients fit in this category (active hepatitis)." He asked Starzl whether "we should consider the possibility of immunosuppressing a patient who contracts hepatitis. . ." J. Garrott Allen, of Palo Alto, California, asked of the hepatitis carrier transfusion donor "How does such an individual manage to harbor the infectious agent of hepatitis . . . for so many years without himself developing evidence of liver disease?" He thought the concept of tolerance was inescapable "tolerance of the carrier for the virus and tolerance of the virus for the carrier." Patients with hypo- or agammaglobulinemia receiving multiple pooled plasma and blood transfusions did not get hepatitis. Few dialysis patients and transplantation patients die of hepatitis "but this is not true of the staff taking care of these patients . . . With a normal immune response, they slowly produce antibodies, and eventually four to eight weeks later, there is a 'confrontation' of the virus with the antibodies in the hepatic cells that leads to cellular destruction." He, too, had wondered about treating hepatitis with immunosuppressive agents. Alan G. Birch, of Boston, had reviewed the "data on 37 cases of clinical hepatitis which occurred on our dialysis and transplant unit during a 16 month span in 1969 and 1970", 14 in dialysis patients out of 150, 13 in 70 transplanted patients and 10 cases in 80 exposed staff. He agreed that "The dialysis and transplant patients have mild cases . . . whereas the cases in the staff have been far more severe clinically, and one dialysis nurse and one patient's wife had succumbed from hepatic failure." When hepatitis in the transplant patient was diagnosed, it was their policy "to decrease or discontinue Imuran . . . and we have discontinued Imuran for 20 to 380 days, for an average of 160 days, in 12 such patients." Three or four patients who had been Au positive, became Au negative in the three to six months after Imuran was discontinued. They had used no other immunosuppressive drugs but had increased the prednisone dose slightly, had seen only three episodes of rejection "in a total of 1700 days at risk off Imuran." They wondered if the deranged hepatic function or another factor might produce a protective effect. Starzl, closing, answered Dr. Najarian that he did not favor withdrawal of Imuran when serum hepatitis occurred in transplant patients. He did fear that immunosuppression would result in chronic Australia antigenemia which might have serious long-term consequences. He was inclined to think with Dr. Allen that immunosuppression might, in fact, lead to tolerance of the virus. He appeared to think that the most exciting thing about the effect of withdrawal of Imuran in the Peter Bent Brigham patients described by Birch was that it "is heartening to see in the human that the rate of continuing graft function after discontinuation [of Imuran] has been higher than that in the experimental animal, or more specifically, the dog."

* * *

Richard E. Wilson, of Boston, Associate Professor of Surgery, Harvard Medical School, and by invitation, C. L. Hampers, D. S. Bernstein, J. W. Johnson, and John P. Merrill, *Subtotal Parathyroidectomy in Chronic Renal Failure: A Seven-Year Experience in a Dialysis and Transplant Program*, reported their experience with subtotal parathyroi-dectomy in 28 patients in a period of seven years, during which 237 patients had received renal transplants. Eight of the parathyroidectomies were done before the onset of hemodialysis, 18 during hemodialysis and two after renal transplantation. All of the patients had elevated alkaline phosphatase and serum calcium although in only 19 was the serum calcium above 10.6 mg./100 ml. Renal osteodystrophy was almost invariable, radiologic changes in the bone in 24 of the 28, nephrocalcinosis in 8, metastatic soft tissue calcification in 10, and vascular calcification in 14. Four patients had duodenal ulcer. Twenty-four patients had bone and joint pain and 17 had severe itching. Nausea, vomiting, and abdominal pain were serious symptoms in four patients. Symptoms were progressive in all of the patients and commonly accompanied by a muscle weakness, which was often relieved by the subtotal parathyroidectomy. The operation involved the resection of a half to two-thirds of one gland and all of the other three. In 26 of the patients, there was chief cell hyperplasia in all glands. In one patient there was a single adenoma, the other three glands being normal. One patient who also had multiple myeloma had four normal glands. All patients but one with multiple myeloma "had virtually complete relief of their hyperparathyroid complaints." Cystic bone disease recalcified within six weeks, metastatic calcification was "often completely absent after 2 months" but vascular calcification reversed slowly, if at all. Itching and gastrointestinal symptoms were relieved within 24 hours of parathyroidectomy and bone and joint pain and pain from soft tissue calcium deposits were relieved within a week to ten days. Improvement in weakness and the return of general well being was evident in most patients. "The indications for subtotal parathyroidectomy in this series were: 1) persistent and symptomatic hypercalcemia in prospective renal transplant patients [10], 2) pathologic fractures secondary to renal osteodystrophy in uremic patients [4], 3) symptomatic hyperparathyroidism including bone pain, ectopic calcification and intractable itching in patients on chronic dialysis [12 patients], and 4) progressive and symptomatic hypercalcemia in patients with well-functioning renal transplants [2].

Discussion

David M. Hume, of Richmond, said that he was in almost complete agreement, the chief difference being that ". . .we do not have a chronic dialysis program *per se*. All of our patients on long-term dialysis are candidates for transplantation." All of his parathyroidectomies but one had been done before transplantation, much as in Wilson's series and he cautioned that "in most instances, the transplant will correct the abnormalities within 6 weeks. If the abnormalities were not corrected within this period of time, then parathyroidectomy should be done." Patients required large amounts of calcium and vitamin D after parathyroidectomy "because the patients have such severe hungry bone syndromes that they develop tetany. . ." Thomas L. Marchioro, of Seattle, said that in their series of 59 transplant patients, 18 had persistent hypercalcemia which usually disappeared within six months but in seven patients persisted as long as two years, elevated parathormone was demonstrated, and subtotal parathyroidectomy was performed. All showed parathryroid hyperplasia and had prompt falls in serum calcium. He suggested "that the most rational test to determine whether parathyroidectomy should be done is parathormone levels." Edwin L. Kaplan, of Chicago, expanded on the hyperparathyroidism "during chronic renal dialysis or following renal transplantation . . . This phenomenon has been called 'tertiary hyperparathyroidism', a term which implies that a hyperplastic gland has become autonomous, i.e., not suppressed or regulated by an elevated serum calcium concentration . . . these parathyroid glands may not be autonomous in most cases . . . the hypercalcemia may reciprocally follow phosphorus diuresis which commonly occurs following successful renal transplantation. With time . . . in most instances both serum calcium and immunoreactive parathyroid hormone will return to normal." Wilson, closing, referred to tertiary hyperparathyroidism as a "semantic problem. We and our pathologists consider tertiary hyperparathyroidism to be the situation where three of the glands show hyperplasia and the fourth appears to show an adenoma . . . We have tried to avoid using this terminology in these patients, because we believe this is secondary to the stimulus of the hypocalcemia in these patients." He agreed with the expressed reluctance to perform parathyroidectomy in posttransplant patients, and in fact both of their posttransplant parathyroidectomies should have been performed before transplant, since the patients were severly hypercalcemic. Disagreeing with Marchioro's final comment, he said, ". . .we do not believe that the level of parathyroid hormone itself . . . is the critical feature, because it's not only how much hormone is being produced, but the effect of this on the end organ." Both magnesium and calcium in the dialysis bath produced a temporary drop in serum parathormone, and serum calcium.

* * *

It is illustrative of the changed character of the programs of the American Surgical Association in which bone surgery was so prominent in the early years, that it should be 13 years after Charnley's introduction in England of total hip replacement that Frank E. Stinchfield, of New York, Professor and Chairman, Department of Orthopedic Surgery, College of Physicians and Surgeons; Director of Orthopedic Hospital, Columbia Presbyterian Medical Center, and by invitation, Eric S. White, *Total Hip Replacement,* presented the first paper on this subject before the Association. The essential features introduced by Charnley were, "A metal-to-plastic rather than metal-to-metal joint surface . . . with a small diameter femoral head . . . the acetabulum is deepened in order to medially displace the center of rotation and the weight-bearing axis . . . A self-curing cement, methylmethacrylate, is used to bond both the acetabular and femoral components to endosteal bone." The long-term reaction of the tissues to the methylmethacrylate was still unknown but in Stinchfield's dog experiments ". . .histologic sections 6 months after implant show normal bone function directly adjacent to cement, with no residual fibrous lining." He employed a lateral approach to the hip joint, with osteotomy of the greater trochanter "to minimize muscle dissection to allow easier dislocation and to facilitate adequate acetabular exposure." The trochanter was divided from the femur with a Gigli saw which was again used to divide the neck of the disarticulated femur, removing the head. The acetabulum was deepened with special reamers and the polyethylene acetabular socket cemented in place with methacrylate. The medullary canal was reamed and the femoral prosthesis cemented in place, the hip reduced and the greater trochanter wired in its new position. Currently, Stinchfield restricted his operation to patients 60 years of age or over with unilateral hip disease, somewhat younger ones with bilateral hip disease and ". . .pain is the primary indication for surgical treatment while limited range of motion and gait disturbance are only secondary considerations." History of infection in the joint was an absolute contraindication to operation, and the operation was to be abandoned if granulation tissue or pus containing bacteria were seen in the wound of a patient who had previously been operated upon. Between April 6, 1969 and May 1970, they had performed 100 hip replacements in 93 patients, observed now six to 18 months. Patients died of unrelated causes after discharge from the hospital, but no operative deaths are mentioned. Relief of pain, often dramatic, was uni-

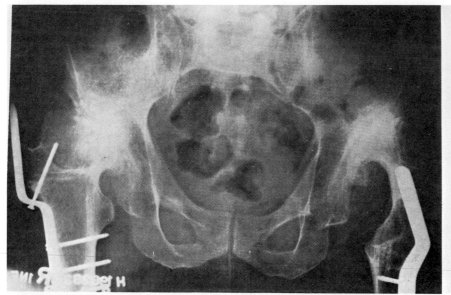

FIG. 4A. J. B., is a 56-year-old man with osteoarthritis secondary to congenitally subluxated hips. Five years ago he underwent bilateral osteotomies but did not obtain permanent relief from pain. At the time of evaluation for LFA, he had Grade 3 pain and was unable to work.

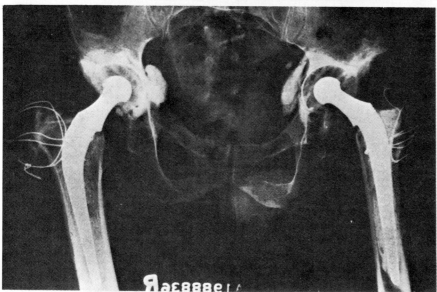

FIG. 4B. The failed osteotomies were converted to low friction arthroplasties. At one-year followup, he has returned to work as a traveling salesman and walks with no pain and no aids.

Stinchfield reported his first 100 total hip replacements mentioning no operative deaths, decrease or elimination of pain in all and marked improvement in function. Adding the next 100 patients, too early yet for postoperative evaluation, pulmonary embolism had occurred in 15, urinary retention in 83, urinary tract infection in 36, gastrointestinal bleeding in three. There had been 12 recognized episodes of thrombophlebitis, 10 deep wound hematomas, two subluxations, one dislocation and no wound infections.

Frank E. Stinchfield and Eric S. White, *Total Hip Replacement.* Volume LXXXIX, 1971.

versal. Most patients had a striking range of motion. Fifteen patients had pulmonary embolism after operation. Two patients subluxated the prosthesis and one patient dislocated it. There were no deep wound infections. The high incidence of pulmonary embolism and phlebitis [based on their first 200 patients] prompted them in their next 120 patients to employ Dextran-40 prophylactically in 60, and not in 60. There was no difference between the two groups in the number of episodes of thrombophlebitis and pulmonary embolism. Charnley's high wound infection rate had led him to introduce a laminar air-flow operating room for implant operations. The Stinchfield group relied upon "strictest aseptic technic in order to eliminate any potential source of intraoperative wound inoculation". There were ten hematomas of which two resulted in superficial infections. They had been employing prophylactic antibiotics usually with penicillin-G. Stinchfield concluded that "The early results of our low friction arthroplasty series are very encouraging. We believe that total hip replacement is here to stay, but we know that this procedure carries with it the potential of many and major complications."

Discussion

The newly elected President, Francis D. Moore, of Boston, asked whether Paget's disease was an indication for the operation and when did Stinchfield use a [Smith-Peterson] cup, if ever? Was there a possibility of late sepsis, blood borne infection carried to the bone injured by the plastic. Kenneth W. Warren, of Boston, asked whether the laminar air-flow emphasized by Charnley was important and "Do you use local antibiotic spray or irrigation during the operation?" Edwin W. Salzman, of Boston, said that in 169 patients with "Vitallium mold arthroplasty", they compared "efficacy of agents affecting platelet function with warfarin for the prophylaxis of venous thromboembolism. In that study, dextran and aspirin were each as effective as warfarin, which was significantly more effective than the control." It seemed to them that the incidence of thromboembolism was higher with total hip arthroplasty than with the cup arthroplasty. Stinchfield, closing, said that in five patients with Paget's disease the operation eliminated hip pain but not the pain of Paget's disease in the bone itself. As for the cup arthroplasty, he continued to employ it in younger patients from 20 to 55 years of age, and when there had been previous infection. Thus far they had not seen late infection in their two-year experience but he thought "that when infection occurs it probably is introduced at the time of operation and is not blood borne." He repeated that they had not found laminar air-flow to be essential. As far as thrombophlebitis and anticoagulation were concerned, "in the total hip replacement patient, we fear hematoma more than thromboembolism . . . Anticoagulation may cause bleeding and hematoma—which could lead to infection. Therefore, we do not routinely anticoagulate the total hip patients."

* * *

[Harvey Cushing and Walter Dandy had felt as strongly about their operations for VIII nerve tumor as about anything, Cushing championing the "safer" intracapsular enucleation and Dandy the definitive complete extirpation, capsule and all. Papin and Horrax (1949, Volume LXVII) had reviewed the controversy and come down strongly on Dandy's side.] Now, in the first mention of the widely expanding application of the microscope to operative surgery, Robert W. Rand, of Los Angeles, Professor of Neurological Surgery, UCLA School of Medicine, *Suboccipital Transmeatal Microneurosurgical Resection of Acoustic Tumors,* brought the Fellows abreast of the current state of the art. He quoted Cushing's 1917 statement "I doubt very much, unless some more perfected method is devised, whether one of these tumors can safely be enucleated", made in the very year that Dandy presented the first successful total resection of an acoustic neuroma. Clinical neurological examination was substantiated by refined and special audiometric examinations but "The Pantopaque cisternography technic is probably the most definitive test in the diagnosis of acoustic tumors" although "Certain vertical and basal laminograms of the internal auditory canals should be obtained initially and will show major or subtle changes in about 75% of patients with these neoplasms." [This was of course just on the eve of the development of computerized tomography.] Less irritating and almost as effective was "Tomography of the posterior fossa during pneumonencephalography. . ." Vertebral angiography was occasionally employed. Rand had, seven years before, developed "The suboccipital transmeatal operation . . . as a modification of Dandy's original acoustic tumor operation . . . Total removal of acoustic tumors regardless of size can be accomplished in a single stage preserving function of noninvolved cochlear, vestibular, and facial nerves . . . accomplished by a microsurgical dissection within the internal auditory canal after the posterior wall had been removed completely by cutting and diamond drill resection under the binocular surgical microscope." Patients operated upon with semi-sitting posture and pin fixation of the head had been given "The usual diuretic agents, including either intravenous urea or mannitol, and intravenous dexamethasone . . . at the commencement of the operation." A suboccipital craniectomy was performed. Lower cranial nerves were freed from the tumor and then with the drill, the petrous bone was cut away "Starting at the edge of the porus acousticus and working laterally" under the binocular microscope. The "noninvolved vestibular and cochlear nerves" could be preserved during the resection of small tumors. Dissection of the tumor from the brain stem was the most critical portion of the operation. The facial nerve was to be separated from the tumor capsule by sharp dissection. Large tumors might be de-

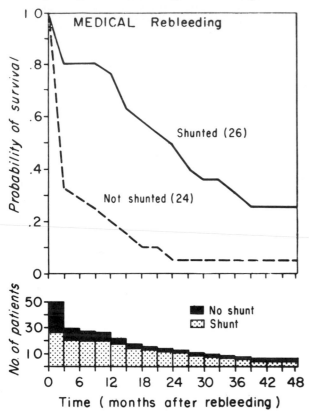

FIG. 4. Analysis of probable survival among rebleeders within the original Medical Group illustrates greater mortality (67%) in the first 3 months of rebleeding patients who were not or could not be shunted. The mortality among rebleeders who were shunted (Medical Group LTS) was by comparison only 20% during the same period. This advantage is maintained although the overall death rates for both groups are higher than for the Medical Group who did not rebleed. What part of the difference in survival between these two groups can be attributed to either operation or differential selection to those shunted, cannot be determined from these data since treatment allocation was not random.

Of the 77 original patients scheduled for "medical" treatment, 50 rebled. Twenty-four of these were not shunted and 26 of them were shunted, at the option of the individual investigator. The shunted patients enjoyed a much better rate of survival. While there was no randomization, review of the protocol showed no obvious prejudice in selection.

Francis C. Jackson, Edward B. Perrin, W. Robert Felix, and Albert G. Smith, *A Clinical Investigation of the Portacaval Shunt:* V. Survival Analysis of the Therapeutic Operation. Volume LXXXIX, 1971.

compressed from within the tumor, small tumors could be removed intact. He tabulated 29 operations with two deaths,- both in tumors greater than 4 cm. in diameter. The facial nerve was sacrificed in three and repaired in two. In the two deaths, both in large tumors, "irreversible edema occurred causing medullary failure." In those two patients, the dura had been tightly closed, "Perhaps a dura graft should have been used to allow more room for the cerebellum", a practice which he had subsequently adopted. The facial nerve was only sacrificed when it was directly invaded by the tumor. Two patients developed stubborn postoperative rhinorrhea, ultimately controlled by "free muscle grafts put into the middle ear". Rand showed a motion picture of the operation.

* * *

The results of the Veterans Administration controlled clinical studies of the portacaval shunt, *A Clinical Investigation of the Portacaval Shunt:* V. Survival Analysis of the Therapeutic Operation, was presented by Francis C. Jackson, of Washington, D.C., Director of Surgical Service, Veterans Administration Office; Office, Clinical Professor of Surgery, Georgetown University School of Medicine, and by invitation, Edward B. Perrin, W. Robert Felix, and Albert G. Smith. It was estimated that in the 25 years since the initial shunts performed by Whipple and his associates, some 10,000 such operations had been performed in the United States. While the beneficial effect upon subsequent variceal hemorrhage had been accepted, there was dispute about the ultimate survival of shunted patients. A series of prospective controlled clinical studies suggested "that while long-term survival of non-bleeding cirrhotic patients is *not* improved by portacaval shunts used prophylactically, emergency shunting operation may provide a more satisfactory immediate survival." The present study was undertaken for "controlled assessment of shunts used electively for previous bleeding in stabilized patients. . ." The report was based upon 78 patients randomized into the shunt group and 77 into the medical treatment group. Eleven of the patients who were scheduled to be shunted declined and were treated medically and behaved much as the entire nonoperative group did. Of the 77 patients treated medically, 50 rebled and of these, approximately half were shunted and half not, depending upon the preference of the investigator. The rate of failure of the shunt was 8% and the rate of rehemorrhage in shunted patients was 8%. Ten years after the beginning of the study, 64% of the medical group patients were dead and 44% of the shunt group. Death rate of patients over 40 years of age in the medical group was significantly higher than those under 40. This difference with age was not seen after shunting, suggesting that only younger patients have a better chance of surviving with frequent bleeding episodes unaccompanied by portacaval shunt. Bleeding varices accounted for 32% of the medical deaths and 7% of the shunted group deaths. "Death primarily from hemorrhage was four times greater when the patient could not be, or was not, shunted." Four deaths from variceal bleeding in the shunted patients occurred in the immediate postoperative period and in all four patients, autopsy disclosed the shunts to be thrombosed. Hepatic failure and encephalopathy were more lethal in the shunted patients than the nonshunted,- 67% versus 39% mortality of those affected. Mortality with encephalopathy in diabetic cirrhotics was 100%. At the time of the evaluation, "Only 36% of the entire Medical Group have survived while 57% of those originally randomized for portacaval shunts are living. "Encephalopathy after portacaval shunt occurs as often as in the control. However, it is significantly more lethal and is a continuing threat to life despite the absence of variceal hemorrhage and irrespective treatment. Encephalopathy among diabetic cirrhotics is uniformly fatal." In his final conclusions, Jackson did say "the stabilized cirrhotic patient has a more favorable opportunity for a prolonged survival if he receives a portacaval shunt", although his statistical tables and grafts were hedged by such statements as "the observed difference between the two curves suggests no statistical significance by existing tests."

Discussion

C. Gardner Child, of Ann Arbor, supported "Dr. Jackson's evidence that portal decompression is a good operation for patients with cirrhosis of the liver whose survival is threatened by recurring variceal hemorrhage." He displayed his own figures for patients in A, B, and C groups, good, intermediate and poor risks, ". . .the good risk patients live longer after portal decompression than do those in the intermediate and poor risk groups." In the good risk patients, side-to-side and end-to-side shunts showed no difference in survival. It was not clear whether there was any difference in the intermediate group but there was a "statistically significant difference between the end-to-side and side-to-side shunt in poor risk . . . patients with little hepatic reserve. We are now convinced that the poor risk patient

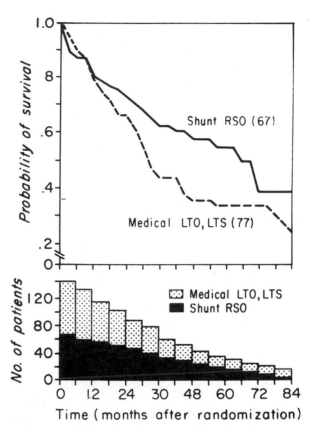

FIG. 8. The most meaningful survival data assessing the role of portacaval shunt in patients with bleeding varices compares survival curves for the Shunt Group RSO and the combined Medical Groups (LTO and LTS). A consistent advantage is observed for the Shunt Group RSO after the first year. The estimated probability of survival for the Shunt Group RSO is 55%, and for the combined Medical Group (LTO and LTS) is only 34% although the magnitude of the difference decreases considerably over the next 2 years. The observed difference between the two curves suggests no statistical significance by existing tests. It appears that the portacaval shunt is responsible for increasing the length of survival among these bleeding cirrhotics.

[Despite the sophistication of the study and the involvement of a biomathematician, the authors still attributed an increased survival to the shunted patients, in spite of their statement that there was no statistical significance to the difference between the two curves.]

Francis C. Jackson, Edward B. Perrin, W. Robert Felix, and Albert G. Smith, *A Clinical Investigation of the Portacaval Shunt:* V. Survival Analysis of the Therapeutic Operation. Volume LXXXIX, 1971.

should have both his liver and his splanchic bed decompressed [i.e., side-to-side shunt] . . . I am convinced as is Dr. Jackson that there is a very real salvage by portal decompression in patients with portal hypertension and bleeding varices." Clarence Dennis, of Brooklyn, commented upon the procedure performed in his department by R. J. Adamsons, who added to an end-to-side portacaval shunt a side-to-end anastomosis of the gastroepiploic artery to the reopened umbilical vein "which, of course, empties into the left branch of the portal vein." Operation had been performed in 11 patients, "The postoperative course has been smooth in all eleven patients, and no patient is suffering from ascites or encephalopathy on unrestricted protein intake." Ronald A. Malt, of Boston, said that in the Boston interhospital liver group, after three-and-a-half years, there was a 56% survival in patients with an end-to-side anastomosis, a 20% survival of those medically treated but no difference between the side-to-side anastomosis and the medical treatment "confirming our clinical impression at the Massachusetts General Hospital that patients in general do better with an end-to-side rather than a side-to-side portacaval." W. Dean Warren, of Miami, said that he now had 23 patients with his distal splenorenal shunt followed up to four-and-a-half years with only one instance of encephalopathy. He said that Dr. Jackson's figures showed a better survival for the shunted group than had been seen previously in the prophylactic shunt study and asked why. Jackson, closing, said they had no answer as to which shunt was better. He had cooperated with the Boston group and agreed with their recommendations concerning prophylactic shunts, "the portacaval shunt is not recommended in the established cirrhotic who has never bled." As for Warren's procedure, a controlled study was worth undertaking, but "When I approached him, and I asked, 'Dean, would you allow us to randomize your operation?' he replied, 'Oh, my God, no!'"

The Business Meetings

The 1971 meeting took place in Boca Raton, Florida, March 24, 25, and 26, President William D. Holden in the Chair.

For the first time, in order to provide more time in the presentation of papers, the various committee reports "that customarily in the past have been given verbally by this Association's representatives to other agencies have been printed and have been distributed to each member of the Association at the time of registration." [The reports made every year at the First Executive Session, as the first item of business on the first day, before any scientific presentations, were those of the Treasurer, Recorder, representatives to the various Surgical Boards, to the Board of Governors of the American College of Surgeons, to the Society for Medical Research, to the National Research Council, were frequently lengthy, accompanied by slides, etc. In substitution for that the reports were reproduced and made available at the back of the room.] There were still only 32 papers presented because the time liberated by the

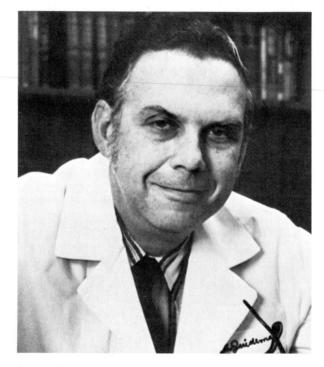

George D. Zuidema, 1928—. M.D. Johns Hopkins, 1953. Internship to Chief Resident, Massachusetts General Hospital, 1953-1959. Assistant Professor to Associate Professor, University of Michigan Medical School, 1960-1964, Warfield M. Firor Professor and Chairman, Department of Surgery, Johns Hopkins, 1964—. His scientific interests have been in the fields of hepatic physiology and portal hypertension. His heavy concern over the social and economic problems involved in medical care and his remarkable effectiveness in administration made him a natural choice for Chairman of SOSSUS—Study on Surgical Services for the United States. From 1970-75, he headed the study,- securing much of the massive funds needed for its support, guiding the numerous committees headed by distinguished, sometimes fractious chairmen, and brought the study to conclusion and its data to publication.

omission of the numerous reports was taken for a discussion of the work of the Committee on Issues.

The Program Committee, F. Henry Ellis, Jr., Chairman [a Thoracic Surgeon], commented that "This year . . . there was a marked reduction in the numbers of cardiovascular papers accepted—two as opposed to five a year ago—and no papers on cardiac subjects, and no papers on noncardiac thoracic surgical problems." The first five papers of the program were given on the first morning following the Presidential Address.

The second morning began with the discussion of the work of the Committee on Issues on SOSSUS. President Holden said that ". . . as many of you know from announcements that have been made in the Bulletin of the American College of Surgeons, shortly after this study was initiated last April the Council joined with the Regents of the American College of Surgeons for several reasons . . . most important, to obtain as broad a base of support for this study within the surgical community as was possible . . . The Chairman of the entire study, to whom this Association owes an incredible debt of gratitude for his efforts, is Dr. George Zuidema, Director of Surgery at Johns Hopkins University. . ." The work had been divided up among ten subcommittees as follows: "1. Academic Manpower, Dr. Robert Zeppa . . . 2. Undergraduate, Graduate, and Postgraduate Manpower, Dr. Francis Moore . . . 3. Allied and Auxiliary Manpower, Dr. William Anlyan . . . 4. Organization, Financing, and Delivery of Surgical Services, Dr. Robert Chase . . . 5. Statistical Subcommittee, Mr. George Sideris . . . 6. Biomedical Research, Dr. Marshall Orloff . . . 7. Government Relations, Dr. Walter Ballinger . . . 8. Community Relationships, Dr. Merle Musselman . . . 9. Legal and Ethics, Dr. Henry Schwartz . . . 10. Professional Interrelationships, Dr. Jack Cole."[-see Appendix D]

It was announced that the practice was to be continued of binding the business portion of the *Transactions* and the Presidential Address separately from the Scientific Proceedings. The Fellows adopted the changes in the Constitition proposed the previous year, to increase the active membership of the Association to 350 Fellows from 300 by yearly increments of no more than ten, to create a category of Corresponding Members "from among those foreign surgeons whose professional status in their own country and whose scientific contributions to the discipline of surgery are comparable to those of Active Fellows of the Association", to create the American Surgical Association Medallion for Scientific Achievement as an award, made only occasion-

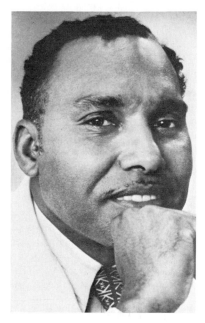

Samuel Lee Kountz, 1930—. M.D. University of Arkansas, 1958. Internship to Chief Resident, Stanford University, 1958-65. Bank of America-Giannini Fellowship in Surgery, Stanford University School of Medicine and Postgraduate Medical School, Hammersmith Hospital, London, England, 1962-63. Instructor to Assistant Professor, Stanford University, 1965-67. Assistant Professor to Professor, University of California, San Francisco, 1967-72, in charge of Transplantation Program. Professor and Chief, Department of Surgery, State University of New York Downstate Medical Center, Brooklyn, New York, 1972-78. At the University of California, San Francisco, he had established a major renal transplantation program and with Belzer introduced the kidney perfusion and preservation system which revolutionized transplantation of cadaver kidneys. An able investigator and surgeon and a superb human being, Kountz was on the way to the creation of a strong and effective department when he was stricken by a neurologic catastrophe.

ally "to those individuals whose scientific contributions have been worthy of the highest recognition the Association can bestow." The sites and dates of future meetings were announced through 1982.

Robert Sparkman had studied the problem of publishing a complete set of the Minutes of the American Surgical Association and had found that if there were 500 subscribers, volumes could be printed for $30 a set. [Sparkman was authorized to proceed and himself guaranteed the cost for which he was ultimately reimbursed from the sale of the volumes.]

Secretary Shires reported that the applications of new members had been properly completed by and large and usually with the right number of reprints,- three of each of the three most important papers,- but was unable to refrain from remarking that "the most interesting were those which contained the reprints of papers written by the Secretary".

In the discussion of the SOSSUS report, Drs. Altemeier, Spencer, and others expressed a sense of urgency and of fear that while statistical data were being collected, Congress would move to legislation which would make the data irrelevant when finally collected and published. Possibly in response to this, at the Final Executive Meeting, the Council recommended the establishment of a subcommittee "on pending legislation to report on urgent issues; that this Subcommittee be appointed by the President of the American Surgical Association and the Chairman of the Board of Regents of the American College of Surgeons, who will be ex-officio members of it; that the Subcommittee be authorized to secure a full-time legislative information officer in Washington, and that the Subcommittee be authorized to use the staff of the American College of Surgeons where necessary; that the Subcommittee be authorized to secure funds, and that the Subcommittee send reports regularly to the Director of the American College of Surgeons, the President of the American Surgical Association, and to the Chairman of the Committee on Issues of the American Surgical Association." This action of the Executive Committee needed no confirmation by the Fellowship.

Twenty four new members were elected, among them, Samuel L. Kountz.

Officers elected were President, Francis D. Moore, of Boston; as Vice-Presidents, Clarence Dennis, of Brooklyn, and Merle M. Musselman, of Omaha; Secretary, Tom G. Shires.

XC

1972

The 1972 meeting took place at the Fairmont Hotel, San Francisco, April 26, 27, and 28, President Francis D. Moore, of Boston, Moseley Professor of Surgery, Harvard Medical School; Surgeon-in-Chief, Peter Bent Brigham Hospital, in the Chair.

President Moore, *Freedom and Organization,* was speaking at a time "of unprecedented pressure on the Congress to legislate changes in the practice of medicine and the delivery of medical care." He predicted, correctly, that between then and the time of the election in November 1972, ". . . most of the rhetoric will be devoted to crisis recognition rather than problem solving . . . There will be few politicians who wish to set sail on these stormy waters until they know which way the wind is blowing." Tight Federal control of the practice of medicine would likely require a socialist form of government, and if ". . . the work of hospitals, the activity of staff, the number of residents trained, the operations a man must do every week to earn his pay . . ." were to be controlled, government would have three methods of implementing its programs, ". . . a system of fiscal inducements, imposition of a system of penalties, or by direct employment in which control is implicit." He said, with an almost wistful reference to the halcyon early days of the research grants program of the National Institutes of Health, "Fiscal inducement introduces subtle control that gradually loses its subtlety with the passage of time. We have seen this evolution in twenty-five years of Federal research finance, in which an initially rather free system of Grants and Peer Review has now evolved

into one of highly directed research, contract control and essentially the design of biologic science by committees meeting in Rockville, Maryland." The Association had already expressed its concern, and undertaken to analyze the problem, in SOSSUS. He thought it important ". . . to identify and isolate a few salient points that are particularly important to the patient and to surgical care, to agree upon them if possible and then to offer affirmative solutions that lie in the private sector and by voluntary effort . . . the medical profession should clean up its own back yard . . . Our alternatives are simple: we must do it ourselves or it will be done for us. If we wish to maintain our freedom, we must get organized." He had three proposals. With respect to the validation of staff credentials he said that ". . . American Surgery places itself in a publicly vulnerable and indefensible position if we establish complex American Board examination procedures to determine the quality of care a man might give to his patient, but then do nothing to assure patients that they will receive that sort of care." The founders of the American Boards of Surgery "purposely avoided any sort of regulation as to who should perform surgery in this country, confining themselves to the examination process alone. They were unaware that later years would demonstrate that a majority of those persons who failed to pass those examinations persist in the practice of surgery anyway. They were likewise unaware that hospital trustees would continue for forty years to give surgical privileges to untrained staff!" The American College of Surgeons, the American Surgical Association, and the ten Boards of Surgery had not taken ". . . a strong public stand on the question of whether or not the responsibility of the open anesthetized tissue dissection in the treatment of human illness should be confined to those who have passed their examinations." He proposed that, under the aegis of the Joint Commission on Accreditation of Hospitals, the credentialling effort be mounted essentially by reviewing the mechanisms and actions of the hospital staffs in reviewing ". . . the fitness and training status of their members in order to maintain accreditation for the hospitals." The second problem was the national control of the production of surgical specialists "After forty years of attention to quality of residency training we must now look also to quantity . . . A national agency should formulate guidelines as to the ideal relation of specialists to population. Data now emerging from SOSSUS will provide such a base for surgery . . . By simple computer programming it is possible to predict how many residents should be produced in any five-year period so as to maintain something close to an optimal ratio, as based on population projections . . . the Residency Review Committee established by the American Boards . . . should approve only that number of residencies established by the national guidelines so as to provide an ideal number of residents. *Quality* training and *restraint* in the performance of surgical operations should be the central criteria." The third matter, a surgical placement service, he considered ". . . the most difficult of the three. No one can force a surgeon—or his wife—to live where he (or she) does not wish to live." He proposed a voluntary National Surgical Placement Service which would match surgeons with opportunities and needs. "No surgical placement service can force relocation or push people around, nor should it try. If the government tried to do this, it would only produce massive resistance; far better to do it voluntarily through the operation of a National Placement Agency in which everyone has confidence. We recently learned that even in Russia, in a completely controlled society, there is a severe problem in locating physicians in rural ares. There is no use abandoning our voluntary system!" [As noted in the Minutes of this meeting, Council was empowered "to move forward in cooperation with other national societies and agencies, as appropriate, so as to implement a national policy for staff credentialing and accreditation, a national policy for the monitoring and control of the flow of residents, and a National Surgical Placement Service."]

* * *

Total parenteral hyperalimentation, employing a continuous infusion of amino acids and hypertonic glucose through a nonreactive plastic catheter inserted in the superior vena cava had swept the country as the result of the publications from the University of Pennsylvania of Stanley J. Dudrick, Jonathan Rhoads, and others over the previous three years. Now from the Department of Surgery and Harrison Department of Surgical Research, School of Medicine, University of Pennsylvania, Stanley J. Dudrick, W. MacFadyen, Jr., T. Van Buren, L. Ruberg, and T. Maynard, all by invitation, *Parenteral Hyperalimentation*, Metabolic Problems and Solutions, discussed their studies in ". . . more than 1300 seriously-ill patients receiving long-term total parenteral nutrition . . ." The hypertonic glucose was initially to be administered slowly, and progressively increased, avoiding blood glucose levels above 200 mg./100 ml. or substantial glycosuria. It had been observed that "Prolonged severe glycosuria can lead to the development of hyperosmolar, non-ketotic hyperglycemic coma." The sudden appearance of glycosuria might ". . . precede the clinical manifestations of sepsis by several hours". In most patients insulin production rose to handle the increased glucose load, but occasionally exogenous insulin was required. Exogenous insulin did "not suppress production of endogenous insulin . . . via the negative feedback mechanism of other endocrine organs . . ." so that a patient initially requiring insulin might by increasing his own insulin production presently go into insulin shock. The sudden interruption of glucose infusion might produce rebound hypoglycemia so that ". . .the infusion must never be interrupted for infusion of blood, fat, or other fluids." The hydrolysates of fibrin and casein, the common sources of parenteral nitrogen, had the disadvantages "of containing large amounts of di- and tripeptides and variable quantities of non-essential amino acids". Particularly in patients with compromised renal or hepatic function, it was preferable to employ solutions of essential L-amino acids. The electrolyte contents of commercial products varied. The crystal amino acid solutions contained the chlorides of amino acids so that it was possible to produce hyperchloremic metabolic acidosis. If sodium or potassium were to be added additionally they were to be added, therefore, as the bicarbonate or lactate of sodium, and the phosphate or acetate of potassium, to avoid an excess of chlorides. Hyperammonemia had been observed, especially in premature infants, and in patients with liver disease, but had "not been a significant complication of protein hydrolysate infusions in patients with normal liver function." Hypophosphatemia had been seen in some patients receiving solutions containing no calcium or phosphorus, and in general, calcium gluconate and potassium phosphate were added to all parenteral hyperalimentation formulae. Patients on prolonged intravenous alimentation showed derrangements of serum lipids. Others had reported, especially in infants, "the syndrome of scaly skin, hair changes, anemia, thrombocytopenia, increased red cell fragility, increased capillary permeability, and impaired wound healing . . ." The addition of intravenous soybean oil emulsion—intra-lipid—had solved that problem. Although the problems of intravenous alimentation in patients with renal failure had not been solved, Dudrick and associates, in nephrectomized beagles, had demonstrated that blood urea nitrogen could be maintained at a much lower level with hypertonic glucose and essential amino acids than with voluntary feeding or with intravenous glucose alone.

* * *

M. F. Brennan, M. H. Goldman, R. C. O'Connell and R. B. Kundsin, all by invitation, and Francis D. Moore, The President, *Prolonged Parenteral Alimentation: Candida Growth and the Prevention of Candidemia by Amphotericin Instillation,* shared the general concern over ". . . the frequent occurrence of sepsis associated with total parenteral feeding . . . the high incidence of septicemia with various Candida species." Their preventive technique consisted of "the introduction and flushing through of 0.6 to 1 ml. of a 1 mg./ml. solution of amphotericin, followed by the instillation of the same quantity, which is left for a minimum of 5 minutes before reconnecting to the nutrient mixture. This therapy has effectively prevented Candida growth *in vivo* and *in vitro* when performed twice a week by a physician at the time the delivering tubing is changed and the skin is cleaned." Prior to instituting this regimen they had had four instances of Candida septicemia in 28 patients on intravenous hyperalimentation, mean duration of 36 days. The 12 patients treated by the regimen described had had no Candidemia, and one of the previous patients who had had five episodes of Candidemia "was maintained for a further 460 days on intravenous feeding using the flush routine twice per week. In this patient we have continued to be able to demonstrate Candida by culture from skin, vagina and fistula tracts, at varying times, but there has been no further Candidemia, and the line has not had to be withdrawn because of sepsis." They assumed that the catheter lumen was a continuous source of entry for the organism.

Discussion

Clarence Dennis, now of Bethesda, Maryland, said he had a 30-year experience "with feeding by highly flexible superior vena cava catheters of hypertonic glucose solutions . . .", primarily in patients with ulcerative colitis and Crohn's disease. They had noted "that the insulin requirement drops in the first 4 or 5 days, and can thereafter be abandoned." It was important for the catheter to be in the mid-superior vena cava. Lloyd D. MacLean, of Montreal, said that over a two-year period they had lowered their "Candida infection rate from one of the highest in the Western world to an acceptable level",- from 33% in their first 20 patients to zero currently. The measures they employed to achieve these changes were "changing leaking administration sets, many of which are available on the market . . . recapped the bottles mechanically . . . abandoned the use of Millipore filters . . . used the subclavian line only for the administration of the hyperalimentation solution, but never for measuring the CVP or drawing blood." Henry T. Randall, of Providence, Rhode Island, had had 14 cases of Candida septicemia in 17 months, but ten of the patients had not been on intravenous alimentation, although most of them had been on chemotherapy, and "Investigation into all the Candida infections showed a common denominator, the prolonged use of broad spectrum antibiotics . . . Thirteen of 14 had been on for more than 2 weeks." He suggested that the result of prolonged use of broad spectrum antibiotics might be to colonize the patients with Candida after which the blood stream infection occurred through the catheter. James D. Hardy, of Jackson, Mississippi, made a point of recalling ". . . that in 1948, Drs. Jonathan E. Rhoads and C. Martin Rhode were maintaining dogs by the continuous infusion of 50% glucose and protein hydrolysate into the superior vena cava . . .". Studies in his department by Richard C. Miller and James B. Grogan had shown that ". . . 31% of the infusion systems were contaminated at some point, only ten systems had sporadically positive cultures on the patient's side of the bacterial filter, and none of these ten patients developed sepsis." Three patients developed confirmed sepsis "one with *E. coli* and two with Candida. Only in the case of coliform sepsis was the organism also found in the filter system, and Candida, although found in two patients' blood, was not found in their fluid or filters . . . this suggested that the ingress of these organisms might have been by a route other than that of contaminated infusate." David V. Habif, of New York City, supported Dr. MacLean's observations on the basis of results at the Harlem Hospital where an incidence of five Candida infections in 200 patients on intravenous alimentation was reduced to zero in the next 200 when ". . . the infusion system was kept closed at all times and the use of topical antibiotic around the catheter was discontinued . . ." George H. A. Clowes, Jr., of Boston, alone discussed Dudrick's metabolic studies. Referring to the studies of Blackburn, at the Boston City Hospitals, with the use of peripherally administered isotonic amino acid solution, Clowes said this had reversed the negative nitrogen balance in sick patients, had not met the patient's caloric requirements, but "the patient is converted to a lipid-using condition instead of an amino acid-using condition. This stops the excessive wastage of protein." Dudrick, closing, said they cultured their catheters as they were withdrawn and in the last 160 consecutive central venous catheters, "18 grew organisms. Eight patients, or 5%, had sepsis and a positive bacterial or fungal blood culture before the catheter was inserted, and the same organism was subsequently recovered from the catheter." In four patients, with sepsis prior to catheterization, a different organism was grown from the catheter than from the blood. Six patients with no prior infection had positive catheter blood cultures at the termination of central venous feeding. The overall contamination rate was 11.25%, "3.75% not having had previous evidence of sepsis nor any other focal area of infection that we could identify as the primary focus. In these patients, the catheter or the technic must be incriminated . . ." He underlined the role of the preparation of the fluid in producing contamination.

* * *

J. Wesley Alexander, and J. L. Meakins, by invitation, from the Department of Surgery and the Shriners Burn Institute, University of Cincinnati Medical Center, *A Physiological Basis for the Development of Opportunistic Infections in Man,* advanced the striking "hypothesis that abnormalities of neutrophilic function appear to be the most important variable of immunological defense relating to the development of opportunistic infections in man." Alexander's test of neutrophil antibacterial function consisted in the addition of a measured bacterial suspension of staphylococcus aureus to a leukocyte suspension which was incubated for four hours after which an aliquot was taken for culture to determine the number of colonies. From this they derived the neutrophil bacterial index, ". . . dividing the average of the numbers of bacteria not killed by the neu-

trophils from each normal control into the number of bacteria not killed by the subject during the 4 hours incubation period", the rise in the index associated with the time of clinical recognition of sepsis. The defect was not one of phagocytosis. In burn or transplant patients, "bacteria are phagocytized and killed by burn neutrophils at a normal rate for the first hour, without further killing . . . leukocytes phagocytize normally and degranulation appears to be intact, thus implicating one or more intraleukocyte bactericidal mechanisms, notably the enzymes contained in lysosomal granules. Within neutrophils, there are a multiplicity of bactericidal mechanisms with different specificities, and bactericidal efficiencies for four separate organisms were observed to vary at different times . . . an abnormality of any single intraleukocyte bactericidal mechanism can not be expected to explain the spectrum of acquired abnormalities which have been observed. Bacteria have been noted to multiply within burn neutrophils, associated with an arrest of the bactericidal mechanisms after one hour, to produce an intracellular infection. While inside leukocytes, the bacteria are protected from the lethal or inhibitory effects of antibiotics." Alexander made no suggestion as to the mechanism of production of the defect or its correction.

Discussion

Basil A. Pruitt, Jr., of San Antonio, said that at the Army Burn Unit infection was still the most common cause of death in burn patients. He asked whether the age of the leukocyte had been investigated. President Moore asked whether antibiotics themselves affected leukocytic activity. J. Wesley Alexander, closing, said that they had been unable to relate "the apparent age of neutrophils to their function . . .", and to President Moore replied that "we have done several studies in experimental animals which would indicate that antibiotics, in themselves, do not cause an inefficiency of killing by the neutrophils."

* * *

G. Tom Shires,- the Secretary,- Professor and Chairman, Department of Surgery, University of Texas, Southwestern Medical School, Dallas, and by invitation, J. N. Cunningham, C. R. F. Baker, S. F. Reeder, H. Illner, I. Y. Wagner, and J. Maher, *Alterations in Cellular Membrane Functions during Hemorrhagic Shock in Primates,* had introduced to the study of the shock problem "The current uses of ultramicroelectrodes to monitor transmembrane potential difference . . . and . . . microaspiration technics to evaluate ionic changes in the interstitial fluid bathing the cells . . ." Baboons were bled to within 25% to 30% of their calculated blood volume, "Skeletal muscle membrane potential (PD) was obtained . . . by impalement of individual skeletal muscle cells with standard Ling electrodes . . . prepared from borosilicate glass capillary pipettes pulled to a tip diameter of approximately 0.2 microns and filled under vacuum with a solution of 2M KC1-0.5M KNO_3. Each electrode was housed inside a thin bore [sic] #18 hypodermic needle and mounted on a movable rack and pinion to allow percutaneous insertion into the anterior muscle mass of the upper thigh or anterior tibial compartment of the baboon's hind limb." They felt that their data "confirms the existence of an altered physiologic function of the cell membrane of skeletal muscle cells as a result of the low flow state produced by severe prolonged hemorrhagic shock." Membrane depolarization occurred with sustained shock, and they calculated a concomitant 49% decrease in extracellular water and a 6% increase in intracellular water. The serum potassium concentration increased significantly after prolonged shock and the sodium concentration in intracellular water increased significantly as well. Their data indicated ". . . that skeletal muscle cells may be a major site of fluid and electrolyte sequestration following severe, prolonged hemorrhagic shock." Studies by others had suggested "similar changes in the intracellular mass of neurons in the brain . . . in response to hypovolemic shock . . . an increase in cellular water content of both cellular and connective tissue components following hemorrhagic shock . . . connective tissue may be the site of some sodium and water sequestration." As for the cause, "The exact mechanism for the production of electrolyte changes as well as the marked diminution in extracellular water which occurs following hemorrhagic shock is not known. It appears that they may well represent a reduction in the efficiency of an active ionic pump mechanism or a selective increase in muscle cell membrane permeability to sodium or both."

Discussion

Arthur E. Baue, of St. Louis, tended to agree. Shires' studies had been *in vivo*, and Baue had "measured cell membrane transport directly, but at the present time this can only be done *in vitro*." Cooled liver slices from a normal rat would take up the sodium, which went into the cells; when the tissue was

rewarmed the sodium was progressively extruded and the sodium content decreased, "Tissue from an animal in late shock has lost this capability. Sodium goes up with cooling, but when the tissue is rewarmed the sodium pump is not activated. Sodium is not extruded. Thus the sodium pump is not working. The reverse of this occurs with potassium . . . This adds further evidence for Dr. Shires' concept that the active portion of the Na-K pump is not working with severe prolonged shock." Shires, closing, accepted the support, "Dr. Baue's work has been going along simultaneously with ours, and I think we are at least ending up with the same common denominator; and that is, there is remarkable interference with energy exchange in response to shock."

* * *

D. Emerick Szilagyi, of Detroit, Chairman, Department of Surgery, Henry Ford Hospital, and by invitation, R. F. Smith, J. P. Elliott, and M. P. Vrandecic, *Infection in Arterial Reconstruction with Synthetic Grafts,* reviewed their experience with 3,347 arterioplastic operations over a 20-year period. Significant infections occurred in 1.9% of cases with synthetic prostheses, including referred cases, 0.4% of autogenous vein grafts, 0.2% endarterectomy, and 0.4% with arterial allografts. Over 90% of the prostheses were the woven Dacron tubes developed by Szilagyi. The incidence of wound infection with prosthetic implants varied by the site of the infection, 0.7% for femoro-femoral grafts, 3.0% for femoro-popliteal grafts, 1.0% for intrathoracic, carotid, renal, and other grafts. "The single most common source of infection was the inguinal skin; the second most common source was the perforation (erosion) of a hollow viscus." In the last 12 years the femoro-popliteal grafts had been almost entirely with saphenous vein grafts, so that the infection rate was lower for that reason. The overall incidence of severe infections was 1.7% in 1955 to 1960, 2.1% in 1961 to 1965, and 1.1% in 1966 to 1971. "The low incidence in the aorto-iliac area, as compared with the femoro-popliteal incidence, suggests that the extent of dissection in terms of area traversed, and bulk of implanted foreign substance (the prosthesis) are less important in potentiating the process of infection than are the proximity to inguinal and genital areas, the amount of skin surface adjacent to the incision and of the subcutaneous tissue exposed, and length of exposure . . . intra-abdominal infections were, in general, very scarce." The lag before the clinical appearance of the infection was sometimes extraordinary, "In about a fifth of the cases this time lag was over 12 months, and the maximum length was 60 months . . . A strong clue as to the true sequence of events was the observation that in the femoropopliteal cases the time lag of onset was usually very short. When the infection is due to contamination in course of operation, as it must be in these cases, the clinical onset was instantaneous. On the other hand, the longest delays were noted in cases of visceroprosthetic fistulas. This would suggest that these sources of contamination require a prolonged length of time for development and for ultimate emergence." Neither his data nor anyone elses indicated whether prophylactic antibiotic administration was useful and with so low an infection rate, several thousand cases in a controlled protocol, over several years would be required to establish the virtue of prophylactic antibiotic administration. Szilagyi found his infection rate was as low or lower than that of others employing prophylactic antibiotics. On the other hand, the recognition that 23 of the 40 significant infections had their sources in the inguinal skin, and that in 18 of them the offending organism was staphylococcus aureus seemed justification "to say that in those vascular operations in which the groin has to be opened, the prophylactic use of antibiotics effective against this particular organism promises a significant decrease of the risk of wound contamination." Antibiotics might also be used in patients "with particularly poor body hygiene, with an uncorrectable depression of the immune defense mechanism of the body, and those with ruptured aortic aneurysm." Given the disastrous effects of infection, he preferred to employ antibiotics. He had arrived at a common sense selection of the operative treatment of the established infection ". . . not all infected prostheses require removal. If the periprosthetic infection is a lingering one of low virulence; if the anastomotic lines are not involved; and if there is no evidence that the pseudointima harbors bacterial colonization, that is, if there are no clinical manifestations of septicemia (in particular, metastatic abscesses distal to the graft site), an attempt to save the implant is justified. The proof that the prosthesis ought not to be excised is rarely obtainable on clinical grounds, and almost always requires surgical exploration. Surgical exploration . . . for this purpose must meticulously avoid any maneuver that would threaten the extension of the infectious involvement. When the circumstances that favor salvage of the graft have been ascertained, the exposed portion of the graft is debrided, covered with appropriate tissue, and provided with means for drainage and in-

termittent antibiotic irrigation. If the infection is low grade but proof is present that the pseudointima or a suture line is involved, the prosthesis must be replaced . . . In all other cases not included in the above two categories, the removal of the prosthesis is mandatory. If the removal of the graft would lead to ischemia threatening life or limb . . . usually the case, it must be preceded by the construction of a remote bypass as a new blood conduit. The infected implant is then excised in a second operative session, with complete avoidance of contamination in the field of the new blood channel . . . Whenever in doubt . . . the assumption must be made that the sacrifice of the graft and the establishment of the bypass are mandatory, and the operative plans must be made accordingly."

Discussion

Thomas J. Whelan, Jr., of Washington, D.C., said that nine years earlier at Walter Reed they had "reported seven cases of infected Dacron grafts, in which we obtained sound healing by local, aggressive and early management with operation, topical antibiotics, systemic antibiotics, and . . . the placement of viable, autologous tissues around the graft . . . If the graft is the site of a grossly suppurative process and infection involves the anastomotic suture line, removal of this graft, with or without extra-anatomic or remote bypass . . . is the treatment of choice."

* * *

Lester W. Martin, by invitation, from the Children's Hospital Universtiy of Cincinnati, *Surgical Management of Total Colonic Aganglionosis,* presented his experience with nine infants with Hirschsprung's disease in which the entire colon was aganglionic. The ileum was divided where ganglion cells were found on biopsy, brought down and anastomosed to the rectum at the anus as in the Duhamel technique. The right and transverse colons were resected and a long anastomosis was made between the descending colon and the ileum lying along side it, to provide a large reservoir. The long side-to-side anastomosis, the length of the descending colon, was done by the usual anastomotic techniques, the spur, between the ileum anastomosed to the rectum and the rectum, was necrosed with a spur crushing clamp. One child died, of sepsis and multiple anomalies, three months after operation, eight of the others did well, one had recurrent diarrhea. Martin made the observation that "It is possible to retain a portion of the colon even though aganglionic, and to incorporate it into the intestinal tract [the principle of the Duhamel operation]. The colon, reintroduced into the intestinal tract in this manner, clinically appears to retain some capacity for reabsorption. When half the circumference of the intestinal tract contains ganglion cells, this appears to be sufficient to propel the fecal stream."

Discussion

Orvar Swenson, of Chicago, opened the Discussion, agreeing that children who had such total aganglionosis of the colon could be salvaged. He had used his own operation for it with good results, and demonstrated slides of two 20-year follow-ups. Eric W. Fonkalsrud, of Los Angeles, said that the prior mortality of Hirschsprung's patients had been 67% or higher, that intravenous hyperalimentation had been a great help and that he had "found that the mechanical stapling instrument which Dr. Ravitch introduced a few years ago for the modified Duhamel procedure has been of great assistance in constructing the long anastomosis which Dr. Martin showed us in his illustrations. [F. M. Steichen, J. L. Talbert, and M. M. Ravitch: *Primary Side-to-Side Colorectal Anastomosis in the Duhamel Operation for Hirschsprung's Disease. Surgery* 642:475–483, 1968. Ravitch, on a mission to the U.S.S.R. in 1958 for the National Research Council, had purchased there one of the stapling instruments being developed in the U.S.S.R., and had launched in Baltimore a program of laboratory and clinical investigation, one result of which was a series of stapling instruments for abdominal and thoracic surgery, which by the mid-70's were widely accepted and used. None of Ravitch's papers on stapling, as such, were presented before the Association.] By placing this stapling device in several different locations one can actually complete this very extensive procedure within minutes and provide a sturdy anastomosis." At what age would Dr. Martin do the definitive procedure, and did he have much difficulty with diarrhea "when he carries the anastomosis down as low as he indicates, taking a portion of the internal sphincter"? Martin, closing, said that he had used the stapler and liked it well, but that in one child the septum had regrown and had to be redivided. As for time, he thought most of the children needed ileostomy and rehabilitation before the operation could be undertaken, and then frequently in stages, the first stage being ". . . to bring the ileum down to the rectum and apply the clamp." All the children had diarrhea for a period of time following operation but in the long run it was not a serious problem.

* * *

Lawrence W. Way, W. H. Admirand, both by invitation, and J. Englebert Dunphy, of San Francisco, Professor and Chairman, Department of Surgery, University of California, *Management of Choledocholithiasis,* had analyzed the records of 200 consecutive patients who had undergone exploration of the common duct for presumed choledocholithiasis, between 1960 and 1969. In 70% of the patients, stones were found in the common duct, and in 65% of the 160 cases in whom choledochotomy was done at the time of cholecystectomy. There were five deaths, 2.5%, two of them after re-exploration for retained common duct stones. Fifty of the common ducts were explored because of palpated stones, with 98% positive yield; 17 for cholangitis with jaundice, a 94% yield; and 23 because of the operative cholangiogram with a 50% yield, but only one of six common ducts yielded a stone when the indication was a visibly dilated duct and only one of nine when the indication was the presence of small stones in the gallbladder. Pre-exploratory operative cholangiography had not been routine. Fourteen patients were found on postoperative cholangiograms to have retained stones. In five of them, operative cholangiograms had not been done after common duct exploration, and in three the cholangiograms had been misinterpreted. Eight of the patients had been operated upon, six were being observed ". . . for development of symptoms." A group of 22 patients not represented in the 200 choledochotomies on which the report was based, had been treated "by infusing a bile salt solution into the T-tube in an attempt to chemically dissolve or disrupt the stones." Stones were eliminated in 12 of those 22. Attempts at instrumental removal with a Dormia ureteral stone basket had been made in five patients, the six months before the meeting, and the stones removed in three.

Discussion

Joel W. Baker, of Seattle, supported operative cholangiography "even where stones are *known* to be in the common duct, a preliminary x-ray should still be made before common duct instrumentation in order to demonstrate the function of the spincter of Oddi . . . By its use the extravagant resort to open common duct instrumentation is avoided and at the same time unsuspected stones are occasionally discovered." In their previously reported study of

1500 cholecystectomy patients ". . . 373 ducts, suspect because of small stones in the gallbladder or moderate dilatation of the duct, were spared unnecessary exploration. In 24 patients completely unsuspected stones were recovered from the ducts. Sixteen patients were spared a second operation by the completion cholangiogram, and two more underwent a second operation, because the surgeon, tired or disbelieving, ignored a positive completion cholangiogram . . . the most significant thing we learned was that the operative cholangiography in this comparative follow-up study, although not perfect, proved *even* more dependable than open choledochostomy in defining the innocence or guilt of the common and hepatic bile ducts." Bernard Gardner, of Brooklyn, commented on his use of heparin for irrigation of the common bile duct in the dissolution of gall stones . . . based on a series of experiments in which we were able to demonstrate that the negative charge supplied by heparin was most likely absorbed in the micelle and produced an increase in the dispersion of the micelles in bile." He had treated six patients successfully with intracholedochal heparin, 25,000 units in 250 cc. saline every eight hours given as a continuous drip. Philip Sandblom, of Lund, Sweden, said "In Sweden we have routinely used the preoperative cholangiography for more than 25 years, and have found it to be of great value . . . The incidence of common duct stones in cholelithiasis is, perhaps, a little bit higher than yours—about 20% . . . so uniform that if a center reports less we suspect them of leaving some stones behind . . . We depend so much on the operative cholangiogram that we, with Dr. Baker, think that it should always be done as the first procedure . . . a good cholangiogram . . . should tell the exact number, size and location . . ." Lawrence W. Way, closing said that the pre-exploration cholangiogram frequently underestimated the actual number of stones.

* * *

Stanley O. Hoerr, of Cleveland, Past Chairman, Division of Surgery, the Cleveland Clinic Foundation, and by invitation, John T. Ward, *Late Results of Three Operations for Chronic Duodenal Ulcer:* Vagotomy-Gastrojejunostomy, Vagotomy-Hemigastrectomy, Vagotomy-Pyloroplasty, had respectively 161, 127, and 177 patients in the three groups, and an additional 25 patients who had had gastric resection alone, usually as an emergency procedure for massive hemorrhage. The mortality rate was 0.7% for vagotomy-gastrojejunostomy, 1.2% for vagotomy-pyloroplasty, and 3.9% for vagotomy-hemigastrectomy. The long-term results in terms of

patient satisfaction were almost identical for all three operations, with about 10% unsatisfactory results in each. Proved or probably recurrent ulcer occurred in 3.3% of the vagotomy-hemigastrectomy, 11.9% in the vagotomy-pyloroplasty, and 13.5% in vagotomy-gastrojejunostomy. The recurrent ulcers were manifested from almost at once to 16 years after operation. Vagotomy-gastroenterostomy required a second operation only 1.7% of the time if the original operation had been done for obstruction, but in 15.4% of the patients if the original operation had been done for hemorrhage. Hoerr said that he favored "vagotomy-drainage as an initial definitive operation, accepting a significant incidence of recurrent ulcer and second operation, noting that the final results will be about the same as those for vagotomy-hemigastrectomy (or vagotomy-antrectomy). Vagotomy with the Finney pyloroplasty seems to produce better results than vagotomy with the Heineke-Mikulicz pyloroplasty." Vagotomy-antrectomy was the preferred operation in the presence of active bleeding.

Discussion

William H. ReMine, of Rochester, Minnesota, had the figures of a Mayo Clinic review of patients operated on from 1955 to 1965, now with a seven- to 17-year follow-up. Of the 1,648 operations there had been 265 vagotomy and pyloroplasty, 215 vagotomy and antrectomy, 227 vagotomy and gastroenterostomy operations. Currently, the Jaboulay was their preferred type of pyloroplasty. There was less than 1% operative mortality with the vagotomy and drainage operation, and 1% with vagotomy and antrectomy. Including the emergency procedures [as Hoerr had], their overall operative mortality was 2.6%. From the functional standpoint, the operations were all equivalent in the results but while the incidence of recurrence with the vagotomy and antrectomy was 2% it was ". . . five times as great with vagotomy and pyloroplasty—10%. I think this is the significant point of the entire study." John Goligher, of Leeds, England, said ". . . it has been shown that each operation has its particular advantages and disadvantages, and, depending on what weight you attach to these respective pros and cons, you can total up the score to show that all operations are equal or that one operation is better than others . . . as well as selecting patients for antrectomy, presumably by gastric secretory studies, it is equally important—perhaps more so—to select the patients that are *un*suitable for antrectomy . . . the patients with deeply penetrating posterior wall ulcers, which are likely to give rise to technical difficulties and dangers if resected. For, whatever dispute there may be about the merits of the different operations for duodenal ulcer, I think there is general agreement that the most disastrous consequence is the death of the patient." Their usual operation had been truncal vagotomy and pyloroplasty, "But I must say that, like Dr. ReMine, we have been very depressed with the results of this operation and so in the last 3 years we have actually gone in for even more minimal operation, and have adopted the operation of highly selective vagotomy . . . it deprives the upper two-thirds of the stomach—the parietal cell mass—of its vagal innervation, but retains the vagal supply to the antrum and the pyloric sphincter via the nerves of Latarjet; and this has the advantage that it maintains normal emptying of the stomach, so that it is not necessary to do a drainage operation . . . Many surgeons would express grave misgiving about leaving an innervated antrum like this, and will wonder what the long-term effect will be. All I can say is that our acid studies have shown that there is as much reduction of acid after this operation as there is after truncal vagotomy and pyloroplasty . . . We have done 120 highly selective vagotomies now without drainage, and have never had to go back to establish drainage subsequently. These have all been done in the last 3 years, so obviously I cannot give you any long-term assessment of this operation . . . the results to date have been most encourging with no proven recurrences, virtually no diarrhea and a good functional state . . . I would like to warn you that it is technically a somewhat difficult maneuver. It is rather finicky going up along the lesser curve, and I can seldom do these operations in less than 2 hours, whereas an ordinary vagotomy and pyloroplasty would, of course, take only a half hour or so." John R. Brooks, of Boston, said, "The heart of the problem . . . lies in testing a duodenal ulcer operation for its effect on the triad of mortality, of morbidity after operation, and on the rate of ulcer recurrence. In our hands, we believe at the moment that the balance of this triad is in favor of simple truncal vagotomy and pyloroplasty." They had 250 truncal vagotomies with pyloroplasty in the decade 1961-71, for duodenal ulcer. The mortality for the elective group was 1%, for the massive bleeders was 13% [previously, 21% for subtotal gastrectomy for massive bleeding]. In 136 followed patients, there were seven proved recurrent ulcers,- 5%. Jack M. Farris, of Los Angeles, said his operation of choice continued to be truncal vagotomy, and the Jaboulay pyloroplasty. J. Lynwood Herrington, Jr., of Nashville, found it "very difficult to currently accept a 10-15% rate of recurrent ulceration with truncal vagotomy and pyloroplasty. According to my judgement this is a bad score." If vagotomy and pyloroplasty was reserved for the poor-risk patients, and vagotomy-antrectomy performed for the rest, the mortality for vagotomy-antrectomy would be very little different than that for vagotomy and pyloroplasty. "During the past 25 years, our overall mortality with vagotomy-antrectomy in over 3,000 patients is 1.7% and when done on an elective basis it is 1.0%." H. William Scott, Jr., of Nashville, reported further on the prospective study of "'old-fashioned' elective vagotomy, not the highly selective procedure which Dr. Goligher referred to . . ." combined with either gastrectomy or pyloroplasty. They now had follow-up studies up to five years in 104 patients. There had been no deaths, two patients with antrectomy had developed recurrent ulcers and no ulcers had developed in the pyloroplasty patients. Stanley L. Hoerr, closing said that they were watching with interest the English experience with highly selective vagotomy. He reminded the Association of Sir Heneage Ogilvie's story, "The duodenal ulcer questionnaire was sent to all patients who had been treated for fracture; when the replies came back, about 20% would have been regarded as very poor results of duodenal ulcer surgery if they had had it done." He agreed with Herrington that vagotomy-antrectomy "is a very good operation for duodenal ulcer, but temperamentally I do not like to do an operation which is more extensive than required in 95% of the patients . . . In Dr. Herrington's skillful hands, the operation may be as safe as vagotomy and pyloroplasty, but I know that for myself after all these years, I would probably lose an occasional patient that I would not otherwise if I persisted in doing a vagotomy and antrectomy."

* * *

Bolek Brant, Josef Rosch, by invitation, and William W. Krippaehne, of Portland, Professor and Chairman, Department of Surgery, University of Oregon Medical School, *Experiences with Angiography in Diagnosis and Treatment of Acute Gastrointestinal Bleeding of Various Etiologies:* Preliminary Report, attributed to Margulis, Heinbecker, and Bernard in 1960, the first visceral arteriographic demonstration of a bleeding cecal arterio-venous malformation. Since the experimental demonstration in 1963 and the clinical use in 1965 by Nusbaum and Baum of percutaneous selective visceral arteriography in the demonstration of bleeding [see Volume LXXXVII, 1969], the use of the technique had become widespread. The effects of vasopressin on the visceral circulation had been known since 1928, and Nusbaum and Blakemore in 1967 had reported the infusion of vasoactive substances into the superior-mesenteric artery, first in dogs then in patients. Krippaehne and associates had studied angiographically 42 patients with massive, acute gastrointestinal hemorrhage in the previous two years with only one imcomplete diagnosis. The only complications were two infections at the arterial catheter site, associated with septicemia, and relieved by catheter removal and antibiotics, and in a third patient, a hematoma of the groin. Pitressin was administered for venous variceal bleeding. Patients with arterial bleeding were infused with epinephrine except for one successfully infused with pitressin. In 11 of the patients, the bleeding was from varices, and in 31 the bleeding was arterial. Of the 11 patients bleeding from varices, seven were controlled with pitressin infusion and did not bleed again during that hospital admission. There were six failures in nine peptic ulcers. There were no failures in an assorted group of one marginal ulcer, one Mallory-Weiss syndrome, three colonic diverticula and one ileal ulcer. In 16 patients bleeding from stress ulcers or gastritis, there were five failures. It had been known that systemic,- intravenous,- injection of vasopressin had been successfully used in controlling variceal bleeding, but the large doses employed caused adverse cardiovascular reactions. Intraarterial infusion required much smaller doses and caused no significant cardiac or renal effects. Their own experimental studies showed equivalent diminution of superior mesenteric arterial blood flow in the dog with either epinephrine or pitressin intraarterially. The infusions were sometimes continued as long as 48 hours, and in no case did ischemic necrosis of the viscera result. Currently they considered pitressin to be the drug of choice for both arterial bleeding and bleeding from varices.

Discussion

David B. Hinshaw, of Loma Linda, California, was enthusiastic about the technique, and pitressin was his usual vasoconstrictor drug. Leslie Wise, of St. Louis, said that in 68 cases their diagnostic accuracy had been only 50%, but they had no serious complications. He made no mention of the use of vasoconstrictors. William S. Blakemore, of Philadelphia, said that the work of Nusbaum and Baum in the laboratory stemmed from ". . . information on organ catheterization from Scandinavian investigators." If bleeding was not demonstrated they could be confident that the patient was not bleeding at the time. They preferred surgical pituitrin for arterial bleeding. They had had only one patient in 50 who did not respond to infusion for variceal bleeding. In arterial bleeding, the percentage of response had not been as high, usually because of failure to catheterize the specific vessel required. Pituitrin should be "continued for 24 to 48 hours after bleeding has been controlled because of the incidence of recurrent bleeding which is a greater risk to the patient than properly monitored infusion for this extended period." They had some success with the use of vasodilator drugs ". . . in uncommonly occurring cases of nonocclusive mesenteric intestinal ischemia, seen with advanced heart failure and digitalis therapy." Had the essayists had any difficulty with catheterizing the superior mesenteric artery or the inferior mesenteric artery? Marshall J. Orloff, of San Diego, said that in some several hundred patients they had been enthusiastic over the diagnostic use of the technique, but expressed ". . . continuing uncertainty about the therapeutic advantages of pharmacologic agents infused into the splanchnic circulation." Would the patient who stopped bleeding have stopped without the pharmacologic agents? How often do they fail to get the catheter into the artery for infusion? His experience, and the general experience, had been that the infusion of pitressin stopped bleeding from esophageal varices in 88% of patients but ". . . no one yet has commented on the effects of this approach on over-all mortality." He was amazed at the low complication rate of the Oregon group. Their own complication rate with cirrhotics, particularly in respect to hematoma of the groin, was high. President Moore asked Dr. Krippaehne to comment whether he had "added the infusion of some small, soft clot through the catheter in patients who would not respond to pharmacology?" Krippaehne, closing, said he was not able to answer from their limited experience what the effect on survival of cirrhotics would be. They had had technical difficulty in catheterizing a specific vessel in only one patient with a huge liver. Some of the patients had indeed had massive bleeding which stopped after infusion. The infusion of an autologous clot, which Dr. Moore asked about, had been successfully employed by injection into a bleeding artery in one patient. "In patients with platelet deficiencies and bleeding from gastritis, we have infused platelets directly through the catheter into the arterial supply from which the bleeding small vessels received their major blood supply. This has resulted in cessation of bleeding."

* * *

Theodore Drapanas, of New Orleans, Professor and Chairman of the Department of Surgery, Tulane University School of Medicine, *Interposition Mesocaval Shunt for Treatment of Portal Hypertension,* had three-and-a-half years before begun "a prospective evaluation of a large diameter Dacron graft interposed between the superior mesenteric vein and the vena cava for management of variceal hemorrhage due to cirrhosis of the liver and portal hypertension." He had performed the operation in 25 patients and had follow-up studies of graft patency in 15, in all of whom the grafts were patent, and additionally in three patients,- two operative deaths at seven and 30 days, and a late death at 14 months, all of whom had patent grafts. Interposition vein grafts between the portal vein and the inferior vena cava had been performed as early as 1951 when Yeoh and Eiseman had employed, between the portal vein and the inferior vena cava, a Teflon graft which eventually occluded. Resende-Alves, in Brazil, in 1963, had successfully employed a Teflon shunt between the superior mesenteric vein and the vena cava, and Foster had an excellent experience with Teflon shunts between the portal vein and the vena cava. Lord, in 1970, had reported successful use of Teflon in mesocaval shunts and by 1971 reported eight of nine shunts patent after one to five years. Raymond C. Read had employed venous mesocaval homografts in 1970 and had had 12 long survivals. Drapanas had found large-sized Dacron prostheses satifactory and preferred to avoid the problem of finding a venous graft of adequate size. Portal pressures in his experience were reduced by 50% or better and he made the statement that ". . . mesocaval shunts are as effective in protecting against subsequent variceal hemorrhage as are direct portacaval shunts." The technique was technically easy, simpler than the mesocaval shunt of Marion and of Clatworthy "who mobilize the vena cava and swing it into the side of the superior mesenteric vein", and avoided the possibility of leg edema. The interposition shunt was much easier than the standard portacaval shunt and more rapidly performed. It was in effect a side-to-side shunt at a distance from the porta hepatis. They had had postoperative ascites in only a single patient. Portacaval shunts resulted in an incidence of encephalopathy varying in different reports from 15% to 50%. The splenectomy and vein division operations failed to prevent the threat of recurrent hemorrhage although avoiding encephalopathy. Warren's distal splenorenal shunt had apparently been free from postoperative encephalopathy but it was a technically difficult procedure. With the meso-

caval shunt Drapanas had two operative deaths, in 25 patients, all of whom were selected because they were poor risks, and one late death due to acute hepatic failure, no recurrence of bleeding, and no postoperative encephalopathy, and patent shunts in all the 15 patients studied, and the three patients autopsied. Drapanas concluded that the operation was extremely effective, easily performed, permitted continued perfusion of the liver, and he was now ready to recommend the operation for good risk patients.

Discussion

Gilbert S. Campbell, of Little Rock, said that from "our Veterans Administration Hospital . . . Raymond Read and Bernie Thompson . . . At the vascular society meeting 2 years ago . . . presented their results in eight patients undergoing mesocaval interposition with vena caval homografts." More recently, they had been using the patient's own jugular vein and now had 18 such patients. They had three early postoperative deaths, two of the 15 long-term survivors died of hepatoma, the grafts open in both. Only one patient had rebled,- from alcoholic gastritis. "Hepatic encephalopathy has not been a problem . . ." Campbell himself preferred interposition of the jugular vein autograft between the vena cava and the portal vein rather than between the vena cava and the superior mesenteric vein. Jere W. Lord, Jr., of New York, emphasized the much lower operative mortality of Drapanas' operation as opposed to portacaval shunts because it was simpler and quicker. Lord believed that Drapanas had settled the question as to whether the shunts would stay open. Lord's group [see page 1279, Volume LXXXVI, 1968] had performed 25 such shunts, and of 13, who were followed a year or longer, 11 were proved to be patent. They had used Teflon for the shunts. Drapanas agreed that emergency shunts should be avoided. W. Dean Warren, of Atlanta, disagreed with the statement Drapanas had made that his operation left the liver to be perfused, doubted with the sharp drop in portal pressure that the liver would in fact be perfused by the portal vein, and commented that the one venogram which was shown to illustrate the forward flow in the portal vein was not very convincing, "In fact, Dr. Gil Campbell commented that his oratory was much sharper than his venograms." Warren thought ". . . this is an important paper. In the first place, this greatly simplifies the technic of doing a side-to-side that will be applicable for emergency procedures, which has been, in most series of recent vintage, the prime indication for the use of an end-to-side portacaval shunt. Secondly . . . those patients not suitable for a distal selective splenorenal shunt fall into two groups, those with ascites and those with high intrahepatic pressures and little portal flow to the liver . . . This technic gives us the side-to-side decompression, which, as Dr. Drapanas pointed out, gives the best control of ascites and will also control bleeding very beautifully." He added [probably not even tongue-in-cheek] "The third point is that this shunt is easy to close. If severe encephalopathy ensues, there is a growing tendency to attempt to close the shunt and reconstitute some other type procedure without diversion of portal flow from the liver. We have just done this at Emory with Dr. Robert Smith who performed a selective distal splenorenal shunt and closed the mesocaval shunt. Dr. Richard Varco, who, by his own admission is one of the Nestors of American surgery, said, 'The only trouble with the distal splenorenal shunt, Warren, is that you took an easy operation and made it look hard.' " The mortality in their initial 12 cases was 50%. They had had 30 additional cases, two operative deaths, and they had had no patients admitted to the hospital with encephalopathy, and no bleeding from varices. Frank C. Spencer, of New York, was puzzled by the rare appearance of late encephalopathy, "How can this shunt differ physiologically from a standard mesocaval shunt? The Columbia Presbyterian group in New York reported several years ago that the frequency of encephalopathy after mesocaval shunts was similar to that after portacaval shunts. The report today, however, shows a much lower frequency." Drapanas, closing, said to Dr. Campbell that while the venous autograft or homograft was useful, using the patient's own jugular vein increased the operative time. Dr. Lord's results were almost identical to Drapanas' and confirmed the low mortality and the 90% patency. To Dr. Warren he said that those were forward angiograms, made by superior mesenteric and celiac artery injections. He agreed with Warren that total diversion of blood from the liver might be bad for it and his shunt was in effect a side-to-side shunt which did "permit prograde flow to the liver in some patients." He could not answer Spencer's question as to why the patients with the Marion-Clatworthy shunt developed encephalopathy and his and Dr. Read's, and Dr. Lord's did not. "Nevertheless, I would remind you that spontaneous encephalopathy does occur, even without shunts, for many of these patients do have progressive severe liver disease." Drapanas commented finally, "Dr. Francis Jackson's statistics

which were presented at this Association last year and which we quoted in the manuscript indeed show that although one can protect against hemorrhage with a portacaval shunt, after about the second year there is no difference in survival between the shunted and non-shunted patients; the shunted group is dying of liver failure and encephalopathy, and the group non-shunted is dying of hemorrhage. The important point is, they are both dead at about the same rate after the second year. We believe that we ought to do better than that and we are trying."

* * *

[The end of the period of rising expectations was in sight, but funding still existed and efforts were continuing in massive programs to develop an implantable artificial heart. While there was still a race between the supporters of the implantable artificial heart and the supporters of homotransplantation, despite an enormous amount of heavily funded work, the implantable heart remained beset by numerous difficulties. The cardiac transplantation program, apart from the special technical problems of cardiac transplantation, although it had already met with much greater success than the artificial heart program, was proving to be beset with more difficulties, certainly, than renal transplantation. Three successive papers pointed all this out.]

John C. Norman, of Boston, Associate Professor of Surgery, Harvard Medical School, and by invitation, F. A. Molokhia, L. T. Harmison, R. L. Whalen, and F. N. Huffman, *An Implantable Nuclear-Fueled Circulatory System:* 1. Systems Analysis of Conception, Design, Fabrication and Initial In Vivo Testing, indicated the complexity of their cooperative approach by listing the sponsoring organizations as ". . . the Department of Surgery of Harvard Medical School, the Cardiovascular Division of the Sears Surgical Laboratories, Harvard Unit, Boston City Hospital, and the Thermo Electron Research and Development Center, Waltham, Massachusetts, and the Medical Devices Applications Program of the National Heart and Lung Institute, Bethesda, Maryland." Their preamble pointed out the complexity of the problem involved in such ". . . mission-oriented research which presents a series of complex multidisciplinary problems. Each must be solved simultaneously within severe weight and volume constraints . . . a multiplicity of parallel approaches . . . integration of biologic and physical disciplines . . . traditionally . . . interfaced . . . continuing cooperation and interaction between federal, industrial and university interests." Multiple institutes and laboratories were required, and the

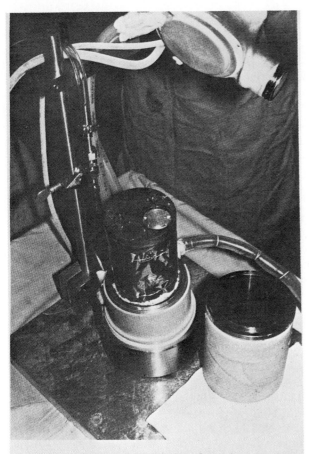

Fig. 9b. The fuel capsule has been inserted into the power source which is at room temperature.

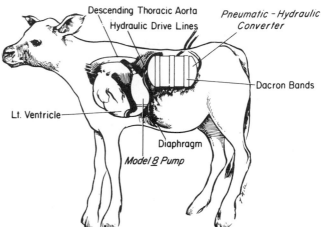

Fig. 11. Functioning system in the calf.

The power source was a 120 Gm. [at $1000/Gm.] Pu-238 fuel cell, 1.28 inches by 2.00 inches which served to drive the miniature steam engine, weighing 24 ounces. The engine vaporization required only one drop of water. The electricity for the logic circuit was obtained by thermoelectric conversion. The silastic pump was hydraulically compressed and capable of a 100 ml. stroke volume at 90 beats per minute.

John C. Norman, R. A. Molokhia, L. T. Harmison, R. L. Whalen, and F. N. Huffman, *An Implantable Nuclear-Fueled Circulatory Support System:* 1. Systems Analysis of Conception, Design, Fabrication and Initial In Vivo Testing. Volume XC, 1972.

traditional step-by-step sequence of problem solution would have required an interminable stretch-out of the development process, so that since 1965 they had "employed a modified systems analysis and development approach in which all subsystems are considered concurrently." Basic to their program had been the use of a nuclear powered pump, the cooling of the pump by the circulating blood with ". . . the entire body surface area as an extended form of heat exchanger . . ." A valveless vapor cycle engine had seemed attractive, powered by ". . . the radioisotope decay heat from a 52 thermal watt Plutonium-238 fuel capsule . . . converted into hydraulic power for driving the Model VIII Left Ventricular Assist Pump by means of this unique implantable steam engine." The miniature steam engine weighed 24 ounces and was electronically controlled from the pumping chamber of the assist blood pump, the signals from which were "processed by a miniature logic unit". The electric power for the logic unit was supplied by a thermoelectric module.

The plutonium fuel capsule measured 1.28 inches by 2.00 inches and reached a temperature of 1000°F. It required 120 Gm. of Pu-238 the cost of which was currently $1000/Gm. The fuel capsule was "designed to withstand corrosion, high impact, crush pressures, cremation and the maximum credible accident temperature of 2400°F." The left ventricular assist pump transferred the blood from the apex of the left ventricle to the descending aorta. A Dacron-reinforced silastic bladder ". . . rolls under the action of a metal pusher plate attached to the drive mechanism." The bladder was contained within a stainless steel housing. The drive fluid circulated "through the plenum, transferring heat rejected from the engine module to the blood . . . The plenum chamber is insulated with closed-cell polyurethane foam to maintain the prosthesis surface temperature below 43°C." The half-life of the fuel was 89.0 years, the design life of the system was ten years. "During the first *in vivo* 8-hour test the left ventricular assist device stroke volume was 100 ml./beat and the calf's rectal temperature was 98°F."

Discussion

The Discussion was opened by Clarence Dennis, Chief of the Medical Devices Application Branch at Bethesda. He commented that "The problems are far from solution. For instance, Dr. Willem Kolff's recent brilliant accomplishment in the 2-week survival mechanical heart was terminated by problems of incompatibility of blood with the materials used. Bio-compatibility indeed appears to be the most challenging problem still to be faced." Benson Roe, of San Francisco, said that Dr. Smail in his laboratory, employing a pneumatically driven pump "invented by Mr. Paul Davis" had a system which was "mechanically simple, requiring no complex external control or electronic apparatus." He showed a motion picture of a calf with such an implanted device, on the sixth day after operation, "The portability and the automaticity of the device is demonstrated by this calf seen here exercising on its sixth postoperative day. Those are scuba tanks carrying the air supply, but you can see that the output demands are met by the variable output response of the automatic pump." David P. Boyd, of Boston, said that "The ingenuity of the hydraulic principle seemed quite remarkable, but the thought of an internal temperature, no matter how insulated, of 500° to 1000°F. is a bit awesome". Stating that "In the laboratory many years ago we could destroy virtually all the right ventricular musculature and surviving animals maintained cardiac output and their response to stress". He asked ". . . if this could not be more than an assist, but could do the whole job with the simple addition of an appropriately calibrated A.S.D." Raymond Heimbecker, of Toronto, asked "how far away the clinical application might be, and . . . what might be the ultimate cost per patient . . . ." John E. Connolly, of Irvine, said that "The early preliminary success with the plutonium atomic powered pacemakers in patients in France, even though the power source is much less than it is in this instrument, does prove that this is a reality." Dr. Norman had shown that his power sources could be successfully shielded and he was on the way to solving the problem of an implantable power source, one of the basic requirements. The other two problems were trauma to the blood, and the need for heparin. Connolly was optimistic enough in congratulating Norman to ". . . predict that the totally implantable heart problem will be solved, perhaps,

within this decade." Norman, closing, said that they were fascinated with Roe's device. To Dr. Boyd he said that with a large enough cardiac output through the pump, the endogenous heat was dissipated. He was not very explicit in answering the question about cost, "The current cost is rather substantial. However, if our coal supply is to be exhausted in 150 years, obviously we will need sources of power. As nuclear generators assume their rightful place in terms of supplanting our power supplies, the whole concept becomes more fiscally feasible." [This was seven years before the near-nuclear catastrophe, at Three-Mile Island near Harrisburg, Pennsylvania which, it appeared to some, threw the future of the nuclear energy industry into question.] He was cautious about predicting the time of solution of the remaining problems. If they could maintain their present momentum and were successful as they had been in the previous eight years "it is quite possible that we could talk in terms of clinical applications of units like this by the end of this decade. It may well be the end of the next decade."

* * *

Norman was followed by E. Dong, Jr., R. B. Griepp, E. B. Stinson, all by invitation, and Norman E. Shumway, of Stanford, Professor of Surgery, Stanford University School of Medicine, *Clinical Transplantation of the Heart.* They said that "Despite significant and widespread interest in mechanical devices, design factors for control, power, and biocompatible materials, cost of production for energy sources, and reliability make the issue of a total replacement device real only on a time scale of a decade, if indeed that soon. On the other hand, heart transplantation is available now." Their experiments with the technique of cardiac transplantation went back to 1959 and since then they had worked on the problems of "cardiac preservation, diagnosis of rejection, hemodynamics despite denervation, and selective immunosuppression", and "The technical feasibility of heart transplantation had also been demonstrated in humans along with the occasional long-term surviving patient." Cardiac transplantation had been under a cloud "in part due to the initial massive failure when introduced clinically." A good deal of progress had been made since then. The patients selected were those for whom no more could be done medically. Histocompatibility grading was ". . . no longer mandatory". During removal of the donor heart ". . . the superior vena cava is divided between ligatures, the inferior vena cava at the diaphragm, the pulmonary artery at the bifurcation, the aorta close to the innominate artery, and the pulmonary veins at their entrances to the left atrium." At the same time, the recipient's heart was removed "by transecting the atria dorsal to the atrial appendices and the great vessels distal to the valvular commissures." In the implantation, the atria were sutured first, then the aorta, and then the pulmonary artery. A pacemaker wire was sutured to the surface of the ventricle. Initially immunosuppression had been with azathioprine and prednisone, then with azathioprine, prednisone, and antilymphocyte serum, and currently with azathioprine, prednisone, and antithymocyte globulin. Dipyridamole and Coumadin had been employed since January 1970. Cardiac rejection was treated with actinomycin D, increased doses of prednisone, and systemic heparinization. Rejection was indicated by ECG changes ". . . decreased voltage, right shift in axis, right bundle branch block, and atrial arrhythmias", as well as by such clinical signs as "diastolic third and fourth heart sounds, decreased precordial impulse, and decreased fullness of the pulse . . . Hypotension, hepatomegaly, fatigue, anorexia, and a gain in weight." Signs of left heart failure appeared very late, the signs listed did not all appear and "As a practical matter, the decreased voltage tends to be the major parameter for assessment of rejection." Forty-two patients had undergone transplantation, 33 for arteriosclerotic heart disease, the remainder for "idiopathic myopathy". Two of the patients had had two transplantations, 16 patients were still alive, three in the hospital, 12 of 31 at risk had survived one year, seven of the 20 at risk had survived two years, two of 14 at risk had survived three years. Twenty-six patients had died, three of them within two days of operation, of right heart failure and low cardiac output, associated with severe pulmonary arteriosclerosis. Four patients died two weeks to two months after transplantation "from unrelenting cardiac rejection." In ten patients the primary cause of death was infection, or infection with rejection. Aspergillus, Nocardia, and Candida infections had become a problem since the advent of antithymocyte globulin. Twenty-one patients of the 42 had left the hospital but three very shortly returned to the hospital and died. Thirteen of the remaining 18 returned to work or housekeeping and all were "physically active without cardiac symptoms." They believed that ". . . cardiac transplantation should be reconsidered as appropriate therapy for advanced heart failure due to irreparable myocardial disease. Using the proper selection criteria . . . the operation can have a low operative mortality. Recognition that pulmonary vascular arteriosclerosis is a contraindication to transplantation has eliminated immediate mortality. Screening for cytotoxic antibodies has . . . avoided hyperacute rejection . . . improved myocardial function is prompt and uniform . . . documented by angiographic and hemodynamic studies in the first and second years after transplantation . . . physical, social and vocational rehabilitation achieved by the group as a whole irrespective of the improved cardiovascular status. In contrast, a study of valvular patients has demonstrated the failure of some . . . to return to work despite improved cardiovascular function." They made the telling point that ". . . the death of all but one untransplanted patient in less than 95 days after completion of workup reflects the fact that myocardial function was extremely compromised in this group of patients." Their one-year survival figure had increased "from the initial 22% to the current 50%." [The initial flurry of enthusiasm to which Dong had referred had produced a long line of disasters and most of the cardiac surgeons had retired from the field leaving it to Shumway and a few others.]

* * *

Samuel L. Kountz, of Brooklyn, Professor and Chairman, Department of Surgery, Downstate Medical Center, New York State University, and Folkert O. Belzer, of San Francisco, Associate Professor of Surgery, University of California, *The Fate of Patients after Renal Transplantation, Graft Rejection, and Retransplantation,* reviewed the eight-year San Francisco experience with 403 transplants in 336 patients. Fifty-four patients had secondary grafts, nine had three grafts, three received four grafts, and one patient received five grafts. The overall mortality was 21.8% during the eight-year period. Deaths occurred from intercurrent disease, from infections in the absence of clinical rejection crisis, from infections in patients treated for rejection by increased steroid dosage, and deaths occurred after patients were returned to chronic hemodialysis. The key to preventing death from infection during severe rejection episodes requiring large doses of cortisone was "to remove the graft early if large doses of immunosuppressive drugs are required to maintain graft function." This policy dropped the mortality rate due to infection from 30% in 1964 to 7% in 1971. Retransplants were similarly removed if massive doses of immunosuppressive drugs were required to maintain graft function. "Improvement in graft survival has not paralleled the improvement in patient survival", except for the improvement with cadaver kidneys when the Belzer perfusion apparatus was introduced. Graft survival was 100% in 32 identical twins, and after two years there was no difference in graft survival in ". . . HL-A non-identical siblings, parents, children, or cadaver donors. Immunosuppressive drugs have not improved the survival of grafts from related donors during the past 5 years nor of cadaver grafts in the last 3 years . . . 81% of patients in the last 18 months have been successfully treated by employing retransplantation with a mortality equal to or less than that for chronic hemodialysis.

Discussion

Richard E. Wilson, of Boston, agreed that ". . . most transplant groups have embarked on this concept of retransplantation, rather than death by overtreatment." Their experience had shown that "people with cytotoxic antibodies against Lymphocytes of greater than 10% of a pool of 40 normal people, had a 36% graft survival at 6 months . . . Those who do not have such nonspecific antibodies had an 89% 6-month survival . . .". Thomas C. Moore, of Torrance, said that, impressed by the ease with which the Belzer perfusion apparatus permitted the San Francisco group to employ cadaver kidneys, they had developed a similar system in Los Angeles. In 13 months, they had preserved 187 cadaveric human kidneys from 110 donors and transplanted 156 of them. David M. Hume, of Richmond, agreed upon the importance of separating patient survival from transplant survival. "If one retransplants freely and stops treating rejections early, the patient survival will improve . . ." [He had made this statement forcefully at the Boca Raton Meeting in 1966, Volume LXXIV]. His experience had been similar to Kountz's. Some of the patients were immunized, could not be retransplanted, leaving ". . . a residue of untransplantable, nephrectomized, living patients . . ." In his series there continued to be a difference between related living donor and cadaver donor transplants. Joseph E. Murray, of Boston, suspected that the fact that there was no difference in the Kountz-Belzer series with kidneys from whatever source except identical twins suggested "the excellence of their tissue typing and donor procurement." He asked about the quality of life in the survivors, whether there were increasing numbers of malignancies, and whether they stopped immunosuppression as soon as infection appeared. "We have adopted the policy of discontinuing immunosuppression because of the relentless nature of these infections." John S. Najarian, of Minneapolis, said that so far as con-

cerned patient survival "hemodialysis in the best centers results in about a 15% attrition rate the first year, and about 10% every year thereafter . . . attrition of people who have received transplants . . . is very small. Dr. Kountz's figures are around 5 or 6% a year. Our own figures are about 5% a year . . ." In his own hands in the four years since he had been using ALG, the cadaver results of 76% survival of first transplants at three years were not nearly as good as living related donor figures, and periodic biopsies showed much better preservation of the human related kidneys than of the cadaver kidneys. His own retransplantation rate was about 10% and he obviously thought the 20% retransplantation rate of Kountz and Belzer to be high. "Is it because they are quitting too soon? They treat two rejection crises, and then they are ready to take the kidney out, while we treat three. Are you giving up too soon with the use of immunosuppressive therapy on two rejection crises?" Willard E. Goodwin, of Los Angeles, said that in the past at San Francisco ". . . the psychiatrists . . . had emphasized the importance of using living, unrelated donors, who gained psychiatric benefit from giving kidneys." They had opposed this at UCLA and rarely used living, unrelated donors. How did Drs. Kountz and Belzer feel about that? Paul S. Russell, of Boston, agreed that HLA identical siblings were the ideal donors and that many of them did not require steroid treatment at all. "Fifty per cent of siblings will share only one of the two relevant chromosomes, thus differing by . . . one haplotype from the recipient . . . clearly better donors than those who differ by both chromosomes . . ." Had Dr. Kountz separated the non-HLA identical siblings for degrees of compatibility? President Moore said that in this tenth anniversary year of the operation "the International Registry shows at the present time that there have been approximately nine thousand of these operations done throughout the world." Samuel L. Kountz, closing, said of the sensitization effect of previous transplants "If one has an adequate supply, it is possible to find a kidney for which the recipient is not sensitized, and we do find that patients who have rejected a graft are much more sensitive than those who have not rejected a graft." They had done 90 sibling transplants typed for 20 HLA antigens, "the HLA identical siblings show 100% survival for up to 8 years. The one-haplotype siblings show an 85 to 95% survival . . . the two haplotype siblings . . . those who have two-haplotype mismatch do not do as well—40% survival. We have observed in the past year, when we dropped our HLA standards and selected all donors, that our results in living, related donors did indeed become worse." The answer to Dr. Murray's question was that "Since we remove all grafts that are not functioning well, more than 95% of our patients who have transplants are gainfully employed and live normal lives . . ." As for Goodwin's question, "We began a program of living, unrelated donors because we did not have a reliable technic for procuring cadaveric kidneys. Since we have an excellent technic for procuring cadaveric kidneys, we feel that living, unrelated donors are no longer justified; and we abandoned the program over 3 years ago. However, our psychiatric study demonstrated that many of these individuals indeed donated their kidney out of altruistic reasons."

The Business Meetings

The 1972 meeting took place at the Fairmont Hotel, San Francisco, April 26, 27, and 28, President Francis D. Moore in the Chair.

At the First Business Session, President Moore announced that the membership had ". . . a remarkable opportunity; namely, that of purchasing the authentic photocopies of the minutes of this Association going back 1880. They have been found in trunks and attics and have been compiled for the first time by Dr. Shires and Dr. Sparkman. They are available in this form near the front door at the bargain price of $50."

A number of small groups, Editorial boards, etc., had been planning their meetings around the meeting of the American Surgical Association and President Moore announced ". . . the Council at the January meeting wanted to caution the Fellowship, hopefully, not to hold other conflicting business meetings of editorial boards or other things of that type that conflict with the actual contents of the program itself this year. In the last 2 or 3 years there have been portions of the program when many of the Fellows were tied up with conflicting business meetings. The early mornings, midnights, and evenings are, of course, free; and let us not have other meetings during the program." [The number of such meetings has not decreased. However, for the most part, the injunctions of Council have been heeded.]

At the Second Business Session, before lunch on the third day, among the recommendations of Council were change of the name of the Committee on Issues to the "Joint Committee on Study of Surgical Services in the United States", and the creation of Senior Fellowship for the group of Corresponding Fellows.

The President and Secretary had been in-structed to "in the next year investigate a mechanism for a history of the American Surgical Association to be written [the first discussions with the Fellow eventually charged with the responsibility for the History were held just before the banquet at the Chateau Frontenac, in Quebec, at the 1975 meeting] and to be written in time for completion and presentation at the 100th Anniversary of the American Surgical Association in 1980."

The Council had once more received a request concerning certification in pediatric surgery and recommended that the Association "recognize the serious problem posed by the proliferation of new, separated Specialty Boards for examination and certification in a wide variety of special skills or fields of surgical care . . . the Council would, therefore, urge that the American Surgical Association urge the American Board of Surgery to give consideration to a solution [for pediatric surgery] that would provide a model for additional requests, should they arise in the future. This would provide that the American Board of Surgery, having passed and certified a candidate on the basis of its regular examination procedure, then offer an additional certificate of special competence in the specialty surgery, such as Pediatric Surgery, as based on an additional examining procedure given or arranged by the American Board of Surgery.

The Committee on pending legislation, Drs. Hanlon, Longmire, Rhoads, Moore, Dunphy, chaired by Altemeier, was to be "moved out of the SOSSUS Committee, and . . . become a joint American Surgical Association—American College of Surgeons Ad Hoc Committee." The SOSSUS reports ". . . annually, or at the close of the study . . ." were to be approved by the Council of the Association before submission to the Department of Health, Education and Welfare.

Francis Moore's Presidential Address had said that surgery must "clean up its own back yard" and now William A. Altermeier moved ". . . that Council be empowered to move forward in cooperation with other national societies and agencies, as appropriate, so as to implement a national policy for staff credentialing and accreditation, a national policy for the monitoring and control of the flow of residents, and a National Surgical Placement Service," [June 15, 1979, Dr. Moore, asked to comment on the present status of his three proposals, wrote.- ". . . validation of staff credentials . . . I believe . . . has been implemented both by hospitals and by trustees and to a minor extent by the JCAH . . . a national control of surgical specialists . . . has not come to pass. It has been threatened, but absolutely nothing has been done about it. The "GEMINAC " commission was supposed to do something about this, but it seems to me to have fizzled out. However, this has been a good example of where voluntarism won out over any sort of centralized legislative control. There has been a slight diminution in certain Board certification rates in surgery. There has been a little bit more sensible control of surgical specialty production. Urology has, particularly, looked at this in a numerical way, trying to tailor specialist production to national needs . . . as to a surgical placement, absolutely nothing has been done . . . curiously enough, it is not so much a matter of locating places that need a surgeon severely, so much as it is a question of being able to warn young surgeons who are looking for a place to settle and make a living about particular localities which are too heavily over crowded by young people in their specialties."] Dr. Altemeier's motion carried.

The Honorary Fellows elected that year were Professor Maurice Ewing, Victoria, Australia, and Professor Boris Petrovsky, Moscow, U.S.S.R., the incumbent Minister of Health and a cardiac surgeon. For the first time Corresponding Fellows were elected and that initial list consisted of Sir Brian Gerald Barratt-Boyes, of New Zealand; Professor Roy Calne, of Cambridge; Professor Daniel J. du Plessis, of Johannesburg; Professor Andrew Patrick Forrest, of Edinburgh; Professor Lars Erick Gelin, of Göteborg, Sweden; Professor Kasarn Chartikavanij, of Bangkok; Professor Andrew Kay, of Glasgow; Professor Maurice Mercadier, of Paris; Dr. Jose Patino, Bogota; Dr. Nen K. Yong, of Kuala Lumpur; and Dr. Keijo Sano, of Tokyo, Japan. The officers elected were Jonathan Rhoads, of Philadelphia, President; K. Alvin Merendino, of Seattle, and Chester McVay, of Yankton, South Dakota, Vice-Presidents; G. Tom Shires, of Dallas, Secretary.

XCI

1973

The 1973 meeting was held April 25, 26, and 27 at the Century Plaza Hotel, Los Angeles, California, President Jonathan E. Rhoads, of Philadelphia, Professor of Surgery, University of Pennsylvania School of Medicine; Director, Department of Surgery, Pennsylvania Hospital, in the Chair. The year had seen the deaths among others of Claude S. Beck, the neurosurgeon who had done so much in the treatment of heart disease by his contributions to electrical defibrillation, his studies of techniques for improving circulation to the heart, and his constant insistence on the possibility of resuscitation after cardiac arrest or fibrillation; Edward D. Churchill, who was President in 1947, with his contributions to pericardiectomy, individual ligation of the hilar structures in pulmonary resection and his distinguished service to Harvard and to the Army in the Mediterranean Theater; John H. Gibbon Jr. who had been President in 1955, the persistent and ultimately successful developer and first successful user of a pump oxygenator; and I. S. Ravdin, the driving force for years at the University of Pennsylvania, and virtual creator of its strong department of surgery and laboratory of surgical research, who had been President in 1959.

Addressing the Association on *The Quality of Surgical Scholarship,* President Rhoads explained that "My reason for selecting this topic for emphasis is a fear that the quality of scholarship in surgery has been slipping and that in a broader sense the M.D. degree has been demeaned in our time." In point of fact, while making a plea for research, scholarly analysis, precision and breadth of knowledge of languages, he devoted most of his address to the current national scene. He commented on the shortening period of education and training, the effect of Medicare, Blue Cross and Blue Shield plans, his hopes for SOSSUS, the indications from SOSSUS that "the present rate of production of surgeons, if continued, would produce a higher surgeon to the population ratio than the present M.D./population ratio by the year 2000 . . . based on projections of a higher population growth rate than now exist", the formation of the Liaison Committee, ". . . for the first time in the U.S.A., there has been established a central agency which might make effective recommendations concerning the number of residency opportunities that will be accredited in each field." He hoped that the addition to the Association of Corresponding Fellows would introduce into the program strong papers from abroad. The programs of the Association had indeed been "a tremendous force for quality in surgical scholarship." He thought that some form of recognition of the surgical scholar might be useful and though it might be logical, he feared there was no likelihood of turning back to the era of Bachelors of Medicine, Masters in Surgery, Doctors of Medicine era. He proposed "a small Ad Hoc Committee be established to study this problem and report its findings and recommendations to the

Association" to recognize "the student who has the ability, the ambition, the energy, and the determination to become a contributor to productive scholarship in our field . . ." A traveling surgical scholarship awarded for the best paper presented each year by a nonmember under 45 might be another effort of the Association. Some of these activities might require funds and the committee was looking into the establishment of a tax exempt foundation for that purpose. He closed feelingly with a quotation from the first President of the Association, Samuel D. Gross, "Whatever of life and of health and of strength remain to me, I hereby, in the presence of Almighty God and of this large assemblage, dedicate to the cause of my Alma Mater, to the interest of medical science and to the good of my fellow creatures."

* * *

D. Emerick Szilagyi, of Detroit, Chairman, Department of Surgery, Henry Ford Hospital and by invitation, J. P. Elliott, J. H. Hageman, R. F. Smith, and C. A. Dall'Olmo, *Biologic Fate of Autogenous Vein Implants as Arterial Substitutes:* Clinical, Angiographic and Histopathologic Observations in Femoro-Popliteal Operations for Atherosclerosis, accepted autogenous vein grafts as "the most nearly ideal arterial substitutes" but felt that remarkably "little is known about their biologic fate after implantation in humans." They had performed 377 autogenous venous bypasses in the lower extremity, 316 of them femoro-popliteal and 61 more, to branches of the popliteal artery. All patients had had repeated postoperative arteriograms, either translumbar or femoral. In addition, they had 21 anatomical specimens, eight of them obtained at autopsy, 13 during a time of reoperation. Angiography showed stenoses at or near the suture line which they thought to be either due to suturing defects or to trauma by instruments, readily recognizable aneurysmal dilatations, usually fusiform, occasionally saccular and multiple. Fibrotic valves were occasionally recognizable. The commonest change was "a wavy narrowing of the lumen, interpreted as intimal thickening" and the second most common was atherosclerosis, "The angiographic appearance consisted of an irregularity of the luminal surface, often associated with local dilatation of mild degree. In more advanced instances the irregular luminal outline assumed the morphological characteristics seen in atherosclerotic arteries: the hunchback contour of a typical atheroma." The anastomotic stenoses were obviously seen soonest and atheromatous changes

and changes attributed to trauma near the anastomosis were the most likely to be progressive. The normal saphenous vein "is thick-walled and very rich in smooth muscle and elastic tissue elements." As time went on, the graft showed "a diminution of the smooth muscle fibers", there was an ingrowth of vessels into the adventitia and the outer media, but it was intimal thickening and atherosclerotic degeneration which were most significant and commonest,- ". . . some degree of intimal thickening is present in all grafts". Presumably as "a response of the subendothelial venous wall—the subendothelial collagen and smooth muscle fibers—to the altered hemodynamic conditions in the lumen", there occurred "an overgrowth of the subendothelial elements, mainly the subendothelial smooth muscle fibers." Narrowing of the distal outflow tract was accompanied by the deposition of fibrin on the intimal surface of the distal portion of the graft, and such fibrin layering progressed rapidly. "The atherosclerotic changes are both grossly and microscopically quite amazingly similar to those seen in arteries . . . fibrotic plaques . . . lipid infiltration . . . with an . . . atherosclerotic complex with its amorphous necrotic center, underlying collagen base, and ulcerated intimal surface, usually covered by a layer of fibrin clot." The changes were usually diffuse and sharp localization suggested "some local mechanical factor" as the application during operation of an occluding clamp. "The older the specimen the more likely to show the change and the more severe the degree of change. About 80 percent of the implants examined two years or more after implantation showed evidence of atherosclerosis." About half of the defects, those due to areas of anastomotic techniques or injury to the grafts by clamps were preventable but Szilagyi considered atherosclerotic and intimal thickening changes inevitable and perhaps ultimately universal. The development of these changes was slow, "atherosclerosis evolves very slowly, taking 4 to 6 years for development to a threatening degree. Subendothelial hypertrophy is also a progressive alteration and it follows a similarly insidious course." It was inescapable, Szilagyi said, that "the primary cause of the atherosclerotic involvement is hemodynamic . . . Since in the same individual a peripheral vein will be totally immune to the process of atherogenesis . . . but becomes fairly readily involved in the atherosclerotic process when it is placed on the arterial side of the circuit . . ." He was concerned about the implications of the study for saphenous vein aorto-coronary bypasses. "The vein material is the same, the surgical technical steps are alike, and the hemodynamic fac-

In all his 377 autogenous venous bypasses in the lower extremity Szilagyi had obtained repeated postoperative arteriograms and from autopsy or reoperation had obtained 21 anastomosis specimens. The illustration shows the frequency of the venous changes seen in arteriograms. Microscopic changes characteristic of atherosclerosis were seen in 80% of the specimens after two years. He thought the changes inevitable, progressive, and the result of the strain of arterial pressure. He was concerned about the implication for coronary bypasses.

D. Emerick Szilagyi, Joseph P. Elliott, John H. Hageman, Roger F. Smith, Carlo A. Dall'Olmo, *Biologic Fate of Autogenous Vein Implants as Arterial Substitutes:* Clinical, Angiographic and Histopathologic Observations in Femoro-Popliteal Operations for Atherosclerosis. Volume XCI, 1973.

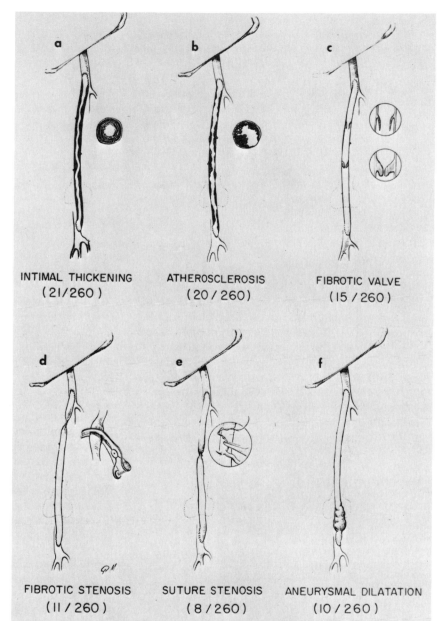

Fig. 2. Schematic representation of morphologic changes of venous autografts seen in angiograms.

tors are similar. The differences are mainly qualitative and relate to the blood pressure relationships, tissue environment and the distal hemodynamics. Unfortunately all the differences are in the disfavor of the aorto-coronary procedure. The arterial blood pressure is higher, the tissue bed in which the graft is placed is less receptive . . . and the arterial outflow circuit is greatly constricted." He suggested that this might mean that the changes seen in femoro-popliteal venous bypasses would be seen "with an accelerated tempo of development" in aorto-coronary bypasses.

Discussion

Jere W. Lord, Jr., of New York City, confirmed Szilagyi's findings. They had seen fibrotic stenosis of the intima and in about 2%, the valves remained open and fused to the opposite wall. Like Szilagyi, he advocated angiographic study for any symptoms and reoperation as needed for local lesions. H. William Scott, Jr., of Nashville, long interested in experimental atherosclerosis, had implanted the jugular veins of dogs in their own abdominal aortae, then placed them on high cholesterol diets. After seven to 12 months, "in five of the eight only minimal atheroma was found in the host aorta. In contrast, in each of the venous grafts which remained patent (one was occluded), there was severe atheroma of diffuse degree consistently present. In controls on ordinary regular diet, vein graft and host aortas showed no disease." They concluded that under the conditions of their study, "the autogenous venous graft implanted in the systemic arterial circuit has a greater avidity for atheroma than does the host artery." Paul Nemir, Jr., of Philadelphia, said that the principal difficulties with the vein graft were at the inflow or the outflow, the body of the graft usually being minimally involved. Szilagyi, closing, said that obviously a low-fat diet after venous implant would be wise, "we recommended it but I doubt that we can effectively enforce it." He suggested that in addition to other factors, the "warm ischemia time" was important and that "All efforts should be made . . . not to remove the vein from its bed until all its tributaries had been carefully tied, and the moment the vein is mobilized it should be cooled in a glucose solution of about 2–3° C."

* * *

Marion S. DeWeese, of Columbus, Professor and Chairman, Department of Surgery, University of Missouri, and by invitation, R. O. Kraft, W. K. Nichols, H. H. Six, and N. W. Thompson, *Fifteen-Year Clinical Experience with the Vena Cava Filter,* had in 1957 begun using a network of sutures crisscrossing the vena cava as a net to trap emboli and now were reporting their experience with 112 patients. Ligation of the vena cava to prevent pulmonary embolism had been introduced by John Homans in 1944. Streuter and Paine (1953) as well as Pualwan (1954) had studied temporary ligation of the vena cava with catgut. Moretz (1954) had employed a removable metal clip to occlude the vena cava and subsequently, in 1959, a permanent Teflon vena cava clip. Spencer, in 1960 "introduced the concept of vena cava *plication*" [DeWeese's sutures crisscrossed the lumen of the vena cava without changing the configuration. Spencer's sutures tacked the walls of the vena cava together at intervals.] Miles (1964), Adams and J. DeWeese (1966), Taber

and Lam (1965) had all explored extraluminal serrated clips. Barkett, Wright, and Greenfield, (1969) "developed an extraluminal prosthesis with tapering channels which permit laminar blood flow." Sensening (1965) and Ravitch (1966) had "studied compartmentation of the vena cava with a mechanical vascular stapler." Recently, methods had been developed for placing "filtering or occluding devices . . . within the inferior vena cava by transvenous jugular or femoral routes",- Mobin-Uddin (1967), Eichelter and Schenk (1968), Pate (1969), Hunter (1970), Moser (1971), Greenfield (1973), employing various expandable metal or plastic devices, or balloons. From October 1957 to October 1972 DeWeese's group had placed their filter in 112 patients. Ten deaths occured within 30 days of operation but in six of the patients, the filter "was placed during the course of an operation which was indicated by another catastrophic illness." None of the deaths were due to pulmonary embolism. Seventeen more patients had died during the study period, none of them from pulmonary embolism. In their follow-up studies, embolism was suspected in 18 patients and proved by lung scan, angiogram or both in seven. Twenty-six percent of patients had edema of the extremities "related to operation or to the antecedent phlebitic process" and an additional 10% had edema which was thought to be due to cardiac or renal disease. Inferior vena cavagrams in the follow-up period were obtained in only 32 patients, and together with autopsy findings, showed patency of the filter in 71%. Five of the seven patients with repeated small embolism had secondary ligation of the vena cava, "However, three of them continue to have intermittent chest pain of the type which led to their secondary caval ligation." A renal transplant patient, in whom at the time of pulmonary embolectomy, a filter was placed in the vena cava, above the transplanted renal vein, was still well three years later. Ordinarily the filter was placed below the renal veins.

Discussion

Lester R. Bryant, of Lexington, Kentucky, said that since Mobin-Uddin had joined their department, they had given up the Spencer vena cava plication technique and employed "the transvenous method of vena caval interruption with . . . the Mobin-Uddin vena caval filter". There had earlier been episodes of migration with the 23 mm. filter. With the currently employed 28 mm. filter, migration had not occurred in 70 consecutive implantations. Lazar J. Greenfield, of Oklahoma City, de-

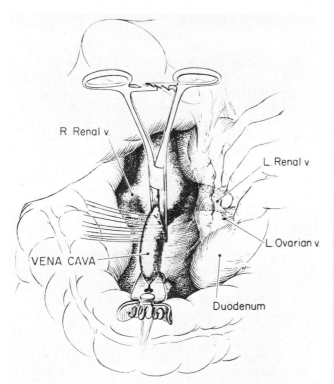

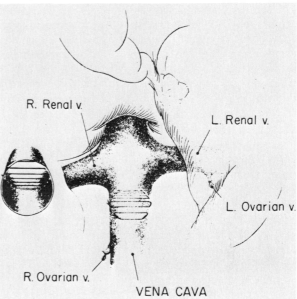

FIG. 3. Vena cava filter has been completed and both ovarian veins have been ligated.

FIG. 2. Construction of vena cava filter at infra-renal level with interrupted vascular sutures.

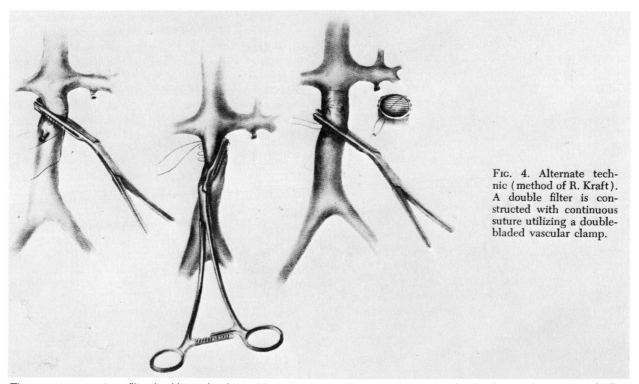

FIG. 4. Alternate technic (method of R. Kraft). A double filter is constructed with continuous suture utilizing a double-bladed vascular clamp.

The vena cava suture-filter had been implanted in 112 patients. There had been no deaths from pulmonary embolism but embolic accidents were proved in seven and suspected in 11 more. 26% of the patients had leg edema not on a cardiac or renal basis. Of 32 venograms 71% showed patency.

Marion S. DeWeese, Richard O. Kraft, W. Kirt Nichols, Herbert H. Six, and Norman W. Thompson, *Fifteen-Year Clinical Experience with the Vena Cava Filter*. Volume XCI, 1973.

scribed his transvenously inserted filter "composed of stainless steel in a cone shape with a very fine recurved hooks which allow fixation within the wall of the vena cava." The geometry of the cone shaped arrangement of wires made it "possible to fill 70% of the depth of the cone with thrombotic material without introducing any significant impairment of flow through the vena cava . . . . The filter device is placed on a carrier catheter and inserted through a femoral venotomy. We have used this approach as a complement to the catheter technic for removal of pulmonary emboli. Thus, following use of the vacuum cup catheter to remove thrombotic material from the pulmonary arteries we can complete the procedure by insertion of the cone device." DeWeese, closing, said "The transvenous methods leave me a little bit anxious because of their failure to protect against emboli from the gonadal vessels. This is a concern which justifies futher investigation."

* * *

Samuel R. Powers, Jr., Professor of Surgery, Albany Medical College; Professor of Bioengineering, Rensselaer Polytechnical Institute, and by invitation, nine others, *Physiologic Consequences of Positive End-Expiratory Pressure (PEEP) Ventilation,* had analyzed "some of the physiologic consequences of increased airway pressure on ventilation, cardiac output and on the peripheral utilization of oxygen." In the posttraumatic respiratory distress syndrome, with increased shunting of blood through non-ventilated portions of the lung, the arterial oxygen tension could usually be elevated by the use of the mechanical ventilator, particularly with positive end-expiratory pressure (PEEP). Powers' previous study had in "33 severely injured patients, including 73 separate alterations in the level of PEEP, indicated that in roughly 1/3 of these an increase of PEEP resulted in a worsening rather than an improvement in the calculated shunt. In some patients PEEP produced a reduction in oxygen delivery to the tissues and a fall in tissue oxygen consumption." The data from their present studies indicated that the use of PEEP might have "at least three separate physiologic consequences . . . an increase in the number of ventilated alveoli as evidenced by an increased functional residual capacity, a change in cardiac output and a redistribution of blood flow within the lung from regions that are well ventilated to regions of poorer ventilation." In the majority of patients, there was "a fall in the calculated pulmonary shunt and an increase in arterial oxygen concentration" and an increase in FRC "indicative of a further ex-

pansion of already open alveoli as well as . . . an opening of previously nonventilated alveoli". However, oxygen delivery to the tissue depended on "the product of arterial oxygen concentration and the cardiac output" and "In one-half of this series, PEEP produced a fall in cardiac output." A third of the time the fall in output outweighed the improved arterial oxygen content as previously noted experimentally by Uzawa and Aschbaugh in 1969. The reduction of cardiac output had been attributed to "a decrease in the filling pressure of the right heart. Increased airway pressure will be partially transmitted as an increase in intrathoracic pressure so that the net right ventricular filling pressure . . . will decrease." In addition, Powers indicated that an improved arterial oxygen content might result in an increase in peripheral resistance decreasing the return to the right heart at the same time that the "direct compressive effect on the pulmonary capillaries" of PEEP would increase pulmonary vascular resistance. Their own studies suggested that the increase in pulmonary vascular resistance was the most important of these. They thought that the reduced cardiac output seen in their patients could, in some cases, have been avoided by "more vigorous intravenous fluid therapy". Increased cardiac output was seen in some patients following the application of PEEP depending upon whether pulmonary vascular resistance was decreased or not. Management of patients was best accomplished "when facilities for the measurement of FRC, cardiac output, pulmonary vascular resistance as well as blood gases are available . . . Ideal ventilatory therapy is demonstrated by an increase in tissue oxygen consumption."

Discussion

Thomas F. Nealon, Jr., of New York City, said that investigating the increase in pneumothoraces with the use of PEEP at their hospital, they had found that "there was only a quarter per cent incidence in those patients who were ventilated with pressure ventilators, which increased to 7% when volume ventilators were used and . . . increased to 17% when PEEP was included . . . at the thoracic meeting last week, there were several reports in which the incidence of pneumothorax with PEEP ran as high as 20% . . . it is very important to be aware of this catastrophic event and unless it is recognized immediately, and decompressed, pneumothorax can be a fatal complication. However, it certainly should not discourage the use of this very valuable technic." George H. A. Clowes, Jr., of Boston, mentioned that "perhaps the way to avoid having to use PEEP is to start using a respirator earlier in the patient's course . . . if on breathing air a patient's arterial blood oxygen tension [septic, injured, post-shock patients] is less than 65 mm. Hg, we will intubate him, start him on a respirator and regulate the blood gases . . . . It is my impression that we have nearly halved the number of serious shunt problems on our general surgical service." The septic patients had to have a high cardiac output and could not tolerate its sharp reduction by the use of PEEP. Powers, closing, said that pneumothorax had been relatively infrequent in their unit ". . . and we believe this has to do with the form of the inflation-pressure pulse rather than its magnitude. If the respirator delivers a very short inspiratory phase then a high peak pressure will result, whereas one can deliver the same quantity of gas with a more prolonged inspiratory phase. End-expiratory pressure can be used without developing a high peak pressure . . . we never permit a patient who is having positive end-expiratory pressure to be alone in the room. A nurse or a physician is there every 60 seconds of every 24 hours a day. If this is recognized and a chest tube is put in place, there is no reason to discontinue the same level of positive end-expiratory pressure." He attributed to Clowes "the original report on the very high cardiac outputs in patients in the post-injury state" and agreed with him on the early use of the respirator "Our house staff has become so expert and does these things so early that we now have difficulty getting patients to study." He made one other practical point "Our data suggest that oxygen delivery is the factor which determines oxygen consumption. The most important determinate of oxygen delivery is the hemoglobin level. It makes little sense to try and increase the Po_2 of a patient a few millimeters with a potentially dangerous modality when oxygen delivery can be increased by much greater amounts by the simple addition of a blood transfusion."

* * *

Philip R. Allison, of Oxford, England, Nuffield Professor of Surgery, University of Oxford, an Honorary Member, *Hiatus Hernia:* (A 20-Year Retrospective Survey), presented his own long-term results over 20 years in 553 patients who were operated upon for hiatus hernia, out of 898 seen with the condition. Of the total 95 were paraesophageal and 801 were sliding. Allison's original operation [reduction of the hernia, attachment of the phrenoesophageal ligament to the edge of the diaphragmatic opening, gentle approximation of the

crura with heavy sutures] was applied alone in 332, with a gastrostomy or vagotomy or a cholecystectomy in 85. There were 39 Heller-type operations and 24 Leigh Collis or similar operations. Sixty-seven patients required resection for stricture. [The very brief published paper must have been word for word the paper he delivered. The results of the various operations are for the most part lumped together.] "When the patients were reviewed radiologically, the presence of a stomachal pouch above the diaphragm, no matter how small, or the presence of reflux from stomach to esophagus, tested in exactly the same way as before operation, were taken to indicate recurrence. By these rigid standards, radiological recurrence was found in 33% of paraesophageal hernia and in 49% of sliding hernia." He made the point that ". . . the recurrences increased steadily in the years after operation—thus in group A [the 153 patients he operated upon himself, excluding the 221 operated upon by his associates] there were 27 recurrences in the first year, 28 between 1 and 5 years, 15 between 5 and 10 years and 11 after 10 years. Very similar figures were found in group B." It was obviously necessary then to follow patients for a long time. Obesity was a factor in the development of hiatus hernia and "It was noted at the time of survey that many patients, immediately freed from symptoms, had grossly overeaten and become obese, despite strict warnings to the contrary." Radiological recurrence was not equivalent to recurrence of symptoms. Forty-three patients with radiological recurrence had been "completely freed of all symptoms in some degree, 86 showed that cardiac function was competent." Most of the patients who had return of symptoms "volunteered that they were mild and not to be compared with their discomfort before operation" but with characteristic candor, Allison said that ". . . this statement must be interpreted in the light of other factors such as the diminution of the severity of discomfort with advancing years, the anxiety of patients to please those who have looked after them, and the philosophy of those who 'learn to live with their troubles.' "

Discussion

The Discussion was opened by Lucius D. Hill, of Seattle, who stressed the importance, in any corrective operation, of restoring the esophageal sphincter pressure. While deferentially stating that "Undoubtedly we are not performing the Allison procedure, as he depicted, in this country. We are certainly not performing it as well as he does", he recited Woodward's damaging analysis measuring reflux "by pH and pressure determinations . . . and his group as you know, indicated a 54% persistent reflux and 39% anatomical recurrence in 127 patients. Other institutions throughout the country reported a similar experience." Hill said that of 80 patients with his own median arcuate repair "by pre- and postoperative pH and pressure studies", there was a mean increase of 6.97 mm. Hg in the esophageal sphincter pressure after operation. He had followed his patients as long as 13 years and the results appeared to be reproducible, for "Other centers, as far away as Santiago, Chile, utilizing this procedure, have had a low recurrence and a high degree of correction of reflux", citing also the report of Thomas and Hall from the University of California, in San Francisco, "79 patients operated upon over a 6 1/2 year period with no anatomical recurrence and a correction of reflux as measured by pH and sphincter pressure studies in 93% of the patients." Hill concluded by saying gracefully that "I am certain that few centers in this country are performing the Allison technic as Professor Allison himself does it. I suspect if we could make the trip to Oxford and observe Professor Allison first-hand, that we too could come up with a high degree of reproducibility." Conrad Lam, of Detroit, on the other hand, had been employing the Allison repair for 20 years in more than 500 patients and "we have had no valid reason to change the technic, although some distinguished colleagues have proposed different operations. The previous discussant, Dr. Hill, has suggested that the defect be approached through an abdominal incision and that the stomach be sutured to the arcuate ligament. Others have advised us to wrap the stomach around the lower part of the esophagus to prevent reflux. One of these operations [Belsey's] bears the name of one of Michigan's fine motor cars—the Mark IV [a Lincoln automobile]." Allison had presented his rather substantial, radiological and symptomatic recurrence rate without explanation, apology, or in fact any characterization at all, although perhaps his feelings can be inferred from his wry remark in closing the Discussion, "I would also like to say what a great relief to me and how pleasant it was to hear him [Hill] say in his last sentence that if he came to Oxford he would be able to produce such a high degree of reproducibility instead of a high degree of recurrence.!"

* * *

John L. Sawyers, of Nashville, Professor of Surgery, Vanderbilt University; Chief of Surgery, Nashville Metropolitan General Hospital, and J. Lyn-

wood Herrington, Jr., Associate Clinical Professor of Surgery, Vanderbilt University School of Medicine, *Superiority of Antiperistaltic Jejunal Segments in Management of Severe Dumping Syndrome*, stressed the characteristics of the condition they were discussing which differentiated it from other postgastrectomy disorders, "Symptoms of vasomotor imbalance manifested by weakness, faintness with an intense desire to lie down, palpitation, pallor and profuse perspiration are dominant while the gastrointestinal symptoms of postprandial cramping, abdominal pain and urgent diarrhea are less prominent. Ingestion of carbohydrates, especially sweet liquids, initiates these symptoms which are similar to the effects experienced by patients having an insulin reaction." They stressed the fact that mild dumping was not rare and that most such patients had transitory symptoms, reasonably well controlled "by dietary measures which limit carbohydrates and restrict fluid intake with meals. However, a few patients, less than one per cent in our experience, have severe dumping symptoms with resultant excessive weight loss, anemia, weakness, abdominal discomfort and occasionally uncontrollable diarrhea." They understood the symptoms to result "after a part of the stomach is sacrificed and is lost as a storage organ, and from alteration or removal of the pyloric emptying mechanism." Schoemaker, of the Hague, was said to have performed the jejunal interposition first in 1911 and S. Hedenstedt, in Scandinavia, and in particular, F. A. Henley, in England, with more than 300 patients, had employed the interposed isoperistaltic loop between gastric remnant and duodenum for the relief of the dumping syndrome. Sawyers and Herrington had employed that operation with great success in patients with the afferent-loop syndrome, but in 10 patients with the early postprandial dumping syndrome, had had no excellent results, two good results, three fair results and five poor results. They had then gone to the "double plicated iso-antiperistaltic jejunal pouch interpolated between the gastric remnant and duodenum, as described by Poth [1964]" in 12 patients, most of them followed up to 12 years, and only one as little as three years. They had four excellent results, three good results, two fair results and two poor results and made the general observation that the patients who had had a high gastric resection initially did better than those who had had a generous gastric remnant. In all the interposition operations, it was important to be sure that the vagus had been divided. Poth had advocated a single antiperistaltic jejunal segment interposed between the gastric remnant and the duodenum in 1957 and Schlicke, Sanders, and Jordan, had subsequently reported its use. Sawyers and Herrington had performed this operation in 28 patients with 20 excellent results, six good results, one fair and one poor. Once more, it was important to divide the vagus if it had not been done at the original operation. An 18 cm. segment had proved unsatisfactory in one patient who then did well after the segment was removed and a shorter segment interpolated. In their hands, a 10 cm. loop proved to be best. Jordan had reported that a 6 cm. segment was inadequate. They reported with obvious relish a patient "of unusual interest. This man originally had truncal vagotomy and pyloroplasty performed. He developed severe dumping symptoms and later underwent antrectomy with Billroth I gastroduodenostomy. There was no improvement after this operation and the patient went to London where Francis Austin Henley inserted an isoperistaltic jejunal segment between the gastric remnant and duodenum. Dumping symptoms persisted. When he was referred to us, we merely reversed the Henley isoperistaltic segment. He is now considered to have a good result." They considered that the 10 cm. reversed segment best achieved the aim of remedial operations for dumping which was "to restore the reservoir function of the stomach and to prolong gastric emptying time." They were unable to explain "the good results reported by others using an isoperistaltic jejunal segment" which in their hands produced no delay in gastric emptying, lacking "The pyloric valve-like mechanism of the reversed segment . . ." The double limb jejunal pouch created a satisfactory gastric reservoir but, particularly if there had been only a modest gastrectomy, stasis occurred and the pouch tended to dilate. Both Woodward and Lawrence had seen the same problem develop in their triple looped jejunal pouches.

E. R. Woodward, of Gainesville, said that he and Hastings in 1954, had "first used a three-limb jejunal pouch as a replacement for a subtotally resected stomach with severe dumping, and as luck would have it, our very first patient had a brilliant result . . . We proceeded to treat a total of 12 patients . . . from 1954 to 1963 and only once did we duplicate this result". The patients developed the symptoms of retention and dilatation of the pouch which Sawyers had described and Woodward had removed or "drastically revised" most of the pouches. The interposed Henley loop had given good results with the chronic afferent loop syndrome but had been less satisfactory for dumping. It was his experience "that if there is a relatively large gastric remnant, a simple Billroth II to Billroth I conversion gives reasonable symptomatic improvement." He concluded by saying ". . . that the best treatment for this horrendous problem is prevention. As Dr. Dragstedt always likes to say, 'the stomach is a very handy organ to take to the dinner table with you!' " Walter H. Gerwig, Jr., of Santa Barbara, California, was unapologetically enthusiastic about his results with the isoperistaltic jejunal segment which he had performed in seven patients out of a total of 600 undergoing gastric operations in a 20 year period. There were long follow-ups in six of the patients, with good results in five. Whereas Sawyers had used a jejunal segment no longer than 25 cm. "ours have all been longer than that." Carl Schlicke, of Spokane, Washington, reminded the Fellows of Alton Ochsner's remark, "The ultimate condemnation which he was able to invoke was that any operation which for the relief of its sequelae might require, as he put it, that most unphysiologic of all procedures, the interposition of a reverse intestinal loop, must be basically unsound." Nevertheless, Schlicke had reported just that procedure in a single patient 10 years before applied with great success to a very ill patient. Despite that success, he had done the operation only three more times and he was fearful ". . . that it may become more widely attempted than can be really justified." He had employed the isoperistaltic loop solely for patients with regurgitation of bile and alkaline gastritis. The reversed jejunal loop for dumping, he thought, was a measure of desperation when all else had failed and he was "truly concerned that with all that has been written about this operation, of late . . . it may become more widely attempted than can be really justified." Walter Lawrence, Jr., of Richmond, whose triple pouch Sawyers had mentioned, took this opportunity "to retract something that we reported some 10 years ago regarding remedial operations for the dumping syndrome." While his initial patients had all done very well in their two-year follow-up, continued observation had shown as in Woodward's experience that "the pouch got bigger, and reoperation was sometimes required." Having pronounced this *mea culpa,* he said "I really appreciate the opportunity to be able to give you this follow-up without having to go through the embarrassment of writing a paper about it!" George L. Jordan, Jr., of Houston, said that "it is rather amazing than disturbing that only 25 to 30% [of gastrectomy patients] have these symptoms . . . most of these symptoms are controlled by medical therapy and only the occasional patient needs an operation." He agreed with Sawyers that too rapid emptying was the problem and the antiperistaltic loop corrected this satisfactorily. "We have been performing this operation now for about 12 years and we agree it is rarely indicated. Our experience is not extensive. It includes 11 patients, but the results also are good." They had done it in a variety of ways, one of which was to anastomose the end of the stomach to the side of the jejunum. Edgar J. Poth, of Galveston, in his characteristically categorical way said of his "substitute gastric pouch with an antiperistaltic outlet fashioned from a long segment of jejunum. This jejunal substitution pouch should be reserved for use when more than 85% of stomach has been resected and a simple reversed segment would be inappropriate unless placed distal to the duodenum in the proximal jejunum." He pointed out that the longer jejunal pouch shown by Jordan in his slides applied "the major portion of the jejunal segment to the end or lesser curvature side of the residual gastric pouch to increase the gastric volume. The remainder of the jejunal segment is used to supply an appropriately long, reversed section between the enlarged gastric pouch and the duodenum." Poth had published this in 1957. With this technique, the reversed segment "should seldom exceed 5 cm." K. A. Merendino, in the Chair, calling on Sawyers to close, asked him how he measured his segment. Sawyers summed up the general consensus as favoring 10 cm. antiperistaltic jejunal segments. Although Woodward had mentioned success with conversion from the Billroth II to Billroth I, "We tried this several years ago but were not successful in relieving many patients of their symptoms." Gerwig, and Henley before him, had satisfactory results with long isoperistaltic limbs, perhaps because their segments were longer than those employed in Nashville. "We have avoided long isoperistaltic segments for fear of stasis and kinking in the jejunal loops." The measurement was of the bowel on tension, the ruler placed "midway between the mesenteric and antimesenteric border of the bowel." Once more, he said that "very few patients need remedial operation. Most patients with dumping syndrome can be satisfactorily controlled by manipulation of their diet. However, there are a few patients who are severely incapacitated with marked weight loss because they are afraid to eat. They cannot carry on their livelihood. These patients are greatly benefited by remedial operation."

* * *

James W. Kilman, by invitation, H. William Clatworthy, Jr., of Columbus, Professor of Surgery, Division of Pediatric Surgery, Ohio State University Medical School, and by invitation, William A. Newton, Jr. and Jay L. Grosfeld, *Reasonable Surgery for*

Rhabdomyosarcoma: A Study of 67 Cases, described their earlier experience with rhabdomyosarcoma at the Columbus Children's Hospital as dismal. Before 1967, of 29 children with rhabdomyosarcoma, 58% died within one year of diagnosis and only four,-14%,- survived for five years. In 1965, they began combining prophylactic chemotherapy and radiation therapy "similar to that employed in Wilms' tumors" in association with "initial and complete removal of all gross tumor". More recently in association with Children's Cancer Study Group A [the sixties had seen the development of multi-institutional cooperative therapeutic studies of this kind under the aegis of the National Institutes of Health], they employed a regimen of cyclic chemotherapy with actinomycin D, vincristine sulfate and most recently of all, cyclophosphamide. Prior to 1967 when operation was employed, it was usually extremely radical. "Since the adoption of the protocol in 1967, it became very obvious that reasonable operation, including complete excision of the tumor as possible, resulted in as good a survival rate as radical operation used with prophylactic chemotherapy and radiation therapy. The standard surgical procedure used has been extensive local resection with an attempt to conserve as much normal tissue as possible. No amputations have been performed for extremity lesions since 1967. For pelvic lesions, anterior exenteration with diverting ileal conduit cutaneous ureterostomies have been used for most of the tumors of the bladder and prostate. We have not performed prophylactic pelvic inguinal or periaortic lymphadenectomies. Head and neck lesions have in general been treated by radical neck dissection only if involved nodes were present." Survival had been vastly improved and it was striking that three of nine patients, who had only a biopsy in addition to chemotherapy and irradiation, were survivors, 86% of those with incomplete excision, and all three undergoing repeated local excisions, as well as 80% with "complete" excision and 86% with radical excision. They concluded "*Reasonable* surgery seems as good as radical surgery as far as survival is concerned as long as adequate radiation therapy and the routine administration of multiple cyclic chemotherapeutic agents are used."

Discussion

Willard E. Goodwin, of Los Angeles, rose "to speak in favor of *ureterosigmoidostomy* for urinary diversion in children, instead of ureteroileocutaneous diversion, because I think that this type of diversion improves the quality of the patient's life." He showed the pyelograms of a boy upon whom he had performed "radical excision of the prostate seminal vesicles, bladder and bulbous urethra" ten years before, employing actinomycin and radiation as well and performing a ureterosigmoidostomy ". . . he is a healthy, active young man who swims, water skis, and rides his motorcycle without the necessity of wearing an external urinary collecting device." [The paper from Columbus had cited this as the first successful operation for rhabdomyosarcoma of the prostate.] Joseph E. Murray, of Boston, wished "to confirm this report of curability of rhabdomyosarcoma in children". They had had no cures with "radical cranio-orbital resection for recurrent rhabdomyosarcoma" but when they added chemotherapy and radiation therapy, they had six long-term survivors, out of seven. The Boston Children's Hospital experience with the combined therapy of rhabdomyosarcoma in children was like Kilman's, 75% survival. He took issue with use of "the term, 'reasonable,' surgery. I would presume that all surgical treatment is reasonable. If the authors wish to avoid the term 'radical', it is their prerogative, but I would hope that all surgical treatment is adequate, thorough, and complete. Nor can I subscribe to the authors' thesis that multiple local excisions is an acceptable way of handling any tumor. One surgical resection should be sufficient, and it should be adequate and thorough. It should encompass the local tumor, and in the current state of knowledge, it should be performed in conjunction with complete chemotherapy and irradiation therapy as indicated for the specific tumor." Kilman, closing, responded to Murray. "We have meant by multiple procedures that biopsy was usually the first procedure that was done and this was followed by extensive excision as was felt indicated. It is interesting . . . that practically 80 to 90% of the resection lines of the tumors . . . show microscopic tumor and a good number obviously of these patients are long-term cures even with tumor in the line of resection at the time of the reasonable or radical surgical procedure."

* * *

Donald L. Morton, of Los Angeles, Professor of Surgery, and Chief, Division of Oncology, University of California; William L. Joseph, Alfred S. Ketcham, and Glenn W. Geelhoed, all by invitation; and Paul C. Adkins, Professor and Chairman, Department of Surgery, George Washington University School of Medicine, *Surgical Resection and Adjunctive Immunotherapy for Selected Patients with Multiple Pulmonary Metastases* , analyzed in 60 consecutive patients the therapeutic possibilities of thoracotomy and resection for metastatic pulmonary lesions, at the Surgery Branch of the National Cancer Institute, the Thoracic Surgical Service of George Washington University Hospital, and the University of California at Los Angeles. While it might be thought that "the presence of pulmonary metastases would indicate disseminated malignancy uncontrollable by surgical treatment . . . many patients dying with pulmonary metastases have no other foci of disease detectable upon autopsy . . . the five-year survival rates in patients undergoing surgical resection of metastatic pulmonary lesions are often better than results obtained followng surgical treatment of primary bronchogenic carcinoma . . . the results of surgical resection for patients with multiple metastases rival those reported in patients with solitary lesions." Twenty-seven of the patients had bilateral multiple lesions, 33 had unilateral multiple lesions. They performed 87 thoracotomies in all, one patient having a simultaneous bilateral thoracotomy. Most of the metastases were removed by wedge resections, the number in one lung varying from three to 28. They did perform 13 lobectomies and three pneumonectomies. There was a single death in 87 thoracotomies. In the last three years of the study, 19 patients had "adjunctive immunotherapy . . . using a vaccine prepared from irradiated autologous tumor cells mixed with BCG." During the same period of time, if doubling time, as judged by serial roentgenogram, was less than 20 days, there was a modest increase in survival compared to nonoperative patients. The survival improved significantly when the tumor doubling time was 20 to 40 days and still more when the tumor doubling time was over 40 days. The increased survival with operative treatment was statistically significant. The validity of the increased survival with immunotherapy was not yet determinable. The significance of the correlation between tumor doubling time and survival was suggested by the fact that "studies of complement fixing antibody titers in patients with metastatic sarcomas . . . found a good correlation between a high titer of antibody and a slowly growing sarcoma. Patients with pulmonary metastases who had titers of 256 or greater usually had tumor doubling times of greater than 40 days, whereas patients with tumor doubling times of less than 20 days had little or no detectable antisarcoma antibody in their serum." Determination of tumor doubling time required X-rays at two and usually at four weeks, and in the presence of multiple metastases, it was the rate of growth of the fastest growing metastasis that counted. The technique of multiple wedge resection was important. Time was taken to

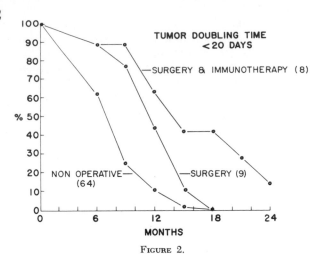

FIGURE 2.

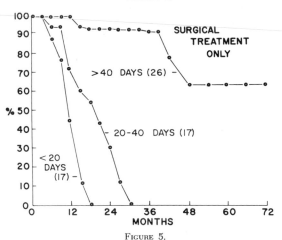

FIGURE 5.

In metastatic pulmonary tumor doubling times of less than 20 days, there is an apparent improvement in survival with multiple resection and a still greater improvement in survival if multiple resection of pulmonary metastases is combined with immunotherapy. With increase in doubling time from less than 20 days to more than 40 days, Morton's Figure 5 shows the striking relationship of tumor doubling time to survival. Of the operated patients followed more than five years with tumor doubling times of greater than 40 days, 63% were still alive and "Most patients in this group are free of disease at 5 years after surgical resection . . . despite the fact that 14 of these 26 patients had bilateral pulmonary metastases and underwent bilateral thoracotomies."

Donald L. Morton, William L. Joseph, Alfred S. Ketcham, Glenn W. Geelhoed and Paul C. Adkins, *Surgical Resection and Adjunctive Immunotherapy for Selected Patients with Multiple Pulmonary Metastases.* Volume XCI, 1973.

identify and mark with a suture each single metastasis before any were removed. Most metastases in human, as in animal tumors, were subpleural. "We have found that the mechanical stapling device is an extremely useful instrument in patients who need multiple wedge resection. Its use is facilitated if the metastasis is outlined with clamps such as Bouie hemorrhoid clamps. The excision is performed with the mechanical stapling device beyond the clamps. This insures an adequate margin of normal lung parenchyma beyond the metastases . . . local recurrence of metastases at the suture line has been kept to a minimum . . . we have had only one incident of local recurrence and two incidences of missed metastatic lesions that require additional thoracotomies in the 26 patients with tumor doubling time greater than 40 days who have survived for long periods."

Discussion

Edward J. Beattie, Jr., of New York, said, as Morton had, that the primary tumor must be under control and without other areas of metastasis. Two years ago they had reported from Memorial Hospital "a series of 29 patients with pulmonary metastases of osteogenic sarcoma . . . In 22 patients, it was possible to remove all of these tumors. In those 22 patients, we have now done 61 thoracotomies, removed over 150 metastases, and six of 22 are well 5 years after amputation." They were hoping that immunotherapy and chemotherapy might improve the present situation which was that "It is possible to cure one of six with amputation; perhaps another 20 to 25% with pulmonary surgery alone . . . " Donald L. Morton, closing, once more emphasized the utility of the multiple wedge resections, the habitually subpleural location of metastases and the usefulness of the mechanical stapling device. In one patient they had removed as many as 27 metastases from one lung and 28 from the other.

* * *

William I. Wolff and Hiromi Shinya, both by invitation, from the Department of Surgery, Beth Israel Medical Center, New York City, *A New Approach to Colonic Polyps,* made the first presentation before the Association of the use of the flexible fiberoptic colonoscope which had been developed in Japan, and was only coming into use in the United States. The instrument could be passed to the cecum. General anesthesia was not required, fluoroscopic assistance was infrequently required. Lesions could be biopsied and polyps could be completely removed. They had performed "2,000 colonoscopic examinations . . . with insignificant morbidity and without mortality." When the colon was distended with air, it was found that in fact most polyps,- 90%,- were pedunculated. Polyps less than a half a centimeter in diameter were inevitably benign. In 26 months, they had removed 499 colonic polyps larger than that from 350 patients, as many as five in one patient. Most of the polyps were less than 2 cm. but some were as large as 5 cm. in diameter. One patient bled moderately for two days and stopped spontaneously. One patient had a "minimally symptomatic perforation" after resection of a sessile polypoid carcinoma, ". . . the patient did very well on conservative management, and when the bowel was segmentally resected 4 weeks later the pathologist could find no evidence of residual tumor." Of the 499 polyps, 17 were carcinomatous, 15 had atypia or carcinoma in situ or superficial carcinoma. They required histologic invasion through the muscularis mucosae to consider the lesions as "clinically malignant". The 17 malignant polyps were found in 16 patients, of whom three were not operated upon and thus far endoscopy had shown no recurrence. Thirteen of the patients were operated upon. In one, the surgeon could find no lesion to resect and follow-up colonoscopy showed no lesion. Of the 12 colons resected, seven showed no residual tumor. There was lymph node metastasis only in a single patient and this patient had "in addition to a malignant polyp, an endoscopically recognized and biopsied adjacent small ulcerating adenocarcinoma." They commented on the importance "of not overlooking an early cancer while attention is focused on the polyp and its removal. We have encountered a number of such incidences . . . The increased incidence of cancer with polyps is well-documented. In the literature, satellite polyps have been reported in association with 25% to 50% of colon carcinomas . . . it has been stated that the patient with multiple polyps is twice. as likely to develop a colon cancer as the patient with a single polyp. Morson claims that of patients who have had a colon resection for cancer those whose specimens showed polyps in addition to the cancer have twice the chance of developing another, metachronous colonic neoplasm." Their polyps more frequently showed mixtures of adenomatous and villous features "than is generally appreciated . . . Definite malignant changes were observed in 6.8% of polyps . . . clinically significant malignant change, manifested histopathologically as 'invasive' cancer, was present in only 3.4% . . . Endoscopic polypectomy can be regarded as almost total biopsy and permits complete and unhurried pathologic study of the entire lesion . . . Selected 'malignant' polyps may not require any more endoscopic removal."

Discussion

Judah Folkman, of Boston, commented, in a child with occult bleeding, on the intraoperative use of the colonoscope which illuminated one by one the vascular malformations which were responsible. Claude E. Welch, of Boston, expressed gratitude "to Drs. Wolff and Shinya for their contributions to this rapidly expanding field . . . their great generosity in demonstrating their technics to so many people. Among others from our institution, Dr. Steven Hedberg sat at their feet for a few days and has developed the procedure at the Massachusetts General Hospital." They had removed 123 polyps, 11 of which contained cancer, ten of them villous adenomas and one an adenomatous polyp. He agreed with Wolff that cancer occurred in 8 to 10% of the polyps removed but "In contradistinction to his findings . . . we have not found colonoscopy-polypectomy quite as safe a procedure. One patient bled severely during a diagnostic colonoscopy because of rupture of the spleen. Three others have had rather severe bleeding. Two have had perforations. The patient with the ruptured spleen and the two with the perforations required laparotomy while the other complications were treated in a conservative fashion." They had discovered some polyps even 2 cm. in diameter which had been missed by barium enema. J. E. Dunphy, of San Francisco, said that "Dr. Theodore Schrock from our department spent a substantial period of time with Dr. Wolff", had performed 300 colonoscopies and removed polyps from 70 patients with one bleeding episode after polypecotomy as the single complication. Colonoscopy had enabled them to make definite diagnoses when x-rays were merely suggestive and had been useful "in the appraisal of patients with a variety of stages of Crohn's disease". For polypectomy, he urged that the "use of this instrument should be concentrated in the hands of a few members of the staff who are quite willing to devote the time and acquire the expertise and skill to do it safely and well. I believe this instrument is going to essentially eliminate the need for abdominal laparotomy in the control of polyps." Francis D. Moore, of Boston, had sent Dr. Paul Sugarbaker to study with Wolff and Shinya and he had now performed 355 colonoscopies, removing 109 polyps, all on patients in the operating room. None of the patients had positive carcino-embryonic antigen studies, even those in whom the polyp was malignant. They had had one espisode of bleeding requiring operation and two free perforations. In 14 patients, they had been able to make the differential diagnosis between carcinoma and diverticulitis when X-ray was inconclusive.

* * *

Coronary revascularization was now being widely employed and its place in pre-infarction angina, evolving myocardial infarction, and myocardial infarction with myogenic shock were under evaluation. E. D. Mundth, M. J. Buckley, R. C. Leinbach, H. K. Gold, W. M. Daggett, all by invitation, and W. G. Austen, of Boston, Professor of Surgery, Harvard Medical School; Chief General Surgical Services, Massachusetts General Hospital, *Surgical Intervention for the Complications of Acute Myocardial Ischemia,* said that the indications for management and surgical intervention in chronic myocardial ischemia were "reasonably well defined" but not yet so for acute myocardial ischemia. Over the previous four years, they had treated 116 patients with acute myocardial ischemia which they divided into five categories, "1) myocardial infarction with cardiogenic shock [80 patients], 2) evolving myocardial infarction [8 patients], 3) impending myocardial infarction [12 patients], 4) myocardial infarction with impending extension [9 patients], 5) refractory ventricular tachyarrhythmias [7 patients]." They had employed intra-aortic ballon pressure cardiac assist in all 80 patients with cardiogenic shock since the shock had persisted "despite medical therapy". "The peak hemodynamic effect of IABP appears to occur within 24 to 48 hours after institution . . . Angiography was undertaken urgently with the adjunct of

continuing IABP in 52 patients. Thirty-five patients were judged operable and 17 patients inoperable." All 16 patients not studied angiographically died of cardiogenic shock despite IABP "in our later experience, the decision regarding IABP-dependency was made within 24 hours, when possible. With hemodynamic IABP dependence, operation was recommended if the angiographic anatomy was deemed operable. Where operation was refused, IABP-dependent patients, uniformly died despite continued IABP." Of 35 patients operated upon, 33 had saphenous vein coronary bypass grafts, two patients had infarctectomy only and 17 patients had both bypass grafts and infarctectomy. Infarctectomy was indicated for "the presence of a paradoxically bulging acute aneurysm which appears to interfere with left ventricular dynamics . . . presence of a thinned out necrotic infarct in which rupture appears imminent . . . localized infarct associated with recurrent ventricular arrhythmias." In five patients, the interventricular septum was found ruptured, and the defect was repaired, without patch. Two of the patients survived. Two patients survived mitral valve replacement necessitated by rupture of the papillary muscle. Thirteen patients of the 35 survived to be discharged from the hospital and ten,- 29%,- were alive one to three years later. Three of the ten patients successfully weaned from IABP and discharged, died of myocardial infarctions within a year. They were now undertaking coronary bypass in such patients after recovery from the myocardial infarction. Of the ten long survivors of urgent operation, "eight have had excellent functional results, being able to work without angina or cardiac failure." Eight patients in whom myocardial infarction was precipitated by coronary angiography, had immediate coronary artery revascularization, three of them developing fibrillation and requiring cardiac massage on the way to the operating room, one of them surviving, now for two years. The other five patients all survived bypass and had excellent results. Of impending myocardial infarction, they said that "clinical studies have well documented an intermediate syndrome of acute coronary insufficiency which, if prolonged, progresses to frank myocardial infarction",- pain continuing more than 30 minutes, electrocardiographic ST and T wave changes of ischemia associated with pain episodes, no evidence of evolution of infarction as determined by serial electrocardiograms or enzymes. "Because of the marginal hemodynamic status of these patients and the risk of coronary angiography with ongoing myocardial ischemia, IABP was introduced in 11 of the 12 patients. IABP effectively abolished pain, reversed electrocardiographic ST and T wave changes of ischemia and improved the altered hemodynamics in nine of the 11 patients . . ." One patient, the patient in whom IABP was not instituted, who had not been recognized as having an impending myocardial infarction, had some difficulty after operation and required IABP temporarily. All patients survived revascularization. Nine were now completely free from angina. Angina had recurred in three, and in two of them severely. They were convinced that "The use of IABP has clearly facilitated management of this critically brittle group of patients in terms of safe angiographic study and safe induction of anesthesia. Revascularization surgery in this group of patients with acute myocardial ischemia has proven to be effective and of no greater operative risk than elective revascularization surgery." In myocardial infarction with impending extension marked by "Recurrent pain of myocardial ischemia in the recovery phase of acute myocardial infarction" their nine patients all had significant hemodynamic deterioration. Two of the patients developed cardiogenic shock and signs and symptoms of impending extension were reversed by use of IABP. In eight instances, angiocardiography was performed with IABP. In the one instance in which IABP was not employed, early in their experience,- "the study was complicated by ventricular tachycardia, hypotension and new infarction." Seven of the patients had double bypasses and two had triple bypasses. One of the latter, who also had infarctectomy, succumbed. One other patient succumbed to renal failure, seven patients were alive and free from angina two months to one-and-one-half years after operation. Of the seven patients with refractory ventricular tachyarrhythmias after myocardial infarction, four were in shock and required IABP. "Six of the seven patients in the acute group underwent resection of the recent infarction and this procedure was combined with revascularization in two. In the remaining patient, revascularization only was performed." Four patients required IABP before operation and all required it after operation. Four of the seven patients survived, three of them with excellent results. They were enthusiastic about IABP which they considered to have "been shown to temporarily reverse acute myocardial ischemia and has been an important adjunct in the management of these patients . . . hemodynamically effective, minimally invasive and relatively safe . . . Prompt identification of complications of acute myocardial ischemia and *early* surgical intervention is recommended for selected patients. Significant salvage and symptomatic improvement in this critical group of patients can be expected."

Discussion

J. M. Matloff, of Los Angeles, reporting from the Cedars-Sinai Medical Center, commented on 86 patients seen with pre-infarction angina treated operatively or not by physician preference. Of the 29 treated nonoperatively, there were 11 deaths within one month of admission,- 38%. Of 57 operated patients there were three deaths,- 5%. Six of eight patients in cardiogenic shock, had survived aortocoronary bypass without resection of the infarct. There had been no survivors in the four patients in the group requiring infarctectomy or mitral valve replacement. He emphasized that early operation improved the chance of survival and the postoperative left ventricular functional status so that ". . . we are encouraged to be very aggressive with early revascularization in patients with acute cardiac ischemia."

* * *

Floyd D. Loop, by invitation, Donald B. Effler, of Cleveland, Head, Department of Thoracic and Cardiovascular Surgery, Cleveland Clinic Foundation, J. A. Navia, W. C. Sheldon, and Laurence K. Groves, all by invitation, *Aneurysms of the Left Ventricle:* Survival and Results of a Ten-year Surgical Experience, reported the results in a staggering series of 400 ventricular aneurysms resected in a ten-year period from January 1962 through April 1972. The operations were undertaken 90% of the time for angina pectoris and congestive heart failure, 7% of the time for ventricular tachycardia and in a few patients because of systemic embolism from mural infarcts. They had 226 patients who had left ventricular aneurysmectomy alone, with 19 deaths, less than 10%,- and 174 patients additionally had myocardial revascularization or valve operations. In general, the mortality was no higher in those patients having revascularization, but it was 25% in those eight patients having valve replacements or closure of ventricular septal ruptures. In terms of the quality of the results, 91% of the survivors of simple aneurysmectomy had marked improvement and 74% of the patients with revascularization. During the decade under study, they had progressively increased the frequency of revascularization procedures and the operative mortality had progressively declined from 20% to 6.8%. Fifteen percent of the patients had died after discharge from the hospital, usually from cardiac causes. They concluded that "The literature indicates that fewer than 20% of cardiac aneurysm patients receiving conservative treatment will live 5 years after the precipitating infarct. In contrast, actuarial survival curves from this series show that 76% of the patients treated surgically are alive 4 years postoperatively."

Discussion

Frank C. Spencer, of New York City, said what was on everyone's mind ". . . this is the largest series of left ventricular aneurysms ever reported. The results are impressive . . ." Denton A. Cooley, of Houston, reminded the Association that ". . . in 1959 before this Association I reported the cases of six patients who survived ventricular aneurysmectomy with cardio-pulmonary bypass. Prior to that time, the only series of cases reported were those of Dr. Charles Bailey in which he had used a closed technic with surprisingly good survival statistics." Cooley made the interesting comment that "When valve damage does occur one has a unique opportunity to replace the mitral valve through a generous ventriculotomy as is seen in this operative photograph. A posterior ventricular aneurysm is opened widely with replacement of the mitral valve from below the annulus. One must reorient his thinking so the prosthetic valve is not upside down." They had had an overall hospital mortality of 15.5% in their 232 patients, 16.4% in the 134 aneurysmectomies alone, and 14.3% in the 98 with coronary bypass procedures. "Usually those patients who did not have concomitant bypass had the most serious lesions. Before 1969 bypass was never performed with aneurysmectomy." Their bypass rate was 14% in 1969, 94% in 1971, 74% in 1972. The mortality was 15% in the first three years and in 1972 was 8%. They compared their results with those of "a medically treated group reported in 1954 by Schlicter, Hellerstein and Katz" with a five-year survival of ten-year while Cooley's five-year survival was 55% and ten-year survival 37%. In his closing comments, Loop remarked, concerning the choice of patients, that the patient with ". . . diffuse myocardial impairment outside the aneurysm area can rarely be restored by even the most aggressive surgical treatment" and interestingly that "We have made no attempt to preserve the anterior descending coronary artery in patients with classic anterior aneurysms. We consider this artery a lost vessel because it traverses the aneurysm wall anteriorly and perfuses only scar tissue in the anterior one-half of the interventricular septum . . . the best long-term results are in patients who have cardiac aneurysms and oth-

erwise normal left ventricular contraction, or the aneurysm patient who has some semblance of preserved ventricular contractility with a coronary obstruction that is amenable to a bypass graft . . . the venous autograft combinations have not increased morbidity or mortality in cardiac aneurysm patients . . ."

* * *

The first from the new category of Corresponding Fellows to present a paper, Sir Brian G. Barratt-Boyes, of Auckland, New Zealand, Professor of Surgery, University of Auckland; Surgeon-in-Charge, Cardiothoracic Surgical Unit, Green Lane Hospital, and by invitation, J. M. Neutze, *Primary Repair of Tetralogy of Fallot in Infancy Using Profound Hypothermia with Circulatory Arrest and Limited Cardiopulmonary Bypass:* A Comparison with Conventional Two Stage Management, defined the latter as ". . . to palliate severely affected infants with the tetralogy of Fallot by performing either a Waterston or a Blalock anastomosis, and to delay second stage intracardiac repair until 4 or 5 years of age." They compared their results in two consecutive periods, 1960–1969 and 1970–1973, in the first of which they had performed the palliative operation in severely cyanotic tetralogy infants under two years of age,- a Blalock or a Pott's anastomosis in the first years and a Brock, blind pulmonary valvotomy when these failed,- in the latter years of that period, employing a Waterston intrapericardial aortopulmonary anastomosis. In that first series, with a total of 44 patients, seven infants required a second palliative procedure because the first was unsatisfactory. The mortality was 50% in infants below four months of age, but approximately 10% in the remainder of the infants. They did not seem to be getting better results in the infants done later in the series than in the infants done earlier in the series. In addition, there were problems after discharge from the hospital, ". . . an occasional late death . . . Incomplete relief of cyanosis, failure to thrive . . . recurrent respiratory infections . . . cerebral abscess" with a late mortality of 6%, and there was still to come the mortality of the second stage definitive operation. Thirty-three of the infants had survived palliation, 24 of these had undergone the second stage repair, with two deaths, both in the extremely high risk condition of "absence or occlusion of the left pulmonary artery". From 1970 to 1973, they undertook primary definitive intracardiac repair of 24 tetralogy infants with severe progressive cyanosis or cyanotic spells, the youngest child four weeks of age. Operation was performed under deep hypothermia with circulatory arrest and limited cardiopulmonary bypass, surface cooling "to approximately 25°C" was followed, after exposure of the heart, by brief cold perfusion. At temperatures between 18 and 24°C, both the cavae and the aorta were occluded. In the more recent cases, external cooling was used to bring the temperature down to 22°C and perfusion to lower the temperature to 18 or 19°C prior to arrest. The arrest time varied from 38 to 67 minutes. The ventriculotomy was transverse unless the angiocardiogram indicated severe outflow tract hypoplasia. If an outflow patch was required it "always extended across the pulmonary valve ring and, when the bifurcation of the pulmonary trunk was also narrowed, into one or both of its branches." An outflow patch was employed in six of eight infants under four months of age and in only four of the 17 beyond four months. The ventricular septal defect was closed with a woven Teflon patch. Rapid rewarming to 35°C was achieved with the heat exchanger and cardiopulmonary bypass. "Right and left atrial pressure lines and ventricular pacing wires were positioned prior to chest closure." The single hospital death had occurred 36 hours after operation in a six-week-old infant who had had severe hypoplasia of the outflow tract. Autopsy showed "no pulmonary cause" for the progressive severe cyanosis which the baby had manifested. Assisted ventilation was employed for 12 to 24 hours in the eight infants up to three months of age but in only five of the 17 over that age. No patient had tracheostomy. Two patients had temporary complete heart block. One patient had a single postoperative seizure. None showed evidence of cerebral injury. "On subsequent clinical assessment the cardiac status of all survivors has been good without evidence of a residual ventricular septal defect and in the three patients who have been recatheterized to date, the data are confirmatory." The arguments concerning a two-stage or one-stage procedure centered around the mortality of the initial one-stage operation since as they and McGoon at the Mayo Clinic had shown, "the late mortality following shunt surgery is relatively low, at 6% in our series and 4% in the Mayo Clinic series; and the risk of repair is not significantly increased by a previous Waterston or Blalock shunt." The major mortality in infants was in those with severe outflow tract hypoplasia, often the very ones requiring operation before four months of age, and Boyes said his own results suggested that these patients could be operated upon successfully. In the New Zealand series and in Starr's series from Oregon, definitive

operation in the first two years of life seemed to carry no increased risk of morbidity or of incomplete repair. [Despite the impressive evidence in favor of the primary definitive operation in infancy, Barratt-Boyes contented himself, in the published paper, with a dispassionate statement of the comparative results of the one-stage definitive operation and the staged operation. No Discussion is recorded, perhaps explained by the fact that in his reference to the work of others employing primary definitive operation in infants, Barratt-Boyes had been able to mention only Starr, whose series included only a single child under four months of age, whereas Barratt-Boyes' startlingly successful series included eight children less than four months of age, including the six-week-old infant who represented the only death in the 25 infants; 24 of them had undergone primary total correction, the 25th, had undergone the only palliative operation during this time period, a Waterston operation at five months of age and was successfully corrected at 13 months of age.]

* * *

W. A. Altemeier, of Cincinnati, Christian R. Holmes Professor and Chairman, Department of Surgery, University of Cincinnati, who had been President in 1970; and by invitation, R. P. Hummel, E. O. Hill, and S. Lewis, *Changing Patterns in Surgical Infections,* suggested that "Various stressful forces imposed upon microorganisms during the past 30 years have produced reactions in the microbial world which, in turn, have influenced the pattern and nature of infections seen in the practice of surgery." Between 1942 and 1956, some "two-thirds of the surgical infections were caused by the gram-positive cocci . . . the *Staphylococcus aureus,* the *Beta Streptococcus,* and the *Pneumococcus.*" Subsequent changes, particularly after 1965 included "An increasing incidence of gram-negative infections with a relative decrease in gram-positive infections . . . Superimposed . . . infections . . . during antibiotic therapy . . . increasing incidence of gram-negative infections by bacteria formerly recognized as having little or no virulence . . . an increasing number of infections with L-forms and other atypical bacterial forms . . . Infections by fungi and viruses . . . growing awareness of the importance of gram-negative anaerobic infections produced principally by the *Bacteroides.* . . Cyclic variations in *Staphylococcal* resistance to penicillin . . . Changing patterns of *Staphylococcal* phage types." The gram-negative infections in the Cincinnati area now accounted for two-thirds of infections, which they suggested "seemed to be related to the widespread and intensive use of antibiotics, the rapid extension of new and complex surgical operations and diagnostic procedures to elderly and other high-risk patients, changes in host resistance, and a number of iatrogenic factors." *E. coli, Aerobacter aerogenes, Proteus, Pseudomonas aeruginosa* were most commonly responsible and in 53% of the cases, originated in the urinary tract. In 80% of cases, the serious surgical infections "developed while patients were on antibiotic prophylaxis or therapy for other infections." An example of the emergence of infections from bacteria thought previously to be of minimal virulence was that due to *Serratia marcescens*. Like secondary infections, *Serratia marcescens* infection occurred in patients already or previously on antibiotics, "often in large dosage." *Serratia marcescens* infection carried a 40% mortality. The "'L' and other atypical forms were found in the blood or thrombi in all cases in a study of 54 patients with thromboembolic disease", and never in patients randomly selected at the same time for control. As for the possible causes of the increase in gram-negative infections, they pointed out that ". . . of 398 cases of gram-negative septicemia . . . three-fourths of the patients in this series acquired this complication in the hospital, and their prognoses were poorer." The source of the gram-negative septicemia was from the urinary tract in more than 50% of the cases and in almost 50%, the onset "was related to urinary tract instrumentation or operation." Nosocomial infections, they thought, were related to the fact that "Current surgical practice frequently required prolonged or frequent use of prolonged urinary bladder catheterizations, complex diagnostic procedures, prolonged intravenous therapy, tracheostomies and respiratory assistance." They were particularly concerned about infection introduced by intravenous catheters. With respect to fungi, they said that infections with *Candida* had "recently emerged as a major threat to survival of severely burned patients at the Cincinnati Unit of the Shriner Burns Institute." The change in the drug resistance of organisms, particularly the staphylococcus aureus had bearing on the problem. "In 1943, 96% of the strains of hemolytic *Staphylococcus aureus* . . . were found to be highly sensitive to penicillin." That figure dropped to 51% by 1950. There was a suggestion that the trend was reversing, and striking variations were found from year to year. The resistant strains of staphylococcus accounted for only 23.8% of the infections in 1968 and during the last quarter of 1970, there had been no resistant strains isolated. "The periods of high resistance of the *Staphylococcus aureus* to penicillin were associ-

ated with changes in the patterns of infection in that the lesions were more resistant to penicillin and were greater in number." During the periods of higher penicillin resistance, there was an increased incidence of staphylococci which could not be phage-typed, and there had been a coincident change in penicillin resistance.

Discussion

Basil A. Pruitt, Jr., of San Antonio, referring to the "microbial opportunists which are increasingly common and increasingly difficult to treat" said that at the U. S. Army Institute of Surgical Research,- Burn Unit,- they had "observed a similar emergence of gram-negative bacteria ordinarily of low virulence. At the present time, *Providencia stuartii* is the bacterium most frequently recovered from our burn patients", had proved to be invasive, could be recovered from the blood, and in less than 3% of the patients, was sensitive to antibiotics. "Many of our patients arrive with this bacterium on their burn wounds . . . we are confident that it is not an organism peculiar to our Institute." They had "also noted a tenfold increase in fungal colonization and a fourfold increase in fungal invasion in our burn patients." Altemeier replied that he had encountered septicemia with *Providencia stuartii* in only three cases, in "the epidemic of infections we had following continuous intravenous therapy associated with thrombophlebitis". He predicted an increase in the number of staphylococcal infections in the next five years with an increase in the incidence of resistant organisms. "In the second quarter of 1972, the percentage of resistance in our staphylococcal population was six-tenths of one per cent. During the first quarter of 1973, however, this resistance has risen to 28% and there is evidence now that we are on the upswing again of another bout with our old adversary, the *Staphylococcus aureus.* "

* * *

R. L. Nichols, P. Broido, both by invitation; Robert E. Condon, of Milwaukee, Professor of Surgery, Medical College of Wisconsin; S. L. Gorbach, by invitation; and Lloyd M. Nyhus, Warren H. Cole Professor and Head, Department of Surgery, University of Illinois, *Effect of Preoperative Neomycin-Erythromycin Intestinal Preparation on the Incidence of Infectious Complications following Colon Surgery,* compared detailed bacteriologic studies of the stools of ten patients treated by their standard regimen of low residue diet, magnesium sulfate by mouth, saline enemas, and three doses of 1 gram neomycin, and 1 gram of erythromycin base, with stool studies in ten patients similarly prepared except for the antibiotics. In patients without antibiotics "Cultures of colon aspirate . . . produce luxuriant growth of both aerobes and anaerobes . . . similar to those normally found in stool." In the patients prepared with the addition of neomycin and erythromycin, the stools "showed suppression of aerobes and anaerobes in each case . . . compared to those of the non-antibiotic prepared patients, the difference in total anaerobes, total aerobes, coliforms, streptococci, bacteroides, and peptostreptococci was highly significant (p 0.001). There was no evidence of overgrowth of staphylococci or fungi in either group." Three of the ten with mechanical preparation only developed wound infections but none did of the ten receiving neomycin-erythromycin. Ninety-eight colon resections in two hospitals were studied retrospectively, 69 of the patients had had neomycin-erythromycin base, 16 had had mechanical preparation only, 13 had had either neomycin alone or neomycin-sulfathalidine or kanamycin. All colon anastomoses were performed by an open technique. No wound sepsis was observed in the 69 patients receiving neomycin-erythromycin base. Five infections occurred in the other 29 patients. "No surgeon had more than one wound infection, and no type of resection seemed more likely to result in infectious complications in this relatively small series." Infection was usually due to E. coli with some involvement of bacteroides. Six of eight wound infections were in patients who had had no antibiotic preparation, one in a neomycin-sulfathalidine preparation, one in a preparation with neomycin alone. They concluded that "elective colon resection should be approached with adequate preoperative mechanical and oral antibiotic preparation; the addition of routine systemic antibiotics appears to be an unwarranted and unrewarding measure."

Discussion

Oliver H. Beahrs, of Rochester, Minnesota, said that "In the earlier part of the decade of the 1930's the mortality associated with colonic surgery was 20% or higher . . . after introduction of chemotherapeutic agents and subsequently the antibiotics, mortality was reduced to 5% or less. The single factor that stands out as a basis for this more favorable experience is the availability of these drugs: Sulfonomides and antibiotics." On that basis, they had continued to use antibiotics for bowel preparation "irrespective of reports that their use exposes the patients to risks especially that of entero-colitis . . . In 1956 we began to use neomycin and oxytetracycline . . . for 36 hours preoperatively". In 520 cases, 83% had received that preparation, 17% had not, "With the standard preparation the hospital mortality rate was 1.5%; in the other 4.7% . . . Wound complications in patients receiving neomycin and terramycin was 2.5% while in those not receiving these drugs it was 10% . . . With the standard preparation 18 in 520 patients developed entero-colitis, all were treated successfully without mortality and in only one case was hospitalization prolonged." William A. Altemeier, of Cincinnati, said that in the "Five-university hospital ultraviolet study [which had failed to show any beneficial effect of ultraviolet light in the operating room], the incidence of infection in cecostomy and colostomy was 19.3%, colectomy with anastomosis 10.3%, and abdomino-perineal resection 11.6% regardless of the type of bowel preparation or antibiotic therapy . . . For many years I have not used antibiotic bowel preparation, but have relied instead on the intravenous administration of penicillin and tetracycline as the factor of antibiotic protection for the patient . . ." He repeated the observations concerning occurrence of staphylococci in the stool which he had made before [Volume LXXXII, 1964, page 1192]. Isidore Cohn, Jr., of New Orleans, believed with Dr. Beahrs that preoperative intestinal antisepsis was important, but it was "obvious that there are a number of people in this room who do not agree. Unfortunately, most of us have feelings based upon emotion rather than solid fact." There had not yet been a prospective randomized study to determine the facts. He agreed that mechanical cleansing was important. He agreed the erythromycin-neomycin was "a very fine combination for the bacteriological control of the colonic flora. On the other hand, we reported . . . and still believe, that this is *not* a good combination to use for the routine preparation of the large bowel for the simple reason that it contains erythromycin. This reduces our options for anti-staphylococcal activity that we like to have if we do get into trouble." He had had very little experience with staphylococcal entero-colitis. He commented on the small size of the patient population study by Nichols and his colleagues. Frederic Herter, of New York, said that in 1970 at Columbia-Presbyterian, there had been 46 postoperative infections in 350 open operations on the colon,- 13.1%, due mainly to E. coli and bacteroides. He had come to the conclusion that "Neomycin or kanamycin alone are inadequate protection against the anaerobes and we have suggested the addition of Sulfathalidine or bacitracin, as have many others". Clindamicin was more effective against bacteroides than any of the other agents and he wondered whether it should not be used in the prophylactic regimen. R. Cameron Harrison, of Vancouver, said that "In dogs, we have used the technique described by Mark Ravitch in which the anastomosis is covered with a thin silastic or plastic membrane to prevent protective adhesions and raise the actual leak rate to permit statistical evaluation. I, personally, have not been sufficiently impressed by the data to use large bowel antibiotics clinically, so I was extremely surprised when Drs. Letwin and Cohn, who are doing this study, found that with the sulpha and neomycin large bowel preparation preoperatively, the anastomotic leak rate under these experimental conditions was halved almost irrespective of what technic or suture was used." Robert E. Condon, closing, answered Altemeier's concern about staphylococcal superinfection, "overgrowth of staphylococci, when a combination of antibiotics, including an aminoglycoside and either an erythromycin or a lincomycin group drug was used" did not occur. He agreed with Dr. Cohn that a large controlled prospective clinical trial was required. The aminoglycosides, in answer to Herter, probably were responsible, with prolonged usage, for the "development and subsequent overgrowth of resistant strains of bacteroides and other anaerobes." They used clindamicin as a therapeutic drug but had not used it in the prophylactic regimen.

* * *

Frank J. Veith, of New York, Professor of Surgery, Albert Einstein College of Medicine; with S. K. Koerner, S. S. Siegelman, M. Torres, P. A. Bardfeld, L. A. Attai, S. J. Boley, T. Takaro, all by invitation; and Marvin L. Gliedman, Professor and Chairman, Department of Surgery, Albert Einstein College of Medicine, *Single Lung Transplantation in Experimental and Human Emphysema,* commented on the brief survival of most humans with lung transplantation. The clinical failure of single lung transplants in emphysematous patients had been "attributed to the physiologic setting in which a transplant with normal vascular resistance, airway resistance and compliance exists in parallel with an emphysematous lung which has a high vascular resistance, a high static compliance and a high expiratory airway resistance." They had set about testing this thesis. Death occurred "from respiratory insufficiency produced mainly by a serious ventilation-perfusion (V/Q) imbalance . . . characterized by underventilation of the transplant despite the fact

that it has been receiving most of the pulmonary blood flow." They had produced bilateral emphysema in dogs by use of a ventilator in which the micronebulizer contained a solution of papain, the treatment repeated three to five times in the course of three months. Emphysema was successfully produced in three surviving dogs, and a left lung allotransplantation performed, the donor being an unrelated pure bred beagle from the same colony. Immunosuppression consisted in the use of azathioprine, prednisone, and rabbit anti-dog thymocyte serum. Ventilation and perfusion scans, and arterial blood gas determinations were made periodically. In nine other dogs, they had produced unilateral, right-sided emphysema, by instillation of the papain into the isolated right bronchial tree, and in 11 such animals performed similar allotransplantation of the left lung. Two of the three dogs with bilateral emphysema survived the immediate posttransplant period. One died at eight days of rejection and one at 12 weeks of a massive gastrointestinal hemorrhage. The transplanted lung appeared normal at autopsy. Eight of the 11 dogs with right lung emphysema were chronic survivors of left lung autotransplantation. Three dogs, with severe unilateral emphysema, died within three days. The ventilation perfusion scans usually showed some decrease in perfusion of the transplant initially, returning to the normal level one to two weeks after operation. Ventilation in the early period was always impaired, sometimes to a greater degree than perfusion and similarly usually returned to the preoperative levels of the left lung within one to two weeks. Late studies showed that the transplanted lung received most of the blood flow and "appeared to be ventilated more rapidly than the larger emphysematous right lungs". They reported two emphysematous patients in whom they had performed single lung allotransplants. A 53-year-old man who had required ventilatory assistance with a respirator and a tracheostomy tube for three years "was able to breathe comfortably without ventilatory assistance and without a tracheostomy . . . From 1-6 months after right lung transplantation . . ." he had what were considered to be multiple episodes of rejection and after six months of gratifying palliation "died suddenly and unexpectedly 6 months after transplantation from a massive hemoptysis which arose from the erosion of a small vessel at a poorly healed corner of his bronchial anastomosis." A 57-year-old woman, who, before operation, had a PO_2 of 40 mm. Hg and a CO_2 of 70 mm. Hg. breathing room air, died 16 days after operation with a progressive pulmonary infiltrate in the transplant and falling oxygen tensions, after ten days of steady improvement. "Postmortem examination revealed extensive pneumonic involvement of the transplant . . . thought to be, in part at least, related to aspiration of infected necrotic bronchial mucosa secondary to ischemia of the transplant bronchus." They considered that their animal and patient experiences indicated that "single lung transplants do *not* produce obligatory V/Q imbalances in emphysematous recipients. This fact and the clear palliation afforded one patient help justify further cautious clinical trials with this procedure."

No Discussion was recorded.

* * *

Thomas E. Starzl, of Denver, Professor of Surgery, University of Colorado School of Medicine; Chairman, Department of Surgery, Denver Veterans Administration Hospital, and eight others, *Portal Diversion for the Treatment of Glycogen Storage Disease in Humans,* now nine years after Starzl's 1965 first report of portacaval transposition in the human, for glycogen storage disease, presented their results in seven of their own patients and one from Bristol, England, as well as new experimental studies. The aim was, by portal diversion in children with hepatic glycogen storage disease, "to make dietary glucose more readily available to peripheral tissues, to coincidentally deglycogenate the liver, and to palliate other complications such as acidosis." Portacaval transposition, originally developed by Gardner Child, "was used in order to avoid the potential hazards of Eck fistula . . . it was suggested in our original report and in subsequent ones by Hermann and Mercer [1969] and ourselves [1969] that an end-to-side portacaval anastomosis probably would be just as effective and that certainly it would be technically safer by virtue of omission of the second venous anastomosis. The simpler procedure of portacaval shunt has been used in all subsequent cases that have appeared in the literature, as well as for the last five cases in our series . . ." Folkman, in Boston, had shown "that a further reduction of operative risks in patients with glycogen storage should be possible by parenteral hyperalimentation and consequent preoperative amelioration of hepatomegaly, acidosis, and other metabolic abnormalties." There was now a world total of 13 patients with a 9-1/2 year follow-up for their first patient. Riddell's Bristol, England, patient who had migrated to Canada, had been studied in Denver. In two of the three patients with portacaval transposition, the flow of vena cava blood into the liver was found obstructed postoperatively, presumably due to thrombosis and a third patient died after operation "when the liver

was unable to transmit the rerouted vena caval flow, causing hepatic swelling and uncontrollable acidosis." The patients with end-to-side portacaval shunts all had simple postoperative courses although there were mild changes in the liver enzymes. The children had shown astonishing acceleration in growth, and increase in bone age. There was a postoperative decrease in hepatomegaly initiated in some cases by the preoperative hyperalimentation. The kidney was known to have decreased in size in at least four patients. Symptomatic hypoglycemia had been eliminated by operation in three patients and improved in two, and in the two long-term survivors, the glucose tolerance test showed an "increased hyperglycemic response to the ingested sugar." In patients with Type I disease, there was "a dramatic improvement of the hyperlipidemia". Histologically the hepatocytes decreased in size and the amount of fat in the cytoplasm of the liver cells increased. Liver glycogen concentration was not affected but the hepatocytes decreased in size, "accounting for the reduction of liver size in most of the cases without a major alteration in glycogen." Preoperative studies showed "a high incidence of preexisting coincidental liver disease . . .", particularly in Type III patients "portal diversion should have an important role in carefully selected cases of glycogen storage disease". They referred briefly to new animal work of their own "which suggests that the effects of portacaval shunt are due more to the rerouting of pancreatic hormones around the liver than to the bypassing of alimentary glucose."

Discussion

W. Kirt Nichols, Columbia, Missouri, and Dr. Hugh Stephenson had performed a side-to-side portacaval shunt for Von Gierke's disease upon a 31-year-old male after he had developed melena and esophageal varices. He now "manifests some evidence of diabetes with persistent hyperglycemia . . . should he now be managed as a diabetic?" Liver biopsy had demonstrated fibrosis and increased glycogen. Judah Folkman, of Boston, said that "Children with glycogen storage disease suffer primarily because caloric intake gets trapped as glycogen in the liver and cannot escape as glucose. These children have hypoglycemic seizures. Their parents are often up all night feeding them. They have acidosis. They have muscle wasting and above all, they do not grow, as Dr. Starzl pointed out. Dr. Starzl was the first to realize, actually, in 1963, that diversion of portal blood around the liver might make more glucose available to the peripheral circulation after each meal and he carried out the first portal diversion for this disease." Folkman emphasized the value of hyperalimentation in anticipation of the portacaval shunt. "What is the mechanism besides redirection of glucose into the bloodstream? Dr. Starzl's elegant studies indicate that redirection of insulin directly into the vena cava without passage through the liver, also plays a role; that insulin in this situation may itself be a growth stimulant . . . in fact, the tissue culture literature of recent years is filled with papers showing that insulin or insulin-like proteins have specific growth stimulating properties . . . but, the importance of insulin in the growth of our patients did not occur to me as it did to Dr. Starzl."

The Business Meetings

The 1973 meeting was held April 25, 26, and 27 at the Century Plaza Hotel, Los Angeles, President Jonathan E. Rhoads, Professor of Surgery, the University of Pennsylvania School of Medicine; Director, Department of Surgery, Pennsylvania Hospital, in the Chair.

It was announced that at President Rhoads' suggestion the SOSSUS report would be read at a breakfast meeting, instead of at a regular session,

and there was therefore room for 34 papers on the program.

At the Second Executive Session, on Friday, a By-laws change was recommended that "The Secretary, Treasurer and Recorder will hold office for six months beyond the election of their successor" to permit them to complete the records of their final meeting. The Council recommended that the American Surgical Association become incorporated "to establish dues and assessments as tax deductible. The Association has never had an Internal Revenue established status since its founding in 1880." The Council also recommended that there be organized "an educational foundation to qualify under Section 501.C3 of Internal Revenue Service in order that gifts and bequests made for the support of the educational, scientific and philanthropic purposes of the foundation be tax deductible."

The entire slate of 27 new members was elected, as well as Honorary Fellows, Lord Arthur Porritt, of England, Professor John Loewenthal, of Sidney, Australia, and Professor Jan Louw, of Capetown, South Africa. Officers elected were Henry William Scott, Jr., of Nashville, President; Mark M. Ravitch, of Pittsburgh, and Allen M. Boyden, of Portland, Oregon, as Vice-Presidents; and G. Thomas Shires, of Dallas, Secretary.

XCII

1974

The 1974 meeting was held at The Broadmoor, Colorado Springs, Colorado, on May 1, 2 and 3, H. William Scott, Jr., of Nashville, Professor of Surgery and Head of Department of Surgery, Vanderbilt University School of Medicine; Surgeon-in-Chief, Vanderbilt University Hospital, in the Chair.

Among those who had died in the preceding year were Philip R. Allison, of Oxford, the distinguished Honorary Member, and David M. Hume, of Richmond, Virginia, one of the pioneers in transplantation and in the modern evolution of pituitary endocrinology. He died flying a plane back from a professional visit to Los Angeles, crashing in the San Gabriel Mountains.

President H. William Scott, Jr., *Professional Freedom and Governmental Control,* described the paradox that at a time of "the high standards of surgical practice and quality care which have established American surgery in a position of leadership throughout the world in the view of most of our professional peers abroad . . . American surgeons have a tarnished image . . . our professional freedoms, as well as our pluralistic system of medical and surgical care are in jeopardy as never before in the history of our nation. The principal source of the attack on our professional freedom is not located in Peking, Hanoi or Moscow . . . the headquarters is in Washington, D.C." He described the minimal involvement of the federal government in medical care before World War II, "The U.S. Public Health Service had a well developed national program . . . in the important areas of preventive medicine, sanitation, communicable disease control, biologic standards and vital statistics. The armed services maintained their own medical corps . . . Their disabled veterans were cared for in a small number of Veterans Hospitals which were essentially old soldiers' homes." The huge Veterans Administration Hospitals which had developed since World War II, "Despite the myriads of bureaucratic inefficiencies . . . and the criticism that it has been the single most expensive program for delivery of medical care the world has ever known . . . have provided good in-patient medical and surgical rehabilitative services to over 16 million of our population during the period 1946 through 1973 . . . a majority of 170 V.A. Hospitals have become firmly affiliated with medical schools and as teaching hospitals have provided strong support to the university programs of education and research." The incorporation in 1953 of the U.S. Public Health Service into the Department of Health, Education and Welfare had been viewed with alarm, but "in the next 18 years the promotion of research and the financing of research facilities, investigators, research trainees and technicians by the U.S. Public Health Service and other programs of H.E.W. achieved a level never before dreamed of by our scientific community. The guiding policies which were employed were wonderfully fair . . . opposed directed research, promoted individual ingenuity and

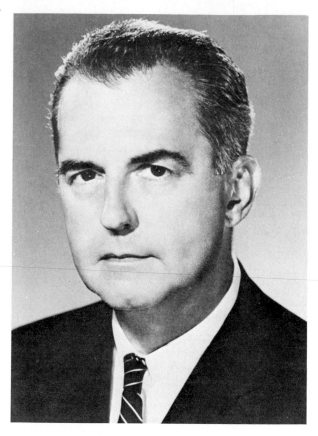

H. William Scott [c. 1960] 1916- . President 1974, and of the American College of Surgeons 1976. M.D. Harvard, 1941. Training in Peter Bent Brigham, Children's Hospital Program, 1941-45 (Resident, Children's Hospital, 1943-45); Fellow in Neurosurgery, Brigham-Children's Hospital, 1945-46; thence to Johns Hopkins as Assistant Resident and Resident, 1946-47; Instructor, Associate Professor of Surgery, Johns Hopkins, 1946-52; Professor of Surgery and Chief of Department, Vanderbilt University School of Medicine, 1952- . Early contributions were in cardiac surgery, before extracorporeal circulation, first successful closure aortic-pulmonary window, first complete correction of tetralogy of Fallot (under inflow occlusion!). Massive systematic studies on production, prevention and relief of experimental atherosclerosis, and effect in animals and man of jejuno-ileal bypass (Scott shunt). An effective, persistent, systematic and logical worker, his publications are marked by thoroughness, and symmetry. As with a number of other Presidents, the combination of great ability and capacity for work with charm and gregariousness, has led to high office in numerous surgical organizations.

freedom of choice in problems for investigation and methodology to be used and developed a healthy competitive system for applicants under an excellent

program of peer review." The Hill-Burton Hospital construction program "had provided federal funds for the construction of some 336,000 beds. In some communities these hospitals improved the quality of medical care by providing good facilities for the well qualified local physicians and surgeons and by attracting others with good qualifications. In many communities, however, the effect was the opposite. The availability of excellent facilities encouraged local staff members without the qualifications of training and experience to undertake management of problems, especially surgical problems, far beyond their capabilities." The balance, for the first 20 years after World War II, Scott thought was favorable, "In retrospect this relatively healthy symbiosis between the voluntary medical sector and the governmental medical programs of the 1950's and 60's brought many advantages for patients and physicians alike and enhanced the strength of American medicine . . . forestalled the omnipresent socialistic pressures for governmental take-over of all medical care as had happened in 1948 in Great Britain." The Medicare-Medicaid legislation enacted in 1965, "Despite the humanitarian motives of the social planners and the liberal politicians . . . have been decidedly mixed blessings and have deluged physicians and hospitals with bureaucratic red tape . . . have actually had the effect of increasing the cost of medical care. The outright discrimination against teaching hospitals, residents in training and the practicing clinicians in teaching hospitals [by contesting their right to accept Medicare surgical fees] has shaken the financial stability of many of our leading institutions . . . have had the effects of moving both Medicare patients and teaching physicians away from university centers." The inflationary impetus of the expenditures for health care had created new problems, "The concomitant massive governmental spending of both the Johnson and Nixon administrations supporting the Viet Nam war, building huge deficits and promoting rampant inflation, was apparently not as impressive to economy-minded Congressmen as were the rapidly rising costs of Medicare and Medicaid." He commented on the size of the expenditures for "health care", 10.4 billion dollars in 1950, of which 3.3 billion dollars—20% "came from the public treasury. By 1973 the total health care bill was 94.1 billion dollars and 31 billion or thirty-seven per cent derived from public funds. For fiscal year 1975 the budget proposed for health spending by Mr. Nixon is 35.5 billion dollars of which 20.7 billion is requested for Medicare and Medicaid." The result, combined with the undocumented charges [which Scott placed in quotation marks] of "doctor shortages", "our archaic system of medical care", "the health care crisis", led to an avalanche of new policies and restrictions. "Under the guise of economy in federal spending the hatchet men of the Nixon administration have harshly terminated the productive period of symbiosis between the private medical sector and the federal government. [One does not recall a more direct criticism of the incumbent administration in Washington by a President of the American Surgical Association. Watergate was rapidly accelerating towards its climax at the end of that summer. One recalls that at the banquet at this meeting, after a senior Canadian, Angus McLachlin, of London, Ontario, had, in the custom of the Association, toasted the Queen, President Scott indicated to the First Vice-President that it was his turn to arise and toast the President of the United States. The Vice-President responded sotto voce that he would not toast Richard Nixon, nor the office of the President of the United States which Nixon had dishonored. It was significant that when the Vice-President then rose and toasted the United States of America, the vast majority of the Fellows jumped to their feet to join in the toast with enthusiasm, having obviously waited with keen interest to see what sort of toast would be offered. To at least one observer the obvious implication of this response in such a bastion of "the establishment" as the American Surgical Association, most of whom had surely voted for Nixon, was that Nixon could not survive.] Their abrasive changes in federal policy have included drastic cuts and impoundments of funds appropriated by Congress for research and research facilities; the ruthless phasing out of training grants, fellowships and many other programs for scientific manpower production; elimination of Hill-Burton Hospital construction, the Regional Medical programs, public and allied health personnel education, general research support grants for medical schools, capitation grants for schools of nursing and many other previously sponsored health programs. Further, the President's Office of Management and Budget has proposed as an 'economy' the elimination of the excellent peer review system at the National Institutes of Health, and as an alternative suggested that the review and award of contracts and grants be solely by NIH scientists and staff. The recent trend toward targeted and contract research at NIH must reflect these bureaucratic pressures." Of the 1972 Public Law 09-603, "popularly known as the Bennett Amendment to the Social Security Act, [which] established the Professional Standards Review Organization (PSRO)", Scott said, "While the underlying theory of PSRO is to improve the quality of medical care, the fundamental issue is economic. With billions of dollars being spent by the government to purchase medical care, some form of review and audit is essential for accountability and good business procedures." By the physician operated review mechanism, Scott thought "medicine can in part control its own destiny in utilization of government resources in fulfillment of its broad mission. It can also become hopelessly enmeshed in bureaucracy." He viewed with great concern the replacement of wage and price controls by the establishment of "a free market for all *except* the health industry . . . the greatest threat ever to the continuation of voluntary non-profit hopitals . . . The Bill not only places hospitals totally under federal control, but places them under the direct and unfettered control of the President and his advisors . . . It is the assumption of complete dictatorial power over all aspects of the health field. This Bill is, and of a right ought to be, unconstitutional. In my opinion, it has closer resemblance to *ein Ausrufung* sent to the Reichstag about 1936 by Adolf Hitler than to a proposal for law in the Congress of the United States." [The law was not enacted.] Scott spoke of the seven Bills which had been introduced into the Congress designed to establish national health insurance, stating that they had "implications for American physicians, surgeons and their patients which are most ominous." He quoted with approval from the book by Harry Schwartz, ". . . the American Medical Care System with its four million workers, its more than 200 million patients and potential patients, its incredible array of specialized skills and equipment, and its billions of dollars of capital investment is quite simply the most complicated industry in the United States. To suppose that we know enough to improve it through radical changes imposed upon this system in a brief period is fantasy more appropriate to an LSD trip than to sober legislative deliberation." He agreed with Schwartz' comments about the lack of unity, organization and effective political influence of medicine and the two most reasonable criticisms of the present system, "the high and rapidly increasing cost of medical care and . . . the difficulties of access to this care in some areas and for some population groups." Scott listed as the cardinal tenets, on which he thought all could agree, "allegiance to the free enterprise system . . . the strongly American tendency to 'plan for a rainy day' . . . the fee-for-service basis . . . the free choice of physicians and of patients . . . the use of public funds to subsidize the health care of the poor . . . the use of public subsidy to defray catastrophic expenses of injury and illness." The first step was to "put our professional house in order", implementing the suggestions of Francis Moore made in his Presidential Address two years earlier, supporting the work of the SOSSUS Committee to provide the information for decisions about the future, the establishment of a conjoined committee of the American College of Surgeons and the American Surgical Association, for "implementation and action" of recommendations to put the house in order. And, finally, the "American Surgical Association needs to become an organization of political activists . . . We have been aloof, superiorly patrician and naively lacking in political clout for 94 years! . . . The American Surgical Association has primary concern for the betterment of medical and surgical care of patients in this country and not primary concern for its own welfare. We have deep concern that much of the health legislation currently proposed would, if enacted, worsen the delivery of medical and surgical care in America and restrict the professional freedom of American physicians and surgeons."

* * *

Henry Buchwald, Richard B. Moore, both by invitation, and Richard L. Varco, of Minneapolis, Professor of Surgery, University of Minnesota Medical Center, *Ten Years Clinical Experience with Partial Ileal Bypass in Management of the Hyperlipidemias,* reviewed their experience with partial ileal bypass in 126 hyperlipidemic patients, of whom the first had been operated upon in 1963. "The retrospective and prospective studies of atherosclerotic risk incriminate the circulating cholesterol concentration as a prime risk variable in the etiology of atherogenesis. The lipid-atherosclerosis hypothesis postulates that the circulating cholesterol concentration acts as an exponential influence on the individual's potential for developing atherosclerosis." It had not been shown that lipid lowering would reduce the risk, and their goal "in the laboratory and in our clinical research has been to test the validity of the lipid hypothesis by the means of the partial ileal bypass operation, a technique designed for maximum reduction of plasma lipid levels." They added that a national cooperative program under auspices of the National Heart and Lung Institute was currently underway. "Partial ileal bypass differs substantially from jejuno-ileal bypass. The jejuno-ileal bypass operation, in which the proximal 40 cm of jejunum are anastomosed to the distal 4 cm of ileum, attempts alleviation of morbid exogenous obesity. With better than 90% of the small intestine bypassed, the therapeutic goal is weight loss. Lipid reduction is a valu-

able and accompanying benefit. The jejuno-ileal bypass usually produces diarrhea, can induce serious electrolyte imbalance, and has been associated with hair loss, arthritis, nephrolithiasis and liver failure. Partial ileal bypass short-circuits only the distal 200 cm of small intestine, or one-third the small intestinal length, whichever is longer . . . partial ileal bypass, though associated with diarrhea at times, is not responsible for the problems mentioned above . . . does not cause significant weight reduction." They had expected small bowel bypass to "interfere with the entero-hepatic cholesterol cycle . . . similarly influence the entero-hepatic bile acid cycle." In their patients the "cholesterol absorption" was reduced an average of 60%, and this seemed permanent. Excretion of fecal steroid and of bile acids was greatly increased, again apparently permanently. Cholesterol synthesis was increased 5.7-fold and cholesterol turnover increased 3-fold. The miscible cholesterol pool decreased one-third. Preliminary prolonged dieting produced a 41.1% decrease in serum cholesterol. The combination of diet and operation produced a 53% decrease. In Type IV, hypertriglyceridemic patients, the plasma triglycerides were decreased 52.6%. Only one patient had died in the hospital and there had been 13 late deaths. The hospital death was from myocardial infarction in a patient who had had three prior infarctions. Eleven of the 13 late deaths were of myocardial infarction, one was from cerebral vascular accident and one from infectious hepatitis. There had been four instances of late intestinal obstruction requiring operation. Although, with the distal ileal bypass they had given all of their patients 1,000 mg of vitamin B_{12} every two months, they and others had noted "a return of B_{12} absorptive capacity ten years after bypass in certain individuals . . ." Of 55 patients with angina pectoris, 26 had complete remission, 18% had marked improvement, 25% reported moderate improvement, and in some patients serial arteriographic studies had shown regression of atherosclerotic plaques. They concluded that "partial ileal bypass is the most effective means for lipid reduction available today; it is obligatory in its actions, safe, and associated with minimal side effects."

Discussion

T. E. Starzl, of Denver, lauded the paper as "part of a landmark accomplishment of the Minnesota group, whereby they have influenced lipid metabolism by changing the intestinal continuity, and which work has been supported by the brilliant studies of Scott and his associates from Vanderbilt [producing a severe atherosclerosis in experimental animals by appropriate high cholesterol diets and studying the effect of a variety of manipulations. [See Scott's discussion of Szilagyi, 1973, Volume XCI, page 1374.] Starzl suggested that portacaval shunt might be an alternative approach, "You may remember from our last year's presentation the profound lowering of the secondary hyperlipidemia of glycogen storage disease after end-to-side portacaval shunt." He had performed such a shunt in a child with "the lethal syndrome of Type II primary homozygous hyperlipidemia, or idiopathic hypercholesterolemia, which has been generally conceded to be relatively refractory to the Buchwald-Varco bypass." At 11 years of age, the child had an almost lethal myocardial infarction. Operation produced a spectacular lowering of the serum cholesterol, her angina pectoris ceased, her heart failure regressed, her aortic murmur receded and she appeared well 14 months after the shunt. He closed by emphasizing, "our really conservative attitude about portacaval shunts for this indication, because of the potentially devastating side effects of portacaval shunts. We did one case 14 months ago, and have not done a second one since. With this long a follow-up we will now go ahead with more cases." William V. McDermott, of Boston, said that the Buchwald-Varco experience led them "to consider this procedure in another relatively rare group of patients, those with intractable pruritus from a variety of causes, whether primary biliary cirrhosis, secondary uncorrectable biliary cirrhosis, giant cell hepatitis, and other." They had a single experience, "a young boy with giant cell hepatitis, uncontrollable in any other way . . . who did respond dramatically in terms of correction of his symptoms from the utilization of this procedure." Richard R. Lower, of Richmond, asked only whether Buchwald had compared operation with drug therapy. Buchwald, closing, said he had reviewed the published data concerning diet and drug therapy of the hyperlipidemias. By dietary management the net reduction of cholesterol was only 6 or 7% and drug therapy 25 to 30%, the drugs were not uniformly effective, and "It is also unrealistic to expect lifelong adherence to strict dietary protocol or a regimen of expensive drugs, especially by younger and asymptomatic individuals." He looked forward to Starzl's future reports and suggested that in the future "a spectrum of operations" might be employed depending upon the specific hyperlipidemia involved.

* * *

The recent optimism about the likelihood of developing an implantable mechanical heart had subsided, and the few premature attempts at implantation in humans of cardiac-assist devices, had not been repeated, but serious laboratory investigation continued. W. S. Pierce, J. A. Brighton, W. O'Bannon, J. H. Donachy, W. M. Phillips, D. L. Landis, and W. J. White, all by invitation, and John A. Waldhausen, of Hershey, Professor and Chairman, Department of Surgery, The Pennsylvania State University College of Medicine, The Milton S. Hershey Medical Center, *Complete Left Ventricular Bypass with a Paracorporeal Pump:* Design and Evaluation, had developed an implantable left ventricular assist device which had been successful in calves for as long as eight months of continuous operation. It was their view that intra-aortic balloon pumping was effective in the treatment of cardiogenic shock [Waldhausen's life was soon to be saved in this situation by the use of the intra-aortic balloon], but the device provided "minimal, albeit at times adequate, assistance to the failing heart." Left atrial to aortic bypass relieved the heart of a major part of its work and provided better support of the circulation, but ". . . *maximal* reduction in left ventricular work requires ventricular decompression, not readily attained with left atrial bypass." They had developed "a sac-type pump with an inlet and outlet cannula, a pneumatic power unit, a synchronization unit, and appropriate monitoring apparatus. The sac-type pump consisted of a flexible segmented polyurethane sac contained within a thin, vacuum formed, polycarbonate shell." The pump was placed outside the chest. "The two cannulae were passed out through separate incisions in the left 6th intercostal space." Blood was drained from the ventricle through a ball-type valve by a polyurethane cannula and entered the descending aorta through a Dacron graft with another ball valve. The external pneumatic power unit delivered alternate positive and negative pressure to the space between the sac and rigid chamber, directed by a "synchronization unit of our own design . . . which sensed the R-wave of the EKG, provided a delay, and then energized the solenoid valve to initiate pumping." In the first six calves, the device functioned continuously for an average of six weeks, delivering approximately 3 L/min. Three of those calves died of emboli, one of sepsis, one of pneumonia and one when the inlet tube in the pump disconnected after two-and-a-half months. The synchronization unit had been employed only in the last four calves. Flow rates of 5.0 to 10.2 L/min were achieved, and perfusion continued for an average of six weeks. One calf died of intestinal obstruction,

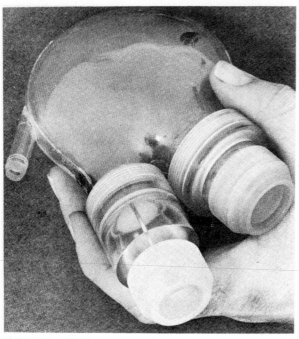
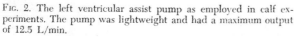

FIG. 2. The left ventricular assist pump as employed in calf experiments. The pump was lightweight and had a maximum output of 12.5 L/min.

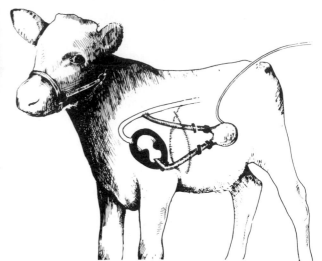

FIG. 3. The assist pump filled from the left ventricular apex and ejected into the thoracic aorta. The pump was positioned on the left side of the calf in the paracorporeal position.

Inside the rigid polycarbonate shell was a flexible segmented polyurethane sac. The small tube led to the pneumatic pump which applied alternating positive and negative pressure between the bladder and the housing. The ball valve can be seen in the outlet tube which was connected to the aorta by a Dacron graft. The inlet, also with a ball valve, connected to a wire-reinforced segmented polyurethane cannula which was inserted in the apex of the left ventricle. The inflow and outflow tubes emerged between the ribs, and the pump's chamber was on the outside in the "paracorporeal position". A synchronization unit, sensitive to the R-wave of the EKG, controlled the pumping. They had been able to employ continuous pumping in one calf for over eight months.

W. S. Pierce, J. A. Brighton, W. O'Bannon, J. H. Donachy, W. M. Phillips, D. L. Landis, W. J. White, and John A. Waldhausen. *Complete Left Ventricular Bypass with a Paracorporeal Pump:* Design and Evaluation. Volume XCII, 1974.

another of pulmonary insufficiency, a third of bleeding through a "frayed experimental vascular graft", and one from infected and occluding left atrial thrombus. In one calf, the pump did not function for six hours and laminated thrombus developed within the cardiac sac of the pump. During pumping the peak ventricular systolic pressure of the calves was 40-45 mm Hg., while the systemic arterial pressure was at normal levels of 100/60 to 120/80 mm Hg. "The aortic valve did not open except during daily tests to verify proper transducer calibration. No aortic valve pathology has subsequently been observed in the calves." They could not say "whether prolonged decompression will lead to 'disuse' atrophy of the left ventricle." They had designed their pump "with particular attention to providing an extremely smooth, seam-free, blood contacting surface, good washout, and a high flow rate." All animals had full anticoagulant therapy and three calves did not develop thromboembolic complications. "We have not employed fabric or cell lined sacs because of concern regarding delamination and progressive tissue buildup."

Discussion

The single discussant, Harris B. Shumacker, of Indianapolis, regretted having to say that the work which he and his colleagues had been doing in this area "is, at the moment, not going on." He remained optimistic in spite of the problems, "All that is required to extend this beautiful study of long-term assistance to total replacement is a lot of hard work on the part of a great many people, and some good original thinking." W. S. Pierce, closing, said that much of the work in the field had been devoted to the type of lining of the device to be used, "About five years ago the use of devices with smooth linings was pretty much abandoned for a variety of flocked or fabric linings. We have never been convinced that the smooth lining was not better. The studies we have performed to date have all employed segmented polyurethane, with as smooth a blood contacting surface as possible." He commented further that the external "paracorporeal" location of their pump "permits removal of the device without requiring an additional operation, which is particularly important in ill patients having marginal left ventricular function."

* * *

Marc R. de Leval, by invitation; Dwight C. McGoon, Professor of Surgery, Mayo Graduate School, University of Minnesota; Robert B. Wallace, Professor and Chairman, Department of Surgery, Mayo Medical School and Mayo Clinic; Gordon K. Danielson and Douglas D. Mair, both by invitation, *Management of Truncal Valvular Regurgitation,* stunned the audience, as much by the implication that their experience with this complicated anomaly was sufficient for them to be concerned with details, as by the operative feats involved. McGoon, Rastelli and Wallace, in 1968, had recorded the first successful repair of truncus arteriosus. Their operative experience was now with 71 patients, since September 1967, and the present paper concerned the tricuspid valve, in the truncus, which became the aortic valve. Insufficiency interfered with intraoperative coronary perfusion through the aortic root, and after operation presented a threat of unknown magnitude. Their patients ranged in age from 12 months to 19 years. While the "typical decrescendo diastolic murmur", and angiographically demonstrated regurgitation allowed anticipation of valvar insufficiency, these findings were a poor guide to the degree of insufficiency. The operation was succinctly described, "The first step is to separate the pulmonary artery (or pulmonary arteries) near its origin from the truncus and to close the resulting truncal defect. During the second step, a longitudinal ventriculotomy is made in the basal portion of the free wall of the right ventricle . . . The ventricular septal defect is then closed so that the aorta receives blood only from the left ventricle. The final step is to insert a valved conduit between the right ventriculotomy and the pulmonary artery." The conduit, initially homograft aorta with its valve, was now a Dacron tube, with an incorporated porcine aortic valve. A number of techniques had been tried to deal with intraoperative aortic insufficiency, and they had now come to temporary suture of the valve cusps, ap-

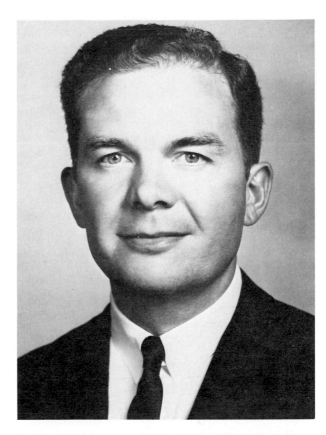

Dwight C. McGoon, (c. 1965) 1925- . M.D. Johns Hopkins 1948. Training at Johns Hopkins 1948-1954. The first Hopkins Resident in Surgery to join the Mayo Clinic. Quiet, modest, a masterful technician achieving results in the "standard" operations of cardiac surgery ranking with the world's best, presenting in some areas of complicated congenital anomalies a dazzling and almost unique experience which has led to his being termed "Mr. Surgery-of-the-Impossible" in congenital heart disease. A quiet perfectionist in speech, manuscript and operation, characteristically he withdrew absolutely from the operating room when he recognized the initial manifestation of a motor impediment.

proached through the right ventriculotomy and ventricular septal defect, after the pulmonary artery had been cut away and the aorta repaired. The sutures in the valve cusps were cut away just before completion of the closure of the ventricular septal defect. This technique was employed in 11 patients with regurgitation, all of whom survived operation, one dying suddenly 17 months later. Of eight other patients with regurgitation, three died early and two died late. Of the 52 children without regurgitation, 21 died early and one died late. At the initial operation they had replaced the incompetent truncus valve with a Starr-Edwards valve in three patients,

TABLE 1. *Overall Experience*

Year	Total No. of Patients	Type of Surgery*	No. of Patients	Operative Mortality No. of Operative Deaths	% Mortality
1968	14	SCB	11	2	
		DCB	3	2	28.6%
		TCB	—	—	
1969	31	SCB	6	0	
		DCB	22	2	6.5%
		TCB	3	0	
1970	73	SCB	12	0	
		DCB	58	8	10.9%
		TCB	3	0	
1971	152	SCB	23	0	
		DCB	59	6	6.5%
		TCB	70	4	
1972	178	SCB	21	0	
		DCB	63	1	2.2%
		TBC	94	3	

* SCB: single coronary bypass
DCB: double coronary bypass
TCB: triple coronary bypass

The mortality of the NYU Group in elective bypasses done without adjunctive procedures had dropped to 2.2% at the same time that they had almost eliminated the single coronary bypasses and increased the proportion of triple coronary bypasses. No patients with chronic congestive failure were operated upon, but "patients with substantial injury of the left ventricle from previous infarction were consistently operated upon. "For the past two years," the commonest procedure had been a triple bypass,- left internal mammary and anterior descending coronary, and saphenous vein grafts to the circumflex and right coronary arteries. They had a 77% five-year survival and an 81% survival, excluding deaths from non-cardiac causes.

F. C. Spencer, et al. *The Long-Term Influence of Coronary Bypass Grafts on Myocardial Infarction and Survival.* Volume XCII, 1974.

accounting for three of the six deaths in patients with incompetent valves. Currently they thought the insufficiency frequently mild enough to be tolerated, and preferable to the risk and consequences of valve replacement, though recognizing that replacement of the valve might become necessary. [An addendum states that after the meeting, in two boys with severe insufficiency and cardiac failure they had, at the time of the initial operation, replaced the truncus valve with a Starr-Edwards valve. Both "recovered more slowly than normal but in each the early result has been excellent".]

[The reception of this paper indicates one of the problems inherent in evaluating Discussions at past meetings. The 1st Vice-President, who presided, recalls almost pleading for discussion of this astounding experience. Many of the great cardiac surgeons of the day were present, but in the light of this display of skill, detailed understanding, and a massive and brilliantly successful experience with a rare lesion by McGoon and his group, not one could be persuaded to rise. The record merely fails to show any discussion.]

* * *

F. C. Spencer, of New York, Professor and Chairman, Department of Surgery, New York University School of Medicine; Director of Surgery, Bellevue Hospital and New York University Hospital, and seven others by invitation, *The Long-Term Influence of Coronary Bypass Grafts on Myocardial Infarction and Survival,* had performed their first coronary bypass in February 1968, and made the interesting point that "the number of operations rapidly escalated to create the serious logistical question about how many bypass operations could be done annually with the institutional resources available. The decision was made to perform no more than 200-300 operations each year." The result was that "the patients operated upon have been automatically selected to some degree as those most seriously disabled with angina, while those with lesser disability were either advised to be operated upon at another hospital, or else operation was not recommended." The present report dealt only with elective operations, excluding "Emergency procedures, operations for pre-infarction angina or myocardial infarction, and those combined with excision of ventricular scars and aneurysms or insertion of prosthetic valves . . ." The indication for operation was "angina incapacitating the patient from normal activity despite the best medical therapy possible." Protracted congestive heart failure was the only contraindication to operation. An angiographic diagnosis of significant coronary obstruction required narrowing by more than 60-70%. Failure of the artery to fill beyond the obstruction was not a contraindication to operation, and "The only angiographic contraindication to operation was an artery with multiple areas of diffuse obstruction throughout its course." They used a disposable bubble oxygenator primed with an electrolyte solution. "Most anastomoses were performed during induced ventricular fibrillation." They had been using aortic occlusion and ischemic arrest less and less, and almost always vented the left ventricle. The saphenous graft was removed, and placed in a 4° C. solution before the bypass was started in most of the patients included in the present report, but "For the past two years the left internal mammary artery has been regularly used, with the most common procedure being a triple bypass with anastomosis of the left internal mammary artery to the anterior descending coronary, and vein grafts to the circumflex and right coronary arteries." Blood flow measurements immediately after bypass ranged from 20-30 ml/min to 60-80 ml/min. Their results had improved from 28.6% mortality in their first 14 patients,- 1968,- to 2.2% in the 178 patients operated upon in 1972. Most of the deaths were from myocardial infarction or low cardiac output. Subclinical myocardial infarcts, recognized by electrocardiographic and enzyme changes and without clinical signs, occurred in 6-10% of patients. Of the 420 patients in the study period, surviving operation, angina was completely relieved or significantly improved in 329 of 382 followed,- 86% of the entire group, and worse than before operation in 2%. Asymptomatic patients were reluctant to have follow-up angiography, and in some of the 201 patients restudied, the study was done because of the reappearance of angina. "When angina returned after being absent, it was almost always found that either a graft was occluded or severely narrowed. Very rarely was disease in another artery found as the explanation." While the patency rate of internal mammary grafts seemed higher, follow-up was still brief. Overall patency for all vein grafts inserted was 72%. "These data probably represent some of the lowest patency rates that can be expected with vein grafts, for at operation an aggressive policy was pursued of attaching grafts to most arteries explored, even those diseased and as small as 1 mm internal diameter." Of the 201 patients studied, there were 17 in whom no grafts were patent, of whom three had no angina, nine had some improvement and in the others, angina was as before or worse. ". . . impaired ventricular function and an elevated end-diastolic pressure was not associated with a high late mortality. This supports the policy of operation upon such patients, realizing that ventricular function will probably not improve but further injury may be prevented." Thirty-two of the 420 patients surviving operation in the study group had subsequently developed a myocardial infarction. They calculated the probability of surviving five years without an infarction to be 73%, their overall five-year survival was 77%, including all deaths, operative, noncardiac, etc., and 81% excluding deaths from noncardiac causes. A Cleveland Clinic study of 590 nonoperated patients had shown a five-year cardiac mortality of 34%,- a survival of 66%, compared to the present cardiac survival of 81%, and Spencer thought his patients had more widespread coronary disease than the Cleveland Clinic study patients. [In 1978 (Volume XCVI) he was able to report that his five-year survival was actually 88%.] Spencer indicated that the objective should be "a method of coronary bypass grafting that will produce a consistent patency rate of at least 80% five years after operation."

Discussion

The Discussion was opened by Donald B. Effler, of the Cleveland Clinic. He differed with Spencer's preferred selection of patients with both myocardial impairment and angina, "We believe that the man with the normal ventricle and with severe angina and threatening disease is probably more deserving of surgery than the man who has already had multiple insults to his ventricle." Dr. Mason Sones, at his clinic, had made a retrospective study of patients [since 1967] who "had good ventricles, but had coronary disease described as single, double, and triple vessel . . ." Unoperated upon, 20% of the single vessel disease patients died within five years, 40-45% of those with double vessel disease and 70% of those with triple vessel disease, "All as a result of their coronary artery disease. This is certainly an unimpressive testimony for medical therapy because all of these patients were private patients and all were given the benefit of the best we had to offer from the standpoint of modern medical treatment." Since "1967, when Rene Favaloro did our first interposed saphenous vein graft, 4600 patients were operated upon with bypass graft techniques by the end of 1972. In the past year, there has been an additional group of 1573 patients—this is the 1973 record—and as mentioned by Dr. Spencer, the mortality rate with experience gets lower and lower. There were exactly 15 deaths in this 1973 group, giving us a mortality of slightly less than 1% overall." He was inclined to agree about the promise of the mammary-coronary anastomosis, 464 of which had been done at the Cleveland Clinic in 1973, with or without an additional vein graft. None of those patients had died and the postoperative myocardial infarct rate was less than 4%. Graft patency rate, in general, was "in the neighborhood of 80%" as determined by postoperative angiographic study [1100 such in 1972], Effler pointing out, as Spencer had, that patients with symptoms were the most likely to agree to restudy. Most patients were angina-free after operation. Currently they performed double or triple grafts in 65% of patients. [The Cleveland Clinic group seemed less aggressive than Spencer in proposing more and more grafts,- double grafts were commoner than triple grafts, and more grafts than three had become progressively less common.] David C. Sabiston, Jr., of Durham, North Carolina, commented upon the computer study at Duke of

CORONARY ARTERY REVASCULARIZATION

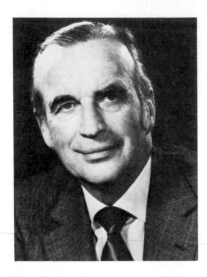

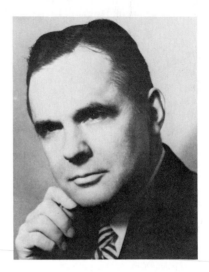

Donald B. Effler, 1915- . M.D. University of Michigan 1941; training Walter Reed, Gallinger Municipal, George Washington University, Washington, D.C., and Cleveland Clinic; Chief, Department of Thoracic and Cardiovascular Surgery, Cleveland Clinic, 1949-75; Chief Cardiac Surgeon, St. Joseph's Hospital, Syracuse, N.Y., 1975- . Insouciant, and blandly brash. Serially explored techniques of myocardial revascularization and had a period of great enthusiasm for the Vineberg procedure, performed with great skill and in large numbers, and subsequently evaluated the direct attack with patch grafting. After Dudley Johnson's 1969 report demonstrating that multiple bypassing anastomoses could be made to both coronary arteries, Favoloro's successes with aorta-coronary bypasses, in Effler's Department, led to a colossal clinical effort. The entire myocardial revascularization program at Cleveland Clinic has from the first been based on and made feasible by Mason Sones' development of coronary angiography, in the same institution.

Frank Cole Spencer, 1925- . M.D. Vanderbilt 1947 (age 21); Training Johns Hopkins 1947-55 (UCLA 1949-51); Instructor to Associate Professor Johns Hopkins 1954-61; Professor of Surgery, University of Kentucky, Lexington, 1961-66; Professor and Chairman, Department of Surgery, New York University, 1966- . Attracted attention by his reports of successful treatment of arterial injuries in the Korean War, with the Marines (in an interlude in his residency years). Prodigious worker, remarkably orderly and disciplined intellect. With Bahnson made multiple contributions to open cardiac surgery, coronary perfusion, postoperative monitoring with catheters implanted at operation. Early (1963) demonstrated feasibility of direct internal mammary-coronary anastomoses, enthusiastically embarked on a coronary revascularization program. His analyses of the relief of angina and prolongation of life by coronary revascularization were an effective counter to the discouraging report of the Veterans Administration cooperative study.

781 patients with angina pectoris, confirmed by coronary arteriography, 402 treated medically, 379 operated upon. "At the end of the second year, the survival rate for all patients in the study was slightly higher in the surgically treated group, but it is impressive that twice as many of the survivors in the surgical group are now completely free of pain." Studying 169 matched patients with three vessel disease, "At the end of the first two years, 76% of the medically treated group had survived, whereas in the surgically managed group the survival was 90%", and he expected the improvement to be more striking with the passage of time. John L. Ochsner, of New Orleans, said that "With proper preparation of the internal mammary, one can achieve as much as 300 cc of free flow per minute." Postoperative angiograms of their patients showed a vein bypass oc-

cluded or narrowed in 29% [of an unspecified number], whereas of 88 internal mammary anastomoses, two were narrowed and one was "occluded during the study, by a catheter that dissected the internal mammary". Jack A. Cannon, of Phoenix, [perhaps prejudiced by his early personal investment in coronary endarterectomy] challenged Spencer's use of the word "curative", "I note that after *palliative* surgery to the arterial tree at *any* level, subsequent atherosclerotic involvement has been recorded in *any* type of reconstructive endeavor. This involvement includes endarterectomy, homologous arterial bypass, Dacron bypass, and autologous vein bypass. I ask Dr. Spencer, how does he envision the possibility of a curative result from a palliative surgical endeavor?" He challenged Spencer's conclusion that the use of the internal mammary artery would give superior results, "I suggest that his improved results may be more related to the improved technique afforded by the use of the operating microscope and even the steady-handed, near-sighted young surgeon in performing these meticulous anastomoses, rather than some mysterious quality of the difficulty harvested, tenously and uncertainly prepared, frequently damaged internal mammary." He asked about the flow measurements in the reconstructed vessels [mentioned in the published paper, but apparently not in the spoken presentation]. He asked, given the striking results of the Buchwald-Varco ileal bypass mentioned earlier at the meeting in reducing the serum triglycerides, and the fact that "Human races with no incidence of atherosclerotic disease show serum cholesterol levels in the 100-150 range with serum triglycerides of a correspondingly reduced level . . . Should ileal shunt for the prevention of this disease in patients with potentially lethal coronary atherosclerosis be considered as implied by the results of Dr. Varco and his group?" Spencer, closing, paid tribute to the contributions of Effler and the group at the Cleveland Clinic. He thought Effler's suggestion that double bypass might be all that would be required was plausible, and suggested, "one reason for the very low mortality reported by Dr. Effler's group may be the relatively short bypass time with most patients." He was enthusiastic about the capacity of the Duke computer program for filtering out special subgroups who had special risks. He shared Dr. Ochsner's enthusiasm for the use of the internal mammary artery, "I consider the mammary probably an ideal graft, except it is difficult and tedious to mobilize in some patients because of its size and friability" and particularly applicable to isolated occlusion of the anterior descending coronary artery, "a group often not operated upon because of the favorable prognosis . . . however, the operative risk approaches zero, the relief of symptoms is dramatic, and the patency shown by several groups over a year after operation with the internal mammary artery is over 95%. Hence [to Dr. Cannon], the operation very closely approaches 'a cure'." They had had no failures with single bypass grafts for isolated disease of the anterior descending coronary. He agreed with Cannon about the importance of the underlying atherosclerosis, but "The grim fact at present is that nothing in medical therapy has yet strongly influenced the course of atherosclerosis when evaluated in randomized studies over a period of five years." He emphasized the need of the "careful accumulation of significant data over a long period of time . . . there are probably at least five million American males with significant occlu-

sive disease of the coronary arteries, who would be theoretical candidates for a prophylactic bypass graft . . . Hence, the great responsibility for careful accumulation of data in reaching a clear decision is evident."

* * *

It was 44 years [Volume XLVIII, 1930, see page 686] since the first presentation of the Trendelenburg operation for pulmonary embolism before the Association. Now Lazar J. Greenfield, Professor and Chairman, Department of Surgery, Medical College of Virginia; and by invitation from the University of Oklahoma, [where Greenfield's work had begun before he succeeded to Hume's chair] Marvin D. Peyton, Phillip P. Brown and Ronald C. Elkins, *Transvenous Management of Pulmonary Embolic Disease,* reported their experience in ten patients with the passage of a catheter, from the femoral vein into the pulmonary artery, holding the embolus against the cup tip of the catheter by constant suction as the catheter was withdrawn, a technique which they had first proposed five years before. The catheter was double lumen with a balloon to permit isolation of the pulmonary artery branch, interrupting flow into it completely, and injection of contrast material to guide the approximation of the cup-device at the end of the catheter to the embolus. They had employed the technique in ten patients, five of whom were living and well, one of whom had died a month after the procedure. As Greenfield said quite candidly, ". . . the results of catheter embolectomy have not improved the survival rate which at 50% is comparable to the collected experience with 306 cardiopulmonary bypass cases through 1971 reported as 51.6% survival rate by Turnier *et al*", and some series had reached a 70% survival rate with cardiopulmonary bypass. Because of the problem of recurrent pulmonary embolism, they had developed a vena caval filter device to be inserted at the time of embolectomy [a device not unlike two old-fashioned lady's wire hairpins nesting at right angles to each other with recurved tips pointed to engage the wall of the vena cava]. They had placed the device in 16 patients, two of whom died of the pulmonary embolus.

Discussion

Marion S. DeWeese said that Greenfield's results were "equal to, or better than, most of those recorded in which open operation employing cardiopulmonary bypass have been utilized." He was impressed by the cone-shaped transvenous filter. He expressed some concern about the possibility that Greenfield's transvenous technique might be applied "by surgeons and nonsurgeons alike, and especially by those nonsurgeons who are conversant with cardiac catheterization techniques. I have been a little alarmed by the great interest which some cardiologists have shown, in that they seem anxious to perform the procedures themselves." Greenfield said that since the femoral vein and all its branches had to be exposed, he doubted the cardiologists would undertake the procedure. There were still numerous problems with the catheter, it was not foolproof. They always injected contrast material as the catheter was being inserted and had seen no evidence that they had displaced the thrombus with the catheter.

* * *

Eric W. Fonkalsrud, of Los Angeles, Professor of Surgery; Chief, Division of Pediatric Surgery, UCLA School of Medicine; and by invitation, Nate A. Myers, from the Royal Children's Hospital, Melbourne, Australia; and Max J. Robinson, *Management of Extrahepatic Portal Hypertension in Children,* reported the combined experience of the UCLA Hospital and the Royal Children's Hospital, Melbourne, from 1948 to 1973, in 15 children from UCLA and 54 from Melbourne, with extrahepatic portal venous thrombosis. Whereas there were 338 variceal bleeding episodes, it was striking that only two patients had died of bleeding, both of whom lived in remote communities inaccessible to medical care. "Portal vein thrombosis is primarily a mechanical problem, with hemorrhage as the only major risk to the patient. In contrast to the high mortality for patients with intrahepatic disease who experience variceal bleeding, the mortality rate is extremely low for patients with PVT", and others had made the same observation. Bleeding episodes were preceded "by an upper respiratory tract infection more than 70% of the time." Ingestion of aspirin had preceded a number of major bleeding episodes. The hemorrhage in children was usually self-limited and emergency procedures were rarely required. They had occasionally performed "balloon tamponade, intra-arterial pitressin infusion, variceal ligation, or gastric division . . .", and all such patients had subsequently bled again. In neither hospital had an emergency shunt ever been performed for bleeding from portal venous thrombosis. Only seven children died. Four of them were among the 20 who had undergone a previous splenectomy "and each died with sepsis, one from pneumococcal infection." Nineteen of the 20 children who had splenectomy alone rebled, and 17 were ultimately reoperated upon. All of

the 22 patients with variceal ligation rebled, and 20 of them were reoperated upon. Fifteen of the 17 patients with gastric division rebled and ten of them were reoperated upon. Gastrectomy with colon interposition was done only twice and one patient rebled. Nine children had cavomesenteric shunts, four of them rebled and three were reoperated upon. Six children had splenorenal shunts, three rebled and one was reoperated upon. Six children had makeshift shunts, all of them rebled, and four were reoperated upon. Three children had splenic transposition, two of them rebled and one was reoperated upon. They agreed with Clatworthy, "that a shunt with a diameter of less than 1 cm is unlikely to remain patent and that shunt procedures should be deferred until the patient is eight years of age." There were numerous postoperative complications, "ascites, intestinal obstruction, wound infection, intestinal perforation, hemorrhage, and jaundice." Seventy-eight operations of a total of 164 "were performed to treat complications of previous operations other than bleeding." They concluded, ". . . that a few children with PVT may be managed very satisfactorily and safely without operation despite recurrent variceal bleeding. Bleeding episodes generally became less frequent as the patients increased in age and became less susceptible to respiratory infections. When bleeding continues to recur with moderate frequency, a planned portal-to-systemic venous shunt would seem justified, provided that a shunt with a diameter of more than 1 cm can be constructed . . . There was no significant difference in the incidence of hemorrhage in nonoperated patients as compared to operated patients in this series, with follow-up extending into late adolescence."

Discussion

H. William Clatworthy, Jr., of Columbus, Ohio, said the information here provided had been hard to glean from the literature, he hoped that it might be possible in the future to separate out those in whom the shunt was necessary and would prove effective. In the literature, he had been able to find 418 cases of extrahepatic block, "There were 53 deaths (12%), which compares closely with the 10% in this series. Twenty-three of these review cases (5%) died of hemorrhage; 22 (5%) died from operations, and 8 (2%) died of hepatitis, which may be presumed to be associated with repeated blood transfusions." At Columbus, they had done 21 shunts in 36 patients, had only four unoperated patients and three treated by splenectomy alone. Twelve of their shunts had been successful while nine of the patients had rebled, the experience going back to 1953. Patients had been followed up to 21 years. "I do think we are becoming more conservative. We now have a number of children we're following. We feel we should not give up shunts, though, because this procedure cures the patient—if it's done on the proper patient." John H. Foster, of Nashville, had followed 21 children since 1950, two had died after splenectomy alone and one after an unsuccessful makeshift shunt; seventeen children had a portal systemic shunt and one had transposition of the spleen into the left hemithorax, and all were alive and well; four with thrombosed splenorenal shunts had subsequent mesocaval shunts, and all shunts were now patent. He agreed that patients could be managed nonoperatively until they were large enough for successful shunt, "The question posed by Dr. Fonkalsrud is 'why not treat these children by non-operative measures if it can be done successfully?' In my opinion the answer is that it is not wise to continue each year to give these children three to six units of blood indefinitely." Jeremiah G. Turcotte, of Ann Arbor, said that in their experience, "some children continue to bleed frequently and massively even if they have not had previous operations. Others develop massive splenomegaly and become symptomatic with this. We certainly would agree that probably not all children need to have shunts constructed, but the clinical course of some patients will be such that a shunt is indicated." They had performed mesocaval shunts in 11 children with portal vein thrombosis, in two of whom the shunts thrombosed in the postoperative period, "the others have remained open for as long as ten years with no long-term morbidity . . . we would recommend that in carefully selected patients mesocaval shunts be constructed in children under the age of 13." William P. Mikkelsen, of Los Angeles, said "As patients grow older, and as they pass the age of 20, they seem to stop bleeding and in a few of these the varices disappear. In the successfully shunted child, as the years go on, BSP retention steadily increases, and some of these children have a fetor hepaticus. I just wonder, when they have been followed long enough, whether they may develop encephalopathy later on in life." Thomas V. Santulli, of New York, said the experience presented paralleled that of Voorhees at Baby's Hospital, Columbia-Presbyterian Medical Center. They never performed emergency shunting, sedated their bleeding children very heavily, never permitted aspirin, "and the hemorrhage usually stops." In the "long-term follow-up in these children, with no matter what type of shunt procedure, the very high incidence of encephalopathy and neuropsychiatric ab-

normalities has been most discouraging. Indeed, it is almost 100% if the follow-up is long enough." Charles Gardner Child, III, of Ann Arbor, was aware "of Dr. Arthur B. Voorhees' discouraging report of children followed up to 20 years after portal decompression. Many of these ultimately developed severe emotional and neurological disturbances. At Michigan we cannot duplicate this experience but then our patients have not been followed for long periods of time." Fonkalsrud, closing, urged that it was better not to perform a shunt at all than to perform a makeshift or a small shunt. The shunt should be 1 cm in diameter, and "It is rare that a child under 8 years of age with portal vein thrombosis will have mesenteric or splenic veins of sufficient size to perform a successful shunt . . . shunts or other portal decompressive operations should rarely be attempted on children under 8 years of age." They had not yet seen a child with true encephalopathy.

* * *

W. Hardy Hendren, of Boston, Director, Division of Pediatric Surgery, Massachusetts General Hospital; Associate Clinical Professor of Surgery, Harvard Medical School, *Urinary Tract Refunctionalization after Prior Diversion in Children,* directed attention to the large group of children who had urinary diversion in infancy for lesions now technically correctable. He displayed a series of tours de force of technical virtuosity in taking down ileal loop diversions, loop ureterostomies, cystostomies, end-ureterostomies, and nephrostomies in one or in staged operations, at the same time correcting the underlying ureterocele, ureteral reflux, vesical outlet obstruction, etc. The figure illustrates the complexity and the ingenuity of the procedures. He emphasized the difficulties and complexities of the techniques, suggesting "that these cases should be relegated, at least for the present time, to those relatively few surgeons in each region whose practice affords a large and continuing experience in major reconstructive pediatric urology." In any case, ". . . many children are subjected to urinary diversion who could be treated by direct reconstruction . . . many previously diverted cases can be refunctionalized if bladder innervation is intact." Even in children who would ultimately require transplantation, reconstruction might be considered because "the quality of life will be better in those years before transplantation . . . it is easier to maintain sterility in a closed urinary tract . . . a patient with a functioning bladder is a more suitable candidate for transplantation than one with a diversion." [Hendren's paper

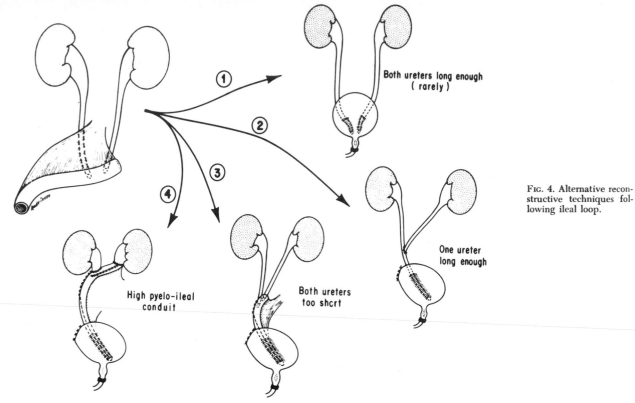

FIG. 4. Alternative reconstructive techniques following ileal loop.

① Both ureters long enough (rarely)

② One ureter long enough

③ Both ureters too short

④ High pyelo-ileal conduit

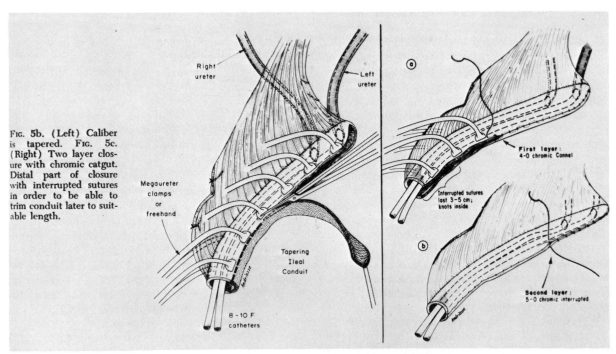

FIG. 5b. (Left) Caliber is tapered. FIG. 5c. (Right) Two layer closure with chromic catgut. Distal part of closure with interrupted sutures in order to be able to trim conduit later to suitable length.

Right ureter

Left ureter

Megaureter clamps or freehand

Tapering Ileal Conduit

8 - 10 F catheters

First layer: 4-0 chromic Connel

Interrupted sutures last 3-5 cm; knots inside

Second layer: 5-0 chromic interrupted

In a wide variety of conditions, Hendren demonstrated that the original urinary diversion had either been unnecessary or that the necessitating cause was now susceptible of correction. The illustrations demonstrate the variety of ways in which the patient with an ileal loop could be "undiverted" and the caliber of the bowel reduced, if the bowel was to be reinserted into a closed urinary tract.

W. H. Hendren, *Urinary Tract Refunctionalization after Prior Diversion in Children.* Volume XCII, 1974.

was a long way from Charles G. Mixter's almost primitive discussion of pediatric urology in 1926.]

Discussion

Robert E. Gross, of Boston, opened the Discussion. [Gross did not attend the meetings often. Since his election in 1948 he had presented only two papers. In the years 1948 to 1960, his name appeared in the Register only four times.] He commented on the changes which had occurred in pediatric urology. ". . . what has been done here required a good deal of initiative, clear thinking, and high technical skill in revamping the urinary systems of some of these unfortunate children and getting them back to near normalcy . . . tremendous advances have been made in correction of many of the anomalies we have seen. We have operated hoping to improve things; very often we have ended up by doing two or three operations to try to get things better, and in the end, being somewhat overawed by the whole business, have turned—reluctantly, but we thought, with good advice—to some sort of permanent external drainage of the urine, believing that this gave the best hope for recovery of damaged kidneys and longer life for the individual. It's very refreshing to now see that many of these things which we did in the past in good faith can now be transformed, and patients turned to normalcy, or near normalcy." He praised the "young men who have been through the residency training program and on our staff who have taken a new look at things in this field . . . They have accomplished things which we thought before were impossible." He ended with the extraordinary praise, coming from Robert Gross, "As I reflect on these things, it is very appropriate to recall the words, uttered so long ago by Leonardo da Vinci when he said: 'The brilliant student will certainly outshine his teacher.'" Victor F. Marshall, of New York, said the patient's urinary control was the point to consider, and that eliminated children with myelomeningocele. With some pessimism he said he was concerned, "Will the patient himself and his urinary tract be able to withstand a failure? These patients have already had some sort of a failure, sometimes very severe. The best laid plans and abilities do sometimes fail, and especially so in complex situations." At times he employed autotransplantation as the simplest method of reconstruction. Could Dr. Hendren tell them "which defunctionalized bladders would respond with a good capacity, and any sort of indication as to when they might respond." Willard E. Goodwin, of Los Angeles, said, "The defunctionalized bladder will usually expand with use, but not always; and it may sometimes be necessary to augment the bladder with intestine." He thought Hendren's system of "tailoring" the ileum to reduce its caliber was unnecessary, that if an antireflux procedure was needed in the ileum, it could be simply provided by creating an intussusception. J. J. Murphy, of Philadelphia, noting that a good number of Hendren's patients had begun with urethral valves, reported that an immediate initial attack upon the obstructing lesion could be undertaken, that "Dr. John Duckett at our Children's Hospital of Philadelphia has used this approach in 26 children in the past three years . . . Ten of these children have required no other surgical therapy." John Lilly, of Denver, emphasized that autotransplantation depended on whether the kidney was close enough to the bladder, could be used when there was only a short segment of good ureter, and illustrated two successful cases. J. Hartwell Harrison, of Boston, spoke of the advancement of pediatric urology and all the contributions that "W. E. Ladd, the late Thomas Lanman, Bob Gross, and now Hardy Hendren" had made, and asked ". . . is it time for children's hospitals to have divisions of urology?" [Something, as Harrison well knew, that the Children's Hospital of Boston had resolutely avoided. The urology there was part and parcel of the work of the general pediatric surgeons.] Hendren, closing, agreed that undiversion was not to be undertaken in the presence of a neurogenic bladder. As for evaluating the function of the bladder, this was not really possible in a child who had had a diversion for many years. "The majority of these bladders are very small from long standing disuse. They stretch up to a reasonable capacity very soon after refunctionalization, however." Others [D. I. Williams, London, E. A. Tanagho, San Francisco] had "emphasized that some of these long diverted, contracted bladders may never work in a satisfactory manner. To this date we have not encountered any whose bladder function proved entirely unsatisfactory, although some have been better than others." He had not preformed autotransplantation, which he thought imposed greater risks and was particularly hazardous when the urine was not sterile. Goodwin, he said, had been a pioneer in the field and might "be correct that perhaps it is not necessary to tailor the conduits as we have done . . .", but the slenderized bowel he though propelled the urine more effectively and had less absorptive mucosal surface, as well as permitting more effective reimplantation into the bladder. He agreed with the importance of the primary attack on urethral valves. As for pediatric urology, it constituted "possibly a third of the surgery of infants and children" and there was "great need for a number of men throughout the country to take special interest in this field, just as . . . in other types of pediatric surgery . . . I believe we must gear our residency programs to train those surgeons who are interested in this field, whether they come from parent programs in urology or from pediatric surgery. It is time we stopped having jurisdictional disputes as to who owns the patients and get together to work at doing a better job for these children."

* * *

Lt. Col. Tom R. DeMeester, Lt. Col. Lawrence F. Johnson, and Col. Alfred H. Kent, all by invitation from the Tripler Army Medical Center, Honolulu, Hawaii, *Evaluation of Current Operations for the Prevention of Gastroesophageal Reflux,* presented their detailed studies of 45 patients with esophageal reflux who had undergone Hill, Nissen or Belsey repairs. Allison had emphasized the importance of reflux in producing the symptoms attributed to hiatus hernia [Volume XCI, 1973], but his operation had been associated with a high incidence of symptomatic and anatomic recurrences. Hill had introduced the "posterior gastropexy in which the phrenoesophageal membrane and the cardioesophageal junction are anchored to the median arcuate ligament of the aortic hiatus", and the Belsey Mark IV and Nissen fundoplications "were designed to reinforce the lower esophageal sphincter with a cuff of stomach as well as reestablishing an intra-abdominal segment of esophagus." The Hill procedure as performed in their patients included "a small plication of the lesser curvature of the stomach around the distal esophagus so as to narrow the esophageal gastric junction" [in effect, a partial Nissen]. The Belsey repair, performed transthoracically, "creates a 4 cm segment of intra-abdominal esophagus and buttresses it by a 270° gastric fundic wrap." In the Nissen fundoplication, performed transabdominally, "the gastric fundus is wrapped 360° around the distal 4 cm of the esophagus to maintain it within the abdomen and buttress it at the same time." The Hill and Nissen repairs were performed over a 30 French tube, the Belsey repair over a standard nasogastric tube. In addition to conventional endoscopic and radiographic studies, they performed manometric studies, acid clearance studies,- evaluating the number of swallows taken to return the intraesophageal pH to 5 after the introduction of 15 cc of normal HCL,- an acid reflex test, and finally, in 34 of the patients, 24-hour pH monitoring of the distal esophagus, before and after operation. The best symptomatic improvement was seen after the Nissen repair.

The Nissen and Belsey procedures increased the distal esophageal sphincter pressure over the preoperative level more than the Hill procedure did, "The Nissen procedure placed more of the manometric sphincter below the respiratory inversion point in the positive pressure environment of the abdomen." There was a higher incidence of dysphagia after both the Nissen and the Hill repairs, thought to be due to the increase in the length of the esophagus. "Reflux is most effectively prevented by the Nissen repair, as shown by the SART [Standard Acid Reflux Test] and the 24-hour esophageal pH monitoring, a sensitive measurement of frequency and duration of reflux." The hospital stay [Tripler Army Medical Center] was 20 days for the Belsey and 12 days for the Nissen and Hill. Vomiting was easiest after the Hill, and most difficult after the Belsey and Nissen. They concluded, "that the Nissen repair best controls reflux and its symptoms by providing the greatest increase in DES pressure and placing more of the sphincter in the positive abdominal environment. This is accomplished with the lowest morbidity but at the expense of temporary postoperative dysphagia and a 50% chance of being unable to vomit after the repair." The postoperative studies were made on the average of five months after operation.

Discussion

L. C. Hill, of Seattle, said that "Since we first reported the use of pH and pressure studies in 1961, we have been gratified that this technique has been employed across the country, and we would agree with the authors that it represents the most sensitive method of detecting reflux." He was critical of what he understood to be their performance of his operation, "It was disturbing that they achieved only a centimeter of esophagus below the diaphragm . . . We generally end up with about 3 cm of esophagus below the diaphragm, and have not found that this creates dysphagia." He measured the lower esophageal sphincter pressure intraoperatively and had consistently found it to be substantially raised. "We persist in calibrating and tightening the cardia at operation [by the Nissen wrap!] until we have a sphincter pressure that is in the proper range . . . if the authors would admonish their chief surgical residents to adhere to these simple points of calibration of the cardia and obtaining adequate esophageal length, they would find that the median arcuate repair will correct reflux with a high degree of efficiency . . . there is always a mystique about a foreign, imported product, such as the Belsey and Nissen procedures . . . if the authors would bear these simple techniques in mind the 'home grown' median arcuate repair will look better than the foreign imports." Edward R. Woodward, of Gainesville, Florida, said that indeed the Nissen fundoplication was "considerably more effective in curing reflux esophagitis" than "the old, traditional crural repair . . ." They had had a recurrence rate of 18% with crural repair and 9% with the Nissen fundoplication, over 100 patients of each. They had found that "The resting pressures in the lower esophageal sphincter closely parallel clinical success; namely, they about doubled in patients in whom the esophagitis was cured . . ." While they had found the Nissen procedure "to be a very reliable method . . . the morbidity that we have observed with this procedure has been very real, although, in most patients, temporary; and in our hands we can achieve more satisfied patients with less morbidity using the method described by Dr. Hill." Lloyd M. Nyhus, of Chicago, showed studies in his own patients after the Nissen procedure, with the appropriate pressure changes, reminding the Fellows "that we do not usually repair the crus, and that one-half of the patients in the postoperative period had their esophagogastric junction above the diaphragm", and he thought this required explanation. DeMeester, closing, said that measured on the X-ray film, their patients with the Hill operation had an average of 3.1 cm of esophagus within the abdomen. There was not a one to one correlation between the pressure in the distal esophageal sphincter and competence. The aim of the operation was to restore cardioesophageal competence and that was best measured by pH studies and not by sphincter pressure. They had not seen the morbidity with the Nissen procedure that Dr. Woodward had seen, perhaps because "We do not extend the wrap more than 3-4 cm over the distal esophagus, using only four sutures, and do the wrap over a 30 French gastric tube." He did feel that it was important to increase the sphincter pressure to produce competence, and "if the sphincter pressure is over 20, there is little chance for reflux to occur."

* * *

The question of preoperative antibiotic preparation of patients for colonic surgery had been discussed on a number of occasions, most recently the previous year, and the need for a prospective randomized study pointed out then by Isidore Cohn. John A. Washington, II, and William H. Dearing, by invitation, Edward S. Judd, of Rochester, Professor of Surgery, Mayo Graduate School of Medicine, University of Minnesota; and by invitation, Lila R. Elveback, *Effect of Preoperative Antibiotic Regimen on Development of Infection after Intestinal Surgery:* Prospective, Randomized, Double-Blind Study, provided just such an investigation. Between 1968 and 1971, patients admitted for elective colonic or rectal surgery "were assigned, on a randomized and double-blind basis, to three preoperative medication groups: neomycin (group 1), neomycin plus tetracycline (group 2), and placebo (group 3) . . ." The preparation was otherwise uniform,- residue-free diet for 48 hours, cathartics, tap-water enemas. Judd performed all the operations. The groups had respectively 68, 65, and 63 patients. The distribution of the patients in the three groups by age, sex, and lesion were the same, and the types of resection almost identical. There was a statistically significant decrease in anaerobes in stool culture at operation in group 2 patients. In the neomycin group, there were 28 wound infections; in the neomycin-tetracycline group, there were three infections; and in the placebo group, there were 27 wound infections. No patient had staphylococcal enteritis, or pseudomembranous enterocolitis.

Discussion

Isidore Cohn, Jr., of New Orleans, showed a composite slide of the results from many institutions of "comparative studies of patients with and without preoperative bowel preparation: and except for one single institution, you see that each institution reported a lower incidence of wound infection, peritonitis, and so forth, on patients who were prepared, as compared with the patients who were not prepared." None of these studies had been prospective. The experimental data from laboratory studies were clear and now Judd had a significant prospective randomized study. ". . . we have got a study that answers just about all of the criteria one could ask for, and the result of this study is an indication that preoperative intestinal antisepsis *is* of value by statistical evaluation. That is a very important fact . . . there is only one other prospective randomized study comparable to this. It was reported in the *British Journal of Surgery* in 1971. The results are entirely comparable to those reported today by Dr. Judd." Cohn did not think neomycin and tetracycline represented an ideal combination, although it was one he had used on his service for years. Allen M. Boyden, of Portland, Oregon, said that since the previous year's presentation by Nyhus and associates "of the use of neomycin and erythromycin given only during the 18 hours preceding operation with the essential elimination of pathogens from the bowel, and remarkable reduction in wound infections", he had followed that routine, and since then had had no wound infections after colon resection. Lloyd M. Nyhus, of Chicago, had continued to use the same preparation in 104 additional patients and now had two wound infections and no septicemia. Why did Dr. Judd not use erythromycin? Judd quoted Altemeier as writing to him ". . . I have used tetracycline intravenously just before, during and for 4 days postoperatively for its effect on the bacteroides and the clostridia. You have used the intestinal route, and the results are just as critical to me, and for the same reasons."

* * *

Harry E. LeVeen, of Brooklyn, Professor of Surgery, State University of New York, Downstate Medical Center; Chief, Surgical Service, Brooklyn Veterans Administration Hospital, and by invitation, G. Christoudias, I. Moon, R. Luft, G. Falk, and S. Grosberg, *Peritoneo-Venous Shunting for Ascites,* said that attempts had been made in recent years by others to establish peritoneal shunts but without success. Evaluating both flow-activated and pressure-activated valves, he found that at low flows the flow-sensitive valves permitted reflux of blood and clotting, so that he had settled on the pressure-sensitive valve. He had developed a silicone valve with an opening pressure of 3 to 5 cm of water, which did not leak. The valve functioned in dogs for as long as three months. The pumping action of respiration, the rise of intra-abdominal pressure with the fall of intrathoracic pressure, provided "a pressure differential sufficient to empty the ascitic fluid into the vena cava in ascitic animals and humans." Forced deep respirations exaggerated the differential pressure. Over-infusion of the patient with his own ascitic fluid was not possible "since a significant rise of venous pressure closes the valve and protects against heart failure and pulmonary edema." The valve and the perforated Silastic tubing were placed into the abdominal cavity through a small incision, and the peritoneum closed around the stem of the valve. The Silastic tubing was pulled under the skin of the thorax into the neck and passed down into the jugular vein to the inferior vena cava. After the first 24 hours, a binder was placed about the abdomen and after 48 hours respiratory exercises were begun, with the patient recumbent. At this point LeVeen could report 19 patients of his own and 26 patients of others reported to him. Several of the patients were in the end stage of liver disease and five of them died. "Jaundiced patients in liver failure cannot be helped sufficiently by valve insertion." One of the six anuric or oliguric patients improved his car-

diac output, lost his ascites, and survived. They did not now accept for valve insertion, patients in whom "volume expansion with plasma or blood combined with furosemide does not bring about an increase in urinary output." There were 13 of their own patients and 21 outside patients available for prolonged observation. Two patients required shunt removal because of infection, although both by then had lost their ascites. One-third of the shunts became occluded in a week or two, "after the ascites had completely disappeared. The sudden reappearance of ascites heralds an occlusion of the shunt." A defect in the valve allowing blood to enter it caused the clotting in 90% of the failures and this had now been corrected by a change in the valve. Two patients required two replacements, in one case after three months, but in general "shunts which are patent longer than one month usually remain patent." Thirteen of his own patients had been followed one week to one-and-a-half years with relief of ascites; 21 of the outside patients who had been followed for two weeks to six months, had lost their ascites. Most patients lost about 50 pounds of liquid by weight, and showed an immediate hemodilution effect on the hematocrit, which never quite returned to normal, "indicating that these patients are depleted of red cell mass." The massive diuresis was sometimes accompanied by potassium loss which required intravenous replacement. Furosemide was given repetitively in the first 48 hours to maintain a maximal urinary output. [The presentation was accompanied by extraordinary before and after photographs of the, inititally, massively ascitic patients.]

Discussion

W. R. Waddell, of Denver, said that they had been evaluating a valve designed "for the treatment of internal hydrocephalus" and somewhat different in concept from LeVeen's. The chamber was placed external to the peritoneal cavity with one tube going into the peritoneal cavity and one through the saphenous vein up to the vena cava. The apparatus was made of silicon rubber and the valves were activated by pressure on the chamber. They had used it also in patients with malignant ascites. L. R. Eidemiller, of Portland, Oregon, had employed the LeVeen shunt for ascites in a Budd-Chiari syndrome patient, almost moribund and with hepatorenal failure. The patient recovered dramatically, and was "discharged at 14 days, ascites free, and now five months after operation has nearly normal liver function." LeVeen, closing, said that obviously other valves might be used, but they must be pressure-

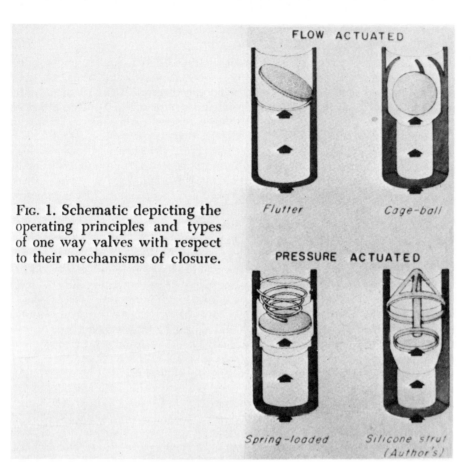

FIG. 1. Schematic depicting the operating principles and types of one way valves with respect to their mechanisms of closure.

FLOW ACTUATED

Flutter   *Cage-ball*

PRESSURE ACTUATED

Spring-loaded   *Silicone strut (Author's)*

LeVeen had determined that at the low flow conditions of a peritoneo-venous shunt a flow sensitive valve was plagued by reflux and clotting. His pressure sensitive valve had an opening pressure of 3-5 cm. of water, and did not permit reflux. He reported 19 patients of his own with massive ascites, and 26 cases of others. Thirteen of his own patients and 21 of the outside patients had lost their ascites.

H. E. LeVeen, G. Christoudias, I. Moon, R. Luft, G. Falk, and S. Grosberg, *Peritoneo-Venous Shunting for Ascites,* Volume XCII, 1974.

activated. The valve Waddell had described was a slit valve, and Waddell provided a pumping chamber,- "A slit valve is a flow-activated valve . . . Such a pump should not be necessary if thrombosis does not occur, and for that reason, one was not incorporated into our system . . . we can always add it; but at this present moment, it doesn't seem necessary."

* * *

Leon C. Parks, Alan N. Baer, Marilyn Pollack, all by invitation, and G. Melville Williams, of Baltimore, Professor of Surgery, Johns Hopkins Hospital, *Alpha Fetoprotein:* An Index of Progression or Regression of Hepatoma, and Target for Immunotherapy, thought that malignancies producing

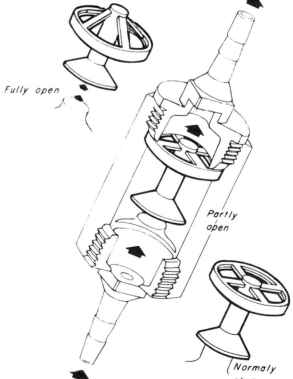

Fully open

Partly open

Normaly shut

FIG. 2. Construction of the valve used by the authors. The valve is held in the normally closed position by tension on the silicone rubber struts.

this albumin-like plasma protein, which was found in the sera of normal adults and in abnormal amounts in the sera of patients with hepatoma and terato-carcinoma and some other tumors, presented the possibility of the evaluation of antibody therapy, because of "the facility with which excellent antisera can be produced . . . the availability of simple, rapid methods for monitoring circulating tumor associated antigen . . . a typically irreversibly fatal disease course . . . the presence of an excellent animal model of the human disease, the BW 7756/C57L murine hepatoma." They found alpha-fetoprotein activity only in patients with hepatocellular carcinoma, not in metastatic GI carcinoma, benign lesions of the liver, acute hepatitis or intrahepatic abscess. The level of AFP showed correlation with the amount of clinical disease present, but in a given patient was an index of his condition, ". . . continued elevation of AFP levels in patients post hepatic resection for tumors appears more likely to reflect residual malignant disease than regenerative hepatic processes." The recurrence of abnormal AFP levels in patients in whom the levels had returned to normal after resection of hepatoma, indicated tumor recurrence at a time when conventional radioisotope scans and arteriograms did not yet show it. In their animal experiments, circulating alpha-fetoprotein "could be cleared by passive administration of an excess of anti-AFP". Anti-AFP as used in their experiments did not affect the tumor growth. Specially prepared concentrated anti-AFP antibody localized significantly in the experimental hepatoma and when it was tagged with the radioisotope, "Hepatomas exposed to anti-AFP_2 contained threefold the amount of radio-activity found in hepatomas exposed to normal IgG while the activity found in other tissues did not differ significantly." The possibility of passive humoral immuno-therapy of cancer by this technique was envisaged.

Discussion

Elton Watkins, Jr., of Boston, asked whether with use of the antibodies they observed "nephrotoxic changes in view of the well known effects of antigen-antibody complexes on the kidney, and in this instance, radioactive antigen-antibody complexes? Such a nephrotoxic effect might interfere with this method as a form of therapy." Donald L. Morton, of Log Angeles, said that "probably all types of tumors secrete unique antigens such as alpha fetoprotein into the blood plasma. The quantity of these circulating tumor associated antigens in the serum are a reflection of the size of tumor burden in

the host and can be used to monitor tumor therapy as so beautifully demonstrated by the authors . . . antibodies highly specific for these tumor associated antigens can be labelled with radioactive isotopes or cytotoxic substances such as diphtheria toxin and the antibody can serve as a lethal missile to carry the toxin directly to the tumor cell." The circulating tumor antigens were also useful in diagnosing and staging malignant disease. "It is likely that the specificity of some of these circulating tumor antigens will be such that the presence of these abnormal antigens in the sera will indicate which patient has a hidden malignancy in their body. But where is the malignant tumor located? It is possible by the use of specific radio-labelled antibodies and radioisotopic scanning devices to determine the exact location of the neoplasm. For example in a woman suspected of having breast cancer because she has a specific breast tumor antigen in her serum, one may determine by radio scanning techniques, not only the involved breast but which quadrant of the breast has the hidden neoplasm . . . it is likely that these techniques will be clinically applicable within this decade."

* * *

T. E. Starzl, of Denver, Professor of Surgery, University of Colorado School of Medicine; Chairman, Department of Surgery, Denver Veterans Administration Hospital; and by invitation, K. A. Porter, C. G. Halgrimson, B. S. Husberg, I. Penn, and C. W. Putnam, *A Decade Follow-up in Early Cases of Renal Homotransplantation,* presented the results in 64 consecutive patients who had undergone renal transplantation, ten years and two months to 11 years and six months earlier, 46 from related donors and 18 from unrelated living donors. Starzl had made a previous report to the Association in 1965, when 36 of the patients were alive 13-1/2 to 30 months after operation. As he said, "The climate between November 1962 and March 1964, when the series was compiled, had overtones of anxiety as well as excitement. Because the degree of success being achieved had not been anticipated by basic immunologists and for that matter was not generally appreciated by clinicians, expressions of criticism and concern were common. [He cited the paper of J. R. Elkinton, Moral Problems in the Use of Borrowed Organs, Artificial and Transplanted. *Annals of Internal Medicine,* 1964]. Even those aware of the encouraging statistics of 1962-1963 conceded that the ultimate prognosis of the renal recipients still living was not predictable, since only very isolated examples of long-term survival had been recorded before this time." [Of his original group of 64 patients, 35 of whom were alive at the time of his 1965 report, 26 still lived.] The 26 patients still surviving, by reference to the data of the American College of Surgeons Registry "account for about half of those in the world who were treated before March 1964 with renal homotransplantation and who remain alive today." While the ten patients who had died since the previous report tended to have subnormal renal function or graft failures ". . . the actual causes of death included 2 or more each of myocardial infarction, hepatitis, or other systemic infections." Although "survival was not obviously related to HL-A tissue match . . . best results were with related kidneys, within which subgroup 24 (52%) of the original recipients are still alive . . . no particular category of consanguineous donor . . . had a marked superiority. Only 2 of 18 nonrelated recipients are still alive." Graft biopsies had been made in all the patients alive in 1965 and "kidneys that were destined to function for a decade tended to have relatively minor histopathologic abnormalities. If serious glomerular lesions were found, the outlook for long graft survival was grave. Vascular lesions had a somewhat less serious import. Mononuclear cell infiltration, tubular atrophy, and interstitial fibrosis proved prognostically to be the least significant." Four of the survivors had undergone retransplantation, one of them three times, the last time in 1972, the first retransplant in that patient having been performed in 1970, seven years after the first transplantation, the longest period after the original transplant before retranplantation. Of the function of the grafts, Starzl was able to say, "On the average, the function of the organs is superb. Only one of the original grafts is distinctly subnormal." Daily doses of prednisone were sufficiently small, "so that only one of the 26 patients (the most recent retransplant) has a Cushing's facies." None of the patients had steroid-induced diabetes. Azathioprine doses had been stable for years in most of the patients. "Over the years, we have had a number of patients discontinue immunosuppressive treatment, usually because of indifference to the tedium of following a therapeutic schedule. One of the chronic survivors . . . in this early series discontinued all medications about 14 months ago without any untoward effect to date. Another recipient . . . who also was brain-damaged from a stroke prior to transplantation, has become an alcoholic in the 11-1/4 years of survival. This patient who has never required prednisone probably discontinued his azathioprine in 1970 or 1971." Although most of the patients had arterial hypertension after transplantation and even for several years

afterward, "With longer follow-up, only one of the 25 survivors who has renal function (and this the retransplant recipient of 16 months ago) has severe hypertension. Four other patients receive small daily doses of antihypertensives." Six of the 36 patients who died after May 1965 developed malignant skin lesions "all successfully treated with conventional means." As for rehabilitation, "The social and vocational rehabilitation amongst the 26 present survivors has been very nearly complete. All 14 of those who were adults (18 or older) at the time of transplantation are employed, frequently in jobs for which they were specifically trained postoperatively. Twelve of the survivors were 'pediatric' patients (ages 3-17). The three-year-old who is now almost 14 is a healthy, but physically stunted school boy. The other 11 have reached adulthood and are college students or job holders." The brain-damaged student who had become an alcoholic was a day field worker. Three of the adolescents, at the time of transplantation, developed necrosis of one or both femoral heads in the early postoperative period. Two had learned to walk adequately, "The third had bilateral total hip replacement performed successfully nine years post-transplantation." Two female patients had had three children and nine patients had fathered 13 children. None of those parents had died. "One of the offspring of a male patient . . . had a meningomyelocele which was surgically repaired." There was justification for greater optimism now than in 1965 when Starzl had said to the Association that ". . . for the present it would seem most reasonable to regard homotransplantation as an effective, but incompletely characterized form of palliative therapy." Late losses occurred more frequently with unrelated donors and it was Starzl's feeling that ". . . improvement in patient survival with the use of unrelated organs under presently employed immunosuppressive regimens, including those using ALG, will require acceptance of a much heavier rate of retransplantation than with consanguineous donors." The expected deaths "from complications of immunologic invalidism" had proven to be a fallacy. After three years, "Except for hepatitis, infection has played no role in the deaths . . ." He acknowledged the increased incidence of malignancies, ". . . a penalty for chronic immunosuppression and the consequent partial loss of immunologic competence, but the resulting neoplasms have usually been treatable by conventional means with the notable exception of mesenchymal malignancies." Their histologic studies of graft biopsies had shown that ". . . the quality of the two year biopsy can predict the functional future of the homografts . . .

glomerular abnormalities were even more discriminating than the vascular ones. A kidney with serious glomerular pathology at two years, had less than a 10% chance of being functional at a decade." While the glomerular lesion might be the autoimmune disease which had destroyed the original kidneys, "the immunologic events of rejection can probably manifest as glomerulonephritis since glomerulonephritis has been seen after animal transplantation or transplantation to humans whose original disease was not autoimmune in nature . . . The prognostic reliability of glomerular pathology is probably as high as it is because it picks up both of the aforementioned main pathways of graft injury."

Discussion

F. O. Belzer, of San Francisco, said they had followed one of Starzl's original patients, "This man is now 11 years post operative, has not missed a day of work, and has never been in the hospital since his transplant." He wished to ask Starzl, ". . . how much can we decrease our immunosuppressive therapy in these long-term patients, and can we ever discontinue these drugs completely . . . seven of our patients did this by themselves and the results were disastrous." One woman who had been doing extremely well had become pregnant ". . . and her obstetrician suggested that she drop her immunosuppressive therapy, which she did without telling us. She delivered a normal child, did well for six months, and then arrived at our hospital with a creatinine of 11. We were never able to reverse the rejection." He doubted that immunosuppression should ever be dropped ". . . below a certain level; and in adult patients we should not drop the Prednisone dose below 10 mg . . . even long-term patients should be followed for the rest of their lives . . . we should emphasize to long-term survivors that the three or four little pills they take in the morning are still the difference between life and death." Richard E. Wilson, of Boston, said that with Dr. Tilney he had reviewed the results of renal transplant, except of those of identical twins, performed at the Peter Bent Brigham Hospital in exactly the same time period, 40 grafts, 19 from living related donors, five from cadaver donors and six from unrelated donors who had had nephrectomy for a Matson arachnoido-ureteral shunt. "None of the cadaver or obligatory unrelated donor kidney recipients transplanted during that time period lived the one year maximum", though one patient done prior to that time period lived for two years on an unrelated transplant. Of the living related donor-recipients, 16 of 19

lived more than one year—84%, eight of the 19 lived more than five years—42%, and seven of the 19 lived more than ten years—37%. "One patient now living over ten years received a second kidney from a cadaver after five years on his first kidney . . . a patient in whom we had tried to stop his prednisone; when we tried to restart it, we could never retrieve the rejecting kidney." They had seen no malignancies develop in these patients. They had had a better one-year survival than Starzl's but a greater attrition in the five and ten-year periods, and wondered "whether there was any selective process, on the basis of tissue typing, in choosing his donor-recipient pairs. We have never excluded any patients, and still don't, for tissue type, just for positive crossmatch." John S. Najarian, of Minneapolis, said that based on actuarial tables with the related kidneys in children, they had a "70% kidney survival at ten years, and practically no attrition between five and ten years . . . The remarkable thing is that 80% of the 100 children are still alive with first, second, and third kidneys. None of the children are presently on dialysis." He suggested that the somewhat better results in children were due to the fact that the donors were predominately parents and that the children were not subject to myocardial infarction and the other causes of death in the adults. Were some of Starzl's early deaths due to excessive immunosuppression?, which would be the case "If the same degree of immunosuppression is given to an A-matched patient as is given to a D- or E- matched patient . . ." He appeared to suggest that the glomerular lesion shown by Starzl might be a recurrence of the original nephritis. T. C. Moore, of Torrance, California, asked "What per cent of the transplants lost after one year were due to rejection? . . . What was the role of early transplant function . . . and long-term survival of patients . . . what is your current feeling concerning the value of splenectomy . . . in the renal transplant patient?" Professor Maurice R. Ewing, of Melbourne, Australia, said they had only just exceeded 200 cases,- and only a handful of those had passed the ten-year mark. All but two or three had been cadaver grafts. They were "deeply disturbed already by the premature development, in the young, of the kind of degenerative changes in the skin with which we are very familiar in the elderly, after exposure over a lifetime to the sun. The incidence of skin cancer in the survivors after four years is 18% . . . many of these patients have multiple skin cancers." The tumors had responded, with one exception, to excision. Lars-Erik Gelin, of Göteborg, Sweden, had an overall 40% graft survival after eight years, 65% in related grafts, but only 18% in the cadaver grafts.

When retransplantation was necessary, they observed that if the retransplantation was performed "while the prior, primary graft still had marginal function, the graft survival was very much superior to the situation when there is an interval between transplantectomy and regrafting . . . What is the mechanism behind this privileged time for retransplantation?" Starzl, closing, said that Gelin's remarks "illustrate the imperfections of treatment as it has been carried out in the last ten or 12 years, and . . . should be a real admonition not to consider this field fully developed." He expected "in the next year or two . . . a very significant advance in immunosuppression, and possibly related to the kind of research work that is being carried out by Monaco and his associates in Boston, in which much more emphasis is being placed on the possiblility of tolerance induction." Professor Ewing's experience, the risk from skin cancers, "is certainly related to chronic immunosuppression." He replied to Najarian that he doubted that over-immunosuppression "led to the loss of those grafts that were still functioning in 1965, because we had already pulled off the heavy immunosuppression that we were using . . . and were in a pattern of light immunosuppression." [The question about glomerulonephritis is answered in the published paper v.s.] To Dr. Wilson he said that "good matching was not a factor . . . in those years, 1962 to 1964 . . . there were no good or even acceptable donor-recipient typing techniques . . . we did not even bother to follow the rules of red blood type matching, which have become recognized to be of such paramount importance . . ." He suggested to the Association that Dr. Wilson's modesty had prevented him from mentioning that "the longest homotransplant survival in the world is a Boston recipient of a fraternal twin kidney treated in 1958. As I understand it, that patient is still alive." As for Belzer's question about stopping immunosuppression, Starzl mentioned the two patients who had stopped immunosuppression without suffering ill effects, "But we certainly have our fingers crossed, because that story that Dr. Belzer has told has been repeated now on many occasions, and usually with dire consequences." To Dr. T. C. Moore's questions, he answered that after one year there was "relative stability" of grafts, that the greatest risk that the transplant recipient faced was not cancer or infection "but slow failure of his homograft with physical deterioration before retransplantation or return to dialysis." He was unable to comment on the relation of initial function to ultimate survival because, "almost all of these kidneys functioned superbly from the beginning." As

for splenectomy, "If you believe basic biology, there is plenty of evidence that splenectomy is a biologic immunosuppressive maneuver", but he doubted that its effect in human transplantation was "provable on the basis of clinical investigation." Concluding, he voiced what many of the audience felt, "This is the first American Surgical meeting that I have ever been to that was not graced by the presence of Dave Hume. It is strange to give a paper on Dave's favorite subject, realizing that his smiling face and swashbuckling emanations are not today, or ever again, going to be working their way to the podium—usually down that aisle—to set up a lively but always good-natured duel. I, for one, have no intention of forgetting our good friend simply because he is not with us today."

* * *

Donald L. Morton, Professor of Surgery and Chief, Division of Oncology, University of California at Los Angeles School of Medicine; F. R. Eilber, E. Holmes and J. S. Hunt, by invitation; Alfred S. Ketcham, Professor of Surgery and Chief, Division of Surgical Oncology, University of Miami School of Medicine; and by invitation, M. J. Silverstein and F. C. Sparks, *BCG Immunotherapy of Malignant Melanoma:* Summary of a Seven-Year Experience, discussed the accretion of information on the subject since "Morton and Malmgren's initial description of tumor associated antigens in human malignant melanomas using immunofluorescent techniques [1969]." There was evidence "that malignant melanomas contain tumor specific antigens which elicit production of circulating humoral antibodies and cytotoxic lymphocytes in patients with melanoma . . . there appears to be a correlation between the clinical status of the melanoma patient and the incidence of antimelanoma antibodies in their sera. Patients with a localized melanoma were more likely to have antibody in their sera than those patients with disseminated disease." Morton and others had reported studies with BCG immunotherapy of malignant melanoma in 1970. The patients presently reported had been seen at the Surgery Branch of the National Cancer Institute from 1967 to 1970 or at UCLA from 1971 to 1974. "The patients selected for immunotherapy had documented recurrent melanoma, known residual disease, or a high risk of developing recurrence." Patients were evaluated immunologically with DNCB and "four common microbial recall antigens . . . mumps . . . PPD . . . Varidase . . . and Monilia antigen . . ." BCG was injected into intracutaneous or subcutaneous melanoma nodules. In patients with Stage II melanoma, three to six weeks after operation BCG was given intradermally either alone, or at the same time as injections of irradiated tissue culture melanoma cells. The same procedure was followed with Stage III disease "following resection of gross disease at distant metastatic sites. . . . Direct injection of metastatic melanoma lesions limited to skin resulted in 90% regression of injected lesions and 17% regression of uninjected lesions in immunocompetent patients. Approximately 25% of these patients remained free of disease for 1 to 6 years. Direct injections of BCG into nodules of patients with subcutaneous or visceral metastases resulted in a lower incidence of local control and no long term survivors . . . palliative surgical resection of large metastatic lesions to lower tumor burden followed by BCG immunotherapy significantly improved the results although many patients still developed recurrent disease." They had undertaken a study with the use of BCG alone or mixed with allogeneic melanoma cells after regional lymphadenectomy in patients with regional lymph node metastasis. "The overall tumor free rate for the entire group of 67 patients is lower at all points in time when compared to 34 patients seen at UCLA during the same time interval who did not receive BCG immunotherapy." The patients had not been randomized but chosen solely on the basis of "distance from UCLA and their willingness to participate in an investigational protocol." There were complications with BCG immunotherapy, "Intratumor injection with BCG frequently resulted in fever, chills, localized abscesses, and sinuses that drained for long periods of up to 3 months. Regional lymphadenitis was frequent. Occasionally a systemic infection occurred with associated granulomatous hepatitis." Others had observed fatal anaphylactoid reactions with repeated large doses of BCG. "Patients who had marked malaise and an influenza-like syndrome following BCG therapy generally responded promptly to Isoniazid administration." As opposed to intratumor injections, intradermal injection was usually tolerated very well "with low incidence of hepatic dysfunction and only mild fever and malaise for short periods following vaccination", although localized lymph node enlargement occasionally occurred. They felt "that intralesional BCG immunotherapy is the treatment of choice for patients with metastatic malignant melanoma limited to the skin . . . Stage III melanoma patients with visceral metastasis and large bulky subcutaneous metastasis . . . should be managed by a combination of surgery to reduce tumor burden, chemotherapy to further lower tumor burden and adjuvant immunotherapy to maintain remission." They considered "most exciting . . . the possible application of BCG immunotherapy as an adjunct to the definitive surgical treatment of patients with Stage II malignant melanoma and a poor prognosis because of metastasis to the regional nodes." Their early results were encouraging and they were embarking on a properly constructed clinical trial of randomized and properly stratified patients.

Discussion

Edward T. Krementz, of New Orleans, took occasion to remind the Association that "In 1957, the late Dr. Oscar Creech, Dr. Bob Ryan, and I introduced the treatment of melanoma with chemotherapy by perfusion which improved the survival rates for melanoma of the extremities." With Stage I, 80% of the patients were free of disease at five years, 76% at ten years, and 57% at 15 years. For Stage II, the figures were 38, 32, and 23%. In 45 patients with satellite lesions of the extremities followed for five to 15 years, six of 27 with negative nodes were free of disease and five of 18 with positive nodes. They too were using BCG and "We have one patient who failed to respond to perfusion who now is disease free for almost four years following injection of satellites with BCG similar to the method described by Dr. Morton." He "emphasized the toxicity, morbidity, and mortality occurring with BCG. There have been at least two reported deaths from the use of BCG in patients with malignancy and low resistance to infection . . .", and two more not yet reported. Joseph C. Fortner, of New York, said they had a similar program underway at Memorial-Sloan Kettering Cancer Center, with similar results but not quite so high a response rate. Of 55 patients with unresectable melanoma treated by BCG inoculation of the tumor, 19 had complete regression of all injected nodules, which occurred only in immunologically competent patients with melanoma confined to skin and lymph nodes. Two of 30 patients in whom only some of the tumor nodules were injected had regression of all the disease, including the uninjected nodules, and were now clinically free of disease, one after two and one after three years. Their randomized study had been underway only a year-and-a half, "The time for recurrence in the BCG-treated group is longer than the controls. These data are very preliminary . . ." Anthony P. Monaco, of Boston, commented that "the best way to immunize a rabbit was to incorporate an antigen in an inflammatory focus . . . directly injected into the skin . . . the best way to elicit the expression of a delayed response is by placing antigen in the skin . . . this could . . . explain why the skin nodules that aren't injected are so vulnerable to the enhanced immunity, and therefore regress." He thought that the destruction of skin nodules by perfusion might "set up the inflammatory focus, and . . . encourage or facilitate the immunizing mechanism." It was the experience of transplant investigators that the attempt to form an enhancing antibody "which facilitates the survival of the graft, rather than destroying it" sometimes produced the opposite effect "namely, accelerated rejections of our graft . . . On the other hand, occasionally we get enhancement of the graft, which would be exacerbation of melanoma growth. So I would like to ask Dr. Morton: Does he ever make the melanoma grow more fast, rather than slower?" Morton, closing, pointed out that Krementz was dealing entirely with extremity melanoma, which carried a more favorable prognosis than melanoma in the trunk, but agreed of perfusion that "for intracutaneous disease in extremities it is very useful and we use it if BCG doesn't work." He said that he agreed with Monaco that skin lesions regressed and those elsewhere did not because of "something to do with the rich lymphatics of the skin." Of enhancement he said that it was "only seen if these immunologic maneuvers are performed prior to or within a few days of the time of tumor transplantation. If the immunologic maneuvers to achieve enhancement are delayed one week or more, enhancement is not achieved and in fact the tumor or organ grafts are rejected in a normal manner . . . once cell mediated immunity has been turned on for at least one week, it is generally not possible to achieve immunologic prolongation of tumor or organ allograft survival." In animals they had been able to achieve enhancement if "the animal has never been exposed to the tumor before and the BCG is given in large doses at the same time as the tumor is transplanted . . . quite a different phenomenon from what one sees in man with a malignancy, because most human neoplasms have been *in situ* for long periods of time (1-10 years) and cancer patients already have an on going immune response against the tumor antigens in their neoplasms . . . Perhaps that is why we have not seen any clear cut instance of enhancement following BCG immunotherapy."

The Business Meetings

The 1974 meeting was held at The Broadmoor, Colorado Springs, Colorado, on May 1, 2, and 3, H. William Scott, Jr., in the Chair.

At the Second Executive Session, the Secretary's report of the actions of Council included the comment that the sale of the reprinted past Minutes had gone well. Owen Wangensteen was to be invited to write a history of the American Surgical Association [The Council were not aware and Wangensteen had not informed them, that he and Mrs. Wangensteen, his capable collaborator, had long been engaged in a great work on the history of surgery, which was ultimately published in 1979 and would have had to have been set aside had he undertaken the charge to write the history of the Association.] and Mark Ravitch was invited to present a paper on medical history at the 1976 Annual Meeting of the Association, the country's bicentennial year.

The American Surgical Association Medallion for Scientific Achievement had been presented in 1969 to Lester R. Dragstedt at the meeting. The 1973 award to Robert E. Gross was at a special meeting in Chicago convened by President Scott at a large dinner at the University Club during the meeting of the American College of Surgeons, presumably because Gross had been unable to attend the Los Angeles meeting, and not at a meeting of the American Surgical Association. The Council proposed that in the future the nomination be made by "the five (5) most recent past presidents of the Association", to the Midwinter Meeting of the Council so that the Secretary could have the "medallion appropriately prepared . . . and will notify the recipient so that the medallion may be presented at the next Annual Meeting of the Association." The purpose was to "let Honorary Fellows and any future recipient of the medallion be presented with somewhat more ceremony at the meeting following their election."

The change in the Constitution proposed the previous year was approved, to the effect that the Secretary, Treasurer, and Recorder hold their offices six months after the election of their successor so as to permit them to complete their records.

The entire list of 29 new Fellows proposed was elected, as well as Corresponding Members, Åke Senning, of Zurich; Fernando Paulino, of Rio de Janeiro; G. B. Ong, of Hong Kong; Viking Bjork, of Stockholm; Richard Welbourne, of London; and David Innes Williams, of London; and Honorary Member, Charles Dubost, of Paris.

Elected as President was William H. Muller, Jr., of Charlottesville; Vice-President, Richard Warren, of Boston, and Fraser N. Gurd, of Ottawa; as Secretary, James V. Maloney, Jr., of Los Angeles.

XCIII

1975

The 1975 meeting was held at Le Chateau Frontenac, Quebec City, Canada, on May 7, 8 and 9, President William H. Muller, Jr., of Charlottesville, Stephen H. Watts Professor, Chairman, Department of Surgery; Surgeon-in-Chief, University of Virginia Medical Center, in the Chair.

President Muller devoted his address, *United We Stand,* very largely to the legislative and federal actions in progress. The previous summer, Congress had before it, "12 bills supporting some type of national health plan" supported by federal, private or combined funds. President Ford had promised to "veto all new spending programs, including National Health Insurance" so that a year's delay at least might be expected. A number of the new health care bills contained provisions for regulatory measures which would reach deeper into medical practice. The malpractice problem was becoming more and more burdensome and the bills before Congress to alleviate it left much to be desired. There was proposed legislation in Congress affecting both medical education and manpower distribution, actually going so far as to fix "the number of first-year residency positions at a level of 155% of the estimated number of graduates from U.S. medical schools, with reduction by steps to 125% over a period of three years." The bill was aimed, in part, at limiting the number of foreign medical graduates in house staff positions and apparently would "fix . . . the number of specialty residency programs and, eventu-

ally, the number of residency programs within each specialty." It was not clear how the reduction in residents in training would be achieved.

Muller was pleased that with the Association's new 501.C3 Internal Revenue status, the Association could become politically active. "It falls on the shoulders of the profession to assume a truly aggressive leadership role and to resolve our major health problems before this is done by others in what might be an unpalatable manner. I believe that the profession has rallied to a great degree, especially during the past five years or so, in an effort to accomplish this, but it may well be too little and too late."

* * *

John F. Burke, of Boston, Associate Professor of Surgery, Harvard Medical School; Chief of Staff, Shriners Burns Institute; W. C. Quinby, C. C. Bondoc and A. B. Cosimi, by invitation; Paul S. Russell, John Homans Professor of Surgery, Harvard University School of Medicine; and S. K. Szyfelbein, by invitation, *Immunosuppression and Temporary Skin Transplantation in the Treatment of Massive Third Degree Burns,* started with the thesis that "An extensive, full thickness burn continues to be a lethal injury, not because of the burn itself but because the extent of normal skin available for donor sites is insufficient to provide skin graft closure in a period short enough to prevent death from malnutrition

1418

and sepsis." In patients with "massive third degree burns (total burn area 80% Body Surface Area or greater with a third degree burn component of 70% or greater)" with 0.5% silver nitrate dressings, maintaining the patient in a plastic "protected environment", excision and wound closure by grafting began on the second or third day and continued every two or three days. Autografts were immediately placed on the excised wounds, to the extent that was possible. Third degree burns of the face and hands were not excised, but the eschar was allowed to separate spontaneously. Penicillin was given to all patients for three days, and thereafter no antibiotics except for specific indication. Additional skin, as needed, was provided from tissue typed family donors or from cadavers, the patients being placed on an immunosuppressive regimen, either with Azathioprine,- the first five patients,- or antithymocyte globulin,- the next six patients. Of the 11 patients with total burns ranging from 81% to 92% and full-thickness destruction ranging from 70% to 90% of the body surface, seven survived and returned to their ordinary school. In the past, the mortality with similar burns had been 100%. Graft takes were 95% to 100%. All of the surviving patients had their wounds completely closed by a combination of autograft or allograft by the third or fourth week postburn. The final replacement of the allografts with autografts required considerably longer, mainly because of "the limited autograft donor sites available and the increasing length of time between croppings as the number of croppings of a single donor site increased . . . Unlike the graft take following primary excision, secondary grafting seldom approached 100%. In the seven patients surviving, autograft wound closure to within 5% of the body surface required 60-102 days . . ." The scalp, which was usually unburned, was the most reliable donor site and regenerated rapidly to permit numerous recroppings. The allografts all seemed clinically to have escaped rejection at the time they were finally excised, but histologically "showed evidence of 'mild' or 'early' rejection beginning as early as three weeks following allograft."

Discussion

Francis D. Moore, of Boston said, at the Peter Bent Brigham they had used allografts in two patients, in one obtaining the skin from a fraternal-identical twin whose skin never did have to be removed. He reminded the Association of Emile Holman's experience 50 years earlier with mother-to-child homografts, his discussion of rejection, auto-

immune disease, etc. Bradford Cannon, of Boston, was impressed with the results and said, "Moral questions are constantly in mind, especially in the extensively burned child with hands and face involved and I emphasize hands and face. Are our efforts justified if the family is disrupted by the return of this severely handicapped, disfigured child to its midst. What will the suicide rate be in the teenaged disfigured child? One recalls the high rate of suicide in the cerebral palsy victims in their late teens. The answers are not ours to give, but society may ultimately have to make the decision about the salvage of these children." Joseph E. Murray, of Boston, was struck by the "striking diminution of degree of post-graft contracture in the patient that Dr. Burke presented." He wondered if the homografts were somehow responsible. Basil A. Pruitt Jr., of San Antonio, seemed to be questioning the reality of the success reported, "We are all aware of the difficulty of early accurate assessment of burn depth and have often been fooled by areas that looked like partial-thickness injury which were actually full-thickness and vice versa. Was there histologic verification of the depth of the burns, since they are usually mixed second and third degree in character?. . ." J. F. Burke, closing, said they used tissue typing when family donors were used and selected the best HLA match even if there was ABO incompatibility. The moral problem was a real one. But it was also "very disturbing to us to note that all patients with massive third degree burns die unless transplanted. With the small number of patients we have treated most of them survived and all survivors are back in school . . . The prospect for living a normal life isn't as black as one might assume . . ." He agreed that the scarring was less than with autografted skin but he didn't know why. To Pruitt, he said that, to be certain that they were not excising living tissue, they shaved the burn repeatedly, "sequential eschar excision" six-thousandths of an inch thickness layers at a time "until we get to viable tissue where excising is stopped. The viable surface following sequential excision is sometimes in the dermis and sometimes in the fat or muscle."

* * *

Marshall J. Orloff, of San Diego, Professor and Chairman, Department of Surgery, University of California, and by invitation, Sun Lee, A. C. Charters, III, E. Grambort, L. G. Storck, and D. Knox, *Long Term Studies of Pancreas Transplantation in Experimental Diabetes Mellitus,* produced diabetes mellitus in inbred rats by intravenous administration

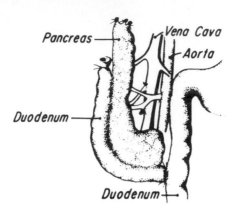
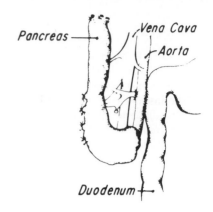

Fig. 1. Microvascular surgical technique of heterotopic pancreaticoduodenal transplantation and of duct-ligated pancreas transplantation showing the operations in the recipient.

Pancreaticoduodenal Transplant

Duct Ligated Pancreas Transplant

Sun Lee had developed and reported in 1971, the techniques of transplantation of the pancreas in rats, with microvascular anastomoses. Both kinds of transplant between rats of the same inbred strain produced good function and correction of diabetes, preventing the renal and the ophthalmic changes which long-term diabetic rats developed. Ligation of the pancreatic duct was performed at the time of the isolated pancreas transplant. The end results were as good as with a pancreaticoduodenal transplant, and the immediate mortality lower. Both transplants were effective in spite of the fact that the venous drainage was directly into the vena cava.

Marshall J. Orloff, Sun Lee, A. C. Charters, III, David E. Grambort, L. G. Storck, and Dale Knox, *Long Term Studies of Pancreas Transplantation in Experimental Diabetes Mellitus,* Volume XCIII, 1975.

of alloxan, and, with unoperated, and sham operated, controls, performed pancreaticoduodenal transplants from rats of the same strain, age and sex, or transplants of the whole pancreas with its ducts ligated. In both groups of transplanted animals the venous drainage of the pancreas was into the vena cava. In the isolated pancreas transplants, the pancreatic duct was ligated at the time of transportation. The diabetic controls rarely survived beyond 18 months, and remained constantly hyperglycemic. The transplanted animals all "had an immediate and permanent reduction of the blood glucose level to normal for the two-year study period." There was no difference between the two types of transplant. Similarly, the control animals had a low serum insulin level, and transplantation of the pancreas with or without the duodenum "produced an immediate and persistent rise in serum insulin to levels that were significantly higher than those in the control groups at all times during the study. The absolute levels of serum insulin in the transplanted animals gradually declined over the two-year study period, similar to what has been observed in the normal Lewis rat as it ages." The control diabetic rats lost weight, did not regain it until six months later, and then gained weight slowly. The transplanted rats regained their preinjection weight within a month and then gained

weight at the normal rate. When the grafts were ultimately removed, the animals reverted to the diabetic state. The control rats developed renal lesions much like those of Kimmelstiel-Wilson's Disease, and the eyes showed cataracts, corneal changes and retinal disease. The peripheral nerves showed severe demyelinization. These changes were "in large measure" prevented by transplantation. These were, of course, inbred animals, and Orloff said "Whether or not similar results can be achieved with pancreas allografts beset by the familiar problems of immunologic rejection remains to be determined. To date, 45 pancreas allografts have been transplanted in human subjects. Only two patients are currently alive with functioning grafts. The longest survivor of a pancreas allograft is living 2.8 years after transplantation. While control of hyperglycemia clearly has been accomplished, reversal or stabilization of the vascular complications of diabetes has not yet been established. The results of the present study provide hope that such may be possible."

Discussion

Keith Reemtsma, of New York, turned the discussion to transplantation of the islets themselves by which, in isologous strains "Dr. Collin Weber in our laboratory at Columbia" had reversed diabetes in animals with the interesting finding, as opposed to the situation in normal or control diabetic animals, that "the insulin and glucagon levels are all elevated in these islet recipients twelve months following transplantation." Walter F. Ballinger, II, of St. Louis, had also worked with islet of Langerhans transplantation and, although his animals, both rats and monkey, were normoglycemic for as long as two years, they had diabetic glucose tolerance curves. He agreed that "The goal is to restore some sort of glucagon-insulin-islet balance in order to prevent the long range complications of diabetes." He had not seen in animals the diabetic complications that Orloff had described. Marshall J. Orloff, closing, suggested that his studies, uncomplicated by immunosuppression and immunologic rejection "demonstrated that during the full lifespan of a diabetic rat, which might be comparable to some 60 or 70 years in the human being, the diabetes was relieved by the whole organ." The glucose tolerance tests in their animals gave normal responses. The pathologic changes in untransplanted diabetic animals were not seen for the first nine or ten months, and became quite prominent in the second year. He took no position on whether islet cell transplantation or whole organ transplantation was the best approach.

* * *

Orvar Swenson, of Miami, Division of Pediatric Surgery, University of Miami, [to which he had retired from his position as Professor of Surgery at Children's Memorial Hospital, Chicago], J. O. Sherman, J. H. Fisher, and E. Cohen, by invitation, *The Treatment and Postoperative Complications of Congenital Megacolon,* had reviewed the records of 501 patients whom Swenson and his associates had treated at the Boston Children's Hospital from 1947 to 1950, the Floating Hospital in Boston, 1950 to 1973, and the Children's Memorial Hospital, 1960 to 1973. "Final evaluations were obtained by traveling to various parts of the United States and Mexico and holding clinics so that these patients could be interviewed and examined. Questionnaires were not used." Swenson gave the story of the original development of the operation. "In 1945 there was no cure for patients with congenital megacolon. We were fortunate to have observed three children who had colostomies performed and who were completely relieved of their symptoms. The patients requested that the colostomies be closed and the children were treated medically but, within 6 months, there was a complete recurrence of symptoms. The colostomies

were reopened and the patients were again relieved of their abdominal distention and severe constipation. We could only conclude that the distal colon contained a physiological block, for there was no mechanical obstruction. We then studied that distal colon by multiple balloon recordings and demonstrated that in the rectosigmoid and rectum there was no peristalsis, while in the proximal colon there was normal peristalsis. Barium enema examination revealed a narrow distal colon with massive dilatation proximally. The next step in this line of reasoning was that removal of the distal narrow malfunctioning colon and substituting for it the proximal dilated but physiologically intact colon should be curative." [The published paper after this brief introduction, and the entire oral presentation, were essentially devoted to complications of the operations.] There was a 4.6% wound infection rate, usually attributed to a pre-existing colostomy. There was only a 0.4% infection rate in the 286 who did not have a preoperative colostomy. There were six dehiscenses. Twenty-four patients,- 5%,- developed leak of the anastomosis, and six of them died. Four of the leaks occurred in the 16 patients who had Down's Syndrome. Thirteen patients developed mechanical intestinal obstruction requiring operation within a month of the Swenson procedure. In all, sixteen patients,- 3.3%,- died during the hospitalization in which the resection was performed, half the deaths in infants less than four months of age,- thought to be a significant factor. "We no longer perform a resection on patients less than 6 months of age or on patients who weigh less than 20 pounds." A postoperative rectal stricture developed in 30 patients,- 6.2%,- but only seven required a second operation. "Temporary late soiling after resection occurred in 64 patients (13.3%)." In ten of these, the soiling persisted permanently. Two-hundred-eighty-two patients interviewed at least five years or more after operation were evaluated for the final result. Normal bowel habit was reported in over 90%. Ten patients still soiled. Two patients had a permanent colostomy and two had permanent ileostomies. One patient had developed ulcerative colitis and required a total colectomy. Urinary incontinence or impotence were denied by all patients. One patient had nocturia if he drank in the evening. The etiology was unknown, but it seemed to be associated with colonic obstruction. For a time, Swenson had performed sphincterotomy for patients with enterocolitis, but "our initial enthusiasm was lost because no significant benefit was obtained . . . The disease is common both before and after the treatment of congenital megacolon and must be diagnosed early to prevent dehydration, shock and death. Treatment is simple and effective and consists of frequent rectal irrigations with warm saline solution for two to three days." The children who had enterocolitis before operation had a significantly increased risk of developing it after the operation. Enterocolitis might develop immediately after operation or late. Enterocolitis after operation was commonest in the first year and, after the fifth year, was never severe enough to require hospitalization. Swenson referred briefly to the Duhamel and Soave operations and their variations, commenting on the reports, "These are small groups of patients and consequently not suitable for a meaningful comparison with our results . . . The one helpful bit of information that has improved the treatment of congenital megacolon, was that the aganglionic distal colon was a physiological block. We still believe that the most enduring good results are obtained when this is removed and not partially left in place."

Discussion

Clifford D. Benson, of Detroit, mentioned 155 patients operated upon for Hirschsprung's disease from 1960 to 1973 in Detroit at the Children's Hospital in Michigan, but said nothing of his results. he asked Swenson whether, for low aganglionosis of the rectum discovered in the newborn, a submucous myotomy might be advisable. Thomas C. Moore, of Torrance, California, mentioned Hirschsprung's disease in one of identical twins so proved by HLA and MLC typing. Alexander H. Bill, Jr., of Seattle, was concerned about the cause of the enterocolitis, not quite satisfied that partial obstruction was the answer. [The discussers had, for the most part, focused on small areas of the presentation of a lifetime of work by the man who had shown how the disease could be cured, in the presentation of which he had spoken mostly of problems. The next discusser arose to be sure that the lesson was not missed]. Mark M. Ravitch, of Pittsburgh, said "I hope this dry, statistical, computer designed, brutally frank review of complications doesn't obscure for this sophisticated audience the fact that this is a historic milestone. There are not many times in the history of surgery when a fatal disease is analyzed by clinicians and studied in the laboratory, who immediately arrive at a successful clinical solution and then carry that through for a lifetime study and now present in very low key the negative aspects of this enormously successful experience." Orvar Swenson, closing, returned, to the question of sphincterotomy, "you

know, if you look back on your publications over the years, you'd like to eradicate some of them. One of them is a paper that we had on sphincterotomy. It simply has not worked out as well as we thought it would and our enthusiasm has waned." They had seen identical twins with the disease and also seen identical twins in whom only one had the disease. Obstruction was not the only answer for enterocolitis since babies with a colostomy sometimes went on to develop enterocolitis.

* * *

Marc I. Rowe, of Miami, Professor of Surgery and Pediatrics; Chief, Division of Pediatric Surgery, University of Miami School of Medicine, and by invitation, D. M. Buckner, and S. Newmark, *The Early Diagnosis of Gram Negative Septicemia in the Pediatric Surgery Patient,* commented on the frequency of septicemia resulting from the survival of small premature infants, the use of invasive monitoring and therapy, and the congregation in neonatal centers of infants suffering from a variety of septic and nonseptic conditions, the increased number of personnel involved in the treatment magnifying the opportunities for infection. A prospective study involved 93 postoperative infants and children studied by "limulus lysate assay . . . to detect circulating endotoxin. Fibrin degradation products were measured by the staphylococcal clumping and protamine sulfate tests. White blood cell count and platelet count were measured" in all patients. Levin and Bang, in 1964, had developed the use of the lysate from the amebocyte of the horseshoe crab, Limulus polyphemus, as a sensitive test for endotoxin. This had been widely used. In the present study it proved accurate in detecting gram negative septicemia, but with both false negatives and false positives and substantial methodological difficulties. Gram negative septicemia might produce disseminated intravascular coagulation, and the protamine sulfate and staphylococcus clumping tests measured the fibrin degradation products which resulted. "At last one of these two tests was positive in 79% of the babies with gram negative bacteriemia, but 32% of babies and 35% of children with major trauma or operation had at least one test positive for degradation products. The test was also frequently positive in patients with gram positive septicemia" so that the tests were "not specific enough to serve as an aid in the early detection of gram negative septicemia in pediatric surgical patients . . . we found that the most rapid, simple and accurate method for the early detection of gram negative septicemia appears to be serial platelet counts. All the infants and children with positive blood cultures for gram negative bacteria had a platelet count below 150,000. None of the infants or children with a negative blood culture, ruptured or non-ruptured appendicitis, or gram positive septicemia had platelet counts below 150,000." Beller and Douglas had made the observation in 1973 that platelet counts were low in patients with abortions. Corrigan, in 1974, in infants and children with medical illness, had found decreased platelet counts even more frequently in children with gram positive than with gram negative septicemia in contrast to the results of the present study. Endotoxin injected into rabbits resulted in thrombocytopenia and platelet aggregation, and there was abundant clinical and experimental evidence "that endotoxin reacts with platelets, resulting in platelet aggregation. The aggregates are then trapped in the microcirculation and vasoactive substances are released into the plasma. The effect of platelet microemboli and vasoactive substances are thought to account for some of the clinical and pathological findings in gram negative septicemia." The fall in platelet count could be extremely rapid, as much as 220,000 in 24 hours suggesting "that thrombocytopenia is not the result of decreased platelet production, but either destruction or trapping of platelets", and there was no evidence for consumptive coagulopathy. The practical conclusions were that serial platelet counts should be done with an electronic counter on patients at risk, that a fall in platelet count should prompt a blood culture and a search for the source of infection and possible withdrawal of intravascular catheters, "A fall in platelet count below 150,000 is strong presumptive evidence of gram negative septicemia", and antibiotic therapy should be undertaken. Conversely a rise in platelet count suggested that therapy was effective, while persistently low platelet counts suggested that therapy was ineffective.

Discussion

Basil A. Pruitt, Jr., of San Antonio, studying burn patients, had found that in those with disseminated intravascular coagulation both fibrinogen and platelets were low, whereas in patients who were infected without DIC, the platelets alone were low. In the infected burned animal, the platelets fell "from the earliest postburn time on." Fibrin degradation products did not serve as an index to the appearance of infection in a burn whereas low platelet count did. What happened to the fibrin split levels in Dr. Rowe's patients after therapy? Rowe, closing, agreed "that the thrombocytopenia that develops as a result of gram negative septicemia is not a part of dissemi-

nated intravascular coagulation. Thirty-one percent of the patients who had thrombocytopenia had negative quantitative tests for fibrin degradation products. Only two of the patients with gram negative septicemia in our series developed DIC who had thrombocytopenia. The most chilling aspect was that because of the low platelet counts, we got nervous and gave them massive platelet transfusions and those patients rapidly developed disseminated intra-vascular coagulation and those were two of our mortalities."

* * *

Åke Senning, Professor of Surgery, Head of Surgical University Clinic A., Zurich, Switzerland, a Corresponding Fellow, *Correction of the Transposition of the Great Arteries,* described his modification of the venous diversion technique for correction of transposition of the great arteries, originally proposed experimentally by Albert, 1954, in dogs [under normothermic inflow occulsion!] and made possible by Mustard, 1964, with his pericardial baffle. Redirecting venous flow by baffles of pericardium or of plastic resulted in a significant incidence, in later life, of obstruction to systemic and pulmonary venous return in the small noncompliant atrial chambers. Both of these "can largely be avoided when a maximum of vascularized auricular tissue is used to inverse the venous flows on atrial level." In children "following a previous Hanlon-Blalock septectomy, a modified atrial inversion technique has been used. No atrial tissue is excised and a minimum of patch or no foreign material is used." By mobilizing the remnant of the atrial septum with a bold incision "through the coronary sinus into the Vena magna cordis to the base of the left atrial appendage along the mitral ring" a flap was produced between the mitral valve and the orifices of the pulmonary veins requiring, in his first technique, only a small patch of Dacron to bridge the gap between the caval orifices, directing the flow to the mitral valve. In his second operation, instead of using a small prosthetic patch, a pedicled flap of the external atrial wall was employed. Of 50 patients operated upon by Method I, 45 survived, 33 out of 35 with simple TGA, and 16 of 20 with complicated TGA. Method II led to 16 survivals out of 19 operations, seven out of eight for simple TGA and six out of eight for complicated TGA. He said that "It seems logical to use the heart's own living tissue when inverting the venous flow on atrial level in infants and children with TGA. The reconstructed chambers can be expected to grow with the patient and to adapt themselves to the flow conditions in the heart . . . the pseudo-

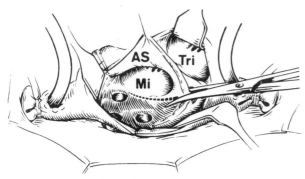

FIG. 1c. The coronary sinus and V. magna cordis are incised. Mi: mitral valve.

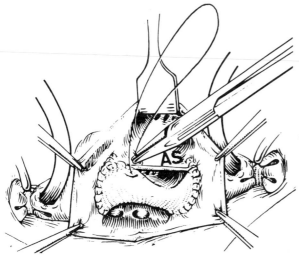

FIG. 1g. The suture of the patch continued around the caval vein orifices and to the reattached atrial septum.

intimal pannus and shrinkage of the patch is avoided. Non-compliant walls are minimized and by approximating the caval vein orifices there is a more direct flow from the caval veins through the atrial septal area." The use of Method II required a pliable and healthy right atrial wall which was not always present after the previous Hanlon-Blalock procedure, in which case, Method I had to be employed.

Discussion

William W. L. Glenn, of New Haven, Connecticut, described a satisfactory 12-year result after his performance of the Senning I. Aldo R. Castaneda, of Boston, commenting upon the anatomical complexity of the procedures, said "As surgeons in 1975, we're barely starting to understand the Senning I Operation. It's probably going to be 1985 or so before we understand the Senning III Operation." He had tried the Senning II but had found it difficult to

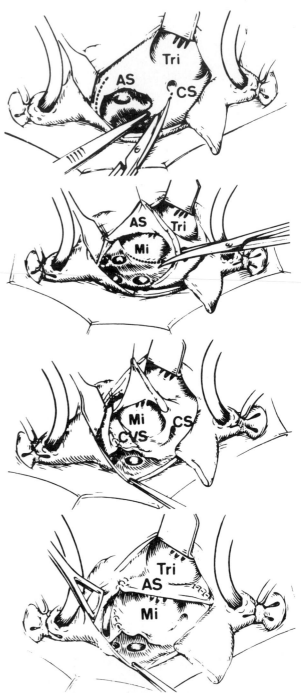

FIGS. 2b to e. (top to bottom) The atrial septal rest is detached from behind. C.S. and V. magna cordis incised along the mitral ring. The coronary vein flap sutured forming a septum anterior to the left pulmonary veins (compare with Fig. 1d). The atrial septum reattached in front of the caval orifices.

use in infants, although he had applied it satisfactorily and wanted to ask "if perhaps the technique cannot be used in infants within the first four

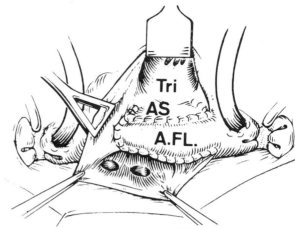

FIG. 2g. The suture continued along the CVS around the superior caval vein orifice and to the reattached atrial septum (AS) has completed a new septum for atrial inversion.

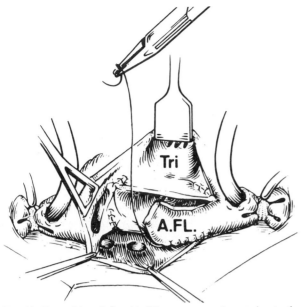

FIG. 2f. The atrial wall flap (A Fl) suture started posterior to the inferior caval orifice runs to the CVS.

◄ To avoid late obstruction to the systemic and pulmonary venous return and the construction of small non-compliant atrial chambers such as occurred with "significant incidence" when the Mustard operation was performed with a pericardial or synthetic cloth baffle, Senning in his Method I, (1c and 1g) boldly mobilized an internal atrial flap and then required only a minimal Dacron patch to divert the systemic venous flow into the mitral valve.

In his Method II, (2b-2e) a pedicled flap of the external atrial wall was used to divert the venous flow, in a repair made entirely with local tissues. He had operated on 50 patients by Method I, 33 of 35 with a simple TGA survived, and 14 of 17 with complicated transpositions survived. He had employed Method II in 16 patients, seven of eight with simple TGA survived, and six of eight with complicated TGA.

Åke Senning, *Correction of the Transposition of the Great Arteries.* Volume XCIII, 1975.

months of life." Senning, closing, said that, in fact "the average age in the group of patients with a [synthetic] patch has been five years. The median age of the 16 patients without patch is four years, varying between four months and 22 years." His first patient, operated in 1958 "was recatheterized in Poland two years ago and he has absolutely normal function . . . there is no sign of tricuspid insufficiency . . . he has a practically normal contraction curve of both auricles. In our series we have not been able to do recatheterization of the patients so we do not know what the function of the atrium is."

* * *

Gordon N. Olinger and J. Po, by invitation, James V. Maloney, Jr., of Los Angeles, the Secretary, Professor of Surgery, UCLA School of Medicine; Chief, Division of Thoracic Surgery; Donald D. Mulder, Professor, Department of Surgery, UCLA Medical Center, and by invitation, Gerald D. Buckberg, *Coronary Revascularization in "High" Versus*

"Low-Risk" Patients: The Role of Myocardial Protection, said that coronary bypass "in stable patients with satisfactory ventricular function is performed widely with an acceptable small incidence of postoperative mortality, myocardial infarction, and depressed cardiac performance requiring pharmacologic or mechanical support." On the other hand, patients with decreased ejection fractions, ventricular tachyarrhythmias, preinfarction angina, evolving myocardial infarction, and recent infarction with extension, considered bad-risk patients, showed "a considerable increase in both mortality and morbidity." Their thesis was that "the conduct of coronary revascularization based on known principles of myocardial protection . . . allows safe revascularization even in the "high-risk" patient." They had done 50 consecutive coronary bypasses in each group from January 1972 to September 1974. "The following principles were used in all patients to minimize ischemic injury: 1) avoidance of pre-bypass hypo- or hypertension, 2) limitation of ischemic arrest to less than 12 minutes, 3) avoidance of ventricular fibrilla-

tion, and 4) prolongation of total bypass as necessary to repay the myocardial oxygen debt." The results in the two kinds of patients were identical. Postoperative inotropic support was required in 10% in each group. A new postoperative infarction developed in 10% of each group. There was a 2% mortality in the high-risk group and a 4% mortality in the low-risk patients. They concluded that "These results are comparable and indicate that optimum myocardial protection allows safe revascularization in the 'high-risk' patient." Admittedly, the high-risk patients were "more vulnerable to ischemic myocardial injury during operation" and it was the surgeon's responsibility to prevent this injury. "Ischemic damage results from an imbalance between myocardial oxygen demand and oxygen supply . . . the 'high-risk' patient has an extremely limited capacity to tolerate even minor imbalances . . . In the absence of supply/demand imbalance postoperative myocardial infarction should not result unless there is a graft closure due to technical problems during anastomosis . . . or to inadequate graft flow because of poor distal run-off . . . Postoperative mortality and morbidity should not be increased in 'high-risk' patients if meticulous attention is directed toward protecting the heart against ischemic damage during operation."

Discussion

John A. Waldhausen, of Hershey, Pennsylvania, expressed some disagreement. "Dr. Buckberg and Dr. Maloney have convinced all of us that ventricular fibrillation is bad for the hypertrophied heart. I do not feel this is necessarily true in the non-hypertrophied ventricle." He used ventricular fibrillation and moderate hypothermia. In 85 consecutive cases, the Hershey group had a single death, and that from a noncardiac cause, many of the patients having been operated upon as emergencies and almost a quarter having a low ventricular ejection fraction. ". . . this operation is safe and sound if done properly, whether done with brief, hypoxic arrest or with ventricular fibrillation and hypothermia." Frank C. Spencer, of New York, had been using techniques almost identical to those presented. His mortality in patients with "bad ventricles", as indicated by an elevated end-diastolic pressure had decreased from 20% in 1971 to less than 5% in 1974. He stressed ". . . maintenance of adequate perfusion pressure, hypothermia, limitation of duration of ischemia to less than 15 minutes, adequate decompression of the left ventricle, and avoidance of long periods of ventricular fibrillation." Not only could

operations be done with a low mortality in patients with impaired ventricular function, but life was prolonged. "This slide shows an actuarial curve of the 60 patients over a period of 24 months, with a survival rate of 85% compared with a normal population of 95%. This 85% survival at two years is of particular importance because several reports with non-surgical therapy have found the expected mortality of patients with bad ventricles approaches 25-30% within two years . . . severe impairment of ventricular function, rather than being a contraindication to operation, is actually a strong indication for operation." He asked why myocardial infarction should develop during a bypass operation and whether, in fact, the patient with a "bad ventricle" should not have a "prophylactic bypass" even in the absence of symptoms. William E. Neville, of Newark, New Jersey, agreed with Dr. Buckberg's emphasis in another publication upon maintaining not only a high flow rate but a blood pressure of at least 75 mm Hg during perfusion "to prevent subendocardial ischemia during bypass." Neville reported experiments in dogs showing that the lactic dehydrogenase and acid phosphatase in cardiac muscle rose sharply during normothermal anoxic arrest or fibrillation, but not during anoxic arrest or fibrillation under hypothermia. Watts R. Webb, of Syracuse, New York, said that they were having more trouble with patients who were bad-risk because of obesity, age or heavy cigarette smoking, and not particularly those who had poor ventricular function. He questioned how the diagnosis of postoperative infarction was made. "About two years ago, our cases were analyzed by our cardiologists who found we were having a 16% incidence of new infarction by virtue of the squiggles on the EKG. Yet by clinical definition or anything else resembling a clinical infarction, about 2% showed something that could be classified as infarction." How did the UCLA group prevent hemorrhagic infarction occurring in patients with acute occlusions of more than six or eight hours, ". . . any time we try to get past this time, we convert an ischemic infarct into a hemorrhagic infarct and this has been disastrous." Gordon Olinger, closing, repeated to Waldhausen the message "that we still caution against fibrillation even though it is a successful procedure in the lion's share of patients that are being done with this technique." Olinger agreed with Spencer, "it's not so much an issue of how short we can make the bypass but how safe we can make it." They still had not arrived at the best method. The heart frequently continued to beat for a few minutes after aortic cross-clamping. "This is dis-

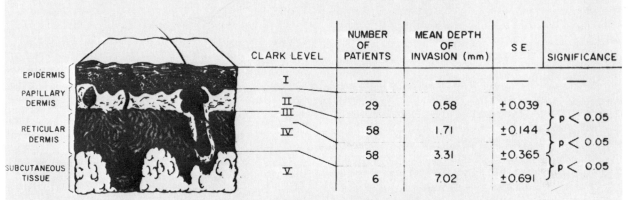

FIG. 1. Measurement of the microinvasion of primary melanoma is given according to each Clark's level.

In melanoma a correlation existed between depth of invasion (Clark's levels) and incidence of nodal metastases at elective node dissection. This incidence was 5% at Level II, 4% at Level III, 25% at Level IV and 75% at Level V. The measured depth of invasion (Breslow), added prognostic insight to each Clark's level; the minimal invasion at which nodal metastases occurred was 0.6mm for level II, 0.9mm for Level III, 1.5mm for Level IV and over 4mm for Level V.

Harold J. Wanebo, Joseph G. Fortner, J. Woodruff, B. MacLean, E. Binkowski, *Selection of the Optimum Surgical Treatment of Stage I Melanoma by Depth of Microinvasion:* Use of the Combined Microstage Technique (Clark-Breslow), Volume XCIII, 1975.

turbing because we know that the heart continues to beat, albeit slowly, and continues to require oxygen that is not being delivered." The diagnosis of postoperative infarction was primarily electrocardiographic. He thought they might have avoided hemorrhagic infarcts by getting the patients to the operating room rapidly. All of the patients done "in an intrainfarctional state in this series" had had angiography prior to the onset of that infarct.

* * *

Harold J. Wanebo, by invitation; Joseph G. Fortner, of New York, Professor of Surgery, Cornell University Medical College; Chief, Gastric and Mixed Tumor Service and Director of Surgical Research Memorial Hospital for Cancer and Allied Diseases; and by invitation, J. Woodruff, B. Mac-Lean, E. Binkowski, *Selection of the Optimum Surgical Treatment of Stage I Melanoma by Depth of Microinvasion:* Use of the Combined Microstage Technique (Clark-Breslow), presented a study of 306 patients with malignant melanoma of the extremities seen in the decade 1954 to 1964. In Stage I melanoma, was wide local excision adequate? Was the morbidity of prophylactic lymph node dissection

warranted? Patients with Stage I melanoma had a "20% to 25% incidence of microscopic nodal metastases." It had been postulated that "Survival is better in patients with Stage I melanoma who have lymph node dissection compared to those treated by wide excision only . . ." and that there was some benefit in prophylactic lymph node dissection for what proved to be microscopic node metastases rather than in lymph node excision when nodes became palpable. On the other hand, others said that four-fifths of the patients did not require operation and there is "no significant difference in survival figures between wide excision with and without elective node dissection, and survival rates are not significantly impaired by treating nodal areas expectantly." They had combined the histologic landmarks of W. H. Clark's 1969 histologic staging system with the direct measurement of the depth of invasion introduced by A. Breslow in 1970. They closed with their final recommendation "On the basis of this material and considering the results of other published studies one might consider the following as an acceptable surgical approach for Stage I melanoma of the extremities, wide excision alone should suffice for primary Stage I melanoma of the extremities classified as Clark Level II and measuring less than 0.9 mm in depth. Prophylactic node dissection in addition to wide local excision (either as continuous or discontinuous dissection) should be done for all primary melanomas classified as Clark Level III to V, for lesions showing 0.9 mm of invasion or greater at any Clark Level, and for all melanomas typed as nodular melanoma."

Discussion

William S. McCune, of Washington, D.C. presented a series of 54 patients followed 25 to 30 years. Of those with enlarged and positive lymph nodes, 27 were dead and one was alive, the deaths from malignant melanoma occurring over a period of 25 years, and the one surviving patient had a brain tumor, possibly metastatic. Of patients with lymph nodes not clinically enlarged but containing metastases, two were alive and seven were dead. Of patients with nodes which proved to be negative, ten were alive and seven were dead. Breslow was at George Washington School of Medicine, and there found "The thickness is easier to measure than the Clark measurements, which vary somewhat with the different pathologists . . ." Patients with lesions of thickness less than 0.76 mm all survived five years with or without lymph node dissections. Of patients with lesions 0.76-1.5mm, 70% survived with or without lymph node dissections. However, with lesions 1.5mm in thickness or greater, 64% of those with lymph node dissection were alive after five years, but only 31% of those without lymph node dissection. "So in this group we feel lymph node dissections are definitely indicated." Hiram C. Polk, Jr., of Louisville, Kentucky, questioned the statistical validity of Wanebo's study, thought multiple variables should be considered, particularly the "immunologic responsiveness of the given patient which may be the missing factor in all of our analyses." John W. Raker, of Boston, said "The survivors of the 206 melanoma patients who were the subject of the original analysis reported by Clark and Mihm are still being followed at the Massachusetts General Hospital", and there are now more than 500 patients followed ten years or more, which "in this unpredictable disease . . . seems to give a more realistic picture of results than shorter intervals." The accrued ten-year survival of Level II patients was 80%. They agreed that "Of the parameters we can measure, the depth level of malignant melanoma invasion into the skin is the most useful in prognosis." There were indeed differences among melanomas. "The concept that certain malignant melanomas

may remain superficial for a protracted period before deep invasion occurs, is now well documented. Lentigo maligna-melanoma only invades after decades, superficial spreading melanoma only after years, but nodular melanoma almost at once." Donald L. Morton, of Los Angeles, said that it was their policy to perform lymph node dissection for Levels III, IV, and V. Pathologically positive but clinically negative nodes occurred in 16% of Level III and 45% of Level IV patients. Wanebo, in closing, said that in their experience too, "patients whose melanoma measured less than 0.76mm in depth did not have lymph node metastasis and had a disease-free five year survival."

* * *

C. Barber Mueller, of Hamilton, Ontario, Department of Surgery, McMaster University School of Medicine, and, by invitation, Wendy Jeffries, *Cancer of the Breast:* Its Outcome as Measured by the Rate of Dying and Causes of Death, presented to the Association what many obviously regarded as a disturbing interpretation of the analysis of the causes of death in 1,552 patients with carcinoma of the breast followed for 15 years. Data from this and other sources showed that "80-85% of all women who die after developing cancer of the breast die of their breast cancer. Modification of the time of dying (rate of dying) or cause of death should be used as objectives of management rather than 5-year survival figures." It was his thesis that "Despite all therapeutic efforts, this disease's death rate has remained fairly constant over the past several decades. However, reported 5-year survival rates during the past 50 years have gradually improved because of earlier case selection, revised staging, or more aggressive therapy." Mueller's gloomy analysis suggested "The forces of mortality due to cancer of the breast seem to be operative over a long period of time (at least 15 years). The percentage of women dying of their breast cancer seems to be a fixed proportion of those at risk in any year, unchanged throughout at least 15 years, except for the small group with early rapid mortality during the first 2 to 3 years after diagnosis. The women over 70 years of age experienced a higher proportion of death due to competing risks . . . presumably because the required exposure to their carcinoma was of insufficient duration and the mortality forces due to competing risks had increased sufficiently to overtake the shorter exposure to mortality forces of the carcinoma . . . It has been customary to attribute a positive effect to any therapeutic modality used in cancer management when death curves due to the cancer approach the natural death curve or normal life expectancy. This explanation is now open to reinterpretation, at least at the time when the competing risk rate exceeds the rate characteristic of cancer of the breast, as in the older-age group. Since death for an overwhelming number of individuals was attributed to cancer of the breast, it appears that treatment may have little or nothing to do with the cause of death. No data are presented which answer whether a therapeutic influence may affect the rate of dying and justify the use of 'delay of death' as an appropriate end point." Mueller found that ". . . the likelihood of dying is no different in the 15th year than in the 3rd year after diagnosis . . . The rate of dying is approximately 8% per year in the group at risk . . ." And his final statement with respect to breast cancer treatment was that it should "Treat the cancer only when and where it is known to exist . . . Not be proposed as a means of influencing either time of death or cause of death. Measurements of quality of life should be established and should constitute the only realistic objectives of treatment."

Discussion

Claude E. Welch, of Boston was obviously unable to accept this pessimistic report. He showed a slide made in 1937, with Dr. Ira Nathanson, on the life expectancy of cancer of the breast, with and without operation, showing the advantage of treatment. Mueller's current figures showed much better results after treatment. "I would submit to you that there is a definite difference then between what happened 40 years ago and what is happening now." Francis D. Moore, of Boston, agreed that "80-85% of women who died after getting this disease will die of the disease." He emphasized the significance of the quality of life in evaluating results. From their own study, "we found that death delay was both possible and justified. The trouble was that the delay was really too short." In late cancer, "we could change the half-times from 0.6 years to 3.0 years if the patient were a responder to the combination of oophorectomy, adrenalectomy and 5-FU, so that we were changing slopes in a way that was significant." Benjamin F. Rush, Jr., of Newark, New Jersey, said that the application of Mueller's log normal plot to untreated patients yielded a half-life of 2.6 to 2.7 years, "quite different from the half-life of the total group . . . how does one reconcile the difference?" He mentioned new data on current efforts, "As you are aware, Urban, for instance, has reported that for lesions measuring 3-15 mm, he had had no deaths at

five years in this selected group and at ten years only one death in 44 patients and no local recurrences." Jonathan E. Rhoads, of Philadelphia, showed his uncertainty. "The surgical approach to cancer is to operate early enough to eradicate it and where metastasis has occurred in breast carcinoma—distant metastasis—the case is declared non-operable. The data showing that the death rate in the second five years is essentially the same as it is in the first five years . . . would seem to belie the idea that one very often gets around the whole cancer and gets it all out . . . one goes back in his thinking to the study that Warren Cole and several others did on cells circulating in the bloodstream . . . wonders whether cancers haven't disseminated . . . there have been showers of cancer cells through the body long before the tumor really becomes palpable . . . a tumor of a centimeter which is perhaps as small as you frequently feel them . . . you already have had so many multiplications of a cell—perhaps 50 times—that it's not biologically a small tumor, then what are we doing? I tend to accept Dr. Welch's view that we are doing some good. I know it's possible to deposit, that you're simply moving the time before diagnosis to the time after diagnosis, but I find that hard to accept as a total explanation for the difference in the lines that he showed. I wonder then if what we are doing isn't really to remove enough of the tumor so that it increases the individual's chance of resistance and in this way, adds a period to her life." Mueller, closing, said of Welch's slide, that he was comparing 100 cases against the 1,500 Mueller studied, "which requires some tough statistical manipulations." As for the apparent improvement in results after 40 years "All you may have shown is that you've done a little early diagnosis or better staging in the treated group rather than different treatment." He agreed with Moore's emphasis on the change in half-life. "The concept of delay of death is a useful concept, I think, in terms of any management objective and the idea that we ever cure anybody is probably not so, and ought to be eliminated from our vocabulary." Rush had questioned the value of retrospective studies as always evaluating the past rather than present techniques. Mueller, who of course had been using such material, defended the value of the material accumulated, for the most part, since World War II, and [although he had gotten some of his statistics from the prospective surgical adjuvant breast cancer studies], said "Prospective problems are horrendous since we all have emotional hangups about what we would like to do and how we want to treat patients. The ability to get any hundred surgeons to do exactly the same thing, as do the basic scientists in the laboratory, is almost unethical and immoral, if not extremely impractical and impossible." To Rhoads, he said, "I don't know about those circulating cells. I'm fascinated by them. I think the disease of cancer must be a systemic disease. We usually see only the first local manifestation and we then treat the local tumor. Therefore my recommendation is that you only treat that cancer wherever you find it, whether it's in the breast, the axilla, or the lung. Please don't go hunting for it if you don't know it is there and subject the patient to treatment for something you don't know they have." [Mueller's fatalistic and pessimistic approach to cancer, so directly opposed to the vigorous "if we can do the right operation early enough, we can cure cancer" approach, which dominated the expressions of surgical attitude during the earlier years of the Association, still caused bemused smiles of discomfort and a shaking of heads in the audience].

* * *

George E. Block, of Chicago, Professor of Surgery, Coordinator of Clinical Oncology, University of Chicago, and by invitation, Elwood V. Jensen and Theodore Z. Polley, Jr., *The Prediction of Hormonal Dependency of Mammary Cancer,* presented their studies in 359 primary breast cancers and 214 metastatic breast cancers upon the significance of the estrogen receptor proteins in the development of which Jensen had played such a significant part. None of the 42 patients with negative estrogen receptor determinations experienced an objective remission to ablative endocrine therapy. "Only one of 6 patients with negative determinations benefited from additive hormonal therapy: 4 of 6 patients with positive determinations benefited from additive therapy". They concluded that "The estrogen receptor content of the primary tumor indicates the hormonal dependency of the tumor and may be used to predict the response to endocrine treatment when recurrent disease appears . . . Those patients whose tumors lack a critical amount of estrophilin have little chance of benefit from either endocrine ablation or hormone administration . . . A biochemical explanation for the correlation of estrogen receptors and clinical response to additive therapy is not obvious. While the mechanism of this correlation with ablative therapy is presumed to be the removal of endogenous estrogen production by the host, no such simple and attractive thesis is readily available as the rationale for additive therapy. The exogenous steroid hormones may compete for receptor binding, or the presence of receptor may characterize a tumor in

which a biochemical lesion is produced by the addition of steroid hormones." Thus far, the tumor receptor pattern seemed to be a consistent feature of a given tumor during the life of the patient. They felt that "estrogen receptor is a practical, reproducible, and reliable determination that should be available to major centers accepting the responsibility of treating patients suffering from mammary cancer." They proposed that estrogen receptor content might "serve as a guide to patient selection for elective or 'prophylactic' castration" and proposed a clinical study to that effect.

Discussion

Richard E. Wilson, of Boston, agreed with the need for a biological "discriminant so as to select patients for ablative therapy" and thought that perhaps the 17-keto steroids and 17-hydroxy steroids and the estrogen output might be evaluated as his studies and those of Heywood [of London] had suggested. What was the feasibility of determining estrogen receptivity in patients returning with metastases? Were there "variations in ER-positivity with any given patient's tumor burden, possibly indicating different cell populations?" He felt the additive effect of chemotherapy, specifically 5-FU should not be ignored. John R. Benfield, of Los Angeles, was as "convinced as I'm certain you are that patients whose breast cancers are negative for estrogen receptors as defined are so unlikely to respond to endocrine therapy that this should not be the primary therapeutic approach when metastases appear", but the quantitative "dividing line between negative and positive . . . will change as greater experience is achieved." Persijn, of Amsterdam, had shown negativity or positivity to be constant in two or more separate biopsies of 31 patients but inconstant in 15 patients. "When I was a medical student, Dr. Huggins challenged me to look at microscopic slides of various breast cancers to tell him which ones were endocrine sensitive. Naturally, I could not do so . . . The answer to the Huggins' question is finally forthcoming and I congratulate Dr. Block and his co-workers for carrying on the tradition of leading research in tumor endocrinology at the University of Chicago." Loren J. Humphrey, of Kansas City, Kansas, said that a number of other receptors had been found in cancers and that Slicer and Van Nuy "have shown that normal parenchymal cells have hormone dependent and independent cells". Had Dr. Block's group "tested the surrounding so-called normal breast tissue from these patients for estrogen receptors?" What about progesterone receptor studies? Block, closing, responded that "the receptor we are talking about here is a receptor that Dr. Jensen found to be in the cytosol fraction. When it unites with estrogen, it migrates into the cell nucleus where the estrogen has its major action. It is not a surface receptor [like the other receptors Humphrey mentioned]". They did not know as yet whether progesterone receptors were the same protein as estrogen receptors. They had investigated normal mammary and other tissues, and "Practically all human tissue contains some of this protein receptor . . . significant receptor content is associated basically with the reproductive system and secondary sex characteristics . . . it is a quantitative difference that is important." The fibro-adipose tissue of breast had practically no receptor in it. Block agreed that in the absence of "significant amounts of receptor in recurrent tumor, chemotherapy via triple drug or quadruple drug therapy should be the first treatment of choice and that we should not subject the patient to a hormonal manipulation. Whatever that manipulation may be, there is at least a 93% chance that it is doomed to failure." As for consistency, 23 patients showed sustained patterns of estrogen receptor content during the course of their disease, but four did not. In one patient with "asynchronous breast cancers 60 months apart" one cancer "had absolutely no receptor . . . while the other contained a significant amount . . .". They could do the "receptor analysis on 200 mg of tumor . . . in a patient with a pleural effusion or ascites, we can drain off the fluid and find 200 mg of cells that we can freeze and then subject to the estrogen receptor test."

* * *

Samuel A. Wells, Jr., D. A. Ontjes, C. W. Cooper, J. F. Hennessy, G. J. Ellis, and H. T. McPherson, all by invitation, and David C. Sabiston, Jr., of Durham, James Buchanan Duke Professor of Surgery and Chairman, Department of Surgery, Duke University; Surgeon-in-Chief, Duke Hospital, *The Early Diagnosis of Medullary Carcinoma of the Thyroid Gland in Patients with Multiple Endocrine Neoplasia Type II*, were discussing the tumor described by Hazard, Hawk, and Crile in 1959, which had been found now to account for five to ten percent of all thyroid malignancies and to present "either sporadically or in a familial pattern inherited as a Mendelian dominant trait and associated with parathyroid hyperplasia and pheochromocytoma(s). This syndrome has been referred to as multiple endocrine neoplasia, type II (MEN-II)." Not all patients developed all three components, but almost all developed medullary thyroid carcinoma, the most life-

threatening manifestation. Medullary carcinoma arose from the "C" cells of the neural crest and was shown to be able to secrete "ACTH, prostaglandins, histaminase, serotonin, and thyrocalcitonin (TCT)." Thyrocalcitonin had proved to be a marker for the presence of medullary carcinoma of the thyroid, and "an elevated serum concentration of this hormone often provides the diagnosis of MCT before the lesion is palpable clinically or is demonstrable by thyroid scanning. Calcium, glucagon, and pentagastrin have all been shown to stimulate the secretion of TCT from medullary carcinoma cells . . ." The thyrocalcitonin assay determination was by radioimmunoassay of plasma. Pentagastrin proved in their hands to be a much more potent stimulator of thyrocalcitonin secretion than was calcium infusion. Pentagastrin stimulation combined with selective venous catheterization was "a very sensitive method for diagnosing primary medullary carcinoma of the thyroid gland," the elevation occurring "only in the catheterized thyroid vein and not in the peripheral vein. They had screened 40 members of a kindred with multiple endocrine neoplasia type II. In four patients, the pentagastrin stimulation had produced a diagnostic elevation of thyrocalcitonin in the peripheral blood. In none of these patients was there a thyroid nodule palpable externally and all had a negative I^{131} thyroid scan, and all four were found at operation to have a macroscopic bilateral medullary carcinoma of the thyroid. In a fifth patient, the peripheral venous TCT elevation with pentagastrin was not diagnostic, but the elevation in the thyroid vein was. There was no palpable thyroid nodule externally and the I^{131} scan was negative. The thyroid at operation showed no macroscopic disease, but " 'C' cell hyperplasia" microscopically. It was their practice "to perform pentagastrin stimulation tests yearly in all children above the age of 10 years . . . with a family history of multiple endocrine neoplasia type II" and to perform total thyroidectomy if the TCT level in the peripheral plasma was 1.0 ng/ml or greater. If the level was between 0.5 and 1.0, they recommended selective thyroid venous catheterization and pentagastrin stimulation. "The pentagastrin test is an extremely sensitive means for diagnosing medullary carcinoma of the thyroid gland. Its combination with selective venous catheterization technics provides a powerful tool both for diagnosis of medullary carcinoma and localization of metastatic foci."

Discussion

Melvin A. Block, of Detroit, had been utilizing intravenous pentagastrin, following earlier reports from Duke, and agreed that it was "the most sensitive test now available for the detection" of medullary thyroid carcinoma. Perhaps the test was too sensitive. One patient, 11 years after a total thyroidectomy for medullary carcinoma, had an elevation of thyrocalcitonin to 3.8 ng/ml after intravenous pentagastrin. Timothy S. Harrison, of Ann Arbor, Michigan, said that applying the test to 36 patients with pheochromocytoma, some of them thought to have been sporadic, they found occult medullary thyroid carcinoma in two, and this was now established as a screening test, for all members of MEN II families and for all patients with pheochromocytoma. Benjamin F. Rush, Jr., of Newark, cited a family with Sipple Syndrome in whom they had explored three siblings for pheochromocytoma, and in each found medullary carcinoma of the thyroid metastatic to the liver. They, therefore, explored the thyroid of the four-year-old child of one of the three and found "a medullary carcinoma of the thyroid occupying both lobes as well as a metastatic lesion in the neck." He asked "just when these lesions do begin in the thyroid and whether they may not actually be present in these children from birth." Charles Eckert, of Albany, said that five "patients with medullary carcinoma who have had total thyroidectomy over five years ago, who have no evidence of disease at present, have elevated levels of calcitonin in their blood without prococative tests" confirming, he thought, Melvin Block's observation that the test might be too sensitive. Samuel A. Wells, Jr., closing, said that when after operation, a patient whose calcitonin had returned to negative, "suddenly develops an elevated level of thyrocalcintonin following pentagastrin stimulation, we perform selective venous catheterization pentagastrin stimulation in an attempt to localize the site of recurrent disease. If it appears to be localized to the neck, then we feel that the patient should undergo repeat neck exploration with resection of recurrent tumor . . . the test is very sensitive and will detect the presence of disease long before it is detectable by clinical or radiological means . . . those individuals who have definite but very minimal elevations of pentagastrin . . . recurrent lesions will be small and perhaps difficult to locate surgically." [He seemed clearly to be stating that Block's and Eckert's patients did indeed have metastases]. He agreed with Harrison that pentagastrin stimulation tests should be performed on patients with pheochromocytoma, especially those with bilateral lesions. He was not sure of the answer to Rush's question about the age at which medullary carcinoma appeared. However, thus far, "All the children in our series who have the diagnosis of

medullary thyroid carcinoma made by pentagastrin stimulation and who have subsequently undergone total thyroidectomies have been negative to pentagastrin stimulation since their surgery . . . a short follow-up time . . ."

* * *

Lester F. Williams, of Boston, Professor of Surgery, University Hospital; Director of Surgical Services, Boston City Hospital, and Jack Wittenberg, by invitation, *Ischemic Colitis:* An Useful Clinical Diagnosis, But Is it Ischemic? [went partway toward demonstration of the truism that when the title of an article is phrased as a question, the answer is in the negative.]. Boley, in 1963, reporting five patients with "reversible vascular occlusion of the colon" emphasized the milder end of the spectrum of vascular disease of the colon, the other end of which was "colonic infarction secondary to accidental arterial ligation during surgical procedures." Marston and Morson from England, in 1966, "reported on 16 patients who manifested three stages of a spontaneous disease which they labeled ischemic colitis." They agreed that "ischemic colitis has become a well recognized clinical entity. Although neither the histologic material nor the barium studies are specific by themselves, the total clinical picture is now considered specific." It "is an acute colonic process occurring in either males or females of an average age of 70 years" manifested by mild abdominal pain, significant, and usually bloody, diarrhea. Barium enema or X-ray demonstrated an acute ulcerative process "or an exudative process manifest on barium studies as thumbprinting with the associated secondary characteristics of transverse ridging, spasm, or rigidity and on endoscopic examination as hemorrhagic bullae." Histologically, there was "an acute mucosal process with extensive submucosal edema and/or hemorrhage." There might be inflammation, but "the absence of bacterial colonization is not uncommon." It was remarkable that "The extent of the process is determined by the first examination since progression to other segments of bowel is quite unusual." Endoscopy and radiography demonstrated rapid changes within five to seven days "Progression to healing or to mild stricture is anticipated in the majority of patients", and the left colon was involved in some 73%. The pain was less severe than with extensive bowel ischemia. The patients tended to be normotensive. Although the lesion was usually in the distribution of the inferior mesenteric artery, there was no occlusion of the vessels in 95% of the cases, whereas with extensive bowel ischemia, shock and electrolyte imbalance, as a rule the superior mesenteric artery was occluded in 50%. The prognosis of segmental ischemic colitis was "fair to excellent" and with an extensive bowel ischemia was "dismal". Probably somewhat over a quarter of the patients had severe degrees of ischemic colitis, in which gangrene or perforation might develop rapidly or in the course of several days. While sufficient blood might be lost to require a transfusion, they were aware of no patient who required emergency resection to control bleeding. Resection was ultimately required in all patients with the severe form, but there was no agreement as to how rapidly operation should be undertaken except in the most fulminating cases. Occasionally a fibrotic stricture might result which presented no organically significant obstruction. Ischemic colitis did occur in patients under 50, and with equal frequency in those with a history of contraceptive medication and those without such history. The spontaneously occurring condition was indistinguishable from that produced by division of the inferior mesenteric artery except for the doubled incidence of severe disease in the latter. Angiography, unexpectedly, and contrary to their earlier published opinion, was not very helpful. ". . . 69% of the occlusive group had mild disease whereas 53% of the non-occlusive patients had mild disease . . . Survival occurred in 65% of those with occlusive and in 66% of those with non-occlusive disease . . . when the patients are divided according to the presence or absence of arterial occlusion on the basis of angiograms, the clinical reflection of the ischemic colitis process does not differ . . . occlusion or non-occlusion is not the basis upon which one can establish either severity or therapy." The experimental studies of Boley and succeeding investigators indicated that the same results could be produced "whether one uses arterial ligation, venous ligation, microsphere injection or partial occlusion complicated by hypotension . . . mechanical interference with colonic blood supply can reproduce the entire spectrum of ischemic colitis . . . changes in the luminal pressure within the colon can influence colonic blood flow in terms of volume flow to the colon, of distributional flow within the colon wall or of nutritional flow to the colon . . . repeated increases in colonic pressure can induce prolonged decreases in flow with the flow decreases persisting after the luminal pressure increases are removed" possibly explaining the occurrence of ischemic colitis proximal to colon carcinoma. However, selective arteriography in proven cases, with good visualization of distal vessels had failed to show small arterial occlusions or venous occlusions and, in some cases, suggested hyperemia, nor did they think that arterial spasm was a factor. "We are forced to conclude on the basis of this review that an ischemic process as the basis for ischemic colitis seen in most patients is not yet established since a detailed evaluation of the blood supply to the involved colon is not consistent with spasm or occlusion." [Curiously, the histologic status of the vessels in the bowel wall is not discussed.] The final sentence of the paper states that "To date no one has established the presence of poor blood flow to the involved colonic wall in a human patient with ischemic colitis. Thus one must question whether or not the pathogenesis of the clinically useful designation, ischemic colitis, includes ischemia."

Discussion

David B. Skinner, of Chicago, said that, in dogs and in monkeys, placing "an occlusive clamp temporarily across the base of the pedicle . . . a bowel loop at the splenic flexure . . . for 6-10 hours, depending on the duration of the occlusion, the full range of different lesions can be seen. When the clamp is released arterial pulsation is restored. An arteriogram shows patent vessels. Some of these bowel loops go on to gangrene and necrosis, some enter an intermediate stage with stricture or bleeding, and some make a complete recovery with persistent hyperemia in the bowel wall for several days." Hypoperfusion was capable of producing the same changes, and Skinner suggested a decrease in cardiac output as the commonest cause of ischemic colitis. It was the healing process which was hyperemic and might be characterized by bleeding and subsequently stricture. His own patients had usually shown severe cardiac disease or a previous myocardial infarction. He took issue with Williams, "We propose that this condition is aptly named. We can demonstrate all these lesions in animal studies by a temporary episode of ischemia which is followed by a reparative process which becomes hyperemic. Since the etiology in this model is ischemia, until we find some other cause I believe that the title of ischemic colitis is correct and can be supported by experimental data." James D. Hardy, of Jackson, Mississippi, agreed. "I think that ischemia has a great deal to do with 'ischemic colitis' and I align myself with Dr. Skinner and his remarks". He cited a case of "a benign cicatrizing inflammatory lesion" resulting from resection of a lumbar aortic aneurysm. Paul S. Jordan, Jr., of Houston, cited a case of a patient with chronic heart failure and begun on digitalis, who suddenly developed symptoms of acute abdomen, and had a localized infarction of the splenic flexure. "We are impressed by the experimental work of Dr. Eugene Jacobsen who has demonstrated so well the decrease in blood flow to the bowel as a consequence of vaso-constrictive effect of digitalis." Edward E. Mason, of Iowa City, Iowa, had seen thumbprinting as a result of severe chemical colitis from clindamycin. Kenneth G. Swan, of Newark, New Jersey, said the problem with determining whether the lesion was ischemic or not was "the interpretation of our only available technique for measuring flow to this organ during the disease process . . . angiography. Clearly it is a poor tool at best." Williams, closing, said that "On an emotional basis I agree with the discussants that this must be ischemia. However, I must stress that to date this ischemia has not yet been documented in patients." In cases of "extensive disease", they had been able to show "precipitating illness, chronic congestive heart failure, digitalis toxicity . . . These are not prominent features of these patients with ischemic colitis, although there is an occasional patient . . . in whom ischemic colitis is incidental to other severe disease." Digitalis had certainly been demonstrated to induce changes in the splanchnic circulation, and they had seen extensive bowel disease after digitalis, but not ischemic colitis. They had seen clindomycin colitis but without thumbprinting. He agreed with "Dr. Swan's suggestion that angiography is not a secure way to show flow."

The Business Meetings

The 1975 meeting was held at Le Chateau Frontenac, Quebec City, Canada, on May 7, 8, and 9, President William H. Muller, Jr., in the Chair.

The SOSSUS project had been completed. The large work was in press, and the business meeting was given over to a detailed discussion of the salient points of the report.

At the second business meeting the Fellows accepted the proposal made at the previous meeting to permit selection of Honorary Fellows and the occasional recipients of the Association's Medallion for Scientific Achievement at the mid-winter meeting of the Council so they might be present at the following meeting of the Association in the Spring.

Secretary, James V. Maloney, Jr., made an interesting financial report. "It has been the long tradition in the Association that the Secretary's office is provided with $2500 to pay for the expenses of operating the Association. Investigation during the past year of other organizations of approximately the same size as this Association, some of which have

hired professional management services and others of which have not, suggests that the actual cost of running an association of seven hundred members is approximately $20,000 per annum. It is appropriate that I, as the new Secretary, pay tribute to Dr. Shires and his assistant Mrs. Ila Fite who served this organization so well for so long. The remarkable Dr. Shires was simultaneously secretary, chairman or president of a half dozen other organizations. Two things are apparent: Dr. Shires is a man of great talent; and he and his department have been subsidizing the Association to a very great extent. Recognizing the steady escalation of costs due to inflation, Council recommends the following: that the Association pay the actual expenses of all officers, with the Secretary being limited to the expenditure of $10,000 per year; that dues be raised from $75 to $100 per year; that guest registration be increased from $20 to $30 per year; that the initiation fee be increased from $50 to $100 per year,"

It was proposed that the number of Honorary Fellows be raised to 45.

Malpractice insurance had become prohibitively expensive in the state of California, and there had been what amounted to a walk-out of surgeons throughout the state. In moving that the excuses of Fellows for nonattendance which had been tendered by mail and telegram be accepted, Maloney jibed "It was interesting that we received a number of telegrams from the members in San Francisco indicating that since they were employees of the University of California they were the only ones in the Bay Area who were covered by malpractice insurance. Since they are doing all the operating, they are unable to attend this meeting."

Council had proceeded with the incorporation of the Association as a corporation under the Internal Revenue Service Code.

The Joint Commission for Accreditation of Hospitals had been pressing hospitals to "delineate" the privileges of surgeons, going so far as to suggest that there be a list of permissible operations for each surgeon on a given staff. ". . . Council has previously expressed its objection to the so-called 'laundry list', a specific list of operative procedures prepared in advance which a surgeon is said to be competent to perform. Council so recommended against such a list because of the medico-legal dangers that such a list presents. We have during the past year been assured, or reassured to learn that the Joint Commission has specifically recommended against such a 'laundry list' unless it be the option of the local hospital."

Council recommended "that a fellow with a

THE RITUAL OF CONGRATULATION

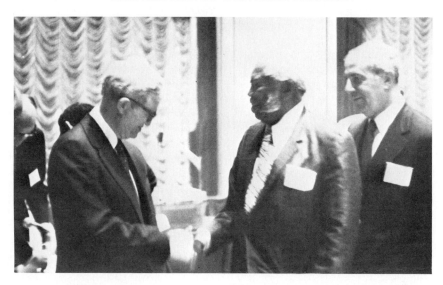

After the election of the President and his remarks of acceptance (and the outgoing President, announcing his successor's accession upon hearing the report of the Nominating Committee to the Fellows, has at times had to be reminded that a vote was in order) Fellows ascend in line to the platform to congratulate the new President.
James D. Hardy, of Jackson, Mississippi, is being congratulated by Matthew Walker, of Nashville, Tennessee, as Paul Nemir, Jr., of Philadelphia, waits in line.
  (Photography: Henry T. Bahnson, M.D., Pittsburgh)

special appreciation of the history of the American Surgery, a man of scholarly distinction and a man fluent in our native tongue be nominated to write the history of the Association. The committee to select a man is Dr. H. William Scott, Jr., Dr. Jonathan E. Rhoads and Dr. Francis D. Moore."

Dr. William P. Longmire, Jr., reporting for the Committee on Government Affairs, commented that the Committee has sent a statement "to all members of legislative committees that were concerned with health legislation" in which ". . . The manpower statistics of SOSSUS were used to support the concept that the number of qualified surgeons in the States is not as over-abundant as sometimes indicated and, before regulating trained surgeons, a mechanism must be developed for regulating the surgical activities of those who do surgery but who are without the generally accepted qualifications of a surgical specialist." They had pointed out the mechanism which had been voluntarily established to coordinate medical education and residency training through the Coordinating Council on Medical Education and the Liaison Committee on Graduate Medical Education and that, before embarking on federal legislation and the federal bureau ". . . con-

trolling residency training . . . we should at least give a chance for voluntary mechanisms to work . . . Federal legislation to regulate control or direct residency training is unnecessary and might prove disastrous." With respect to malpractice, they recommend a dollar limit on liability, a return to the statute of limitations and a system "that compensates the patient and removes the prohibitive cost of malpractice litigation, including some regulation of contingency fees."

With regard to health insurance, they favored "a comprehensive coverage, both basic and catastrophic for the entire population with funding through federal, state and private funds, with the utilization of private health insurance and the maintenance of a pluralistic system of health care delivery."

Jonathan E. Rhoads, as Chairman of the Committee for Definition of Surgical Privileges said they had recommended to serve as guidelines for the Joint Commission on Accreditation of Hospitals, "that surgical privileges should be granted only to physicians who have successfully completed the approved surgical training program which would ordinarily qualify them to cope with the problems from which the patients upon whom they operate appear to suffer." The programs were to be acceptable to the appropriate "member board of the American Board of Medical Specialties" [thus excluding a certain number of self-declared and free-standing boards", viz., "The Board of Abdominal Surgery"]. They recognized that several programs might prepare a surgeon for a field in a given area. There should be an annual operative record of staff and resident physicians. There should be a record of "attendance at professional meetings, postgraduate courses and/or teaching exercises." It was to be expected that, for some operations a given frequency of performance was required to maintain expertise. It was to be emphasized that it was still necessary, at times, to operate for diagnosis and that the preoperative diagnosis might be incorrect and "therefore it remains extremely important that a body of broadly trained surgeons continue in the field of surgery who can cope satisfactorily with the unexpected." Broad training was essential even in the "more specialized fields such as cardiothoracic surgery . . ." In remote and isolated areas, it might be necessary for physicians without special training to perform "certain surgical procedures". SOSSUS had shown that there was a lack of precise information as to the vocational state of activity of even those certified by the Boards, and a motion was made and passed that "each of the ten American Boards of Surgery" be directed to maintain and update files of their diplomates.

The Secretary informed the membership of the existence of the 501.C3 American Surgical Foundation, which allowed the Association active political involvement, formed with the hope that the members would persuade "patients, donors and others who have a particular interest in improving the quality of surgical care in the United States" to make tax deductible donations to the Foundation so that the Association would "be able to continue the kind of work that it has done in connection with SOSSUS and other kinds of activity which would improve surgical care".

Thirty-eight new members were elected. Sir Brian Gerald Barratt-Boyes of Auckland, New Zealand, who had been a Corresponding Fellow, was now elected an Honorary Fellow.

The officers elected were James D. Hardy, of Jackson, Mississippi, President; Vice-Presidents, Henry G. Schwartz, of St. Louis, and Clarence J. Berne, of Los Angeles, James V. Maloney, Jr., continuing as Secretary.

XCIV

1976

The 1976 meeting was held at the Fairmont Hotel, New Orleans, Louisiana, April 7, 8, and 9, with President James D. Hardy, Professor and Chairman, Department of Surgery, and Director of Surgical Research, University of Mississippi Medical Center; Surgeon-in-Chief to the Hospital of the University of Mississippi, in the Chair. That year had seen the death of Theodore Drapanas, Professor and Chairman, Department of Surgery, Tulane University Medical Center [who had been killed in New York in an airplane crash on his way to a special committee meeting for the American Board of Surgery dealing with the advisability of conferring a certificate of special competence in pediatric surgery]. Among the Senior Members who died were Lester R. Dragstedt, recipient in 1970 of the American Surgical Association Medallion for Scientific Achievement, who contributed so much to the physiological understanding and treatment of peptic ulcer disease and established the value of vagal section, and the extraordinary D. W. Gordon Murray, of Toronto, who, often by long margins, had scored first with heparin therapy, renal dialysis, saphenous vein grafts, aortic valve homografts, closure of cardiac septal defects, excision of ventricular infarcts.

As had become the custom for a number of years, President Hardy, *American Surgery—1976,* reviewed the current scene. ". . . vast financial support has been withdrawn—in the form of NIH research grants and research fellowships, federal student loans and scholarships, and direct faculty and institutional subsidies from private sources. The re-

sult has been large scale departure of personnel from medical school research and teaching positions . . . a warning and deterrent to bright young people who may now see medical school employment as risky, often low paid, and also less rewarding in terms of the less tangible satisfactions of teaching that were once so gratifying." Faculty were under pressure. Their teaching quality was monitored and criticized by students. The size of medical schools in many cases had "exceeded the capacities of the physical plant and the faculty" as a result of pressure from a variety of groups, although "the most seductive influence has been the 'capitation grants' from the federal government," and now that the capitation had been reduced and was probably about to be phased out, medical schools were left "with large classes which for political reasons cannot readily be reduced." In capsule, the SOSSUS project with respect to resident training suggested that ". . . unless the number of trainees in some specialties be reduced, a serious surplus of such specialists may develop within the next twenty years . . . One suspects that if the numbers of residency positions were to be significantly reduced, the graduates would be better trained and would come largely from American medical schools." He commented on the frequent English language difficulty of the foreign medical graduates, the poor training they received in the programs which would accept them. Despite the effects of Medicaid and Medicare in terms of the disappearance of the clinic patient, as a result of "judicious compromise" with strict interpretation of the regula-

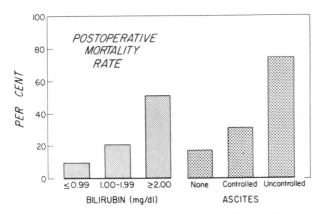

FIG. 2. Correlation of bilirubin levels and ascites with mortality rate.

The influence of bilirubin levels (divided as shown) and of ascites upon rising mortality of portasystemic shunting.
"No patient with a normal bilirubin level and without ascites died after an elective shunting procedure. Even a slight deviation from normality, or an emergency shunt instead of an elective shunt, raised the risk of postoperative death to 1/8, a category that for these operations might be called 'modest risk.' "
R. A. Malt, J. Szczerban, and R. B. Malt, *Risks in Therapeutic and Splenorenal Shunts*. Volume XCIV, 1976.

tions, "The quality of the residency training program has been little impaired," and he felt it perhaps often better, because supervision was closer. "An additional dividend of the inclusion of previously indigent patients under third party coverage, is that it has given junior staff members some access to private patients, without which the young academic surgeon who really wants to operate will not stay long in the teaching hospital" [a point which had concerned McKittrick in his 1966 Presidential Address]. His concern over the "encroachment of federal control" is mainly voiced in the section entitled, *"Showdown Power Politics"*. ". . . I see on all sides evidence that many are eager to assault and to take over American medicine and use it as an instrument of power and prestige—all in the name of improved distribution of medical care . . . I know only too well that American medicine needs to be improved, can be improved, must be improved . . . However, it is not necessary that the government take over the medical profession in this country to achieve this improvement . . . To be strong, we must organize. We must be prepared, if all else fails, to withhold our services from all but emergency patients. If this seems hard, and it is hard, we nonetheless must accept it. In the final analysis, it is our only weapon. The cost must be counted, we must decide the

lengths to which we will go, we must be prepared to face the consequences. But we must win on the vital issues. The political solution of political problems requires political means . . . We can approach enough people only through the members of the American Medical Association. The American Surgical Association has talent, the American College of Surgeons has both talent and muscle, but the American Medical Association has access to the votes." Concrete proposals were, "Support JCAH monitoring of surgical results in hospitals . . . Support the panel review mechanism in malpractice claims . . . Support appropriate residency limitations and further strengthen programs . . . Work with American College of Surgeons to respond to news media attacks . . . Monitor federal encroachment . . . Give superior care to the individual patient."

* * *

Ronald A. Malt, of Boston, Chief, Surgical Gastroenterology, Massachusetts General Hospital; Professor of Surgery, Harvard Medical School, and by invitation, J. Szczerban, and R. B. Malt, *Risks in Therapeutic Portacaval and Splenorenal Shunts*, analysed the records of 120 patients who had undergone portasystemic shunts, 57% of them portacaval shunts, 43% splenorenal shunts, from 1966 to 1973. Their data was computer analysed by a number of sophisticated statistical techniques. Of the portacaval shunts, almost half were done as emergency operations for uncontrollable bleeding. The most significant predictors of operative mortality, death within four weeks of shunting, or any time during the same hospitalization, proved to be serum bilirubin level and the presence of ascites. Patients electively shunted whether splenorenal or portacaval were similar in preoperative physical condition and postoperative mortality rates,- about 20%. The mortality from emergency shunts was 48%, but these patients were more severely ill. [Malt made the astonishing statement that, "Surgical skill does not appear to be an overwhelming determinant of survival rate." There is no indication of how he arrived at this interesting statement. Presumably, he meant "surgical skill" within the visiting and resident staff of the Massachusetts General Hospital. There is the hint of a suggestion that he was implying that Dr. Linton's results were no better than those of the other surgeons at the MGH. "Other studies show no difference in 5-year survival rates between the two kinds of shunts whether the number of surgeons involved is few (Bismuth and Hepp, 1974) or many (Voorhees, Price and Britton, 1970), although the

TABLE 5. *Scale for Predicting Operative Mortality*

Predictor	Points Assigned		
	0	1	2
Bilirubin (mg dl)	≦ 0.99	1.00–1.99	≧ 2.0
Ascites	none	controlled (stable)	uncontrollable
Operative urgency	elective	emergency	—

Score is the sum of points assigned for each predictor: minimum = 0. maximum = 5.

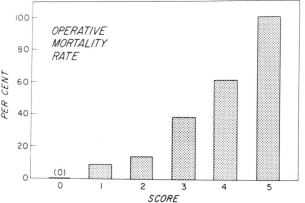

FIG. 3. Mortality rates associated with preoperative score (Table 6).

With Malt's point system, a patient with a bilirubin less than 0.99, no ascites, but uncontrollable bleeding, would have a "predictive score" of one, and less than 10% operative risk. A patient with bilirubin of greater than 2 and uncontrollable ascites, operated upon as an emergency, with a score of five, therefore, would have a 100% operative risk.

R. A. Malt, J. Szczerban, and R. B. Malt, *Risks in Therapeutic Portacaval and Splenorenal Shunts.* Volume XCIV, 1976.

experience of a single expert surgeon may differ from that of surgeons in general (Linton, 1973)." One does not recall whether this statement was made in the oral presentation, if so, it was not challenged.] The physiological status of the patient had more to do with the mortality rate and the incidence of encephalopathy than did the kind of shunt performed. "Preoperative encephalopathy . . . predicts encephalopathy per se rather than operative mortality." They were not able to obtain reliable figures on subsequent episodes of bleeding among the survivors in this retrospective study. "The last review from this hospital found that the incidence and prevalence of gastrointestinal bleeding was greater after splenorenal shunting than after portacaval shunting, but that patients with splenorenal anastomoses tolerated the hemorrhages with less chance of portasystemic encephalopathy." Postoperative encephalopathy increased in frequency as the preoperative predictive score rose, the incidence for splenorenal shunts,- 36%,- and elective portacaval shunts, 46%,- was statistically similar and a figure they considered low. "Eighty-five percent of our surviving patients having had preoperative encephalopathy, had it postoperatively as well. Only 30% of the patients with no preoperative encephalopathy had it later." They summed up as follows, "The totality of data in our study identify no overwhelming balance of one shunt or the other—portacaval or end-to-side splenorenal. An argument could be made in favor of the splenorenal shunt, since patients survived as long as those with portacaval shunts and did at least as well in

terms of encephalopathy despite a longer and more formidable thoracoabdominal operation that per se might be expected to worsen results. Alternatively, since the portacaval anastomosis is easier to do, surer to stop bleeding, and more likely to remain open in the absence of controlled trials, preference for it seems a bit surer except in select circumstances. One of these would be the presence of appreciable hypersplenism . . . because a portacaval anastomosis relieves not more than 60% of cases of hypersplenism associated with portal hypertension." They made no comment about any difference between end-to-side or side-to-side portacaval shunts. They mentioned Inokuchi's coronary-caval shunt, as possibly ideal, but anatomically difficult, and of Warren's shunt said, "Although wholesale endorsement would be premature, the selective or distal splenorenal shunt promises a practical compromise between technical difficulty and excellence of results."

Discussion

The Discussion was opened by Robert R. Linton, of Boston, who prefaced his vigorous disagreement with Malt's paper by saying, "I greatly admire Dr. Malt's skill as a surgeon since he saved my life two years ago after an automobile accident." He decried Malt's emphasis on large caliber portal systemic shunts to prevent recurrent bleeding which completely ignored "the fact that they result in a higher incidence of postshunt encephalopathy and liver failure than smaller caliber shunts." He showed a slide of his own total mortality for five years. In 109 consecutive cirrhotic patients, the mortality was 43% after splenectomies and splenorenal shunts and 64% in 40 patients with end-to-side portacaval shunts. ". . . it is my opinion that what we should be interested in is how long and well are the patients going to live as well as the control of their esophageal varices after shunt surgery . . . if the younger surgeons interested in this symptom complex will learn how to construct these small caliber shunts that I have described, the results will be even better than my splenorenal ones." Donald C. Nabseth, of Boston, emphasized "the importance of an intact clotting mechanism in determining immediate mortality in cirrhotic patients undergoing shunting." In 27 splenorenal shunts they had one operative death and "several close calls from persistent intra-abdominal hemorrhage", all the patients being Child Category B or C, and the survivors subsequently showing no other metabolic defects, so that, "clotting defects, whether existing preoperatively or arising intraoperatively, may be the most important determinant of operative mortality." Dean Warren, of Atlanta, said that, "I actually agree with most of what Dr. Malt says," and devoted most of his discussion to nitrogen metabolism in cirrhosis, and testing with ammonia tolerance curves and blood tyramine levels. He interpreted the Emory experience as supporting "the superiority of portal perfusion of the liver [never once mentioning that he was speaking of his own selective splenorenal shunt], as it relates to chronic systemic encephalopathy and nitrogen metabolism." William V. McDermott, of Boston, on the basis of 500 shunts performed between 1945 and 1974, said, "Our data would tend to agree with Dr. Linton, in that the incidence of encephalopathy is considerably lower, with the splenorenal shunt than it has been with the portacaval shunt, although this perhaps is counter-balanced by the fact that the rebleeding after construction of the splenorenal shunt is considerably higher, perhaps roughly twice that seen in the portacaval." His figures suggested to him that long-term survival was better with the splenorenal shunt, but analysis of preoperative risk factors showed that ". . . the splenorenal group, by chance or by selection, was actually better by these standards than the portacaval; and that probably accounts for the better survival, rather than any intrinsic difference in the shunts themselves." Marshall J. Orloff, of San Diego, said his prospective studies of emergency portacaval shunt performed within eight hours of admission on all bleeding cirrhotic patients "support the conclusions that Dr. Malt presented to us today regarding the predictors of survival." He had found the two most significant factors out of some 70-odd analyzed were the presence of ascites and an SGOT level of 100 or more units, "which was a reflection of acute alcoholic hepatitis and active hepatic necrosis superimposed on chronic cirrhosis." Orloff felt that Malt had not dealt with the question, "Do the large number of so-called poor-risk bleeding cirrhotic patients, including those with ascites or any other predictors of a high mortality rate, have a better chance of survival with portacaval shunt than with any other available form of therapy?" Except in operating for cancer, ". . . in which the recognized high lethality of the disease makes an operative mortality rate of 20% and a 5-year survival rate of 30% quite acceptable, and, in some cancers, really quite excellent . . . surgeons have had almost a reflex abhorrence for an operative mortality rate of 10 to 20% or higher, or a long-term survival rate of less than 60 or 70% . . . cirrhosis with varix bleeding is every bit as lethal as most cancers. Unless the portal hypertension is decompressed, 5-year survival of an unselected population of bleeding cirrhotics is not much more than 5 to 10%. Our studies in 233 unselected patients have shown a 10-year survival with medical treatment of zero, with emergency transesophageal ligation, followed by elective shunt (11%), and emergency portacaval shunt (29%) . . . It is possible by restricting portacaval shunt to only the good-risk patients to obtain a 4 or 5% operative mortality rate and a high long-term survival . . . Dr. Malt and his colleagues did not adopt such a restrictive policy . . . The important objective in the therapy of cirrhosis must be improving the survival of the over-all population with the disease, not selecting a few patients who will have a low operative mortality rate." Malt, closing, declined to joust with Linton saying only, "Dr. Linton is the doyen of portal-hypertension surgery and continues to set the standard to which we aspire." With Nabseth he agreed, "If the patient isn't going to clot, he is not going to survive." Clotting defects were a good predictor, but not as good as some others. Warren had said that in speaking of preoperative encephalopathy he was speaking of chronic encephalopathy. Warren did not consider the patient who developed encephalopathy at the time of a major bleed to have encephalopathy, and Malt made the obvious comment that, "Unless we agree on what we are talking about, we are never going to come to the same conclusions." The SGOT, as Orloff said, was a useful predictor, but again not as useful as the ones they had chosen. His feeling of pessimism is expressed by his concluding statement,

"I am glad that in our hospital the survival rate after medical treatment of ligation of varices is a bit better than it is in California, and that our shunt comparisons don't have to be made with such ominous data. But, certainly, it is true that about 20% 5-year survival rate in untreated patients is the best one can hope for. One could even turn the issue and ask: If the surgical survival rate is only 30 or 40% with all this effort, is that appropriate, or should we be devoting ourselves to some other line of endeavor?"

* * *

Charles Dubost, of Paris, Professor of Cardiac Surgery, Hospital Broussais, [Honorary Member], and by invitation, nine others, *The Surgical Treatment of Constrictive Fibrous Endocarditis*, ascribed the original identification of the condition to Löffler in 1936. The patients had cardiac insufficiency, either right- or left-sided, which proceeded rapidly to death. Angiocardiography showed failure of either or both ventricles to dilate in diastole. Dubost had first operated for this condition in 1971, and now presented a total of five patients. The condition "involved the filling chambers of one or both ventricles, including the papillary muscles and chordae tendinae of the mitral and tricuspid valves" which were usually involved, whereas in none of their cases did the fibrosis involve the atria. "The thickness of the fibrous process varies from 4 to 10 mm. The underlying myocardium presents fibrous lesions which are localized to the subendocardial layer." Involvement of the right side was characterized by "peripheral edema, frequently massive hepatomegaly and ascites." Repeated episodes of pulmonary edema characterized the left-sided form. Auscultation suggested mitral insufficiency and on catheterization, pressures in the atrium and ventricle were equal. "Angiocardiography of the right sided cavities reveals atrial dilatation with stasis of the contrast medium. There is an amputation of the filling chamber of the ventricle with a direct passage between the atrium and the pulmonary artery. On the left side, the ventricular apex is deformed in a characteristic configuration resembling the 'ace of hearts' and there is an associated marked mitral insufficiency with atrial dilatation." Operation, under extracorporeal circulation required atriotomy, excision of the atrio-ventricular valve with its replacement by a prosthesis, and "decortication" of the ventricular wall. "The simplest way to perform the decortication is to resect the mitral apparatus and to incise the fibrous tissue at its junction with the mitral annulus as to find the plane of cleavage between it and the underlying myocardium. The dissection is pursued towards the ventric-

ular apex at first on the posterior wall followed by the anterior wall. It is important to sharply dissect the fibrous bands which join the endocardium shell to the cardiac muscle. Towards the ventricular apex, the adhesions are frequently dense and it is not unusual to find calcifications in this area. At the level of the mitral papillary muscles, it is essential to divide these on their bases which are most often completely fibrotic . . . The mitral valve is then replaced by an artificial valve, either a Starr prosthesis with a silastic ball, a Björk valve, or a heterograft valve." In four patients, the disease was "biventricular" requiring double valve replacements in three and a mitral valve replacement and tricuspid annuloplasty in one. All four did well. A boy with right-sided disease died after 20 months of malfunction of a heterograft valve. Davies had described an endocardial fibrosis in Africans [J. N. P. Davies, 1948] which was probably the same disease as Löffler's fibroplastic endocarditis. The disease could affect Caucasians who "for the most part" had never resided in Africa, "nevertheless, the frequency of the disease in Central Africa has stimulated . . . active epidemiological research, especially in the Ivory Coast."

Discussion

Åke Senning, of Zurich [Corresponding Member], since hearing of Dubost's work the previous fall, had seen and operated upon one patient with the typical left-sided disease. "The mitral valve was replaced and an endocardiectomy was done, as Dr. Dubost had described, and the patient is in very good condition one month later. I think we may find more of these cases . . ." James V. Maloney, Jr., of Los Angeles, said the condition was relatively common in infants, as endocardial fibroelastosis and that, in 1958, his "pediatric cardiologist associate, Dr. Forrest Adams" had tried unsuccessfully to persuade him to resect the endocardium in those children. "We had an epidemic at that time of a disease which we suspected was related to nutritional deficiencies caused by synthetic baby foods. At that time we found, as Dr. Dubost has, that the disease is extremely common in Africa, and is associated with kwashiorkor." Since this valve replacement was not available at that time and would have been necessary, it was probably as well that he had not undertaken the operation. As far as the etiological mechanism was concerned, "In view of the recent work of my associate, Dr. Buckberg, on the demand-supply ratio as a cause of subendocardial necrosis, I think my present speculation would be that this disease is caused by an abnormal demand-supply ratio, probably less than 0.7, related, perhaps, to congenital heart disease, perhaps metabolic deficiency, and perhaps abnormal cardiac function in patients with nutritional disease." Dubost, closing, emphasized "the fact that this disease occurs in both Caucasian and Negro people. The majority of cases occur, probably, in Africa, and for a long time it was believed that Filaria was the cause of the disease, but now it is admitted that this is not true . . . The first description by Löffler of the disease emphasized the importance of the presence of eosinophilia, but . . . eosinophilia very often accompanies many diseases of Africa . . . this disease is of unknown cause . . . occurs in wealthy Caucasians, and in poor Negroes. It makes no difference. It is quite the same, and we had better try to operate on the people early in the evolution of the disease. Now that we know that the disease can be operated, you will find it more often. It looks like a constrictive pericarditis but the angiogram makes the diagnosis different due to the lack of opacification of inflow chambers of the ventricles. So when you see a constrictive pericarditis which is not constrictive pericarditis, it is possibly constrictive endocarditis."

* * *

Marvin M. Kirsh, Douglas M. Behrendt, Mark B. Orringer, Otto Gago, Laman A. Gray, Jr., Lawrence J. Mills, Joseph F. Walter, all by invitation, and Herbert E. Sloan, Jr., of Ann Arbor, Professor of Surgery, University of Michigan Medical School, *The Treatment of Acute Traumatic Rupture of the Aorta:* A 10-Year Experience, had seen 43 such patients in that period, and salvaged 70% of them. Thirty-four of the patients were in automobiles, seven on motorcycles, there was a pedestrian struck by a car, and one had been in an airplane crash. They stressed the meagerness of clinical signs, the importance of radiographic signs, 42 showing a widened mediastinum, 41 an abnormal aortic contour, 14 deviation of trachea to the right, 13 depression of the left main stem bronchus, and 15 a left pleural effusion. Only one patient had shown no radiographic findings. "All but two patients had pseudoaneurysm formation at or near the ligamentum arteriosum." The pseudoaneurysm was located in the descending mid-thoracic aorta in one, in one the aorta was completely obstructed immediately distal to the left subclavian artery. Somewhat more than half of the repairs were with the use of an external shunt "composed of plastic arterial cannulae connected to Tygon tubing" inserted in the ascending aorta and in the distal thoracic aorta. "The aortic tears varied from the small laceration to complete circumferential separation, the latter occurring in 10 patients. Aortic continuity was restored in all patients with a woven graft, even in the cases of incomplete transection." The overall survival in 43 patients was 70%. The mortality in the 37 repaired was seven,- 19%. Five patients died without operation, one in the emergency room, three in the radiology department, and one "8 hours after aortography while awaiting operation." Six of 12 patients with coexisting intraabdominal injuries had celiotomy first,- "Five of the 6 died of exsanguinating hemorrhage from the aortic rupture prior to completion of celiotomy or after celiotomy, but before a thoracotomy could be performed. Retrospectively it was felt that celiotomy could have been deferred in these 6 patients because none of them actually had massive intraabdominal bleeding. In contrast 6 other patients who underwent celiotomy immediately after repair of aortic rupture survived." One patient developed paraplegia.

Discussion

Michael E. DeBakey, of Houston, agreed with Dr. Kirsh in most respects. The patients were most commonly injured in automobile accidents and second most commonly in falls from high construction sites. He agreed that the aorta was best approached by control above and below the aneurysm before approaching the site of rupture. Initially they had used atriofemoral and femoro-femoral bypasses as well as shunts similar to that described by Kirsh but "in the past five years . . . we have discontinued using any of these because we found that we could not reduce our incidence of between 1 and 3% of spinal cord disturbances, particularly paresis or paralysis, by any of the methods we were using. We now approach these lesions directly, applying the occluding clamps, and as expeditiously as possible, repairing the defect. This has provided, as far as we are concerned, equally good results, and I think, probably improves the mortality rate." He gave no overall figures. R. Bryant, of New Orleans, described a 47-year-old man with an aortic aneurysm with calcification, and a history of a serious automobile injury 12 years earlier. They resected the aneurysm, inserting a graft, and the patient did well, but the torn aorta was so firmly healed, that he questioned whether the operation was necessary. William E. DeMuth, of Hershey, emphasized that a number of patients died within minutes of injury, rather than hours. In such, thoracotomy in the emergency room was required. "Several years ago we reported such a patient who was admitted paraplegic with a blood pressure of 50.

We could not hear heart sounds, much less a murmur. We operated upon him immediately without benefit of bypass or shunt, repaired the injured aorta, and within an hour his paraplegia disappeared. We have a healthy truck driver to show for it." Kirsh, closing, said they usually draped the abdomen as well as the chest so that the abdomen could be opened if need be. Alley and others had performed direct anastomoses in ruptured aortas, but the shunts used at Ann Arbor had "prevented adequate mobilization for performing anastomosis." They had known of Dr. DeBakey's resection of thoracic aneurysms without any bypass and the recent report from Alabama and Maryland included 13 patients "who underwent repair of acute transection without the use of shunts and without paraplegia." On the order of 5% of patients with acute aortic rupture went on to chronic aneurysm formation, "these aneurysms do increase in size with time . . . a significant percentage of them rupture, or become symptomatic . . . resection of these chronic aneurysms is indicated."

* * *

Walter P. Dembitsky, by invitation, and Clarence S. Weldon, of St. Louis, Professor, Cardiothoracic Surgery, Washington University School of Medicine, *Clinical Experience with the Use of a Valve-Bearing Conduit to Construct a Second Left Ventricular Outflow Tract in Cases of Unresectable Intra-Ventricular Obstruction,* in two young patients with severe left ventricular outflow tract obstruction encased a rigid metal cylinder in a cloth sleeve, inside and out, for insertion into the left ventricle, attaching the external end to a conventional vascular prosthesis within which was a Hancock porcine valve. The distal end of the prosthesis was delivered through the diaphragm, passed behind the stomach through the transverse mesocolon and sutured to the infra-renal abdominal aorta. The valve was left above the diaphragm in one, below the diaphragm in the other, which was thought to be more satisfactory. Alexis Carrel, in 1910 [see Volume XXVIII, page 423], had attempted a ventricular-aortic shunt and in 1923, Jeger had inserted a valve-bearing conduit which functioned four days in an animal whose ascending aorta had been ligated. Bailey, in 1950 had tried unsuccessfully to create ventricular aortic shunts in dogs with aortic homografts, as had Hufnagel in 1951. Sarnoff, in 1955, reported seven long-term dog survivors with valve-bearing conduits inserted between the apex of the left ventricle and the aorta and Templeton applied the technique clinically some years later in five patients with aortic stenosis,

interposing "a rigid Hufnagel type prosthesis . . . between the apex of the left ventricle and the thoracic aorta". One of them survived 13 years. Bernhard, in 1975, successfully inserted a stainless steel tube for an apical-aortic conduit into a 22-year-old patient, connecting the aortic end of the rigid tube to a porcine, xenograft, glutaraldehyde-treated tissue valve. At the meeting in 1975, Cooley mentioned a patient "in whom he had inserted by direct suture a commercially available Hancock prosthesis between the left ventricle and the supra-renal abdominal aorta", leading to Weldon's interest in the problem. Cooley and Norman had recently reported three more successful cases. The rigid portion of the conduit close to the ventricle was necessitated because, as J. W. Brown had shown [1974], ". . . muscle bundles within the left ventricle will eventually occlude the orifice of a conduit which does not extend into the left ventricular cavity for a minimum of 5 mm. beyond the endocardial surface." In the second patient, they had placed the valve below the diaphragm "because of the strong conviction that no available prosthetic or tissue valve has any durability which approximates normal life expectancy. With the view that such a valve inserted into a child will require replacement in the future, it was felt that such a valve will be more readily accessible when situated in the abdominal cavity. This same reasoning suggests the possibility that apical-aortic shunting may have advantage over valve replacement into the subcoronary position when prosthetic replacement of the aortic valve is required in young children."

Discussion

W. F. Bernhard, of Boston, agreed with "Their use of the left ventricular aortic bypass for unusual left heart obstructive lesions" and agreed also that the apical section of the conduit should be rigid. He showed angiograms of two patients with the porcine valve close to the anastomosis with the thoracic aorta. He was concerned about the suitability of the unstented Hancock graft. One of his patients had developed an obvious diastolic murmur although he remained well. He thought that there was "ample room in the chest for a flexible stent, which would provide support for the commissures and prevent development of xenograft valve regurgitation." John C. Norman, of Houston, agreed that serious problems arose after various operative procedures for "supravalvular, valvular and subvalvular stenoses", and in such patients "following an extended series of bovine experiments lasting in excess of 20,000 hours in approximately 200 calves," they had constructed such double-outlet left ventricles in nine patients. Afterwards ". . . all left ventricular-ascending aortic gradients were markedly reduced, and the deranged left ventricular physiologic indices returned toward normalcy. None of these patients is now receiving Coumadin, and none has exhibited any deleterious effects from the fractionation of the left ventricular output, cephalad and caudad." Their prosthesis was a rigid inlet tube of pyrolytic carbon "with a left ventricular apical sewing ring of Teflon, and a low-porosity graft extension anastomosed beneath the diaphragm to a Hancock prosthesis . . . in turn . . . anastomosed to the supraceliac abdominal aorta." The results in seven of the nine patients were good. The Houston group agreed the Hancock valve should be below the diaphragm. They differed from Bernhard ". . . we have found that the orientation of the apex varied from patient to patient and many times rested on the diaphragm. In some of our partial artificial heart (ALVAD) clinical trials, which we have also begun during the past year, we have found that it is difficult to achieve good cardiac hemodynamics if the left ventricular apex is dislocated by the prosthesis angulating toward the thoracic aorta . . . the left ventricle functions best when its

apex is returned to its anatomic position." They were sufficiently enthusiastic about the procedure to say that "In certain instances, this approach may have advantages over conventional primary aortic valvotomy in infants or valve replacement in adults." Weldon agreed that the design of the prosthesis was certainly not yet complete. The Hancock valve did need support, and taking note of the Houston to St. Louis ratio of nine cases to two, commented "If anybody in the audience missed my acknowledgement of our debt to Drs. Bernhard, Cooley, and Norman, I'd like to re-emphasize it. We, as always, stand in awe of how quickly Dr. Cooley can amass a sizeable clinical trial."

* * *

Donald L. Paulson, of Dallas, Clinical Professor of Thoracic and Cardiovascular Surgery, University of Texas Health Science Center; Chief, Thoracic Surgery, Baylor University Medical Center, and by invitation, Joan S. Reisch, *Long-Term Survival after Resection for Bronchogenic Carcinoma*, presented his personal results in 915 resections for bronchogenic carcinoma over the 25 years, 1945-1969. These patients had been selected from a group of 2,393 with bronchogenic carcinoma, of whom 1,156 [48%] were

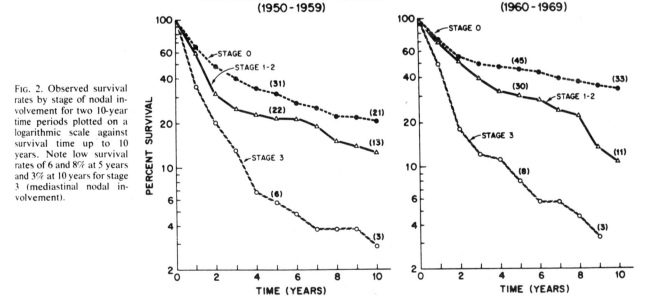

FIG. 2. Observed survival rates by stage of nodal involvement for two 10-year time periods plotted on a logarithmic scale against survival time up to 10 years. Note low survival rates of 6 and 8% at 5 years and 3% at 10 years for stage 3 (mediastinal nodal involvement).

Hilar node involvement. The middle line (Stage 1-2) yielded somewhat poorer survivals than was seen in patients with no involvement of hilar nodes; but mediastinal node involvement, the lower line (Stage 3) showed the poorest survival, 6% to 8% at 5 years,- 3% at 10 years.
Donald L. Paulson, Joan S. Reisch, *Long-Term Survival after Resection for Bronchogenic Carcinoma*. Volume XCIV, 1976.

operated upon, and 1,237 [52%] considered inoperable. Nine-hundred-and-fifteen,- 79%,- of the patients operated upon, had resections, and 241 operations [21%] were simply exploratory thoracotomies. The resection rates of those operable had risen from 61% in 1945-49, 75% in 1950-59, to 90% in the period 1960-69, without change in operative mortality. The operation had changed. In the period 1945-49, lobectomies were only 28% of the operations, 57% in the 50's and 74% in the 60's. The overall surgical mortality for all resections was 6%, for lobectomy 4%, and pneumonectomy 9%. "In the interest of the quality of survival, lobectomy, when applicable, has been considered the operation of choice for both peripheral and central lesions, depending on the location, stage and extent of involvement and objective evidence of benefit to survival. Pneumonectomy has been reserved for the more extensive lesions, with nodal involvement." The survival rates for lobectomy performed in 1945-49 were five years, 19%; ten years, 11.5%; and 15 years, 11.5%. Lobectomies in the 50's yielded survivals of 28%, 20%, and 14.5% and in the 60's, 41%, 28%, and 19%. The survivals for pneumonectomy failed to show any significant improvement in the two time periods, with 15% at five years, 8% at ten years, and 6% at 15 years. The reason for the improvement in survival in successive time periods is plain. "The concept of selectivity for operation, based on complete pretreatment evaluation of the patient, has resulted in improved resection rates and survival figures . . . Resection rates improved from 61% to 90% and the percentage of lobectomies from 28% to 74%." Tumors arising in or beyond the segmental bronchi showed nodal involvement much less frequently, and were more commonly treated by lobectomy than tumors arising in the principal bronchi, but there was no difference in survival for patients with central or peripheral lesions. In patients without nodal involvement and having lobectomy, survivals at five years were 45% for those with central lesions, and 42% with peripheral lesions. In pneumonectomies, the corresponding figures were 21% and 16%. If there was nodal involvement, the survival figures were similar for central and peripheral lesions. Paulson noted, ". . . the highly significant association between histologic type and mediastinal node metastases. In both small cell undifferentiated and adenocarcinoma, a much higher percentage of mediastinal node involvement was found than in epidermoid carcinomas." Between five and ten years after operation, 30% of the patients "died of metastases from the original lesions. After ten years, 41 of 50 patients (82%) died of competing risks other than lung cancer."

Discussion

A. P. Naef, of Lausanne, Switzerland, in 435 pulmonary resections for bronchogenic carcinoma, had mortalities of 8.2% for pneumonectomy, 2.5% for lobectomy, 2.3% for segmentectomy, and 3.4% for sleeve resection. Even wedge resections, which he called "economic resections", had their place. Dr. Davila, of Detroit, cited 6,900 autopsies in a study in which it was found that "among those who had carcinoma of the lung, 51% had lesions in the brain. A number of these were isolated, single lesions in locations which he proposed might be removable." At the Henry Ford Hospital, Knight had 22 patients with carcinoma of the lung and "solitary intracranial metastases either at the time of their thoracotomy or subsequently." 99% survived thoracotomy after craniotomy, with "excellent" symptom-free interval. There were only three survivors of patients having first the craniotomy and then a thoracotomy, but the symptom-free interval in the others had been worthwhile. Mortality in the craniotomies was less than 4%. C. Barber Mueller, of Hamilton, Ontario, presented an analysis very similar to that which he had presented for carcinoma of the breast the year before, and with the same pessimistic note. At Hamilton, Ontario, he and Dr. Herbert Sullivan had collected 594 cases of cancer of the lung. "Three and a half years later, after the last case had been entered, every case was identified as to status, alive or dead, and dead of what cause. Every patient was found. There were none lost to follow-up." It was found that in six months, half the men had died, in a group whose expected longevity was 14 years. Of the entire group, "96% died of their cancer, and another 2.5% died with those physicians who cared for them believing that cancer was a contributory cause." Paulson, closing, went into some detail over the studies of Bergh and Scherstein, and Carlens, in Sweden, concerning the type of nodal involvement "ipsilateral or contralateral . . . perinodal (extracapsular) or intranodal . . . No patient with perinodal involvement lived over two years after resection . . . Survival at 3 years with . . . ipsilateral and intranodal, was better than 50% . . ." Carlens had suggested that contralateral, perinodal involvement should be considered inoperable. In Paulson's series "Only 13 cases (6-8%) with mediastinal node involvement survived 5 years . . . and all of these were ipsilateral, at a low level, and in retrospect we would interpret them as being intranodal. Only 3 such cases survived 10 years, and two cases, 15 years." To Mueller, he had to say, essentially, ". . . that I am a surgeon, and thinking positively, we

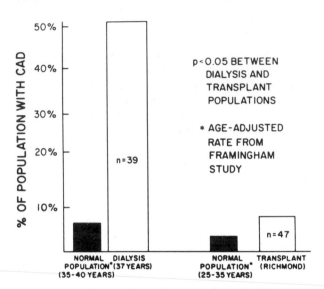

FIG. 2. Comparative rate of clinical coronary disease in U.S. populations at-risk for 10 years.

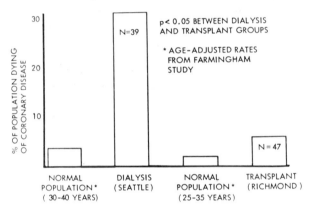

FIG. 3. Comparative death rates from coronary heart disease in U.S. populations at-risk for 10 years.

Arteriosclerotic disease incidence and coronary artery disease in particular was higher in the long-term transplant population than in the normal population, but strikingly lower than in the long-term dialysis population, coincident with a decrease in hyperlipidemia and hypertriglyceridemia, and a sharp decrease in the frequency of hypertension.

F. T. Thomas and H. M. Lee, *Factors in the Differential Rate of Arteriosclerosis (AS) between Long Surviving Renal Transplant Recipients and Dialysis Patients.* Volume XCIV, 1976.

have presented a series of pulmonary resections performed selectively for bronchogenic carcinoma with good long term results."

* * *

F. T. Thomas and H. M. Lee, by invitation, from the Medical College of Virginia, *Factors in the Differential Rate of Arteriosclerosis (AS) between Long Surviving Renal Transplant Recipients and Dialysis Patients,* addressed themselves to the differential survival of renal transplant patients and patients undergoing long-term dialysis. Both the Colorado group and the Richmond group had ten-year survivorships of 45 to 55% of renal transplantations, and from those two groups alone, over 100 patients were entering their second post-transplant decade. "The large majority of these patients have excellent renal function and their life and health are largely threatened by non-renal disease including hepatic disease, cardiovascular disease, non-renal infections and malignancy." They compared their 82 five-year transplant patients with 38 long-term dialysis survivors, most of them from Scribner's group in Seattle. Of the 82, five to 13 years post-transplant survivors, 68 had survived a mean of 9.28 years. The 14 patients dying after five years all had complete autopsies. "The results suggest that long-term transplant patients suffer arteriosclerotic complications at a rate higher than the normal age-adjusted population but far lower than comparable dialysis populations reported from other centers." At mean follow-up of ten years, "only 2% of recipients had died of arteriosclerotic complications", an annual rate of attrition of 0.2%. Starzl's Denver series was similar,- beyond ten years post-transplant the arteriosclerotic related risk was 1.21% per year, and there had been only two arteriosclerotic deaths in patients transplanted prior to 1965. Whereas Scribner's Seattle group "reported an especially high incidence of arteriosclerosis in female dialysis patients at long-term follow-up of about 50%", in the Richmond transplant series "no arteriosclerotic complications during a mean at-risk period of 10 years was seen in the female population" so that ". . . the female transplant population may be especially well-favored over a 10-year period." Correction of the data for sex and age did not significantly affect the differences, nor were there obvious differences in patient selection. Most patients on dialysis had hypertension. Most transplant patients were hypertensive before transplantation and for the first two years thereafter, when the hypertension began to ameliorate and "At 5 years post-transplant, only 17% of patients are hypertensive and by the 7th post-transplant year over 90% of patients are normotensive with less than 15% . . . on anti-hypertensive medications. At present, we achieve an 80% incidence of normotension by 2 years by use of anti-hypertensive agents so that both our current transplant population as well as these early recipients experienced normotension throughout most of their post-transplant course." The nephrectomies performed on the transplantations "may have been a factor in the high incidence of normotension seen." Whereas other groups had reported that the hypertriglyceridemia of renal failure was not modified by successful renal transplantation, the Richmond group had found the triglyceride levels to be normal in 77% of recipients five years post-transplantation. Most of the other studies had determined the triglyceride levels in the first two years post-transplantation. More than half of the Richmond patients had tended to be hyperlipemic for two to five years post-transplant when, in some 80% of patients, the serum lipids tended to return to normal levels, and at ten years 85% of the patients had normal lipid levels. They pointed out that "A long standing policy of minimizing steroid doses post-transplant has been in force in the Richmond unit for at least 10 years. This policy was developed as a result of the basic tenet that a large proportion of post-transplant complications are due to steroids and the feeling that a state of iatrogenic Cushing's disease . . . was associated, per se, with a 50% mortality over a 5-year period." Their steroid dosage was half that of the patients in two studies reporting a high rate of hyperlipidemia after transplant. They concluded that ". . . these results suggest that the superior survival of transplant patients over dialysis patients already evident at the 10-year mark will widen further during the second post-transplantation decade . . . No major risk factor appears on the horizon for the transplant recipient at the 10-year follow-up . . . We predict that the transplant recipient entering the second post-treatment decade will enjoy a favored survival in contrast to his dialysis counterpart and that a major factor in this favorable outlook will be a relatively low rate of arteriosclerotic complications as follow-up progression enters the second decade."

Discussion

Richard L. Simmons, of Minneapolis, saying ". . . the rest of the transplant world is still playing variations on the themes elucidated at Richmond" went on to comment about "the special case of the juvenile diabetic, who seems to die almost 100% of the time after the first two years on hemodialysis . . ." One hundred and seventy-eight of 198 diabetic transplant patients were alive at least four years and only 10% "who survived the first three years have since died",- 20 patients,- of whom only six died of atherosclerotic disease. "This should be compared with the high incidence of cardiovascular deaths reported by Dr. Scribner." Looking at the entire population of 571 patients transplanted since 1968, there was only one fatal myocardial infarct in the 436 non-diabetics, a 9.6% incidence of myocardial infarction in the diabetics and a 6.7% incidence of fatal infarctions. Strokes, for the most part due to cerebral aneurysms, affected 2.5% of non-diabetic patients and 2.9% of diabetic patients. Peripheral vascular disease had not caused any limb loss in non-diabetics, but in the diabetics, 18 fingers, eight toes and 11 lower extremities had been lost. Richmond and Minneapolis saw fewer cardiovascular complications than other transplant centers and he wondered whether there was a population selection problem. Richard E. Wilson, of Boston, wanted to know whether this was a reversal of arteriosclerosis or a prevention of progression. He asked, "What is the relationship of the length of dialysis to the lethality of arteriosclerosis? . . . how many of those long term patients had other factors . . . such as hyperparathyroidism?" Jay C. Fish, of Galveston, Texas, also suggested that patient selection might have been the basic factor in the differential rate of arteriosclerotic deaths. In their home dialysis program, they had an eight-year mortality rate of 20% or 2.5% per year, one third of the deaths being due to the consequences of arteriosclerosis,- a death rate from arteriosclerosis of 0.8% per year. Lars-Erik Gelin, of Göteborg, Sweden, said they had a yearly mortality among transplant patients of 4 or 5%, and in Europe, the annual death rate from dialysis was 10%, the major cause of death in both cases being cardiovascular. He suggested that "this progressive cardiovascular disease is related to a metabolic disturbance evoked during the uremic period, rather than to the immunological situation of the transplanted patient or to the immunosuppressive medication. The secondary hyperparathyroidism of uremia might very well constitute such a relationship." Thomas, closing, was pleasantly surprised that the Minnesota results in the diabetics, with respect to arteriosclerosis, were so good. He agreed with the implication of Wilson's point that the relative advantage seen in transplantation over dialysis, was "not a reversal of arteriosclerosis, but, rather, a prevention of further progression by elimination of two very high risk factors." He did not think the length of dialysis or patient selection was a factor. He had no data about the role of parathyroid disease but agreed that it deserved study. In regard to Fish's comments, he said, "There are many different figures for survival at various dialysis and transplant centers. I think . . . our feeling has grown more over the years that the figures which are most meaningful are those which are actual figures observed over an actual per-

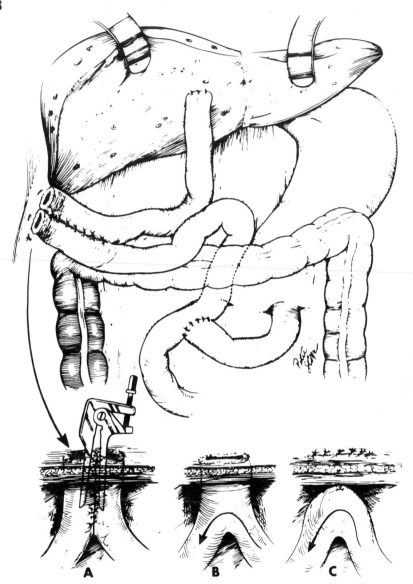

FIG. 1. Illustration of modified hepatic portoenterostomy procedure employing a Mikulicz anastomosis in the Roux-en-Y intestinal segment. Insets show subsequent management of Mikulicz enterostomy.

Lilly had modified Kasai's operation by introducing the Roux-en-Y and temporary Mikulicz enterostomy of the extrapolated loop draining the liver in the hope of avoiding cholangitis which was common when the liver was drained directly into the alimentary stream. There were no operative deaths in their 16; five infants never drained bile, 11 drained bile but four of these had progressive cirrhosis, and the other seven had large firm livers. Their longest good result thus far was in one child who at four years showed "no apparent stigmata of his disease".

John R. Lilly and Norman B. Javitt, *Biliary Lipid Excretion after Hepatic Portoenterostomy.* Volume XCIV, 1976.

iod of time, and not actuarial statistics", and the only two groups which had long-term figures large enough to achieve statistical significance were Starzl's and their own and they were in agreement.

* * *

John R. Lilly and Norman B. Javitt, by invitation, from the University of Colorado, *Biliary Lipid Excretion after Hepatic Portoenterostomy,* performed the procedure in 16 infants since 1974 [Kasai, of Japan, in 1968, first made available, in English, the operation of hepatic portoenterostomy, (dissection of the porta hepatis until frozen section confirmed the presence of tiny ducts, then anastomosis to the bowel) which he had been performing for infants with biliary atresia. The operation had met with great skepticism in the United States, but among others, Lilly and Bill had expressed some optimism]. The biliary tract was drained out to the wound through an extrapolated loop brought out in gunbarrel fashion with the loop connecting to the Roux-en-Y intestinal reconstruction so that the fistula could be readily closed by the Mikulicz technique. They hoped in this way to avoid cholangitis and utilized the total biliary fistula to study the hepatic output. Eleven of the patients had sustained bile drainage with progressive increase in bile volume and the concentrations of bilirubin and biliary lipid in the excretions correlated well with the subsequent return toward normal. There were no deaths, five infants never drained bile. Despite the bile drainage, four patients had progressive cirrhosis, manifested by hepatosplenomegaly and ascites, and one of them had esophageal variceal bleeding. Livers of the other seven were all enlarged and the two that had been biopsied showed continuing, but lesser degrees of hepatic fibrosis than before operation. Lilly and Altman had said [1975] "the reason for the unpredictable outcome of surgery was that biliary atresia was an ongoing obliterative process of varying severity involving both the intra and extra hepatic bile ducts . . . hepatic portoenterostomy would relieve simply one manifestation of the disease . . . extrahepatic biliary obstruction, and would not affect the . . . course of the intrahepatic process." Lilly felt his present findings supported that concept.

Discussion

Eric W. Fonkalsrud, of Los Angeles, agreed, "It is becoming increasingly apparent that we should consider biliary atresia as a form of perinatal sclerosing cholangitis, rather than congenital malformation . . . there is almost never a dilatation of the intrahepatic ducts above the obstruction in patients with extrahepatic atresia, perhaps because of this inflammatory reaction in the liver." What was the rationale for the success of portoenterostomy, "if the intrahepatic ductal system is not patent at the time of operation." Two of his own patients over four years of age had clear sclerae and low serum bilirubins, "but very large livers and . . . some ascites." Alexander H. Bill, of Seattle, likewise accepted the cholangitis, atresia, cirrhosis sequence. He held in addition that "there have been 5 or 6 well-authenticated cases in which babies have been explored for biliary atresia, and found to have normal cholangiograms with open ducts, and they have had hepatitis. Those 5 or 6 children have died of biliary atresia, proven at autopsy." Lilly, closing, said, "Rose bengal studies in patients with sustained bile drainage have shown good excretion of the isotope into the gut after surgery. Transhepatic cholangiography has been successful in about 25% of the cases, and has shown a patent bilio-enteric anastomosis." Long-term outcome would depend upon "the sever-

ity of the residual liver damage." He agreed that there was ongoing inflammatory disease of the bile ducts.

* * *

Charles F. Frey, by invitation; Charles G. Child, III, of Ann Arbor, Professor of Surgery, University of Michigan School of Medicine; Director of Surgery, Wayne County General Hospital; and William J. Fry, of Dallas, Professor and Chairman, Department of Surgery, University of Texas [where he had only recently transferred from Michigan], *Pancreatectomy for Chronic Pancreatitis,* presented their results in 149 patients who had had pancreatectomy for pancreatitis. "Nineteen patients underwent pancreaticoduodenectomy; seventy-seven, 80-95% distal resection; and fifty-three, 40-80% distal pancreatic resection. There were 3 operative deaths and 30 late deaths 6 months to 11 years post pancreatectomy." Over the years, splanchnicectomy had been discarded because with time the pain recurred. Sphincterotomy or sphincteroplasty "once widely applied by Doubilet" had been confined to a very narrow group of patients, and "the use of longitudinal pancreaticojejunostomy [Puestow] is restricted to patients with multiple sites of stricture in a dilated pancreatic ductal system . . . In recent years, the operations most commonly employed in the management of chronic pancreatitis and its complications have been proximal or distal resection of the pancreas as practiced by Guillemin, Mercadier, Leger, and Child, or a procedure to drain a dilated ductal system or pseudocyst." There was enough experience now to define the role of each of the procedures in the management of chronic pancreatitis. Of the 63 patients with a history of pseudocyst, 36, who had had 55 prior operations, underwent pancreatectomy because of recurrence of the cyst, for pain, or for hemorrhage. The other 27 patients with pseudocyst underwent pancreatectomy as a primary form of treatment,- seven for an acute hemorrhage into the cyst demonstrated arteriographically. Of the 86 patients without a pseudocyst, 41 undergoing pancreatectomy had had 61 prior operations. "The choice between pancreaticoduodenectomy or distal pancreatectomy was based on the principal site of inflammation whether proximal or distal in the gland, the size of the common bile duct, the inability to rule out carcinoma and the patency and size of the pancreatic duct." Recently, operative pancreatography had been performed routinely. In the 19 pancreaticoduodenectomies, there was one operative death and two late deaths. Just under half the patients were alive and working well. In the 53 patients who underwent 40-80% distal resection, there was one operative death, four late deaths not a result of the pancreatitis, four late deaths related to pancreatitis. A little over 50% were alive and working well. Of the 77 patients undergoing 80-95% distal resection, one died of operation, nine late deaths were unrelated to pancreatitis, and 11 related to pancreatitis. Just under 50% were alive and working well. The non-alcoholic patients did much better than the alcoholic patients. Diabetes occurred more than twice as often after 80-95% distal resection, as after 40-80% resection or pancreaticoduodenectomy. Steatorrhea was most troublesome after pancreaticoduodenectomy and least after 40-80% resections. Patients with 80-90% distal pancreatic resection had the most marked weight loss. "Eighty to 95% pancreatectomy is technically a much easier procedure to perform but is much more radical than pancreaticoduodenectomy in the mass of pancreatic tissue excised and the high incidence of exocrine and endocrine insufficiency which results. The incidence and severity of diabetes, steatorrhea, peptic ulcer disease, pre and postoperative weight change, and late deaths are all sequelae which adversely reflect on the usefulness of the 80-95% resection for control of pain . . . we are now more conscious of the desirability of conserving pancreatic tissue and avoiding imposition of a diabetic state on a group of mostly alcoholic patients who do not adhere to a regular diet or follow instructions regarding their insulin regulation . . . the institutionalization of 4 patients with organic brain damage from problems associated with insulin management justifies our skepticism as to the capacity of the alcoholic to manage his diabetes . . . we tend to recommend pancreaticoduodenectomy when the major site of inflammation is in the head and uncinate process of the pancreas . . . believe that a major distal pancreatectomy under these circumstances is ill advised, particularly if the patient is an alcoholic . . . We see no major advantage to longitudinal pancreaticojejunostomy when compared with 40-80% distal pancreatic resection."

Discussion

Hiram C. Polk, Jr., of Louisville, discussed the importance of preoperative knowledge of duct anatomy by endoscopic retrograde pancreatography. Lester F. Williams, of Boston, added "In those patients with severe pancreatitis who can be shown *not* to have a pseudocyst or a dilated duct that is amenable to some sort of drainage procedure, is it not reasonable to do resection earlier than we have done?

. . . What role should the presence of nutritional depletion . . . play in the definition of severe pancreatitis? . . . does this suggest a need for resection when dilated ducts or pseudocysts cannot be drained?" William H. ReMine, of Rochester, Minnesota, rose "to support Dr. Frey in everything he said." In their figures, 85% of good results was obtained for resection of the tail or tail and body, and about the same for internal drainage of the pseudocyst. They had performed the Whipple operation only seven times with five good results, ". . . an operation that should be strictly confined to those lesions directly involving only the head of the pancreas." Total pancreatectomy was performed only three times with one good result. The long-term patients ultimately become diabetic even if not diabetic at first after operation. How did Dr. Frey manage ". . . the stump of the pancreas following distal resection?" Kenneth W. Warren, of Boston, agreed that the operation should be tailored to the patient and they had done 180 Whipple procedures for chronic relapsing pancreatitis at the Lahey Clinic, and "today, with a large, dilated duct . . . we're doing fewer of these . . . yet it does have a place." William P. Longmire, Jr., of Los Angeles, said for a time they had been resecting the disease, "Recently our attempts have been directed more toward trying to preserve the function of the gland, and to improving the drainage procedures, so that we can eliminate the extensive resections that we have previously been performing." He agreed with Dr. Polk about the usefulness of retrograde endoscopic pancreatography in performing "lateral pancreaticojejunostomy". He emphasized, "the importance of opening the branch of the duct of Wirsung that passes into the uncinate process . . ." In addition, he performed a duodenotomy and sphincterotomy removing all the calculi from the duct, performing a sphincteroplasty and pancreaticojejunostomy in the same patient. Maurice P. Mercadier, of Paris, France, had treated some 600 cases of pancreatitis over 23 years. He preferred pancreatectomy because "of the impossibility of draining the duct system by means of an anastomosis between the duct of Wirsung and a part of the digestive tract", and because of the late stage of the disease he usually saw. Operations of choice were "distal pancreatectomy when the sclerosis is at the tail of the pancreas, or left hemipancreatectomy when the tail and the body are involved . . . very rare; proximal pancreatectomy by Whipple's operation when the sclerosis is located at the level of the head of the pancreas." For distal or hemipancreatectomy, he generally added a Roux-en-Y loop of the pancreas to the jejunum. The all but total pancreatectomy he found more difficult to perform than total pancreatectomy, but on the basis of the complications of the "diabetes and hypoglycemia, steatorrhea and weight loss, malnutrition and even tuberculosis" in the alcoholics he had "reached the point where I consider total pancreatectomy an unwise operation." Frey, closing, agreed about the value of preoperative retrograde pancreatography, agreed with Williams about the value of an elemental diet or parenteral hyperalimentation in the preoperative management of patients. He would not favor earlier operation. In the 40-50% resections, they usually ligated the pancreatic duct and sewed the end of the pancreas over it. In nearly 95% resections, they merely ligated the duct. They did not implant the end of the pancreas into the bowel in either case. They performed a truncal vagotomy and pyloroplasty in patients known to be hypersecretors.

* * *

The interest in parietal cell vagotomy had spread from Europe. It was agreed that the procedure was the least hazardous ulcer operation, but there was uneasiness about the end results. G. A. Hallenbeck, of La Jolla, Chairman, Department of Surgery, Scripp's Medical Group, and, by invitation, J. J. Gleysteen, J. S. Aldrete, R. L. Slaughter, from the University of Alabama School of Medicine, Birmingham; *Proximal Gastric Vagotomy:* Effects of Two Operative Techniques on Clinical and Gastric Secretory Results, had operated upon two series of patients by proximal gastric vagotomy. In the first series, A, of 39 patients, Hallenbeck cleared only the distal 2 cm. of the esophagus, as well as the entire lesser curvature of the stomach down to the "crow's foot", preserving the nerves of Latarjet. In the second series, B, as a result of persistent or recurrent duodenal ulcers in the first series, he modified his procedure by clearing the distal 5 to 7.5 cm. of the esophagus of any possible nerve fibers,- 19 patients. The patients were similar in all respects. 15% of patients in series A had proven duodenal ulcer in follow-up, 6% of those in series B. Follow-ups were, however, somewhat longer in series A. Insulin tests

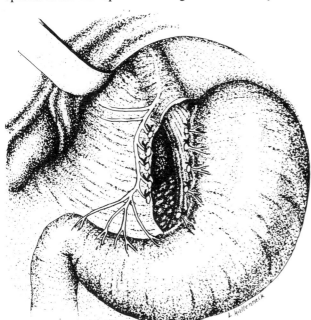

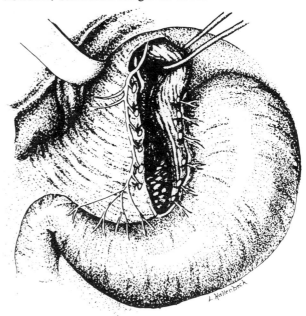

FIG. 1. Proximal gastric vagotomy as performed in Series A (see text). The periesophageal dissection is limited to the distal 1 or 2 cm of the esophagus.

FIG. 2. Proximal gastric vagotomy as performed in Series B (see text). The distal 5 to 7.5 cm of esophagus is skeletonized.

Figure 1: Group A Patients. Hallenbeck cleared only 1 or 2 cms. of esophagus of vagal nerve fibers, preserving the nerves of Latarjet and denervating the lesser curvature down to the "crow's foot" as shown in his Figure 1. 17 patients, duodenal ulcer proved in 15% on follow-up.

Figure 2: Series B,- The operation modified only by clearing 5 to 7.5 cm. of esophagus of vagal fibers. The result of the additional esophageal dissection was a sharp improvement in results,- 19 patients, 6% proven ulcers.

G. A. Hallenbeck J. J. Gleysteen, J. S. Aldrete, R. L. Slaughter, *Proximal Gastric Vagotomy: Effects of Two Operative Techniques on Clinical and Gastric Secretory Results.* Volume XCIV, 1976.

after series A often showed incomplete vagotomy, and rarely did in series B. There was good correspondence between the "postoperative acid secretory response to insulin-hypoglycemia and recurrent ulceration . . ." Hallenbeck remained cautious in his final appraisal, "Although most of our patients with recurrent ulceration, as well as some who have not yet experienced recurrence, retained high acid secretory responses to hyperglycemia indicating inadequate vagotomy and although it is logical to propose that the incidence of recurrent ulceration should be greater in these patients than in those with adequate vagotomy, other factors such as obstruction and the as yet unmeasurable individual resistance to peptic ulceration must be involved as well." He emphasized the need for "standardized operative techniques if results of PGV done by various workers are to be comparable."

Discussion

J. Lynwood Herrington, Jr., of Nashville, said that he and John Sawyers had been performing their dissections high on the esophagus from the first, and emphasized the "criminal nerve" of Grassi which had to be excised on the splenic side of the esophagus. Herrington and Sawyers, together with Hallenbeck and Woodward of Gainesville, had been "randomizing vagotomy-antrectomy" with parietal cell vagotomy over some 30 months. Sawyers and Herrington had done 68 parietal cell vagotomies with no deaths and no recurrent ulcer in the 34 months, and in another series, they were comparing gastric-selective vagotomy and parietal cell vagotomy. There had been no deaths in any, dumping had occurred in 20% of patients with antrectomy and truncal vagotomy, 26% of patients with gastric selective vagotomy and pyloroplasty and in no patients with parietal cell vagotomy, although that group had had 3% incidence of diarrhea. Patients with obstruction, some patients with massive bleeding or large posterior ulcers "do not qualify for parietal cell vagotomy." Had Dr. Hallenbeck employed parietal cell vagotomy for benign gastric ulcer? Considered extending parietal cell vagotomy distally? Paul H. Jordan, of Houston, could "accept as fact that parietal cell vagotomy is associated with fewer side effects than any other gastric procedure for the treatment of duodenal ulcer. However, what value would this be if the recurrence rate was inordinately high . . . to the point of being unacceptable? . . . In our own series of over 150 cases the recurrence rate is now 4%" at four years. They had been denervating the distal 4 cm. of the esophagus, but others had much

higher recurrence rates. Careful studies like Hallenbeck's were necessary to evaluate the procedure. "It is important that this painfully slow, but careful acquisition of data be performed, even if the general application of the operation is delayed. The alternative is that the operation risks being discredited before its maximal potential for the treatment of duodenal ulcer is known." James C. Thompson, of Galveston, Texas, thought the results seemed clearcut, but still a bit early. ". . . it is imperative that this procedure be limited to those centers that are willing to carefully follow their patients by periodic secretory studies . . . to avoid some of the vicissitudes that have followed with the changing fads in ulcer surgery." He urged that the Hollander test be abandoned,- "I know that is heresy",- and any insulin test as well, ". . . it's a hazardous stimulant; there are more than 10 reported cases of death, and for every death reported there may be many more that were not reported . . . the information we get from insulin is readily available from other secretory stimulants. I think pentagastrin and Histalog maximal stimulation tests will give nearly the same information, and with almost no risk at all . . . We have been told that the Hollander test gives an evaluation of the integrity of the vagus nerves, and that's simply not true. If you do a complete antrectomy, without touching the vagi, you will have a negative Hollander test in about 30% of individuals." Kenneth Eng, of New York, said that since 1973 they had performed 30 proximal vagotomies, with no deaths. One patient had failed to show the expected decrease in acid secretion, was reoperated upon, found to have an intact "criminal nerve". Lloyd M. Nyhus, of Chicago, said, "I had the pleasure of watching Dr. Dragstedt perform a truncal vagotomy. He stressed at that time the necessity of meticulous dissection of the lower end of the esophagus to assure total vagotomy. This is the message of Hallenbeck and Goligher. It appears to me that we have come full circle." He reported long-term follow-up studies showing recurrence of ulcer in 28% of patients after truncal vagotomy and drainage, and in less than 2% after truncal vagotomy with antrectomy, "There is little question that the partial gastrectomy protects many patients from the sequelae of incomplete vagotomy. He said this had led surgeons to be careless about their vagotomy technique,- ". . . parietal cell vagotomy must be performed with the same meticulous attention to detail originally taught to us by Dragstedt for truncal vagotomy." Hallenbeck, closing, said he had not employed proximal gastric vagotomy for gastric ulcer, but Goligher, in Leeds, and Hedenstedt, in Stockholm, had employed it with excision or oversewing of the gastric ulcer. He did not see any reason to extend the vagotomy more distally. He agreed with Dr. Thompson about the Hollander test "there is no use using the insulin test at the present time", but he had not known that when starting the study.

* * *

H. Harlan Stone, of Atlanta, Professor of Surgery, Emory University School of Medicine, and by invitation, C. Ann Hooper, L. D. Kolb, C. E. Geheber, and E. J. Dawkins, *Antibiotic Prophylaxis in Gastric, Biliary and Colonic Surgery,* made the sweeping charge, about the problem of the prophylactic use of antibiotics that "Only the animal experiments of Burke and relatively sophisticated clinical trials by Polk, Ledger, and a few others have given any true insight as to the benefits of such a program. All other supportive reports have primarily been emotional claims, based upon either poorly or totally uncontrolled scientific evidence." Over a period of 20 months, 400 consecutive patients "admitted for elective operations of the stomach, biliary tract, and/or colon" had been enrolled in the study. All colon patients received 1 gm. of oral neomycin every four to six hours for two days prior to operation as well as 500 mg. of erythromycin base every six hours for 24 hours before operation. Each patient, including the colon surgery patients "was given an intramuscular injection of either antibiotic (1 gm. of cefazolin) or placebo (equivalent volume of diluent) on the evening before operation, on call to the operating room and on that same evening after return to either the ward or the intensive care unit, on the morning of the day following surgery, and again during the evening of the first postoperative day." A quarter of the patients had their antibiotic initiated 12 hours before operation, a quarter, one hour before operation, a quarter, one hour after operation, and a quarter received no antibiotic at all. The cefazolin levels in the portal vein blood and the peripheral venous blood taken during operation were not significantly different, tissue levels of cefazolin were 40% higher if the drug had been given eight to 12 hours before operation than if it had been started an hour before operation. There was a higher incidence of intraperitoneal sepsis if antibiotics were given only after operation or not at all, particularly in the colon cases, but there was no difference between the 8 to 12 hour preop or one hour preop dose in this regard. Antibiotic given after operation was no better than no antibiotic. The effect on wound infection was strikingly more impressive than the effect on intraperitoneal sepsis. Wounds were cul-

tured at operation. No wounds had culture-proven contamination. Seven percent of those with antibiotic prophylaxis developed wound infection, and 29% of those without antibiotic protection. [Despite the evidence that antibiotic therapy given before operation significantly affected the rate of wound infection, Stone, curiously, restricted his indications for such prophylactic use] "Whenever: 1) the consequences of wound infection are uniformly disastrous, even though the occurrence of this sepsis is uncommon; 2) the incidence of wound infection is great, yet seldom does it . . . threaten life or limb; and 3) the patient has such an extreme impairment in host defense mechanisms that any infection, no matter how minor, has a propensity for becoming systemic and thereby fatal."

Discussion

Paul Nemir, Jr., of Philadelphia, said that they used antibiotics preoperatively in colon surgery, and in major vascular procedures and went on to stress the value of antibiotics in prolonged low-flow states

Table 3. *Wound Infection*

Area of Operation	Antibiotic Begun				Totals
	8–12 hr Preop	1 hr Preop	1–4 hr Postop	Never Given	
Gastric	22	27	24	23	96
Infected	1	1	4	5	11
Incidence	5%	4%	17%	22%	11%
Biliary	29	31	33	38	131
Infected	1	0	3	4	8
Incidence	3%	—	9%	11%	6%
Colonic	54	47	46	43	190
Infected	3	3	7	7	20
Incidence	6%	6%	15%	16%	11%
Totals	100	100	100	100	400
Infected	4	3	14	15	36
Incidence	4%	3%	14%	15%	9%

400 consecutive patients admitted for elective, gastric, biliary or colonic surgery received injection of either a placebo or 1 gm. of cefazolin, at one of the times indicated in the Table, as well as the night after operation and each of the succeeding two days. The colon patients, additionally, received a neomycin-erythromycin preparation. While there was some relation between the time of administration of the first dose of cefazolin, and intraperitoneal infection, the effect on wound infection, as shown in the Table, was striking. This jibed with the observation that tissue levels of cefazolin were 40% higher in those patients receiving the drug 8-12 hours before operation than in those receiving it one hour before operation.

H. Stone, and others, *Antibiotic Prophylaxis in Gastric, Biliary and Colonic Surgery.* Volume XCIV, 1976.

to protect the injured bowel from bacterial invasion. Jere Lord, Jr., of New York, said in "clean arterial surgical procedures and clean major general surgical procedures" they employed lavage of the wound at the beginning and end of the operation. He had now a prospective study underway, but could report an earlier retrospective study with neomycin for two or three years, then kanamycin 0.1% and keflin 0.2%. He had previously observed "that a continuous drip of neomycin solution through an in-dwelling catheter would salvage, occasionally, an infected arterial prosthesis or an infected endarterectomized artery." Prior to 1969, a consecutive series of 400 arterial procedures had resulted in two in-hospital infections and four late infections, three weeks to 10 months after discharge. In 185 consecutive clean major general surgical operations, there had been three in-hospital wound infections. Since they had been using the lavage, there had been 420 consecutive arterial procedures with no in-hospital infections, and one late infection,- after four months. In 215 general surgical procedures since 1971, there had been no in-hospital or late wound infections. Emerick Szilagyi, of Detroit, discussed his 1972 2,125 vascular operations without antibiotic prophylaxis. 75% of the infections originated in the groin wounds and 75% of the infections were *Staphylococcus aureus.* "We adopted a rigorous protocol of antistaphylococcal prophylaxis of pre-, intra- and immediate postoperative intravenous administration of methicillin, very much according to the principles expounded by Burke." He stated positively that "in spite of the universal use of antimicrobial prophylaxis, no properly conducted, i.e., double blind, randomized, prospective study had been published on this problem." Summarizing his own patients, using his own historic controls, with synthetic prostheses the rate of wound infection dropped from 1.7% to .09% with prophylaxis and in venous grafts from 6.4 to 2.0%,- highly significant differences. Both "the results suggest strongly, but cannot be put to proof, that antimicrobial prophylaxis in these cases reduced the incidence of wound infection." Dan W. Elliott, of Pittsburgh, had made a prospective controlled, randomized study of infection after biliary tract surgery, with and without prophylactic cephaloridine. Cephaloridine sharply lowered the incidence of infection after biliary tract operations, but he pointed out that 85% of bile cultures are sterile, and patients with such cultures had a 1% postoperative infection rate or less, whereas "wound infection rates of 27 to 40%, including . . . intraabdominal abscesses and blood stream sepsis occurred in . . . patients with common duct stones, obstructive jaundice of any cause, or

acute infected cholecystitis, operated upon as an emergency." Preoperative antibiotics were of special benefit in such patients. William A. Altemeier, of Cincinnati, referred to the ultraviolet study in which "the incidence of infection for hernioplasty was 1.9 . . . thyroidectomy, 2.2; hysterectomy, after transection of the vagina, was 6.1; cholecystectomy . . . 6.9%; partial colectomy, 10; subtotal gastrectomy, 10.1; appendectomy, 11.4; nephrectomy, 17.3; and radical mastectomy, 18.9." Prophylactic antibiotic therapy was recommended, "In the clean-contaminated type of operation in which the gastrointestinal or respiratory tracts are entered without significant spillage, or with spillage; gastrointestinal and respiratory tracts not entered, when transection of the appendix or cholecystic duct is considered clean-contaminated, in the absence of acute inflammation; entrance into the genito-urinary or biliary tracts in clean-contaminated, in the absence of infected urine or bile; and then, minor breaks in technique . . . a period of 6 hours is critical . . . if antibiotic therapy is delayed for as long as 6 hours, one can anticipate marked reduction in the prophylactic effect—6 hours after contamination of tissues by infecting bacteria." Stone, closing, said to Dr. Nemir that in low-flow states the delivery of the antibiotic is impaired, and that in any case, he wondered whether that was not therapeutic rather than prophylactic. He thought Lord's program of topical antibiotics useful if the antibiotic penetrated the tissues. Dr. Elliott's point was somewhat weakened, he said, by the fact that one does not always know when a cholangiogram is going to show a common duct stone.

* * *

John M. Buckingham, F. M. Howard, by invitation; Philip E. Bernatz, of Rochester, Professor of Surgery, Mayo Medical School; W. Spencer Payne, E. G. Harrison, Jr., Peter C. O'Brien and Louis H. Weiland, by invitation, from the Mayo Clinic and Mayo Foundation, *The Value of Thymectomy in Myasthenia Gravis:* A Computer-Assisted Matched Study, reviewed a series of 563 patients treated for myasthenia gravis without thymoma, of whom 104 had undergone thymectomy. Blalock's 1939 report had initiated the surgical attack on myasthenia gravis by thymectomy, but the results were still in dispute and there had been no randomized prospective study. Their bias was frankly stated, "With the certain knowledge that such a study would not be entertained in our institution and in an effort to improve retrospective review, we have selected matched groups of medically and surgically treated patients with computer assistance." Satisfactorily matching 80 of the operated patients with 80 unoperated patients, they found complete remissions in 27 of the thymectomy patients and only six of the medically treated patients. Of the operated patients, 26 were improved, of the medical group, only 13. There were 21 dead in the surgical group, 11 of myasthenia,- the operative mortality was 6%. Forty-seven of the medical group patients had died, 34 of myasthenia. Deaths in half of the surgical group were due to myasthenia gravis and in three-quarters of the medical patients. "Keynes, of Great Britain, was an early and firm advocate of thymectomy, and Clagett and Eaton, of this clinic, supported the concept" [they did not mention the fact that Blalock after a very energetic program of intervention had lost interest in the operative therapy of myasthenia gravis as being too unpredictable]. The influence of the histology of thymus upon the prognosis had been differently interpreted. MacKay "correlated the presence of thymic follicular hyperplasia with a good response to surgery and its absence to a poor response." Genkins, and Alpert, "found that delayed remission after thymectomy was related to the presence of thymic hyperplasia and that patients with more germinal centers in their thymus survived longer. In our study the longer survival of patients with severe hyperplasia was statistically significant." Previously, reports had suggested that young females with myasthenia gravis of short duration had the best choice of operation, but the present study would suggest "that the guidelines for surgical treatment should be liberalized. The survival of patients 30 years of age or older treated by thymectomy probably does not differ from that of patients 30 years of age or younger, but both groups, regardless of sex, had considerably better survival rates than patients treated medically."

Discussion

Earl W. Wilkins, Jr., of Boston, reporting on the collaborative study between Massachusetts General Hospital and the New York Mount Sinai Hospital group, compared 267 patients undergoing thymectomy to the 417 treated non-operatively, and as in the Mayo Clinic study, none of the patients had thymoma. Improvement in the "medical group" was 28%, in the thymectomized patients over 80%. "Our total of remission or improvement . . . is 76%, which compares very favorably with the figures reported today. Our total death rate is 14%, which, as I calculated from the protocol, was identical with theirs. There is no question that their computerized

study is a far better approach to comparison of the thymectomized and the conservatively treated patients than ours, but I would ask the authors: Is this good enough? Have we totally eliminated bias? Have we totally disproved the possibility—as Henry Beecher, our chief of anesthesia, used to challenge us—'is this a placebo operation?' . . . the time, indeed, has come for a prospective randomized study, and I would suggest that a broad collaborative effort would speed the accomplishment of this information." W. H. Muller, Jr., of Charlottesville, Virginia, accepted that the Mayo Clinic series had shown "survival is significantly longer in patients who have had thymectomy than in those treated medically, and . . . the data just shown by Dr. Wilkins of the combined study of the Mount Sinai Hospital and the Massachusetts General Hospital . . . indicated that the patients treated surgically do much better than those treated medically. All of this is of great importance because of the general dissatisfaction with the results of thymectomy throughout the 1940's and 50's. Dr. Blalock himself felt very confused about this operation some 10 years after he first performed it. In fact, Sir Geoffrey Keynes . . . chided his colleagues by saying: 'There seems to be a tendency among the writers of leading articles in journals of this country to try to discredit the surgical treatment of myasthenia gravis with douches of cold water drawn from the Mayo Clinic cistern . . .' " Keynes' remission rate at that time was about 41%, Blalock's, in Baltimore, and Clagett's at the Mayo Clinic, were 8 to 15%. Muller's group had found the use of large dose corticosteroid therapy along with cholinesterase inhibitors, brought the patients to operation almost at a normal state and largely eliminated the morbidity and mortality. "We believe that nearly all myasthenic patients should have thymectomy, and that virtually all will develop remission, if one waits long enough. That may be as long as 10 years, until the long-lived thymocytes, which have been shown by immunofluorescent studies to persist for quite long periods of time, disappear, and the immune competence of the B-cells is no longer maintained." Philip E. Bernatz, closing, could only agree that "There is no question that a well-designed randomized prospective study is in order . . ."

* * *

Max R. Gaspar, of Long Beach, Clinical Professor of Surgery, University of Southern California, and by invitation, H. J. Movius, II, J. J. Rosenthal, D. Anderson, *Comparison of Payne and Scott Operations for Morbid Obesity*, compared 45 patients operated upon by the Payne operation with 45 undergoing the Scott operation. Movius performed the Payne procedure, and the others performed the Scott. In Payne's procedure, 14″ of jejunum was joined end-to-side 4″ from the ileocecal valve. In the Scott procedure, 12″ of jejunum was joined end-to-end to the terminal 6″ of ileum and the distal end of the bypassed loop of small intestine vented into the transverse colon or sigmoid. Scott had abandoned the Payne procedure because of inadequate weight loss, "attributing that to hypertrophy, dilatation and elongation of the proximal jejunum and to elongation of the terminal ileum with reflux into the bypassed ileum probably being the most important factor." Starkloff found that with the Payne operation 20% of his patients "reached a weight plateau too early. . . ." Woodward, after initially agreeing, found no difference between the two procedures. Diarrhea usually became tolerable after either operation after two years, without difference between the two procedures, nor were there differences "in the incidence of nausea, vomiting, weakness, loss of sex drive, hair loss, thirst or rectal problems." With the Payne operation, two patients developed urinary calculi, as eight of the Scott patients did. The figures for arthritis were respectively, two and five. "Electrolyte disturbances were frequent in both groups with hypokalemia being most prevalent." There were no in-hospital deaths, but six deaths at home [no statement is made as to which operations were responsible for the deaths]. The weight loss was relatively comparable for the first two years, but the Scott patients lost a little more weight, and after two years, there was more of a tendency for regaining weight in the Payne group. They thought that a 45 cm. total intestine length was appropriate, not more than 15 cm. of ileum nor less than 22 cm. of jejunum. Scott patients did a little better, but the operation took a little longer and was a little more dangerous. They surmised "that the Payne configuration with 30 cm. of jejunum and 10 cm. of ileum might be ideal". The younger patients did better than older ones, and "more intelligent and well motivated patients do better than the less intelligent and less well motivated."

Discussion

J. Howard Payne, of Los Angeles, said that hypertrophy, hyperplasia, elongation of the bowel and reflux in the bypassed segment did occur in certain instances and there might be a weight gain. He showed a slide of extraordinary hypertrophy of the villi of the jejunum ten years after operation in a pa-

tient who had had an inadequate weight loss after his operation and asked why the same thing would not occur after the Scott operation. He thought reflux into the bypassed ileum might prevent anemia or B_{12} deficiency, that about 65% of the patients had a very satisfactory result, and 10% were failures. In general, he had very satisfactory maintenance of large weight losses for many years. H. William Scott, Jr., of Nashville, said after his first 11 Payne operations, he had done 175 by the end-to-end technique to avoid reflux into the bowel and its absorption. He had originally used Payne's 14″ of jejunum and 4″ of ileum, had gone to 12″ and 12″ in his end-to-end anastomoses, dropped down to 12″ and 6″ and reverted to 12″ and 8″. The 12″ and 6″ and 12″ and 8″ patients had "gotten down into a range closer to ideal weight, and have had better results in general." With the shorter lengths, 35% of the patients had had good results. He did not discuss complications. Edward R. Woodward, of Gainesville, said patients with the end-to-side shunt shed 30% of their original weight in 12 months, thereafter some patients became grossly malnourished and others had leveled off at an undesirably high weight. Regaining weight had been uncommon. Reoperation in patients who had failed to lose weight, had been quite unsatisfactory,- "it is purely an empiric operation, and there are some patients who will simply outeat any shunt you put in them." In general, he was satisfied with the end-to-side shunt as to "the functional weight, consistent with reasonable health, adequate drop in serum lipids, adequate control of hypertension, and so on. And we feel that the quicker, simpler operation is adequate." Gaspar, closing, said, "These operations are being done in many community hospitals and often without the team approach which is so necessary. Dr. Payne has estimated that 5,000 to 15,000 such operations have been performed." He had seen elongation and hypertrophy of the jejunum after both operative procedures. It was important to get the patient down to a functional weight rather than an ideal weight. "Although Dr. Scott was not satisfied with the eleven Payne operations which he performed, I thought his patients plateaued out quite well. I believe he abandoned the Payne procedure prematurely."

The Business Meetings

The 1976 meeting was held at the Fairmont Hotel, New Orleans, Louisiana, on April 7, 8, and 9, President James D. Hardy in the Chair.

At the first Business Meeting for the first time

appears notice of the Trustees of the American Surgical Association Foundation,- "The Foundation Trustees, including myself [J. D. Hardy], Dr. Maloney, Dr. Ballinger, Dr. Warren, Dr. Ravitch, Dr. Merendino, Dr. Gerbode, Dr. Alton Ochsner, and Dr. Jonathan Rhoads." At the Business Meeting on the second day, the Secretary, James V. Maloney, Jr., gave the report of Council. At the midwinter meeting the Council had elected to Honorary Fellowship, in accordance with the new procedures, Professor Maurice Paul Mercadier, of Paris, and Professor R. B. Welbourne, of the Hammersmith Royal Postgraduate Medical School, London. Mercadier was in attendance and had been fully introduced by President Hardy at the first Business Meeting. Maloney made a fulsome apology to Mark M. Ravitch for the fact that his paper for this meeting, at the time of the Bicentennial of the United States, which had been commissioned by Council at the 1974 meeting, had been omitted from the program.

Further to obscure the issue, in a delightful monologue, Maloney referred to it as a paper on the history of the American Surgical Association, confusing it with the formal History of the Association that at the Quebec meeting Ravitch had been charged to prepare for the 1980 meeting. [Secretary Maloney] ". . . in some remote past issue of the *Transactions* of this Association, it is recorded that the Council, in anticipation of the Bicentennial Year of this nation, invited the Association's most distinguished historian, Mark M. Ravitch, to devote a period of years preparing a history of American Surgery to be presented at this, the Bicentennial Meeting of the Association. The Secretary of the Association, being unaware of both the invitation and how Dr. Ravitch had spent every waking moment for the past ten years, failed to inform the Program Committee and the printers. We were unaware of this, at least until recently. I recall, as a matter of fact, precisely the moment of awareness. [Laughter] It occurred three weeks ago, about sixty seconds after the postman in Pittsburgh delivered the printed program to Dr. Ravitch's office. [Laughter]

"Now, despite the Council's experience in dealing with delicate matters, this is a situation which was considered a real challenge by Council. Consideration was given to our reading Dr. Ravitch's paper by title, having him present it during the coffee break, [laughter] or to a private audience in the Presidential Suite. [Laughter] All of these alternatives were really considered inadequate to the recognition of Dr. Ravitch's decade of labor.

"It then occurred to the Council that, with ma-

jor surgical events occurring practically daily at the present time, and with the fact that the 200 years are not really up until this coming July 4, Council in what had to be considered a masterstroke of ex post facto reasoning, [laughter] concluded that even though Dr. Ravitch might be willing to speak at this meeting, [laughter] he could not possibly write a history of 200 years of American surgery with the high standards of completeness which are demanded by this Association of its essayists until some time after the national birthday on July 4. [Laughter] Therefore, Dr. Ravitch's special address will appear on next year's program. [Laughter and applause]"

The Secretary also announced that "President Hardy has been in contact with the Director of Philatelic Affairs of the U. S. Postal Service regarding the possibility of a centennial stamp issue honoring American surgery."

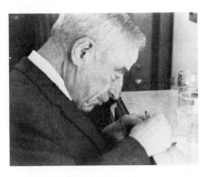

Leo Eloesser, 1881-1976. A. B. University of California, 1906. M.D. Heidelberg, 1907. Trained in Heidelberg, Berlin, London and San Francisco City and County Hospitals, presently becoming Professor of Surgery at Stanford and Chief of the Stanford Service at the hospitals. A small man, he was a great outdoorsman. As his comments at meetings show, he had broad interests in surgery but his special interests were in Thoracic Surgery - the Eloesser operation, a variant of the old Estlander procedure. He had an extraordinary life - a musician and linguist and remarkably independent thinker, he volunteered to help the German war wounded in the First World War, leaving Germany with the sinking of the Lusitania, volunteering in the U. S. Army and becoming Chief of Surgery at Letterman General. He organized and headed a field service unit supporting the Republican Army in the Spanish Civil War and after World War II, served for a time with the Chinese Communist Army. After retiring to Mexico, he returned annually for the meetings of the American Surgical Association and the American Association of Thoracic Surgery. Dr. Bahnson's photo beautifully captures his appearance, his rigid spine hunched forward, the hooded eyes seemingly closed. Yet he was attentive, rose to comment from time to time, sharply and succinctly in a clear and powerful voice, never succumbing to the garrulousness of other oldsters, remembering names, faces, and associations, interested in what was current.

(Photograph courtesy of Henry T. Bahnson, M.D., Pittsburgh)

The Ad Hoc Committee on the advancement of surgical scholarship, Dr. John Najarian, Chairman, suggested, and Council supported, "efforts to obtain funds for a surgical scholarship program permitting promising young surgeons to obtain support to further their careers in academic surgery." Council pointed out that "the current income from dues and initiation fees pays only a portion of the costs of operating the Association, the deficit being made up by officers and members who serve the association both loyally and generously" [see Maloney's report of previous year]. Council recommended increase of the initiation fee from $100 to $300, half to be placed in an endowment fund in the American Surgical Association Foundation, increase in annual dues from $100 to $140, a constitutional amendment requiring Senior Members to pay dues to age 65, rather than 60.

Council was hurriedly recommending elimination from the Constitution of the provision that "Any Fellow who has been a member in good standing for ten years may become a life member of the Association by the payment of two-hundred and fifty dollars."

Members had objected to the travel time involved in getting to the relatively inaccessible Homestead and The Greenbrier. The Secretary was in-

structed to "investigate other resorts which provide similar atmospheres and amenities, but which have immediate access to major airports."

The Constitutional proposal made at the previous meeting, to increase the number of Honorary Fellows to 45 was accepted. 20 new Fellows were proposed and all elected, and 49 new names proposed for consideration for the first time the following year.

The third award of the American Surgical Association Medallion for Scientific Achievement was made to Owen H. Wangensteen; the two previous recipients having been Lester R. Dragstedt and Robert E. Gross.

Officers elected were, Claude E. Welch, of Boston, President; Vice-Presidents, Harwell Wilson, of Memphis, and Carl Schlicke, of Spokane, Washington; Secretary, James V. Maloney, Jr.

It had always been the custom to ask two Fellows to escort the President-elect to the Chair. On this occasion, President Hardy designated as one of these, Leo Eloesser, of Tacambaro, Michoacan, Mexico, Clinical Professor Emeritus of Surgery, Medical Department, Stanford University. Eloesser, a Fellow for just 40 years, then 95 years of age, died before the next meeting.

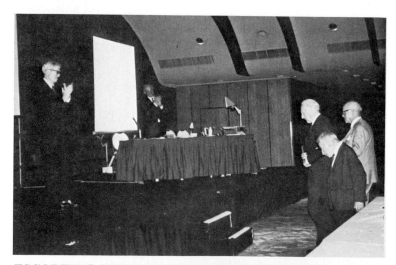

ESCORTING THE NEW PRESIDENT TO THE PLATFORM

1976 – The Fairmont Hotel, New Orleans, La.

By time honored tradition, the single nominee for the office of President, having been named and elected by voice vote [and at least twice, the President has failed to call for the vote], the outgoing President calls on two Fellows to escort the new President to the Chair. Here, President James D. Hardy and Secretary James V. Maloney applaud as newly elected President Claude E. Welch approaches, "supported" by Leo Eloesser and Marshall K. Bartlett. The small screen by the table, at which President or Vice-President, Secretary and Recorder sit, serves for the projection of the names of the essayists and discussers,- written with a wax pencil on clear plastic,- on the projector at right of the table.

Photograph courtesy of Robert S. Sparkman, M.D., Dallas, Texas

XCV

1977

The 1977 meeting was held at the Boca Raton Hotel and Club, Boca Raton, Florida, March 23, 24, and 25, Claude E. Welch, of Boston, Clinical Professor of Surgery Emeritus, Harvard Medical School, in the Chair. Among those who had died in that year were the incredible Leo Eloesser, in his 95th year. A native San Franciscan but a graduate of medicine in Heidelberg and trained principally at Heidelberg under Czerny and others, and at Kiel, he had served in the Medical Corps in the German Army in World War I until the sinking of the Lusitania when he joined the Medical Corps of the United States Army, had served with the Spanish Republican Army in the Spanish Civil War and in both Nationalist and Communist Chinese armies. He had been at the meeting the year before. There had also died, Emile Holman, who had been Halsted's resident at Hopkins. His coming to Stanford in 1926 had ushered in a brillant career for the institution. David H. Patey, of the Middlesex Hospital, the distinguished British Honorary Fellow, had died, whose technique of modified radical mastectomy had been widely accepted.

The Presidential Address, *Surgical Competence in a Changing World,* having gotten over the now almost obligatory annual viewing with alarm, devoted itself largely to the competence and qualifications of surgeons. Board certification and membership in appropriate societies were no longer regarded by the public as sufficient, and indeed "There must be methods by which continuing rather than one-time competence may be assured . . . Continuing competence depends on each individual, but must be supplemented by the efforts of the profession, by government regulations, or by a combination of the two." He spoke of peer review mechanisms, already numerous and said that "*Formal examinations* almost surely will be the method chosen by the Specialty Boards as a basis for recertification just as they have been used for certification in the past. All 22 Specialty Boards have started to implement either voluntary or mandatory recertification." The Medical Societies of 16 states required of their membership evidence of continuing medical education and the legislature of 15 states had passed laws requiring a reregistration "and, as a condition, either specify continuing medical education or give powers to the state boards of registration to demand it if they so desire." State boards of registration had been viewed with "some disdain by the public and by the profession itself" however, they had recently been acquiring new powers and could be enormously important if a Federal Board of Registration was not created. Pressure from the public and from the Massachusetts Medical Society had resulted in the establishment in that state of a new Board of Registration and Discipline in medicine which reregistered physicians every two years, could discipline doctors, "identify and rectify substandard levels of practice and had a broad power to 'adopt rules and regulations governing the practice of medicine in order to promote the public health, welfare and safety' ". There had been established a Joint Underwriting Association for malpractice insurance. Medical tribunals, established to hear all claims of malpractice, had discouraged many complaints and resulted in the dismissal of many others. In a 12-month period, two licenses had been revoked and two other physicians had resigned under pressure. Actions against 25 other physicians were in progress. The Board had established rules and regulations providing for "the yearly requirement that 50 hours of continuing medical education be established as a condition for reregistration . . . the development of a new type of license that restricts the type of practice . . . the construction of an accurate data base that can serve as a directory for health manpower." Statements were under consideration concerning such matters as the practice of acupuncture, regulations governing physicians' assistants, "the performance of specialized procedures such as open heart surgery." Welch listed all of the usual arguments for and against continuing medical education admitting that "absolute proof of the value of CME is hard to substantiate. Yet, after an annual meeting of the American College of Surgeons what person can escape without some visual memory of the method by which a difficult technical problem may be handled or can fail to remember some statements from the platform that change his concepts of proper care?" The problem with the restriction of type of practice had never been squarely faced by the medical profession "it is accepted as a truism that a good surgeon must first be a good physician; on the other hand, it has never been proposed that a good physician must first be a good surgeon." He thought the only way that practice could be logically restricted would be "by peer review of individuals at the local level . . . if the privileges of a person are limited in any one hospital because of lack of training or ability, such restrictions should be applicable to all the hospitals in which he practices. Mandatory reporting of such restrictions to the Board of Registration will indicate the magnitude of this problem; at the present time it is completely unestimated . . ." Restriction of a license by state boards, obviously could be contested on legal grounds but it was thought "if such specifications are established for the benefit of the public, it is unlikely that any appeal on the basis of constitutionality would be effective." Welch had obviously played a key role in these developments in Massachusetts as he intimated, "President Scott has urged this Association to become an organization of political activists [Volume XCI, 1973]. Perhaps this report will serve as a personal testament, proving that each one of us has an individual as well as a collective responsibility. Let us all keep our fingers in the dike."

* * *

[From McGill University, Lloyd MacLean, in 1975, reported in a preliminary study "a significant correlation between altered skin test reactivity (anergy and relative anergy) and subsequent development of sepsis and related mortality."] Now, with five associates, *Delayed Hypersensitivity: Indicator of Acquired Failure of Host Defenses in Sepsis and Trauma,* Lloyd D. MacLean, of Montreal, Surgeon-in-Chief, Royal Victoria Hospital; Professor and Chairman of Surgery, McGill University, presented the results of a detailed investigation in 354 patients from the surgical wards and the Surgical Intensive Care Unit of the Royal Victoria Hospital. This was a consecutive series of surgical patients excluding only those at low risk for infection, such as hernia repair, thyroidectomy, etc. Patients were skin tested by intradermal injection of each of five recall antigens: PPD, mumps test antigen, candidin, trichophytin and streptokinase-streptodornase, as well as a control solution of buffered diluent. In 40 anergic and 15 relatively anergic patients, neutrophil chemotaxis was appraised. Additional studies were neutrophil bactericidal function and lymphocyte function as indicated by E-rosette assay, mixed leukocyte culture and cell-mediated lympholysis. There were three groups of patients, those tested preoperatively, those tested after an operation for a major trauma and those who underwent no operation. "Of the 218 patients tested preoperatively, 26 (12%) had altered cutaneous responses with a significantly higher rate of sepsis 19% (p < 0.025) and of mortality 35% (p < 0.001) than did the 192 normal responders. Similarly, of the 75 patients initially tested following major trauma and/or surgery, 64 (85%) were anergic or relatively anergic with an associated high rate of sepsis (70%) and a 28% mortality rate (p < 0.001). Amongst the 61 patients not operated upon, the incidence of sepsis (25%) and death (40%) in the 20 patients with abnormal responses was also statistically different (p < 0.001) from that in the 41 normal responders." Serial testing of the patients showed that "The anergic and relatively anergic patients whose skin test failed to improve had a mortality rate of 74.4%, whereas those who improved their responses had a mortality rate of 5.1% (p < 0.001)." In "the 97 patients who had preoperative tests and serial tests post-operatively . . . eliminating patients who were infected or seriously injured at the time of first testing, there was no mortality or sepsis if the patients remained normal or improved their reaction (83 patients) . . . four of eight who were anergic or relatively anergic preoperatively and remained so following surgery, developed sepsis and five died . . . in the remaining 6 patients whose responses worsened postoperatively, four had septic complications and all 6 died." Neutrophil chemotaxis studied in patients with altered responses, either anergic or relatively anergic, showed significantly less stimulated and random migration of neutrophils in patients with altered responses, but improved significantly in those patients whose cutaneous responses improved. "Incubation of normal cells in anergic serum when compared to incubation of autologous serum reduced stimulated migration of normal neutrophils significantly . . ." While "the phagocytic and bactericidal function of neutrophils is not significantly abnormal [in anergic patients]. . . there is a statistically significant relationship between numbers of bacteria not phagocytized or not killed and the distance migrated by these same neutrophils." The mixed lymphocyte culture studies, studies of cell-mediated lympholysis and response to a blastogenic factor produced no significant results. "In anergic patients, the total number of lymphocytes was reduced by a third and the total T-cells by almost 50%." There was a "reduction by 30% in number of rosetting cells produced by incubation of normal lymphocytes in anergic serum." They concluded that "Serial testing of skin reactivity, at weekly intervals, is a very sensitive guide to the adequacy of management and prognosis . . . . Delayed hypersensitivity has usually been viewed as a reflection of cell-mediated immunity. This branch of the immune response is thought to relate to tumor resistance, transplantation immunity and resistance to fungal, viral and intracellular bacterial infections. Survival in patients with cancer has also been associated with skin test responsiveness [Eilber and Morton, 1970] and *in vitro* T-cell numbers. Anergic patients have had more rapid progression of their disease and earlier detection of metastases. The sepsis in the anergic patients we described was caused by common gram-negative rods and gram-positive cocci, traditionally controlled by humoral and phagocytic mechanisms." So far as concerned reversal of the anergic state, MacLean indicated chiefly the necessity for maintaining general nutrition and early and appropriate use of total parenteral nutrition.

Discussion

Hiram C. Polk, Jr., of Louisville, complained that, in his own work as in these studies, ". . . these tests do not become abnormal in such a sufficiently early manner as to be helpful in the early diagnosis of impending infection. It does pick out those patients in the elective situation which are genuine high-risk individuals, but from a point of view of looking at a patient and seeing whether these signs might be helpful as to who's brewing septic complications or not, they really don't become sufficiently abnormal far enough in advance of the clinical signs to be very helpful." He asked whether the McGill group had had experience "with transfer factor, which has the capability of altering some of these abnormalities in a beneficial way for these very ill patients?" John A. Mannick, of Boston, said that "We have recently described the recovery from the serum of similar traumatized and septic patients of a peptide fraction, which is suppressive of lymphocyte activation at relatively low concentrations, and is also suppressive of E-rosette formation when applied to normal lymphocytes in tissue culture medium." Had Dr. Meakins and Dr. MacLean characterized the material in the serum of their anergic patients. Mannick had found in his own work that the lymphocytes from anergic patients repeatedly washed in culture medium would respond normally. How did Meakins and MacLean prepare their lymphocytes? George H. A. Clowes, Jr., of Boston, said, in comparing the plasma of septic and of normal animals or patients they found "that rabbit muscle incubated in the plasma of normal patients responds normally to insulin and other metabolic stimuli . . . if we incubate that same normal skeletal muscle with plasma from a septic animal, or patient, these responses are inhibited." He asked whether this and Mannick's observations about washing indicated that there was a circulating polypeptide. The active fraction of plasma in their septic patients in these studies had shown a material of 4,000-7,000 molecular weight. The production or activity of the material could be inhibited by peptidase inhibitors. Meakins, closing, said that they had not used transfer factor, that they had not characterized the serum factors which produce inhibition in E-rosettes or neutrophil chemotaxis, although others had suggested that there might be multiple inhibitors. They had not employed multiple washings of the kind Mannick asked about. He felt ". . . that we are able to define those patients who are at risk for sepsis, either preoperatively or in the postoperative period, and that sequential skin testing is at the present time the most sensitive measure that we have easily available to identify and follow those patients with acquired abnormalities of host defense and therefore at risk for either present or continuing sepsis." [Jacob Fine, of Boston, at the exciting 1955 meeting in Philadelphia (when cardiovascular surgery was in center stage), *Host Resistance to Bacteria and to Bacterial Toxins in Traumatic Shock*, studying the problem in an entirely different way, concluded that animals in shock tolerated massive infection or injection of bacterial toxins less well than normal dogs, that as shock continued there was a progressing decline "in potency of the phagocytosis-promoting factors in serum . . . and a rapid disappearance of Properdin from the blood . . . within four to six hours . . ." and that "The therapeutic objectives in shock should include not only replacement of blood volume deficit, but all available methods to suppress bacterial activity", including "measures to preserve cellular integrity in general, since impairment of enzymatic processes involved in antibacterial defense begins early in shock. Hence the necessity for blood volume therapy at the earliest possible moment in hypovolemic shock."]

* * *

R. Y. Calne, of Cambridge, England, Professor of Surgery, University of Cambridge, Corresponding Fellow and by invitation, P. McMaster, B. Portmann, W. J. Wall, and Roger Williams, *Observations on Preservation, Bile Drainage and Rejection in 64 Human Orthotopic Liver Allografts,* had developed a technique of liver preservation "which permits up to 8 hours of safe storage without any complicated machines and we have been able to transport 22 livers by air and road from other institutions to our own unit." It had recently become possible in England to remove livers from "heart-beating cadavers". "The initial cooling of the liver is performed *in situ* through the portal vein with gravity drainage of Hartmann's solution at 4°. After infusion of 1.5-2 litres of this solution the flush is changed to an ice-cold protein fraction with additives. Seven hundred milliliters of this solution are infused through the portal vein and another 300 ml via the hepatic artery. The liver is then stored in ice-cold saline in a sterile container surrounded by ice." A marked reduction in early postoperative complications of biliary fistula and obstructed bile drainage resulted from "a new method of biliary drainage . . . using the vascularized gallbladder as a conduit between the donor and recipient common ducts." In the past, half of their patients and half of those in the Denver series, "have developed serious biliary tract complications and this figure would probably be higher if patients succumbing in the earlier postoperative period had survived longer." The poor blood supply of the lower end of the donor common duct and anastomotic tension were considered to be the principal problems. Starzl, since 1973, "has favoured using a long Roux loop to avoid ascending infection and anastomosing this to the gall bladder or the com-

mon bile duct. We feel that the objective of biliary drainage should be to preserve the sphincter of Oddi, to provide a wide anastomosis with a good blood supply, to have no sump for the accumulation of biliary sludge and to have ready access to the biliary ducts for irrigation and diagnostic radiography." In 24 of the last 29 cases, Calne had used a technique which satisfied these objectives. The donor common duct was trimmed back close to the cystic, divided obliquely and then anastomosed to the side of the gallbladder, thus removing dependence upon the often unsatisfactorily narrow cystic duct. The fundus of the donor gallbladder was then anastomosed to the distal stump of the recipient common duct. The limbs of the T-tube in the gallbladder passed up through the anastomosis into the donor common duct and down through the anastomosis into the recipient common duct. Formation of biliary sludge was not an uncommon occurrence in liver recipients. A considerable contributor to the sludge appeared to be collagen, "The shedding of collagen from the lining of intra- and extrahepatic ducts probably follows ischemic necrosis", although conceivably it was the result of rejection. The immunosuppression employed was with azathioprine and prednisolone. For the first three days, cyclophosphamide was given instead of azathioprine. "Two patients were weaned completely off Prednisolone, and maintenance therapy of immunosuppression in most patients has required less drug dosage than patients with kidney grafts. In contrast to the Denver practice, we do not now use antilymphocyte globulin." Rejection was difficult to diagnose and needle biopsies were undependable. "A positive leukocyte migration test in the presence of deteriorating liver function and a normal T-tube cholangiogram is assumed to indicate rejection and a short course of increased steroid dosage is commenced." Despite the numerous complications, "patients who have been discharged from hospital have often done extremely well. They frequently require less steroids than renal transplant patients and therefore do not have such severe cushingoid features. One hundred and three of the patients in Starzl's series were transplanted a year or more ago. Thirty of them or 29% have survived for at least one year after liver replacement . . . most of the patients who reach the one year mark continue to do well thereafter. Thus, half of the Denver one-year survivors are still alive. 15 patients have reached the two year mark, eight have reached three years, and there have been four five-year survivors. The longest survivor in their series and in the world is now more than seven years post-transplantation . . . living at home, attending

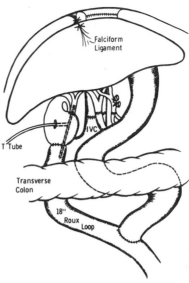

FIG. 3. Gall bladder conduit technique used when the recipient common bile duct is unsuitable. The fundus of the gall bladder is anastomosed to a long Roux loop of jejunum. (By courtesy of the World J. Surg.).

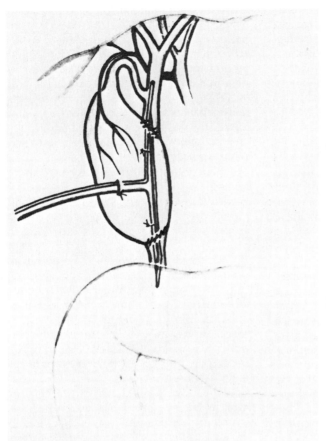

FIG. 1. Pedicle graft conduit with donor gall bladder. Hartmann's pouch is anastomosed to donor common duct and fundus anastomosed to recipient common duct. Irrigating T-tube is inserted with irrigating arm through upper anastomosis. Blood supply to gall bladder is carefully preserved. (By courtesy of the Br. Med. J.).

Calne postulated "that the objective of biliary drainage should be to preserve the sphincter of Oddi, to provide a wide anastomosis with a good blood supply, to have no sump for the accumulation of biliary sludge and to have ready access to the biliary ducts for irrigation and diagnostic radiography." The mobilized donor gallbladder with its blood supply intact was in effect interposed between the stump of the donor common duct above and of the recipient common duct below, and the two arms of the T-Tube in the gallbladder passed through these two anastomoses, permitting the well-vascularized gallbladder to bridge the gap in the common duct without tension, at the same time that the biliary pathway was freed from dependence upon the uncertain cystic duct. If the recipient common duct was unavailable or unsuitable, a Roux loop of jejunum was employed as shown in Calne's Figure 3.

R. Y. Calne, P. McMaster, B. Portmann, W. J. Wall, Roger Williams, *Observations on Preservation, Bile Drainage and Rejection in 64 Human Orthotopic Liver Allografts,* Volume XCV, 1977.

school and has normal liver function. Two other five-year survivors are also entirely well, but the fourth one died a few days short of the six year mark of chronic rejection and partial biliary obstruction." Of the total 64 transplants in the Cambridge series, 11 resulted in death in the first week, (all before 1975), 29 more by six months, (19 of those before 1975) six died between six months and one year, three died after one to five years. Out of the entire group, 15 were at present alive, the earliest grafted in February, 1974, but ten had gone less than one year. "Between June 1975 and May 1976 our results for liver grafting have been better than those obtained with cadaveric renal transplants . . . It is likely that many patients have been overtreated with immuno-suppressive drugs and this has been responsible for some of the infective complications and may in theory have impaired the development of active immunosuppressive mechanisms . . . now that survival has improved, it has become clear that uncontrollable rejection of the allografted liver in man is much less severe than that experienced with kidney transplants." In only four patients was rejection considered "a major cause of death".

Discussion

Joseph G. Fortner, of New York, was not enthusiastic about the use of the gallbladder as a conduit. In the 14 liver transplants performed at Memorial Sloan-Kettering Cancer Center "we have found . . . that an end-to-side choledochojejunostomy really is, in our hands, at least, the best way to have biliary drainage, and thus cope with one of the big problems." They had done seven heterotopic or auxiliary liver grafts "One patient is living and well more than four years after transplantation, a little boy with biliary atresia. One patient lived eight months, and one lived three and one half months." Paul S. Russell, of Boston, said Calne had discussed some of the technical difficulties in the present state of organ availability. Calne had improved preservation techniques "but you will note that they are still rather limited, and still far from what we can do with kidney transplantation." Most interesting was "the special quality of the liver in respect to rejection . . . I think it's true that the liver is rejected with less vigor than are many other organs . . . it may be suggested that the liver is less rejectable than is the kidney, which is less rejectable than is the heart, which is much less rejectable than is skin." Had Dr. Calne, "any idea at all as to what the mechanism for the striking difference in behavior of livers on transplantation as compared to the other organs might be"? Joseph E. Murray, of Boston, while urging credit to Starzl and Calne, "for bringing clinical liver transplantation into actuality" reminded the Fellows that "both of the authors will recognize the experimental prototype which Dr. Francis D. Moore established in the late fifties in the laboratory at Harvard Medical School; and I believe it was there that Dr. Calne received some of his first stimulus in the field of liver transplantation." He agreed with Russell about the hierarchy of rejection of organs. Calne answered Fortner only that the gallbladder technique "in our hands . . . has produced much better results. I think it must wait time to be proven, but every other technique that's been used in any large series has been unsatisfactory." He had no answer to Paul Russell's question on the mechanism of acceptance of the liver but did have some information,- "Liver cells, hepatocytes, have

less transplantation antigens than kidney cells. They have SD-antigens, but not LD-antigens. The liver has a unique lining of the endothelium with Kupffer cells, which changed to recipient type after six months in two human cases that have been studied. This could be relevant. We don't know if the liver has a major influence on the recipient's immune system, or whether the liver itself is less susceptible to rejection, possibly it's a combination of both these factors." He was "delighted to have the opportunity to pay homage to Dr. Moore for having worked in his department, and getting my first interest in liver grafting at the Brigham, and being associated with Dr. Murray for many years in experimental and clinical transplantation."

* * *

The Bicentennial Paper, Commissioned by the Council several years earlier, and overlooked by the Program Committee at the 1976 meeting, as Secretary Maloney had pointed out at length at the Business Meeting, was presented now, *Surgery in 1776,* Mark M. Ravitch, of Pittsburgh, Professor of Surgery, University of Pittsburgh; Surgeon-in-Chief Montefiore Hospital. What had been written of surgery in those days was the surgery of war and of wounds. The Bicentennial paper concluded "it is hard to tell whether Jones, Shippen, Morgan, Warren, and their colleagues would be more astonished by the witchcraft of today's radio communication and helicopter evacuation, or by a surgeon's general anesthesia, blood replacement, precise operative technique, careful hemostasis, and the control of the hideous problem of infection. They would have felt almost at home with trench foot, frost bite, the diarrheal diseases, and venereal infections, then, as now, an accompaniment of military life. They might have been surprised that we have sometimes chosen to go so far afield in our search for the loci of battle. And I would hope that with 200 years of reflection in the grave, it would have occurred to them that a civilization which produced so many miraculous advances ought long since to have elaborated a society in which military surgery would be only a subject for historians."

* * *

P. E. Oyer, E. B. Stinson, R. B. Griepp, all by invitation, and Norman E. Shumway, of Stanford, Professor and Chairman, Department of Cardiovascular Surgery, Stanford University School of Medicine, *Valve Replacement with the Starr-Edwards and Hancock Prostheses:* Comparative Analysis of Late Morbidity and Mortality, had been led by "a substantial incidence of thromboembolic and hemorrhage complications" with the Starr-Edwards caged-ball valve to evaluate the Hancock glutaraldehyde-fixed porcine xenograft. The numbers were large. There were 435 Starr aortic valves and 251 xenografts, 515 Starr mitral valves and 338 xenografts, 121 double Starr valves and 88 xenografts. The patients in each group, with either valve were very nearly identical in age, sex distribution, New York Heart Classification or Cardiac Catheterization data. This was not a prospective randomized study, the Starr-Edwards experience beginning much earlier than the Hancock xenograft experience, with an overlap in the middle years. It was stated that "The operative techniques for aortic and mitral valve replacement have undergone only minor modification during the course of this study . . . The mitral valve was approached through a left atrial incision immediately posterior to the interatrial groove. The aortic valve was exposed through a low oblique aortotomy . . . Myocardial protection during periods of aortic crossclamping was assured by continuous topical irrigation of the heart, and intermittent lavage of the interior of the left ventricle, with 1.9% saline cooled to 4° . . . Total cardiopulmonary bypass times and aortic crossclamp times were similar for comparable patient groups." Patients with Starr-Edwards valves "were treated with warfarin sodium indefinitely. Approximately one-half of the patients undergoing xenograft mitral valve replacement received anticoagulant therapy during the first three months postoperatively, beginning on the day of chest tube removal. The remaining patients undergoing mitral valve replacement with xenografts received no postoperative anticoagulation". A quarter of the xenograft aortic valve patients received "short-term anticoagulant treatment". For special indications, "Those patients . . . judged to be at high risk for late thrombo-embolism were placed on anticoagulants indefinitely . . . [viz.] patients who exhibited significant amounts of intracardiac thrombus formation." This amounted to "0.4% of all aortic xenograft valve patients, 17% of all mitral xenograft patients, and 1.4% of all double xenograft patients." For the aortic valve replacements, the hospital mortality was 6.9% for the Starr-Edwards valve and 6.4% for the xenograft valve. Late mortality with the Starr-Edwards valve was 6.3% per patient year and for the xenograft valve patients 3.4% per patient year. Thromboembolism with the Starr-Edwards aortic valve was 6.0% per patient year and with the xenograft, 2.6% per patient year. "The linearized rate of *fatal* emboli in the Starr-Edwards group was 0.5% per patient year, while no fatal emboli occurred

among patients receiving the xenograft valve." Valve failure was 1.8% per patient year for the Starr-Edwards valve and 1.1% for the xenograft valve. "anticoagulant-related hemorrhage . . . occurred at a rate of 5.7% per patient year in the Starr-Edwards aortic group. In addition, these patients were subject to a 0.7% per year risk of *fatal* hemorrhage." In patients with xenograft aortic valves, the risk of hemorrhage was 0.7% per patient year and there had been no fatal hemorrhages. The risks of endocarditis were 1.2% per year for the Starr-Edwards valve, 1.4% for the xenograft valve, a difference considered not significant. For mitral valve replacement the operative mortalities were 8.6% and 9.7% [all figures are given as Starr-Edwards preceding]. The mortality rates were 7.9% per patient year and 4.5% per patient year, thromboembolism, 10.9% and 4.1% per patient year. "The rate of occurrence of *fatal* emboli in the Starr-Edwards group was 1.0% per patient year. No patient in the xenograft mitral replacement group sustained a fatal embolus." Of the 24 thromboemboli occurring in the xenograft valve group, 16 occurred within the first three months after operation. Valve failures were 2.6% per patient year and 1.7% respectively, anticoagulant related hemorrhage 5.5% and 1.4% and fatal hemorrhagic events 0.9% and 0.2% The endocarditis rates were 0.4% per patient year and 0.2% per patient year, not significantly different. For double valve replacements the mortality was 7.5% and 10.2%, the late mortalities 7.8% and 6.2%, the difference not being significant. The relative frequency of thromboembolic events was 6.6% per patient year, and 3.1% per patient year, and again, all three of the embolic events with the xenograft valves occurred in the first postoperative month while the 28 thromboembolic events occurring among the Starr-Edwards patients were evenly distributed over 6.9 years. The valve failure rates were 1.0 and 3.1% per year,- not significantly different. Anticoagulant related hemorrhage rates were 4.1% per patient year and 1.0% per patient year, no fatal hemorrhages among the xenograft patients, 0.2% per patient year fatality for anticoagulant hemorrhage in the Starr-Edwards valve group. The endocarditis rates were not significantly different, 0.9% per patient year and 1.0% per patient year. Their analysis, they said "confirms in several aspects the superiority of the xenograft bioprosthesis in comparison to the Starr-Edwards models we have previously employed. Although we recognize that more recently introduced permutations of Starr-Edwards valves are reported to have significantly fewer associated complications, the older noncloth-covered models 1260 and 6120 valves [those employed by the Stanford group] have continued in widespread use for nearly ten years." Among their own patients, the survival rate with xenograft valves in both positions was better than that of similar patients with Starr-Edwards noncloth valves, and compared favorably with Starr's own reports for the "cloth-covered composite seat prosthesis", although it was acknowledged that "preoperative patient-associated variables are primary determinants of late mortality and . . . comparison in inter-institutional data may be misleading when preoperative patient status is not statistically similar." The thromboembolic rate had been much lower for xenografts and ". . . we have observed no fatal thromboembolic events in any patient who has received a xenograft aortic or mitral valve in 947 patient years of observation . . . The importance of anticoagulant therapy during the initial two or three months postoperatively was not fully appreciated early in our experience with xenograft valves. It is reasonable to assume that our recently adopted policy of prescribing short-term anticoagulation for all patients receiving xenograft valves should eliminate some of these early embolic events." The Stanford group counted transient episodes of cerebral ischemia as embolic incidents. Starr did not always include those. The present xenograft valve seemed to have overcome the problem with earlier valves which at the end of two or three years had "an unacceptably high rate of valve failure . . . tissue degeneration with consequent valvular regurgitation. Occasionally, valve tissue disruption occurred suddenly with catastrophic result . . ." Their period of observation had now been over five-and-a-half years, "During this time only three proved primary tissue failures have occurred in 667 patients. All occurred in xenografts in the mitral position." One was "an idiopathic perforation" of a single leaflet and the other two were stenoses caused by dense fibrin deposits. So far as they knew, there had been "no known instances of hemolysis in patients receiving xenograft valves in the absence of periprosthetic leak. We have noted this complication in approximately three percent of our patients receiving Starr-Edwards prostheses" though this never required valve replacement. The final statement of their summary is "The Hancock xenograft bioprosthesis appears, therefore, to be the valve of choice."

* * *

O. W. Isom, by invitation; Frank C. Spencer, of New York, Professor and Chairman, Department of Surgery, New York University School of Medicine; and by invitation, E. Glassman, P. Teiko, Arthur D. Boyd, J. N. Cunningham, and G. E. Reed, *Long-Term Results in 1375 Patients Undergoing Valve Replacement with the Starr-Edwards Cloth-Covered Steel Ball Prosthesis,* reported their eight year experience ending December, 1975, during which time 90% of the patients had received the prosthesis in question. The earlier high operative mortality ". . . has progressively decreased, with experience, to the range of five to eight per cent in most major centers in the past two to four years." The numerous different valves ". . . ball valves, disc valves, and different forms of tissue valves . . ." were generally hemodynamically equivalent. "The principal problem with prosthetic valves throughout had been thromboembolism and the need for anticoagulants. The exciting findings with the porcine xenograft reported by several groups in the past five years, with its freedom from thromboembolism and the necessity for anticoagulation, prompted this detailed review of our experiences." They had a 97% follow-up of the 1187 patients surviving valve replacement. At operation, "Mean perfusion pressures were usually maintained during bypass at a level similar to that existing beforehand . . . the prosthesis was inserted with mattress sutures of 1-0 Dacron routinely buttressed with Dacron pledgets. For the past several years, the routine use of pledgets for *all* sutures has virtually eliminated the problem of perivalvular leakage . . . In most instances, coronary perfusion was employed during aortic valve replacement . . . In the past two to three years . . . hypothermic ischemic arrest (myocardial temperature below 20 to 25°) with potassium cardioplegia has been frequently used . . . During mitral and tricuspid valve replacement, intermittent aortic cross-clamping for periods less than 15 minutes at 24 to 30°, followed by three to five minutes of perfusion was used . . . For the past four to five years, coronary artery lesions have been bypassed with saphenous vein grafts if significant stenosis were found on coronary angiography. With tricuspid disease, replacement has been used less and less in recent years, finding a posterior leaflet annuloplasty satisfactory in the majority of patients . . . In December, 1970, a trial of terminating anticoagulation was evaluated stopping it one year following mitral valve replacement and three months following aortic valve replacement. This promptly resulted in an impressive increase in the frequency of thromboembolism, rising in patients with mitral valve replacement from two to three per cent to 22%; so anticoagulation was routinely reinstituted. With aortic valve replacement, embolic complications were less frequent; patients were left without routine anticoagulation until 1975 . . . because reports from several groups demonstrated benefit with anticoagulation, the policy of routine anticoagulation was restarted for patients with aortic prostheses." In eight years of the study, the overall operative mortality dropped from 28.5% to 9.6%. The aortic valve replacement mortality dropped from 33% to 7%. The combined aortic and mitral replacement held steady at over 20%. The five-year survival following isolated aortic valve replacement was 70%, seven-year survival 64% and following mitral valve replacements, the survivals were 71% and 64%. Following combined aortic and mitral valve replacement, the five-year survival was 47%. The incidence of embolism in patients with aortic valve replacement was 3% per year. The incidence of embolism after mitral valve replacement was 4% per year. There were four fatal cerebral emboli in the aortic valve patients and six in the mitral valve patients, three deaths from anticoagulant related hemorrhage in the aortic valve patients and five in the mitral valve patients. Prosthetic endocarditis occurred in 5.7% of all surviving patients, and carried a mortality of 23% for antibiotic therapy and 44% if the valve was replaced. Hemolysis requiring transfusion or iron therapy occurred in 5% of the patients and was usually transient, only five patients,- 0.24%,- requiring reoperation on that basis. Their overall conclusion was that ". . . these data reveal that the Starr-Edwards cloth-covered steel ball valve has remained a durable prosthesis in spite of the complications of thromboembolism and endocarditis."

Discussion

Albert Starr, of Portland, described "the current choice that we now have in valvular prosthetic substitutes. On the one hand, we have bioprostheses capable of acting hemodynamically in a satisfactory manner with a low incidence of thromboembolism, without the need for long-term anticoagulants; on the other hand, the durable type of mechanical prostheses." Prostheses should be available in the operating room ". . . so that a prosthesis can be chosen for a patient, depending upon the patient's requirements and his ability to take anticoagulation." Cloth wear did occur and it had been their experience that "in about three out of four patients who have reoperation following aortic valve replacement with a cloth-covered valve, we see cloth wear, perhaps asymptomatic." Since 1972 when using a cloth-covered type of prosthesis they used a modification of the valve which Spencer's group had employed ". . . the track valve". With the noncloth-covered valve, 98% of the patients surviving had not required

replacement; with a cloth-covered valve, at six years 91% had escaped replacement. The track valve in the mitral position "seems to provide us with a prosthesis that has the durability of the noncloth-covered valve . . ." In the aortic position by ten years, only 8% of the noncloth-covered valves had had to be replaced but 15% of the cloth-covered valves. The track valve at the end of four years seemed to be equivalent to the noncloth-covered valve, and had the added advantage that it seemed to have the same "low incidence of thromboembolism" that the cloth-covered valve had. "I believe we have to focus our attention on the permanent type of prosthesis that will not be susceptible to mechanical derangement . . . and I believe that the track configuration does add this to the cloth-covered valve, and retains the low thromboembolic rate of that type of prosthesis." James R. Malm, at Columbia Presbyterian Hospital, had placed 848 ball valve prostheses, "mainly of the Starr-Edwards type, but 200 of the Cutter-Braunwald type" and had a smaller experience with the Hancock xenograft valve. The xenograft experience, now into the third year, showed less than 2% of embolic events per year "the mitrals receiving anticoagulants for a three-month period; only three surgical valve-related complications, and no valve failures." He concluded that "first of all, the prosthesis, and particularly the track valve, is a very noisy valve, and patients do object to the click. The very low incidence of embolus in the xenograft, the lack of need for long-term anticoagulation, and the rather excellent long-term survival make this a very desirable prosthesis." Charles R. Hatcher, Jr., of Atlanta, in two-and-a-half years had implanted 250 Hancock valves at Emory University Hospital. Aortic valve replacement was with a 4% operative mortality and a 1% late mortality. Mitral valve replacement, 9% and 2%, and multiple valve replacement, 6% and 4%. Only 16 patients were placed on anticoagulation therapy,- because of marked left atrial enlargement, chronic atrial fibrillation or known atrial thrombus. He said nothing about embolic events but noted that "The major disadvantage of the porcine heterograft has been the high gradients noted in recatheterization of some of the smaller-size valves in either position in certain of our patients. We therefore at present use a No. 29 or larger mitral valve and a No. 23 or larger aortic valve. If necessary, the aortic root is enlarged by carrying a transverse aortotomy through the noncoronary sinus and a few millimeters into the anterior leaflet of the mitral valve." Dwight C. McGoon, of Rochester, Minnesota, raised questions concerning the comparisons made ". . . with the realization that none of us have been able to achieve true randomization, or true comparability." He had understood that in their earlier experience with Starr-Edwards valves, the Stanford group had also been employing homograft valves in some patients and ". . . although they have assured us that the groups are comparable in terms of age and other categorizations, I would like to know how selection was determined, as to whether a patient received a Starr-Edwards valve or a homograft valve during the time when the prosthetic valve experience was being accumulated . . . Certainly, if the tissue valve, namely, the Hancock valve and its similar types, has an Achilles' heel, it must be with respect to its durability. And I question whether the comments that it provides an improved long-term patient survival and satisfactory durability can be justified on the basis of an average follow-up of 1.2 years for the aortic valves and 1.8 years for the mitral valves." Oyer answered McGoon that the homograft experience at Stanford had predated his arrival there and indeed the homograft patients tended "to be younger patients who were felt to have a longer survival outlook" although their physiologic studies were no different than those of patients receiving Starr-Edwards valves. The xenograft patients had not been selected in any way, "Virtually all patients undergoing valve replacement at Stanford now receive xenograft prostheses." In the last two or three years, "It is true that coronary bypass grafting was performed more frequently in conjunction with valve replacement . . ." Although the data were from consecutive series of patients, he believed "this sort of data from a single institution is still frequently more instructive than that generated from comparison of interinstitutional data, since patient-associated variables, major differences in operative technique, etc., may enter in and are much more difficult to control and evaluate." Dr. McGoon was right about the brief average follow-up of the xenografts but this low figure resulted because of the large number of new patients being added with extremely short follow-ups, and their maximum follow-up was five-and-a-half years for the mitral xenograft. "Although there are admittedly relatively few patients followed this long postoperatively, the fact that we have seen only three primary tissue failures in this entire series, and only one of these was actually a tissue disruption is, I think, extremely encouraging . . ." The gradient mentioned by Dr. Hatcher had been more of a problem with the aortic than with the mitral valve and "There is now available a modified orifice valve for placement in the aortic position." Isom said they had not employed the track valve at New York University "because of

the increased thrombogenicity of the valve off anticoagulants." He was inclined to agree with Dr. McGoon's point, ". . . both these series started in 1974. We are certainly encouraged by the data generated since 1971 from Stanford . . . However, if you took our patients and just started following them since 1971 and 1972, our survival curves would be very similar to that obtained by the California group. Our emboli would be very similar. I would also point out that a lot of things have changed in the past four or five years, and some of the improvements that we see in survival and in complications may be due to improved techniques."

* * *

John E. Connolly, Professor and Chairman, Department of Surgery, University of California at Irvine, and by invitation, J. H. M. Kwaan, and E. A. Stemmer, *Improved Results with Carotid Endarterectomy*, analyzed a series of 290 patients operated upon between 1968 and 1972. Loucks, in Peking in 1936 had resected an occluded internal carotid artery with reported relief from intermittent attacks of right hemiplegia and aphasia, Carrea, Molins, and Murphy in 1951 in Argentina had anastomosed the external carotid artery to the internal carotid artery distal to the stenotic lesion, reporting that operation in 1955. Strully, in New York, in 1953 had unsuccessfuly undertaken thromboendarterectomy of the carotid bifurcation. DeBakey performed such an operation successfully in the same year but did not report it until 1975. In 1954 in London, Eastcott, Pickering and Rob excised an obstructed carotid bifurcation and reanastomosed the common and internal carotid arteries, inaugurating the modern attack upon carotid occlusion. Connolly's first 188 endarterectomies, from 1960 to 1972, "were performed under general anesthesia with the use of an internal shunt, 5000 units of heparin, and arterial pressure and gas monitoring with induced hypercarbia. Stump pressures were not recorded . . . There were three deaths, three post-operative hemiplegias, and two complications of transient limb weakness." In the 102 carotid endarterectomies performed from 1973 to 1975, local anesthesia was employed, arterial pressure and blood gases were monitored by an intra-arterial catheter, normocarbia was maintained and 5000 units of heparin administered intravenously. Stump pressures were recorded in these patients, ". . . there was no death, no hemiplegia, and no complications of transient limb weakness." A Javid shunt was employed in 20 of the 102 patients, "either on the basis of stump pressure below 25 mm

Hg or the loss of motor ability or consciousness on five minutes of trial clamping of the internal carotid artery. Those shunted had stump pressures ranging from ten to 70 mm Hg with a mean of 20 mm Hg while those not shunted had stump pressures ranging from 25 to 85 mm Hg. with a mean of 53 mm Hg. Five patients lapsed into unconsciousness despite internal carotid stump pressure of 30, 30, 34, 36, and 70 mm Hg respectively . . . This experience seriously questions the reliability of carotid stump pressure as the sole determinant to identify those patients who require intraoperative shunting." The 10 to 20% incidence of cerebral ischemia with clamping of the carotid led some operators to employ shunts in all patients. Others, including Connolly and his associates, were selective because "the technique of shunting itself has its own complications . . . clotting within the shunt, embolization of clots from within the shunt, air introduced through the shunt, dissection of a distal internal carotid artery intimal flap or dislodgement of atherosclerotic material by insertion of the shunt, the need for the higher or more proximal incision in the internal carotid artery to place the shunt above the diseased core, and finally the lack of an operative field unobstructed by the shunt." Jugular venous oxygen saturation as an indication for the use of a shunt, had proved unreliable because "it is more a reflection of global hemisphere perfusion and interhemispheric mixing of venous blood." Constant electroencephalographic monitoring did seem to be useful. The effects of hypercarbia and hypocarbia had been disputed and Connolly now strove to maintain normal range of Pco_2. Crawford, DeBakey, and Blaisdell, in 1960 had been the first to describe "internal carotid artery . . . back pressure or what has commonly become known as the stump pressure". Various investigators had used the level of stump pressure to determine whether intraoperative shunting should be employed or not, and with varying degrees of satisfaction. Others relied on carotid occlusion and observation of the patient although it occurred that patients who tolerated a test occlusion during operation developed postoperative neurologic deficits. Connolly was led, overall, to conclude "carotid endarterectomy without a shunt is technically easier and avoids possible complications of the intraluminal tube itself . . . only one or two patients in ten require a shunt, particularly if such patients can be reliably identified . . . Visual assessment of back flow, electroencephalographic monitoring, and venous oxygen saturation determinations are not exact methods for such patient selection . . . Internal carotid back pressure or stump pressure is a useful intraoperative tool but

cannot be depended upon absolutely . . . The only proven absolute method to assess the safety of carotid endarterectomy without shunting is continuous neurological monitoring of the patient in the conscious state . . . Carotid endarterectomy can now be performed under local anesthesia without difficulty in almost any patient by adjunct use of Innovar and Sublimaze . . . Continuous arterial pressures and blood gas determinations are mandatory . . . The patient's Pco_2 must be in normal ranges . . . to assure optimal contralateral cerebral perfusion."

Discussion

Jesse E. Thompson, of Dallas, had used local anesthesia previously and now was operating under general anesthesia entirely. "One of the chief causes of operative-related strokes is embolization from a necrotic plaque during manipulation of the artery. This can occur under local or general, with or without a shunt, and bears no relationship to anesthesia. It is prevented by gentleness in surgical technique . . . Dr. Connolly prefers to operate on his patients awake, so that he can insert a shunt if the patient develops a neurologic deficit . . . we have observed on occasion that a patient who develops a deficit may not reverse the deficit after the shunt is inserted, and ends up with a permanent neurologic deficit." Inhalation anesthetics particularly halothane produced "a decrease in cerebral vascular resistance, with a resulting increase in cerebral blood flow . . . a reduction in the cerebral metabolic demands for oxygen, by about 30% on the average . . . general anesthesia is in itself a good means of cerebral protection. However . . . one either uses no shunt, and risks a certain incidence of stroke, uses a shunt routinely, or uses a shunt selectively, based on the EEG or the level of carotid stump pressure. Routine shunting and selective shunting based on EEG and stump pressures have given excellent results, with the same low incidence of mortality and strokes as Dr. Connolly has shown with local anesthesia." Thompson had a 20-year experience with 1259 operations and, ". . . in the last 14 years we have used general anesthesia and routine shunting, which presents no technical problems when one becomes familiar with the technique". In 987 recent operations upon patients with transient cerebral ischemia, ". . . the operative mortality has been 0.7%, largely of cardiac origin. The incidence of operated-related strokes, both transient and permanent, has been 1.6%." W. Sterling Edwards, of Albuquerque, New Mexico, agreed that Connolly's 102 endarterectomies with one death and no neurological residua "is certainly a remarkable feat, and will be hard to exceed." Were the results attributable "mostly or entirely, to the use of local anesthesia and only using a shunt selectively? . . . It's been reported by many vascular centers that carotid endarterectomy results progressively improve with the experience of the team . . . most of the postoperative deficits that occur are due to intraoperative emboli, either too vigorous manipulation of the carotid arteries or from debris or air remaining in the lumen when blood flow is restored . . . much of the improvement in the reduction of neurologic complications on busy vascular services has been due to reduction in these mechanical causes of intraoperative emboli, as well as to improved monitoring of the adequacy of cerebral blood flow . . . I would suspect . . . in Dr. Connolly's situation, that not only has better monitoring improved his results, but that better technique has been employed." Paul Nemir, Jr., of Philadelphia, said "There is good evidence that embolization from an ulcerating plaque is a more common remediable cause of TIA's than hemodynamically significant stenosis. We recently completed a study of the plaques removed in just over 200 operations. Ulcerations ranging from one centimeter in diameter to microscopic size were present in 72% . . . and our indications for operation have widened." He utilized an internal shunt routinely, with general anesthesia "but the impressive results reported in this paper, especially with respect to the total absence of neurologic complications, is strong encouragement for returning to local anesthesia." Louis L. Smith, of Loma Linda, California, had like Connolly been employing shunting in selective cases in 269 patients from 1972 through 1975, 63 of the operations bilateral. Studying Pco_2 and stump pressure, they had failed to "find a correlation between the Pco_2 level and the stump pressure in those individuals experiencing a neurologic deficit . . . roughly one half of 50 mm Hg or greater." Edwin J. Wylie, of San Francisco, agreed that carotid reconstruction was easier without a shunt in the way. He had given up operation under local anesthesia 15 years earlier. "Carotid operations under local anesthesia are distressing to both the patient and to the surgeon. In addition, the value of general anesthesia in reducing cerebral metabolic demand is sacrificed. In our subsequent experience we have found that stump pressure determination is a completely reliable technic. I think there are two fallacies in the conclusion from this paper . . . The first . . . the assumption that the strokes reported in this series were the result of clamp ischemia. There are other

causes of post-operative stroke, the most common being embolization from excess manipulation of the carotid bulb . . . The second . . . concerns the selection of the level of stump pressure that indicates adequacy of collateral hemispheric blood flow. In an earlier published report we had settled upon a level of 50 mm Hg mean, a higher level than the one used by Dr. Connolly's group . . . In the past two years, 423 carotid operations were performed. There were 350 patients whose stump pressures exceeded 50 mm Hg and none of these were shunted . . . two patients (0.6%) developed hemiparesis . . . One . . . the result of avulsion of the distal internal carotid artery and the other . . . in a patient with crescendo TIA and an existing neurologic deficit which worsened postoperatively . . . Stump pressures continue to be the most reliable index for determining the need for intraoperative shunting." Max R. Gaspar, of Long Beach, California, had started out with local anesthesia 20 years earlier ". . . often a harrowing experience . . ." If shunts were to be used every time, "I agree with Dr. Thompson that it really is easier to do a leisurely operation on the carotid with a shunt in place. We use them routinely. In our last 100 patients there was one death due to myocardial infarction, there were two transient neurological deficits lasting less than two hours and one that lasted several days and then cleared completely . . . everybody eventually uses a shunt at least some of the time, and I think we all should be able to use it very well all of the time." Connolly, closing, agreed that manipulation of the artery was a common cause of neurologic complications. He questioned some of the assumptions made about the benefits of general anesthesia and in any case, "Innovar and Sublimaze have made it possible to operate under local anesthesia safely and conveniently with a sedated but conscious patient." His series was not large enough to predict that his next hundred patients would do as well as the last hundred, but "our change to the use of local anesthesia has given us an absolutely safe method of determining when a shunt is required." As for the safety of given levels of stump pressure, a wide range of "safe levels" had been reported. Fifty mm Hg was probably safe in most cases, but not invariably. As for his own practice, "If no unconsciousness or motor changes are noted during the trial carotid crossclamping but occur during the endarterectomy procedure, we can always insert a shunt at that time. This is possible because we continue to talk to the patient and assess the neurological status during the operation . . . it doesn't mean that we make one final decision right at the beginning of the operation as to whether we are going to use a shunt or not." The 20% frequency was sufficient to ensure expertise for the team including trainees.

* * *

[In the continuing effort to reduce the mortality from cancer on the assumption that the earlier the cancer was found, the better would be the cure rate,- an assumption made from the earliest days of the Association,- tumor clinics for periodic examination of patients for a wide range of possible cancers, and screening programs aimed at case finding of specific cancers in specific population groups, had been increasingly employed since World War II.] D. Panoussopoulos, J. Chang, by invitation, and Loren J. Humphrey, Clinical Professor, University of Missouri Medical School at Kansas City [the Screening Center having been operated by the Departments of Surgery and Radiology, Kansas University Medical Center, where Humphrey had been Chairman of the Department of Surgery], *Screening for Breast Cancer,* focused attention on "the cancer which developed during the interval between visits to the detection center." Their study base consisted of 10,000 women ages 38 to 78 screened by physical examination performed by a nurse-clinician, mammography and thermography. A non-interval cancer was one detected by any of the three examinations, an interval cancer was one which "developed or was recognized after a negative screening visit of the patient and prior to the recommended subsequent examination." 536 patients had been recommended for biopsy after a screening visit, only 326 of these had biopsies performed and of these, 65 were positive. Of the 65, 63 had been advised on the basis of mammography, which gave it an accuracy rate of 97%. There were 24 interval cancers, reducing the "mammographic accuracy for detection of early breast cancer to 73%." Women who developed interval cancers were somewhat younger than the women developing non-interval cancers,- body weight and breast size were little different. Estrogens were being taken by 33% of women in the interval group and 17% in the non-interval group. The benefit of mammography remained great for those in whom it diagnosed a cancer,- the patients, on the basis of the 1974 paper of Wanebo, Huvos, and Urban, having a 95% survival rate. But the fact remained that one-third of the breast cancers were not detected by the screening process.

Discussion

John S. Spratt, Jr., of Louisville, Kentucky, estimated "that some breast cancers are so acute that they can go from inception of the cancer to the death of the host in as brief a period of time as 120 days. Other breast cancers are so chronic that the patient might live 23 years with no treatment at all. These chronic cancers, obviously, would be picked up by the annual mammography, while the acute cancers would be interval cancers . . . all breast cancers with doubling times of less than 17 days would be interval cancers . . . at least five per cent of all breast cancers fall in this acute category." He commented on the publicly expressed concern over the cancerogenic effect of radiation of the breast ". . . many arguments regarding the biological effect of radiation on the induction of breast cancer can be answered by the accurate and diligent monitoring of cohort-specific interval cancer rates. A rate rising faster than could be accounted for by the aging of the cohort might, for example, mandate an early cessation of mammography. A falling rate would support the continuance of screening mammography." W. W. Shingleton, of Durham, North Carolina, said that at Duke, they were "in the fourth year of this screening project . . . there have been 10,000 women who have been screened on three occasions" [indicating an annual screening]. The Duke group had detected 70 cancers and had found "nine so-called interval cancers." The concern about the effect of irradiation of the breast arose from data based on the experience in the Health Insurance Plan of New York study, "This study is about ten years old, and the techniques, including the amount of radiation used for the mammogram, was quite different than that being used in the demonstration projects today." Dr. Oliver Beahrs, "who is a member of this organization" was chairing a committee "to look at all the data from the twenty-seven screening clinics around the country. This will be data . . . on 270,000 women . . . who have undergone multiple screenings." J. D. Lewis, of Milwaukee, Wisconsin, where they had screened 10,000 women for over four years, had recommended 801 biopsies, 486 had been performed, and there had been 85 cancers, 27 of them minimal, *in situ* cancers, and they had 18 interval cancers. However, six of the 18 cancers "were lobular carcinoma *in situ,* and two were *in situ* intraductal carcinomas . . . So that the distribution of invasion in this group really is not . . . in our experience . . . much different than that in our cancers found on screening." He asked Humphrey the stages of the interval cancers found in Kansas City. They had also found a progressive drop-off in the number of cancers and the number of interval cancers in Milwaukee. Was the situation the same in Humphrey's experience? Originally, 20% of the cancers were found on physical examination only and there were still 12% of the cancers found by physical examination when mammography was considered negative. He asked Humphrey "In those patients in whom you have recommended biopsy, but no biopsy has been done, has there been any significant incidence of development of carcinoma during that particular interval?" Benjamin F. Rush, Jr., of Newark, said they too had the same percentage of interval cancers. In the first two years, their examinations had all been done by residents "we switched to a single physician who did all examinations for the following year. This made no difference whatsoever . . . in the incidence of the interval cancers . . . we're still struggling with whether these represent misses on the part of the mammographist and the physician examining the patient—or are they, lesions, as has been suggested by Dr. Spratt, which have emerged because of rapid growth in the intervening period?" They had had the same incidence as Humphrey of patient refusal to undergo biopsy. "Our estimate from those patients who actually did have biopsies done would be that at least a third of them have cancer. The fact is that these patients inform us that their own physicians have advised them not to go through with the biopsy, for a number of reasons, perhaps the most common being that physical examination in the physician's office was negative." William Stahl, of New York, was a consultant for the Health Insurance Plan of Greater New York, ". . . granddaddy of the screening programs", the program had been in being 14 years, 30,000 women selected as a study group matched with 30,000 controls, "who still don't know who they are, nor do their physicians." Twenty thousand of the 30,000 women selected had accepted screening and been followed for five years. He presented data "up to the present time." Mammography at the time of the study, was not quite as good as that currently available. "The group with interval cancers had the same death rate as the control group. Perhaps this implies something about the types of cancers that these people had. They don't seem to be better or worse than the people who had no screening at all." The interval cancers were found more than two months after screening "and a roughly equal distribution then through the eighth month, with a marked increment in the last four months." They were all then detected by physical examination. Various questions arose. Were there two kinds of interval cancers, missed cancers, and rapidly developing cancers? Were nurse-clinicians missing cancers? Should physical examination be performed every six months? Fourteen years after the selection of the groups in the HIP study, there had been 507 cancers in the study group and 509 cancers in the control group. In the study group, there had been 91 deaths and in the control group, 128 deaths. Michael R. Coates, of Torrance, California, said that at the Harbor General Hospital, they were doing all of their biopsies under local anesthesia feeling that patients were being scared away from biopsy because of the requirement of general anesthesia, although he recognized the possible difficulties in finding the small "screening lesions" under local anesthesia. Brock E. Brush, of Detroit, asked about the relation of mammographic accuracy to the histologic character of the tumors. They had found that with lobular carcinoma, the accuracy of mammography was low. James V. Maloney, Jr., of Los Angeles, said "A recent publication from a major university breast screening clinic involving 20,000 patient visits reported the discovery and early treatment of approximately 50 cancers. The five year survival rate was in excess of 90%. The authors concluded, therefore, that breast screening clinics were a valuable aid to the early diagnosis and treatment of this disease, and made possible better long-term results. Some 40 interval cancers, which were mentioned almost parenthetically, had a survival rate one half that customarily reported in large series of breast cancers. I reworked the data, combining the two groups, and found that the average survival rate of the entire group was identical to what we all obtain. This means to me that the women who has her tumor discovered at . . . a routine visit to a breast screening clinic almost by definition has a tumor with a long doubling time. The woman who discovers her tumor in the interval between visits is very likely to have a tumor with a short doubling time. I therefore conclude that a breast screening clinic is a cute method of separating tumors with fast and slow doubling times. . . . Dr. C. B. Mueller, of this fellowship . . . showed [Volume XCIII, 1975] that of all patients who originally had a diagnosis of breast cancer, 96% . . . ultimately die of that tumor . . . they die at a rate of seven and one-half per cent per annum . . . the recurrence rate in the third year following the discovery of the tumor is identical to the recurrence rate in the fifteenth or the twentieth year following the discovery of that tumor." Maloney summed up his deflating analysis, "Although it is true that treatment, surgical or otherwise, affects the survival rate favorably, the most spectacular apparent therapeutic results, and I emphasize 'apparent therapeutic results,' are achieved by devices such as screening clinics, which allow the surgeon to select for treatment tumors with slow doubling times, and claim credit not due him for good five-year results." Humphrey agreed, he said, with Spratt, "I think within this group there are those that have a short doubling time, and they probably are the interval cancers. The histologic differences were not at variance in the two groups. There were some that were lobular carcinoma *in situ* . . . the thing that spurred this investigation was a conversation with Dr. Hamblin Letton. He told me he had a patient who had a negative screen and in two months came in with a large, six centimeter mass, and had bony metastasis . . . And it may well be, Dr. Maloney, that we as surgeons are benefitting from those who have a long doubling time . . . we may be adding their survival on the front end by getting them that much earlier." He agreed that perhaps the nurse-clinicians might be better trained and encouraged more frequently to ask for confirmation of their examinations by the physicians. He refused to make any overall recommendation, obviously thought the screening clinic should continue and said "The one point that I want to make in closing . . . is that while we missed, in this study, one third of the patients that had cancer in the screening process, of those 10,000 only 0.3% developed an interval cancer."

* * *

W. C. Johnson, W. C. Widrich, J. E. Ansell, A. H. Robbins, all by invitation, and Donald C. Nabseth, of Boston, Professor of Surgery, Tufts University School of Medicine; Lecturer in Surgery, Boston University School of Medicine; Director of Surgery, Boston Veterans Administration Hospital, *Control of Bleeding Varices by Vasopressin:* A Prospective Randomized Study, had embarked upon an evaluation of the relative merits of vasopressin given by percutaneous superior mesenteric artery catheter or by peripheral vein. After 16 months and 25 patients, the study was terminated because of two serious complications with the arterial catheter [catheter dissection-occlusion of SMA in one, septic femoral pseudoaneurysm to the other]. Oliver, in 1895, had noted the vasopressor effect of pituitary extracts. Clark had noted the resultant decreased portal pressure in 1928. Kehne, Hughes and Gumpertz, 1956, had controlled variceal bleeding successfully in two patients with a single intravenous bolus of vasopressin, and subsequent reports had indicated frequent initial success but severe systemic effects and some rebleeding. Nusbaum and others introduced continuous infusion of vasopressin into the superior mesenteric artery. In their interrupted study at the Boston

Veterans Administration Hospital, 14 patients had had vasopressin infused through the SMA catheter, and 11 through a peripheral vein. The vasopressin was administered at the same rate by either route, 0.4 u/min. until bleeding stopped or for 24 hours, the dose halved for the second 24 hours and halved again for the third 24 hours. Arrhythmias and bradycardias required drop in the initial dose to 0.2 u/min. The results were essentially identical. In seven patients in each group, bleeding was controlled during and after vasopressin administration. Three patients in the SMA group rebled. Two patients in each group required the addition of the Sengstaken balloon to control bleeding and two patients in each group exsanguinated. The 30-day survival rate for the 25 patients was 64% and 20 months later, 48% were alive. "The best prognostic factor of long-term survival was the initial response to vasopressin therapy. Of the 14 patients whose bleeding was controlled during and after vasopressin therapy . . . 11 patients survived. Of the 11 patients who were classified as Temporary Control, Combined Control or exsanguination, only one patient is alive in the 6 to 21 month follow-up period." Nusbaum, Younis, Baum, and Blakemore, in 1974, had reported 98% success in control of bleeding with superior mesenteric arterial infusion of vasopressin. However, it had been Johnson's earlier experience that half of those patients rebled. The site and mechanism of action of the Pitressin were still argued about. Johnson and Nabseth concluded that there were no specific advantages of intra-arterial therapy, that it carried specific hazards. "We have found the continuous infusion of vasopressin to be useful in the treatment of massive gastroesophageal variceal bleeding. It is our impression that the intravenous route is as effective as the direct intra-arterial route and we now employ it almost exclusively."

Discussion

William S. Blakemore, of Toledo, [who, then from Philadelphia, had been a co-author of the Nusbaum report] thought the arterial catheterization technique complications excessive, that the cardiac arrhythmias occurred on twice the recommended dose ". . . it was recommended, and has always been, that the dosage intra-arterially be monitored by repeat angiography after a short interval of initiating treatment" and he wanted to make it clear that the arguments in this situation in any case, "should not be confused with the rationale for use of this for other modalities, such as drug infusion, superselective catheterization . . . selective embolectomy, all of which are still under trial . . ." The series, he thought, was too small to answer any questions. Marshall J. Orloff, of San Diego, called the study, "yet another nail in the coffin of selective mesenteric intra-arterial vasopressin therapy for bleeding esophageal varices." He had contended for seven years, and other investigations had shown in laboratory and clinical studies, "that infusion of vasopressin into the mesenteric arteries is not significantly different from infusion of vasopressin into a systemic vein, in terms of the effect on portal pressure, control of bleeding varices, and systemic side effects." He thought there were "very few indications" for mesenteric intra-arterial vasopressin for variceal hemorrhage and that intravenous vasopressin was extremely effective in obtaining initial hemostasis. "During the past 15 years we have given systemic intravenous vasopressin by single bolus injection to every patient admitted to our hospital with bleeding esophageal varices within one hour of entry into our emergency room . . . intravenous vasopressin controlled the varix hemorrhage initially in about 95% of the patients." He employed the time gained only in preparing the patient for immediate portacaval shunt within his eight-hour time limit. Harry H. LeVeen, of Brooklyn, had "studied the selective use of vasoconstrictors by putting them into the peritoneal cavity, where they belong . . . those vasopressor materials will be absorbed into the portal circulation and, hopefully, destroyed by the liver." Norepinephrine was the vasopressor most rapidly destroyed by the liver. "My preference for the treatment of acute esophageal variceal bleeding would still be intraperitoneal norepinephrine . . ." W. C. Johnson, closing, said their original dosage of 0.4 unit per minute of Pitressin had evolved from their study of the previous four years, "the higher dosage achieves an early control in most of our patients, and the dosage can be lowered to 0.2 unit/min. for maintenance of bleeding control." They had had no evidence of gastrointestinal ischemia in their patients and thought the initial dosage level was safe. Cardiac output was reduced by vasopressin infusion but there was usually not a significant depression of urinary output.

* * *

Kenneth P. Ramming and Jean B. deKernion, by invitation, from the Department of Surgery, Division of Oncology and Urology, UCLA School of Medicine and Sepulveda Veterans Administration Hospital, *Immune RNA Therapy for Renal Cell Carcinoma:* Survival and Immunologic Monitoring,

traced the mediation of immune reactions by lymphoid ribonucleic acid to Fishman and Adler in 1961. In a number of systems, it had been demonstrated that "RNA from the lymphoid tissues of specifically immunized donors" incubated with nonimmune lymphoid cells produced "an immune response in the RNA-treated cells identical to that which had been induced in the RNA donor." Because, occasionally, spontaneous regression of metastatic renal-cell cancer occurred, and growth patterns were sometimes erratic and appearance of metastases might be remote from the time of removal of the primary tumor, it had been speculated that this tumor might "be responsive to immunologic tumor-host factors." In the present experiments, since the patients frequently were first seen subsequent to the removal of their tumors, the usual source of renal cell carcinoma was tumor from another patient. The prepared RNA, extracted from the spleen and nodes of a sheep injected with tumor was not, as in the animal models, incubated with lymphocytes, but lyophilized RNA was resuspended in sterile saline and injected intracutaneously "about the lymph node-bearing areas of the groins or axillae." The study initially undertaken attempted to see whether in the first phase there would be any untoward reaction to the treatment. When survivals began to seem significant, a retrospective study was undertaken to provide historical controls. In no patients did metastatic disease disappear. Of the 29 patients, all with metastatic disease, 11 failed to respond at all but seven patients exhibited what was considered a partial response, "a measurable regression of less than 50% by x-ray or palpation, or stability of previously growing lesions for a minimum of three months." In the minimal residual disease group, no patient had developed a recurrence during a mean observation time of 18 months. A comparison with the historical controls, showed significantly better survival for the RNA patients with metastatic disease confined to the lungs, compared to the controls. "Such a statistically significant difference in survival between RNA recipients and control patients was not observed when survival of groups of patients with metastases to any other organ site outside the lungs was compared." They concluded that "RNA therapy may be of value in selected patients with metastatic renal cell carcinoma, and is an adjunct to definitive surgery" particularly in the group of patients with "minimal residual disease . . . there have been no recurrences in any of the nine patients in this group, several followed almost up to three years, a mean observation period of 18 months. It is in this area that there is a suggestion of therapeutic promise with immune RNA that can only be established by further observation and carefully controlled, randomized, prospective trials."

Discussion

Charles F. McKhann, of Minneapolis, picturesquely described the three approaches "currently in use for clinical immunotherapy. The first . . . active, nonspecific immunotherapy, in which one essentially is trying to turn up the floodlights in the entire room on the immune response, including that portion of the immune response directed toward a tumor. The materials most frequently used for this are BCG and C. parvum. The second is active, specific immunotherapy . . . trying to put a spotlight on the tumor itself, leaving the background dark. The material for this must be tumor cells, or antigen preparations from the tumor cells . . . the third . . . we have been hearing about today, is the transfer of immunity from one individual to another . . . the Robin Hood technique . . . taking from the 'haves' and giving to the 'have-nots'." The patient "cured" of melanoma, for instance, could be such a donor, but adds some danger to himself since it was not known whether he was really cured or not and to remove a "significant portion of his immune capacity" might actually place him at risk. "The approach that we have heard today sidesteps this very nicely by creating a new have . . . the sheep . . . and inducing the immune response in the sheep, and then transferring that back to the patient who needs it." McKhann asked whether the essayists thought the immune RNA was really specific "or is it acting as a nonspecific immunostimulant, much as BCG does?" and if it really was specific, what was the danger of "transferring back to the patient immunity against many normal cellular antigens, creating essentially an immunological backlash and a severe auto-immunity situation? . . . the sheep who receives these cells receives not only renal cell carcinoma antigen, but also a plethora of normal human antigens which are present on the same cell. It is unlikely that the sheep distinguishes between these." John A. Mannick, of Boston, enjoyed the presentation "for a number of reasons, not the last of which is the fact that it was almost exactly 15 years ago that I was privileged to present a description of the transfer of cellular immunity mediated by immune RNA to this society. [Volume LXXX, 1962] The presentation at that time, I recall was greeted with complete silence, and I suspect that this was at least partly due to the fact that no one there, including me, had any idea about practical applications of this system." Subsequently,

he and Egdahl "suggested that this RNA-mediated transfer of immunity might be useful in the induction of tumor immunity in experimental animals and, potentially, people, but it was five years after that before Ramming and Pilch at the National Cancer Institute were able to show that this, indeed, was possible in animal systems." Employing the technique of Mannick's original experiment, his colleagues, Deckers and Wang with a chemical-carcinogen-induced mouse tumor injected into guinea pigs and the mouse lymphocytes then incubated with guinea pig RNA had shown in tissue culture the effective killing power of such mouse lymphocytes against the mouse tumor. Deckers and Wang had shown that the lymphocytes of a mouse in whom the tumor was growing could be stimulated in the same way [he did not mention the effect on the mouse's tumor]. Kenneth P. Ramming, closing said to McKhann that they did not know whether the RNA was specific for tumor or not but thought there was a degree of specificity. They had certainly seen no evidence of autoimmunity in their patients as the result of the injections.

* * *

R. J. Stoney, W. K. Ehrenfeld, by invitation, and Edwin J. Wylie, of San Francisco, Professor of Surgery, Vice Chairman, Department of Surgery; Chief, Vascular Surgery Service, University of California, *Revascularization Methods in Chronic Visceral Ischemia Caused by Atherosclerosis,* said that the direct transabdominal attack on the vessels themselves had been unsatisfactory and the direct transabdominal incision of the aorta and transaortic endarterectomy had similarly frequently been difficult. They described a thoracic retroperitoneal approach which gave "Unrestricted exposure of the aorta and its visceral and renal branches . . . from the distal thoracic segment to the aortic bifurcation." The aorta was incised longitudinally to the left of the celiac or SMA orifices "with a transverse hockey stick incision at each end of the aortotomy. This creates a trapdoor which can be swung back carrying with it the orifices of the stenosed or occluded arteries. The intima on the undersurface of the trapdoor is separated from the media saving the visceral artery endarterectomy until last." Making traction from the aortic side on the specimen within the artery and continuing to dissect it "the atheromatous intima eventually separates from the normal distal intima." They had seen no difficulties, subsequent occlusions or thromboses because of "the ledge of thickened intima at the distal end of the aortic endarterectomy." Lesions of the celiac, superior mesenteric and inferior mesenteric artery were reached by the same technique and in five patients associated renal artery stenosis was corrected by extending the aortotomy. In a total of 35 patients operated upon for chronic visceral ischemia, Wylie's group had employed a variety of types of reconstructions, also employing arterial grafts, saphenous vein grafts and Dacron grafts. They suggested that "in some patients with two vessel (celiac and SMA) disease, reconstruction of the celiac artery alone may be all that is required to relieve visceral ischemic symptoms, provided the IMA is undiseased. The use of Dacron grafts from the undiseased distal thoracic aorta to the transected celiac artery . . . easily performed through a transabdominal approach, proved to be the most successful and durable technique to accomplish this objective." They were reluctant to advocate single artery revascularization for multiple visceral artery disease "One of the two deaths in this series occurred in a patient with two vessel disease who had a celiac reconstruction only. Damage to the gastroduodenal artery interrupted the collateral channel and resulted in visceral infarction . . . in these young patients with a unique and apparently rapidly progressive form of aortic atherosclerosis, we believe the preferable operation is one that removes the diseased intima in the aorta and all of the involved branches. These objectives were accomplished in the patients who underwent transthoracic endarterectomy using the transthoracic retroperitoneal approach." There were 12 of those, five of whom also had their renal arteries operated upon, and in two, the inferior mesenterics as well. One died of hepatitis, the others were all considered cured.

Discussion

Gilbert S. Campbell, of Little Rock, commented that the syndrome had been described by "J. Englebert Dunphy, in 1936. Dr. Dunphy was an assistant resident at the Peter Bent Brigham Hospital at that time, and he recognized that chronic intestinal ischemia caused abdominal angina and may eventuate in gangrene of the intestinal tract." Campbell showed slides of a patient with a celiac artery occlusion whom he and Hugh Burnett had treated by interposing a saphenous vein bypass between the right common iliac artery "and a marginal artery about two millimeters in size" with striking clinical and radiographic results. John E. Connolly, of Irvine, California, thought the classical picture was that of celiac artery involvement "at its takeoff from the aorta." In the superior mesenteric artery it is a napkin-ring deformity about one and one half centimeters distal to its takeoff from the aorta." He showed an example of a prophylactic operation on the superior mesenteric artery in a patient who was not yet asymptomatic, at the time of an aorto-iliac endarterectomy for extremity claudication, and said he had done such prophylactic operations on eight occasions. He employed a saphenous vein to connect the superior mesenteric artery to the limb of the prosthetic graft. He indicated that he felt the trapdoor method would be inapplicable to most patients and perhaps dangerous "in the average surgeon's hands" and was inclined to think that vein bypasses would be preferable into the distal mesenteric vessels as they had turned out to be elsewhere. Frank G. Moody, of Salt Lake City, thought this operative approach represented "a tremendous advantage". He asked about the relief of symptoms. R. J. Stoney, closing, said that although as in Campbell's case, the superior mesenteric artery appeared solid, the atheroma was confined to the proximal two or three centimeters, the rest of the plug being a removable "organized tail thrombus." To Connolly, he said bluntly, ". . . your suggestion for performing prophylactic operations on asymptomatic patients would seem to be unnecessary and often risky meddling. Aortography for patients with aorto-iliac or renal artery disease often demonstrates asymptomatic occlusion of one or more visceral branches, usually the superior mesenteric artery. In the 20 years that such patients have been under continuous follow-up in our hospital, we have yet to encounter a patient who subsequently developed symptoms of visceral ischemia or infarction. I am also concerned over advocacy of long vein grafts . . . since our experience parallels that of Dr. Rob, reported in 1966, in which 60% of the vein grafts subsequently failed. To Dr. Moody, he answered that the symptoms recurred only in those patients in whom there was "postoperative arteriographic evidence of reocclusion, an event most commonly encountered in the grafts of patients with saphenous vein grafts."

* * *

Lester W. Martin, of Cincinnati, Professor of Surgery and Pediatrics, College of Medicine, University of Cincinnati, and by invitation, C. LeCoultre, and W. K. Schubert, *Total Colectomy and Mucosal Proctectomy with Preservation of Continence in Ulcerative Colitis*, attributed the philosophy of the operation and the operative technique to Ravitch and Sabiston, in 1947. Soave, in 1963 reported the same technique for Hirschsprung's disease for which it had already been used in Brazil by several investigators. Martin had a series of 17 patients undergoing total colectomy for chronic ulcerative colitis in whom he had tried to preserve rectal continence. The rectal mucosa was required to be free of gross disease. From the abdomen, "A circumferential incision is made through the muscular wall of the colon just below the peritoneal reflection. Dissection is then continued downward separating the muscular wall of the rectum from the mucosa and the submucosa . . . The resulting mucosal cylinder can be dissected free all the way to the anus." The tube of rectal mucosa was everted and delivered outside the anus, as much of the colon as remained was resected, the ileum mobilized, brought down through the intact musculature of the rectal canal and anastomosed to the anorectal mucosa. He then performed a diverting ileostomy. The results "in general have been encouraging with no deaths, and only two failures. It is now ten years since our first patient's operation. He has two to three stools daily, has complete control, and is a full-time college student." Patients had frequent watery stools for a time, sometimes required as long as 12 months "for adaptation, after which patients have complete control of two to eight semiformed stools daily. All 17 patients recovered and are currently free of disease." The two failures resulted from pelvic sepsis and both patients had permanent ileostomies. Two patients still had their diverting ileostomies. The other 13 all had complete bowel control. "Our experience with 17 patients with chronic ulcerative colitis demonstrates that it is possible to perform a total colectomy with mucosal proctectomy and preserve anorectal continence."

Discussion

Mark M. Ravitch, of Pittsburgh, opened the Discussion, saying that as Martin had indicated "Dr. Sabiston and I did this in dogs about 30 years ago, and we have applied the procedure now to ulcerative colitis, polyposis, long pullthroughs for long segment villous adenoma, and even for people with a destroyed rectum from lymphopathia venereum . . . the first patient we performed this on had ulcerative colitis. He did beautifully. he's done beautifully ever since. I've never done that well again with a patient with ulcerative colitis. In polyposis it would seem to be that if you do the operation well technically, the patient will be continent and will be happy for ever, although it may take a while. Dr. Soper in Iowa and others have now considerable experience with this operation for polyposis." He was concerned about

Martin's description of the rectum as normal. He thought Martin's technique was superior "We were doing originally our submucosal stripping entirely from below. I remember Harry Shumacker writing me a long time ago saying he tried it from above . . . these people are continent . . . In our experience the attainment of total continence has required from three weeks to nine months, with continence appearing earlier during the day, and then finally at night . . . In adults, given the superiority of our methods of handling ordinary ileostomy today over those of a couple of decades ago, and with the advent of the Koch ileostomy, I'm not as certain that the game is worth the candle, but this is a very impressive and encouraging series." Martin, in closing, agreed that the operation was even easier and more satisfactory in children with polyposis, much more difficult in ulcerative colitis, where he employed preoperative parenteral alimentation and at operation a complimentary ileostomy. The rectum probably was not truly normal but if it was seriously diseased, he thought the patient should have subtotal colectomy "and establishment of an ileostomy . . . with preservation of the rectum in the hopes that at some future time, the rectal disease may become sufficiently quiescent to permit mucosal proctectomy."

* * *

J. A. Hunter, W. S. Dye, Hushang Javid, all by invitation; Hassan Najafi, of Chicago, Professor of Surgery, Rush Medical College; Chairman, Department of Cardiovascular-Thoracic Surgery, Rush-Presbyterian-St. Luke's Medical Center, and by invitation, M. D. Goldin and C. Serry, *Permanent Transvenous Balloon Occlusion of the Inferior Vena Cava,* agreed that "The majority of patients with venous thromboembolism are successfully treated with anticoagulant therapy." When anticoagulant therapy was contraindicated or failed, the available techniques for ligation or plication of the inferior vena cava "are associated with significant morbidity and mortality . . . have the great disadvantage of requiring that anticoagulant therapy be interrupted." Judging "that it is not possible to insert a transvenous filter that will remain predictably patent", they had devised a balloon catheter which could be inserted through the jugular vein, accurately positioned with the aid of venography through the catheter, and the balloon inflated in the vena cava. "The distensible vein permits the balloon to develop a diameter greater than the I.V.C. proximal to the occluder." Tugging on the balloon with the inserting catheter demonstrated it to be securely

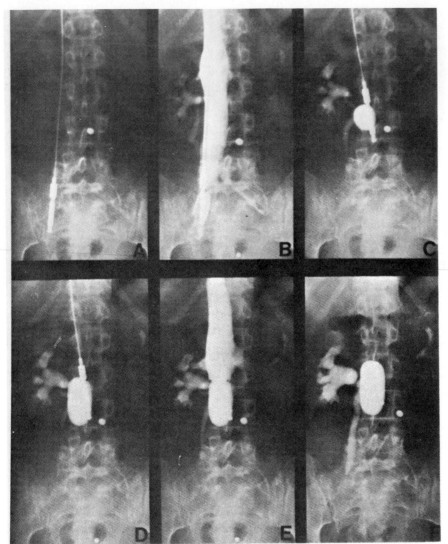

FIG. 4. Series of x-rays during balloon placement: (A) Catheter in right iliac vein. (B) Venogram shows anatomy and left iliac thrombus. (C) Balloon inflation between iliac and renal veins results initially in round shape. (D) Balloon elongates as it is molded by I.V.C. (E) Venogram confirms adequate size and proper position of balloon. (F) Catheter separates and is withdrawn.

When anticoagulant therapy was inadvisable, or had failed, in the prevention of pulmonary embolism, and disliking the ligations and compartmentations, the Presbyterian-St. Luke's group devised a balloon catheter which could be inserted through the jugular vein, accurately positioned fluoroscopically, the balloon inflated to occlude the vena cava, the catheter disengaged and the balloon left there. In their 60 patients, there were two failures from the procedure and no subsequent emboli. "One patient had an unstable balloon removed by flank incision . . . the other patient had pulmonary embolectomy of . . . embolized venous clots from the legs and the balloon remnant . . . Both of these patients recovered."

J. A. Hunter, W. S. Dye, H. Javid, H. Najafi, M. D. Goldin and C. Sperry, *Permanent Transvenous Balloon Occlusion of the Inferior Vena Cava,* Volume XCV, 1977.

lodged. The catheter, detached from the balloon, was then left occluding the vena cava. Since July 2, 1970, they had placed the balloon in 60 consecutive patients, at first restricting the technique to patients too ill for conventional I.V.C. interruption. Twenty-nine of the patients were on anticoagulant therapy at the time and remained so without interruption. Transient hold-up in the right renal vein was the most common technical difficulty "readily overcome by partial inflation of the balloon, which shifted the catheter tip off the lateral venous wall permitting it to move into the distal I.V.C. . . . Despite the fact that most patients were quite ill, and 11 were on drug support to maintain cardiovascular adequacy, only a single patient had a significant decline in blood pressure when the I.V.C. was occluded. In this instance, the balloon was deflated, colloid was given through the outer catheter of the instrument, and the balloon reinflated. With an augmented blood volume, I.V.C. occlusion was well-tolerated." In five patients, intracaval thrombus was recognized by venogram and isolated in the distal I.V.C. by the balloon, the partially inflated balloon being employed in two of them to move the clot into the distal I.V.C. There was no mortality attributable to the procedure, and no subsequent pulmonary embolism. The 29 patients who were on anticoagulant therapy had no complications. One patient had an "unstable" balloon removed by a flank incision, and an I.V.C. ligation was done. Another patient had pulmonary embolectomy for "embolized venous clots from the legs and the balloon remnant . . . Both of these patients recovered and were discharged from the hospital in good condition." The balloon failures "were traced to specific defects in the balloon assembly design." The instrument had been redesigned and this had not occurred again. Thirty-two patients had phlebitis with edema before balloon occlusion. Four of 29 patients who were on anticoagulants had worsening of the condition of their lower extremities after occlusion. Nine of 25 patients who were not on anticoagulants had worsening of their edema. There were nine hospital deaths from the basic underlying disease with autopsy in all "and in every instance, the balloon occluder was in its original and proper position." The figures on edema of the legs indicated the value of combining heparin administration with occlusion. The balloon ultimately deflated spontaneously and became "encased in a fibrous capsule which permanently obstructs the vena cava."

Discussion

Frank C. Spencer, of New York, was convinced "that this technique prevented pulmonary emboli" but was particularly struck by "the absence of hypotension following inflation of the balloon. Following complete occlusion of the vena cava, several reports have described a lowering of blood volume from trapping of blood in the lower extremities with resulting hypotension. This has precipitated serious sequelae in critically ill patients." He suggested that the phenomenon had been due to "hypovolemia or to the concomitant effects of anesthesia on compensatory mechanisms for sudden changes in blood volume." He asked whether there were any indications for direct approach to the vena cava or could the balloon always be used. Hunter, in closing, agreed that the absence of physiological effects was because the patients were not anesthetized. In the single pa-

tient in whom hypotension had occurred, deflation of the balloon and blood volume augmentation had provided immediate relief. As to selection of patients, "At present we use balloon occlusion as the method of I.V.C. interruption whenever the circumstance of the patient makes it desirable to avoid surgical or anesthetic trauma. The technique may also be chosen for the heparinized patient, when we wish to combine the advantages of I.V.C. interruption with anticoagulant therapy."

* * *

Ward O. Griffen, Jr., of Lexington, Professor of Surgery and Physiology, Chairman, Department of Surgery, University of Kentucky, and by invitation, V. L. Young, and C. C. Stevenson, *A Prospective Comparison of Gastric and Jejunoileal Bypass Procedures for Morbid Obesity,* had undertaken a randomized prospective evaluation in which a 90% gastric exclusion with a Roux-en-Y reconstitution was compared to a jejunoileal bypass performed as an end-to-end anastomosis between 30 cm. of jejunum and 25 cm. of terminal ileum, the bypassed segment of small bowel being decompressed by an end-to-side ileocolostomy. There were 32 patients in the gastric group and 27 in the jejunoileal group. "Stapling devices were used routinely in these procedures although all staple lines were oversewn where appropriate . . . There were no immediate postoperative deaths in either group and one patient in each group has required a takedown of the bypass procedure." The gastric takedown patient, one of the two in that group who had had an anastomotic leak, had developed an almost completely obstructed gastrojejunostomy. "The patient in the jejunoileal group who required reanastomosis lost 116 kg in one year and developed jaundice, ascites and peripheral edema." There had been one late death in each group. The death in the jejunoileal group was in a patient who developed severe liver disease and refused reanastomosis. "The patient in the gastric group who died was readmitted three months after the bypass procedure for observation. Two days after admission she collapsed and could not be resuscitated. The clinical impression was pulmonary embolus, but none was found at autopsy." Ten other of the jejunoileal patients and four of the gastric bypass patients required rehospitalization. Three of the latter for repair of an incisional hernia and one for fistula after an anastomotic leak. The principal immediate difference was in the two anastomotic leaks in the gastric patients and the absence of any leaks in the jejunoileal shunts. The gastric bypass led to three incidental splenectomies. The gastric bypass patients had nausea and vomiting; the jejunoileal shunt patients had troublesome diarrhea and excessive potassium loss. Four of the jejunoileal shunt patients had kidney stones, none of the gastric patients did. No patient undergoing gastric bypass developed liver disease. Two of the jejunoileal shunt patients did, one died of it and the other required a takedown of the shunt. The weight loss pattern showed no difference with the two operations. At one year, the mean weight loss was 51 kg for the gastric bypass and 57.9% kg for the jejunoileal bypass. Griffen admitted that the gastric bypass procedure was "somewhat more demanding technically . . . definitely has a finite learning curve both to obtain the correct size in the gastric pouch and the diameter of the gastrojejunostomy opening and to eliminate technical errors. Once the technique of gastric bypass is learned, it would appear to be superior to jejunoileal bypass in that it has the same weight loss capability, fewer long-term sequelae, and no evidence of the development of significant liver disease."

Discussion

Henry Buchwald, of Minneapolis, congratulated Griffen on the first comparative study in this field. He thought that Griffen's jejunoileal shunts, leaving 55 cm. were too long. "We leave 40 to 45 cm, as does Dr. H. William Scott. This five to ten centimeter difference is critical and, I believe, may account for the jejuno-ileal bypass patients in Dr. Griffen's series losing no more weight than his gastric patients. In our experience, we have found a far more significant weight reduction after the intestinal bypass procedure." He agreed that 75% of jejunoileal bypass patients showed worsening hepatic histology at the end of a year but they tended to improve sequentially up to five years and "Far more critical, is the fact that only five per cent of jejunoileal bypass patients exhibit clinical liver failure." [The audience might well have considered this figure as an argument against the use of the intestinal shunt.] He hoped Dr. Griffen would extend the number of his patients and the years of follow-up and see whether perhaps different operations should be done for different individuals, whether the gastric pouch distended with time. "Experience has shown that the gastric bypass can probably be outeaten; whereas, it is only rare that the jejuno-ileal bypass can be outeaten." Edward E. Mason, of Iowa City, mentioned a modification of the gastric operation being done in the Twin Cities, particularly by Dr. John Alden. A very high gastroenterostomy was done and the stapling machine was placed across the stomach just below the gastroenterostomy and adjusted to leave a 100 ml. gastric pouch. The stomach was not divided. Alden had done 200 such operations with no mortality and an average operating time of 67 minutes. William V. McDermott, Jr., of Boston, said that "the apparent advantage of the intestinal bypass in achieving greater weight loss is illusory, inasmuch as the amount of fat loss is nearly identical in the two procedures, and the excess recorded weight loss following intestinal bypass is due to associated depletion of lean body mass, as measured in our metabolic unit . . . a metabolically undesirable side effect which occurs minimally after gastric bypass . . . the gastric bypass is unquestionably . . . a more difficult technical procedure. Anastomotic complications have been reported repeatedly; but we have felt that these are due mainly to the ischemia of the small gastric pouch." Lloyd D. MacLean, of Montreal, asked whether Griffen would agree "that, what determines an excellent result may not, in fact, have been controlled in this type of study; that is, intelligence of the patient, family support, income, and motivation to succeed, no addiction to other than overeating, and, particularly important, the change in dietary habits after intestinal bypass . . ." With jejunoileal shunt, if the patients were losing more than 20 pounds a month, he admitted them to the hospital for fear of liver failure, treating them with 5% casein hydrolysate intravenously. He asked Griffen whether it was not too early to know what the end result of gastric bypass would be and whether he did not agree that intractable diarrhea was commoner in the end-to-end than end-to-side jejunoileal shunts. John Halverson, of St. Louis, had data to support Griffen. At Washington University, 101 jejunoileal bypass patients, they had no in-hospital deaths, five late deaths, numerous complications, six patients with liver failure, had restored intestinal continuity in 21% of the patients over a period of four years, in half the patients for liver dysfunction and electrolyte imbalance. Cesar Gomez, of St. Louis, had reviewed 173 gastric bypass patients with "only one death and very few serious postoperative problems . . . however, transient nausea and vomiting occurred in nearly all the patients, almost always associated with overeating." None of the patients had metabolic problems or dumping or diarrhea, and "the incidence of marginal ulceration was low". Ward O. Griffen, in closing, said there was, indeed, a definite learning curve to the performance of the gastric operation. To Buchwald, he said that the patients could not outeat the operation if it was done correctly. The pouch should not hold more than 60 ml. of fluid and the anastomosis be no larger than 1.2 cm. He agreed that "there is no question that the gastric bypass patients do not lose the lean body mass that the jejunoileal patients do, and I think that is the key to the difference in the weight loss." His gastric patients had been going three years, he would continue to observe them.

* * *

John L. Sawyers, of Nashville, Professor of Surgery, Vanderbilt University; J. Lynwood Herrington, Jr., Associate Clinical Professor of Surgery, Vanderbilt University, and by invitation, D. P. Burney, *Proximal Gastric Vagotomy Compared with Vagotomy and Antrectomy and Selective Gastric Vagotomy and Pyloroplasty,* now presented data from the study they had mentioned in discussion at previous meetings. Proximal gastric vagotomy performed in 174 adult men with chronic duodenal ulcer, intractable to medical therapy, was randomized against truncal vagotomy with antrectomy, and selective gastric vagotomy with Finney pyloroplasty. All operations were elective though some of the patients had had bleeding episodes in the past. The proximal gastric vagotomy was performed down to the "crow's foot", approximately 7 cm. from the pylorus, and the dissection continued cephalad on the esophagus at least 5 cm. above the esophagogastric junction. There were no deaths in the proximal gastric vagotomy-selective gastric vagotomy plus pyloroplasty trial, and one death from pulmonary embolism after proximal gastric vagotomy in the comparison with truncal vagotomy and antrectomy. There were three minor wound infections in all, one persistent obstruction of the Billroth I anastomosis after antrectomy, which required gastrojejunostomy for relief. "Epigastric fullness and early satiety occurred in 15 patients (17%) who had PGV, but no patient required reoperation." Employing the well-known Visick classification, interpreted as Visick I, excellent; II, good; III, fair; IV, poor, the proximal gastric vagotomy gave 80% Visick I in the one trial and 78% in the other, the vagotomy and antrectomy, 56% Visick I, the selective vagotomy and pyloroplasty, 73%. The poor results were 4% and 3% in the PGV groups, 6% in the vagotomy and antrectomy group, and 3% in the selective gastric vagotomy and pyloroplasty. Dumping occurred in 0 and 3% of the PGV, 22% of the others, diarrhea in 2% and 0 of the PGV groups, 18% and 3% in the others. Reflux gastritis occurred in 0 and 3% of the PGV groups, 4% and 5% of the others. There had been two recurrent duodenal ulcers, one after proximal gastric vagotomy and one after selective vagotomy with pyloroplasty. After proximal gastric vagotomy, there had been two gastric ulcers. Griffith and Harkins, in

1957, had performed proximal gastric vagotomy in dogs and Holle and Hart, in 1967, had first performed it in patients with a drainage procedure. Amdrup, and Johnston and Wilkinson had subsequently employed the procedure without drainage operations. Amdrup had recently tabulated six retrospective studies in which the ulcer recurrence rate in proximal gastric vagotomy was 1 to 9%, dumping, 0.4% to 7%, and mild diarrhea, 0 to 2%. Goligher had reported 306 proximal gastric vagotomies for duodenal ulcer with no operative deaths, a 2% proven ulcer recurrence rate, an additional 3% suspected recurrence and reported a Visick I and II grading of 81%, higher than after other operations he had used for duodenal ulcer. The long-term effectiveness of proximal gastric vagotomy in controlling ulcer was as yet unknown. They drew no conclusions and expressed no philosophy.

Discussion

Professor S. Hedenstedt, of Stockholm, said that, without randomization, in Stockholm they had operated on 600 patients and considered proximal gastric vagotomy "without drainage . . . the safest operation now for duodenal ulcer." They had had no mortality in 500 uncomplicated cases of duodenal ulcer. In 50 acute bleeding ulcers, they had lost eight patients. They considered that 90% of the results were excellent or good. The basal stimulated acid output remained depressed after five years in his patients. With some it tended to rise slowly with time, although thus far, this had not been associated with any increase in recurrence rate. He asked when the pylorus seemed stenotic how Sawyers and Herrington resisted the temptation to perform a pyloroplasty and how they explained the increase in acid with time. His group had had some intraoperative complications, 1% esophagus rupture, 1% spleen rupture with mortality, had Dr. Sawyers seen such complications? James C. Thompson, of Galveston, said recurrent rising acid secretion was the worry. "The report of David Johnston of a 90% positive Hollander at four years is frightening, although in his series, there were no recurrences in that same group of patients." In any case, Thompson had given up the use of the Hollander test ". . . mainly because it's dangerous, and it doesn't supply you any information that you can't get from some other source." He now measured "the actual response to intragastric food." He asked about the reported occurrence of necrosis of the lesser curvature and whether it was associated with splenectomy depriving the stomach of collaterals. Lloyd M. Nyhus, of

DUODENAL ULCER, GASTRIC PHYSIOLOGY
AND THE VAGOTOMISTS

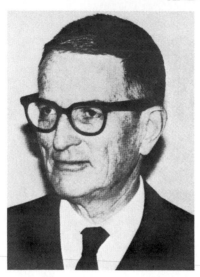

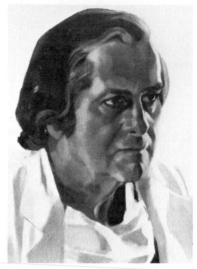

Henry N. Harkins, 1905-1967. M.D. Rush 1930; Intern, Presbyterian Hospital, Chicago; Resident, University of Chicago 1931-38; Guggenheim wanderjahr 1938-39 (he was characteristically fond of saying he visited 14 countries and of enumerating the clinics in which he worked); Henry Ford Hospital 1939-43; Associate Professor, Johns Hopkins 1943-47; Professor of Surgery and first Chairman of the Department, University of Washington, Seattle, 1947-64. A contrasting combination of ambition and self-deprecation, almost unreasonably candid and honest, an assiduous worker in the laboratory and prolific writer,- his books *Surgery of the Stomach and Duodenum,* and *Hernia,* both with Nyhus, are standard authorities and superlative. He put to experimental study numerous facets of gastric physiology, acid production, bloodflow, etc., evaluated, then tried, clinically, selective gastric vagotomy, studied highly selective (parietal cell) vagotomy, perhaps the first to do so, but did not employ it clinically. Gave his life to found a department of surgery, dying of a coronary occlusion, water skiing at a surgical department picnic.

J. Lynwood Herrington, 1919-. M.D. Vanderbilt 1945; Training Vanderbilt and St. Thomas Hospitals; Clinical Professor of Surgery, Vanderbilt University, Leonard W. Edwards, in Nashville, had early accumulated a massive and impressively successful experience at the Edwards-Eve Clinic with antrectomy-vagotomy, and with H. W. Scott's arrival at Vanderbilt, there began the long and fruitful collaboration in the evaluation of the successive operations for duodenal ulcer, Scott and Sawyers at Vanderbilt and Nashville General Hospital, and Herrington and now Sawyers, as well, at St. Thomas. Herrington, a widely experienced gastric surgeon has had a particular interest also in the reparative, reconstructive procedures for the treatment of sequelae to ulcer operations. Has a keen sense of history, and a rapid-fire platform delivery which assures maximal content in minimal time.

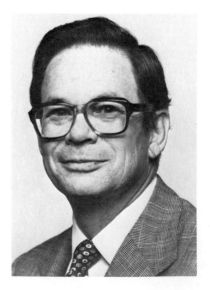

Paul H. Jordan, 1919-. M.D. University of Chicago 1944, where he was a student of Dragstedt; Training at St. Luke's, University of Illinois, Hines V.A.; NIH Fellowship at Karolinska Institute, Stockholm 1958-59; Instructor to Assistant Professor UCLA 1953-58; Assistant Professor, University of Florida 1959-64; Professor of Surgery, Baylor College of Medicine, Houston 1964-. Broad interests in surgery of trauma and surgery of the gastrointestinal tract, judicious evaluator of the types of vagotomy and adjuvant procedures in controlled clinical trials in patients with duodenal ulcer.

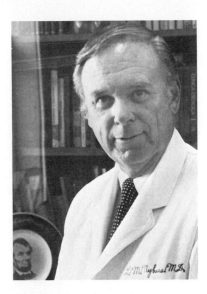

Lloyd M. Nyhus, 1923- . (Recorder 1976-) M.D. 1947 Medical College of Alabama; Training University of Washington, Seattle 1955; Guggenheim Fellow 1955-56 with Sandblom in Lund and Illingworth in Glasgow; Instructor to Professor, University of Washington 1954-67; Professor and Chairman of Surgery, University of Illinois, Chicago 1967- . Student and close collaborator of Harkins, has continued systematic clinical and laboratory evaluation of the problems of duodenal ulcer and groin hernia. Scholarly, thorough, candid, prolific writer and editor, active on the international scene.

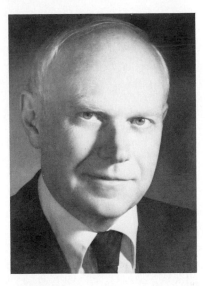

John L. Sawyers, 1925- . M.D. Johns Hopkins 1949; Intern, Johns Hopkins; Residency training Vanderbilt; Instructor to Professor of Surgery, Vanderbilt 1958-1969. Under H. W. Scott's leadership and with Herrington from the Edwards-Eve Clinic, has major role in the serial evaluation in controlled comparative trials of operations for duodenal ulcer,- subtotal gastrectomy, truncal vagotomy with drainage or antrectomy, parietal cell vagotomy, currently emerging as a principal advocate of parietal cell vagotomy.

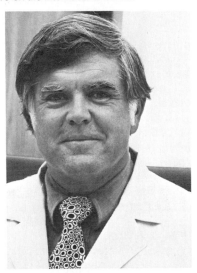

James C. Thompson, 1928- . M.D., University of Texas, Galveston 1951 and internship 1952; Residency, University of Pennsylvania 1952-59, to Assistant Professor of Surgery 1961-63; Associate Professor of Surgery, UCLA to Professor 1963-70; Professor and Chairman, Department of Surgery, University of Texas, Galveston 1970- and Professor of Physiology and Biophysics. Colorful, witty, iconoclastic, and a major contributor to gastric physiology; widely respected for his thorough and admirably scientific studies of the biochemical characterization, measurements, and function of gastrointestinal hormones in health and disease.

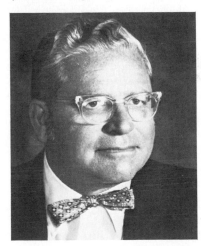

Edward R. Woodward, 1916- . M.D. University of Chicago 1942 to Resident in Surgery 1952; Instructor, University of Chicago 1952-53; Assistant to Associate Professor of Surgery, UCLA 1953-57; Professor and Chairman, Department of Surgery, University of Florida, Gainesville 1957- . Dragstedt's resident at the University of Chicago and his disciple in the study of gastric physiology. In one of those moves which warms the heart, and proves mutually profitable, invited the "retired" Dragstedt to join him in Gainesville in 1967, where until his death in 1975, Dragstedt ran a productive laboratory, stimulating students, house officers, graduate students and faculty. Woodward's laboratory and clinical efforts and contributions have been in the problems of esophageal reflux, and operations for morbid obesity—as well as in peptic ulcer.

Chicago, commented on the patients with early satiety ". . . because we are ignorant, truly ignorant of the precise dissection at the 'crow's foot'. If we don't dissect far enough distally, we are not going to reduce acidity sufficiently. Contrariwise, if we cut too many nerves of Latarjet at the crow's foot, we may get gastric stasis." [He seemed to be suggesting that they had, in fact, gone too far distally.] Nyhus asked "What will be the long term results? This is totally unknown at the present." He looked to a longer follow-up. J. Lynwood Herrington, Jr., closing, said that they had, in addition, operated upon 25 patients with perforated ulcer and done a proximal gastric vagotomy with no operative mortality. They had operated on a few patients with pyloric obstruction, passed a Maloney dilator through into the duodenum for dilatation, with good results. To Thompson, he said that they too, had abandoned the Hollander test but were concerned that, with a meal of beef extract, after proximal gastric vagotomy the acid did rise. They had not seen necrosis or slough of the lesser curvature and thought it was probably due to direct injury to the stomach with instruments. He agreed "the unanswered problem at present with proximal gastric vagotomy is the likelihood of recurrent ulcer. In those centers where the operation is being done correctly the recurrence rate is two to five percent over a follow-up now extending from five to almost eight years", most of the ulcers recurring within a year or two. They had not used the procedure for benign gastric ulcer but were planning to extend it to ulcers with perforation, obstruction, and bleeding.

The Business Meetings

The 1977 meeting was held at the Boca Raton Hotel and Club, Boca Raton, Florida, March 23, 24, and 25, President Claude E. Welch, in the Chair. The newly elected Honorary Members were Sir Andrew Kay, of England, Professor G. B. Ong, of Hong Kong, and Professor Lars-Erik Gelin, of Göteborg, and in spite of the arrangements to have the elections and make the notifications at the time of the winter meeting of the Council, only Gelin was able to be present.

At the Second Business Session, by an amendment proposed the previous year and accepted this year, Active Fellows were automatically to be placed on the list of Senior Fellows at age 60 and excused from dues after age 65. The opportunity of becoming a life member by the payment of $250 and being thereafter excused payment of all dues was withdrawn.

Council announced that the 1980 Centennial Meeting which was to have been held appropriately in Philadelphia was moved to the Hyatt Regency House, Atlanta, Georgia, "representing a change from the Bellevue-Stratford Hotel in Philadelphia, the demise of which, under Chapter 11 of the Federal Bankruptcy Act is attributed to an infectious disease" [this was the outbreak of Legionnaire's Disease, an acute respiratory infection which resulted in a number of deaths in American Legion conventioneers who had stayed at the Hotel and was ultimately decided to have probably been disseminated from the air conditioning system. The Hotel, in fact, has survived after long being closed, has been completely renovated, is open and will, in fact, be functioning at the time of the Centennial Meeting]. The Association heard with interest that it "was the subject of a subpoena by the Federal Trade Commission, as were 40 other surgical associations and boards in connection with the Federal Trade Commission's allegation of restraint of trade against the American Medical Association. At the request of the Secretary, the Association is excused from appearance at a public hearing in Washington, and answered to the specifications of the subpoena in writing."

The American Medical Association in the opinion of the Council of the American Surgical Association and the Regents and Director of the American College of Surgeons had very largely moved to control the Liaison Committee on Graduate Education by virtue of housing, staffing, and underwriting it. Now William H. Muller, Chairman of the Board of Regents of the American College of Surgeons, reported to the Association, stating that "The Liaison Committee on Graduate Medical Education has designated itself as an accrediting body for all residency programs, a role that has been actually served by the Residency Review Committees in recommending approval or disapproval of residency training programs. Moreover, the Residency Review Committees are incorrectly presumed to be capable of speaking to policy matters affecting their composition and function when such matters are within the authority of the sponsoring organizations of the Residency Review Committees. Thus the Liaison Committee on Graduate Medical Education in matters of policy ignores the ultimate power base for the Residency Review Committees; that is, their sponsoring organizations." The Council had approved, and now offered to the Fellowship for their decision, a series of resolutions, correcting what was considered to be the attempt at moving control of residency training programs from the sponsoring specialty organizations to what was, in effect, a bureaucratic arm of the AMA. Feuding on this matter had been going on for some time at an increasing tempo. The Council of the Association and the Regents of the College felt strongly on the matters. The resolutions all carried.

All of the 26 candidates proposed were elected at the meeting. President Welch then announced the decision of Council to make Robert M. Zollinger, of Columbus, Ohio, the fourth recipient of the Association's Medallion for Scientific Achievement.

Officers elected were David C. Sabiston, of Durham, North Carolina, President; John A. Schilling, of Seattle, Washington; and Robert S. Sparkman, of Dallas, Vice-Presidents; Lloyd M. Nyhus, of Chicago, Secretary.

XCVI

1978

The 1978 meeting was held at the Sheraton-Dallas Hotel, Dallas, Texas, April 26, 27, and 28, President David C. Sabiston, Jr., of Durham, James Buchanan Duke Professor of Surgery and Chairman, Department of Surgery, Surgeon-in-Chief, Duke Hospital, in the Chair.

President Sabiston's address was devoted to a marvelous sketch of the character and contributions of his teacher, Alfred Blalock [forbearing to mention that he was the fourth Blalock Resident to be the Association's President].

* * *

Layton F. Rikkers and eight others, by invitation, and W. Dean Warren, Professor and Chairman, Department of Surgery, Emory University Hospital, *A Randomized, Controlled Trial of the Distal Splenorenal Shunt,* took up the challenge which they had previously [see page 1239, Volume LXXXV, 1967] presented to others to evaluate the efficacy of what had come to be known as the Warren shunt, compared to what Warren called "nonselective" shunts. He opened with a statement of the current understanding of the effects of shunting, "The role of portasystemic shunts in the management of cirrhotic patients who have hemorrhaged from esophageal varices remains controversial. Four prospective, randomized trials have been conducted to determine the effects of totally diverting shunts (end-to-side and side-to-side portocaval shunts) on liver function and survival [Jackson's Veterans Administration study, Mikkelsen's West Coast Study, the Boston Hospital group's study, and a British study]. Although three of the studies show prolongation of survival in shunted patients when compared to medically treated controls, in no instance is the difference statistically significant. While medically managed patients have a high fatality secondary to recurrent variceal hemorrhage, surgically treated patients have an accelerated rate of death from hepatic failure. In addition, some of these studies, as well as others, indicate that quality of life following a portocaval shunt is impaired because of an increased incidence and severity of portasystemic encephalopathy. A probable explanation for these adverse effects of shunting procedures is their elimination of hepatic portal perfusion. Several experimental studies [Marchioro, Starzl] have suggested that splanchnic perfusion of the liver is essential for optimal hepatic function. Portal blood appears to contain hepatotrophic factors which maintain hepatocyte integrity and capacity for regeneration. Another detrimental effect of total portal diversion is shunting of intestinally absorbed nitrogenous substances, normally extracted by the liver, into the systemic circulation. It has been hypothesized that some of these compounds may be cerebral toxins and play a role in the pathogenesis of encephalopathy." Warren claimed for his distal splenorenal shunt ". . . selective decompression of esophageal varices through the gastrosplenic component of the splanchnic circulation and maintenance of superior mesenteric venous perfusion of the liver." The trial at Emory University Affiliated Hospitals had begun in 1971, and entry into it terminated in 1976, so that all patients had been followed for a minimum of two years and for an average of four years. All patients had documented cirrhosis with one major upper gastrointestinal hemorrhage, no significant ascites at the time of surgery, and "no appreciable hepatocellular necrosis or inflammation on current liver biopsy". The Warren shunt was done on 26 patients and nonselective shunts on 29 [one other patient insisted on having the Warren shunt, and in two patients the Warren shunt proved technically unfeasible]. The "nonselective" shunts, most of them with Dacron prostheses, were 18 interposition grafts between the superior mesenteric and left renal veins, six mesocaval grafts, two side-to-side splenorenal anastomoses, one end-to-side renosplenic, one splenocaval, and one end-to-side portocaval. "The distal splenorenal shunt operation consisted of anastomosis of distal splenic vein to left renal vein, ligation or suture closure of proximal splenic vein, and interruption of left gastric, right gastroepiploic, and umbilical veins." There were three postoperative deaths in each group, five from hepatic failure, one from infected ascites and sepsis. Ten patients undergoing Warren shunts and eight of the others had expired by the conclusion of the study. The Warren shunt patients died somewhat later,- mean 26.7 months vs. 12.8 months, and that difference was statistically significant although differences in mortality or longevity for the two groups were not. There was a striking difference in the incidence of encephalopathy, 52% for the nonselective shunt and 12% for the Warren shunt, five of the 15 patients with conventional shunts being "totally disabled by encephalopathy". More of the Warren shunt patients returned to heavy drinking after operation. Angiography or autopsy proved five nonselective shunts and two Warren shunts to be occluded. One Warren shunt patient and two in the other group bled subsequently of duodenal ulcers in the presence of patent shunts. One Warren shunt patient died of "upper gastrointestinal hemorrhage of unknown etiology in a remote community . . . the only fatality secondary to hemorrhage in the trial." So far as the effect upon the liver was concerned, "None of the conventional liver function or hematological tests were consistently altered by shunt surgery in either group." However, the Child's score and the maximal rate of urea synthesis after a challenge of casein by mouth, both "significantly deteriorated in nonselective pa-

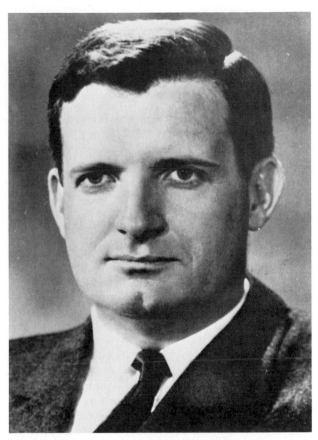

David C. Sabiston, Jr., (c. 1964) 1924-. President 1978. M.D. Johns Hopkins 1947, Intern through Resident 1947-1953, Assistant Professor to Professor 1955-1964, Professor and Chairman, Department of Surgery, Duke University 1971-. Early interested in relief of atherosclerotic coronary artery disease, established nature of appropriate operation for coronary-pulmonary fistulae, with Wagner introduced RAI tagged micro-aggregated human albumin for lung scanning in diagnosis of pulmonary embolism. An extraordinarily well-organized and efficient worker, he has made his Department at Duke one of the strongest in the nation. The successive editions of his *Textbook of Surgery*, and *Gibbon's Thoracic Surgery*,- co-edited with F. C. Spencer,- have had enormous success.

tients between the preoperative and early postoperative evaluation . . . In contrast, the selective procedure had no apparent deleterious effect on either Child's score or MRUS . . . in the early interval following surgery." Compared later after operation, the Child's score was significantly affected after both operations [they lacked late data on the MRUS]. Visceral angiography "revealed maintenance of hepatic portal perfusion in 14 of 16 selective patients and one of 20 nonselective patients, and "Late post-operative studies" had altered the figures to five of 12 Warren shunts and two of 15 others, not a significant difference. However, in the non-Warren shunts, hepatic portal perfusion occurred only when interposition grafts were totally occluded, "Two separate mechanisms, portal vein thrombosis and formation of new portasystemic collaterals, appeared to be responsible for loss of hepatic portal perfusion following distal splenorenal shunt." Two patients developed portal vein thrombosis, one abruptly and one progressively. Other Warren shunt patients without hepatopetal portal flow all had new collateral pathways. Comparing the persistence of portal perfusion of the liver with hepatic function and encephalopathy, Warren was able to say "Patients with continuing splanchnic perfusion of the liver into the late postoperative interval show a statistically significant superiority over those without hepatic portal perfusion with respect to nearly every test of hepatic function, nitrogen metabolism, and cerebral function . . . In fact, no patient with hepatopetal portal flow developed either clinical or EEG evidence of portasystemic encephalopathy. He interpreted his results as indicating that ". . . if progression of liver disease is the main factor limiting survival, type of shunt performed probably has little influence on this variable. However, if the liver disease is quiescent or can be made stable by removing the responsible hepatotoxin, e.g., alcohol, and recurrent variceal hemorrhage is the factor limiting survival, the selective shunt may provide for both a more encephalopathy-free and longer life . . . the distal splenorenal shunt, especially when its objective of maintaining hepatic portal perfusion is achieved, results in significantly less morbidity than nonselective shunting procedures."

Discussion

Watts R. Webb, of New Orleans [who had succeeded Drapanas as Chairman of the Department at the Tulane Medical School], sharply attacked Rikkers' presentation of Warren's material, ". . . I think the most intriguing aspect of today's report is the very novel way in which he has developed his data. The control group scrambles three different procedures and all are called total shunts. The short, broad mesocaval shunt usually remains patent as a partial shunt, while the mesorenal shunt—longer and poorly positioned—usually thromboses, and is a nonshunt. Second, in comparing portal perfusion to nonportal perfusion in the effect on the liver, he's actually thrown failure of the Warren shunt into the control group, and I don't think this is a valid concept." Reduced function was "more of a reflection of the continuing hepatic disease, than of the nature of the shunt or decompression. He reports that the Warren shunt does not alter portal pressure, yet a high percentage of them still lose their prograde flow, which again emphasizes that this probably is due to the progressive liver disease rather than the shunt." Webb presented the Tulane experience, begun by Drapanas in 1968 and continued by James Dowling, of 132 patients, only 18 of them Child's Type A,- ". . . and essentially all of those that Dr. Warren talked about today would be in the A group. The rebleeding is very low, none in the A, only 4% in the B. Encephalopathy . . . none in the A group, comparable to the 11% encephalopathy rate presented today; 16% in the B group; and about 35% of those in the C group. Operative mortality is under 10% . . . concentrated in the C group, and the total related mortality over a ten-year cumulative period is less than 20%. There are, additionally, four other deaths all due to suicide, which emphasizes the psychosocial aspect of this particular disease." Late patency was demonstrated in 90% of 73 patients studied, "and all patients who had preoperative prograde flow and had a patent graft likewise had postoperative prograde flow." His summation was in direct contradiction, and a challenge to Warren, "I find it very difficult to accept the advocating of a procedure that is difficult, time-consuming, and has a learning curve with a very high mortality. It is a disconnection, rather than a shunt, doing very little for portal hypertension. It increases the incidence of ascites, and is applicable only for Class A patients, who hardly need the procedure. This is in contrast to a procedure which a ten-year experience shows to be simple, rapid, relatively bloodless, easily learned and effective in controlling portal hypertension and variceal bleeding. It prolongs life, and it drastically reduces the incidence of encephalopathy and ascites. I hope that at the next presentation Dean Warren makes he'll put this in proper perspective." Robert Zeppa, of Miami [who had, of course, been associated with Warren when he began the distal splenorenal shunt work in Miami, before moving to Atlanta], rose to Warren's defense, ". . . Dr. Rikkers has presented the definitive study demonstrating the superiority of selective shunting in reproducible physiological terms." Zeppa now had a series of 118 patients in whom there had been only two postoperative deaths. He demonstrated a statistical analysis to show that the problem of survival was so heavily affected by continual alcohol abuse that ". . . one will never be able to compare these operations until we get a randomized study of the nonalcoholics . . . I do believe we can support the theory, on the basis of protein testing and serial electroencephalograms, that the patients who have survived at the three-year level have no change in this parameter." John Terblanche, of Cape Town, South Africa [who had been spending a year at the Mayo Clinic], referred to his experience with injection sclerotherapy for the control of variceal bleeding. They had undertaken a prospective randomized controlled clinical trial in August 1975, "All comers and all risk grades were included." It was still too early to discuss survival, but in the injection group, "we have been able to eradicate varices by repeated-injection sclerotherapy in all survivors, and once the varices had been eradicated there was no further recurrent variceal bleeding." Two patients each developed a single variceal channel subsequently, which was successfully injected. "On the other hand, the control patients [conventional medical management] have continued to have recurrent variceal bleeds." William V. McDermott, of Boston, said that it had initially been possible to predict that the operation would achieve "selective decompression of esophageal varices", that "portal perfusion of the liver would be maintained, and perhaps portal-systemic encephalopathy minimized", that the shunt would not be effective in the presence of intractable ascites,- "this had proved to be true, in many instances",- and that it would be no more effective,- 50%,- in reversing severe pancytopenia than "any other decompressive shunt which leaves the spleen *in situ.*" The Boston Interhospital Liver Group had attempted a randomized study, but of 53 patients, "35 were rejected for randomization for various reasons, the most prominent of which were ascites, severe pancytopenia, retrograde flow, previous bouts of severe pancreatitis, splenic vein abnormalities . . . and a number of other miscellaneous causes." The remaining 18 patients had been followed only a year and none in either group had had encephalopathy, and "there has been only one bleed, in a patient with a thrombosed distal splenorenal shunt." This was, therefore, a very difficult problem to study. He thought the incidence of encephalopathy would rise with time but would probably be lower in the selective shunts, and "I would visualize this selective shunt as being useful in selected patients". Donald C. Nabseth, of Boston, rose ". . . as a supporter of the Warren procedure, but with some reservation. Our experience with a series of 25 patients has shown distal splenorenal shunts to be superior to the portacaval shunt or the mesocaval shunt . . . However, late hemodynamic studies on certain of our pa-

tients have shown reversal of portal flow." He asked whether portal flow might not be reversed in more of the selective shunt patients as time went on, "If this occurs, perhaps their freedom from encephalopathy will significantly depend on their capacity to increase their hepatic arterial flow, as Burchell and associates have shown in patients with portacaval shunts." Carlo E. Grossi, of St. Vincent's Hospital, New York [where Rousselot had migrated from Whipple's Spleen Clinic at Presbyterian to set up a similar program], said that "the real rates of morbidity and mortality don't show until the fifth or eighth year after operation. We feel that 70% incidence of encephalopathy for the total shunts is inordinately large" and attributed this to diagnosis by "laboratory malfunction or EEG evidence". Their group had shown "that the postshunt increase in hepatic arterial flow seemed to be the only, single factor associated with survival and incidence of encephalopathy that was significant upon analysis . . . probably due to the decreased arteriolar resistance induced by the shunt. This implies an "improved oxygenation of liver cells, with better function." He asked, "Could total hepatic blood flow be estimated in this group of patients before and after, so that we might discover why there is this decrease in encephalopathy with the Warren shunt?" Warren, closing, responded to Watts Webb's attack in kind, "We sent our angiographer to Charity Hospital, and he went over their records, and there is not a single proven case of perfusion of the liver with a patent mesocaval interposition graft. It is a perfusion/confusion picture where they inject the liver at the same time as the intestine, and the blood is coming out of the liver . . . It gives the impression of perfusion of the liver, when it actually is not. I would be very grateful if Dr. Webb would explain the difference between putting in an 18 mm. Dacron graft between the vena cava and the superior mesenteric vein, or the mesenteric vein and the renal vein . . . The physiology of that escapes me . . ." Warren said they did not restrict themselves to Class A [Child], "the only ones that we turn down are those with acute, tense ascites . . ." [although in fact the laboratory values given for the patients suggested that they were in or close to Class A]. Of Zeppa's remarks, he said, "He has probably worked with more cases than anybody in the world, as he was on the original team, with John Ploman and me, that developed this procedure. Although he didn't give you time enough to record in your minds that figure, nonalcoholic cirrhotics have a 90% five-year survival." Warren agreed with Dr. Terblanche that "sclerotherapy is an advance in an adjunctive therapy", and they were attempting to use it at Emory. They had not, like McDermott, rejected patients with hypersplenism for distal splenorenal shunts, "Every one of them has hypersplenism . . . There is no reason to turn them down, if you understand blood control during operation . . . Acute tense ascites is a contraindication to the procedure, not just the presence of ascites . . ." They had a proven patency rate of 95% at Emory. He agreed with Nabseth that the progressive development of collaterals decreased the hepatic perfusion and suggested that with "percutaneous catheterization of the portal vein . . . we think we can occlude some of those collaterals, and maintain flow for a longer length of time." He agreed with Grossi about the importance of the arterial flow. At Emory, they were now seeing,- and they had done over 90 distal splenorenal shunts,- a higher proportion of cirrhotics who were not alcoholics, and in the entire group of 90 patients, there were only two hospital deaths, and "In that are included at least six or eight emergency shunts. Most of the patients had ascites, or had had it just prior to the shunt; and dating back to 1971, there are still only 10 deaths in that group." In a typical Warren combination of humor and good-natured brashness, he said, in closing, "that a total shunt is a total shunt, and it doesn't matter if it goes to the right, into the vena cava, or to the left, into renal vein. Dr. Webb, I'm going to work with you on this; you just have patience. It bypasses the liver; the portal blood does not get there . . . The big problem is the one that was highlighted last, and that is the loss of portal flow through continued portal hypertension and development of collaterals."

* * *

Perhaps nowhere in surgical practice were prophylactic antibiotics more regularly used than in peripheral vascular operations, yet it had been repeatedly pointed out that there had never been a properly mounted prospective randomized clinical trial of the efficacy of such antibiotics. Now, Allen B. Kaiser, Karl R. Clayson, Joseph Mulherin, Jr., Albert C. Roach, Terry R. Allen, William H. Edwards, all by invitation, and W. Andrew Dale, of Nashville, Professor of Clinical Surgery, Vanderbilt University, *Antibiotic Prophylaxis in Vascular Surgery*, attempted to correct this deficiency. Over a period of 18 months, 565 patients undergoing arterial reconstructive procedures were entered into the study. Since the first 103 patients undergoing carotid or brachial artery procedures showed no infections, patients undergoing operations on those vessels were dropped from the study, leaving 462 with operations upon the abdominal aorta and arteries of the lower

extremities. The operations were all elective and patients with wet gangrene or cellulitis were excluded. The cefazolin or placebo were given "with the on-call medications and postoperatively every six hours for four doses", with an additional dose during operation if the procedure lasted beyond four hours. The wound infection rate for the 462 patients was 0.9% with cefazolin prophylaxis and 6.8% without it. There were only four infections of a graft in the entire study, and all four were in the placebo group. It was important that "Wound infections harboring cefazolin-resistant pathogens were no more frequent in the patients receiving cefazolin prophylaxis than in patients receiving placebo", and patients receiving cefazolin never yielded cefazolin-sensitive organisms in their cultures. The infection rate in abdominal aortic resection was 2.6% under cefazolin protection and 11.8% without it. For aortofemoral bypass, there were no infections with cefazolin and 2.1% (one of 47) with the placebo. For the femoral to lower leg bypass, there was one infection in 105 operations under cefazolin (1%), nine infections in 103 in the placebo group (8.7%). It was discovered midway through the study "that a number of patients had received a hexachlorophene-ethanol skin preparation as contrasted with a povidone-iodine-containing skin preparation used in the majority of the patients." There were seven infections in 68 operations done with hexachlorophene-ethanol, none of them in the patients receiving cefazolin. There were 394 operations done under povidone-iodine with 11 infections, two in the cefazolin patients and nine in the placebos, the respective percentages being 1.0% and 4.5%. They considered that "The results were conclusive: wound infections occurred significantly less often following perioperative cefazolin prophylaxis and no adverse effects (phlebitis, rash, antimicrobial resistance) were related to the 24-36 hours of cefazolin use." The small total of four graft infections for the entire study, although they were all in the placebo group, was not significant, but "a consistent trend of more infections in the placebo group was observed with the Class I and Class II infections [soft tissue only]. The total infection rate for abdominal incisions was 4.9%, 1.2% for cefazolin protected patients, 8.2% for the patients given placebo; the total infection rate for groin incisions was 0.6%, none in the cefazolin patients and 1.1% in the placebo patients; total infection rate in the leg incisions was 3.1%, 0.9% for the cefazolin group and 5.4% for the placebo group. Given the significant difference in infection rates when the wounds were considered together, the authors and monitors were unwilling to continue the study in order to accrue additional Class III infections to prove the point statistically." They noted a much lower rate of infection in groin wounds than was generally reported in the literature, "meticulous care of the groin area has been emphasized for years and probably accounted for this low infection rate." The high infection rate in the group whose skin had been prepared with hexacholorophene-ethanol was striking and significant. As in previous studies, staphylococcus aureus was the commonest organism, and that confirmed the wisdom of the use of a cephalosporin. They, therefore, recommended the prophylactic use of cefazolin and povidone-iodine in vascular reconstructive surgery.

Discussion

Wiley F. Barker, of Los Angeles, was grateful to the authors, "for presenting the objective data to justify what many of us have been doing on the basis of their prior advice several years ago, with good apparent results, but most of us haven't had the documentation." He quoted the recent experience of St. Mary's Hospital, London, provided him by Sir H. H. G. Eastcott [with Pickering and Rob, the author of the landmark first paper on the successful correction of arteriosclerotic obstruction of the carotid bifurcation]. In a seven-year study at St. Mary's Hospital, they had cultured the nasopharynx of patients. Those patients with pathogens on culture were given the appropriate antibiotic on-call to the operating room, the other patients received none. ". . . there were five graft infections in the patient group that seemed to be less at risk [and therefore given no antibiotic], whereas there were no graft infections in the 76 from which pathogens were grown." Since then they had treated 139 patients with floxicillin in this way "and have had only one instance of an infected graft; the patient is thought to have been already infected at the time of operation, as the patient was moribund, with a leaking aneurysm, in established renal failure." Robert E. Condon, of Wood, Wisconsin, said that "Prior to this morning's presentation" there had been some experimental evidence and no accepted clinical evidence to justify routine antibiotic practice in peripheral vasculoarterial surgery. While describing it as a "well-designed, prospective, blinded, well-controlled clinical trial", he actually questioned the validity of the study. "The infection rate in the placebo group over all was about 6%. Surprisingly, many of those infections involved, not the groin wound, but the abdominal wound where the infection rate was about 8%." Even without the hexachlorophene-alcohol skin

preparation patients, their infection rate was 4%. "These infection rates seem to me to be a little high for clean elective surgery, and since the conclusion of the study supporting the administration of prophylactic antibiotics really depends primarily on the infection rate in the control group, I'd appreciate it if Dr. Mulherin or Dr. Dale could give us some further information about the infection rate in the placebo group, in comparison with their previous experience. Is the infection rate experienced in this study representative of their previous experience with vascular procedures, or is it some kind of unusual phenomon, related only to the study, and perhaps not truly representative of the infection risk in patients undergoing vascular grafts?" Emerick Szilagyi, of Detroit, repeating, as he had at previous meetings, that antibiotic prophylaxis in this field was "a nearly universal practice" and that there was "a reasonable body of evidence in support of its rational selective employment", said that "The report we have just heard is an account of the first attempt to provide . . . the ultimate proof of its value—that is, a randomized, prospective, double-blind evaluation . . ." Like Condon he seemed to question the validity of the study, "I find it regrettable that the authors included in the overall statistical treatment of the results the trivial degrees of infection. What one is exclusively interested in is the incidence of infectious involvement of the prosthetic implant . . . The decision to interrupt this study before the estimated size of the clinical sample had been reached was unfortunate. Although, by the application of standard techniques of testing significance, a striking difference can be shown in favor of the prophylaxis group, one has doubts about the practical value of this demonstration. The zero incidence of infection in the prophylaxis group is unrealistic, and the rather high incidence of serious infections involving the grafts in the placebo group is disturbing. One suspects the operation of factors that, because of the small size of the sample, are not reflected in the statistical manipulation . . . to achieve the goal of the study one would require a sample size of 500 to 1000 in each group. In brief . . . this valuable study has given us important new information in support of the selective . . . use of antimicrobial prophylaxis, but owing to the sample size, it has not provided the definitive answer which we have been looking for." Hiram C. Polk, of Louisville, came down unequivocally on the side of the authors, ". . . I would disagree with Dr. Szilagyi, in that I really believe this is as careful a clinical study as can be done in this area. It represents and supports the idea of common practice, good laboratory data and even common sense . . .

the investigators here chose one of the known effective, proven drugs, I believe, which Dr. [Harlan] Stone shared with this group two years ago . . . so that it is a valid trial. They have an effective drug. Their conclusions are valid. I always find that in retrospect people question infection rates in control groups when they seem somewhat higher than we like to remember as our own rate. In general, when we have looked objectively on our service, the infection rate has been of the magnitude that has been described by the authors here today." W. Andrew Dale, closing, said to Dr. Szilagyi, "Only four grafts were infected; the graft infection rate was 0.9%, and not 4%. We believe the overall rate of infection of 3.9% is good, and that the graft infection rate of 0.9% is better, and especially note that no graft in a patient treated with cefazolin became infected." [There was no such statement in Szilagyi's discussion as published. One would suppose that in fact he had made an error,•and hearing Dale's correction from the platform, corrected the transcript of his discussion sent him by the Recorder. Evidence of this sort of editing recurs in the *Transactions* and often leads to puzzling non sequiturs.] Dale said that both the propriety and the possibility of conducting such a study had been challenged some years before and he was glad to see that patients would cooperate, that studies could be undertaken, "We are encouraged to turn from empiricism to controlled-study research in other areas as well."

* * *

James D. Hardy, of Jackson, Professor and Chairman, Department of Surgery, and Director of Surgical Research, University of Mississippi Medical Center, *Surgical Management of Cushing's Syndrome with Emphasis on Adrenal Autotransplantation,* said "the results of treatment of pituitary dependent adrenocortical hyperplasia producing Cushing's syndrome are reasonably satisfactory . . ." despite the complexities of the physiologic relationships involved in the production of the condition, ". . . whereas the altered clinical picture in Cushing's syndrome is due specifically to the secretion of excess cortisol by the adrenal cortex . . . the subtleties of hypothalamic stimulation of ACTH release in Cushing's disease, effected by the corticotrophin (ACTH) releasing factor (CRF), are complex . . . there is an increasing body of opinion that the higher centers, and specifically the cerebral cortex, may play a major role in the pathogenesis of pituitary dependent Cushing's syndrome . . . it appears possible that excessive release of CRF by the hypothalamus can produce pituitary hyperplasia and nodularity . . .

the fact that some patients with Cushing's disease exhibit continued psychiatric disturbances long after 'eucortisolism' has been achieved by adrenalectomy is of interest in this connection." He presented "consecutive series of 22 patients of whom 16 had bilateral adrenocortical hyperplasia (13 females), four, benign cortical adenoma (all females) and two cortical carcinoma (both males)." He excluded patients with ectopic ACTH-secreting tumors. Three of the patients with adenomas were cured, one died of postoperative respiratory insufficiency and sepsis. The two men with adrenocortical carcinomas already had liver metastases and both ultimately succumbed. There was one in-hospital death of anuria secondary to intraoperative hemorrhage. There were now 12 surviving patients who had had bilateral adrenal hyperplasia, "several have some degree of psychiatric disturbance, and four increased pigmentation. One patient developed a large chromophobe adenoma of the pituitary (Nelson's syndrome . . .) with acute onset of blindness 15 years after subtotal adrenalectomy; hypophysectomy permitted substantial visual recovery." Their first patients underwent subtotal adrenalectomy and "Beginning in 1962, we began performing total intra-abdominal adrenalectomy in Cushing's disease, with auto-transplantation of adrenal tissue into the thigh. In our opinion, subtotal adrenalectomy should probably be abandoned." Of their eight subtotal adrenalectomy patients, one was alive and well, one had developed Nelson's syndrome, "three patients are well but have psychiatric problems." Their first transplant had been performed because of the necessity in a treated patient for re-exploration to remove a portion of adrenal left behind which "had achieved a parasitic arterial blood supply . . .", so that in the first transplantation, "the left adrenal gland was transplanted to the right thigh with the gland's central vein being anastomosed to the distal end of the divided saphenous vein." It was hoped that this might "avoid the necessity for life-long replacement therapy . . . diminish the likelihood or the degree of excessive skin pigmentation which occurs after adrenalectomy in some patients . . . and . . . reduce the possibility of the development of . . .'Nelson's syndrome'. . ." The first and second transplants survived, although at biopsy, in the second, the vein was found to have thrombosed, and subsequently it was found not necessary to perform venous anastomoses at all, ". . .the adrenal gland was simply hand-sliced and the multiple slices were inserted into pockets prepared in the sartorius muscle. The site of each insertion was marked with a black silk suture cut long for ready visualization at the time of subsequent biopsy

. . . progressively thinner slices have been used." The results varied from minimal graft function to "recurrent Cushing's syndrome due to marked enlargement of virtually all the adrenal slices implanted into the sartorius muscle . . ." Irradiation of the pituitary had been employed, but effected remissions in only one-quarter to one-half the patients and had the disadvantages of "uncertain control of the hypercortisolism, late recurrence in some patients temporarily improved, interference with the secretion of growth hormone and normal development in young people, and impairment of prolactin secretion in young women who may want to have children." It was best reserved for older patients or recurrences after subtotal adrenalectomy. The commonest treatment was now total adrenalectomy, which involved "a fairly extensive operation, permanent dependence on steroid replacement unless adrenal autotransplantation is elected, development of excessive pigmentation in some patients, and late development of a chromophobe tumor of the pituitary which may impair vision and even become malignant . . . the anterior approach . . . may result in pancreatitis . . . while the posterior approach limits exposure." Surgical attack directly upon the pituitary "has logic and appeal. Cushing early described the pituitary basophil adenoma as the cause of Cushing's disease, and the suspicion has always persisted that many patients with Cushing's disease harbor a basophil adenoma. Recently, with improved methods of diagnosis and surgical approach to the pituitary, it has become clear that basophilic microadenomas of the pituitary are indeed present in many if not most patients with Cushing's disease." The insecticide DDD had been found to produce "selective destruction of the zona fasciculata and zona reticularis in the adrenals of dogs while to a considerable extent sparing the zona granulosa". Several investigators had employed it successfully in treating Cushing's syndrome. Franksson, in Scandinavia in 1956, had reported adrenal autotransplantation combined with total intra-abdominal adrenalectomy, and Hardy had collected published reports of 18 such operations. Hardy had had functioning tissue in all eight of his patients, one who had been off steroid therapy since 1972, one for two months, and one for one month, and 13 of the reported patients had been able to stop steroids, so that ". . . some degree of 'take' of the transplant may be expected in almost every patient, but with marked variations in 'success' among patients, regardless of the operative technique employed." Dramatic proof of the function of the transplants was afforded by one of Franksson's patients in whom excision of the transplant produced adrenocortical insufficiency, and two reported patients who developed Cushing's syndrome due to hyperplasia of the transplants reversed by excision of the transplants, this being true, as well, of one of Hardy's cases. It had thus been established that adrenal transplants could survive and function and none of the patients had thus far developed Nelson's syndrome with a chromophobe adenoma. On the other hand, the transplants had not prevented the development of skin pigmentation in some of the patients.

Discussion

Edwin L. Kaplan, of Chicago, said that they had had one adrenal transplant at the University of Chicago with minced adrenal cortex, "This patient still requires steroid therapy. However, there is a very nice gradient of both cortisol and aldosterone, which is higher in the arm of the transplant." Frank Glenn, of New York, had had 113 patients with Cushing's disease operated upon at The New York Hospital, 60 of them with hyperplasia and 52 of those had had total adrenalectomy. Although their longest follow-up was now 28 years, "replacement therapy leaves much to be desired from the patient's viewpoint", and he was hopeful of Dr. Hardy's technique. William H. ReMine, of Rochester, Minnesota, commented "I don't know that we've ever really gotten away from Cushing's original premise that these problems were caused by pituitary tumors, but because of frustrations in making the diagnosis of the tumor there, we have treated the end product of the disease, and I think we're now getting back to what was originally described . . . the result of more sophisticated means of diagnosis at the present time, with spiral tomography and carotid arteriography." By 1950, they had had an experience with over 300 cases of subtotal adrenalectomy, 15% of whom had ultimately developed pituitary tumors. In the last four-and-a-half years, his colleagues at the Mayo Clinic had performed 250 transsphenoidal removal of microadenomas of the pituitary of all kinds, with a 1.1% mortality. Since 1974, using spiral tomography and carotid angiography for diagnosis, they had treated 18 patients by transsphenoidal removal of microadenomas for Cushing's syndrome, 16 had had a complete remission, no tumor was found in one, but found at autopsy when the patient died of diverticulitis, one was unrelieved by removal of the tumor but relieved by subsequent radiation. Of DDD, he said, "In our experience, this is totally useless. It makes patients terribly sick and in the end they die of their disease anyway." He asked Hardy why he was so sure the recurrence in one case was coming from the transplant and not from residual disease in the abdomen [Hardy's published paper provides a very detailed account of the transsphenoidal hypophysectomy experience including that of the Mayo Clinic, but he apparently had not mentioned it in the presentation]. J. Hartwell Harrison, of Boston, said it was "significant and appropriate that Dr. James Hardy should bring to us this first description of autotransplantation of the adrenal [which it was not and which Hardy had not claimed it was]. To my knowledge, he was the first person to carry out successfully autotransplantation of the kidney." They had done 61 total adrenalectomies and 13 subtotal adrenalectomies, in seven of these the remnant became hyperplastic and required a second operation. They had tried transplantation of adrenal slices in the muscle without success. They had treated "106 patients with Cushing's disease, and 18 patients with Nelson's syndrome, by stereotactic Bragg peak proton hypophysectomy. In patients with pituitary-dependent Cushing's disease, clinical remission occurs in 65%, but another 20% are improved to the point that no further therapy is involved . . . Replacement therapy was necessary in only 13% of these patients . . ." Philip Sandblom, of Lausanne, Switzerland [where he had "retired" from Lund and was working at the University], said that studying wound healing in patients with varying disease, he found it less than half of normal in patients with Cushing's syndrome. He asked whether special precautions were taken for closing the wound to prevent dehiscence. Hardy, closing, emphasized the fact that "it is often literally years— nine in one patient, seven in another—before the plasma levels of 17-hydroxycorticosteroids are normal in these adrenal autotransplant patients. And that's not really too surprising, when one realizes that it often takes years for Cushing's disease to develop . . ." To Dr. Re-Mine, he said that the patient with recurrent Cushing's syndrome after transplantation might well have had hypertrophy of the remnant within the abdomen, "but when we took those eight so-called 'adenomas' out of the thigh, the plasma 17-hydroxycorticoid level dropped from 23 mcg/% down to 10 mcg/%. We believe that additional 'adenomas' remain in the thigh . . . data published in the world literature fully support function of the transplants." To Sandblom he said that they had taken no special precautions with the wounds and had had no dehiscences.

* * *

Jesse E. Thompson, of Dallas, Clinical Professor of Surgery, University of Texas Southwestern Medical School, and by invitation, R. Don Patman and C. M. Talkington, *Asymptomatic Carotid Bruit: Long-term Outcome of Patients Having Endarterectomy Compared with Unoperated Controls,* considered "Carotid endarterectomy . . . highly effective in the treatment of patients with transient cerebral ischemia since symptoms are relieved in most instances and the incidence of subsequent strokes is markedly reduced . . . However, . . . The indications for endarterectomy in patients with asymptomatic carotid bruits . . . have not been clearly defined." They had now had an experience with 1,286 carotid endarterectomies on 1,022 private patients for syndromes of cerebrovascular insufficiency, since April 1957. In 1965, "struck by the finding that among 16 patients with asymptomatic bruits not operated upon, five sustained frank strokes without episodes of transient ischemia", they undertook to follow "two series, an operated group and a non-operated control group . . . over the years." In 270 patients with asymptomatic mid-carotid bruits, they had performed endarterectomy upon 132 when first seen, and followed 138 without initial operation. Those operated on initially were patients with harsh bruits, patients about to undergo major operation upon other systems, patients who had had arteriograms and were found to have more than 50% reduction in caliber of the internal carotid, particularly if there was a suggestion of an ulcerated plaque. In the earlier years, many of the referring physicians advised their patients against arteriography, and many patients declined spontaneously. "If there is any bias in selection of patients for therapy, it would appear to favor the non-operated group as being at *less* risk for stroke. . . . 72% of the deaths among the operated patients and 48% of those in the non-operated group were due to cardiac disease . . ." The 132 patients operated upon [167 sides] had a zero operative mortality, there were two patients with transient neurologic deficits and two patients with permanent mild deficits, related to operation. In the subsequent follow-ups, the operated group of 132 patients had six TIA's, three non-fatal strokes and three fatal strokes. Of the 138 unoperated patients, 37 had TIA's, 21 had non-fatal strokes, and three had fatal strokes. The operated patients had a mean follow-up of 55 months, and the non-operated patients a mean follow-up of 45 months. Javid and associates, in 1970, studying the natural history of growth of carotid atheromas, found an increase of more than 25% per year in a third of the lesions, less than 25% in a fifth, while progression to stenosis or thrombosis occurred in 7%. Other studies had shown an increased risk of TIA's in patients with asymptomatic bruits, and it was accepted that TIA's "have been shown in a number of studies to be forerunners of actual strokes in 30-35% of cases followed three to five years or longer." Ocular pneumoplethysmography, ultrasonic scanning, and orbital Doppler studies were noninvasive techniques for screening patients with asymptomatic bruits to determine the need for angiography, which should particularly be done for harsh and bilateral bruits. The specific indications then for endarterectomy were ". . . bilateral stenoses . . . unilateral stenoses with contralateral occlusion . . . stenosis in the artery to the dominant hemisphere . . . known progressive atherosclerosis elsewhere in the peripheral vasculature, especially in younger patients . . . contemplated major operation of another sort . . . a markedly ulcerated plaque."

Discussion

Charles G. Rob, of Rochester, New York, agreed in toto except that he warned that stenosis of the external carotid artery, which was unimportant, might give a loud bruit. In his experience, "a completely asymptomatic internal carotid bruit is quite rare. After we have examined and interviewed such a patient, we usually find that they have symptoms which have not been noted before, either by the patient or his doctor." Thompson, closing, agreed that patients after operation "will frequently tell you that they do feel better in many respects and did have some symptoms of which they were not aware preoperatively."

* * *

John W. Braasch, of Boston, Clinical Assistant Professor of Surgery, Harvard Medical School; Chairman, Department of General Surgery, Lahey Clinic Foundation; and by invitation, Louis Vito and F. Warren Nugent, *Total Pancreatectomy for End-Stage Chronic Pancreatitis,* reported the Lahey Clinic experience from 1952 to 1976 with 26 total pancreatectomies for chronic pancreatitis, the published world literature listing 53 other cases. Twenty-three of the patients had had a total of 62 previous operations. All had severe pain and were using narcotics, nine had been jaundiced, 11 had what appeared to be steatorrhea, 25 had marked weight loss and 12 were diabetic. All patients but one had an associated gastrectomy of some extent, six had vagotomies, and 19 had splenectomy at the time of pancreatectomy. There were no in-hospital deaths or any deaths within 60 days of operation. There were numerous in-hospital complications in 14 patients, including four biliary fistulae, two intra-

abdominal abscesses, one intraperitoneal hemorrhage. Twelve patients had died, among them two of marginal ulcer, two of hypoglycemia, two of fever and seizures and one found dead in bed. "All of these patients were subject to insulin reactions . . . two patients who died had a deteriorated mental state, probably due in part to chronic hypoglycemia." Ten of the patients were relieved of their severe epigastric pain, although two continued on alcohol and three on narcotics. Their indications for total pancreatectomy were "a failure to control pain with ampullary procedures in patients with ampullary disease, with lateral pancreatojejunostomy in patients with dilated pancreatic ducts, and with partial or subtotal resection in patients with small duct disease." The operation "should include an adequate gastric resection with truncal vagotomy to avoid jejunal ulcers and other causes of upper gastrointestinal hemorrhage." They mentioned the possibility of "reimplantation of the patients' own islet cells [reported the year before by Najarian's group] . . . If this technique becomes clinically useful, subtotal or total pancreatectomy in one stage would be the preferred approach."

Discussion

William P. Longmire, Jr., of Los Angeles, had performed some type of resection in 30 of 78 patients who had been operated upon for chronic pancreatitis, 20 of them distal resections, of whom 12 had had more than an 80% resection and ten of whom had undergone proximal or total pancreatic resection. "Although in the past the majority of our patients have been treated by a lateral pancreaticojejunostomy, or by less than an 80% distal resection . . . the diseased head of the pancreas . . . is responsible for maintaining the smoldering inflammation in the gland . . . treatment of our recent patients has usually involved a proximal resection." When performing a pancreaticoduodenectomy for benign disease, it was possible to save the pylorus and often enough of the distal pancreas to prevent diabetes. They had injected the patient's own islets into the portal vein recently, but without success. William H. ReMine, of Rochester, Minnesota, said their last report of total pancreatectomy for all causes numbered 68 cases, of which five were for pancreatitis. The longest survival of those was eight years. "It's our policy now not to try to do total pancreatectomy on these patients if we can possibly avoid it . . . We now try to go to splanchnic block because these people are going to continue drinking . . . and I urge you to follow Dr. Braasch's advice and not submit them to total pancreatectomy. If you can accomplish a splanchnic block, they can be comfortable and they can go back to work." George L. Jordan, of Houston, commented that Braasch's was the largest series of total pancreatectomies on record for chronic pancreatitis, and like others showed that total pancreatectomy for pancreatitis was safer than it was for carcinoma. Jordan had done only two total pancreatectomies for chronic pancreatitis, the patients had both survived for some time, but had innumerable problems with hypoglycemia, with septic complications, and died of complications of these. Louis Vito, closing, said they shared Longmire's concern about the head of the pancreas and six of their patients had first had a Whipple operation without relief. He agreed with Dr. ReMine "that total pancreatectomies should be avoided." At the Lahey Clinic they had abandoned splanchnicectomy because it had not been very successful. In short, total pancreatectomy was a last measure, to be performed "after all else fails".

* * *

The newspapers and the editorial columns of medical journals had been filled with comment resulting from the Veterans Administration Cooperative Coronary Artery Study which failed to show any improvement after coronary revascularization, except in operations for left main coronary artery stenosis. George C. Kaiser, of St. Louis, Professor of Surgery, St. Louis University School of Medicine; Hendrick B. Barner, Denis H. Tyras, John E. Codd, J. Gerard Mudd, by invitation, and Vallee L. Willman, Professor of Surgery and Chairman, Department of Surgery, St. Louis University, *Myocardial Revascularization:* A Rebuttal of the Cooperative Study, had operated upon 550 patients from January 1972 through December 1974. Excluding patients from the analysis on the same basis as those excluded from the VA study, and excluding also the 54 with left main coronary stenosis, of whom none had died and on whom the results of the VA Study had also been very good, they came up with 345 patients, followed for an average of 56.9 months, with a 96% complete follow-up. Most patients had been readmitted for coronary angiography and left ventriculography. They had eight operative deaths, 2.3%, compared to the VA 5.6%,- a significant difference, "clearly affects long term statistics, especially when considering the low early mortality in the non-operative group of 310 VA patients." The 95% four-year survival of their patients was superior to the 85% survival of the VA operated patients and 86% of the VA medical patients." Angina pectoris was

absent or markedly improved in 91% of their patients at four years, and 90% at five years. "This consideration is not addressed in the VA reports to this time." Perioperative myocardial infarction occurred in 8.4% of their patients, 18% of the VA patients. The annual rate of myocardial infarction in their patients over five years, including perioperative infarctions was 3.4% per year, excluding them it was 1.8% per year. Kaiser and Willman's cumulative graft patency was 87% at one and 84% at three years, "Both are better than the VA patency rate of 71% at a mean of one year. All grafts were patent in 76% of SLU patients at one year and 71% at three years, while only 54% of VA patients had all grafts patent at an average of one year." There was no difference between the two studies in patients with single vessel disease and patients with double vessel disease. The four-year survival of the SLU patients was 97%, the VA medical survival 87%, surgical 83%. "The SLU four-year survival is essentially that of a matched population." For triple vessel disease, the SLU four-year survival was 92%, the VA medical group 74%, the VA surgical group 89%, essentially similar to the SLU group. The VA Study has suggested that coronary artery bypass grafting had no effect upon prolongation of life except in left main coronary artery disease, but had not "addressed the problem of reduction of myocardial infarction, nor the permanence of relief of angina pectoris." Furthermore, completeness of revascularization was generally considered to be significant in influencing longevity after operation. In the SLU patients, "Complete revascularization was accomplished at operation in 272 patients (79%) and was persistent at one year in 147 patients (44%)." The VA Study had not yielded data on completeness of revascularization. Kaiser suggested that "The statistically superior survival of this [SLU] group, over the comparable VA patients treated operatively, suggests that incomplete revascularization in these patients may have been one of the factors responsible for their less favorable results . . . A major criticism of the VA study has been that the operative mortality (5.6%) was high, and the graft patency low (71%). Considering the good long-term survival of their control group of operative candidates treated without operation, they acknowledged that in order to demonstrate a significant difference in favor of CABG, lower operative mortality, improved graft patency, and more complete myocardial revascularization would be necessary . . . Considering the generally good prognosis of all patients entering the VA study, with a yearly loss of less than 4%, it may well take a much longer period than five years to differentiate the effects of treatment upon long-term survival."

Discussion

John Norman, of Houston, said that "the major contribution of the . . . Veterans Administration report . . . has been to elicit substantial, well-grounded and documented rebuttals, such as that just presented." The Houston group had done aortocoronary bypass grafting in 12,310 patients. There was a 92% three-year survival, and a 79.6% nine-year survival, their operative mortality had decreased from 9.1% in 1968 to 1.7% in 1,516 cases in 1977, without excluding the high risk cases that the VA Study had excluded. Frank C. Spencer, of New York, said that at the Colorado Springs Meeting four years earlier, he had projected a five-year survival in the New York University cases of about 80% in 450 patients. They had recently updated their data, "The slopes of the actuarial survival curves are strikingly similar to those of Dr. Kaiser, in sharp contrast to the VA study." Their average mortality for 1968 had been 5%, but their one-year survival 92-93%, and after the first year was "very flat, not changing from either graft occlusion or progression of atherosclerosis. As does Dr. Kaiser's data, it parallels a matched population group. It is unlike the VA's figures, which steadily go down, both for medicine and surgery, for unknown reasons." He had 88% of patients alive at five years, including the initial operative mortality. Currently the operative mortality was 1-2%. Spencer went through a number of calculations based upon "The only known fact . . . that there are about 600,000 deaths each year, with a male to female ratio of 4:1; hence about 500,000 males die each year from coronary disease." If the death rate from coronary disease was as little as 2% a year, a figure frequently given in medical textbooks, an incredible portion of 50% of the adult male population would have to be affected, so that the death rate was surely substantially higher. ". . . the spectrum is very broad, depending upon the capacity of collateral circulation to develop. Clearly, a number of people with good collaterals don't need an operation. It's equally clear that with left main disease, triple vessel disease or bad left ventricles, an operation is very badly needed . . . the problem is . . . who needs it and who doesn't need it . . . At the present time, with the available knowledge, whom would he [Dr. Kaiser] consider for operation and whom would he recommend for medical therapy?" Raymond Read, of Little Rock, Arkansas, who had been the first author in the Veterans Ad-

ministration report, emphasized as Kaiser had, "that surgery significantly benefited patients with left main disease with a probability of 999 chances out of a thousand." However, Kaiser's 2.3% mortality was not only better than that of the VA Cooperative Study group, but than reported at the same time from a number of other centers, and his graft patency was similarly higher. As for survival, ". . . we find that Dr. Kaiser had a remarkable 97% survival rate at three years, which suggests that if you include the mortality of surgery, he had a loss per year of only 0.2%. Now, a white male aged 50 years in this country has a 1% chance of dying each year; so that these people, following surgery, only have an attrition rate of one fifth normal." Furthermore, analyzing of the VA group, in comparison "with the classical studies from Duke, Baylor and Cleveland in the literature, we find that the VA Study group is not that abnormal in regard to left main disease, triple vessel disease, and other characteristics. In fact, it does show a severe degree of coronary artery disease being operated on." How to explain Kaiser's "very fine results"? "We can always ascribe them to superior surgical skill . . . The final examination may well be that when Dr. Kaiser went down to the record room and did his retrospective analysis in the hospital files in St. Louis, they came up with a series of patients that do not match the study group that was prospectively randomized way back in 1972 by the VA. This problem of matching patients with coronary artery disease and angina has been carefully worked on by the Duke group, and they pointed out that even with a computer, where they have 87 variables of patient characteristics, they couldn't set up two groups of comparable patients with medically and surgically treated coronary artery disease . . . it's very difficult to match one group against another." Kaiser, closing, responded to Read's spirited defense. He showed a slide indicating the similarity of the patient groups in numerous respects, and said as well, "These data were not derived retrospectively from the record room. In our department, records of all the patients that have received CABG at St. Louis University since 1970 have been kept current." He appeared to have caught Read redhanded, "Dr. Read, you have shown us published series to which you have compared the VA Cooperative Study results today. This comparison was also published in your report of the Cooperative Study (in the *Journal of Thoracic and Cardiovascular Surgery* in January 1978). I have reviewed these original published reports. The majority either included patients that would have been excluded from the VA Study or were series of patients treated before 1972, a period which the VA Study excluded because of the operative mortality of 16%." A question asked in the editorial columns of *The New England Journal of Medicine* of the VA Study was "If the mortality rate were reduced by one-half, and if the graft patency rate were improved 15%, would the survival of patients treated with CABG be improved." Kaiser answered that question, "Our experience with a similar group of patients operated upon at a similar time indicates a mortality rate of one-half and a 15% greater graft patency rate. This is associated with a greater survival."

* * *

F. H. Ellis, Jr., of Boston, Chief of Thoracic and Cardiovascular Surgery, New England Deaconess Hospital and Section of Thoracic and Cardiovascular Surgery, Lahey Clinic Foundation; and by invitation, H. K. Leonardi, L. Dabuzhsky, and R. E. Crozier, *Surgery for Short Esophagus with Stricture: An Experimental and Clinical Manometric Study*, had undertaken manometric studies in cats and in patients, evaluating the relative antireflux capacities of the Collis-Belsey and Collis-Nissen operations. Resection of esophageal strictures secondary to reflux esophagitis had been replaced "by procedures of lesser magnitude, such as the Thal-Nissen, the Collis-Belsey and the Collis-Nissen procedures." The Collis-Belsey had been particularly popular [F. G. Pearson, H. C. Urschel, Jr.], but its antireflux effect in this had been challenged [R. D. Henderson, Orringer and Sloan]. In the cat circumferential resection of the lower 2 cm. of the esophageal musculature was performed to invite reflux, the stomach was incised longitudinally to extend the esophagus for 3 cm. by a lesser curvature tube,- the Collis operation. To this was added in some animals a Belsey fundoplication and in others a Nissen fundoplication. Manometry showed that the Collis gastroplasty produced no improvement in the lower esophageal sphincter function compared to animals in which the LES had been excised by myectomy and no other procedure performed. The Collis-Belsey and Collis-Nissen both increased the amplitude of pressure in the high pressure zone, the Collis-Nissen procedure significantly more so. Collis-Belsey did not restore competence measured by the pH reflex test while the Collis-Nissen did very successfully. Of 20 patients with short esophagus, hiatus hernia and stricture, 11 had a Collis-Belsey procedure and nine had a Collis-Nissen. The pressure studies in the patients showed that "The Collis-Nissen procedure produced pressures of greater amplitude and length than did the Collis-Belsey operation and these differences were

statistically significant. While the ability of the two procedures to restore a normal adaptive response of the HPZ appears to be comparable, the Collis-Nissen procedure was more effective in preventing reflux than was the Collis-Belsey procedure, for none of the patients so treated had a positive pH reflux test postoperatively, while all but one of the patients studied after the Collis-Belsey operation exhibited a positive response to the pH reflux test." The clinical results of operation conformed to the functional tests. Of ten Collis-Belsey patients available for follow-up, six had good or excellent results, four required repeated postoperative dilations,- poor results,- one of them subsequently undergoing resection and colon interposition. As for the Collis-Nissen operation, only one of nine patients required continued dilation, the remaining eight were considered good to excellent results. "On the basis of our experimental and clinical data . . . we believe the evidence supports the superiority of the Collis-Nissen procedure over the Collis-Belsey and continue to prefer its use in carefully selected patients with short esophagus and stricture resistant to conventional efforts at peroral dilation."

Discussion

Alan P. Thal, of Las Vegas, said, "We have adopted a somewhat different approach than Dr. Ellis' and first reported it exactly ten years ago at this meeting [referring to the Thal fundic patch applied to the split-open esophagus to widen the strictured area, placing a skin graft over the applied gastric surface, if the esophageal defect was a large one]. He had done ten cases in the last five years, adding a "valvuloplasty . . . calibrating the reconstructed neoesophagus around a #30 Maloney dilator." Only one case, with the stricture at the level of the aortic arch, had required dilatation. They used the same fundic patch for "emetic perforation of the esophagus". F. Griffith Pearson, of Toronto, Ontario, referred to the recent reports of Lucius Hill on intraoperative pressure monitoring, "Using his own repair, Dr. Hill has identified a critical relationship between the level of the lower esophageal pressure achieved and the clinical result. In his series of 200 patients followed for up to three years, no patient with a postoperative, lower esophageal pressure greater than 15 mm. Hg had symptomatic or radiologically demonstrable reflux." Pearson had evaluated 20 patients with reflux problems "managed by a modified gastroplasty and a Belsey-type of partial fundoplication", and had studied them with intraoperative and postoperative esophageal pressures. "Dr.

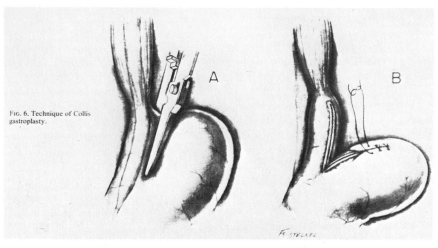

FIG. 6. Technique of Collis gastroplasty.

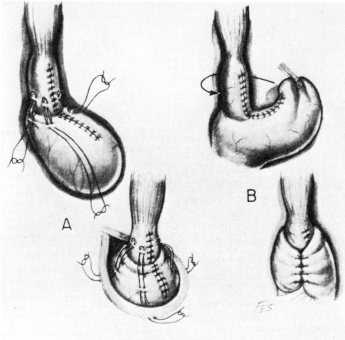

FIG. 7. Techniques employed in performance of Collis-Belsey (A) and Collis-Nissen (B) procedures.

In 11 patients the Collis-Belsey procedure was performed and in nine the Collis-Nissen. In either case, the esophagus was extended by dividing the stomach longitudinally alongside a #40 Maloney dilator passed into the stomach, using the anastomosing stapler which cut the stomach and at the same time placed two rows of staples on either side of the cut. Ellis' Figure 7 shows techniques of the Belsey intussuscepting fundoplication and the Nissen wrap-around fundoplication. Of ten re-evaluated Collis-Belsey patients, four had poor results, requiring repeated dilations and one had undergone resection and colon interposition. Of nine re-evaluated Collis-Nissen patients, eight had good to excellent results, one required continued dilation.

F. H. Ellis, Jr., H. K. Leonardi, L. Dabuzhsky, and R. E. Crozier, *Surgery for Short Esophagus with Stricture:* An Experimental and Clinical Manometric Study. Volume XCVI, 1978.

Hill, reporting on 200 patients records a postoperative pressure which is more than three times the preoperative level, records an incidence of symptomatic reflux of less than 5%. In our own series of patients, the postoperative lower esophageal pressure is more than double the preoperative value, and we have observed an 11% incidence of postoperative symptomatic reflux. Orringer, reporting on 75 patients managed by gastroplasty and partial fundoplication, observed a postoperative elevation of about 1.5 times the preoperative level, records a 19% incidence of recurrent reflux. Henderson, reporting on 35 patients managed by gastroplasty and partial fundoplication actually observed a drop in lower esophageal pressure after this repair, records the highest incidence of postoperative reflux at 45% . . . the differences in percentage increase in lower esophageal pressure after repair in these various reports are logically explained by technical differences in the operative procedure done and are reflected in the quality of the results obtained." The acid reflux test was the most sensitive, but did a total absence of reflux under strain with the patient prone "indicate normal physiology? I suspect not. It may well be that any operation which totally prevents reflux under all conditions designed to induce reflux is likely to have associated adverse effects such as the inability to burp or still worse the inability to vomit." Pearson had accumulated experience with "220 patients with complex reflux problems managed by modified Collis gastroplasty combined with a Belsey type of partial fundoplication. One hundred and four of these patients had peptic stricture with acquired shortening and 65 had had one or more prior hiatal repair . . . Complete clinical follow-up is available on 96% of these patients . . . from one to 15 years following repair. No patient has been reoperated on because of recurrent symptomatic reflux. The incidence of significant symptomatic reflux, requiring medical therapy, is just under 5%, and the overall incidence of symptomatic reflux of even minimal degree is 11%." Harold C. Urschel, Jr., of Dallas, had been employing the Collis-Belsey procedure first for strictures and then for complicated cases of hiatus hernia with reflux or those thought to be likely to recur. In some 200 patients, "Four patients have had demonstrated reflux in the postoperative period. Only one patient, however, has been symptomatic following this procedure . . . Patients with stricture have to have an occasional dilatation." He criticized Ellis' series as small and the follow-up as brief. Ellis, closing, agreed with Pearson that technical factors within the operations might be involved in the varying results, as well as possible differences in the types of patients. Pearson and Urschel had been speaking of "a wide variety of conditions, while this report is concerned only with stricture. If the stricture continues to require dilation postoperatively, the operation was not a success and a 40% failure rate of the Collis-Belsey operation over a period of fifteen months is not success in my mind."

* * *

Lilly had discussed hepatic portoenterostomy for biliary atresia before the Association at the 1976 meeting, and now R. Peter Altman, by invitation, from the Department of Surgery, George Washington University and Children's Hospital, National Medical Center, *The Portoenterostomy Procedure for Biliary Atresia: A Five Year Experience*, discussed the 43 patients they had operated upon in that fashion since 1972, 31 of them younger than 12 weeks at the time of operation. Twenty-six of the patients had atresia of the entire extrahepatic ductal system. In 12 the gallbladder, cystic duct and common bile duct were patent to the duodenum, but the hepatic ducts were fibrous. He described the technique of exposing the ducts in the hilum, "the most reliable anatomic landmark for identification of the fibrous ductal remnants has proven to be the superior aspect of the left portal vein as it courses toward the left lobe of the liver. The hepatic artery is extremely variable in its relationship to these ducts and is therefore less reliable as a landmark. After placement of the 6-0 stay sutures at the lateral margins of the fibrous ductal tissue investing the hepatic ducts, this tissue and ducts are transected and submitted for immediate frozen section examination . . . While the ductal tissue is examined by frozen section, the intestinal phase of the operation is begun." The reconstruction Altman favored was the Roux-Y with a double-barreled Mikulicz diverting enterostomy, which Lilly had favored as well,- 18 patients,- an ordinary Roux-Y had been performed in 11 patients. The fundus of the gallbladder had been sutured to the portal structures in seven patients, a technique which "while theoretically attractive, has been associated with a disappointingly high rate of complications." A single child of the 43 operated upon died of the operation. In the children with jejunostomies a catheter in the hepatic limb yielded a "few ml of bile as early as the second or third postoperative day." More than 30 ml of bile a day was predictive of sustained bile drainage, and bile output between 120 ml and 400 ml per day occurred in infants completely relieved of jaundice. "Such volumes are attained by the end of the first month." Rose Bengal

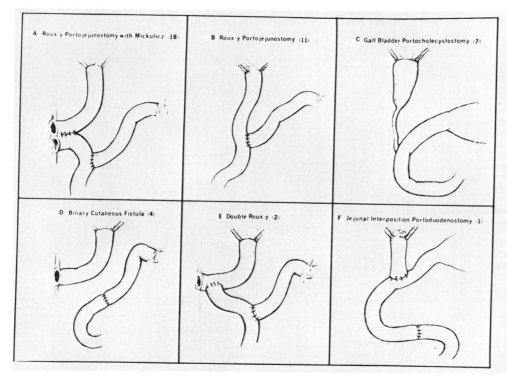

FIG. 3. Surgical procedures for correction of biliary atresia. (A) Roux-en-Y portojejunostomy with Mikulicz diversion (18 patients). (B) Roux-en-Y portojejunostomy without external vent (11 patients). (C) Portocholecystostomy (7 patients). (D) Biliary cutaneous conduit with jejunojejunostomy end-to-end (4 patients). (E) Double Roux-en-Y construction (2 patients). (F) Jejunal interposition with end-to-end jejunojejunostomy (1 patient).

The Roux-Y procedure used most frequently, with the double-barreled jejunostomy in the Roux limb draining the liver, permitted immediate evaluation of the production of bile, and was thought to minimize the likelihood of ascending cholangitis. Sixteen patients of the 43 were alive and jaundice-free. No statement was made as to the number of children in whom the double-barreled jejunostomy had been closed.

R. Peter Altman, *The Portoenterostomy Procedure for Biliary Atresia:* A Five Year Experience. Volume XCVI, 1978.

scan was used to determine bile excretion in children without an external fistula. The serum bilirubin remained elevated for four to six weeks after operation, and their analysis of the content of the bile confirmed Lilly's previous report to the Association. Reoperation was performed in 18 patients, the original operation having been performed in eight infants elsewhere. In all patients, the lumen of the common hepatic duct was found to be completely obliterated. If there were large ductules in the excised tissue from the porta hepatis, there was a high incidence of success. There was extended bile drainage in 29 patients, of whom 16 were surviving and jaundice free. Five were alive with jaundice, six were dead with jaundice. Two died of unrelated causes, jaundice free. Of 14 who had brief or no bile drainage, ten were dead of liver failure and four were alive, but with liver failure. They were careful in their interpretations. They could confirm Kasai's claims and the confirmation of others that "the portoenterostomy procedure when performed on infants less than three months of age will favorably alter their clinical course . . . Nonetheless, the role of the portoen-

terostomy for infants with biliary atresia has remained clouded, in part because of varying results. In fact, a conclusion reached as a result of this study is that provision of bile drainage does not necessarily mean 'cure'. Despite bile drainage, progressive cirrhosis has plagued many of these infants." He agreed with the import of the discussion of Lilly's paper at the 1976 meeting, "that biliary atresia is a dynamic postnatal obliterative process . . . The microscopic ductular patency at the liver hilus regularly seen in the very young infants is probably lost at about three months. This dynamic phenomenon may account for the discrepancy in operative results between patients operated upon before and after three months of age . . . In spite of the diminutive ductal size (30-200 micra) adequate bile egress occurs to allow hepatic decompression. In some, but not all of the patients, the accompanying biliary cirrhosis moderates and improves . . . some patients retain adequate hepatic parenchymal reserve to remain jaundice free and grow and develop normally . . . other infants have followed a modified, but unremitting downhill course leading to liver failure and death despite bile drainage." Reoperations had been performed after failure of initial operation and nine such children had had extended bile drainage after the second operation.

Discussion

Eric W. Fonkalsrud, of Los Angeles, agreed that anastomosis to the intestine rather than to the gallbladder was preferable. Since an anastomosis would be done in any case, he was not sure there was any point in a frozen section of the material acquired out of the hilum. Had Dr. Altman seen demonstrated histologic improvement in the liver after portoenterostomy? What about portal hypertension? Did the jejunostomy prevent infection? Marshall J. Orloff, of San Diego, asked whether earlier operation, say at three or four weeks of age, would "limit the amount of damage that the disease process produces and, therefore, improve the prognosis, or would earlier operation not have any effect on the outcome?" Alexander H. Bill, of Seattle, pointed out that half of the affected children were not jaundiced at birth, and presented slides interpreted as showing inflammation which caused the fibrosis and closure of the ducts. The original process in the liver sometimes improved and sometimes did not. It was not known how to prevent the disease. Altman, closing, said that in fact inflammation "was not a common finding. Of the 43 patients, inflammatory reaction was seen in only about half", and there was no correspondence between the extent of the inflammatory reaction and outcome. Dr. Bill's point about the absence of jaundice at birth in 50% of the cases was the answer to Dr. Orloff's question about operating at three or four weeks, "These infants often are unrecognized until they are a month old, and sometimes older than that." But indeed, Altman wished the pediatricians were more energetic about establishing definitive diagnosis on one-month-old infants with jaundice. Orloff was correct in his "surmise that patients who were operated early do better. This has been shown in Kasai's work and appears to be true in our own experience", ten weeks appearing to be the dividing point. They had biopsied 14 of their patients at six months and at one year. In most patients fibrosis of the liver had progressed, but in some six they had demonstrated, "if not improvement, at least histologic stabilization." In either case, the growth and development of the babies were normal "so whatever is left in the way of liver function is adequate to support growth and development, and all the synthetic functions of the liver are retained." They had seen some portal hypertension,

but only a single shunt, mesocaval, had been performed. "Cirrhosis and portal hypertension are clinically apparent in many patients, but shunt procedures, fortunately are not going to be necessary for most." Ascending infection and cholangitis remained a problem, "We're waiting longer and longer to close these ostomies because after the first year or year and a half the severity and the incidence of infection are decreased, and that's because there are greater bile flow and less bile stasis . . . these venting procedures, while not the whole answer, are useful."

* * *

Clifford W. Deveney and Karen S. Deveney, by invitation, and Lawrence W. Way, of San Francisco, Professor and Vice Chairman, Department of Surgery, University of California School of Medicine, *The Zollinger-Ellison Syndrome—23 Years Later,* had had 27 patients with the syndrome between 1955 and 1970 and an additional 38 between 1971 and 1977. The demonstration that the secretagogue produced by the tumor was gastrin, and the development of radioimmunoassay technique for detection of gastrin in the serum by Gregory in 1967, and the subsequent demonstration that gastrin release could be stimulated by administration of calcium or secretin or a standard meal had led to earlier and earlier diagnosis. In their patients, "The earlier patients had a higher incidence of virulent ulcer disease (56% vs. 24%), other endocrinopathes (48% vs. 13%), and malignant gastrinoma (44% vs. 25%). In recent years, almost half the patients had borderline basal gastrin values and required provocative testing with secretin for firm diagnosis. Total gastrectomy was performed in 38 patients with two anastomotic leaks and a single operative death. Of 24 patients available for follow-up, "Thirteen . . . maintained their weight without diarrhea or dumping", the others had mild problems of one sort or another. In only six patients was tumor resected for cure and in two of these the tumor resection was incomplete "and both patients died in the postoperative period of ulcer complications." These were in the earlier series and very large tumors. In the four more recent resections, "All four patients experienced an abrupt fall of gastrin levels to normal following resection, and studies 3-40 months postoperatively in three patients demonstrated normal basal gastrin levels and a normal (negative) response to secretin." The other patient was only a month postoperative and her gastrin levels were normal. In three of the successfully resected tumors, the tumor was in the tail, in one it was in the head of the pancreas together with a simultaneous insulinoma and a Whipple resection was performed. "We are much more inclined to consider an attempt at tumor excision now than previously, however, because cimetidine should prevent complications of persistent hypergastrinemia if the tumor is incompletely removed. If there is a chance of cure by resection, this procedure would avoid the risks and morbidity of total gastrectomy, and would eliminate a potentially lethal tumor. We perform resection if a single tumor is found at laparotomy which can be resected with more ease and less morbidity than performing a total gastrectomy . . . Total gastrectomy remains the preferred treatment for most patients with ZES. In our patients this procedure was associated with little postoperative morbidity and a 5% operative mortality. Ninety-five percent of the patients treated this way achieved an adequate nutritional status." Celiac arteriography, performed in 12 patients, showed 60% false negative in the five patients who had thus far been operated upon, and 50% false positive in four patients. Twelve patients with ulcer had been treated with cimetidine, four had marked symptomatic relief, five had moderate improvement, three had little or none. The tumor was considered to be malignant in 18 on the basis of lymph node or hepatic metastases, five of the patients died after their operations of complications of peptic ulcer disease, and one died of carcinoma of the lung. Three died of metastatic gastrinoma, one, two and 11 years later. Nine patients were well from three months to 11 years after diagnosis of the tumor. In the 47 patients whose tumors were thought to be benign, there had been no subsequent evidence to indicate that the tumor was malignant.

Discussion

Bernard M. Jaffe, of St. Louis, said "There's no question that, theoretically, the most direct approach to the management of the Zollinger-Ellison syndrome is resection of the gastrin-producing tumor. For duodenal tumors, this has proven relatively successful, as initially suggested by Dr. Oberhelman and supported by our clinical experience. On the other hand, there has certainly been no uniformity in the response to the resection of even presumably isolated pancreatic tumors." The gastrin levels were not useful in predicting histologic malignancy, nor, "in fact, how virulent the ulcer diathesis is likely to be." Cimetidine, he said, "should not be allowed to become a crutch to permit injudicious resection of otherwise unresectable tumors. Cimetidine offers us a great opportunity to prepare patients for what should be safe and careful elective total gastrectomy." Stanley R. Friesen, of Kansas City,

seemed particularly pleased with the paper because it was "in contradistinction to some of the recent reports in the literature regarding the possibility that cimetidine should be used routinely, long term, in all patients suspected of having Z-E syndrome . . . we should arrive at specific indications for the use of cimetidine and specific indications for the use of surgical treatment." Cimetidine controlled the ulcer symptoms in most patients with a Z-E and tended to prevent complications, but "I think surgical treatment is still indicated in these patients to confirm the diagnosis histologically, to remove the tumor if resectable, and to carry out total gastrectomy, in some patients who opt not to take cimetidine every day for the rest of their lives." Tumor rarely regressed after total gastrectomy and he would not expect tumor to regress under cimetidine treatment. He mentioned the importance of distinguishing Z-E tumor hypergastrinemia from the hypergastrinemia associated with G-cell hyperplasia for which vagotomy and antrectomy was the treatment. James C. Thompson, of Galveston, similarly said "There are now several gastroenterologists who have written that we should treat this disease by medication. It seems to me that they are attempting to seize the therapeutic initiative, largely to spare patients from the vicissitudes of total gastrectomy." But total gastrectomy was different in these patients, "the nutritional sequelae are remarkably small, and often absent. In Galveston, they had performed total gastrectomy on 11 Z-E patients, two of them were working full time as stevedores, and one woman had gone on a diet because she had become obese. They had also seen patients on cimetidine who had had "secretory break-throughs with complications". He suggested a more energetic approach to removing the tumors, and compared them to carcinoid tumors with which the patient could live in harmony for years until a period of sudden tumor growth. Thompson had resected two tumors out of 17 patients, in both of whom the tumor was extrapancreatic, in the omentum. Paul H. Jordan, Jr., of Houston, suggested that there might be patients with less virulent forms of the disease who could be managed entirely by cimetidine. R. Scott Jones, of Durham, asked whether "the failure of response to this treatment is due to some biological phenomenon or is it due to noncompliance?" Way, closing [Deveney had given the paper], repeated that the principal value in resecting the tumor was if there was "a reasonable chance of curing the patient, i.e., when the tumor is solitary and confined to the pancreas. In our opinion, resection is unlikely to accomplish much if there is extrapancreatic spread of tumor, especially if tumor must be left behind." He feared to resort to more aggressive operations, after the failure of which it might still be necessary, for persistent ulcer disease, to perform a total gastrectomy. He agreed with Dr. Jaffe that the absolute gastrin levels bore no relationship to the manifestations of the disease or the nature of the tumor. Like Dr. Thompson, he thought that the principal value of cimetidine was that "it allows the surgeon to prepare the patient preoperatively." To Dr. Jones he said that several of the patients who responded clinically showed a marked drop in acid secretion with cimetidine, and one patient who was a cimetidine failure had a much less striking decrease in acid secretion.

* * *

C. T. Strobel and W. J. Byrne, by invitation; Eric W. Fonkalsrud, Professor of Surgery, and Chief, Division of Pediatric Surgery, University of California at Los Angeles; and, by invitation, M. E. Ament, *Home Parenteral Nutrition:* Results in 34 Pediatric Patients, a decade after Dudrick's demonstration [Growth and Development of an Infant Receiving All Nutrients Exclusively by Vein] and eight years after Scribner's demonstration of the feasibility of chronic maintenance of parenteral nutrition outside the hospital with a semipermanent venous catheter, presented their experience with the latter problem in "children" [six of the patients were under 2-1/2 years, but 16 were 16 years old or older]. Of the 34 patients, 17 had Crohn's disease, six had "chronic idiopathic intestinal pseudo-obstruction syndrome", only one had "congenital short bowel", and one had "short bowel syndrome." The "Broviac" catheter, of Silastic, with a Dacron sheathing near its mid-portion to be positioned just under the skin for tissue ingrowth and fixation, was inserted into the external jugular vein through a cervical incision, passed into the superior vena cava, and the proximal, hubbed end tunneled subcutaneously to emerge through an anterior thoracic stab wound. In some patients the saphenous vein had been used, and proved "safe and reliable". The nutrient solution was 20 or 25% dextrose, 3 or 5% casein hydrolysate,- or 4.25% synthetic amino acids. Intralipid 4 gms/Kg./day was added through a Y connection to supply free fatty acids, or Safflower oil was rubbed into the skin four times daily. The infusion was impelled by an automatic pump, the fluids were made up in the hospital, but except for the small children, the patients took entire care of the catheter and the administration. Administration, 23 to 786 days, had always begun with a two- to three-

week hospital stay. The single death was in a 19-year-old girl with carcinomatosis. All patients showed significant weight gain and most of the smaller ones showed a growth spurt. The patients were encouraged to engage in sports, including tennis and swimming. Nutritional problems were few, and catheter problems not grave. The 34 patients had 48 catheters in all, replacements having been for dislodgement, infection, leak, thrombophlebitis,- after an average of 149 days. There were four minor wound infections and four instances of catheter sepsis—two *Staphylococcus aureus,* and two *Candida apsilosis,* the former responding to antibiotics, the latter recovering upon removal of the catheter. The cost of the nutrient was $1500/month for an infant, $3000/month for an adolescent. [The nature of the underlying illnesses was such as to lead in very few to the possibility of permanent return to good health, and independence of intravenous nutrition.] Nine patients had been off HPN for longer than 200 days, most of them patients with Crohn's disease, for which, although anticipating relapses, Fonkalsrud said, "long term parenteral nutrition promises to be a highly effective" method of treatment.

Discussion

Stanley J. Dudrick, of Houston [who had demonstrated that a Silastic catheter, placed centrally, would permit continuous infusion of hyperosmotic fluids and so satisfy the need for nutrition of surgical patients achieving the ends toward which Ravdin and Rhoads had worked] alluded to the ethical problem in undertaking what might be a permanent intravenous alimentation program in an otherwise doomed child, commenting only that if such alimentation was undertaken it provided great opportunities for biochemical and physiological investigation. Apart from this he confined himself to a series of illustrated success stories, but in concluding stated, "I think in a country that can afford a billion dollar dialysis program, we can certainly afford some kind of catastrophic care for patients who through a quirk of fate lose all or most of their gastrointestinal tract." [The implications of disease-oriented congressionally supported programs, their effect on competition for funds, in the health fields, the abuses arising ..s in quasi-commercial private "dialysis clinics", were causing increasing concern in the scientific world as well as in a government now realizing the U. S. economy could not endlessly support every expenditure for individual health which scientific progress made feasible. The kinship of the philosophy which engendered such programs and that which led to federally directed research and an emphasis on applied research,- "results",- was not difficult to see.] Fonkalsrud extended his "appreciation to Dr. Dudrick and particularly to Dr. Rhoads, for developing the whole technique of intravenous hyperalimentation . . . one of the great developments in surgery and in medicine during the past decade". Particularly impressive in Fonkalsrud's experience had been the result in some patients with massive intestinal resection for Crohn's disease who were "able to resume limited oral feeding" and might presently be weaned from hyperalimentation.

* * *

E. Stanley Crawford, of Houston, Professor of Surgery, Baylor College of Medicine, and by invitation, Donald M. Snyder, Gwen C. Cho, and John O. F. Roehm, Jr., *Progress in Treatment of Thoracoabdominal and Abdominal Aortic Aneurysms Involving Celiac, Superior Mesenteric, and Renal Arteries,* presented a colossal series of 82 of these extensive aneurysms, which Crawford divided into five groups, "Group I (10 patients) involved most of the thoracic and abdominal aorta down to celiac axis. Group II (22 patients) involved most of the thoracic and abdominal aorta distal to left subclavian artery. Group III (20 patients) involved most of the abdominal aorta with lesser involvement of the thoracic aorta. Group IV (18 patients) with involvement of the entire abdominal aorta and, Group V (12 patients) with involvement of lower abdominal aorta and renal arteries." He achieved the extraordinary result of 95% overall survival and 6% paraplegia [five cases, all in Group II]. These results he attributed to three technical measures, "1) graft inclusion without aneurysm resection as advocated by Javid, et al., in the treatment of infrarenal aortic aneurysms, 2) preservation of spinal cord circulation by restoration or maintenance of intercostal and/or lumbar artery circulation as suggested by Spencer in experimental studies in dogs, and 3) reattachment of celiac axis, superior mesenteric, and renal arteries by direct suture of vessel orifices to openings made in the graft, a technique first suggested experimentally by Carrel and Guthrie in 1906 for organ artery reattachment and later in clinical settings by DeBakey, Connolly and others." The large aneurysms involving the descending thoracic and the abdominal aorta were generally exposed by a long thoraco-abdominal incision, going down the abdominal midline to the pubis. He did not employ shunts or hypothermia, relying upon rapid operating and serial occlusion and reattach-

ment of vessels. At the time of reporting, 51 patients,- 62%,- were alive and well, 15 of them having survived five to 17 years. "The patients in this series with extensive aneurysm operations compare favorably with those with more localized simple aneurysm resections." The four patients in whom operation was refused because of other disease, died of aneurysm rupture in seven to 18 months. In the last 22 patients there had been no complications.

Harris B. Shumacker, of Indianapolis, said one could "only gasp with amazement" at the "break with traditional management and so excellent . . . outcome . . . Most of us have feared cases involving the entire descending thoracic and abdominal aorta because paraplegia seemed almost inevitable. They have shown this not to be true. To be sure, their only instances of paraplegia were in this group of 22 cases, but then only in five. Furthermore, their reconstitution of blood flow to intercostal and lumbar arteries seems to have lessened the risk by at least half . . . Others who operate well and without wasting time might see if they can duplicate these fantastic results. Almost certainly, no one who operates slowly and tediously should undertake to do so." John Connolly, of Irvine, California, claiming to speak for those "not as quick and as technically facile as Dr. Crawford" said he always had a "heparinless shunt available." Wakabayashi, in his Department, left the back wall of the distal aorta,- as Crawford did,- but used a nonthrombogenic shunt. With such a shunt, and leaving the back wall of the distal thoracic aorta, "we have been able to operate on 49 lesions of the descending thoracic aorta, 12 of which involved the entire aorta from the subclavian to the diaphragm, without a case of postoperative paraplegia . . . we are not nearly as aggressive as we used to be in attacking the area between the diaphragm and the renal arteries. I'd like to ask Dr. Crawford what evidence he has about percentage of rupture of the abdominal aorta in this area, because obviously there is an increased risk when we have to operate in that area, and we prefer to try to preserve that area if we can and do our operations as two separate operations, an infrarenal and a thoracic . . ." Denton A. Cooley, of Houston, said "Our technique of resecting such lesions is almost identical to the technique presented today. Dr. Crawford did not mention how he managed the left kidney. In our technique we choose to leave the kidney lying in its natural fossa. This requires division of the left renal vein, with reanastomosis at the completion of the operation. We believe it is technically more simple to do the arterial anastomosis when the kidney is

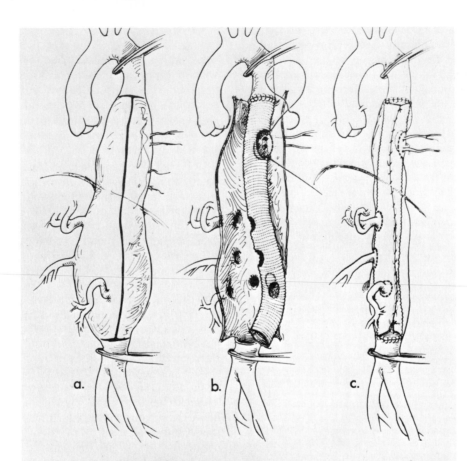

Fig. 13. Diagrams showing graft inclusion and direct vessel reattachment technique as employed in treatment of extensive aneurysm involving descending thoracic and abdominal aorta in which visceral vessel origins are widely separated. (a) The aorta is clamped proximal and distal to aneurysm. The aneurysm is incised longitudinally and transverse incisions made at each end through the anterior half of aortic circumference. (b) Graft is inserted inside aneurysm end to end anastomosis, and opening made in the graft and sutured circumferentially around origins of intercostal arteries. Under appropriate tension openings are sequentially made in the graft and sutured around the visceral artery origins. (c) The distal anastomosis is completed and the aneurysmal wall is sutured around the graft.

In a series of 82 extensive aneurysms, Crawford had a survival of 94%. In 22 of the kind here pictured, a 91% survival, and this the only group with paraplegias,- five out of 22. The drawing shows the use of three techniques to which he attributed much of his success, "graft inclusion without aneurysm resection" [Javid], "preservation of spinal cord circulation by restoration or maintenance of intercostal and/or lumbar artery circulation" [Spencer], reattachment of visceral vessels "by direct suture of vessel orifice to openings made in the graft, the technique first suggested experimentally by Carrel and Guthrie in 1906 for organ artery reattachment, and later in clinical settings by DeBakey, Connolly and others." Closing the aneurysm wall around the graft reduced bleeding substantially, separated the graft from adjacent viscera and was thought to prevent erosion into the gastrointestinal tract.

E. Stanley Crawford, D. M. Snyder, G. C. Cho, and J. O. F. Roehm, Jr., *Progress in Treatment of Thoracoabdominal and Abdominal Aortic Aneurysms Involving Celiac, Superior Mesenteric, and Renal Arteries.* Volume XCVI, 1978.

lying in its natural sulcus, and . . . causes less renal injury, and, therefore, fewer postoperative complications." Did Dr. Crawford find it necessary to remove the spleen? Were there any attendant complications? He thought many of the lesions formerly attributed to ischemia were caused by microthrombi and used small doses of heparin distal to points of distal clamping. Finally, Cooley asked, "if any of the patients in the series who developed paraplegia underwent reimplantation of the segmental vessels. Dr. Crawford, how firmly are you convinced that reimplantation of these vessels prevents cord damage?" Crawford, closing, said to Connolly that "a significant number of cases in this series required operation for rupture of aneurysm proximal to previous infrarenal aortic aneurysm resection." He agreed with the general emphasis that "two of the major factors in the development of paraplegia are aortic clamping and aortic resection." To Cooley, he said, "Reattachment of intercostal and lumbar arteries . . . has reduced the incidence of paraplegia from 38 to 14%. For simplicity, to minimize periaortic bleeding, and to avoid renal vein anastomosis, we prefer to reflect the left kidney forward and to the right. The spleen is removed in about half the cases either for injury or to use the splenic artery for arterial reconstruction. We feel that heparin is contraindicated because it adds to the bleeding problem."

* * *

Harold J. Wanebo, Maus Stearns, and Morton K. Schwartz, all by invitation, from the University of Virginia Medical Center, and the Memorial Sloan Kettering Cancer Center, *Use of CEA as an Indicator of Early Recurrence and as a Guide to a Selected Second-Look Procedure in Patients with Colorectal Cancer,* had found in 358 patients with colorectal cancer and 47 with benign colonic lesions that the carcinoembryonic antigen (CEA) correlated well with stage of disease, levels greater than 5 ng/ml occurring in from 4% in Dukes' A tumors to 65% in Dukes' D tumors and 72% in patients with recurrent or metastatic tumors, and among those, highest in those with liver metastases. The changes in CEA levels after operation ranged rather widely, but tended to fall and "there was a high recurrence rate in patients whose CEA level remained above 5.0 ng/ml postoperatively. Four of 6 patients (67%) with Dukes' B lesions and all of 8 patients (100%) with Dukes' C lesions, whose CEA level remained above 5.0 ng/ml after resection, developed recurrence." In a group of patients followed sequentially, a rapid rise in CEA level often signified liver metastases. In patients with local recurrence, the CEA level rose more slowly and often did not anticipate the clinical signs of recurrence. "In 16 patients the CEA elevation was the major reason for admission for second-look surgery", 13 of them having had Dukes' C and three Dukes' B cancers. They were 4-57 months after operation, and the range of CEA levels was 10-57 ng/ml. Two patients had a negative laparotomy and were assumed to have had false-positive elevations of CEA. Four patients had what was thought to be curative resection at the second-look operation, and the others had palliative resection, or biopsy was performed. One of the "false-positive" patients died of spinal metastases eight months after laparotomy failed to disclose any tumor. Three of the patients resected for cure at the second look were alive without evidence of disease at 15 months,- for a 6 cm. metastasis of the left lobe of the liver, at 12 months for excision of nodule in the pelvic floor, and one who had salpingo-oophorectomy, and subsequently a pulmonary lobectomy, alive at 37 months. Gunderson and Sosin's 1974 update of Wangensteen's second-look series, reported that 52 of 75 patients with second-look operations after abdominal-perineal resections were found to have tumor and only four were converted to a disease-free state. On the other hand, Martin and his colleagues employing CEA levels and a nomogram of specific indications for second-look in 14 patients with colorectal cancer and one with hepatocellular cancer, operated upon and found 12 totally resectable tumors, residual or recurrent. In all of the patients after resection of the tumor, the CEA levels decreased to baseline values. Wanebo was disturbed by the fluctuation of CEA levels in patients without demonstrated recurrence. He would say no more than that "The CEA test provides a method of early detection of recurrence and may permit surgical retrieval in selected patients and earlier initiation of palliation in other patients. The long-term effects in patient salvage remain to be defined."

Discussion

Richard E. Wilson, of Boston, commented that the CEA level in colon cancer was not so specific a biologic marker for malignant disease as were thyrocalcitonin and gastrin [for medullary carcinoma of the thyroid and Z-E tumors]. They too had found transient high elevations at times which were worrying. Simultaneous measurement of circulating immune complexes—CIC—was at times helpful. At the Brigham they had explored 13 patients solely because of rising of CEA levels, and in four of the patients curative procedures were possible. There were no false-positives. Hiram C. Polk, Jr., of Louisville, said that it had been their experience as well "that the CEA examination does have a fair number of false positives—occasionally it's false negative——and it is expensive." They had been attempting by a variety of ways to detect "favorable early recurrent disease" and while that "has yielded significant palliation for a large number of the patients, there's not a single one of them that's been rendered free of cancer for more than five years." John Minton, of Columbus, Ohio, thought "the single most important thing is to detect a slowly rising CEA and repeat this observation. Then do the second look at an appropriate time, before the opportunity for resection of recurrent cancer is gone." In a group of 22 patients with second look operations for rising CEA, six patients were found with resectable local disease, one was now alive after five years, three alive into their third year and two had died. Minton said that elevated CEA and no abdominal findings proved ultimately to be due to bone or brain metastases. ". . . by changing the frequency of CEA evaluation from every three months to every month, we were able to increase the percent of patients who had localized disease at the second-look operation from 25% to 75 per cent." Donald L. Morton, of Los Angeles, was much less enthusiastic. "We have a number of patients who had negative explorations after a positive CEA, that is, a rising CEA as the only indication of recurrence . . . we are now more cautious and make sure that the CEA continues to rise on repeated samplings. We have patients whose CEA has risen to 10, or even 14, before it gradually dropped toward normal. Some of these patients have subsequently remained free of disease for as long as four years . . . it has yet to be shown whether earlier resection of a recurrence, as detected by elevated CEA, will result in a more significant prolongation of the quality and duration of life than the resection done after clinical detection of recurrence."

* * *

Marshall J. Orloff, of San Diego, Professor and Chairman, Department of Surgery, University of California, and by invitation, K. H. Johansen, *Treatment of Budd-Chiari Syndrome by Side-to-Side Portacaval Shunt: Experimental and Clinical Results*, defined the syndrome as ". . . caused by occlusion of the major hepatic veins, often of unknown etiology . . . typically characterized by massive ascites, hepatomegaly and abdominal pain due to intense congestion of the liver. The outcome has almost always been fatal." While there had been a good many individual reports of the use of a variety of portosys-

temic shunts "based on substantial evidence that the valveless portal vein can be converted to an outflow tract by in-continuity anastomosis with the systemic venous system, thereby decompressing the obstructed hepatic vascular bed . . . a thorough trial of side-to-side shunt in the treatment of the Budd-Chiari syndrome has not been conducted, mainly because the condition is uncommon and often the diagnosis had not been made until near or after death." In dogs, "ligation and division of all hepatic veins except the large left hapatic vein . . . which was loosely surrounded by an ameroid constrictor . . . a hygroscopic casein plastic disc . . . containing a triangular opening . . . to accommodate the left hepatic vein", produced "severe hepatic outflow block, portal hypertension and massive, intractable ascites" within several weeks. Following sham laparotomy or end-to-side portacaval shunt, ascites reformed rapidly and persisted until death in all animals. "In striking contrast, only one of the 24 dogs . . . reaccumulated ascites following a side-to-side portacaval shunt", and no cause for that was found. In the animals with side-to-side shunts, the liver regressed in size and was histologically normal though it showed minimal fibrosis. Their six patients had all had onset with abdominal distention increasing progressively in the course of a few weeks, anorexia and progressive weakness, and three of them were mildly jaundiced. All patients had a patent inferior vena cava and were demonstrated on hepatic venography to have occlusion of the major hepatic veins, and one had a patent portal vein. In the five patients the side-to-side portacaval shunt was readily performed; the sixth patient "suddenly developed edema of the lower extremities and trunk, showed extension of thrombus into the IVC with sudden elevation of IVC pressure. An emergency IVC thrombectomy and portacaval shunt was undertaken in a desperate attempt to reverse a rapidly downhill course." That patient, who had polycythemia vera, died in six days, the other five patients had been followed from eight months to seven years, had no ascites, needed no diuretics, had normal liver function tests, and no encephalopathy. "Successful treatment of the Budd-Chiari syndrome due to occlusion of the hepatic veins by side-by-side portacaval shunt, splenorenal shunt or mesocaval H-graft has been accomplished in at least nine patients reported by eight authors . . . all of the patients were relatively young women ranging in age from 18 to 43 years." [Four of Orloff's patients had been men.] In those reported successes, "The underlying condition was polycythemia vera in three, leukemia in one, ingestion of oral contraceptives in one and unknown in four." [In Orloff's cases, four were of unknown cause, one was attributed to oral contraceptives. and one was the case of polycythemia vera.] Appropriately enough, the first successful reported case had been that of Arthur Blakemore, the patient dying of leukemia eight years later. The nine patients when reported were all still surviving or had died of non-hepatic causes. In 11 patients, shunts had failed, either because operation had been unsatisfactory or because the patients had been in extremis. "The results of our experimental studies combined with our small but consistent clinical experience indicate that side-to-side portacaval shunt provides definitive treatment of hepatic vein occlusion and offers the possibility of long-term survival. Early diagnosis and prompt operation appear to be important ingredients of the therapeutic regimen."

Discussion

Arthur B. Voorhees, Jr., of New York, said that he had seen two forms of the condition, the fulminating acute form, usually diagnosed at autopsy, "characterized by a relatively fresh clot involving most of the hepatic outflow tract". They had seen six such, operated on only one, and that unsuccessfully. In some 2,000 patients with portal hypertension seen at Columbia-Presbyterian, they had made the diagnosis of the more chronic condition described by Dr. Orloff in three instances, the first being the patient operated on by Arthur Blakemore in 1948. All three had been operated upon, two successfully. William V. McDermott, Jr., of Boston, said that the pathophysiology was the same "regardless of whether the outflow block is located in the suprahepatic or retrohepatic vena cava, the major hepatic veins, the intrahepatic small venules . . . or is due to the changes secondary to cirrhosis . . ." In some cases, slow recovery occurred with the development of reversal of flow in the portal vein. They had been successful with portal decompression in patients in whom this syndrome had occurred in association with cirrhosis or "with 'bush tea' Senechio poisoning, a peculiar process of obliteration of the smaller hepatic venules . . . due to the ingestion of toxic alkaloids in herbal teas brewed by the natives in the Jamaican highlands." Most fascinating was the absence of encephalopathy in his patients and in Orloff's. William P. Longmire, Jr., of Los Angeles, cited three cases, one with spontaneous recovery, one with block in the vena cava occluding the hepatic veins in which "Dr. Donald Mulder was able to bypass successfully the blockage of the inferior vena cava and hepatic veins with a vascular graft

between the portal vein and the right atrium." The third patient arrived moribund with extensive thrombosis in the inferior vene cava. Harry H. LeVeen, of Brooklyn, never one to mince words, said, "The fact that Dr. Orloff had only one death in six patients proves only that Dr. Orloff can do side-to-side shunts better than most of us. However, he has offered no evidence that this is the correct procedure to use." LeVeen had worked out his peritoneal-jugular shunt on dogs with Budd-Chiari syndrome, in 1976 had "recounted eight cases of Budd-Chiari syndrome . . . Since that time, surgeons throughout the United States have made me aware of a total of 18 cases that have been treated by peritoneo-jugular shunt." One patient with necrotic bowel and peritonitis was "not treatable by this method. All of the other 17 cases were commonplace, ordinary successes . . . I would suggest to you that the simpler peritoneojugular shunt be the procedure of choice." John Cameron, of Baltimore, described a case much like that of Mulder's presented by Longmire, with vena cava obstruction, treated by a long Dacron graft between the superior mesenteric vein and the right atrium, the patient, "now a year-and-a-half post-mesoatrial shunt . . . asymptomatic, without ascites . . . employed and has no difficulties with encephalopathy, as do any of our other patients treated for the Budd-Chiari syndrome." He had found the mesocaval shunt in general much easier in patients with the huge livers of the Budd-Chiari syndrome than a side-to-side portacaval shunt and wanted to "ask Dr. Orloff what the advantages of a side-to-side portacaval shunt are over a mesocaval shunt." Orloff, closing, agreed that no one had extensive experience "even our six patients treated by side-to-side shunt represent the largest single experience reported to date." It was a condition which was fatal in 95% of cases. Spontaneous recovery occurred but was extremely rare, and "the syndrome is known to wax and wane and ultimately to result in the death of most patients." He discussed but did not answer Cameron's question as to the reason for preferring a side-to-side portacaval shunt over a mesocaval shunt. He replied to LeVeen's attack in kind and with interest, ". . . I cannot comment from personal experience on the effectiveness of the LeVeen shunt in Budd-Chiari syndrome since my only experience with this device has been in removing it from a sizable number of patients with cirrhotic ascites who had it inserted by other surgeons and were then sent to us because of complications or nonfunction." He did in any case take issue with LeVeen. LeVeen's dogs did not have hepatic vein occlusion but inferior vena cava constriction "quite different from the condition that is the subject of our report . . . Secondly, his reference to 17 patients that had been 'cured' of the Budd-Chiari syndrome by the LeVeen shunt is purely anecdotal and is similar to much of the other information reported on the LeVeen shunt. If indeed, the peritoneojugular shunt is effective in the Budd-Chiari syndrome, then he should prove it by a systematic study of patients with this condition, diagnosed by accepted criteria and then subjected to long-term follow-up with liver biopsies and measurements of liver function as we have done in our study. I doubt that he can provide such information at the present time . . . I doubt that the LeVeen shunt, which simply returns ascites from the peritoneal cavity to the jugular vein, will be effective in the Budd-Chiari syndrome due to hepatic vein occlusion. The peritoneojugular shunt has no effect on the fundamental problem, which is intense congestion and necrosis of the liver that ultimately leads to death from liver failure or from the complications of portal hypertension, such as bleeding esophageal varices. It is not the ascites that kills patients with Budd-Chiari syndrome, but the intense congestion of the liver. Dr. LeVeen's comments suggest that he does not understand the Budd-Chiari syndrome."

The Business Meetings

The 1978 meeting was held at the Sheraton-Dallas Hotel, Dallas, Texas, April 26, 27, and 28, President David C. Sabiston, Jr., in the Chair.

Among those elected as Honorary Fellows were Professor John Goligher, of Leeds; Sir Rodney Smith, Past President of the Royal College of Surgeons, and very shortly to become Lord Smith of Marlowe; and most interesting of all, Wu Ying-k'ai, whose listing was given as Fu Wai Hospital and Cardiovascular Institute, Chinese Academy of Medical Sciences, People's Republic of China; Director of Fu Wai Hospital and Cardiovascular Disease Institute, Chinese Academy of Medical Sciences, Peking. None of the three was able to attend. Professor Ivan D. Johnston, of Newcastle, the only new Honorary Member able to attend, was introduced by the President.

At the Executive Session on the third day, the Secretary reading the Report of Council announced that the Council had appointed an ad hoc committee to consider revision of the entire Constitution and By-Laws of the Association, "because our present By-Laws and Constitution have been under a process of continual evolution and random amendment for many years. The committee consists of George

W. Stephenson, Clarence Dennis, and Jonathan Rhoads, Chairman."

Under "Item 6, the American Board of Family Practice", the Secretary read, "The Council believes that family practitioners should not do surgery, but only those formally trained and certified in surgery are competent in the early recognition, diagnosis, and treatment of surgical problems. This is a position which [Maloney remarked] your Secretary observes editorially is at variance with the Competition Division of the Federal Trade Commission, which bureaucracy appears determined to achieve what they consider to be the free market over the dead bodies of postoperative patients."

"The Council reinforced the view of the American Board of Surgery . . . that emergency medicine does not constitute a primary discipline" and thus should not be represented by a separate board, but by a conjoined or subsidiary board, "possibly sponsored by the American Board of Medicine, the

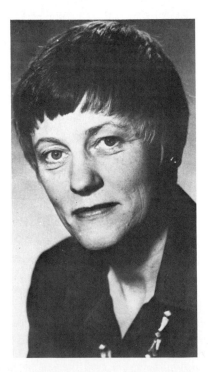

Olga Jonasson, 1934—. M.D. University of Illinois 1958, and Intern through Resident 1958-64. Postdoctoral Fellow, Walter Reed Army Institute of Research 1964-65; Massachusetts General Hospital 1965-66 (Transplantation); Presbyterian-St. Luke's Hospital 1966-69 (Cardiovascular and Thoracic Surgery); Instructor to Professor of Surgery, University of Illinois 1963-1975; Chief, Division of Transplantation Surgery, University of Illinois Hospital 1968; Chief of Surgery, Cook County Hospital 1977—.

THE PRESIDENT'S DINNER, January 20, 1979
Mayo Foundation House

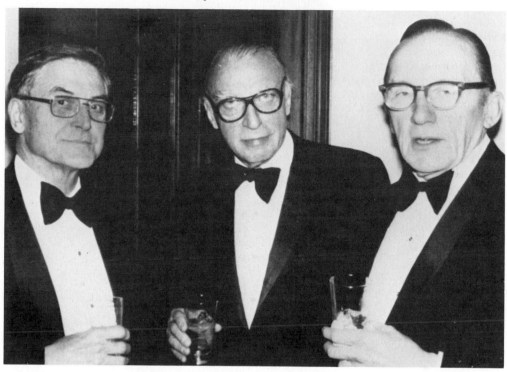

President Oliver H. Beahrs; Mark M. Ravitch, Vice-President, 1974; C. Rollins Hanlon, Secretary, 1969, Director, American College of Surgeons. The President's dinner, perhaps from earliest days, a function of the mid-winter meeting of the Council, was until recently relatively small and intimate, including the Officers and a few specially invited Fellows. In part because of the increasing complexity of the affairs of the Association, and the many committees which it is useful to have meet when the Officers can meet with them, the dinners have become large, and somewhat more formal, if no less congenial. A between-meetings conclave of Officers and Council had been ordained from the first. Dr. Jonathan Rhoads' ad hoc Committee on the Purpose and Functions of the American Surgical Association, reviewing the structure, function and direction of the Association, foresaw the need for additional interim meetings of the Council. Formal interim Council meetings have not been instituted, but meetings of the Advisory Membership Committee and the Committee on Issues with the Officers sitting in, have taken place at the time of the Clinical Congress of the American College of Surgeons for a number of years.

(Photograph courtesy of O. H. Beahrs, M.D., Rochester, Minn.)

American Board of Surgery, and the American Board of Family Practice."

The Council recommended that the Committee on Government Affairs be terminated, and the Secretary announced optimistically that "the Council notes with gratitude that Dr. Ravitch has completed the first draft of Volume 1 of the *History of the American Surgical Association,* and notes that he anticipates completion of this history by the time of the Centenary Meeting in Atlanta in 1980."

Evidence that, in essence, the officers had another meeting a year in addition to the mid-winter one, was included in the report of James D. Hardy,

for the Committee on Issues, "I think one of the things we have achieved is to continue to develop the administrative aspects of the Committee. For example, from now on we will always—I say 'always' meaning in the immediate future, at least in the next year—meet in connection with the American College of Surgeons in a room adjacent to the one being used by the Advisory Committee on Membership. That gives the President and the Secretary and others the opportunity to go from room to room, and to be present and participate in at least a portion of our program that day. In addition, there will be a meeting each January, on the Friday pre-

1512

ceding the Council meeting on Saturday in January."

Among the 22 candidates elected to Active Fellowship was Olga Jonasson.

At President Sabiston's invitation, Claude E. Welch arose and announced the award of the Association's Medallion for Scientific Achievement, the fifth, to Dr. Francis D. Moore, of Boston.

Officers elected were President, Oliver H. Beahrs, of Rochester, Minnesota; Vice-Presidents, Joseph Murray, of Boston, and Charles Rob, of Rochester, New York; Secretary, James V. Maloney, of Los Angeles.

XCVII

1979

The 1979 meeting was held at The Homestead, Hot Springs, Virginia, April 26, 27, and 28, President Oliver H. Beahrs, of Rochester, Professor of Surgery, Mayo Medical School; Consultant in Surgery, Mayo Clinic, in the Chair. Beahrs in his wide ranging inspirational address paid special tribute to the genius, vision and strong principles of the Mayo brothers. Among those who had died that year was Leland S. McKittrick, of Boston, who had been President in 1966.

[The following consideration of the 1979 meeting at The Homestead is necessarily based on the actual manuscripts of the papers and on the unedited transcripts of the discussions, kindly made available by the recorder of the Association, Dr. Lloyd Nyhus. Comparison with the published *Transactions* may show some differences. We all speak from the platform with Churchillian elegance and professional precision. How humbling when the transcript records our all but unintelligible, ill phrased, solecism-filled utterances,- lacking, too, the telling points we had meant to make. The edited discussions often bear a striking resemblance to what the mind's ear of the speaker thought it heard him say. In addition the editor of the *Annals,* in the presumed interest of comity and dignity has been known to delete what seemed to him an excess of passion, acerbity or humor. A comparison between several of the discussions presented here from the stenotypist's transcript and the published *Transactions* is illuminating.]

* * *

G. A. McLoughlin, A. V. Wu, I. Saporoschetz, R. Nimberg, all by invitation, and John A. Mannick, of Boston, Moseley Professor of Surgery, Harvard Medical School; Surgeon-in-Chief, Peter Bent Brigham Hospital, *Correlation between Anergy and a Circulating Immunosuppressive Factor following Major Surgical Trauma,* said that anergy, seen commonly in surgical patients with advanced cancer or nutritionally depleted, was associated with poor resistance to infection and with a high mortality rate. In previous studies, they had found that after major operations, patients often had serum suppressive of T-lymphocyte activation, and that this phenomenon was related to the magnitude of the operation performed. They undertook to "clarify the relationship between anergy and immunosuppressive activity in the serum" by repeated study in 40 patients undergoing elective minor surgery,- inguinal herniorrhaphy,- or major cardiovascular surgery,- 12 aortic aneurysms and 13 coronary artery revascularizations. Delayed hypersensitivity was measured by skin testing with standard recall antigens and the immunosuppressive activity of the serum "was determined by the ability of the patient's serum in 10% concentration to suppress by 50% or more the PHA [phytohemagglutinin] of normal human lymphocytes as compared to pooled normal serum." Before operation, all the patients manifested delayed hypersensitivity and no patient had immunosuppressive serum. None of the herniorrhaphy patients developed anergy or immunosuppressive serum. Thirteen of the patients undergoing cardiac operations became anergic by the third day after operation and 12 of these developed immunosuppressive serum whereas of the 12 others who maintained their delayed hypersensitivity, only two developed immunosuppressive serum. By the 28th day, all patients had recovered their capacity for delayed hypersensitivity and their serum was no longer immunosuppressive. "The occurrence of post-operative anergy and immunosuppressive serum . . . was associated with an increase in post-operative infectious complications . . . and in post-operative days in the hospital." Most exciting of all, ion exchange chromatography, gel filtration and high voltage electrophoresis, of pooled immunosuppressive serum from the anergic patients demonstrated an "electrophoretically homogenous polypeptide-containing fraction not identified in the serum of patients undergoing minor surgery or in normal individuals." The anergic patients had not lost their capacity to mount an inflammatory response since they responded normally to intradermal histamine, none was nutritionally depleted and none had known malignancy, and serum cortisol levels were normal in all patients. "The most obvious explanation for the present observations appears to be that major operative trauma in itself triggers a temporary inhibition of cellular immunity, possibly mediated by circulating immunosuppressive factors . . . the majority, but not all, of the immunosuppressive activity can be accounted for by a polypeptide-like fraction which from its behavior on gel filtration has a molecular weight of approximately 1,000 daltons. This material can be recovered as a homogeneous molecular species by high voltage electrophoresis. The highly basic character of this material on electrophoresis makes it unlikely that it is a conventional polypeptide . . . . This material was not recoverable in detectable quantities by identical fractionation of the serum from normal individuals or from patients who had undergone minor surgical procedures." The modest conclusion was, "Major operative trauma is often followed by the appearance in the serum of a circulating factor or factors suppressive of T-lymphocyte activation."

Discussion

George H. A. Clowes, Jr., of Boston, said he had been "interested in circulating factors of the small nonprotein peptide type that John Mannick has discussed with you this morning." His study suggested that the material in an experimental preparation affected the metabolism of muscle cells, a suppression of their response to insulin, "I can tell you from experience that the same thing happens for protein synthesis and a variety of other parameters that we have measured . . . the bottom line of all this work, and the responses that we're looking at, is protein synthesis. After all, T-cell function depends on its ability to make a protein pretty quickly; and I would say that this probably is the common denominator in all of these matters". John L. Meakins, of Montreal, suggested from their studies [in MacLean's laboratory] that there might be two sets of inhibitors in the Mannick serum. They thought they had found them by Sephadex chromatography and other techniques ". . . at 360,000 and 120,000 molecular weight. More recently, we have found smaller inhibitors . . . I wonder if Dr. Mannick could comment upon the nature of these multiple inhibitors, and whether they are all part of a common, or similar, immunoregulatory system." Donald L. Morton, of Los Angeles, had found that cancer patients with operations which opened either the abdominal or thoracic cavity, developed more immunosuppression than operations of the same duration in which the cavities were not entered. They had found a correlation between blood transfusion and degree of duration of immunosuppression and found that the most immunosuppressed patients were those undergoing cardiopulmonary bypass. However, ". . . if the tumor was completely resected, there was a disappearance of the immunosuppressive factors, so that the patients, even though they might have major trauma—major surgical trauma; that is, an operation involving the thoracic or adominal cavity . . . if the tumor was completely resected, and they were anergic preoperatively, they may very early recover their allergic state during the early postoperative period." Immunosuppression in their patients lasted about the same time as in Dr. Mannick's series ". . . in seven to fourteen days the immune competence and immunosuppressive factors and the ability of the lymphocytes to respond returns quite promptly to normal." He asked whether there was any difference in the degree of immunosuppression between the patients having cardiopulmonary bypass and those having major aortic resections. Stanley M. Levenson, of the Bronx, New York, thoughtfully asked about the specific amino acid composition of the active fraction, ". . . because in the late '40's and early '50's my colleagues and I had described an amino conjugate fraction which appeared in the serum of previously healthy animals who were injured, or previously healthy men who were injured. The concentration of this correlated with the severity of the injury, and, in particular, it was a dialyzable compound, or group of compounds, and increased remarkably in patients with renal dysfunction." He wondered whether the amino acid composition might have been similar to that in Dr. Mannick's compound and whether any of Dr. Mannick's patients had had renal dysfunction with a rise in the fraction. ". . . this perhaps may be one of the explanations why a patient with renal failure is particularly susceptible to infection." Mannick, closing, agreed "that we are just now finding some functions for that myriad of polypeptide molecules that circulate around in everyone's serum, whose function has heretofore been unknown; and I suppose that they represent a few words in the biochemical language that cells use to communicate with one another, and that language has by no means been translated yet." He did not know the relationship between the material he had been talking about and "the factors that Dr. Clowes has been working with". While Mannick's factor had an effect on rosette formation, he didn't know that that meant that it had a metabolic effect on lymphocytes. He was intrigued by what he understood of Meakins' suggestion "that the immunoregulatory system may have some features similar to the complement system; and that is that breakdown products of one activity may, in fact, therefore subsume other activities, and that we may be talking about pieces of molecules that once did something else, and now affect a different cell type",- he could only admit the possibility. To Morton, he said that the bypass and aneurysm patients reacted essentially the same way. To Dr. Levenson, he said that he had been "intrigued by that early paper of his, and he may be right. He may, in fact, have identified this material. I just don't know whether they are similar or not. The amino acid composition of our material I don't think I can give him with any confidence. We do have a sample of this material in the hands of the Molecular Biology Institute at Hoffmann-La Roche, and we hope to have some information about its true nature in a few weeks."

* * *

What seemed to be almost a nostalgic throwback to the programs of an earlier day, Warren E. Enker and Urban Th. Laffer, by invitation, and George E. Block, of Chicago, Professor of Surgery, University of Chicago, Pritzker School of Medicine, *The Enhanced Survival of Patients with Colon and Rectal Cancer Is Based upon Wide Anatomic Resection,* was based upon 216 resections of carcinoma of the large bowel performed from 1966 through 1970. This was an unabashed plea for the vintage Halstedian principle of wide removal of the tumor and draining lymphatic tissues with the pathway in be-

tween, in continuity. "The major principles of the curative operation for large bowel cancer have been established for nearly three quarters of a century . . . en-bloc resection of lymph nodes to the origin of the named arteries supplying the colon and rectum . . . resection of the zone of upward spread in rectal cancers . . . and wide pelvic and hypogastric lymph node dissection . . ." Their position was that "few institutions have consistently applied *all* of these principles to their surgical practice and, more importantly, the concept of radical lymphadenectomy has not received universal application outside of major surgical centers. We are convinced that this latter factor alone is responsible for an unwarranted national pessimism concerning the survival of patients with colorectal cancer. Since the cure of colorectal cancer is almost exclusively surgical, we have chosen to examine the results of our own operative experience in which we have strictly adhered to all of the above principles." Fourteen patients, 6.4%, died within 60 days of operation. The absolute five-year survival for all patients was 52.8% and for those without distant metastases, was 65.3%. For rectal cancer, the total survival at five years was 45.5%; the relative five-year survival "which is tantamount to cure" was 80.4% of all patients with colon cancer and 63.3% of the patients with rectal cancer who did not have distant abdominal spread at the time of operation. The National Cancer Institute figures covering almost 10,000 patients showed "a relative five-year survival of 43 percent for males and 46 percent for females." Their own five-year survival of 45 patients with Stage III tumors was 66.6%, far higher than that reported elsewhere in the country. Of Turnbull's results, they suggested that they were due to the limits of his resection and not to his "no touch technique", thus providing a radical and anatomic lymphadenectomy. They had not used the no touch technique and their results were superior to Turnbull's.

Discussion

The Honorary Fellow from Leeds, Professor John Goligher, rose to comment "with particular reference to their remarks on the use of superradical surgery for rectal cancer." He approached the subject "in a prejudiced frame of mind . . . from . . . (1) my own disappointing experiences in the early 1950's with this sort of operation, with internal iliac adenectomy, and partly also from the report in 1958 by Stearns and Deddish . . . at the Memorial Hospital in New York. They found that it did not enhance the five-year survival rate, and that virtually all the patients who had metastases in the internal iliac nodes that were removed subsequently succumbed, with pelvic recurrence. In fact, the only effect of the operation seemed to be to increase considerably the immediate postoperative complications, particularly in regard to the bladder and sexual function. Now comes this enthusiastic reappraisal of this issue by Dr. Enker and his colleagues, with their clarion call to more aggressive surgery. What are we to believe, and to do? . . . with the utmost respect, I have to say that the improvement in results reported by Dr. Enker with internal iliac adenectomy seems so dramatic, it immediately arouses my suspicion there must be a snag somewhere . . . the number of cases concerned is very small, and the differences observed might well be entirely fortuitous . . . it's not at all clear how patients were selected for dissection or nondissection of these pelvic nodes . . . based entirely on the personal predilection of the surgeon operating, or might it have been due to the heavy involvement of the nodes, making them fixed, so that they were, in fact, irremovable? . . . we cannot be sure that the two series, with and without internal iliac node dissection, were truly similar; and I may add that nothing in my experience of doing many clinical studies of this kind is so important as the absolute similarity of the groups being contrasted . . . a similar criticism applies to the other comparative data in this paper; and also, I hasten to add, to the data in all the other studies of this kind, such as those of Stearns and Deddish, of Dr. Rosi, of Chicago, the recent paper by Dr. Longmire and one of his colleagues advocating the very opposite of this thesis; and, of course, Dr. Turnbull's trial was totally uncontrolled, and I think, of very dubious value." To arrive at the answer would require a "properly controlled, randomized, prospective trial" and an extremely difficult one. "And, of course, it will take at least four or five years . . . in most centers, other than the Mayo Clinic, Mr. President [Oliver Beahrs, of the Mayo Clinic] . . . to accumulate sufficient cases to run such a trial of any validity" and then another five years to evaluate the results. "This is apt to prove rather daunting to surgeons, who would like to see the results a good deal sooner, and who have a very, very natural desire to be in the land of the living and the operating when the final result becomes available." Richard E. Wilson, of Boston, said that at the Brigham, they had reviewed an 11-year experience with colorectal cancer. They found that 67% of recurrences were either distant or distant plus regional and only 35% were regional alone. Recurrence was associated with the size of the tumor and the Dukes' stage plus, particularly, loca-

tion, "For all of the colonic lesions except the rectum, distant recurrence, or distant plus simultaneous regional and distant, led the pattern of recurrence, except for the rectum, where regional recurrence and regional and distant recurrences were similar." And even after abdominoperineal resection, the regional recurrence was equivalent to distant and regional recurrences. "While I believe that the surgical technique must be an important part of the equation, effective systemic therapy will be the most important method of altering the present results in the treatment of this disease; and, unfortunately, we don't have adequate, effective chemotherapy at this time." Jerome J. deCosse, of New York [newly established as the Director of Surgery at the Memorial Hospital], welcomed "a re-affirmation of the thesis that more attentive adherence to well-established surgical principles of resection, particularly an adequate margin of mesentery, will reduce recurrence." The Cancer Commission Survey of the American College of Surgeons reported a five-year survival rate for patients with C lesions of 28%, the National Cancer Institute a five-year survival rate of 35%, the Cleveland Clinic 58%, Memorial Hospital 52%, "and in this paper Enker reports a five-year survival rate of 66.7% and 56.5% for C_1 and C_2 cancers respectively. All advocate aggressive resection." Owen H. Wangensteen, of Minneapolis, reminded the Fellows of his proposal some 35 years before for "near-total or total excision of the large bowel for cancer of the rectum and colon some distance above the spincter." Three of nine patients with such an operation developed cancer in the very small residual portion of the colon and Wangensteen said "There is a distinct advantage in doing a total over a near-total colectomy." [A Fellow was heard to say, "You can't have cancer in an organ that has been removed".] Isidore Cohn, Jr., of New Orleans, pointed out that in 2,000 patients from the Charity Hospital in New Orleans, results were better in those without lymph node involvement and better in those with Dukes A level than Dukes B or C level, and said [without citing any evidence for it] "that it certainly is clear that a more extensive operation is better than a highly confined one. And I would like to go on record as suggesting that we would do better to extend our operative procedure, rather than to confine it, as I think some effort has been indicated in the recent past." Alfred S. Ketcham, of Miami, mentioned the fact that he had recently seen three recurrences in low rectal lesions, which had been removed by somebody using a stapler. "Mr. President . . . You have burdened us today with the bit about our teaching our residents, and in this day and age when some of them know better how to use a stapler than a needle holder, I just bring to our attention that these three recurrences have come in by using the low-lying stapler transrectally . . . that we have now seen three recurrences since Christmas. And I would encourage us to continue to look at quality of survival of our patients, meaning trying to avoid the colostomy, but I just think we've got to take a new look at the use of this stapler for lesions that are one to two inches within the anus." Enker, in closing, acknowledged that the group of patients in whom they studied the virtues of hypogastric lymph node dissection was small. Urinary problems after operation, they accepted as "part of the management of the patient". He commented to Wilson that "I would only accept what the results of systemic treatment are once the United States surgeons have standardized survival based on an adequate operation." As for the stapler, "Dr. Goligher spoke to us in Chicago about the way he used the stapler, approximately six months ago, and I think that this is a model in many respects for the use of the stapler. Once one has accomplished a dissection of the pelvis in all three planes, and is satisfied that one has not coned down to the point of anastomosis to prepare oneself in that regard, and possibly has compromised the extent of the pelvic dissection, if there is sufficient bowel remaining for a staple anastomosis, but one which would be technically impossible for a nonstaple anastomosis, then I think the stapler is of value. But it is the extent of the resection first."

* * *

There was a change in the Program on the next morning. In place of the scheduled paper, which was cancelled [it was heard that the paper had been simultaneously offered to two societies and accepted by both] the President announced that the Honorary Member from Peking, Professor Wu Ying-k'ai [elected to Honorary Fellowship the year before], would speak on cancer of the esophagus. Wu, who had trained at the Peking Union Medical College with Loucks (H. H.) a Fellow of the Association, and had had two years of work at the Barnes Hospital in St. Louis with Evarts Graham, now, *Chinese Experience in the Surgical Treatment of Carcinoma of the Esophagus,* spoke in easy, flawless English, and after a graceful and good humored introduction, presented a total experience from 13 Chinese clinics, of 5,412 cases of carcinoma and gastric cardia between 1940 and 1960. In a more recent series of 778 cases from his own Fu Wai Hospital, 1962 to 1968, 69% of the patients had resectable lesions and that figure had now risen to 80%. "In one series from the county hospital of Linhsien of Honan province, where a number of early esophageal cancers had been operated upon on the basis of frequent population surveys, the resectability rate in a series of 1228 cases was as high as 94.1%." The operative mortality had dropped steadily from 25% in the earlier years to 10% in 1960 and now, 3 to 5%. Their experience with carcinoma of the esophagus in China did not support the widespread pessimism concerning the utility of operation for esophageal cancer. A number of Chinese clinics reported five-year survival rates of around 25% and more recently, 30 to 40%. In the same Linhsien series, there was a 44% five-year survival in 250 resections, and in the very early esophageal cancers discovered during a population survey, there was only one postoperative recurrence in 163 cases, and that one nine years after resection. In his own series of patients operated upon between 1940 and 1961 "the five-year survival rate for cancers of the lower third of the esophagus was 31.3%, that for the gastric cardia was 22.6%. That for the upper and middle third of the esophagus was only 14.3%." Invasion through the wall of the esophagus, in a series from the Peking Medical College Hospitals, dropped the five-year survival rate from 32.6% to 7.3%. Similarly, lymph node metastases dropped survivals in another series from 47.9% to 6.3%. Their general practice was to employ "left posterolateral thoracotomy and a one stage extensive esophagectomy followed by esophago-gastrostomy" removing "the accessible lymph nodes in the mediastinum and in the epigastric region together with the esophagus and the gastric cardia." They insisted upon a free margin of 5 or 6 cm. proximal to the tumor, and even that was frequently inadequate so that now "For cancers of the lower esophagus, the esophagogastrostomy after resection is often performed at the supra-aortic level. In cancers of the middle segment of the esophagus, the esophagogastrostomy following resection is often done at the level of the dome of the pleural cavity, and when the cancer has extended to above the level of the aortic arch, the esophagogastrostomy is to be performed in the neck." Anastomosis was open, with two layers of interrupted sutures and a leakage rate of some 3 to 5%. "During recent years, stapler type suturing apparatus for esophagogastrostomy has been used in several clinics in China." Series of 100 and 275 cases had been reported "of esophageal resections and esophagogastrostomy using the suture apparatus with no anastomosis leakage, but there were a few cases of mild stenosis of the anastomosis stoma in the early postoperative period." At the Cancer Institute of the Chinese Academy of Medical Science, preoperative radiation therapy had been evaluated for lesions of borderline resectability and in 212 such patients, there was a five-year operative survival rate of 31.6% and in 178 a ten-year survival rate of 21.9%. There was no difference in operative mortality. "We are of the opinion that this type of combined therapy is to be recommended for carcinoma of the esophagus of questionable resectability."

Discussion

There was no formal Discussion but Carl E. Lischer, of St. Louis, who had been on the House Staff at the Barnes Hospital when Wu had been there, remembered "When Dr. Wu came to St. Louis . . . Carcinoma of the esophagus was a medical curiosity at Barnes Hospital. I think Dr. Phemister did the first resection of a carcinoma of the esophagus in this country, and shortly thereafter Dr. Graham did one or two cases, and Dr. Womack at his weekly surgical/path conference had a discussion of carcinoma of the esophagus, these two cases, and towards the end of the conference, in a very modest and quiet manner, Dr. Wu said, 'I just happen to have a couple of slides.' So he got up and discussed his own personal experience of some 40 or 50 cases. Well, after that Dr. Graham had the highest regard for Dr. Wu . . ."

* * *

Mark M. Ravitch, of Pittsburgh, Professor of Surgery, University of Pittsburgh; Surgeon-in-Chief, Montefiore Hospital, Pittsburgh, and by invitation, Robert E. Brolin, *The Price of Weight Loss by Jejunoileal Shunt,* said that "The concept of controlled malabsorption, by exclusion from the alimentary stream of measured segments of the bowel, in the effort to correct massive obesity, introduced by Kremen and pioneered and intensively studied by Salmon, Payne, Scott, Varco, their collaborators, and others, and since put widely into clinical application around the world had now has more than a decade of extensive experience." They had performed the Scott type of bypass with end-to-end anastomosis of the residual jejunum and ileum in 64 patients from 1972 to 1978. The review had been undertaken because they had been "impressed by the number of patients who several years after operation complained of lack of strength, still required medication for the control of diarrhea, continued to manifest, or to develop anew, a variety of complications, and sometimes one or another complication would develop late in a patient who had never before had any significant trouble." Evaluation of the worth of the operation by patient satisfaction was difficult, "The depth of the prior unhappiness of these massively obese patients can perhaps best be measured by their ecstasy over their weight loss, ability to buy clothes off the shelf, bend down and tie their own shoes, go swimming with their children, create jealousy in their husbands, and even more by their unwillingness to consider restoration of intestinal continuity." Evaluation of patient satisfaction was particularly difficult "after operations for morbid obesity since the patients are guiltily aware that the obesity was self-induced, and they have more than the usual patient's vested interest in finding that the risks, expense, suffering were all justified." There had been no operative deaths, no anastomotic leaks, no eviscerations, one incisional hernia. Weight loss had been unpredictable. Three of 12 patients with functioning j.-i. lengths of 19 inches or more lost 33% of their original weight at three years, while 33 of 36 patients with lengths of 17 or 18 inches lost 33% of their weight in 18 months. Four patients had had secondary revisions for inadequate weight loss. Thirty-three percent of the patients had early postoperative complications and 70% had readmissions to the hospital for late complications. Fewer than a quarter of the patients followed 18 months or longer had been without complications. Complications included electrolyte imbalance,- chiefly calcium, potassium, and magnesium, 31/64; abdominal distress, 27/64; anemia, 23/64; renal stones, 9/64; hepatic dysfunction, 9/64; anorectal problems requiring operation, 5/64; arthritis, 3/64; lower gastrointestinal bleeding, 3/64; severe psychiatric disorders, 3/64; measured vitamin A deficiency, 2/64. The syndrome known as bypass enteritis,- distention, pain and tenderness, diarrhea, sometimes fever,- was diagnosed in 12 patients, three of whom had unequivocal evidence of disease, one of them with severe changes in a long segment of indurated thickened bypassed bowel, another with numerous deep chronic ulcers in the bypassed bowel, and a third had pneumatosis intestinalis. Particularly alarming was the appearance in five patients of similar unexplained neurologic symptoms including episodic dizziness, staggering, postural vertigo and paraparesis, two of whom had remission of symptoms with peripheral amino acid infusions. Lack of energy, easy fatigability were common even in patients who considered themselves well. There had been four late deaths, two from gross hepatic failure and two unexplained. Seven patients had already undergone restoration of alimentary continuity. The 170 readmissions ranging from four to 57 days, mean 16 days, had been at a cost of approximately $3,000 per 16-day admission [it was explained from the platform by Ravitch that these 1977-1978 cost estimates were already irrelevant for future admissions]. There had been 703 outpatient visits at a laboratory cost of $49 per visit. In sum, of patients who had gone 18 months or longer, 53% had sustained adequate weight loss and were free of major problems. They concluded that "Despite brilliant results in some patients, and satisfactory results in perhaps half, the cost in life, suffering, dollars, and in patient and physician time, the uncertain long-term effects, the unpredictability of weight loss, all place in question the appropriateness of jejunoileal shunt as the remedy for morbid obesity."

* * *

William G. Pace, of Columbus, Professor of Surgery, Ohio State University, College of Medicine, Attending Staff, University Hospital and Childrens Hospital; by invitation, E. W. Martin, Jr., T. Tetirick, P. J. Fabri; and Larry C. Carey, Professor and Chairman, Department of Surgery, The Ohio State University College of Medicine, *Gastric Partitioning for Morbid Obesity.* In 220 patients with morbid obesity, they had stapled the stomach close enough to the esophagogastric junction to make a pouch of between 30 and 60 cc. proximal to the staple line. Two staples from the center of the proximal row and one staple opposite from the center of the distal row of the cartridge were removed before the stapler was applied. This left a passageway of fixed size which just permitted a 9 mm. catheter to be passed. The operation had been performed in 220 patients. There was a single death from pulmonary embolism, ten days after discharge from the hospital. Two patients had fistulae and one patient had a "partial staple line necrosis with leak". There were four severe wound infections and two dehiscences. Two patients required splenectomy and in two patients the stomach was lacerated posteriorly in creating a tunnel for the stapler. "Of the 220 patients, 180 are considered to be successful results (82%), while 40 are considered failures (18%)." They felt that all the failures were the result of early ingestion of solid food or large quantities of liquid with violent vomiting and disruption of the partition. They now required the patients to stay on a liquid diet for eight weeks. Their animal investigation had suggested that after eight weeks, the healing was secure.

Discussion

J. Howard Payne, of Los Angeles, [the Fellow with the longest and greatest experience with operations for morbid obesity] said "Our first experience was in 1956, and our first publication was in 1963. This now represents 23 years of experience, some pretty hard and some not so hard . . . we still see and follow our first patient to undergo surgical therapy for malnutrition/morbid obesity . . . The jejunocolic decompression following the end-to-end anastomosis, the so-called Scott procedure, with the decompression into the colon . . . will produce a problem, and I think, in my opinion, is the primary cause of one of our relatively new problems; namely, pneumatosis intestinalis, or the so-called bypass enteritis." He turned now to the gastric bypass which "has been changed so many times that I can't keep up with it. We are now seeing some serious failures and some serious complications . . . we have continued to do . . . the jejunoileal bypass, utilizing 35 cm of proximal jejunum, anastomosed end-to-side to the distal 10 cm of the ileum, with some minor modifications . . . to prevent reflux into the bypassed segment. We are at this present time quite happy and satisfied with our results . . . satisfactory or excellent . . . 75%; good, 15%; and 10 outright failures. We have not used the stapling machine . . . I do think that the operation investigation should be continued, and it's worthwhile in spite of the cost." H. William Scott, of Nashville, commented on the 225 massively obese patients in whom he had performed his operation with an early postoperative mortality rate of 2%, showing the very satisfactory weight losses, ". . . the greatest sustained weight reduction occurred in patients who had total incontinence small intestine shortened to 45 to 50 cm." They similarly had some 22% of immediate complications in the first 100 patients but "almost eliminated these surgical complications in the last 100 patients . . . Major metabolic complications include oxalate urinary stones in 15% and episodes of the enterohepatic syndrome of hepatocellular injury in 12% of patients. There were four late deaths from liver failure." The hyperoxaluria and urinary stones were a matter of the short bowel and not due to inappropriate absorption from the bypassed bowel whereas "the 'flulike syndrome of nausea, vomiting, hypergeusia, myalgias, and prostration, accompanied by elevation of liver enzymes and later by icterus and hepatomegaly, reflects hepatocellular injury from absorption of toxic metabolites of heavy bacterial growth in the bypassed small bowel." For this, they used Flagyl—micronidazole—and a high protein diet,- if necessary, hospitalization and parenteral alimentation. They had a mean weight loss in their patients of 45 to 50% and reductions in serum cholesterol and triglycerides of 40 to 60% and uniform relief of adult onset diabetes. He said that "With current dimensional considerations, good results have been achieved in 75% of our patients. However, certainly morbidity and mortality risks are significant, and I must agree with Dr. Ravitch that these limit wide application of the procedure. Gastric stapling is indeed an attractive alternative for obese patients who are not hyperlipidemic." Max R. Gaspar, Long Beach, California, described a technique of Dr. Larry Wilkinson, of Albuquerque, "His idea was to plicate the stomach upon itself, and then wrap it with a mesh." Wilkinson had operated on 26 such patients and Gaspar had operated upon seven with satisfactory weight loss and no metabolic complications. He called the operation "a tubular gastric plication . . ." Henry Buchwald, of Minneapolis, started by saying "I believe we are entering a very difficult area for jejunoileal and gastric bypass for obesity. We are now seeing the late complications of gastric bypass." Morbid obesity was a serious problem and a lethal one. Non-medical treatment had a 99% failure rate and in the cost benefit analysis, one had to weigh "the outcome of no therapy". He thought the weight loss, patient satisfaction, decrease in blood pressure, relief of diabetes, lipid reduction, relief of disc disease and traumatic arthritis weighed strongly in a cost benefit analysis. "In our own series of approximately 900 patients with jejunoileal bypass, utilizing a 40 cm jejunum to 4 cm ileum, end-to-end anastomosis, Richard L. Varco and I have seen an excellent weight response and far fewer complications than have been reported by Dr. Ravitch. Our serious complication rate is well under 10%." Of the gastric procedure, he said, "we have done approximately 100 gastric bypass procedures, with no deaths, no wound infection, and good results. We are not anti-gastric bypass, gastroplasty, or gastric partitioning. And I would agree with the authors that 15 patients, one-year follow-up, is insufficient at this time for a data base from which to draw a judgment . . . I would predict that the staple line will disrupt in the future . . . late, not early, in some of these cases . . . that the orifice will widen, and that we will see a failure rate beyond that reported at this time." Hastings K. Wright, of New Haven, said he rose "to insert one more nail in the coffin being constructed by Dr. Ravitch for the jejunoileal bypass . . . It was supposed to be the best of all possible worlds. The glutton could continue to eat to his heart's desire, and all those excess calories were to be swept away in the stool. It's not really true." They had done careful intake and output studies in three patients after jejunoileal shunt on the 2,500 calorie diet and found only 500 calories per day in the stool "This is a loss insufficient to account for the weight documented in our patients, and a loss which is little more than the calorie losses in the stool . . . documented at 12 and 24 months, when weight was beginning to stabilize. Intestinal bypass patients . . . lose weight, probably, because they can't eat . . . Our patients tell us they get very uncomfortable when they eat. They can't describe exactly what it is, but they don't want to eat. If this is so, what advantage is left for the jejunoileal bypass over the Pace procedure?" Edward E. Mason, of Iowa City, said, weight loss with his first gastroplasty [leaving only a small channel in the stomach high on the greater curvature] "which we did in 1971 . . . was about 25 kg at five years. For those that had a second operation to convert them to a gastric bypass, it wasn't much better, and the reason for that was that we didn't make the upper part of the stomach smaller. The patients that were operated upon in 1975 to '78, who had measured small pouches, have had a one-year weight loss of 45 kg, on the average . . . you must have a small upper stomach, less than 50 cc. You must have a small outlet, 12 mm in diameter, we believe. And you must have some method of keeping that small outlet from stretching. And you must have some way to keep the staple line from disrupting. We're using two cartridges now, taking three staples out at the greater curvature of the first set, five from the second set; a 0 chromic catgut is placed through the wall of the stomach at the end of the staple line and tied down around the greater curvature with a No. 32 French Hurst dilator, or an Ewald tube in place, to calibrate this. This is then reinforced with a 3.0 proline seromuscular circumferential suture to help control the size for as long as that suture will stay in place." [Vice-President Rob, in the Chair, announced that Dr. Jonathan Rhoads would be the final discussant. He apologized to a number of others who had indicated that they wished to discuss the papers.] Jonathan E. Rhoads, of Philadelphia, suggested only that he thought that the "short transit time after jejunoileal bypass might prevent adequate methionine release" from food protein which permitted the body to synthesize choline, and he had given patients 3 to 6 grams of methionine per day without any hepatic complications thus far. He thought it might prevent hepatic complications. Mark M. Ravitch, closing, reminded the Fellows that it was Arnold Kremen's paper before the Association some 20 years before concerning his experiments in dogs that had been the start of the interest in operations for obesity and that on that occasion "Philip Sandblom arose to say: 'Yes, there is a doctor in Sweden who had done just exactly this on a patient to lose weight.' And Arnold Kremen got up and said: 'I was hoping nobody would mention that, but as long as it has been mentioned, we've done one too.' And this thing has mushroomed ever since." Ravitch took the position "that, basically, surgery—certainly, operation—is the application of mechanical principles to disease. And we can accept it as axiomatic that any disease which is basically not mechanical in origin will not ultimately be treated mechanically. Some of our most brilliant successes for a time, in the history of surgery, have been with mechanical things; but I don't believe, in the end, vagotomy or gastrectomy or antrectomy, or any of those things, are going to be the right answer to the ulcer problem. The physiological answer ought to be; it's just that the physiologists aren't smart enough to arrive at that." He said to Dr. Wright that he was not driving home a nail in the coffin, "Our abstract ends with a question. The question is: Is the game worth the candle? And for me, right now, I find that I am not able to schedule patients for a jejunoileal shunt, and it may be that I can't face the problems as well as they can face them." He commented also on Pace's paper. Pace had said that to study the effect of the staples on the stomach, they had gone to the laboratory. Ravitch said "instead of going to the laboratory—it would have been more cost effective if he had gone to the library" showing a quotation from a paper some 15 years back in which he "in essence, closed off the stomach and did a gastroenterostomy around it, and we found that just because the staplers are not necrotizing instruments, the pressure isn't destructive, the mucosa stays healed. It doesn't heal mucosa to mucosa, and gradually some of the staples tear out . . . It is perfectly possible that enough of the staples will stay behind to maintain the reduced weight after it had been achieved. This is an interesting attempt, and something needs to be done for these people." Larry C. Carey, in closing, said that "Morbid obesity, like alcoholism, is a disease which leads to other diseases." He had never done gastric bypass and suspected he never would "because of the ravages of the problem that I have been witness to in following the patients that have been done by others . . . Gastric partitioning will very likely not provide the ultimate solution, but it seems to be a logical step in the evolution of the surgical treatment for this disease. I apologize to Dr. Ravitch for not having been aware of his writings in the literature in this regard. We have been for the last two and a half years trying to cull through all of the things that Dr. Ravitch has written, and we obviously haven't gotten to that point. [Laughter] We'll continue the quest. [Laughter and applause]"

* * *

Floyd D. Loop, and six others by invitation from the Cleveland Clinic, *An 11-Year Evolution of Coronary Arterial Surgery (1967-1968),* compared the 741 patients who underwent isolated myocardial revascularization procedures from 1967 to 1970 with the first 1,000 patients similarly operated upon electively *each year* from 1971 through 1978. The median age of the patients had risen steadily from 50 in the earliest years to 56 in 1978. The extent of coronary atherosclerosis had steadily increased. In 1967-1970, single-vessel disease accounted for 56% of the cases "Thereafter the prevalence of multiple-vessel disease rose consistently to a high of 89% in 1978." Preoperative left ventricular impairment showed "A gradual increase in categories of moderate and severe left ventricular impairment . . . in 1977 and 1978. In these . . . years, 13% and 19% had moderate dysfunction and 6% each year had extremely poor left ventricular function manifested by global impairment and markedly elevated LVEDP . . . all had angina as the predominant symptom . . ." The hospital mortality in 1967 to 1970 was 3% and had varied from 0.4% to 1.5% since "Overall operative mortality was 1.1% for 11 years and 0.9% for 1971 through 1978." The number of grafts per patient rose steadily from 1.5 in 1967-1970 to 2.5 in 1978. Perioperative infarction had dropped from 7.1% in 1967-1970 to 1.2% in 1978. Reoperation for bleeding ranged from 4% to 10% without any recognizable pattern. "From 1967 through 1973, stress gastrointestinal bleeding occurred with an incidence of 1.4% to 2.6%. In later years this complication became less frequent; no cases of gastrointestinal bleeding were recorded in 1978." Graft patency improved from 1971 to 1973 over the 1967-1970 experience, thought to be largely a reflection of the "greater use of the IMA [internal mammary artery] graft with its attendant higher patency." Anastomoses to the anterior descending coronary artery had the highest patency. For the first five postoperative years, graft attrition rate was low "Serial vein graft and IMA graft studies were . . . reviewed for 1971–1973 cohorts. Of 144 vein grafts studied serially, 85% were patent at the first postoperative catheterization (mean 14 months) and 76% were open after the second catheterization (mean 56 months). For serially studied IMA grafts, all were patent intially and 54 of 58 (93%) were patent at the second catheterization, a mean interval of 44 months postoperatively . . . Our original contention that the majority of graft closures occur within the first three months and are related to runoff and technical factors holds true; however, late atherosclerotic changes in vein grafts have been reported, usually three or more years postoperatively." The five-year actuarial survival in the 1967-1970 group varied from 85% for triple-vessel disease to 91.6% for single-vessel disease. For the 1971-1973 group, it was 89.8% for triple-vessel disease and 96.5% for single-vessel disease. The overall survival in the 1971-1973 group with complete revascularization was 93.8%; with incomplete revascularization, it was 88.0%. For the years 1967–70, 71, 72, 73, 65% and 69% of patients were free of chest pain. Just over 50% of survivors of the 1971-1973 period were employed five years later. Some 5% of that early group had hospitalization for subsequent infarction. The results had steadily improved in spite of the fact that they found "no shift toward lower risk surgical candidates. In fact, if extent of coronary atherosclerosis, left ventricular status, and age are indices of risk, the trend is toward less restrictive selection policies."

Discussion

David C. Sabiston, Jr., of Durham, North Carolina, who had been President in 1978, reminded the Fellows that "the annual death rate from ischemic heart disease in this country had risen dramatically each year until 1970. At that time, a definite decline in mortality began, and has since continued in a very gratifying trend." This had been due to a variety of factors, just as had the reduction in morbidity and mortality with coronary bypass. Dr. Loop attributed the reduction in perioperative myocardial infarction rates "to the result of the introduction of cold cardioplegia in 1977." Mortimer J. Buckley, of Boston, spoke of the furor in the press about the justification for coronary bypass, ". . . people have said that this material covered a selected group of patients, possibly the lowest-risk group; and his detail showed to us today that the high-risk patient is involved in this surgical practice, and the results are outstanding . . ." Buckley was critical of "the two major random studies in the United States, supporting by federal agencies . . ." The NIH study of unstable angina did not "bring out in close detail that that study involved a 40% transfer of patients from medical treatment to surgical treatment, and they are still kept in the category of medically treated patients . . . Similarly, with the study of stable angina, the VA study . . . brings out an equivalent result with surgery and medicine. There the surgical mortality ran extremely high, compared to those numbers that we have seen today, and the medical therapy did not clearly bring out that over 17% of these were patients transferred from medicine to surgery because of the intractable nature of their problem." He asked

Dr. Loop whether he was doing increasing numbers of grafts in individual patients and was that the reason for his improved survival or was it greater attention to detail of the operation. Nicholas T. Kouchoukos, of Birmingham, Alabama, again emphasized the fact that the improved results were not "due to the selection of a more favorable group of patients for operation." The Birmingham series included "3050 patients operated on during an eight-year interval ending in December of 1977 . . ." In the second four-year interval, there was "a substantial increase in the number of patients with three-vessel disease . . . and a corresponding decrease in the number of patients with single- and double-vessel disease." There was a higher proportion of patients in the second four-year interval with severe depression of left ventricular function. Mortality had steadily declined until in the 750 patients operated upon in 1977 it was 0.9%, "despite an increase in the complexity of the procedure. In 1970, the average number of grafts was 1.3, and in 1977 it had increased to 3.4." They too had had a progressive decline in the perioperative infarction rate. The improved survival of patients with two- and three-vessel disease was directly related to the lower mortality. "The failure to demonstrate the beneficial effect of bypass grafting on survival of patients with two- and three-vessel disease, in a prospective study conducted by the Veterans Administration, and which has generated considerable controversy, was related in a major way to the high early mortality . . . Unless hospital mortality is kept at a minimum, enhancement of survival will not be demonstrated in the subsets of patients with relatively favorable five-year survival rates managed without operation . . . The five-year survival for the patients managed nonoperatively was 80%; and this is a group with a relatively favorable five-year survival. For the patients managed with coronary bypass, grafting, it was 96%, and this difference is statistically significant." Floyd D. Loop, closing, said "we use cold cardioplegia for virtually all of our open heart operations, with the exception of the occasional patient who has single-vessel disease, who requires only a single graft. We use the traditional aortic root method of injection, except for patients who have aortic valve surgery, and then the solution is injected directly into the coronary orifices . . . we believe that cold potassium arrest has revolutionized these operations, and particularly complex operations for combined forms of acquired heart disease." He said to Buckley that "usually our patients who have multiple-vessel disease receive three or four bypass grafts." He concluded that "Today there is no excuse for mediocre performance. Cardiac surgery has been simplified and standardized, and the results of coronary arterial surgery from many groups have shown that it provides effective rehabilitation and improved longevity at least for the first five postoperative years . . . As methods of myocardial protection and management continue to evolve, I am convinced that within our lifetime elective coronary arterial surgery can be performed with no mortality."

* * *

F. T. Rapaport, Professor of Surgery, Deputy Chairman for Research and Development and Chief, Transplantation Division, State University of New York at Stonybrook; and by invitation, R. J. Bachvaroff, N. Mollen, H. Hirasawa, T. Asano, and J. W. Ferrebee, *The Induction of Unresponsiveness to Major Transplantable Organs in Adult Mammals* - A Recapitulation of Ontogeny by Irradiation and Bone Marrow Replacement, sought to avoid the undesirable consequences of standard immunosuppression,- "interference with host defenses against infectious microorganisms . . . non-immunological complications such as gastrointestinal bleeding, diabetes and other metabolic derangements . . . These considerations have stimulated intense efforts to develop techniques of immunological manipulation producing specific allogeneic unresponsiveness without disturbing the remainder of the recipients' cellular and-/or humoral defense mechanisms. Earlier studies in this laboratory have shown that transplantation of allogeneic bone marrow into supralethally irradiated canine recipients, bearing DLA-identical haplotypes derived from the same pedigree origins as the donors, can regularly produce long-term stable chimerism in the recipients without any evidence of graft-versus-host . . . complications. The resulting chimeras were unresponsive to other tissues from the same donor, and tolerated kidney, heart, lung, liver, pancreas and/or skin allografts without any further immunosuppressive therapy. The animals were capable, however, of rejecting allogeneic tissues from other dogs at a tempo and intensity similar to those observed in untreated animals." The transplanted bone marrow cells survived at least four and a half years. These and further studies "have provided convincing evidence of the feasibility of inducing specific unresponsiveness to major transplantable organs in large adult mammals. The applicability of irradiation and bone marrow transplantation to the human situation is severely hampered, however, by the high incidence of graft-versus-host disease associated with the use of allogeneic marrow in outbred populations

even under conditions of donor-recipient identity for products of the main histocompatability complex." The animals were beagles from the Cooperstown colony DLA haplotype and pedigree identity. "A suspension of 3 to 3.5 x 10^9 nucleated bone marrow cells was obtained by needle aspiration of the femora and humeri of each prospective recipient." Material was suspended, strained, and stored at 4° C. The dog was then exposed to supralethal total body irradiation for a total of 1200 to 1400 R of continuous irradiation. At predetermined intervals after irradiation, the dog's own stored bone marrow was returned intravenously. Kidney allografts were varyingly transplanted, before removal of the bone marrow, at the time of bone marrow replacement or 12, 28, or 36 hours after marrow replacement. The recipient's own kidneys were removed two months after transplantation. Only three of 21 animals receiving the graft before irradiation, failed to reject their grafts and were alive now over three years, some of the others showing modest prolongation of survival. Twenty-five percent of 16 kidneys transplanted at the time of marrow replacement were long-term survivors. Kidneys transplanted 18, 28, or 36 hours after marrrow replacement were long-term survivors in over 60% of the cases. Twelve dogs unresponsive to their kidney allografts were studied with skin allografts from the corresponding kidney donor. Five of these animals were unresponsive to the skin grafts, the others showed chronic rejection of the skin grafts from their kidney donor. The rejection of first, second, or third set skin allografts "appeared to have no measurable deleterious effect upon the corresponding kidney allografts, which have continued to survive and function uneventfully in the recipients." The fact that there was an optimal period of time required to elapse "between replacement of autologous marrow and exposure of the host to alloantigens by establishment of vascular connections between the transplanted kidney and the recipient's circulation . . . suggests that at least one, and probably several early cycles of cell generation by the retransplanted hemopoietic stem cells are necessary in order to establish the type of cell population most amenable to the induction of unresponsiveness . . . these data raise the possibility that the early period after irradiation and bone marrow replacement may temporarily recapitulate immunological ontogeny . . . placing the host into a state of responsiveness similar to that shown to be operative in the fetus (or newborn, depending upon the species) prior to the full development of immunological competence." Rapaport's final statement was that "Supralethal total body irradiation and bone marrow replacement can estab-

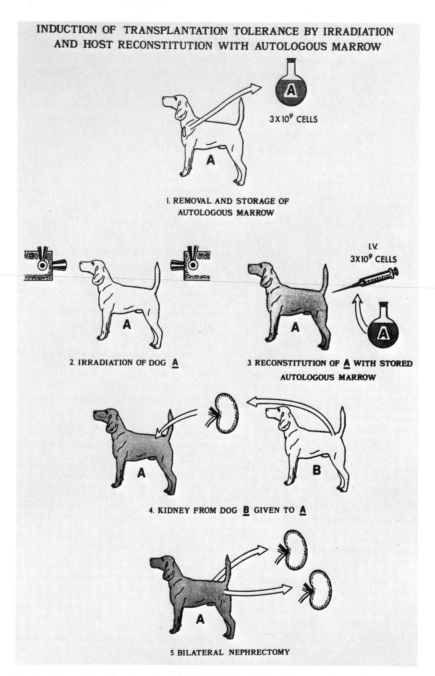

INDUCTION OF TRANSPLANTATION TOLERANCE BY IRRADIATION AND HOST RECONSTITUTION WITH AUTOLOGOUS MARROW

3 X 10⁹ CELLS

1. REMOVAL AND STORAGE OF AUTOLOGOUS MARROW

I.V. 3 X 10⁹ CELLS

2. IRRADIATION OF DOG **A**

3. RECONSTITUTION OF **A** WITH STORED AUTOLOGOUS MARROW

4. KIDNEY FROM DOG **B** GIVEN TO **A**

5. BILATERAL NEPHRECTOMY

With the protocol indicated by the diagram, it was striking that if the kidney was grafted before irradiation only three of 21 did not reject; if the kidneys were transplanted at the time of marrow replacement, 25% of the transplants were long-term successes; if the transplant was made at 18, 28, or 36 hours after irradiation, over 60% were long-term survivors,- without any immunosuppressive drugs.

F. T. Rapaport, R. J. Bachvaroff, N. Mollen, H. Hirasawa, T. Asano, and J. W. Ferrebee, *The Induction of Unresponsiveness to Major Transplantable Organs in Adult Mammals*- A Recapitulation of Ontogeny by Irradiation and Bone Marrow Replacement. Volume XCVII, 1979.

lish in the adult canine host a privileged phase of immunological reactivity during which exposure to alloantigens produces specific long-term unresponsiveness rather than sensitization. The use of stored autologous rather than allogeneic bone marrow for reconstitution of the irradiated recipient eliminates the hazards of GVH complications usually associated with this procedure. This consideration and the apparent capacity of the tolerant host to maintain a long-term state of unresponsiveness without any further immunosuppressive therapy point to the potential relevance of the results to human transplantation."

Discussion

The paper was warmly received. Dr. Joseph E. Murray, of Boston,- "It's just a beautiful presentation . . . However, we must realize that all the results that he shows us are partial, in a way. His controls have one or two survivors. Even in his best experimental series he has a few failures. So we are dealing with a spectrum, and this has always been the result in dog experiments in transplantation . . . even in the early days of Imuran study in dogs, we were only able to get a certain number. We increased our results from 10% to 30 or 40% survival, and it was on this basis that we were able to go into the human." Thomas E. Starzl, of Denver,- "in the early 1950's and early 1960's . . . total body irradiation was used in clinical kidney transplantation. The pioneer work was by Murray and Merrill of Boston, joined later by Hamberger . . . of Paris. Although some patients achieved long survival, the approach was too dangerous to be acceptable. This outstanding paper by Rapaport shows a possible way to reduce or eliminate the terrible risk, while achieving graft survival, somewhat surprisingly, by the simple expedient of marrow reconstitution with autologous cells . . . Felix, have you tried the system with other than these DLA-compatible donors? And how . . . does it work in mongrel kidney transplantation?" David A. Blumenstock, Cooperstown, New York, had done similar studies involving lung transplantation "We think the autologous marrow system has great advantage, in that there's less risk of graft versus host, and rejection, and it does work in both kidneys and lungs part of the time . . . what about less degrees of histo-compatability relationship?" Untreated controls DLA non-identical, i.e., mismatched animals, survived some 13 days. Total body irradiation and autologous marrow in the DLA nonidentical or mismatched animals produced survival up to 27 days ". . . however . . . the addition of

three doses of methotrexate as the only additional immunosuppressive therapy in the posttransplant period changed the picture radically. We have living animals now 336 to 673 days. Of a series of ten animals, seven are alive, and apparently doing well." The pulmonary function of the lungs seemed very good in two of the animals, marginal in others. Richard E. Wilson, of Boston, asked about the cell populations involved, wanting to know "if you have looked at any specific populations of either macrophages or lymphocytes or polys . . . to see if there is any deletion, or what the kinetics of recurrence, or return, of these populations are after this period of total body irradiation." Richard R. Lower, of Richmond, asked "why the delay of such a few hours in transplanting the kidney to the marrow recipient results in such a high rate of failure." Rapaport, closing, agreed that the results were not uniform, "We obviously would not dare advocate this sort of an approach to clinical problems, unless we could get a reproducible 100% result; and we believe that probably the source of the problem is either insufficient or excess antigen being released by the organ that is inducing tolerance to itself. And we are approaching this problem by the usual techniques of either adding antigen or, as Dr. Blumenstock mentioned, trying various judicious doses of immuno-suppression during the early recovery phase." That had a risk because the immunosuppressors might kill early precursor stem cells, which were suppressor cells rather than killer cells and required to induce tolerance. In the hands of his group, the transplantation with which Dr. Blumenstock had succeeded with lungs failed with kidneys in animals between a mongrel partner and a Cooperstown dog, using the very same regimen. He was exploring the factors systematically, "The eventual hope, of course, as pointed up by Drs. Lower and Wilson, is to try and, No. 1, isolate the effector cells which are responsible, and, even more importantly, isolate from these cells the molecular elements which actually mediate the reaction."

* * *

Thoracic Duct Fistula and Renal Transplantation, Thomas E. Starzl, Professor and Chairman, Department of Surgery, University of Colorado Medical Center; Attending Surgeon, Colorado General Hospital, Denver General Hospital; and Children's Hospital; Staff Surgeon, Denver Veterans Administration Hospital, and Richard Weil, III, Lawrence J. Koep, Robert T. McCalmon, Jr., Paul I. Terasaki, Y. Iwaki, G. P. J. Schröter, J. J. Franks, V. Subryan, and C. G. Halgrimson, all by invitation, had employed thoracic duct drainage as an adjunct to standard immunosuppressive therapy. "The rationale for such an approach was provided by the classical investigations by Gowans and his associates in rats. TDD apparently was first tried clinically in 1963 in Saint Louis by Newton and later in Stockholm by Franksson. However, Newton's attempt was not described until 1965, nearly a year after Franksson's first report." Their patients received azathioprine, prednisone, and antithymocyte globulin [although Starzl commented that "The use or omission of ATG was not thought to be an important factor in either the TDD cases or the retrospective controls with which they were compared. When producing our own antilymphocyte globulin (ALG), our cadaveric graft survival was improved. However, during the last several years while using a commercial ATG in a clinical trial, there has been no difference in results with or without this agent."] Half the patients had splenectomy prior to transplantation and a few more subsequently "because of persistent leukopenia which precluded effective treatment with azathioprine." They had found that they did not need to replace the thoracic duct lymph with plasma, "In fact, we have recently found that the lymph sometimes could be discarded for weeks or months on end without adverse effects providing adequate volumes of electrolyte solution were given intravenously." During the time they had been successful with thoracic duct drainage in 40 patients, they had failed with it in two others, in whom they could not find the cervical thoracic duct. In two of the successful cases they had had to find the thoracic duct in the right thorax. An empyema in one of the patients with thoracotomy was the only major complication of TDD. Starzl considered it realistic in most centers to expect a 50% unfavorable outcome of first cadaver kidneys. All of the early reports of TDD claimed benefit and all were abandoned, "The most important reason apparently was the inability to consistently obtain effective lymph drainage, an objection that was almost completely eliminated in our trial. Annoyance to the patients and expense were other factors." However, Walker and Johnson, at Vanderbilt, in 1977 "described the use of TDD for about one month to prepare 50 poor risk patients for cadaveric kidneys. The graft survival 2 to 5 years later was almost 75%, nearly twice as good as in a control group." Others had established that three to four weeks of thoracic duct drainage produced substantial immunosuppression. "TDD in our trial was used differently in that TDD usually was instituted at the time of transplantation instead of preoperatively. Pretreatment in patients without antibodies

was omitted because of the unpredictable availability of cadaveric organs and because of our subsequently allayed fear that TDD could not be maintained throughout long waiting periods . . . After 5 months 22 (88%) of 25 primary cadaveric recipients have life-sustaining renal function either with their first (64%) or promptly inserted back-up (24%) graft. At 5 months the results in the 25 cadaveric cases were almost twice as good as in 25 immediately precedent and similar controls not treated with TDD." However, eight patients needed retransplants, losing their kidneys during the first three or four weeks of posttransplant and post initiation of thoracic duct drainage so that ". . . we now recommend TDD pretreatment. The need for so many back-up grafts has been unnecessarily wasteful of organs, to say nothing of the emotional trauma and extra risks imposed on the recipient . . . With successful transplantation, TDD will usually be discontinued after a total preoperative plus postoperative duration of about 60 days."

Discussion

Allan E. Dumont, of New York, [who had presented thoracic duct drainage before the Association in 1964, Volume LXXXII, p. 1185] said, "Dr. Starzl has shown us very clearly, I think, that it is the removal of thoracic duct lymphocytes rather than lymph-borne globulin, that is critical in the preparation of these patients for transplantation. It is particularly interesting to me that serum immunoglobulin levels fell so rapidly, despite the reinfusion of the antibody-rich lymph . . . these findings appear . . . consistent with the idea that thoracic duct lymph includes a functionally distinct pool of immunologically competent cells, presumably B-cells, which synthesize and release antibody molecules into lymph and into blood." Joseph E. Murray, of Boston, said of thoracic duct fistula, "This is a blunt tool. It is depriving a recipient of all of his mechanisms, or trying to go at him in a blunt way, but it's sharpened by the study of the placing and the timing of the antigen . . . it's time consuming, and it's expensive; it does increase bed occupancy. You have all the problems of centrifugation, reinfusion . . . it will probably not be used by most transplantation centers until it does prove its place in effectiveness." Starzl, closing, agreed with Dumont "that the removal of the cells, in some way that we don't fully understand . . . cuts off the immunoglobulin production, rather than having the effect be because of the removal of immunoglobulin from the thoracic duct limb. The amount of immunoglobulin or, for that matter, proteins in the thoracic duct lymph is only about half of that in the serum . . . so . . . if this were attempted . . . would be best done by peripheral plasmapheresis, since that's where the IgG is that you would want to remove . . . I understand perfectly Dr. Murray's concerns from a perspective, however, that was between ten and fifteen years old. In the very important and great pioneering work done by Murray and his associates in Boston in the '60's, they did report unequivocally improved results with thoracic duct drainage [see Volume LXXXV, 1968] . . . it's always been surprising to me that that procedure was abandoned at Harvard . . . Galveston, and some other places." The problem of the technical difficulty of the collection "was rectified by a young Hopkins surgeon who is with us, named Dr. Larry Koep, who had the bright idea of using a Swann-Ganz catheter for the collections, and he cut the balloon off the Swann-Ganz catheter, and thus created a double lumen, and was able with this new advancement in instrumentation to be able to put those fistulas down into the mediastinum, and to meet many of the objections that had confronted the pioneer workers with thoracic duct fistula . . . there were only two attempts beyond those forty that failed; and that meant that you have a tool now different than ten or fifteen years ago. You have a technique that has a 95% reliability . . . my position is that I believe that pretreatment, now, in view of this panoply of data that we've got . . . that pretreatment with thoracic duct fistulae in our center is being used for all cases, related and unrelated, with the possible exception of double haplotype identical siblings, and that we think it will have a broad, and not a narrow, use in clinical transplantation. Thank you very much."

The Business Meetings

The 1979 meeting took place April 26, 27, and 28, at The Homestead, Hot Springs, Virginia, President Oliver H. Beahrs in the Chair. The President introduced Viking Bjork, of the Karolinska Institute, in Stockholm, one of the three Honorary Members elected by Council at the midwinter meeting. The other two new Honorary Members, Professor Åke Senning, of Zurich, and Professor Lucien Leger, from the University of Paris, were unable to attend.

The Committee on Issues had been concerned in the year just past with cost containment in surgery, a widely publicized and pressing issue [the President of the United States, numerous public offi-

cials and innumerable journal articles, television programs addressed themselves to the subject], and the Breakfast Meeting at 7 o'clock the following morning would focus on that.

At the Second Executive Session on the afternoon of the third day, Dr. Rhoads reported for the Committee appointed the previous year to consider the Constitution and produce "a consistent set of By-laws." Rhoads pointed out that in the first place ". . . incorporation of the Association in California resulted in the Articles of Incorporation becoming the Constitution, so that the document which you have should be headed, simply, 'By-laws'. The word 'Constitution' should be deleted." It had been decided to recommend the elimination of the class of Corresponding Members because, "it was believed that to elect both Corresponding and Honorary members was confusing, and could at times lead to embarrassment." The proposed changes in the Constitution had been distributed and were to lie over for action in 1980. President Beahrs, for the Association, presented Dr. Jonathan Rhoads, the sixth recipient, with the American Surgical Association Medallion for Scientific Achievement.

On this occasion, the meeting had been shifted from Wednesday, Thursday, Friday, to Thursday, Friday, and Saturday because the Hotel had discovered an "overlooked" booking. The Secretary announced for the Council that "The list of future meetings has been adjusted for the withdrawal of The Greenbrier in 1983, and The Breakers in 1986. The Association, because of its continued growth, will find it progressively more difficult to schedule meetings at resort hotels, few of which can really accommodate our progressively increasing size, and many of which, because of their own economic interests, would rather have week-long conventions, and would rather not start meetings in midweek, which causes them occupancy problems and financial loss. We are attempting, as best we can, to deal with this problem."

Treasurer, Walter Ballinger reported that the increase in dues, the increase in the initiation fee, and "most important, the establishment of a registration fee for guests at the Annual Meeting . . ." had served to make the Association's financial position very satisfactory.

Officers elected were, G. Thomas Shires, of New York, President; William G. Anlyan, of Durham, North Carolina, and George L. Jordan, Jr., of Houston, Vice-Presidents; Secretary to succeed J. V. Maloney, W. Gerald Austen, of Boston.

THE LAST PRESIDENT OF THE FIRST CENTURY CONGRATULATES
THE FIRST PRESIDENT OF THE SECOND CENTURY.

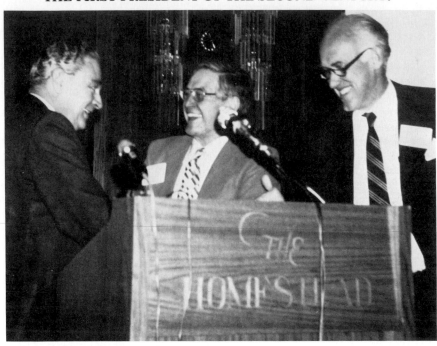

Oliver H. Beahrs, of Rochester, Minnesota, turning the lectern over to G. Thomas Shires, of New York, with the obvious approval of Secretary James V. Maloney, of Los Angeles, at the 1979 meeting at the Homstead, Hot Springs, Virginia.

(Photography: Robert S. Sparkman, M.D., Dallas, Texas)

CODE OF MEDICAL ETHICS OF THE AMA

In the Transactions of the American Medical Association, Volume XXXIII, published in 1882, there appeared the "Code of Medical Ethics. Of the Duties of Physicians To Their Patients, and of The Obligations of Patients To Their Physicians". Dr. Morris Fishbein's, *A History of the American Medical Association, 1847-1947* (Philadelphia, Saunders, 1947), states that the American Medical Association Code of Ethics, first adopted in 1847, was written chiefly by John Bell and Isaac Hays, both of Philadelphia, who acknowledged their close adherence to Thomas Percival's 1803 statement of ethical principles for the Manchester Infirmary. Relevant to the concern which evidently involved particularly some of the New York Fellows of the American Surgical Association, but not fully illuminating as to their specific objections, is the following, from Fishbein. "From time to time after 1847, circumstances developed which made necessary reconsiderations and modifications of the Principles of Ethics. In 1852 there was serious debate over the acceptance of homeopathic doctrines by some members of the medical profession. In 1882 delegates from the Medical Society of the State of New York presented a report which offered a simplified and brief system of medical ethics as a substitute for the national code. This was adopted. Then in June 1882, at the meeting of the American Medical Association in St. Paul, delegates from the Medical Society of the State of New York were refused admission. At that time Dr. Austin Flint wrote a commentary on the Code of Ethics in an endeavor to persuade the New York society to reenact the code of the American Medical Association. So fierce was the battle that a group was formed with the title 'Society for the Prevention of the Reenactment in the State of New York of the Present Code of Ethics of the American Medical Association.' The battle continued with pamphleteering, debate and discussion on both sides. At various meetings of the Medical Society of the State of New York the Code was voted in and voted out, and at one time a conservative group which found it impossible to reenact the national code in the original Medical Society of the State of New York withdrew and organized a rival New York State Medical Association."

It is not immediately clear to what provisions of the Code some of the members of the American Surgical Association objected. Certainly, there would be very little in Article 1—"*Duties of physicians to their patients* " to which objection could be taken. Paragraph 1, "A physician should not only be ever ready to obey the calls of the sick, but his mind ought also to be imbued with the greatness of his mission, and the responsibility he habitually incurs in its discharge . . . Physicians . . . should study, also, in their deportment, so to unite *tenderness* with *firmness,* and *condescension* with *authority,* as to inspire the minds of their patients with gratitude, respect, and confidence."

Nor are there any warning flags in Paragraph 2. "Every case committed to the charge of a physician should be treated with attention, steadiness, and humanity. Reasonable indulgence should be granted to the mental imbecility and caprices of the sick. Secrecy and delicacy, when required by peculiar circumstances, should be strictly observed; and the familiar and confidential intercourse to which physicians are admitted in their professional visits, should be used with discretion, and with the most scrupulous regards to fidelity and honor . . . none of the privacies of personal and domestic life, no infirmity of disposition or flaw of character observed during professional attendance should ever be divulged by the physician except when he is imperatively required to do so . . . indeed . . . professional men have, under certain circumstances, been protected in their observance of secrecy by courts of justice."

Certainly Paragraph 3, still a valid injunction, might have seemed insulting to some, but it is hard to believe that anyone would make it a matter of conscience to record an objection to it. "Frequent visits to the sick are in general requisite . . . But unnecessary visits are to be avoided, as they give useless anxiety to the patient, tend to diminish the authority of the physician, and render him liable to be suspected of interested motives." The advent of governmental reimbursement for medical services has made the last few words more apposite than ever.

The wisdom of Paragraph 4 is certainly debatable, but the language is sufficiently permissive as again not to be objectionable. "A physician should not be forward to make gloomy prognostications, because they savor of empiricism, by magnifying the importance of his services in the treatment or cure of the disease. But he should not fail, on proper occasions, to give to the friends of the patient timely notice of danger when it really occurs; and even to the patient himself, if absolutely necessary. This office, however, is so peculiarly alarming when executed by him, that it ought to be declined whenever it can be assigned to any other person of sufficient judgment and delicacy. For the physician should be the minister of hope and comfort to the sick; that, by such cordials to the drooping spirit he may smooth the bed of death, revive expiring life, and counteract the depressing influence of those maladies which often disturb the tranquillity of the most resigned in their last moments. The life of a sick person can be shortened not only by the acts, but also by the words or the manner of a physician. It is . . . a sacred duty . . . to avoid all things which have a tendency to discourage the patient and to depress his spirits." Obviously, some of this runs contrary to the currently espoused doctrines of full disclosure and informed consent, and points up the occasionally harmful, not to say brutal, effects of a literal application of these doctrines.

Paragraph 5 seems reasonable enough, al-

though, once more, some might take offense at the implication that venality in financial matters might control the activity of physicians,- "A physician ought not to abandon a patient because the case is deemed incurable . . . To decline attendance, under such circumstances, would be sacrificing to fanciful delicacy and mistaken liberality, that moral duty which is independent of, and far superior to, all pecuniary consideration."

Paragraph 6, "Consultations should be promoted in difficult or protracted cases, as they give rise to confidence, energy, and more enlarged views in practice", was certainly widely accepted in practice by the members of the Association, and is only one more evidence of the general acceptance by the profession of the "second opinion" doctrine now being proposed as new and revolutionary.

Certainly Paragraph 7, which enjoins the physician to promote and strengthen ". . . the good resolutions of his patients, suffering under the consequences of vicious conduct", could have been no source of serious objection.

Article II—"*Obligations of patients to their physicians*" has even less in it to which the surgeons of the day would have been likely to object. Paragraph 1, ". . . patients should entertain a just sense of the duties which they owe to their medical attendants."

Paragraph 2 might have been objected to by many practicing surgery in the United States at that time, but hardly by the select members of the American Surgical Association. "The first duty of a patient is to select as his medical adviser one who has received a regular professional education. In no trade or occupation do mankind rely on the skill of an untaught artist; and in medicine, confessedly the most difficult and intricate of the sciences, the world ought not to suppose that knowledge is intuitive." [In fact, 90 years later, President Francis D. Moore, (1972, Volume XC, page 1353) was still urging that "It is a common platitude to say that the medical profession should clean up its own back yard . . . patient has no assurance that the person who carries out a major operation will have demonstrated his fitness to carry out that act by any credentials for his education beyond the M.D. degree and state licensure . . . I would like, therefore, to devote our attention now to three specific proposals for the improvement of surgical care that could be carried out by voluntary national action starting this year . . . These three proposals are: the validation of staff credentials, control of the flow of residency trainees, and the placement of surgical specialists."]

It is possible that the recommendations to the patient in Paragraph 3 might have been seen as going beyond the bounds of necessity in instructing that, "Patients should prefer a physician whose habits of life are regular, and who is not devoted to company, pleasure, or to any pursuit incompatible with his professional obligations." The implication that patients might pass judgment on the personal lives of their surgeons might very well seem objectionable. The assumption by the American Medical Association,- and then by the American Surgical Association,- of this stance of mild purity might well have been offensive, although it does not seem possible that the recommendation of Paragraph 3, so eminently sensible, would be objected to,- "A patient should, also, confide the care of himself and family, as much as possible, to one physician: for a medical man who has become acquainted with the peculiarities of constitution, habits, and predispositions of those he attends, is more likely to be successful in his treatment than one who does not possess that knowledge." The patients were also urged to apply for medical advice even for trivial symptoms or the early stages of serious illnesses because, ". . . it is to a neglect of this precept that medicine owes much of the uncertainty and imperfection with which it has been reproached."

Paragraph 4 counsels patients to ". . . faithfully and unreservedly communicate to their physician the supposed cause of their disease . . . Even the female sex should never allow feelings of shame or delicacy to prevent their disclosing the seat, symptoms, and causes of complaints peculiar to them . . . a patient may sink under a painful and loathsome disease, which might have been readily prevented had timely intimation been given to the physician."

The behavior suggested by Paragraph 5 would have been as welcome to surgeons of that day as of this,- "A patient should never weary his physician with a tedious detail of events or matters not appertaining to his disease . . . he will convey much more real information by giving clear answers to interrogatories, than by the most minute account of his own framing. Neither should he obtrude upon his physician the details of his business nor the history of his family concerns."

By the same token, Paragraph 6 must have been welcome in enjoining upon patients, ". . . obedience . . . to the prescriptions of his physician . . . prompt and implicit . . . Patients should never allow themselves to be persuaded to take any medicine whatever, that may be recommended to them by the self-constituted doctors and doctresses who are so frequently met with, and who pretend to possess infallible remedies for the cure of every disease."

Paragraph 7, on the face of it, is unobjectionable, though it easily presents the possibilities of friction. "A patient should, if possible, avoid even the *friendly visits of a physician* who is not attending him . . . A patient should never send for a consulting physician without the expressed consent of his own medical attendant. It is of great importance that the physicians should act in concert . . ."

Clearly, Paragraph 8, "When a patient wishes to dismiss his physician, justice and common courtesy require that he should declare his reasons for doing", should have been a comfort to the members unless they objected to even the thought that a patient had a right to dismiss them.

Paragraph 9 must have been applauded by all then, as it probably would be today. "Patients should always, when practicable, send for their physician in the morning, before his usual hour of going out; for, by being early aware of the visits he has to pay during the day, the physician is able to apportion his time in such a manner as to prevent an interference of engagements. Patients should also avoid calling on their medical adviser unnecessarily during the hours devoted to meals or sleep. They should always be in readiness to receive the visits of their physician, as the detention of a few minutes is often of serious inconvenience to him." [There might be some objection today to the idea that patients could, in fact, "*send* for their physician", or even in the obvious intimation that house calls could be a regularly expected part of a physician's attentions to his patient.]

Paragraph 10. Surely there is nothing which a surgeon, then and now, could object to in the obviously laudable recommendation that, "A patient should, after his recovery, entertain a just and enduring sense of the value of the services rendered him by his physician; for these are of such a character, that no mere pecuniary acknowledgment can repay or cancel them."

The next section is entitled, "*Of the Duties of Physicians to Each Other, and to the Profession at Large.*" Article I—"*Duties for the support of professional character*", exhorts physicians to "exalt" the standing of the profession, and to "avoid all contumelious and sarcastic remarks relative to the faculty as a body". Diplomas or certificates of proficiency were not to be signed for people whom they had "good reason to believe intend to support and practice any exclusive and irregular system of medicine . . . Greater purity of character, and a higher standard of moral excellence" were demanded than for any other profession, and the physician was ". . . to be temperate in all things, for the practice of physic requires the unremitting exercise of a clear and vigorous understanding; and, on emergencies, for which no professional man should be unprepared, a steady hand, an acute eye, and an unclouded head may be essential to the well-being, and even to the life, of a fellow-creature." None of the foregoing are likely to have been objectionable to the members of the American Surgical Association.

Nor is it likely that Paragraphs 4 and 5 were offensive. Flagrant advertising had largely disappeared, except for that of obvious quacks! Paragraph 4, "It is derogatory to the dignity of the profession to resort to public advertisements, or private cards, or handbills, inviting the attention of individuals affected with particular diseases . . . to publish cases and operations in the daily prints . . . to boast of cures and remedies, to adduce certificates of skill and success . . ."

Paragraph 5, "Equally derogatory to professional character is it for a physician to hold a patent for any surgical instrument or medicine; or to dispense a secret *nostrum* . . . if such nostrum be of real efficacy, any concealment regarding it is inconsistent with beneficence and professional liberality; and if mystery alone give it value and importance, such craft implies either disgraceful ignorance or fraudulent avarice." [Nevertheless, Dr. J. McFadden Gaston, of Atlanta, Georgia, at the 1896 meeting, said he had a secret cure for prostatic hypertrophy, the nature of which he was not at liberty to divulge.]

Article II recommends that "All practitioners of medicine, their wives, and their children while under the paternal care, are entitled to the gratuitous services of any one or more of the faculty residing near them, whose assistance may be desired."

Article III suggests that if a physician requests "some of his professional brethren to officiate for him", because of pursuit of health or other matters on a temporary basis, his brother physicians should see his patients and return his fees to him, "But if a member of the profession neglect his business in quest of pleasure and amusement . . ." the fee should be awarded "to the physician who officiates . . ."

Article IV deals with consultations. Paragraph 1 suggests that consultation requested by the patient with any "intelligent regular practitioner, who has a license to practice from some medical board of known and acknowledged respectability, recognized by this Association, and who is in good moral and professional standing . . ." should be honored, but one "whose practice is based on an exclusive dogma, to the rejection of the accumulated experience of the profession, and of the aids actually furnished by anatomy, physiology, pathology and organic chemistry", could not be "considered as a regular practitioner or a fit associate in consultation . . ." [a position that at this writing the AMA has in essence abandoned, in agreeing with the position of a Pennsylvania Court that a hospital is obliged to send reports of its X-ray examinations to a chiropractor]. The protocol of consultation is detailed. "In consultations, the attending physician should be the first to propose the necessary questions to the sick; after which the consulting physician should have the opportunity to make such further inquiries of the patient as may be necessary to satisfy him of the true character of the case. Both physicians should then retire to a private place for deliberation; and the one first in attendance should communicate the directions agreed upon to the patient or his friends, as well as any opinions which it may be thought proper to express . . . no *opinions* or *prognostications* should be delivered which are not the result of previous deliberation and concurrence." The physician in attendance was to deliver his opinion first, followed by the consultants in the order in which they had been called in; and the opinion of the consultants was not to be binding upon the attending physician. The physicians were enjoined to be punctual in their attendance at consultations. If the consultant arrived and the attending physician did not, the consultant, if he had been called from a considerable distance, might "examine the patient, and give his opinion in *writing* and *under seal,* to be delivered to his associate." Theoretical discussions were to be avoided in consultations, "as occasioning perplexity and loss of time." The discussions in consultation were to be "held as secret and confidential . . . Should an irreconcilable diversity of opinion occur when several physicians are called upon to consult together, the opinion of the majority should be considered as decisive; but if the numbers be equal on each side, then the decision should rest with the attending physician." It was deplorable if physicians could not agree, and disagreement ". . . should always be avoided, if possible, by mutual concessions . . .", or a third physician called in "to act as umpire". When there was difference of opinion, the patient might be invited to select the physician whose advice he would follow and, in any case, the physicians left in the minority, should "politely and consistently retire from any further deliberation in the consultation, or participation in the management of the case." Consultants "should sedulously guard against . . . unsolicited attendance. As such consultations require an extraordinary portion of both time and attention, at least a double honorarium may be reasonably expected." It is not likely that this last judgment would have been objected to. The consultant was to be careful to ". . . observe the most honorable and scrupulous regard for the character and standing of the practitioner in attendance; the practice of the latter, if necessary, should be justified as far as it can be, consistently with a conscientious regard for truth . . ."

Article V dealt with "cases of interference". Consultants were not to pursue ". . . any course of conduct . . . that may directly or indirectly tend to diminish the trust reposed in the physician employed." In social visits to patients of others, ". . . the topics of conversation should be as foreign to the case as circumstances will admit." Physicians ought not to take over the patients recently treated by others, except in emergency, in consultation, or when the patient had been formally "relinquished" or the physician discharged. If a number of physicians were sent for simultaneously, "courtesy should assign the patient to the first who arrives . . . A wealthy physician should not give advice *gratis* to the affluent; because his doing so is an injury to his professional brethren. The office of a physician can never be supported as an exclusively beneficent one; and it is defrauding, in some degree, the common funds for its support, when fees are dispensed with which might justly be claimed." If, in emergency, a physician delivered the patient of another, he was "entitled to the fee, but should resign the patient to the practitioner first engaged."

Article VI enjoins physicians to keep controversy within the profession and out of the public view.

Article VII, "*Of pecuniary acknowledgments:*, would probably be looked upon with suspicion by the Federal Trade Commission today, for it suggests, "Some general rules should be adopted by the faculty, in every town or district, relative to *pecuniary acknowledgments* from their patients; and it should be deemed a point of honor to adhere to these rules with as much uniformity as varying circumstances will admit."

The physician had obligations to the public and the public had obligations to the profession as indicated in the next section. Article I indicated that physicians were to be "ever ready to give counsel to the public in relation to matters especially appertaining to their profession, as on subjects of medical police, public hygiene, and legal medicine . . . quarantine regulations; the location, arrangement, and dietaries of hospitals", etc., be ready to testify before coroners' inquests and courts of justice. "But in these cases, and especially where they are required to make a *post-mortem* examination, it is just, in consequence of the time, labor, and skill required, and the responsibility and risk they incur, that the public should award them a proper honorarium."

There is further concern with remuneration for physicians, and, while "There is no profession by the members of which eleemosynary services are more liberally dispensed than the medical . . . Poverty, professional brotherhood, and certain of the public duties referred to in the first section of this article, should always be recognized as presenting valid claims for gratuitous services . . ." But public or privately endowed institutions, benefit societies or insurance societies could not expect gratuitous services. Physicians were to be recompensed for furnishing "certificates of inability to serve on juries, to perform militia duty", or for insurance or pension claims, etc., except for indigents. Physicians had an obligation because they were "frequent witnesses of the enormities committed by quackery, and the injury to health and even destruction of life caused by the use of quack medicine, to enlighten the public on these subjects, to expose the injuries sustained by the unwary from the devices and pretensions of artful empirics and impostors", and should direct their prescriptions to "druggists and apothecaries", who did not vend "quack or secret medicines". The public should appreciate the virtues and beneficence of the profession and should "make a proper discrimination between true science and the assumptions of ignorance and empiricism."

All in all, the Code of Ethics might be taken as a harmless description of the path of true virtue, yet some members of the Association objected, to the point of losing their membership, perhaps because of the "big brother" aspect, perhaps because of the strictures against dealing with irregular practitioners.

THE GROSS STATUE

At the 1891 meeting, in September, in the Grand Army Building in Washington, D.C., President Claudius H. Mastin, of Mobile, Alabama, suggested that a statue of Dr. Gross be commissioned.

". . . Samuel David Gross stood first in the foremost rank in his chosen branch of the profession, and the high position to which American surgery has attained all over the world is largely due to his example and his teachings.

"Since he has passed away and his life-work gone into history, we fully appreciate his real worth, and therefore it is that his friends and admirers have been inspired to erect a monument to his memory—such a monument as will bear testimony of their gratitude, and be in the future an incentive to those who are to come after us to like noble deeds. To further this praiseworthy enterprise, I suggest that a committee from this Association be appointed to confer with the friends and admirers of Dr. Gross, and with the medical profession of the whole country, to determine the best method to be adopted to secure the requisite amount for the erection of a monument, either of marble or of bronze.

"Such tributes to the memory of distinguished men are common, both in this country and abroad; and when in our own profession a man is found who has done so much to adorn it, it is mete that we should show to the world our appreciation of his works.

"Dr. Gross was probably more widely known and appreciated than any American surgeon of recent years; and when we remember the thousands of his pupils scattered throughout the whole of America—men who sat under his teaching, and who still retain of him the warmest memories—it is not expecting too much when we feel assured of their co-operation in raising speedily, and without difficulty, the requisite amount for the completion of such a monument.

"I do not suggest that this work be done by this Association exclusively, nor would I advise it if it could be. I would prefer to see it done by the profession of the entire country, because Dr. Gross belonged to no exclusive faction, but was a member of the profession at large. It is proper, however, that this Association take the initiative in beginning the movement, and I feel assured that there will not be the least doubt as to the successful issue of the undertaking . . .

"Appreciated and honored as he has been in life, let us now, since he is dead, build to his memory such a monument as will bear witness in after years to the estimate in which the profession of to-day holds its distinguished members.

"If it were asked of me where such a statue should be erected, I would answer: Not at Easton, in the State of Pennsylvania, the place of his birth; neither at Cincinnati nor Louisville, where he laid the foundations of his future greatness; nor even in the city of Philadelphia, where that greatness culminated in all its grandeur—but here, in the city of Washington, the capital of the country which claims him as her own. His name and fame are a sacred heritage to the country at large, and to the profession he loved so well! Then, here in this beautiful city, amid these verdant parks and hard by these massive piles of classic architecture, let us place it; place it among these statues, emblems of a nation's gratitude to her illustrious dead—her statesmen, her warriors, her jurists, her philosophers—build it here, so that in the ages to come, when the youth of the land make their pilgrimages hither, they will behold the monument which their forefathers reared to commemorate the life and character of her greatest surgeon. It will teach them to emulate his example!"

At the Business Meeting on Thursday, September 24, 1891, the *Report of the Committee on the President's Address,* Item No. 3, "They recommend that the President be empowered to appoint a committee with authority to confer with the friends and admirers of the late Professor S. D. Gross, and with the profession at large, for the initiation of a movement on the part of the Association, having for its object the erection of a monument to Dr. Gross, in the City of Washington." The report was accepted. On the fourth day of the meeting, September 25, the President appointed to the Gross Monument Committee J. R. Weist, of Indiana, as Chairman, and 25 members.

The Minutes of the 1892 meeting simply state that Dr. C. H. Mastin, Secretary of the Gross Monument Committee, and Dr. J. R. Weist, the President, made a verbal report and asked power to fill the vacancies on the Committee caused by death.

A detailed report at the 1893 meeting contains the fascinating information that Thomas Eakins, the painter of the great "Gross Clinic" masterpiece, had volunteered to assist.

"The first information necessary to be obtained was the probable cost of a monument appropriate for the purpose and worthy of the profession. To secure this information an extensive correspondence was opened with some of the most distinguished artists, sculptors and painters of America. We found a liberality of spirit and an interest displayed which justified the belief that the work could be as well and cheaply done in this country as abroad; and in addition, we found in the person of Mr. Eakins, of Philadelphia, an artist of great renown, who had been personally acquainted with Dr. Gross, being the painter who produced the great painting of the distinguished surgeon which was on exhibition at the Centennial Exposition of 1876. [see Frontispiece] This gentleman has still in his keeping all the drawings, measurements and models from which he executed that painting, and he now generously offers to place them at our disposal and then to superintend the modeling, casting and erection of the monument, and that too without one dollar of remuneration for his services.

"After diligent and painstaking investigation, by correspondence and personal interviews, we found that a bronze statue, the figure of heroic size, upon a granite pedestal proportioned to the size of the figure, could be made, erected and delivered to the committee for the sum of $12,000—all work to

be done in most artistic style and finish, out of best bronze and granite."

Circulars were widely distributed, and "prominent gentlemen in various States of the Union" were appointed as chairmen of local committees. Dr. Weist and Dr. Mastin, the Chairman and Secretary of the Committee had apparently done all the work, felt a bit put upon and, with a nice example of Ciceronian praeteritio, said "The amount of postage and stationery paid for by your Secretary of the committee has been no small item, but since it has not been his purpose to make any charge for the same, it is not included in expense account, and no mention will be made of it.

"The amount of clerical and other work done by your committee has been executed mainly by its chairman and secretary; and whilst we have no intention of reflecting upon our associates of the committee, we are sorry to be compelled to say we have had very little aid or encouragement in our labors. It has, however, been with a degree of pleasure on our parts, that we have pushed on the work until we now feel assured that success will crown our efforts, and hope and believe that the Fellows of the Association will, ere a great while, see the monument an established fact."

They had spent only $33.34 and that left $4,590.66, which meant that they still had to raise $7,410. Of the money in hand, $3,500 had been pledged by "Nameless Friends of Dr. Gross . . . For reasons which are pertinent to themselves, these subscribers decline to have their names made public until such time as the amount necessary to complete the monument, *minus* the $3,500, has been subscribed." Dr. Weist said that, "Somewhere about one year ago a proposition was made us, by the Medical Alumni of the Jefferson Medical College, Philadelphia, to unite with us and assist in raising the funds necessary to complete the monument. We accepted their offer, and are under the impression that they have collected quite a sum for the purpose, but of what amount we have no report from them."

There was some uncertainty as to where the statue was to go. Dr. Weist says, "As we understood the proposition, we thought it was in reference to assisting us in the completion of a monument *in the city of Washington, D.C.* Since that time a meeting of the Jefferson Med. Alumni have sent us 'A resolution,' which we attach in envelope marked *No. 6.* [no record of that is to be found]" Dr. Weist says nothing about that communication and directly chided the members for the fact that they were still short of the goal for the subscription. Dr. Roswell Park, in moving that the Committee continue with its charge

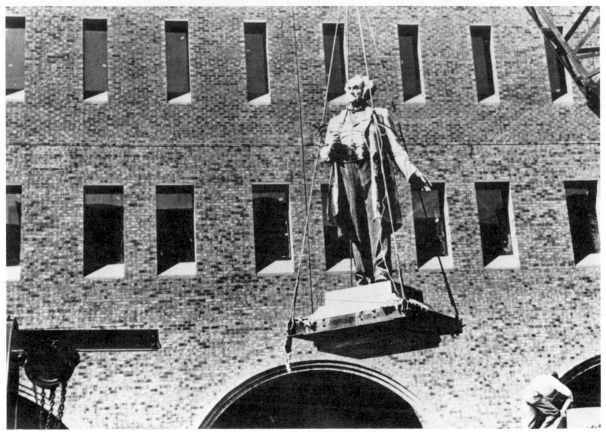

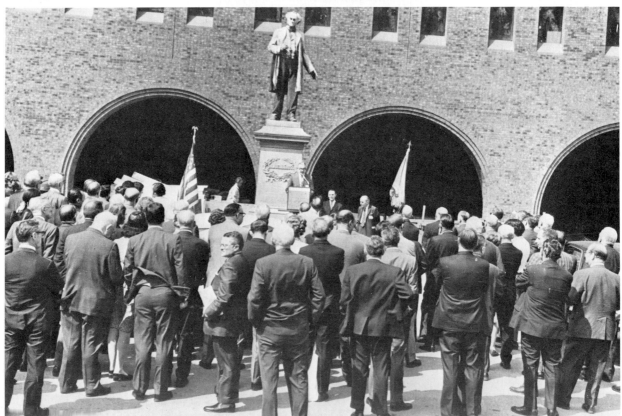

1536

(Continued on opposite page)

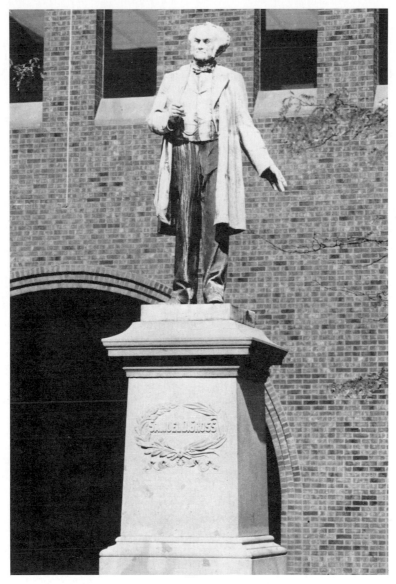

The statue of Samuel D. Gross, Founder of the American Surgical Association, commissioned by the American Surgical Association and the Alumni of Jefferson Medical College, created by Alexander Stirling Calder, originally dedicated May 5, 1897, on the driveway between the Army Medical Museum and the Smithsonian Museum. Removed from that site when the Smithsonian was demolished to make way for the Hirshhorn Art Museum, and scheduled for ultimate relocation in front of the new A.F.I.P. on the grounds of Walter Reed Hospital, it was rescued from a warehouse by the Jefferson Medical College Centennial Celebration Committee (without recorded consultation with the American Surgical Association), transported to Philadelphia, erected on the grounds of the Medical School at the rear of the Scott Library Building and dedicated on May 1, 1970.

(Courtesy of Scott Memorial Library, Thomas Jefferson University)

and handle the matter as it saw fit, added that they should have "permission to erect the proposed monument either in the city of Washington, as at first proposed, or in Fairmount Park, Philadelphia."

The matter is not mentioned in the Minutes for 1894.

At the 1895 meeting in New York, when Louis McLane Tiffany, of Baltimore ["A.M. Cantab., M.D."] was President, Christian Fenger was First Vice-President and Maurice Richardson was Secretary, Dr. Weist read the report of the Committee on the Gross Monument. The Jefferson Alumni had been extremely active in soliciting contributions, "In fact, pecuniarily they have collected more than has

1537

1538

been collected by the Committee of the Surgical Association itself." A year before, having $6,000 in hand, the Committee had announced a competition for the commission to model the statue. ". . . three sculptors submitted four models, which were placed in the Exhibition Hall of the Academy of Fine Arts of Pennsylvania. They were there inspected by the Committee, by members of Professor Gross's family and others, and the Committee were so fortunate as to secure the assistance of Edward H. Coates, Esq., President of the Academy, Prof. R. W. Vonnoh, the Professor of Painting in the Academy, and Mr. St. Gaudens of New York. They finally decided upon the model by Mr. A. Stirling Calder, a photograph of which is exhibited herewith." [Alexander Stirling Calder, a Philadelphian like his famous sculptor father, Alexander Milne Calder (the statue of William Penn atop Philadelphia's City Hall), had trained at the Pennsylvania Academy of Fine Arts and then studied in Paris. He was 25 years old when he began work on the Gross Statue and went on to win many awards and become a leading member of the American academic community. His son, in turn, was the Alexander Calder, whose name is synonymous with sculptured mobiles.] The commission had been given to Mr. Calder, who was then in Paris working on it. "The contract calls for a statue of heroic size, nine feet high, of standard United States bronze, the statue to be completed within two years." It was anticipated that it would be unveiled in Washington when the Association met there. A resolution had been introduced into Congress, ". . . giving permission to the American Surgical Association and the Jefferson Alumni Association to erect the statue on a Government reservation in the city of Washington and making an appropriation of fifteen hundred dollars for the foundation and pedestal. We are very happy to state that, through the active exertions of Messrs. Clark and Adams of the House, and of Morgan and Quay of the Senate, this resolution and appropriation were passed and the appropriation is now available. The designation of the site and the erection of the pedestal will be under the direction of Col. John M. Wilson, U.S.A., the Superintendent of Public Buildings and Grounds." The Treasurer's report for that year indicates that J. R. Weist was reimbursed $51.77 for expenses. The Committee report at this meeting was signed by Weist, Mastin and, now, W. W. Keen.

At the 1896 meeting in Detroit, John Collins Warren in the Chair, Weist, Mastin and Keen presented a detailed report of their Committee. W. W. Keen, one of the original members of the American Surgical Association, had been added to the Committee to represent the Jefferson Alumni Association. This report provides some background for the choice of the artist. One of the original three artists had withdrawn from the competition and three models received from the other two had been inspected at the Academy of Fine Arts by "the President of the Academy, the Professor of Painting in the Academy, Mr. St. Gaudens, sculptor, of New York, Dr. Orville Horwitz [S. D. Gross' son-in-law] and Mr. A. Haller Gross [Gross' attorney-son], representing the family, and Dr. W. W. Keen, representing the committee. Photographs of the models were also examined by the other members of the committee,- Drs. J. R. Weist and C. H. Mastin . . . The clay model was seen last summer by Dr. Keen of the committee, who was much pleased with it, as was also Mrs. Orville Horwitz, Dr. Gross's daughter, who examined it repeatedly. The statue will soon be cast in bronze at Munich. Through the exertions of Senator J. H. Morgan, of Alabama, the Secretary of the Treasury has given permission for the entrance into the United States, free of the fifty per cent. duty which is the tariff rate upon such work." It was now stated that the site selected for the erection was ". . . on the driveway between the Army Medical Museum and the National [Smithsonian] Museum, a point where it will be seen by many thousands annually, and especially by medical men who will visit the Army Medical Museum. The pedestal is to be ten feet high from the base course of the granite to bed-plate of statue, making when the statue is erected, a monument something over twenty-feet high.

"The amount of funds collected up to the present time is $_____ [the figure remains blank in the Minutes!]." The sculptor had already received $2,000 on account. Again it was proposed that the unveiling be at the Washington meeting in May, 1897, and a place for the ceremony had been requested of Congress.

At the 1897 meeting in Washington on May 4, 5, and 6, with J. Collins Warren as President, the Minutes record for the 5th of May:

"AFTERNOON SESSION, 5 P.M.

The American Surgical Association, together with the Alumni of the Jefferson Medical College of Philadelphia and the members of the Congress, with their friends, were present at the unveiling of the statue of the late Prof. Samuel D. Gross, M.D., on the Smithsonian grounds near the Army Medical Museum. The exercises were conducted in the lecture-room of the Army Medical Museum, and were as follows:

Prayer, by Rev. B. L. Whitman, D.D., President of Columbian University.

Presentation of the Statue to the United States Government, by C. H. Mastin, M.D.

Reception of the Statue on the Part of the Government, by Surgeon General G. M. Sternberg.

Address, by W. W. Keen, M.D.

Benediction."

* * *

The statue is, of course, now on the grounds of the Jefferson Medical College in Philadelphia. So little was Jefferson aware of the statue that, as preparations for the Medical School's centennial celebration were underway, an "Initial Report" of the "Committee for the Procurement of the Statue of Samuel D. Gross" of the Alumni Association stated that "the existence of the statue in Washington, D.C., was called to the attention of the Alumni Association by Harold L. Stewart, a member of the Board of Trustees of the Jefferson Medical College of the Thomas Jefferson University, in the fall of 1969." At the request of Dr. Francis J. Sweeney, Jr., Director of the Thomas Jefferson University Hospital, Dr. Stewart on May 7, 1970, put down an account of the genesis of the removal of the statue. "This statue always stood on the lawn of the mall at the rear of the old building at the corner of 7th Street and Independence Avenue in Washington. That building housed the Surgeon General's Library and the Army Medical Museum. Some years ago the Army Medical Museum, now renamed the Armed Forces Institute of Pathology, moved into its new building on the grounds of the Walter Reed Army Medical Center. Later the Surgeon General's Library became part of the National Institutes of Health and moved into its new building in Bethesda now called The National Library of Medicine. All that remained housed in the old building at 7th Street and Independence Avenue were the exhibits of pathologic specimens and visual displays of various diseases that were open to the public and the activities of the section on geographic pathology of the AFIP. Then when our Congress accepted the art collection of Mr. Hirshhorn, it decided to demolish this old building in order to provide the ground upon which to build the new Hirshhorn Art Gallery.

"I had always admired the Gross statue. It is a fine work of art and one of the few statues to physicians in this country. Few people seem to know about it as I learned when I pointed it out on innu-merable occasions to visitors to the city. I had always thought that it should by rights be at Jefferson. Now, when it would certainly have to be moved anyway and maybe put in storage, perhaps permanently, seemed to be the appropriate time to try to secure it for Jefferson.

"Last fall, on the afternoon and evening of September 25, I met with a group of members of the Executive Committee of the Alumni Association of Jefferson Medical College, had dinner with them and later attended the meeting of the full committee. That evening I mentioned the Gross statue to some of those present and asked if they knew its fate during and after the demolition of the old Army Medical Museum building, and whether it might be possible to bring it to Philadelphia. No one knew anything about the statue or its fate but all to whom I talked were interested and it was agreed to ask Dr. Norman J. Quinn, Jr., Chairman of the Centennial Committee, to look into the matter."

Correspondence relating to the destruction of the Armed Forces Institute of Pathology Medical Museum and the salvage of certain objects is contained in the Otis Historical Archives of the Armed Forces Medical Museum. A memorandum of April 18, 1968, "*Subject:* AFIP Medical Museum, Demolition, Request for Reservation and Donation or Sale of Certain Salvage Material; Possession of the Samuel D. Gross Statue", from the office of the Special Assistant for Legal Affairs, reads in part, "1. The Director desired this office to determine a legal course of action to secure two thousand whole red bricks (uncleaned) from the exterior of the AFIP Medical Museum for sale as mementos to pathologists. The Curator of the AFIP Medical Museum desired this office to take action to secure the reservation of certain salvage materials by the Federal Government for the AFIP Medical Museum, and to secure the Samuel D. Gross Statue located on the Hirshhorn Museum site." Subsequently, it was asked that there would be added to the list "seven ventilation grids, one brass bannister, two fireplaces, three doors, complete with frames, hinges and hardware, and the original dedication plaques."

On April 29, 1968, L. L. Hunter, Assistant Commissioner for Design and Construction of the General Services Administration, was able to reply to James L. Hansen, Colonel, MC, USA, Acting Director, Armed Forces Institute of Pathology, "We have your letter of recent date requesting the salvage of certain materials from the AFIP Museum. The detailed list of items you wish to salvage will be included in the contract specifications for demolition of the museum as reservation items. Should the plans for the Hirshhorn Museum and Sculpture Garden continue to develop as presently scheduled, the demolition of the AFIP Museum should occur early in calendar year 1969." It was not as simple as it appeared. A letter of October 18, 1968, indicating that "The AFIP Medical Museum is forced to move prior to 2 January 1969 to make room for the construction of the Joseph H. Hirshhorn Museum and Sculpture Garden", and requesting authority for the removal, storage and relocation of the statue, received the answer from the General Services Administration, that "Since this statue is the property of the National Park Service we suggest that you address a request for same to: Mr. William R. Failor, Superintendent of National Capital Parks . . . We shall be pleased to reserve this statue for your use, along with the other items you requested, provided that Mr. Failor grants your request . . . demolition of the AFIP museum will begin on January 2, 1969." Colonel Hansen wrote to the National Park Service, apparently suggesting that the Gross Statue be moved to the new location of the AFIP at Walter Reed Hospital, and was informed by the National Park Service that a transfer of property would be required. Authority for the transfer was granted, but "There are no funds available within the General Services Administration or the National Capital Parks Services for accomplishment of this action. Total cost of such transfer will be a responsibility of the Armed Forces Institute of Pathology." Colonel Hansen was asked that $1000 "be made available for the movement of the Gross Statue from its current location, to Building 29, National Bureau of Standards, where it will be held in storage until such time as it is further transferred for placement at the newly landscaped site of Building 54." Funds were available and their release was appropriately authorized. A Transfer of Property form dated December 20, 1968,- dangerously approaching the demolition date,- lists the "Quantity of Items - 1", the "Description of Articles - Statue of Samuel D.. Gross (Bronze Standing Figure mounted on a red granite pedestal) Statue located in Reservation No. 3A, L'Enfant Square in the mall". Its value is put at $11,500, its age and condition stated to be 71 years, good. "Justification" was stated to be "Statue is being transferred to Institute to be placed on the immediate grounds of a new wing to be built on to the present AFIP building at Walter Reed Army Hospital. Statue will be placed in temporary storage until construction is completed, approximately summer 1970." There is an additional note which seems to have been typed on the form, "Statue is now being

moved to Bldg 29, Bu Standards Conn. Ave. & Van Ness Sts. N.W., (Moved Dec. 20th, 1968)". The appropriate form dated December 27, 1968, indicates that the statue had been received and was "Located in Tempo Storage Bldg 29, Bu Stand."

As Dr. Stewart noted in his letter, he had asked Norman J. Quinn, Jr., Chairman of the Centennial Committee to look into the matter. Miss Nancy S. Groseclose, Executive Secretary of the Centennial Committee of the Alumni Association, had written Colonel Hansen, the Acting Director of the AFIP, about their interest in the statue. He replied, "Enclosed is the requested photograph of Doctor Samuel D. Gross. Although the statue is greatly in need of a cleaning, this is quite a nice bronze. It was done by A. Stirling Calder of Philadelphia circa 1897. If you have a sincere interest in acquiring this statue, I think before any further negotiations, you should make a personal inspection." Dr. Quinn did then go to Washington on January 15, 1970, meeting with a Major Moss. The initial report of the Centennial Committee states of that visit to Washington, "Dr. and Mrs. John J. McKeown and Dr. and Mrs. Norman Quinn met Col. Cook at 11 am at the Institute. We were introduced to Captain Bruce Smith, M.C., USN. Transportation was provided to the Van Ness Annex and we were introduced to Miss Helen Purtle, Curator of the Museum and Major Frederick E. Moss, legal counsel of the Institute . . . Major Moss then transported the Committee to the statue which was dismantled and located in a nearby driveway. Inspection revealed the following: The statue is bronze and weathered to a blue green color. The statue is approximately 1-1/2 life size and is approximately 10 feet tall." The "Telephone or Verbal Conversation Record" by a Mrs. Buddle from the Executive Office, concerning Major Moss' meeting with Dr. Quinn indicated that transfer of the statue from the Park Service to the AFIP had in fact been completed despite an earlier thought that the papers had never been signed. However, "The statute dedicating the statue provided that it would be erected in the Washington area. Mr. Failor of the Park Service and Major Moss both are of the opinion this statute would bar our giving the statue to Jefferson Medical College unless amended." Major Moss had recommended to Dr. Quinn that he seek the help of his congressman in amending this statute. A Memorandum for Record, by Frederick E. Moss, Legal Counsel, of December 15, 1969, stated that "Several weeks ago we received an inquiry from representatives of the Jefferson Medical School in Philadelphia regarding the possibility of acquiring the statue of Dr. Samuel Gross which formerly had been located on the grounds of the 'Old Red Brick' at 7th and Independence Avenues . . . A review of available records indicated that title and accountability for the statue rested in the National Park Service [subsequently found to be incorrect, an acceptance of transfer was found to have been signed by someone from the AFIP]." But even if the statue proved to be the property of the AFIP, ". . . it does not appear that the AFIP would be authorized to dispose of the statue in this way without referral to the Secretary of the Army. I could find no authority even for the Secretary of the Army to dispose of such property on a permanent basis save by declaring it excess to the needs of the service and going through normal property disposal channels." He had also looked into the possibility of an indefinite loan, but ". . . permissive use of army property by non-governmental agencies and individuals, without statutory authority, can be sustained only if such use serves a definite military purpose, such as morale, or welfare of soldiers . . . Not being able to perceive any direct military benefit from this transaction, I advised the Director at the staff conference on 15 December 1969 of the above situation and recommended that if we desired to have the gift made, or if the Jefferson group wished to purchase the statue from the government, we could act as intermediaries for them to the National Park Service."

A further review of the legal problems involved, this time by the Chief, Tax and Property Law Branch, Procurement Law Division, of the Judge Advocate General's office, resulted in turning up a justification for a loan of the statue to the Alumni Association of the Jefferson Medical College, "In the past, Secretaries of the Army have authorized the use of Army property by persons or organizations outside the Army and other government agencies, based upon the authority implied from 5 U.S.C. 301, 10 U.S.C. 3012, and 10 U.S.C. 4831. Such use has been authorized by the Secretary after he determined that: a. the proposed use to which the property is to be put is at least quasi-public and serves a military purpose; b. the Army reserves the right to immediate possession; c. the Army retains constructive custody and control of the property, and d. the use in the public behalf is permissive as distinguished from an outright transfer." The Judge Advocate General's office saw no legal objection if the consent were obtained from the Secretary of the Army.

On March 25, 1970, the appropriate request went forward, "For Loan of Government-Owned Personalty". The request, dated 25 March 1970, and signed by Bruce H. Smith, Captain, USN, MC, The Director, Armed Forces Institute of Pathology, stated that, "It is the opinion of the Director, AFIP, that there would be public relations benefits which may accrue to the recruitment of military medical personnel. Additionally, the Jefferson Medical College would assume the responsibility for the cleaning, protection and maintenance of the statue during a time that it would otherwise be in storage." The intimation is that the loan was to be temporary and that the statue would be returned when the new building at the AFIP had been completed. A letter of April 7, 1970, from Frank M. Rosenberry, Jr., Office of the Director of Purchasing, Thomas Jefferson University, to Frederick E. Moss, MAG, JAGC, USA, Legal Counsel, AFIP, enclosed "the draft bailment agreement signed by Peter A. Herbut, M.D., President of the Thomas Jefferson University," and reassured the AFIP that "The Samuel D. Gross Statue arrived safely in Philadelphia this past week-end. It is currently in storage awaiting site preparation prior to its being erected and cleaned." It cost $5,568.87 to move the statue and erect it upon its new foundation.

On May 1, 1970, the statue, having been successfully transported to Philadelphia and lowered into place on its pedestal, at the rear of the Scott Library Building, was rededicated as part of the Centennial celebration of the medical school to which Samuel D. Gross had made such a distinguished contribution, and whose alumni had assured the success of the project, originally conceived by the American Surgical Association.

THE AMERICAN BOARD OF SURGERY

The need for formalization of the training, and accreditation of that training, in surgery had been referred to a number of times in Presidential Addresses. At the 1907 meeting in Washington, D.C., President Dudley P. Allen, Professor of Surgery, Medical Department of Western Reserve University, *The Teaching of Surgery* very clearly made a firm recommendation for uniform standards of training, a national examining board, and national certification. "How may a standard of surgical knowledge be established, the attainment of which will gain men general recognition? . . . The American Surgical Association could create itself a national college of surgeons and hold annual examinations. Only those passing this examination would be eligible to Fellowship. The eligibility to such Fellowship and the certification of having passed such an examination would at once give a man a recognized standing." (Vol. XXV, 1907) That proposal probably smacked too much of the structure and functions of the Royal Colleges, and would clearly have threatened the elitist nature of the Association, which was important to many of the Fellows, as the perennial resistance to enlargement of the membership made clear.

President J. M. T. Finney, Associate Professor of Surgery, Johns Hopkins University, at the 1922 Washington meeting, had issued a clear call, to which the Council failed to recommend a response, for the development of a plan ". . . by means of which prospective surgeons may receive adequate training under proper supervision and be properly certified to before beginning the practice of surgery . . ."

And in 1933, for the third time at a meeting held in Washington, the Presidential Address of Arthur Dean Bevan, Professor and Head of the Department of Surgery, Rush Medical College, University of Chicago; Surgeon to the Presbyterian Hospital, stressed the need for standards of training.

He suggested requiring "Three years of training in the specialty in an accepted hospital and under the instructions of a recognized specialist", and hoped "all of our best hospitals" could be induced to require such training as a prerequisite to staff appointment.

At the Boston meeting in 1935, when President Edward William Archibald, Professor of Surgery and Director of the Surgical Department, McGill University; Surgeon, Royal Victoria Hospital; Associate Surgeon, Children's Memorial Hospital, recommended a Board of Examiners in Surgery, Evarts A. Graham, of St. Louis, a recognized leader of the forward element in American surgery, and already engaged in shaking up the tightly entrenched control of the American College of Surgeons under Franklin H. Martin and a group of powerful surgeons antagonistic to "professors", rose from the floor (Vol. LIII, 1935) to introduce the motion which was to result in the creation of the American Board of Surgery. This was in no sense a precocious move, long overdue as it was, and having been preceded by the formation of ten other specialty boards. Graham commented that "Dr. Bevan started the ball rolling in this Association." The American Board of Surgery came into being as a result of the initiative of the Association, but was planned by a committee representing the various regional societies as well as the American Surgical Association. Once the mechanism for organization and approval was set in motion the Association became only one of the sponsoring organizations, although inevitably the representatives of the other surgical organizations were for the most part Fellows of the Association as well. The annual reports to the Fellows, made by their representatives to the American Board, portray in fascinating detail the progress of the Board, the increasing numbers of candidates, the steady rise, for a considerable time, in the numbers of the candidates whose medical degrees had been obtained in foreign medical schools, the changing examination techniques, failure rates, etc., and can be read in the Minutes. For the purposes of this history, it is the foundation of the American Board of Surgery which is relevant.

Evarts Graham, having seized [by prearrangement?] on Dr. Archibald's address, to make a motion, in time honored fashion was made chairman of a committee of six to consider the matter and report to the Association the following year. Other surgical organizations were to be consulted. As Olch says, [P. D. Olch, *Evarts A. Graham, The American College of Surgeons, and the American Board of Surgery;* Journal of the History of Medicine and Allied Sciences, XXVII, 1972] Graham

> wasted no time. Ten days after the meeting, he wrote the five other members: "You are of course familiar with the general dissatisfaction which exists with the existing qualification of Fellows of the American College of Surgeons. The ASA feels that there is an urgent need for the creation of some mechanism by which properly qualified surgeons can be certified to the public." His letter contained a series of key questions and a statement of his views. At this point he apparently had a relatively open mind toward the role of the College in his plans *if* the College had a radical change in its administration. Even though Franklin Martin had died four months earlier, he did not want the authority for certification placed in the hands of a group beholden to one individual, such as the Director General of the College, whoever that might be. The Committee agreed that a more representative body should receive this authority and recommended the other surgical societies be enlisted in the movement to organize the qualifying board and be represented in its final makeup.

> Dr. George Crile, Chairman of the Executive Committee of the ACS, visited Graham and urged that the College assume the functions of the proposed independent certifying board. Dr. Graham firmly opposed this suggestion and warned Crile that the annual meeting of the ACS would be little more than a surgical circus if the College did not participate with the other surgical organizations in the founding of the independent board. The result of this conversation was an agreement to hold a meeting in Chicago at the headquarters of the College in October 1935 with the ASA Committee, the representatives of the Surgical Section of the AMA, and representatives of the ACS.

At the 1936 meeting of the Association, Graham, in a brief paper, *Report of the Committee to Study Further Problems of Postgraduate Surgical Education in General and the Qualifications for Specialization in General Surgery in Particular,* reported for the Committee, which consisted of Graham, Archibald, Elting, Joyce, Orr and Whipple. Graham

said that after "preliminary consideration and correspondence" the members of the Committee thought it "probable that it would be necessary to organize a qualifying board of some sort to take care of the certification of surgeons to the public. It also seemed advisable to obtain the cooperation of the other surgical societies in this movement." The committee of the Surgical Section of the American Medical Association had been appointed: Fred. W. Rankin, Chairman; Henry W. Cave, Brian T. King, Roy D. McClure, J. Stewart Rodman, and Hugh H. Trout, [all but King, members of the American Surgical Association]. Graham did not say at whose instance in the American Medical Association the decision to appoint such a committee had been made. Graham had "discussed the matter with the chairman of the Executive Committee of the American College of Surgeons, Dr. George W. Crile", and a meeting had been held of the committees representing the American Surgical Association, the Surgical Section of the American Medical Association, and representatives of the American College of Surgeons, who were: Drs. George Crile, J. Bentley Squier, Samuel C. Harvey, Irvin Abell, and Bowman C. Crowell. Squier, a distinguished urologist, and Crowell, a pathologist and Associate Director of the American College of Surgeons, were not members of the American Surgical Association. The committee of the American Surgical Association had already "decided that very probably it would be found necessary to organize a qualifying board which should be national in scope." The committee, had therefore prepared a resolution to be presented to this meeting and to the representatives of the three associations.

> A committee appointed by the American Surgical Association to consider the elevation of standards of the practice of surgery and to increase the hospital facilities for the training of young surgeons, proposes that a joint national committee representing the various surgical organizations of the country be formed to discuss and arrange a program for accomplishing those objects. The committee proposes that a national committee of 24 members be formed for this purpose, consisting of six members representing the American College of Surgeons, six the American Medical Association, six the American Surgical Association, two the Western Surgical Association, two the Southern Surgical Association, and two the Pacific Coast Surgical Association. It is hoped that the American College of Surgeons will cooperate in the proposed endeavor by appointing six members to serve on the national committee to organize this work.

At that time, relations with the American College of Surgeons were touchy. Graham had recently challenged Franklin Martin, who with George Crile and W. H. Mayo had tightly controlled College policies. In any case there was strong sentiment in the College leadership that certification was naturally a matter in the College's domain. Rodman, ["History of the American Board of Surgery-1937-1952". J. Stewart Rodman, M.D., J. B. Lippincott Company 1956] states of the meeting Graham refers, to, "The discussion which followed was most interesting, though at times somewhat acrimonious. The representatives of the College of Surgeons stated quite frankly that such a proposal seemed to be unnecessary since the College had long been interested in improving surgical standards. However, it was made clear that this proposal represented a different approach to the problem and was in keeping with the experience of other specialties in which examining boards had been established which already had helped materially to raise the standards of specialties in the fields concerned. After further debate, it became apparent that the majority present favored the proposal. It was agreed that a National Committee, as proposed, be approved." The representatives of the American College of Surgeons did agree, finally, to cooperate and to appoint six members for the proposed "National Committee of 24, to discuss ways and means of creating a suitable organization to take care of the qualification of surgeons." The delegation of the College appointed to this National Committee was Samuel C. Harvey, Chairman, Irvin Abell, Donald Guthrie, Allen B. Kanavel, C. Jeff Miller, and Alexander Munroe. Miller, a gynecologist, and Munroe, a Canadian, from Edmonton, were the only ones not Fellows of the American Surgical Association.

It is only fair to say that the College had indeed been concerned with the problem of postgraduate instruction. The minutes of the Board of Regents for their meeting the year before, on October 19, 1934, show that "Dr. Greenough suggested that small committees of the Board of Regents be appointed to study the work of the Medical Service Board and postgraduate instruction . . . The Director-General moved that the College appoint a committee to study the question of graduate teaching, of which Dr. Samuel C. Harvey, of New Haven, shall be the Chairman, "with the understanding that he nominate for his committee, three men who are practicing surgery in a big way but who are not teachers in undergraduate medical schools, and three men who are doing either undergraduate or postgraduate teaching in medical schools." The members of that committee were Irvin Abell, of Louisville, Kentucky; Donald Guthrie, of Sayre, Pennsylvania; Samuel C. Harvey, of New Haven, Connecticut, Chairman; Allen B. Kanavel, of Chicago, Illinois; C. Jeff Miller, of New Orleans, Louisiana; Alexander R. Munroe, of Edmonton, Alberta; and Allen O. Whipple, of New York. Harvey, Whipple, Miller, and Kanavel were certainly teachers (and operating surgeons) and Abell, and Guthrie, fit the bill of men "practicing surgery in a big way". All but Whipple and Guthrie were members of the Board of Regents of the College.

At the October 29, 1935, meeting of the Regents, (after the meeting with delegations from the American Surgical Association and the American Medical Association Surgical Section), Harvey reported that at the October 23 meeting with Graham and the other two delegations they had received formal submission of "an invitation to the College to act in conjunction with the proposed national committee in the formation of a Board of Surgery. Harvey's committee, after a long review of the methods of training surgeons recommended "that the College co-operate in the formation of a surgical board". Presumably anticipating resistance, and to provide reassurance, the Committee's report stated that "It is not, however, proposed that the College shall in any sense abrogate its right to determine the futures of the candidates for its Fellowship . . . The membership in the College cannot be limited or ensured by an extraneous board" [although, since July 1, 1974, certification by the American Board of Surgery has been a prerequisite to Fellowship in the College, except in unusual circumstances]. The College, Harvey said, would have to adjust "its qualifying procedures so as to test the adequacy of any program for the graduate training for surgery which it sees fit to endorse." Acceptance of the report, moved by Greenough seconded by Abell was unanimous. No hint is given as to the nature of the discussion which led to acceptance of the report concerning which there obviously were serious misgivings. However, at the same meeting of the Regents, Dr. Malcolm T. MacEachern, of the College staff presented a detailed proposal for designation by the College of training program requirements. This envisioned "Regular surveys by an officer of the College or a local liaison committee of all hospitals and clinics which give the suggested courses . . . A central board on training for surgery, which would be responsible for the rating of the various courses, the promulgation of standards, and general reputation of the work." Harvey diplomatically pronounced the suggestions "excellent". There is not recorded any further discussion of MacEachern's plan for assumption by the College of the regulation of training. Instead Kanavel moved the appointment of six men to the "joint committee of twenty-four referred to in Dr. Harvey's report . . . to attain the desirable ends, but that the activities of the group from the College should be safeguarded and freedom of action reserved to the College organization" and the motion carried.

At the February 8, 1936, meeting of the Executive Committee of the Regents, Harvey said MacEachern's suggestions would be "invaluable but . . . it would probably be a mistake to bring into the joint committee a plan which had been approved in full detail, and which would thereby become rather fixed . . . better to bring in broad general principles . . ." He said forthrightly to the Regents that ". . . the business of the large general committee of twenty-four would eventually be . . . setting up qualifying boards and engineering every phase of that situation . . . the business of the College to organize the hospitals to control the training leading up to the qualifying boards . . ." R. B. Greenough, moved approval of MacEachern's report in principle "as a statement of what the College is prepared to do toward elevating the standard of surgery". Dr. Balfour, in the "full discussion of the subject", emphasized the magnitude of the undertaking, "which is striking a new note in the procedure of the College", but Muller, Besley and Greenough saw such a program as a College responsibility. Greenough,- "the College was the only organization which could undertake to organize the residencies in hospitals." Kanavel,- "felt the College should undertake the program", and suggested that Dr. Harvey show Dr. MacEachern's report to the committee of twenty-four, assure them of cooperation and aid in elevating the standards for Fellowship in the American College of Surgery,- but that "if the joint group does establish a qualifying board, while the College would not oppose it, the organization could not take active part in the formation of the board since it would stultify the College and complicate its own endeavors." Dr. Crile, Chairman of the Board of Regents, agreed, "he did not think that the College should enter into the organization or formation of qualifying boards, as that is a function which is already being performed by the College." Harvey said it would be disastrous "to have two bodies each completely independent of the other, and bound therefore to be in conflict . . . much better for the College to be represented on such a board, which would have nothing whatever to do with the requirements for Fellowship in the College . . ." [After numerous guarded and qualifying statements, MacEachern's report was accepted in principle "as a statement of what the College is prepared to do to-

ward elevating the standard of surgery".]

Shortly after came the February, 1936 meeting at the Palmer House, of "the committee of 24", in which the representatives of the American Surgical Association, the American College of Surgeons, the Surgical Section of the American Medical Association were joined by representatives of the Western Surgical Association and the Southern Surgical Association. "The two representatives from the Pacific Coast Surgical Association could not be present. The New England Surgical Society was not invited to send representatives to the meeting of the National Committee because it would have been necessary to wait for nearly a year for that Society to select its representatives."

The representatives of the various societies elected officers of their joint committee: Evarts A. Graham, Chairman; Samuel C. Harvey, Vice-Chairman; and J. Stewart Rodman, Secretary. The Chairman appointed two subcommittees to report on the following day with "a plan for the organization of an American Board of Surgery . . . a plan for increasing the opportunity for training of surgeons", Stewart Rodman, Chairman of the first committee; Samuel C. Harvey, Chairman of the second. The resultant plan for an American Board of Surgery suggested that the details would be worked out by the Board itself. There were already nine boards functioning, in ophthalmology, otolaryngology, obstetrics and gynecology, dermatology and syphilology, pediatrics, psychiatry and neurology, radiology, orthopedic surgery, and urology, and most recently added was the American Board of Internal Medicine. The scheme of organization of the other boards had in general been followed except for one important difference, ". . . the responsibility for the American Board of Surgery will rest with the large national and regional surgical associations." They proposed a board of 13 representing the seven surgical societies mentioned earlier, with six-year terms of office, the initial appointments to be for staggered terms. They recommended the establishment of a Founders Group, which would include all the active and senior members of the American, Southern, Western, and Pacific Coast and New England Surgical associations, also "professors of surgery, clinical, associate and assistant professors of surgery in all Class A medical schools of the United States and Canada", and for the first two years invited men who had had 15 years of practice limited to surgery to make direct application to the Board for certification without examination. They expected that the requirements to be fulfilled for examination would be not less than three years of graduate study beyond internship and two years of study or practice in surgery thereafter. The surgeon should have had an adequate operative experience. The examinations would be "divided into two parts of which one will be written and the other practical, covering bedside work, clinical, and operative features." As for increasing the facilities for training of surgeons, the American College of Surgeons and the American Medical Association "should be asked to form a joint council to organize and carry out a program for the training of surgeons in properly qualified hospitals, setting up such standards as will meet the requirements of the proposed American Board of Surgery. The standards for the proper training of surgeons shall be subject to the approval of the American Board of Surgery . . . certain hospitals not now associated with teaching institutions must be developed to the point of carrying out such training." For this purpose, ". . . such a hospital must have a continuous ward service of non-private patients under the control of a director, or the equivalent of this, who is responsible for carrying out the program of training of surgeons". The nature of the required facilities was indicated. They anticipated that "careful and competent periodic survey of the hospitals designated as suitable for the training of surgeons" would have to be provided ". . . by surgeons who themselves have been qualified by the Board, are of mature judgment and command the respect of those undertaking to train young surgeons." Dr. Graham's report was accepted by the American Surgical Association at the meeting on May 7, 1936. The Association's first representatives to the American Board of Surgery were Evarts A. Graham, Allen O. Whipple and Arthur W. Elting.

On March 29, 1936, Dr. Harvey had reported the full plan for an American Board of Surgery to the Executive Committee of the Regents of the College. He was unable to get from the Regents on that occasion a statement as to whether "the College will co-operate in the formation of the Council", Dr. Crile stating ". . . while the College can co-operate, it must, as in the past, continue to formulate its own standards for Fellowship." The discussion was continued at the full meeting of the Regents on May 10, 1936, three days after the affirmative action of the American Surgical Association. The pulling and hauling within the Board of Regents emerges from the ensuing discussion, with its discreet exchange of opinions, arguments posed as questions, statements of uncertainty which were to be interpreted as indications of a clear preference, all without frontal assault or argumentative declaration—in the familiar manner of men who must continue to work together on other matters whatever their differences on the

matter at hand. By then Harvey could say "the recommendations of the National Committee for the Elevation of the Standard of Surgery were approved by the American Surgical Association, the Pacific Coast Surgical Association, and the New England Surgical Society; that by the late Fall the other associations will also have considered the recommendations, and that by the first of January, 1937, it should be possible to function." MacEachern now presented in detail his studies and recommendations for a College controlled program. Shipley, of Baltimore, and Pool, of New York, expressed interest in Harvey's report and Kanavel, stating that the College should "always maintain its independence, and not be required to submit its acts for approval to any other bodies", nevertheless submitted a resolution approving the proposals embodied in Harvey's report and authorizing the Chairman of the Board of Regents "to name the three nominees [for the College] to serve if, and when, the American Board of Surgery is organized." The motion carried, but the discussion indicates a hope that the actual regulation of training programs for surgeons could be made a College function and in the end MacEachern's detailed description of training programs was accepted,- "in principle". The three initial members of the Board, from the American College of Surgeons, were Erwin R. Schmidt, of Madison; Donald Guthrie, of Sayre, Pennsylvania; and Harvey Stone, of Baltimore.

Clear evidence of the amicable way in which the American College of Surgeons and the American Board of Surgery have come to delimit their respective activities and to collaborate for the good of surgery is seen in the statement in the 1979 pamphlet of the Board, "Recertification in Surgery",

> "The American Board of Surgery and the American College of Surgeons have agreed that the College would continue to provide opportunities for continuing education for the surgeon through its Congresses, postgraduate courses, SESAP and other activities. The Board will not produce nor provide educational materials nor opportunities. The Board will base the greater part of its examination for recertification on the material contained in SESAP, but will not utilize the actual SESAP questions as such. Participation in the SESAP program is therefore recommended but not required by the Board."

One might add, as epilogue to the allusions to the struggle to reform the College, that the efforts of Graham and his colleagues were eminently successful, a vigorous infusion of younger, academically oriented men occurred in the higher echelons, the College outlook on surgical education and research was greatly altered.

SOSSUS

Dr. Jonathan Rhoads was appointed by President Wangensteen as Chairman of the Committee on Issues in 1969. Following Dr. Rhoads' provocative report, Dr. William Altemeier brought this mission sharply into focus in his Presidential Address in 1970, and gave the Association a strong sense of urgency. Dr. William Holden then appointed Dr. George Zuidema as Chairman of a working group. Dr. William Longmire, Chairman of the Board of Regents of the American College of Surgeons had taken a similar step within the College. In the summer of 1970, Dr. J. Englebert Dunphy catalyzed the joining together of these two Associations in the joint undertaking now known as the Study on Surgical Services for the United States. In this effort, initially mounted by two parent organizations, we will now be joined by several other surgical organizations and specialty societies ultimately representing the whole spectrum of American Surgery, and with solid representation from community surgeons unassociated with the academic establishment. [Presidential Address, Francis D. Moore, 1972]

The enormous data gathering study launched by the Association jointly with the American College of Surgeons was reported back to the Fellows annually, as the work progressed. Reference to the origins of the enterprise had been made in the reports of the minutes of the relevant meetings. The huge mass of data, published in one "short" form, and three all-inclusive volumes is a basic document of its time, although, as it was pointed out, with the rapid change of events the data were no longer current when issued, and the bases for projection into the future were changed. A detailed analysis of SOSSUS is beyond the purview of this history, but the major role of the Association in the initiation and funding of the study, the fact that Fellows and Officers, past, current, and future, played determining

roles in the study, all justify the inclusion of this Appendix. Dr. Jonathan Rhoads (President 1973), Professor of Surgery, University of Pennsylvania School of Medicine, has provided a brief overview of the SOSSUS project. *The History of SOSSUS* was written by Dr. George D. Zuidema, Warfield M. Firor Professor of Surgery and Director of the Department, Johns Hopkins University Medical School, specifically for these volumes. Dr. Claude E. Welch, (President 1977) Senior Surgeon, Massachusetts General Hospital; Clinical Professor of Surgery Emeritus, Harvard Medical School, has very kindly permitted us to publish, for the first time, *SOSSUS Revisited,* a personal analysis of SOSSUS and its reception which he wrote in 1978, and decided at that time not to publish, thinking that it "would have stirred up so many fires that were now dying down that I decided in the interest of all concerned it would be better not to publish it". As indicated in Dr. Welch's article, the disagreement was principally over the nature of the data base, and some thereby invalidated conclusions, and was chiefly with the American College of Surgeons, its officials and officers being for the most part, of course, Fellows of the Association, and in some cases officers as well. It seems a valid service to history to publish Dr. Welch's account as he wrote it. Some future history or doctoral thesis devoting itself to SOSSUS will surely quote at length, from the Bulletin of the American College of Surgeons, the serial trenchant analyses of the SOSSUS report, and the challenge to the statistical validity of some sections.

From Jonathan E. Rhoads, April 11, 1978:

When Dr. Wangensteen was President he felt that it was important to review the purposes, activities, and directions of the ASA and he asked me to chair a committee to do this. He was good enough to consult with me on many of the other members, and I was delighted with the composition of the committee as a whole. In the course of our meetings, we concluded that the ASA should interest itself more in the public issues which affect surgery and the teaching of surgery and surgical research than it had customarily done. The formal response of the committee included the recommendation for the establishment of a Committee on Issues. Our early thinking was that this committee might meet periodically and organize a summer seminar for a limited number of members of the Association, along with persons from other disciplines whose counsel might be relevant. Stemming from such a meeting which might last several days or possibly a week would come a report and summary which could likely be presented during the regular meetings of the ASA, possibly as a breakfast seminar.

During the evolution of these plans, Dr. Francis D. Moore had pressed for a similar accentuation of concern with public issues in the American College of Surgeons. Indeed the College always had substantial interest in this field and the impetus for this new thrust came from multiple sources. However, it focused when Dr. Moore was assigned to prepare a report on the subject. As many of the people involved knew each other, and as in some instances individuals were involved both by the American College of Surgeons and the American Surgical Association, it seemed wiser to consolidate the effort. This decision was approved by the Regents for the College and the Council for the ASA and probably by the vote of the members also, though I do not recall this specifically. This resulted in the development of SOSSUS which was set up when Dr. William Holden was President of the ASA. I think it was largely through his good offices that Dr. George Zuidema was asked to chair this joint committee. There were a number of additions to the committee later as it became evident that specific representation from the specialty societies was important.

Dr. Zuidema proposed a number of committees and this plan was approved and the various committees were brought into being. Their names indicate their areas of responsibility. They were as follows:

Subcommittee on Academic Surgical Manpower
Subcommittee on Surgical Manpower
Subcommittee on Allied Surgical Manpower
Subcommittee on Organization, Delivery, and Financing of Surgical Services
Subcommittee on Legal and Ethical Issues in Surgery
Subcommittee on Community-Physician Relations
Subcommittee on Interprofessional Relations
Subcommittee on Surgical Research
Subcommittee on Quality of Surgical Care
Subcommittee on Government Relations

Dr. Moore logically became Chairman of the Subcommittee on Surgical Manpower and proceeded in a very active way to recruit Dr. Osler Peterson from the public health sector of Harvard University to assist with the design of this study. A good deal of the early effort of SOSSUS was to raise sufficient money to carry out a meaningful study. A total in excess of $2,000,000. was raised (though this figure should be checked with Dr. Zuidema), and the largest single portion was the manpower study. This included a questionnaire sent to a wide sample of surgeons across the country and a more intensive study in two or three specific areas where an effort was made to see what the breakdown was in the way individuals spent their time. There was a request for voluntary indication of earnings which as you can imagine was the subject of considerable debate and some criticism. However, enough data were returned to provide a fair indication of the average earnings received in various specialties. Of course there was no way to test the accuracy of the figures completely since income tax returns are confidential. The figures seemed to be reasonably in accord with other voluntary surveys, such as those conducted by Medical Economics.

The net result of these studies was to show that despite the tendency toward concentration of specialists near large medical centers, the general surgeons had distributed themselves fairly evenly throughout the population of the United States. Thus there was seldom a variation of more than two times between the surgeons per hundred thousand of population in the more thinly settled parts of the country from the same ratio in the more thickly settled parts of the country.

The particular subcommittee on which I served on the legal and ethical problems was chaired by our mutual friend, Henry Schwartz, Professor of Neurosurgery at Washington University. I thought he did an admirable job in covering the subject and wrote an excellent report. Dr. Marshall Orloff tackled the problem of Surgical Research and its support and the preparation of personnel for it. Not surprisingly, he concluded that we need more support, both for the preparation of personnel and for research endeavors.

In the course of these efforts the members from the ASA felt that there were certain issues coming before the Congress on which we should be prepared to speak out. The College however had an organized staff with a director who was responsible to the Board of Regents and particularly to the Chairman of the Board of Regents. There was some feeling that this central organization should be the spokesman for the College so that the ASA organized a special Committee on Government Affairs, not to speak for SOSSUS as a whole, but to speak for the ASA. This committee met in Washington on several occasions and had some useful interchanges with congressional staff people, AMA lobbyists, and others who were relevant to our understanding of the Washington scene and knowledgeable about the issues that were then being developed. We had considerable help from John

Pompelli of the College staff who was spending a portion of his time in Washington. All of this resulted in considerably improved understanding of the legislative process on the part of a number of members of the Association which I think to some degree radiated to the Association as a whole.

You are familiar with the breakfast meetings which were held at the ASA and with some of the special programs put on at the College which presented portions of the SOSSUS studies. Taking the SOSSUS study as a whole, I think it did a great deal to throw light on the manpower problem and to dispel an exaggerated feeling that a number of us had that we were training entirely too many surgeons. At the same time, it did point out clearly that if the recent trends had continued, we would be training too many surgeons and a brake was put on this, partly through the knowledge diffused through the medical student public and partly through the Coordinating Committee for Medical Education, the Liaison Committee for Graduate Medical Education, the Boards, and their respective Residency Review committees. In this way, the number of approved spots for surgical residencies has been held down and I believe actually decreased.

The study also showed that if surgical operations were done by certified surgeons, the number of surgeons was by no means too great and pointed out that it would now be possible to move toward a situation in which the informally trained surgeon or those who simply had gained experience through necessity need no longer be looked to as a longterm source of surgical services.

I think that the research needs of surgeons was pointed up as was to some extent the need for surgical teaching time. A good deal of time and effort went into some of the legal efforts and I think our understanding of the American tort laws, as they apply to malpractice, was strengthened and we got a better idea of what would be necessary to diminish professional liability awards, both by decreasing the occasion for suits by keeping better records which could be relied on when suit is brought and in trying to educate the public to have more realistic expectations of their medical members.

* * *

THE HISTORY OF SOSSUS

AN ACCOUNT OF THE ROLE OF THE AMERICAN SURGICAL ASSOCIATION IN THE STUDY ON SURGICAL SERVICES FOR THE UNITED STATES

George D. Zuidema, M.D.

The Study on Surgical Services for the United States (SOSSUS) was a massive undertaking by the surgical profession, to study itself and its role in the future

care of patients in the United States. It was from the beginning unlike any previous study, and its scope was exceptionally broad. I am relatively certain that everyone connected with it in its early days underestimated the problems associated, the scope of the project and the time which would be required to complete it.

The actual beginnings of the study can be traced to January 1969 when Dr. Owen Wangensteen, then President of the American Surgical Association, appointed a committee to be chaired by Dr. Jonathan Rhoads, to study the future course of that organization. Dr. Rhoads' committee delivered its report at the annual meeting of the American Surgical Association in April 1970, and recommended the formation of a Committee on Issues to undertake a broad approach to the major issues facing American surgery. Dr. William Holden was elected President of the American Surgical Association at that meeting, and he met with Dr. George Zuidema to ask him to plan the work of the newly formed committee and outline its task. Dr. Zuidema assumed the chairmanship of that committee and began working closely with Dr. Holden in organizing the study. At almost the same time the Board of Regents of the American College of Surgeons had appointed a steering committee on the distribution and adequacy of surgical care, under the chairmanship of Dr. Francis Moore, with the assignment of studying the distribution and quality of surgical services in the United States. The two organizations became aware of the parallel studies and it soon became obvious there was much to be gained by combining the resources of the two associations. In July 1970 representatives of both organizations met at Washington National Airport and SOSSUS was born. We were helped enormously in those early days by sharing the experience of Dr. Charles Herndon, Professor and Chairman of the Department of Orthopedic Surgery at Case Western Reserve. Dr. Herndon had chaired a somewhat similar systems study of orthopedic surgery and was familiar with both the problems involved in organization and with the central roles of consultants in getting the study financed and under way. Furthermore, the study which had been undertaken by the orthopedic surgeons had experienced difficulties in acceptance by the profession, in large part because the profession had not been fully informed of some of the issues during the period of the study itself and consequently reacted at its conclusion by refusing to accept the group's report. This was an important lesson for SOSSUS for all of us realized that an extensive study of this kind would inevitably result in some differences of opinion and a lack of uniformity in understanding and commitment. We, therefore, from the beginning adopted a policy of delivering regular reports to both the American College of Surgeons and to the American Surgical Association to keep the membership of the two sponsoring organizations fully informed of directions, issues and data as they were collected.

The first meeting of the Committee on Issues, held in July 1970, had been carefully planned. A rough outline of the scope of the work had been prepared with the study objectives, the goals and a list of working committees with prospective chairmen also outlined. A number of consultants and special participants were also present. They included Dr. Carruth J. Wagner, who had been instrumental in developing the orthopedic study, Dr. John Cooper, President of the Association of American Medical Colleges, Dr. C. Rollins Hanlon, Director of the American College of Surgeons, Dr. Richard Wilbur of the American Medical Association, Dr. Vernon Wilson of the Health Services and Mental Health Administration, Dr. Geo. Gehrig of the American Hospital Association and Dr. Kerr White of the Johns Hopkins School of Hygiene and Public Health. Dr. Gerald M. Michael of the Environmental Health Service of the U. S. Public Health Service also served as a consultant and was helpful in the early phases of organization.

The group had a very successful organizational meeting and in addition to outlining the study itself, prepared a schedule which called for publication of the report in March of 1972, a goal which in retrospect seems incredibly naive. Major assignments faced the Executive Committee of the study very early. The first requirement was for fund raising to support the actual investigative phases of the study and to finance its ultimate final publication. To accomplish this, the group approached a number of foundations. It became apparent, however, that the surgical associations had to establish their credibility by supplying some "earnest money" of their own. During the first two years of its operation, members of the American Surgical Association contributed $21,000 derived from personal assessment of its members. During this same period of time, the American College of Surgeons contributed nearly $70,000, and these sums together were instrumental in obtaining unrestricted grants from the Commonwealth Fund, the Richard King Mellon Charitable Trust, the Walnut Medical Charitable Trust, and the Matilda R. Wilson Fund. These foundations were particularly helpful in contributing toward the plan-

ning of the entire SOSSUS study, and making it possible in turn then to obtain support for particular phases and research projects from the National Institute of Health (NIH), the Health Services and Mental Health Administration (HSMHA), the Rockefeller Foundation, the Bureau of Health Manpower Education of the National Institutes of Health, and the Robert Wood Johnson Foundation. Later the Kaiser Family Foundation and the Commonwealth Fund allocated further monies, as did the two sponsoring organizations. The early financing was particularly difficult, however, because of the unique nature of the study which had been proposed, and the fact that each organization which was approached had its own ideas as to what should be studied and how the study should be conducted. The time frame of the SOSSUS project was necessarily extended beyond its original two-year projection for several reasons. First of all, the scope was broadened considerably by our wish to do a thorough and extensive study. This involved each of the ten subcommittees conducting at least one research project of its own.

The entire organization, or course, was run on a voluntary basis, other than the staff office which was established in Baltimore to be responsible for the day-to-day operations. No physician and no member of the Executive Committee ever received more than reimbursement for expenses involved in what proved to be a tremendously time-consuming activity.

At the onset we were told that if the project lasted more than two years enthusiasm would flag and the ultimate completion or the value of the data would be in question. I can only say that those observers had never encountered individuals of the character we ultimately enlisted in the project. During the entire five-year period that the work was undertaken, the intensity of interest and the dedication of all the participants was outstanding. There was a spirit of cooperation and enthusiasm which insured our carrying on to a satisfactory completion.

The study was organized to be conducted under an executive committee which included the chairmen of the SOSSUS sub-committees. Later, representatives from five regional surgical associations and appointed representatives from the surgical specialty organizations were added. Others served by virtue of their positions within either the American College of Surgeons or the American Surgical Association. Ultimately a seven member advisory committee, reporting to the Executive Committee, was established to permit a prompt response to issues which arose and to assist Dr. Zuidema in steering the reports of the ten sub-committees through to an inclusive and representative report. The sub-committees were planned to cover all aspects of surgical work. Consequently one was established on Academic Surgical Manpower, a second on Surgical Manpower and a third was appointed to deal with special aspects of Allied Surgical Manpower. These groups also had special consultants in addition to their surgical membership. A further sub-committee was appointed to review the status of Organization, Delivery and Financing of Surgical Services and others dealt with Legal and Ethical issues, Community-Physician Relations, Interprofessional Relationships, Surgical Research, Government Relations and the Quality of Surgical Care. In all, more than 150 surgeons participated as members of these committees or consultants to them. There were also many contributors from the Federal government and from the other established medical specialties so that all committees had the benefit of experts from a great many fields. The structure of the organization permitted us to maintain close liaison with regional societies and with surgical specialities so that we could be made aware of feelings and projects being undertaken in those areas and in turn their memberships could be fully informed as to the deliberations of SOSSUS. This proved to be an essential ingredient in the success of the enterprise. It was quite obvious that a study of this kind could prove to be highly threatening to many individuals in the practice of general surgery or of one of the specialties, and we set out from the beginning to keep the specialists and particularly the membership of the American College of Surgeons as fully informed as possible. This also provided an avenue for their input to the operation of the study itself so that although it greatly complicated our work, in the final analysis, it was instrumental to our success. Plans for organization of the various components of the study became formalized and each sub-committee chairman identified members of his own working group together with consultants, and began to put together the rough format of his sub-committee's research effort. The Executive Committee met in the Fall of 1970 at the time of the Clinical Congress of the American College of Surgeons and, in addition to talking to several consultants from government, instituted final plans for a national conference which was held in December of that year at the Airlie House Conference Center in Warrington, Virginia. This conference, sponsored by the American College of Surgeons and SOSSUS, was attended by some 70 individuals including the Regents of the American College of Surgeons, the Executive Committee of the study and a number of Washington consultants. The purpose was to intro-duce the group to the study, its goals and objectives and its plan for implementation. Responses to the study were presented by Dr. Bornemeier, President of the AMA, Dr. Wiley Armstrong, President of the NMA, Dr. Roger Egeberg, then Assistant Secretary for Health and Scientific Affairs, DHEW, Dr. Paul Sanazaro, Director of Health Services Research and Development, HSMHA, DHEW, and Dr. Louis Rousselot, Assistant Secretary for Health and Environment, Department of Defense. The conference included a series of workshop sessions dealing with each of the sub-committee charges followed by additional group discussions. Dr. Egeberg underlined a significant problem when he pointed out the urgent needs for involving the profession in a dialogue with government to open the way for the profession to contribute to legislative plans which would affect health care delivery in surgical care in the United States. This raised some real problems, for the study itself had been set up to collect data, and because of the diverse interest and makeup of the two sponsoring bodies, there was great potential for the creation of serious problems in opening discussions with the Federal government. There was concern expressed that SOSSUS would identify itself with government rather than truly representing the sponsoring organizations. On the other hand, it was obvious that unless the professions became involved rather widely in an educational and contributory sense, events would probably move more rapidly than the profession would like. It thus became obvious that the sponsoring organizations needed to be fully informed at all times, and as a first step in this direction the Regents of the American College of Surgeons established a full-scale meeting for the Governors of the College and chapter Presidents, in Chicago on February 6, 1971. At this highly effective meeting the group was told of the scope and nature of the study, and their support for its continuing activities was obtained. The chapter Presidents and Governors met with the sub-committee chairmen and received background reports and detailed planning proposals together with a series of workshops and summary statements. This unprecedented session had rich dividends for it immediately brought the details of the SOSSUS plan to the full attention of the College membership. It was also decided at this time that the surgical community would itself conduct the study rather than hiring a private firm to collect the data. We recognized that this represented a substantially greater expenditure of effort and time, but considered that the net result would be well worth it.

There was a curious aftermath of the Airlie House Conference. Organized surgery had assembled some 70 participants to kick off a national study regarding the delivery of surgical services to the people of the United States. A press conference was announced, at which time it was planned to go into the long-range plans of the group. No press representatives bothered to show up; an indication of the feelings of the press towards surgery at that time.

Plans, however, moved forward. By early 1971 we had raised a total of nearly $130,000 and were able to parcel out small sums to the various subcommittees in order to help them prepare their research proposals. At this time two facts began to emerge and assume increasing importance. It became obvious that if SOSSUS was to speak for all of surgery that the practicing surgeons and the surgical specialties had to be involved, and at this point definitive approaches to the surgical groups began to be made. Also, at this time it was recognized that it would be very difficult for the study to participate in any way with the Congress without jeopardizing its status as a data-collecting agency. As a result, a special Committee on Pending Legislation was established, separate from the SOSSUS project. This committee was appointed by the President of the American Surgical Association and the Chairman of the Board of Regents of the College. Although it frequently reported to the Executive Committee on SOSSUS, it was an independent operation and remained so throughout the duration of the study. Mr. John Pompelli, a member of the College staff, experienced in establishing relationships with congressmen proved to be a valuable source of information and served as a liaison agent for the Committee on Pending Legislation.

Another point of interest dealt with a proposed plan to estimate future developments in medical and surgical care by way of the Delphi technique. The Delphi approach is to select a panel of experts in widely divergent, but related, fields and ask them to predict long-range future developments. By studying a series of these predictions, called probes, it is possible to achieve long-range predictions. This technique had been used in government and was proposed to the SOSSUS executive group as well. The study was actually begun, and initial panels were selected. It proved, however, to be the source of considerable agonizing and uncertainty. The group had enough difficulty with the collection and interpretation of acknowledged information without getting into the complications associated with the prediction of future developments. For these reasons, and perhaps others, the Delphi study was phased out, and from this time on no further attempts were made in

a formal way to establish any attempts at prediction of future needs or developments.

By the Fall of 1971 when the Executive Committee next met, individual studies were well under way, and the Executive Committee began the task of looking ahead and grappling with some rather thorny issues. The first of these dealt with the relationship of the surgical specialities to the sponsoring organizations. Dr. Herndon who had chaired the orthopedic study was well aware of the potential pitfalls here, and wisely advised the group to separate data collection from interpretation-recommendation. Consequently, a policy emerged that the SOSSUS group itself would collect the data and that prior to interpretation or adoption the data would be presented to broadly representative groups including both the parent organizations and the specialty societies. In order to insure solid participation by specialty groups, their representatives were invited to serve as full members of the Executive Committee with, of course, full access to data and reports, with the expectation that they would function as liaison representatives with their sponsoring specialty organizations. The Executive Committee also tackled the difficult subject of review and approval mechanisms. It was obvious at this point that a lot of interest, some of it rather intense, had been generated by SOSSUS's very existence, and since some of the areas under investigation were potentially troublesome, a policy had to be developed. There was little question that factual data should be collected and reported. Government contracts posed some problems in that unless some interpretation were offered there was a distinct risk that the Federal agencies would attach their own interpretation, which might be at variance with the actual situation as seen by the surgical investigators. Consequently, it was decided that broad conclusions could be approved by the Executive Committee and the sponsoring organizations, and then used to develop options and interpretations to meet Federal requirements. It eventually developed that the main thrust of the SOSSUS study would be to gather factual data. This information was then developed into report form and made available to the sponsoring organizations. The report itself included lists of options, and in some instances, some rather obvious recommendations. The approach used, however, made it possible for the report of the study to stand alone rather than requiring the "approval" of an entire sponsoring body. In actual fact, although there was considerable discussion and apprehension, this proved to be less of a problem than was anticipated early on.

SOSSUS was much more than a series of executive committee meetings, however. Probably the best known study was the massive manpower evaluation research undertaken by Dr. Francis Moore and his group of investigators at the Harvard Medical School in the Harvard School of Public Health. They carried out two substantial studies. The first of these consisted of a detailed study conducted within four geographic regions. Data were gathered on the characteristics and credentials of the surgeons performing operations within these regions, as well as their supporting teams. Rates for all operations and for specific operations were determined by specialty, and the work of the surgeons was also characterized by age, by those certified or non-certified, and by work performed in small towns and urban centers. This detailed work was necessary in order to provide a baseline for the subsequent estimate of surgical work performed, as well as possible calculations for future need. The regions selected were not publicly identified but all had the following characteristics: They were sufficiently large in population to approach at least a million; the region was self contained for virtually all of its medical care, and constituted a standard metropolitan statistical area (SMSA) with some degree of urban and rural mix. The area had to offer all levels of care ranging from emergency to tertiary, and the range in the ratio of surgeons to population in terms of high, low and middle range was sought. The regional studies encompassed one area in the southeastern area of the United States, one of the Pacific coast and two in the Atlantic and New England areas. The massive data collected through this portion of the study are reported in great detail within the three-volume final set of SOSSUS report. An excellent summary is included in the short form volume. In general the physicians within these geographical areas were extremely cooperative with the study teams which went into the various hospitals to go over their statistics. One geographic area, however, refused admission of the study group so that ultimately the final report was based on four of these geographic areas rather than five as originally proposed. On the whole it was remarkable that the level of cooperation was as high as it proved to be.

The second major study conducted by the Manpower Evaluation Committee consisted of a questionnaire sent to a sample of approximately 10,000 surgeons. The intention of this effort was to gather data on surgeons' work, their opinions and workloads as well as the characteristics of their practice. The sample was selected from the AMA manpower tapes, and the data collected later proved to give valuable information regarding work patterns and characteristics. The questionnaire study also gave the executive office some difficult moments. The data were collected and analyzed on tapes by Dr. Ivan Fahs in Minneapolis. At one point in the study we were unable to raise the $43,000 necessary to pay Dr. Fahs for his tapes so that the information badly needed by other committees remained in limbo until the money was ultimately raised. Part of the additional funds was raised by Dr. Moore's group and part was loaned by the American College of Surgeons, a loan later forgiven by the Regents at the conclusion of the study.

There were, of course, other studies undertaken by the manpower evaluation group. Members of Dr. Moore's sub-committee looked at medical school input into surgery, trends in surgical practice. A collaborative study, with the American Boards, of application rates for board certification and the fate of the applicants was undertaken as well as a detailed study of the ratio of surgeons to population in all of the major European countries; and a study of the foreign medical graduates in this country, where they go and what they do. There was also a questionnaire study of surgical residents in this country. Both of the questionnaire studies were well received and had an excellent response rate.

Dr. Chase had originally chaired the Organization, Financing and Delivery of Services Committee, but this chairmanship was later switched to Dr. Walter Ballinger at the mutual agreement of both parties and the Executive Committee. Dr. Chase had been very active on the Washington scene and continued to be interested in the development of various legislative proposals and the committee wished to free him to continue that. Consequently, Dr. Ballinger took over this piece of work. His committee with help from consultants and economists also utilized the data from the AMA tapes, and investigated various patterns of surgical practice including prepaid and private practice patterns as well as investigating relationships of surgeons to private insurance carriers, Federal, State and county agencies. There was a project reviewing the role of the Veteran's Administration, conducted by Dr. Francis Jackson. Dr. LaSalle Lafall actively explored the role of the Social Security office. It was originally intended to coordinate much of Dr. Moore's data with Dr. Ballinger's committee, but this proved to be difficult to accomplish.

Dr. Robert Chase headed the committee on Government Relations. It was very difficult to fund this for many reasons, and several aspects of this committee's work were ultimately split off into the free-standing committee on Pending Legislation. Dr.

William Altemeier came to chair this committee.

Dr. Henry Schwartz of Washington University headed a group investigating legal and ethical aspects of surgical practice. This committee was very active in a number of areas including abortion, death, experimental procedures, transplantation, the responsibilities of surgical trainees to their patients and their preceptors, liability and malpractice and the use of auxiliary personnel. Their work was strengthened by the assistance of Dr. William Nick of Columbus, Ohio, both a surgeon and an attorney. In many ways this group foresaw the crisis in the liability and negligence field which later emerged prominently.

Dr. Merle Musselman chaired the committee on Community-Physician Relationships. This committee's deliberations dealt with the field of contemporary sociology and studied the role of the physician in the community and the problems involved in communications between the groups. I would have to say that of all the studies undertaken that this was probably the "softest" area in both its approach and its conclusions. Dr. Ben Colcock later joined this committee and performed yeoman service in bringing the major community and physician issues into focus.

Dr. Marshall Orloff's group at the University of California, San Diego, carried out a monumental piece of work in the surgical research area. They identified the significant research contributions in surgery and the surgical specialities which had occurred during the past 25 years, using a literature search and a questionnaire. Consultants from the specialties also added input into the final decision. The group was able to study not only the funding of surgical research but also to a significant degree to perform a cost/benefit analysis of various types of surgical care. Dr. Orloff concludes his study with an extensive report in which 27 advances in surgery are identified and the historical development of each outlined, with a list of references. This material, included in the large volume of the three volume set of SOSSUS reports, makes for fascinating reading for anyone interested in reviewing the research background of many of these important developments.

Two other manpower committees performed essential service, although neither received quite the national attention that the general Manpower Evaluation Committee received. Dr. Zeppa and his group investigated the status of academic manpower and received an excellent response to their questionnaire surveys. He sought to determine the size and scope of departments of surgery, various options for departmental funding, number of vacancies and the role of research and research grants in both departmental productivity and terms of support for teaching functions. The Allied Surgical Manpower Committee was chaired by Dr. William Anlyan with the able help of Dr. Robert Howard. They had the difficult assignment of examining relationships with the nursing profession, operating room nursing, nurse anesthetists and physicians' assistants. Their work required coordination with other manpower committees, the Legal and Ethics Committee and the Organization, Financing and Delivery Sub-committee Many aspects of their study which surfaced during the investigative period have later proven to be highly significant. Their work will probably continue to grow in importance as recent manpower legislation, trimming back of house staff size and unionization of nursing professionals continue to develop on the national scene.

The final committee was that chaired by Dr. Charles G. Child III with the assignment of examining the Quality of Surgical Care. This, as might be imagined, proved to be an exceptionally difficult problem. The committee began by taking a leaf from the notebook of the maternal mortality studies which developed in the late thirties, and began an examination of "critical incidents" in surgical care. They examined a series of operative procedures in which, under ordinary circumstances, mortality and morbidity were not expected to occur. They then looked at the incidents which did occur and sought to attribute this to problems of technical competence, "patients' disease", community or societal problems or hospital associated difficulties. The study itself, conducted through the voluntary cooperation of three College chapters, was later expanded on a partial basis to a total of six. All critical incidents reviewed by the committee were selected by representatives in participating hospitals, examined locally for a judgment as to the cause of the incident and then submitted to the study. Obviously, this represented a highly selected experience. Yet to our consternation and dismay, when the newspaper reports of the critical incident studies were written, these were translated into direct surgical rates so the headlines would proclaim "18% of surgical deaths claimed due to physician error, etc." Most of the problems with the press related to an article written in Modern Medicine on the Critical Incident study. The factual data included in the substance of the article appear to be fairly accurately reported, but the headings of the various sections of the manuscripts were "creative" and when picked up by the newspapers led to gross inaccuracies and a fair amount of unfavorable, completely incorrect publicity. The approach for the assessment of quality of care appears to be a good one, but the difficulties which developed through misuse and misunderstanding of information were fairly sizeable, and led to one of the major problems which we experienced with SOSSUS.

A word might be said here about the modus operandi. Each sub-committee had been given its assigned task, had outlined its proposed research approach and conducted its study. Each sub-committee undertook to do this after its own fashion, some with very large grants, others on a shoestring budget. Each sub-committee, however, adhered to its own time schedule and national meetings found the individual groups huddling, going over data and planning the next step. The SOSSUS Executive office in Baltimore coordinated activities almost on a day-to-day basis with subcommittee chairmen, and the entire Executive Committee was kept informed by means of large meetings held once or twice a year. The subcommittee chairmen, members of the Executive Committee, representatives from the Board of Regents and from the Council of the American Surgical Association and other consultants were invited to attend these meetings. On these occasions each subcommittee chairman would present a written report which was distributed either on the scene or in advance to all attendees. There would then be an oral presentation giving the status of research projects and a time for questions and answers, and suggestions. After each day's work, the discussions and questions would be summarized, copied and distributed to those attending so that they would be available for further reflection and written comments for the audience, and as a written summary of conclusions for the sub-committee chairmen to work from. This proved to be a remarkably effective method of operation and it gave every participating organization a voice in the deliberations as they went on.

We all realized that it was a matter of critical importance to keep our constituencies informed. For this reason, the American Surgical Association instituted a series of breakfast meetings at the annual meetings, at which time the membership would receive a report from SOSSUS Detailed summaries of activities and research in progress were presented at these meetings so that the membership truly felt a part of the operation. A similar program was held at the Clinical Congress of the American College of Surgeons each year where there was an educational panel as a part of one of the large sessions. This served to keep the fellowship of the College informed as to the directions SOSSUS was taking. In addition each member of the Executive Committee who was a representative of a surgical specialty took his report back to the parent organization and discussed it either in council or in open meetings with the members. In this way the information emanating from the SOSSUS study was effectively transmitted to the constituency as we went along. We sought by this technique to avoid having any unpleasant surprises when the final report came out.

The Executive Committee had an important working meeting in Charlottesville, Virginia, in July of 1974. At this time we were in the process of bringing our work to a conclusion, and it was at this meeting the reports were dissected and analyzed in detail before going into final draft form. A similar meeting was held in January 1975 in Chicago at which time the final drafts were reviewed by the membership of the Executive Committee and the other representatives who had attended, and accepted in final form. The editorial team of Mr. Robert A. Potter and Blair Burns Potter took the last draft form and translated the individual reports into a final uniform text for printing. The manuscripts went to the printer in early 1975, shortly after the last Executive Committee meeting and were distributed later that Spring.

As Director of the SOSSUS project, I had to be acutely aware at all times of a serious and central concern held by all participating organizations and to seek implementation of its conclusions by including a series of recommendations for action. We had to recognize throughout that the use of SOSSUS data and recommendations for action were properties which were reserved by the participating organizations. Each organization dealt with this in a different way. At times the American College of Surgeons held SOSSUS at arm's length, pointing out that it was a study group which although sponsored by the College, did not speak with authority on College policy. In this way the Board of Regents reserved the right to comment on the SOSSUS data, a step which it later took in a most perplexing way. That, however, is beyond the scope of this narration. The American Surgical Association, in an effort to deal with this problem, re-established the Committee on Issues and this group under the chairmanship of Dr. Francis D. Moore convened for the first time in its new incarnation in January 1975 following the final meeting of the SOSSUS Executive Committee. The Issues Committee has met regularly since the end of the SOSSUS project, dealing with various aspects of issues brought to life by the study as well as others which have surfaced since that time. The basic principle adhered to, however, was that SOSSUS was essentially a data gathering effort and the right of interpretation and recommendation was held by the sponsoring organizations.

SOSSUS came to a successful conclusion in July 1975 with the publication of a summary volume and a series of press releases. In contrast to our prior experience with press conferences, these were in general highly successful. Other specialties within the profession took a leaf from the SOSSUS notebook and instituted studies of their own. Several members of the Executive Committee were called to testify before Congress and although testimony in many instances led to discussions of other types of subjects and other issues, nonetheless, the surgical organizations had made their point and had demonstrated their interest and willingness to perform a massive self-examination.

I would like to add two footnotes to this story. The first is a brief word about the role of Monte Firor in the entire episode. I remember very clearly Dr. Firor rising at the 1970 Business Meeting of the American Surgical Association, after the Rhoads Committee had submitted its report and recommended that a Committee on Issues be formed, the recommendation which led to the original conception of SOSSUS. Dr. Firor spoke very eloquently at that time of the responsibilities of American surgery and the American Surgical Association, and his presentation was instrumental in getting the study approved and off the ground. Dr. Firor was appointed to the Executive Committee. Almost before the major portion of the study was done, he had made a major contribution by writing the introduction to the summary volume. This is a remarkable piece of work and set the tone for the entire subsequent project. Dr. Firor was with us throughout the study, and I recall vividly the Executive Committee meeting in Charlottesville in 1973 when he rose, just as we were breaking up into working groups, to remind us it was our duty to accumulate factual information for the Council of the American Surgical Association and the Regents of the American College of Surgeons to work with to enhance the progress of American surgery. He then urged all of us to roll up our sleeves, get down to work, shorten our reports, avoid redundancy and stop editorializing. With that echoing in our minds, we went back to work with the knowledge of his constant urging so helpful in producing the final result.

Another footnote worth mentioning deals with the subject of "unnecessary surgery." The subject came up at one of the Charlottesville Executive Committee sessions at which time we received a report of the second opinion studies which were being undertaken in New York by Dr. Eugene McCarthy with the cooperation of the various departments of surgery at Cornell and NYU. In the course of the discussion the problems of definition surfaced and the general feeling was that it would be almost impossible to get worthwhile data and that the field was so controversial that it would be better left to individual investigators to explore. We ultimately came up with a series of six categories of surgery which under certain circumstances might be "unnecessary". I suspect that in recognizing that this was such a complex and loaded field we probably, in part at least, ducked the issue. I am not sure, looking back, whether any step we would have taken would have been very constructive, however, for the clinical studies and the second opinion programs are still going on and are still highly controversial and, of course, are often misquoted in the press. This is one area, however, where the profession probably could have taken a stronger stand, although at the time I believe that we failed to appreciate what was in store for all of us in this regard.

* * *

SOSSUS Revisited

Claude E. Welch, M.D.

In 1972, two major surgical organizations—the American Surgical Association and the American College of Surgeons—began a comprehensive survey of surgical practice in the United States. The initial impetus for the study had been furnished by the American Surgical Association and its president in 1969, Dr. Owen Wangensteen.

The project was organized with Dr. George Zuidema as chairman and Dr. Francis Moore as chairman of the Subcommittee on Manpower. The work was accomplished with the aid of many committees, the Department of Preventive Medicine, Harvard Medical School, and innumerable individuals. Financial support was obtained by grants from foundations and the government. This report, unique because of its scope, was published in summary in 1975 and was followed a year later by the completed volumes.[1,2] Meanwhile, during this period a method of estimation of surgical workloads devised by Hughes was followed by a series of papers by Moore, et al. that included extensive compilations of data and computer projections.[3,4,5,6,7,8] Today it is possible to appraise the early effects of the Study on Surgical Services for the United States

(SOSSUS). It should be emphasized that this summary represents an individual point of view and does not imply specific approval by the sponsoring societies.

First a few words about the content of the report are in order. Ten subcommittees submitted recommendations. Subsequently some of their statements received relatively little attention. For example, one suggestion that surgeons should cooperate with other professionals and join in local and governmental health planning was received without adverse criticism. One particularly important chapter contained documentation of major contributions of surgical research in the last thirty years. However, attention has been focused particularly on the sections that are concerned with the issues of surgical manpower, of financing, and with the quality of surgical care.

The main thrusts of the report were to suggest that there are too many individuals engaged in the practice of surgery in the United States, that at present approximately a third of them are less than fully qualified by adequate training, that costs of surgical care can be reduced, and that the quality of care is capable of improvement.

The assumption was made—probably not unreasonably—that the quality of surgical care almost certainly can be improved by better education and training of surgeons. While surgeons do learn by on-the-job practice, protection of the public demands that graduate education and patient care should be carried out under strict supervision. For this reason the report looked forward to the rosy day when elective surgery would be done by surgeons who had obtained Board certification or who had other excellent qualifications which testified to a long term of training that theoretically should correspond to superior performance.

The most important objectives that were suggested by the study were:

1. The number of training programs should be reduced and identified more closely with university centers, i.e., "affiliated hospitals."

2. Ultimately, the total number of persons entering practice with Board certificates in general surgery and the surgical specialties should be reduced to provide a total of 1,600 to 2,000 yearly in the next ten years. Though not examined in detail in the report, it is obvious that as a corollary, the total number of persons in training would need to be reduced to an appropriate level.

3. Ideally surgical procedures should be carried out only by individuals with appropriate training, continued activity and proficiency in their fields. In order to attain these goals individual hospital staffs should grant surgical privileges only to well-trained individuals, and should continue to monitor their performances.

4. Academic manpower must be strengthened. Research activities and teaching are in a precarious condition both because of lack of adequate personnel and financial support.

5. Costs must be controlled; such experiments as ambulatory clinics, development of surgical teams in which reliance is placed on non-M.D. members, and prepaid programs furnish possible methods.

6. Quality must be improved by stricter peer review.

Attention recently has been focused on the first three of these recommendations. The influence of SOSSUS can be assessed objectively by data demonstrating changing trends in the number of individuals entering and graduating from surgical programs, the location of these programs and the number of individuals certified by surgical Boards. Before these data are considered it is appropriate to ask what attention has been paid to this report.

The evidence suggests that surgeons have been profoundly influenced by it and that medical students, certain governmental agencies, the public and other professional groups have reacted to it in various ways. These actions perhaps would have occurred in the absence of SOSSUS. However, some of the data in the manpower study were made public long before the final report, and it must be concluded that SOSSUS historically furnished a powerful stimulus and provided the first solid statistical base from which future manpower projections could be made.

Students certainly have received the message from SOSSUS that there are too many individuals performing surgical procedures and that there may be a decreasing demand for young people to enter practice even though they are highly qualified in surgery. However, financial support of primary-care programs in medical schools by the government has provided a more potent stimulus for students to shift away from surgery into family practice. For example, in Harvard Medical School in 1978 only 23, or 14% of the 162 senior students selected general surgery or a surgical specialty for their internship or residency. These figures correspond closely with those of the national intern and residency matching program in 1977 when only 14% of the entire group of 16,574 offered positions were filled by individuals who selected general surgery and an additional 2% by those who selected surgical specialties. Eventually, of course, some graduates who begin in primary care, will transfer into surgical programs, but this figure stands in contrast with a 25% surgical entrance rate covering a large number of medical school alumni over the past 40 years.

From governmental agencies there have been varied reactions. The Congress is 1976 finally abandoned efforts to increase the number of doctors of medicine and declared in PL 94-484 "that there is no longer an insufficient number of physicians and surgeons in the United States" and instituted strenuous restrictions of the number of foreign medical graduates entering the United States. GMENAC (Graduate Medical Education National Advisory Committee to the Secretary of HEW) was established. Fourteen of the 21 members are professionals and the others are public members. The exact duties of this organization never have been clearly defined though presumably they could duplicate those of residency review committees. Up to the present time the committee has held only four meetings so that the scope of its influence is not clear. It does, however, indicate the government's desire to participate and perhaps even to control and to limit the number of surgical residencies in surgery as well as in other specialties. It should be noted that certain governmental programs have required Board certification as a measure of fitness; the Veteran's Administration has required it for certain types of consultants in surgery for almost thirty years.

Meanwhile other agencies of the government have spawned programs that are completely opposed to the recommendations of SOSSUS. The Federal Trade Commission (FTC) in an attempt to preserve free competition, is advocating measures that could destroy the present system of Boards and of credentialing. It seems certain that the FTC has viewed the honest attempt of SOSSUS to upgrade surgery as a method to corral all surgical procedures into the hands of a select few who then could manipulate prices at will. The activities of the FTC could furnish a very serious threat to the production of well-trained surgeons and to the limitation of their numbers and could lead to an unfortunate deterioration in the quality of surgical care. Fortunately there are strong voices in government that support the concepts of SOSSUS. Sooner or later these opposing forces must meet in head-on collision and the problem settled at a national level.

The public knows little of SOSSUS. Essentially the only publicity followed sensational reports in some newspapers that took the figures of the study of critical incidents and extrapolated them in an inaccurate, sensational version that led to the erroneous conclusions that surgeons were responsible for many deaths following "unnecessary surgery". Refutation by Hanlon of the inaccuracies of these allegations need not be repeated in this brief report.[9]

Some professional societies have reacted to SOSSUS. For example, other specialty societies such as the American College of Physicians have flattered SOSSUS by the initiation of similar studies. In this context it may be mentioned that a minor disagreement between the American College of Surgeons (one of the sponsoring organizations) and the final report developed.[10, 11] SOSSUS used slightly different data sources than the College. Furthermore, SOSSUS based its figures on 1969 data and failed to update them to 1975. Some of the basic figures were questioned; in particular there are more individuals in training programs than stated in SOSSUS. Such changes would not invalidate but actually strengthen one of the major thrusts of SOSSUS—that too many individuals are performing surgical procedures. They would, however, indicate that a dramatic reduction in the number of persons certified by Boards to the number visualized by SOSSUS could lead to unappreciated serious dislocations especially in city, county, state and municipal hospitals, where many of the operations are carried out by residents, and a consequent lack of available good surgical care throughout the country. Continuing studies and projections will be necessary to accomplish this transition without jeopardizing health care.

The Joint Commission on Accreditation of Hospitals (JCAH) has heeded the warnings of SOSSUS, namely that if surgical procedures are to be performed by persons well trained in the art, it is necessary that individual hospitals must be more careful about their credentialing procedures. It is the primary responsibility of a hospital to control the individuals who carry out operations. Despite this surveillance, there is some evidence that in certain parts of the country there is a continuing influx of surgeons who have not had adequate training. If the concepts of SOSSUS are to be supported, individual hospital requirements will require continuous reevaluation.

Finally, the profound effects of SOSSUS on surgeons themselves may be shown by available statistics. Since surgeons play the major role in the corresponding residency review committees and in the surgical Boards, SOSSUS provided a strong stimulus to further restrictions in manpower. Data are available for the number of training programs, both in affiliated and nonaffiliated hospitals, on the number of individuals in training, and on the number of Board-certified specialists that are produced. Three sets of figures drawn from the Directory of Approved Internships and Residencies published by the AMA will be used. The year 1970–71 marked the initiation of SOSSUS. Three years later, in 1973–74, just before the effects of SOSSUS were felt, the number of programs reached a high level. The most recent figures for the year 1977–78 demonstrate the effects of SOSSUS. The available data may be summarized as follows:

1. The total number of training programs. SOSSUS recommended a reduction in this number. The total number of programs in surgery and in the surgical specialties was 1,798 in 1970–71, 1,848 in 1973–74, and 1,604 in 1977–78. This represents a decline from the 1973–74 level of 8%. The decrease has been sharper in general surgery where there were 536 programs in 1970–71, 482 in 1973–74, and 401 in 1977–78, or a decline of 25% from the high level of 1970–71. It should be emphasized that in interpretation of these and succeeding data, that, although SOSSUS contributed additional pressure for change, it was the aggressive work of residency review committees that accepted these changes.

2. Reduction in the number of nonaffiliated programs. SOSSUS recommended this reduction in the number of training programs that were not affiliated with medical schools. There were 359 nonaffiliated programs in 1970–71, 212 in 1973–74, and 121 in 1977–78. This represented a decline during this period of 67%. In surgery 75% of the nonaffiliated programs have been eliminated (i.e., from 172 in 1970–71 to 42 in 1977–78). Thus there has been a sharp shift away from the nonaffiliated hospitals to university centers and hospitals affiliated with them. This shift is consistent with the recommendations of SOSSUS. It should be noted that prior to SOSSUS, the Carnegie Report (1970) had recommended a shift from nonaffiliated to affiliated programs.[12] Residency review committees had instituted such changes, that were accelerated by SOSSUS.

3. Reduction in the number of affiliated programs. SOSSUS and residency review committees have considered that the second phase in the reduction of the total number of surgeons will require reduction in the number of affiliated programs. To date there has been much less progress in this particular effort. There were 1,439 affiliated programs in 1970–71, 1,636 in 1973–74, and 1,583 in 1977–78. General surgical programs have remained static; there were 364 in 1970–71, 394 in 1973–74, and 359

in 1977–78. Other important factors have been brought into play that have led to this relatively stable situation. The increased number of medical schools with the requirements for training and the great expansion of cardiac surgery, vascular surgery, and plastic surgery all have been important contributing factors.

4. The number of individuals in training. SOSSUS recommended a reduction in this number. Available data include the number of first-year positions that were offered and filled, and the total number of positions that were also offered or filled. Until recently, since approximately 95% of all offered positions were filled, there was little difference between the offered and filled groups. However, two forces are combining to make an important difference in the near future. The reduction in the number of foreign medical graduates (FMGs) who fill about 33% of all positions, will be exceedingly important. Also, for the first time some outstanding programs have not been able to fill all of their open slots.

Probably the most significant figure in this group, to use to determine trends, is that of the filled first-year positions. This is true because of the long lag period that occurs in the reduction in the number of programs and individuals engaged in them. It requires about four years to discontinue a program and the full effect upon the number of Board-certified specialists will not appear until six to seven years after a first-year position has been created or eliminated. Reservations in the interpretation of these figures also must be made on the basis that many individuals may begin with general surgery and then transfer to a surgical specialty at a later date.

Concentrating upon the number of filled first-year positions, this number was 5,301 in 1970–71, 5,846 in 1973–74, and 5,653 in 1977–78. This is a decrease of 3% from the high level in 1973–74. These reductions, however, have been accomplished chiefly by the elimination of nonaffiliated programs.

There has been a marked difference between the various specialties in this respect. For example, in comparison with the figures of 1973–74 and those of 1977–78, urology has lost 43 residents, or 13%, otolaryngology 27, or 11%, orthopedic surgery 28, or 5%, ophthalmology 40, or 8%, neurological surgery 22, or 15%, general surgery 123, or 5%. Meanwhile there have been ten additional residencies filled in plastic surgery, 12 in thoracic surgery, 6 in colorectal surgery and 62 in obstetrics-gynecology. The rather spectacular expansion of plastic and thoracic programs that was evident prior to 1973–74 has been slowed. The reason for the increase of 6% in the

Ob-Gyn residents is not readily apparent, but the SOSSUS data clearly showed that in all regions of the country studied hysterectomies and obstetrical deliveries were two procedures most frequently performed by noncertified personnel. Possibly there was a need, which now is being filled.

In contrast to the number of first-year positions that are filled, the total positions that have been offered have increased from 17,060 in 1970–71 to 18,481 in 1973–74, to 20,106 in 1977–78. This is an increase of 18% from the 1970–71 figures. The percentage of positions offered in nonaffiliated hospitals has decreased from 18% of the total in 1970–71 to 6% in 1977–78.

In summary, if the total number of positions that are offered is considered, it will appear that there is a continuing expansion in numbers. However, if the first-year filled positions are considered, there are clear indications that this tendency has been reversed. However, this reversal is still modest.

5. The total number of Board-certified surgeons. In SOSSUS it was calculated that the needs of the country could be supplied by an output of 1,600 to 2,000 Board-certified individuals in surgery and surgical specialties per year through about 1985. Actually there were 3,621 certificates awarded in 1972 and 4,306 in 1976. At the later date there were 65,508 "active" certificates in surgery and surgical specialties. These numbers are far in excess of those recommended in SOSSUS.

Corrections need to be made for individuals who have qualified for more than one Board, and for those in government programs, teaching positions and administration. The number of persons actively in surgical practice in 1976 has been estimated to be 60,000.

If it is assumed that all of the individuals engaged today in the first-year programs will continue and become Board-certified, it is apparent that the total number of certificates issued in 1984 would be in the neighborhood of 5,653. The contrast between this figure and that suggested by SOSSUS is apparent.

* * *

In a final appraisal, the effects of SOSSUS have been enormous. Unfortunately there may be a tendency to judge the success or failure of the entire study by a single criterion, namely, whether or not the total number of Board-certified surgeons can be reduced to the figures suggested in the study. The most important recommendation, on the contrary, has been to continue the manpower studies and projections that need to be kept current at least for the next decade.

In this connection, the SOSSUS Report tabulated comparable data for the United States, as contrasted with countries in western Europe, and then with Canada, Australia, and New Zealand. The ratio of certified surgeons plus their residents in practice (the credentialled cohort, as it were) shows a population ratio in the United States that is 50%-100% higher than in most comparable countries, though there are spotty exceptions such as West Germany, Israel, and Scotland, all of which have high surgical ratios.

While surgical Board certification rates are still climbing slowly, there has been a large increase in numbers of internists, radiologists, anesthesiologists and family practitioners achieving certification and entering practice.

There are strong voices raised for and against the drastic reductions in the number of individuals certified by Boards and entering practice proposed by SOSSUS If medical students continue to prefer primary care rather than surgical residencies to the extent that they do in 1978, the total number of applicants for the first-year surgical positions shortly will be closer to 3,000 than the 5,653 that are filled at present. Most of the FMGs in training who now comprise 33% of the individuals in surgical programs will be phased out, and provided that program directors and residency review committees reduce the number of available slots rather than allowing them to be filled with individuals in nonsurgical programs, the number of persons in training could approach that recommended in SOSSUS in a very brief time.

Forces against this restriction include the chauvinistic demands of directors who wish to maintain large programs even in the face of inadequate clinical facilities, the increased number of extensive, time-consuming technical procedures such as those involved in vascular, cardiac, and micro-surgery, and the numerous problems that will arise with a sudden, sharp reduction in numbers of trainees. Furthermore, the low figure is based upon an almost ideal distribution of specialists and of access of patients to them. To this may be added the theoretical consideration that it might be better to have an excess of well-trained surgeons than to have surgical procedures performed by the untrained.

At any rate, SOSSUS started the discussion; it will continue for years to come. The importance of continuing studies, particularly of manpower requirements, cannot be overemphasized. For the public and for medicine and surgery a critical decade lies ahead.

The author extends thanks to the following for their helpful suggestions in preparation of the manuscript: Dr. James D. Hardy, Dr. Francis D. Moore, Dr. William H. Muller, Jr., Dr. David C. Sabiston, Jr., and Dr. George D. Zuidema.

Bibliography

1. *Surgery in the United States: A Summary Report of the Study on Surgical Services for the United States.* The American College of Surgeons and The American Surgical Association. The Short Form Report. Lewis Advertising Company, 1975.
2. *Surgery in the United States: A Report of the Study on Surgical Services for the United States.* The American College of Surgeons and The American Surgical Association. The Long Form Report. Lewis Advertising Company, 1976.
3. Hughes EFX, Fuchs VT, Jacobey FE, et al: Surgical work loads in a community practice. *Surgery* 71:315-327, 1972.
4. Nickerson RJ, Colton T, Peterson OL, et al: Doctors who perform operations. A study on in-hospital surgery in four diverse geographic areas. *N England J Med* 295:921-926 & 982-989, 1976.
5. Hauck WW, Bloom BS, McPherson CK, et al: Surgeons in the United States. Activities, output, and income. *JAMA* 236:1864-1871, 1976.
6. Moore FD, Boyden CM, Sabiston D, et al: The production, attrition, and biological life-time of surgeons in relation to the population of the United States: A look into the future through the clouded computer crystal. *Ann Surg* 176:457-468, 1972.
7. Moore FD: Manpower goals in American surgery. Implications for residency training. Future surgical manpower in the frame-work of total U.S. physicians. *Ann Surg* 184:125-144, 1976.
8. Moore FD, Nickerson RJ, Colton T, et al: National surgical work patterns as a basis for residency training plans. *Arch Surg* 112:125-147, 1977.
9. Hanlon CR: Testimony before Subcommittee on Oversight and Investigations, Committee on Interstate and Foreign Commerce, Washington, DC, Oct. 6, 1977. Pages 87 & 88 of transcript.
10. Haug JN: Misconceptions on surgical residency. *Bulletin of the American College of Surgeons* 61 (Sept.):6-12, 1976.
11. Moore FD, Zuidema GD, Ballinger WF: Surgical manpower and public policy. *Surgery* 83:116-120, 1978.
12. *Higher Education and the Nation's Health. Policies for Medical and Dental Education. A Special Report and Recommendations by the Carnegie Commission on Higher Education.* Hightstown, New Jersey, McGraw-Hill Book Company, 1970.

FELLOWS OF THE
AMERICAN SURGICAL ASSOCIATION

NAME	YEAR OF ELECTION	LOCATION AT TIME OF ELECTION	OFFICES AND YEAR HELD	YEAR OF DEATH
ABBE, ROBERT	1890	New York, New York	Vice-President-1902	1928
ABBOTT, LEROY CHARLES	1951	San Francisco, Calif.		1965
ABBOTT, WILLIAM EDWIN	1957	Cleveland, Ohio		1963
ABELL, IRVIN	1930	Louisville, Kentucky		1949
ABERDEEN, EOIN	1973	Philadelphia, Pa.		
ABRAMS, JEROME S.	1977	Burlington, Vermont		
ACKERMAN, NORMAN B.	1979	Syracuse, New York		
ADAMS, HERBERT DAN	1951	Boston, Massachusetts		
ADAMS, JAMES T.	1978	Rochester, New York		
ADAMS, WILLIAM E.	1943	Chicago, Illinois		1973
ADIE, GEORGE C.	1947	New Rochelle, New York		1976
ADKINS, PAUL CHARLES	1968	Washington, D.C.		
ADRIANI, JOHN	1955	New Orleans, Louisiana		
ADSON, ALFRED WASHINGTON	1933	Rochester, Minnesota		1951
ADSON, MARTIN A.	1977	Rochester, Minnesota		
AGNEW, D. HAYES	1882	Philadelphia, Pa.	President-1888	1892
ALEXANDER, EBEN, Jr.	1970	Winston-Salem, N.C.		
ALEXANDER, EMORY GRAHAM	1928	Philadelphia, Pa.		1930
ALEXANDER, JOHN	1935	Ann Arbor, Michigan		1954
ALEXANDER, J. WESLEY	1973	Cincinnati, Ohio		
ALLBRITTEN, FRANK F., Jr.	1950	Philadelphia, Pa.		
ALLEN, ARTHUR WILBURN	1929	Boston, Massachusetts		1958
ALLEN, DUDLEY P.	1894	Cleveland, Ohio	Secretary-1902–1906 President-1907	1915
ALLEN, HARVEY STUART	1948	Chicago, Illinois		1955
ALLEN, JOSEPH GARROTT	1952	Chicago, Illinois		
ALLEY, RALPH DAVID	1974	Albany, New York		
ALLIS, OSCAR HUNTINGTON	1890	Philadelphia, Pa.		1921
ALRICH, ELTON MEREDITH	1962	Charlottesville, Va.		
ALTEMEIER, WILLIAM A.	1947	Cincinnati, Ohio	Secretary-1958–1964 President-1970	
AMENDOLA, FREDERICK H.	1951	New York, New York		
ANDERSEN, MURRAY NOEL	1966	Buffalo, New York		
ANDERSON, MARION C.	1971	Toledo, Ohio		
ANDREWS, EDMUND	1882	Chicago, Illinois		Resigned?
ANDREWS, EDMUND	1929	Chicago, Illinois		?
ANDREWS, EDWARD WYLLYS	1902	Chicago, Illinois	Vice-President-1924	1927
ANDRUS, WILLIAM DeW.	1939	New York, New York		1951
ANKENEY, JAY LLOYD	1966	Cleveland, Ohio		
ANLYAN, WILLIAM GEORGE	1965	Durham, N.C.	Vice-President-1980	
ARCHIBALD, EDWARD W.	1916	Montreal, Canada	Vice-President-1926 President-1935	1945
ARMSTRONG, GEORGE E.	1901	Montreal, Canada	Vice-President-1911 President-1915	1933
ARTZ, CURTIS PRICE	1960	Jackson, Mississippi		1977
ASHHURST, ASTLEY P.C.	1913	Philadelphia, Pa.	Vice-President-1930	1932
ASHHURST, JOHN, Jr.	1880	Philadelphia, Pa.	Vice-President-1897	1900
AUFSES, ARTHUR H., Jr.	1977	New York, New York		
AUST, JOE BRADLEY, Jr.	1965	Minneapolis, Minnesota		
AUSTEN, WILLIAM GERALD	1967	Boston, Massachusetts	Secretary-1980	
AYCOCK, THOMAS BAYRON	1943	Baltimore, Maryland		1948
BADGLEY, CARL EGBERT	1947	Ann Arbor, Michigan		1973
BAHNSON, HENRY T.	1954	Baltimore, Maryland		
BAILEY, FRED WARREN	1922	St. Louis, Missouri		1964
BAIRD, RONALD JAMES	1969	Toronto, Canada		
BAKER, JOEL WILSON	1951	Seattle, Washington	Vice-President-1961	
BAKER, R. ROBINSON	1976	Baltimore, Maryland		

NAME	YEAR OF ELECTION	LOCATION AT TIME OF ELECTION	OFFICES AND YEAR HELD	YEAR OF DEATH
BAKER, ROBERT J.	1979	Chicago, Illinois		
BALCH, FRANKLIN G.	1920	Boston, Massachusetts		1958
BALCH, HENRY H.	1960	Washington, D.C.		
BALFOUR, DONALD CHURCH	1917	Rochester, Minnesota	Vice-President-1923	1963
BALLIN, MAX	1927	Detroit, Michigan		1934
BALLINGER, WALTER F., II	1965	Baltimore, Maryland	Treasurer-1976–1980	
BANCROFT, FREDERIC W.	1925	New York, New York		1963
BARKER, CLYDE F.	1977	Philadelphia, Pa.		
BARKER, HAROLD GRANT	1960	New York, New York		
BARKER, WILEY FRANKLIN	1964	Los Angeles, Calif.		
BARNER, HENDRICK BOYER	1976	St. Louis, Missouri		
BARNETT, WILLIAM OSCAR	1967	Jackson, Mississippi		
BARROW, DAVID	1906	Lexington, Kentucky		1932
BARTLETT, MARSHALL K.	1958	Boston, Massachusetts		
BARTON, JAMES M.	1882	Philadelphia, Pa.		1926
BATTERSBY, JAMES STANLEY	1967	Indianapolis, Indiana		
BAUE, ARTHUR E.	1971	St. Louis, Missouri		
BAXTER, CHARLES RUFUS	1973	Dallas, Texas		
BAXTER, GEORGE A.	1896	Chattanooga, Tennessee	Forfeited Membership 1903	
BAZIN, ALFRED T.	1926	Montreal, Canada		1958
BEAHRS, OLIVER H.	1967	Rochester, Minnesota	President-1979	
BEAL, JOHN MANN, JR.	1956	New York, New York		
BEATTIE, EDWARD J., JR.	1957	Chicago, Illinois		
BECK, CLAUDE S.	1934	Cleveland, Ohio		1971
BECK, WILLIAM CARL	1955	Sayre, Pa.		
BECKER, WALTER FRANCIS	1967	New Orleans, Louisiana		
BECKMAN, EMIL H.	1915	Rochester, Minnesota		1916
BEECHER, HENRY KNOWLES	1955	Boston, Massachusetts		1976
BEER, EDWIN	1924	New York, New York		1938
BELL, HENRY GLENN	1948	San Francisco, Calif.		
BELL, JAMES	1901	Montreal, Canada	Vice-President-1905	1910
BELZER, FOLKERT O.	1972	San Francisco, Calif.		
BENDER, HARVEY W., Jr.	1977	Nashville, Tennessee		
BENFIELD, JOHN R.	1975	Torrance, Calif.		
BENHAM, SILAS NELSON	1880	Pittsburg(h), Pa.		
BENNETT, GEORGE ELI	1943	Baltimore, Maryland		1962
BENNETT, JAMES E.	1975	Indianapolis, Indiana		
BENSON, CLIFFORD D.	1947	Detroit, Michigan		
BERGAN, JOHN	1974	Chicago, Illinois		
BERK, JAMES L.	1979	Bath, Ohio		
BERNARD, HARVEY ROLLAND	1971	Glenmont, New York		
BERNATZ, PHILIP E.	1975	Rochester, Minnesota		
BERNE, CLARENCE JOHN	1953	Los Angeles, Calif.	Vice-President-1976	
BERNHARD, WILLIAM F.	1970	Boston, Massachusetts		
BERNSTEIN, EUGENE F.	1976	San Diego, Calif.		
BERRY, FRANK BROWN	1940	New York, New York		1976
BESLEY, FREDERIC A.	1915	Chicago, Illinois		1944
BEST, R. RUSSELL	1946	Omaha, Nebraska		
BEVAN, ARTHUR D.	1900	Chicago, Illinois	President-1933	1943
BEYE, HAROLD LOMBARD	1931	Iowa City, Iowa		1936
BIGELOW, WILFRED GORDON	1955	Toronto, Canada		
BIGGER, ISAAC A.	1936	Richmond, Virginia		1955
BILL, ALEXANDER H., Jr.	1972	Seattle, Washington		
BILLINGS, ARTHUR E.	1927	Philadelphia, Pa.		1974
BINNEY, HORACE	1930	Boston, Massachusetts		1956
BINNIE, JOHN FAIRBAIRN	1901	Kansas City, Missouri	Vice-President-1908 Recorder 1916–1919 Vice-President-1920	1936

NAME	YEAR OF ELECTION	LOCATION AT TIME OF ELECTION	OFFICES AND YEAR HELD	YEAR OF DEATH
BIRTCH, ALAN G.	1975	Springfield, Illinois		
BISGARD, J. DEWEY	1938	Omaha, Nebraska		1975
BLACK, BENJAMIN MARDEN	1957	Rochester, Minnesota		
BLADES, BRIAN B.	1948	Washington, D.C.	Recorder 1953–1956 Vice-President-1957	1977
BLAIR, VILRAY P., Sr.	1918	St. Louis, Missouri		1955
BLAISDELL, FRANK W.	1968	San Francisco, Calif.		
BLAKE, JOHN BAPST	1906	Boston, Massachusetts		1943
BLAKE, JOSEPH A.	1902	New York, New York		1937
BLAKEMORE, ARTHUR H.	1946	New York, New York		1970
BLAKEMORE, WILLIAM S.	1964	Philadelphia, Pa.		
BLALOCK, ALFRED	1934	Nashville, Tennessee	President-1956	1964
BLOCK, GEORGE EDWARD	1970	Chicago, Illinois		
BLOCK, MELVIN AUGUST	1970	Detroit, Michigan		
BLOCKER, TRUMAN G., Jr.	1948	Galveston, Texas	Vice-President-1968	
BLOODGOOD, JOSEPH C.	1901	Baltimore, Maryland	Vice-President-1925	1935
BLOUNT, WALTER PUTMAN	1964	Milwaukee, Wisconsin		
BLUMENSTOCK, DAVID A.	1976	Cooperstown, New York		
BOHRER, JOHN VERNE	1940	New York, New York		1945
BOLAND, FRANK K.	1927	Atlanta, Georgia		1953
BOLLING, RICHARD W.	1927	New York, New York		1929
BONTECOU, REED B.	1882	Troy, New York		1906–07
BOSHER, LEWIS C.	1901	Richmond, Virginia		1920
BOTHE, FREDERICK A.	1944	Philadelphia, Pa.		1963
BOTTOMLEY, JOHN T.	1913	Boston, Massachusetts		1925
BOWERS, RALPH F.	1941	New York, New York		1969
BOYCE, WILLIAM HENRY	1969	Winston-Salem, N.C.		
BOYD, DAVID PRESTON	1969	Boston, Massachusetts		
BOYDEN, ALLEN MARSTON	1956	Portland, Oregon	Vice-President-1974	
BOZEMAN, NATHAN	1882	New York, New York	Resigned -1887	
BRAASCH, JOHN W.	1972	Boston, Massachusetts		
BRADFORD, EDWARD H.	1890	Boston, Massachusetts		1926
BRADSHAW, HOWARD HOLT	1949	Winston-Salem, N.C.		1969
BRAMBLE, D. D.	1880	Cincinnati, Ohio	Forfeited Membership -1893	
BRANCH, CHARLES DIGGES	1954	Peoria, Illinois		
BRANTIGAN, OTTO CHARLES	1951	Baltimore, Maryland		
BREWER, GEORGE E.	1900	New York, New York	Vice-President-1914 President-1920	1939
BREWER, LYMAN AUGUSTUS, III	1964	Los Angeles, Calif.		
BREWSTER, GEORGE W. W.	1917	Boston, Massachusetts		1939
BRICKER, EUGENE MYRON	1956	St. Louis, Missouri	Vice-President-1967	
BRIGGS, WILLIAM THOMPSON	1880	Nashville, Tennessee	Recorder-1881–1882 President-1885	1894
BRINDLEY, GEORGE V., Jr.	1968	Temple, Texas		
BRINSMADE, WILLIAM B.	1915	Brooklyn, New York		1943
BRINTON, JOHN H.	1880	Philadelphia, Pa.	Treasurer-1885–1886	1907
BRISTOW, ALGERNON T.	1906	Brooklyn, New York		1913
BROCK, HUGH W.	1880	Morgantown, W.Va.		1882
BROOKS, BARNEY	1925	Nashville, Tennessee	Vice-President-1939	1952
BROOKS, JOHN ROBINSON	1965	Boston, Massachusetts		
BROWDER, E. JEFFERSON	1943	Brooklyn, New York		1976
BROWN, ALFRED J.	1927	Omaha, Nebraska		1960
BROWN, HENRY P., Jr.	1929	Philadelphia, Pa.		1955
BROWN, IVAN WILLARD, Jr.	1959	Durham, N.C.		
BROWN, JAMES BARRETT	1940	St. Louis, Missouri		1971
BROWN, ROBERT BRUCE	1951	U.S.N., San Francisco, Calif.		1977
BRUCE, HERBERT A.	1911	Toronto, Canada		1963

NAME	YEAR OF ELECTION	LOCATION AT TIME OF ELECTION	OFFICES AND YEAR HELD	YEAR OF DEATH
BRUNN, HAROLD	1929	San Francisco, Calif.		1950
BRUNSCHWIG, ALEXANDER	1940	Chicago, Illinois		1969
BRUSH, BROCK EDWIN	1959	Detroit, Michigan		
BRYANT, JOSEPH D.	1895	New York, New York		1914
BRYANT, LESTER R.	1972	Lexington, Kentucky		
BUCHANAN, JOHN J.	1911	Pittsburg(h), Pa.		1937
BUCHWALD, HENRY	1976	Minneapolis, Minnesota		
BUCKBERG, GERALD D.	1977	Los Angeles, Calif.		
BUCKLEY, MORTIMER J.	1974	Boston, Massachusetts		
BUCY, PAUL C.	1949	Chicago, Illinois		
BULL, WM. TILLINGHAST	1882	New York, New York		1909
BUNNELL, STERLING	1948	San Francisco, Calif.		1957
BUNTS, FRANK E.	1900	Cleveland, Ohio	Vice-President-1915	1928
BURCH, JOHN C.	1941	Nashville, Tennessee	Treasurer 1956–1959	1977
BURDETTE, WALTER JAMES	1955	Columbia, Missouri		
BURDICK, CARL G.	1932	New York, New York		1946
BURFORD, THOMAS HANNAHAN	1950	St. Louis, Missouri		1977
BURKE, JOHN FRANCIS	1966	Boston, Massachusetts		
BURNETT, W. EMORY	1947	Philadelphia, Pa.		1979
BURRELL, HERBERT LESLIE	1893	Boston, Massachusetts	Secretary-1898–1901	1910
BUTCHER, HARVEY R., JR.	1961	St. Louis, Missouri		
BUXTON, ROBERT WILLIAM	1949	Ann Arbor, Michigan		1970
BYARS, LOUIS T.	1949	St. Louis, Missouri		1969
BYRD, BENJAMIN FRANKLIN, Jr.	1959	Nashville, Tennessee		
BYRD, WILLIAM ANDREW	1880	Quincy, Illinois		1887
BYRNE, JOHN JOSEPH	1964	Boston, Massachusetts		
CABELL, JAMES L.	1880	Charlottesville, Va.		1889
CABOT, ARTHUR T.	1889	Boston, Massachusetts		1912
CABOT, HUGH	1924	Ann Arbor, Michigan		1945
CALDWELL, FRED T., Jr.	1975	Little Rock, Arkansas		
CALDWELL, GUY A.	1944	New Orleans, Louisiana		
CALLAGHAN, JOHN CARTER	1966	Edmonton, Canada		
CALLOW, ALLEN DANA	1973	Boston, Massachusetts		
CAMERON, JOHN L.	1979	Baltimore, Maryland		
CAMISHION, RUDOLPH C.	1967	Philadelphia, Pa.		
CAMPBELL, ELDRIDGE HOUSTON, Jr.	1950	Albany, New York		1956
CAMPBELL, GILBERT S.	1960	Oklahoma City, Oklahoma		
CAMPBELL, HENRY FRASER	1880	Augusta, Georgia		1891
CAMPBELL, WILLIAM F.	1921	Brooklyn, New York		1926
CANNON, BRADFORD	1949	Boston, Massachusetts		
CANNON, JACK A.	1959	Los Angeles, Calif.		
CANTRELL, JAMES RANDALL	1964	Seattle, Washington		
CAREY, LARRY C.	1972	Pittsburgh, Pa.		
CARMALT, WILLIAM H.	1885	New Haven, Connecticut	Vice-President-1896 President-1908	1929
CARON, WILFRED-MICHEL	1966	Quebec, Canada		1971
CARREL, ALEXIS	1909	New York, New York	Vice-President-1920	1944
CARSON, NORMAN BRUCE	1896	St. Louis, Missouri	Vice-President-1903	1931
CARTER, BURR NOLAND	1935	Cincinnati, Ohio	Vice-President-1950 Treasurer 1951–1955	
CASTANEDA, ALDO R.	1971	Boston, Massachusetts		
CASWELL, H. TAYLOR	1966	Philadelphia, Pa.		
CATTELL, RICHARD B.	1940	Boston, Massachusetts		1964
CAVE, HENRY WISDOM	1934	New York, New York		1964
CERILLI, JAMES	1975	Columbus, Ohio		
CHAFFIN, LAWRENCE G.	1946	Los Angeles, Calif.	Vice-President-1954 Vice-President-1966	

NAME	YEAR OF ELECTION	LOCATION AT TIME OF ELECTION	OFFICES AND YEAR HELD	YEAR OF DEATH
CHANDLER, LOREN R.	1947	San Francisco, Calif.		
CHASE, ROBERT ARTHUR	1965	Palo Alto, Calif.		
CHEEVER, DAVID	1922	Boston, Massachusetts	Vice-President-1935 President-1941	1955
CHEEVER, DAVID WILLIAMS	1882	Boston, Massachusetts	President-1889	1915
CHILD, CHARLES GARDNER, III	1949	New York, New York		
CHRISTOPHER, FREDERICK	1942	Evanston, Illinois		1967
CHURCHILL, EDWARD D.	1932	Boston, Massachusetts	President-1947	1972
CLAGETT, O. THERON	1949	Rochester, Minnesota		
CLARK, DWIGHT E.	1949	Chicago, Illinois		1959
CLARK, EDMUND D.	1926	Indianapolis, Indiana		1937
CLARK, RANDOLPH LEE	1973	Houston, Texas		
CLARK, RICHARD E.	1978	St. Louis, Missouri		
CLARKE, JAMES SPENCER	1965	Albuquerque, New Mexico		1976
CLATWORTHY, H. WILLIAM, Jr.	1960	Columbus, Ohio		
CLEVELAND, RICHARD J.	1975	Boston, Massachusetts		
CLINE, JOHN WESLEY	1967	San Francisco, Calif.		1974
CLINTON, MARSHALL	1920	Buffalo, New York		1943
CLOPTON, MALVERN B.	1920	St. Louis, Missouri		1947
CLOWES, GEORGE H.A., Jr.	1963	Charleston, S.C.		
CLUTE, HOWARD M.	1939	Boston, Massachusetts		1946
CODMAN, ERNEST AMORY	1916	Boston, Massachusetts		1940
COFFEY, ROBERT JAMES	1956	Washington, D.C.		
COHN, ISIDORE, Jr.	1960	New Orleans, La.		
COHN, ROY BARNETT	1957	San Francisco, Calif.		
COLCOCK, BENTLEY P.	1956	Boston, Massachusetts	Vice-President-1969	
COLE, CHARLES KNOX	1896	Helena, Montana		1920
COLE, JACK WESTLEY	1961	Cleveland, Ohio	Recorder-1973–1976	
COLE, RICHARD BEVERLY	1881	San Francisco, Calif.	Forfeited Membership -1887–88	
COLE, WARREN HENRY	1937	Chicago, Illinois	Vice-President-1948 President-1960	
COLEMAN, JOHN SCOTT	1880	Augusta, Georgia	Resigned -1890	
COLEY, BRADLEY L.	1939	New York, New York		1961
COLEY, WILLIAM B.	1898	New York, New York		1936
COLLER, FREDERICK A.	1928	Ann Arbor, Michigan	President-1944	1964
COLLINS, JOHN A.	1974	St. Louis, Missouri		
COLLINS, JOHN J., Jr.	1975	Boston, Massachusetts		
COLP, RALPH	1936	New York, New York		1974
COMINGOR, JOHN A.	1882	Indianapolis, Indiana	Forfeited Membership -1893	
CONDON, ROBERT EDWARD	1971	Milwaukee, Wisconsin		
CONNER, PHINEAS SANBORN	1880	Cincinnati, Ohio	Treasurer-1887–1891 President-1892	1909
CONNORS, JOHN F.	1922	New York, New York		1935
CONNOLLY, JOHN EARLE	1964	Palo Alto, Calif.		
CONWAY, HERBERT	1953	New York, New York		1969
COOLEY, DENTON ARTHUR	1955	Houston, Texas		
COON, WILLIAM W.	1977	Ann Arbor, Michigan		
COOPER, FREDERICK W., Jr.	1950	Atlanta, Georgia		1961
COPE, OLIVER	1943	Boston, Massachusetts	Vice-President-1957 President-1963	
COPHER, GLOVER H.	1930	St. Louis, Missouri		1970
CORDELL, ALFRED ROBERT	1964	Winston-Salem, N.C.		
COTTON, FREDERICK J.	1914	Brooklyn, Massachusetts		1938
COUNSELLER, VIRGIL S.	1939	Rochester, Minnesota	Vice-President-1964	1977
COWAN, JOHN F.	1927	San Francisco, Calif		1929
COWLEY, R. ADAMS	1972	Baltimore, Maryland		

NAME	YEAR OF ELECTION	LOCATION AT TIME OF ELECTION	OFFICES AND YEAR HELD	YEAR OF DEATH
CRAIG, WINCHELL McK.	1941	Rochester, Minnesota		1960
CRAWFORD, ERNEST STANLEY	1962	Houston, Texas		
CREECH, OSCAR, Jr.	1957	New Orleans, Louisiana	President-1967	1967
CRILE, GEORGE, Jr.	1950	Cleveland, Ohio		
CRILE, GEORGE W.	1905	Cleveland, Ohio	Vice-President-1912 and 1919	1943
			President-1924	
CROSS, FREDERICK S.	1971	Cleveland, Ohio		
CULBERTSON, WILLIAM R.	1962	Cincinnati, Ohio		
CUNNINGHAM, FRANCIS D.	1882	Richmond, Virginia		1885
CURRERI, ANTHONY R.	1950	Madison, Wisconsin		
CURTIS, BENJAMIN F.	1896	New York, New York	Resigned -1910	
CURTIS, GEORGE MORRIS	1935	Columbus, Ohio		1965
CUSHING, HARVEY	1906	Baltimore, Maryland	President-1927	1939
CUSHING, HAYWARD W.	1896	Boston, Massachusetts		1934
CUTLER, CONDICT W., Jr.	1942	New York, New York		1958
CUTLER, ELLIOTT CARR	1925	Cleveland, Ohio	President Elect-1948 died Aug. 1947	1947
DaCOSTA, JOHN CHALMERS	1897	Philadelphia, Pa.		1933
DAGGETT, WILLARD M., Jr.	1976	Boston, Massachusetts		
DALE, WILLIAM ANDREW	1966	Nashville, Tennessee		
DANDRIDGE, NATHANIEL P.	1883	Cincinnati, Ohio	Treasurer-1895–1898 President-1904	1910
DANDY, WALTER EDWARD	1925	Baltimore, Maryland		1946
DANIEL, ROLLIN A., Jr.	1948	Nashville, Tennessee		1978
DARIN, JOSEPH C.	1974	Milwaukee, Wisconsin		
DARLING, R. CLEMENT, Jr.	1978	Boston, Massachusetts		
DARRACH, WILLIAM	1917	New York, New York	President-1945–1946	1948
DasGUPTA, TAPAS K.	1976	Chicago, Illinois		
DAVID, VERNON, C.	1923	Chicago, Illinois	Secretary-1932–1936 Vice-President-1938 President-1943	1961
DAVIS, CARL BRADON	1916	Chicago, Illinois		1950
DAVIS, GWILYM G.	1909	Philadelphia, Pa.		1918
DAVIS, HERBERT H.	1949	Omaha, Nebraska		
DAVIS, JOHN HERSCHEL	1967	Cleveland, Ohio		
DAVIS, JOHN STAIGE	1882	Charlottesville, Va.		1885
DAVIS, JOHN STAIGE, Jr.	1917	Baltimore, Maryland	Vice-President-1940	1946
DAVIS, LINCOLN L.	1919	Boston, Massachusetts	Secretary-1928–1931 Vice-President-1932	?
DAVIS, LOYAL	1933	Chicago, Illinois	Vice-President-1942 President-1957	
DAVIS, SAMUEL T.	1880	Lancaster, Pa.		1890
DAVIS, WILLIAM CLAYTON	1972	Omaha, Nebraska		
DAWSON, WILLIAM WIRT	1880	Cincinnati, Ohio	Vice-President-1884	1893
DEAVER, HARRY C.	1912	Philadelphia, Pa.		1931
DEAVER, JOHN B.	1892	Philadelphia, Pa.	Vice-President-1918	1931
DEAVER, JOSHUA M.	1943	Philadelphia, Pa.		1978
DeBAKEY, MICHAEL E.	1946	New Orleans, Louisiana		
DeCOSSE, JEROME J.	1970	Milwaukee, Wisconsin		
DELANEY, JOHN PATRICK	1978	Minneapolis, Minnesota		
DELATOUR, HENRY B.	1910	Brooklyn, New York		1930
DelGUERCIO, LOUIS R.M.	1970	Livingston, New Jersey		
DeMUTH, WILLIAM E., Jr.	1974	Hershey, Pa.		
DenBESTEN, LAWRENCE	1979	Los Angeles, Calif.		
DENNIS, CLARENCE	1946	St. Paul, Minnesota	Vice-President-1972	
DENNIS, FREDERIC S.	1882	New York, New York	Vice-President-1888 President-1895	1934

NAME	YEAR OF ELECTION	LOCATION AT TIME OF ELECTION	OFFICES AND YEAR HELD	YEAR OF DEATH
DePALMA, RALPH G.	1978	Cleveland, Ohio		
DERRICK, JOHN RAFTER	1966	Galveston, Texas		
DETERLING, RALPH A., Jr.	1960	Boston, Massachusetts		
DETMOLD, WILLIAM	1882	New York, New York	Resigned -1888	
DeWEESE, JAMES ARVILLE	1967	Rochester, New York		
DeWESSE, MARION SPENCER	1965	Columbia, Missouri		
DICKSON, FRANKLIN D.	1942	Kansas City, Missouri		1964
DIETHELEM, ARNOLD G.	1978	Birmingham, Alabama		
DILLARD, DAVID HUGH	1970	Ann Arbor, Michigan		
DINEEN, P. A. PETER	1971	New York, New York		
DINGMAN, REED OTHELBERT	1966	Ann Arbor, Michigan		
DINSMORE, ROBERT SCOTT	1935	Cleveland, Ohio	President-1953	1957
DIXON, CLAUDE FRANK	1936	Rochester, Minnesota		1968
DOBELL, ANTHONY R. C.	1970	Montreal, Canada		
DOBYNS, BROWN McI.	1960	Cleveland, Ohio		
DONALD, JOSEPH MARION	1953	Birmingham, Alabama		1961
DONALDSON, GORDON A.	1964	Boston, Massachusetts		
DONOVAN, ARTHUR J.	1975	Pasadena, Calif.		
DONOVAN, EDWARD JOSEPH	1936	New York, New York		1970
DORSEY, JOHN MICHAEL	1954	Evanston, Illinois		
DOUGLAS, JOHN	1924	New York, New York		1938
DOUGLASS, THOMAS CARTER	1953	Chicago, Illinois		?
DOWD, CHARLES N.	1910	New York, New York		1931
DOWNES, WILLIAM A.	1914	New York, New York		1948
DRAGSTEDT, LESTER R.	1934	Chicago, Illinois		1975
DRAKE, CHARLES G.	1977	London, Canada		
DRAPANAS, THEODORE	1964	Pittsburgh, Pa.		1975
DRENNEN, WESLEY EARLE	1924	Birmingham, Alabama		1957
DRIPPS, ROBERT DUNNING	1955	Philadelphia, Pa.		1974
DRUCKER, WILLIAM R.	1965	Cleveland, Ohio		
DUBÈ, EDMOND	1949	Montreal, Canada		1960
DUDRICK, STANLEY JOHN	1973	Houston, Texas		
DUGAN, DAVID, J.	1978	Oakland, Calif.		
DUGAS, LOUIS ALEXANDER	1880	Augusta, Georgia	Vice-President-1881–1882	1884
DUMONT, ALLAN E.	1967	New York, New York		
DUNLOP, GEORGE R.	1968	Worcester, Massachusetts		
DUNN, JAMES H.	1899	Minneapolis, Minnesota		1904
DUNOTT, THOMAS JUSTUS	1882	Harrisburg, Pa.		1893
DUNPHY, JOHN ENGLEBERT	1950	Boston, Massachusetts	Recorder-1957–1961 President-1962	
DuVAL, MERLIN K., Jr.	1961	Oklahoma City, Oklahoma		
EASTMAN, JOSEPH RILUS	1919	Indianapolis, Indiana		1942
EBERT, PAUL ALLEN	1971	New York, New York		
EBERTS, EDWARD MELCHOIR	1925	Montreal, Canada		1945
ECKERT, CHARLES	1958	Albany, New York		
ECONOMOU, STEVEN G.	1967	Chicago, Illinois		
EDGERTON, MILTON T., Jr.	1962	Baltimore, Maryland		
EDMUNDS, LOUIS H., Jr.	1974	Philadelphia, Pa.		
EDWARDS, CHARLES R.	1939	Baltimore, Maryland		1965
EDWARDS, WILLIAM S.	1964	Birmingham, Alabama		
EFFLER, DONALD B.	1959	Cleveland, Ohio		
EGDAHL, RICHARD H.	1963	Richmond, Virginia		
EGGERS, CARL	1930	New York, New York		1956
EHRENHAFT, JOHANN L.	1964	Iowa City, Iowa		
EISEMAN, BEN	1958	Denver, Colorado		
EISENBERG, M. MICHAEL	1974	Minneapolis, Minnesota		
ELIASON, ELDRIDGE E.	1926	Philadelphia, Pa.		1950

NAME	YEAR OF ELECTION	LOCATION AT TIME OF ELECTION	OFFICES AND YEAR HELD	YEAR OF DEATH
ELIOT, ELLSWORTH, Jr.	1901	New York, New York	Vice-President-1923 President-1929	1945
ELKIN, DANIEL COLLIER	1935	Atlanta, Georgia	Vice-President-1942 President-1952	1958
ELKINS, RONALD CHARLES	1979	Oklahoma City, Oklahoma		
ELLIOTT, JOHN WHEELOCK	1893	Boston, Massachusetts		1925
ELLIOT, DANIEL W.	1963	Columbus, Ohio		
ELLIS, FRANKLIN H., Jr.	1965	Rochester, Minnesota		
ELLISON, EDWIN H.	1957	Columbus, Ohio		
ELLISON, ROBERT G.	1967	Augusta, Georgia		1970
ELMAN, ROBERT	1938	St. Louis, Missouri		1956
ELOESSER, LEO	1936	San Francisco, Calif.		1976
ELTING, ARTHUR W.	1911	Albany, New York	Vice-President-1936 President-1938	1948
EMMETT, JOHN M. M.	1950	Clifton Forge, Virginia		1969
ENQUIST, IRVING F.	1966	Brooklyn, New York		
ERDMAN, SEWARD	1926	New York, New York	Vice-President-1939	1966
ESTES, WILLIAM L.	1896	South Bethlehem, Pa.		1940
ESTES, WILLIAM L., Jr.	1927	Bethlehem, Pa.		1971
EVANS, EVERETT IDRIS	1947	Richmond, Virginia		1954
EVE, DUNCAN	1898	Nashville, Tennessee		1937
EVERSON, TILDEN C.	1960	Chicago, Illinois		
FALLIS, LAURENCE S.	1944	Detroit, Michigan		1974
FARRIS, JACK MATTHEWS	1951	Los Angeles, Calif.		
FAXON, HENRY HARDWICK	1954	Brookline, Mass.		1976
FELL, EGBERT H.	1944	Chicago, Illinois		
FENGER, CHRISTIAN	1883	Chicago, Illinois	Vice-President-1896	1902
FERGUSON, ALEXANDER H.	1901	Chicago, Illinois		1911
FERGUSON, COLIN CAMPBELL	1964	Winnipeg, Canada		
FERGUSON, DONALD JOHN	1962	Chicago, Illinois		
FERGUSON, LEWIS KRAEER	1940	Penn Valley, Pa.		1968
FERGUSON, THOMAS B.	1975	St Louis, Missouri		
FIFIELD, WILLIAM C.B.	1882	Boston, Massachusetts		Resigned -1888
FINE, JACOB	1941	Boston, Massachusetts		
FINNEY, GEORGE G.	1947	Baltimore, Maryland		
FINNEY, JOHN M. T.	1899	Baltimore, Maryland	Vice-President-1910 President-1922	1942
FINNEY, JOHN M. T., Jr.	1932	Baltimore, Maryland		1969
FIROR, WARFIELD MONROE	1937	Baltimore, Maryland	Secretary-1943–1948 Vice-President-1951 President-1964	
FISH, JAY C.	1975	Galveston, Texas		
FISHER, BERNARD	1963	Pittsburgh, Pa.		
FISHER, WILLIAM A., Jr.	1921	Baltimore, Maryland		1956
FITTS, CHARLES T.	1977	Charleston, S.C.		
FITTS, WILLIAM T., Jr.	1954	Philadelphia, Pa.		
FITZGERALD, RALPH R.	1943	Montreal, Canada		1956
FITZPATRICK, HUGH F.	1978	Tenafly, New Jersey		
FLETCHER, WILLIAM S.	1979	Portland, Oregon		
FLICK, JOHN B.	1933	Philadelphia, Pa.		1979
FLINT, JOSEPH MARSHALL	1915	New Haven, Connecticut	Forfeited Membership -1923	
FLOCKS, RUBIN H.	1969	Iowa City, Iowa		1975
FOLKMAN, MOSES JUDAH	1969	Boston, Massachusetts		
FONKALSRUD, ERIC WALTER	1971	Los Angeles, Calif.		
FOOTE, MERRILL NEWTON	1965	Brooklyn Heights, N.Y.		
FORBES, WILLIAM SMITH	1882	Philadelphia, Pa.		1905
FORTNER, JOSEPH GERALD	1973	New York, New York		
FOSS, HAROLD L.	1929	Danville, Pa.		1967

NAME	YEAR OF ELECTION	LOCATION AT TIME OF ELECTION	OFFICES AND YEAR HELD	YEAR OF DEATH
FOSTER, JAMES H.	1975	Hartford, Connecticut		
FOSTER, JOHN HOSKINS	1965	Nashville, Tennessee		
FOSTER, JOHN M.	1942	Denver, Colorado	Vice-President-1951	
FOWLER, GEORGE RYERSON	1891	Brooklyn, New York	Treasurer-1898–1906	1906
FRANK, HOWARD ALVIN	1955	Boston, Massachusetts		
FRAZIER, CHARLES H.	1904	Boston, Massachusetts		
FREEARK, ROBERT JAMES	1973	Maywood, Illinois		1936
FREEMAN, LEONARD	1898	Denver, Colorado	Vice-President-1909	1935
FREEMAN, NORMAN E.	1940	Philadelphia, Pa.		1975
FRENCH, LYLE A.	1967	Minneapolis, Minnesota		
FRIESEN, STANLEY R.	1954	Kansas City, Kansas		
FRY, WILLIAM JAMES	1969	Ann Arbor, Michigan		
FRYER, MINOT PACKER	1968	St. Louis, Missouri		
GAGE, HOMER	1910	Worcester, Massachusetts	Vice-President-1924	1938
GAGE, IDYS MIMS	1941	New Orleans, Louisiana		1957
GAGNON, EDOUARD D.	1958	Montreal, Canada		1975
GALE, JOSEPH W.	1939	Madison, Wisconsin		1968
GALLIE, WILLIAM EDWARD	1922	Toronto, Canada	Vice-President-1936 and 1948 President-1948	1959
GANN, DONALD S.	1977	Baltimore, Maryland		
GARDNER, CLARENCE E., Jr.	1949	Durham, N.C.	Vice-President-1965	
GASPAR, MAX RAYMOND	1974	Long Beach, Calif.		
GASTON, JAMES McFADDEN	1893	Atlanta, Georgia	Vice-President-1898	1903
GATCH, WILLIS D.	1934	Indianapolis, Indiana		1962
GATEWOOD	1929	Chicago, Illinois		1939
GAUB, OTTO CARL	1919	Pittsburgh, Pa.		1941
GAY, GEORGE WASHINGTON	1882	Boston, Massachusetts		1931
GERBODE, FRANK LEVEN A.	1951	San Francisco, Calif.	Vice-President-1963	
GERRISH, EDWIN W.	1979	Chicago, Illinois		
GERRISH, FREDERIC H.	1892	Portland, Maine		1920
GERSTER, ARPAD G.	1890	New York, New York	Vice-President-1909 President-1912	1923
GERWIG, WALTER H., Jr.	1955	Washington, D.C.		
GHORMLEY, RALPH K.	1950	Rochester, Minnesota		1959
GIBBON, JOHN H., Jr.	1940	Philadelphia, Pa.	Recorder-1947–1952 Vice-President-1953 President-1955	1973
GIBBON, JOHN H., Sr.	1906	Philadelphia, Pa.	Secretary-1916–1922 President-1926	1956
GIBSON, CHARLES L.	1906	New York, New York	Treasurer-1913–1915 Vice-President-1916	1944
GILCHRIST, RICHARD K.	1941	Chicago, Illinois	Vice-President-1953 Secretary-1954–1957 Vice-President-1958	
GLENN, FRANK	1942	New York, New York		
GLENN, JAMES FRANCIS	1976	Durham, N.C.		
GLENN, WILLIAM W. L.	1961	New Haven, Connecticut		
GLIEDMAN, MARVIN L.	1970	Bronx, New York		
GLOVER, DONALD M.	1946	Cleveland, Ohio	Vice-President-1955	
GOETSCH, EMIL	1928	Brooklyn, New York		1963
GOLDMAN, LEON	1950	San Francisco, Calif.	Vice-President-1969	1975
GOODE, JOHN V.	1949	Dallas, Texas		
GOODWIN, WILLARD E.	1961	Los Angeles, Calif.		
GOTT, VINCENT LYNN	1968	Baltimore, Maryland		
GOULEY, JOHN W. S.	1880	New York, New York	Vice-President-1887	Forfeited Membership 1890
GRACE, JAMES THOMAS, Jr.	1966	Buffalo, New York		1971

NAME	YEAR OF ELECTION	LOCATION AT TIME OF ELECTION	OFFICES AND YEAR HELD	YEAR OF DEATH
GRACE, RODERICK V.	1934	New York, New York		?
GRAHAM, A. STEPHENS	1947	Richmond, Virginia		
GRAHAM, EVARTS A.	1920	St. Louis, Missouri	President-1937	1957
GRAHAM, HENRY F.	1933	Brooklyn, New York		1958
GRAHAM, ROSCOE R.	1932	Toronto, Canada	Vice-President-1941	1948
GRAMLICH, JOHN B.	1977	Cheyenne, Wyoming		
GRANT, FRANCIS C.	1936	Philadelphia, Pa.		1967
GRAY, HOWARD K.	1943	Rochester, Minnesota		1955
GRAYHACK, JOHN T.	1977	Chicago, Illinois		
GREELEY, PAUL WEBB	1949	Chicago, Illinois		
GREENE, W. WARREN	1880	Portland, Maine		1881
GREENFIELD, LAZAR J.	1972	Oklahoma City, Oklahoma		
GREENOUGH, ROBERT B.	1911	Boston, Massachusetts	Secretary-1923–1927 Vice-President-1928	1937
GREGORY, ELISHA H.	1882	St. Louis, Missouri	Vice-President-1885	Resigned 1893
GRIFFEN, WARD O., Jr.	1968	Lexington, Kentucky		
GRILLO, HERMES C.	1968	Boston, Massachusetts		
GRIMES, ORVILLE F.	1955	San Francisco, Calif.		
GRIMSON, KEITH S.	1950	Durham, N.C.		
GRISWOLD, RETTIG A., Sr.	1941	Louisville, Kentucky		1972
GROSS, ROBERT E.	1948	Boston, Massachusetts		
GROSS, SAMUEL DAVID	1880	Philadelphia, Pa.	President-1881–1883	1884
GROSS, SAMUEL WEISSEL	1880	Philadelphia, Pa.		1889
GROSSI, CARLO EUGENE	1973	New York, New York		
GROVE, WILLIAM J.	1961	Chicago, Illinois		
GUERRY, LeGRAND	1922	Columbia, S.C.	Vice-President-1934	1947
GUNN, MOSES	1880	Chicago, Illinois	Vice-President-1883 President-1886	1887
GURD, FRASER B.	1934	Montreal, Canada		1948
GURD, FRASER N.	1963	Montreal, Canada	Vice-President-1975	
GUTELIUS, JOHN R.	1973	Saskatoon, Canada		
GUTHRIE, DONALD	1924	Sayre, Pa.		1958
GUTHRIE, GEORGE W.	1908	Wilkes Barre, Pa.		1915
HABIF, DAVID VALENTINE	1954	New York, New York		
HAGGARD, WILLIAM D.	1916	Nashville, Tennessee		1940
HAIGHT, CAMERON	1942	Ann Arbor, Michigan		1970
HALASZ, NICHOLAS ALEXIS	1969	San Diego, California		
HALGRIMSON, CHARLES G.	1978	Denver, Colorado		
HALLENBECK, GEORGE A.	1958	Rochester, Minnesota		
HALLER, J. ALEX, Jr.	1969	Baltimore, Maryland		
HALLMAN, GRADY L., Jr.	1971	Houston, Texas		
HALSTEAD, ALBERT E.	1909	Chicago, Illinois		1926
HALSTED, WILLIAM S.	1892	Baltimore, Maryland	Vice-President-1914	1922
HAMANN, CARL A.	1907	Cleveland, Ohio	Vice-President-1930	1930
HAMM, WILLIAM GIDEON	1950	Atlanta, Georgia		
HAMPSON, LAWRENCE GARTH	1973	Montreal, Canada		
HANLON, CYRIL ROLLINS	1952	St. Louis, Missouri	Secretary-1969	
HARBISON, SAMUEL POLLOCK	1951	Pittsburgh, Pa.		1976
HARDIN, CREIGHTON, A.	1963	Kansas City, Kansas		
HARDY, JAMES DANIEL	1956	Jackson, Mississippi	President-1976	
HARKINS, HENRY N.	1948	Baltimore, Maryland	Vice-President-1958	1967
HARPER, PAUL VINCENT	1962	Chicago, Illinois		Resigned?
HARRINGTON, FRANCIS B.	1898	Boston, Massachusetts	Vice-President-1913	1914
HARRINGTON, STUART W.	1931	Rochester, Minnesota	Vice-President-1956	1973
HARRIS, MALCOLM L.	1900	Chicago, Illinois		1936
HARRIS, ROBERT I.	1936	Toronto, Canada		1966

NAME	YEAR OF ELECTION	LOCATION AT TIME OF ELECTION	OFFICES AND YEAR HELD	YEAR OF DEATH
HARRISON, JOHN HARTWELL	1955	Boston, Massachusetts	Vice-President-1971	
HARRISON, ROBERT CAMERON	1963	Edmonton, Canada		
HARRISON, TIMOTHY S.	1970	Ann Arbor, Michigan		
HART, JULIAN DERYL	1938	Durham, North Carolina		
HARTE, RICHARD H.	1895	Philadelphia, Pa.	Recorder-1902–1910 President-1911	1925
HARTWELL, JOHN A.	1916	New York, New York		1940
HARTZELL, JOHN BERRY	1949	Detroit, Michigan		1970
HARVEY, HAROLD D.	1949	New York, New York		1973
HARVEY, SAMUEL CLARK	1926	New Haven, Connecticut	President-1951	1953
HATCHER, CHARLES R., Jr.	1973	Atlanta, Georgia		
HAWTHORNE, HERBERT REID	1952	Philadelphia, Pa.		
HAYES, MARK ALLAN	1957	New Haven, Connecticut		
HAYNES, BOYD W., Jr.	1964	Richmond, Virginia		
HEARN, W. JOSEPH	1898	Philadelphia, Pa.		1917
HEATON, LEONARD DUDLEY	1956	Washington, D.C.	Vice-President-1970	
HEDBLOM, CARL A.	1928	Chicago, Illinois		1934
HEGNER, CASPER FRANK	1929	Denver, Colorado		1960
HEIMBECKER, RAYMOND O.	1968	Toronto, Canada		
HEINBECKER, PETER	1937	St. Louis, Missouri		1967
HELMSWORTH, JAMES A.	1963	Cincinnati, Ohio		
HENDREN, WILLIAM H., III	1973	Boston, Massachusetts		
HERMANN, ROBERT E.	1972	Cleveland, Ohio		
HERNDON, CHARLES H.	1969	Cleveland, Ohio		
HERRINGTON, JOHN L., Jr.	1967	Nashville, Tennessee		
HERRMANN, LOUIS G.	1941	Cincinnati, Ohio		1965
HERTER, FREDERIC P.	1972	New York, New York		
HEUER, GEORGE J.	1922	Cincinnati, Ohio		1950
HEWSON, ADDINELL	1882	Philadelphia, Pa.	Forfeited Membership 1887-88	
HIATT, ROBERT BURRITT	1964	New York, New York		
HICKEY, ROBERT C.	1967	Houston, Texas		
HILL, LUCIUS DAVIS, III	1966	Seattle, Washington		
HINMAN, FRANK, Jr.	1967	San Francisco, Calif.		
HINSHAW, DAVID BURDG	1971	Loma Linda, Calif.		
HINTON, JAMES WILLIAMS	1948	New York, New York		1973
HITCHCOCK, CLAUDE R.	1969	Minneapolis, Minnesota		
HITZROT, JAMES MORLEY	1922	New York, New York		1963
HODGE, EDWARD B.	1918	Philadelphia, Pa.		1945
HODGE, H. LENOX	1880	Philadelphia, Pa.		1881
HODGEN, JOHN T.	1880	St. Louis, Missouri		1882
HODGES, R.M.	1882	Boston, Massachusetts		Resigned?
HOERR, STANLEY OBERMANN	1954	Cleveland, Ohio		
HOLDEN, WILLIAM DOUGLAS	1951	Cleveland, Ohio	Treasurer-1966–1970 President-1971	
HOLDER, THOMAS M.	1972	Kansas City, Missouri		
HOLLENBERG, HENRY G.	1949	Little Rock, Arkansas		
HOLMAN, CRANSTON W.	1947	New York, New York		
HOLMAN, EMILE F.	1939	San Francisco, Calif.	Vice-President-1949	1977
HOMANS, JOHN	1889	Boston, Massachusetts		1903
HOMANS, JOHN	1923	Boston, Massachusetts	Vice-President-1938	1954
HOOK, FREDERICK R.	1943	Oakland, Calif.		1955
HOPKINS, ROBERT WEST	1975	Providence, Rhode Island		
HORRAX, GILBERT	1936	Boston, Massachusetts		1957
HORSLEY, GUY WINSTON	1950	Richmond, Virginia		1967
HORSLEY, JOHN SHELTON	1924	Richmond, Virginia		1946
HORSLEY, JOHN SHELTON, III	1975	Charlottesville, Virginia		
HORWITZ, ORVILLE	1899	Philadelphia, Pa.		1913

NAME	YEAR OF ELECTION	LOCATION AT TIME OF ELECTION	OFFICES AND YEAR HELD	YEAR OF DEATH
HOTCHKISS, LUCIUS W.	1909	New York, New York		1926
HOXWORTH, PAUL IRWIN	1953	Cincinnati, Ohio		1973
HOWARD, JOHN MALONE	1960	Philadelphia, Pa.		
HUBAY, CHARLES ALFRED	1964	Cleveland, Ohio		
HUBBARD, JOSHUA CLAPP	1918	Boston, Massachusetts		1934
HUFNAGAL, CHARLES A.	1956	Washington, D.C.		
HUGGINS, CHARLES BRENTON	1937	Chicago, Illinois		
HUGHES, CARL WILSON	1969	Washington, D.C.		
HUGHES, J.C.	1880	Keokuk, Iowa		1881
HUME, DAVID M.	1957	Richmond, Virginia		1973
HUMMEL, ROBERT PAUL	1974	Cincinnati, Ohio		
HUMPHREY, EDWARD W.	1973	Minneapolis, Minnesotta		
HUMPHREY, LOREN J.	1972	Kansas City, Kansas		
HUMPHREYS, GEORGE H., II	1947	New York, New York		
HUMPHREYS, JAMES W., Jr.	1974	Philadelphia, Pa.		
HUN, HENRY H.	1938	Albany, New York		1972
HUNT, THOMAS K.	1972	San Francisco, Calif.		
HUNT, VERNE C.	1938	Los Angeles, Calif.		1943
HUNTINGTON, THOMAS W.	1901	San Francisco, Calif.	Vice-President-1907 President-1918	1929
HUPP, FRANK LeMOYNE	1919	Wheeling, West Virginia		1929
HURWITT, ELLIOTT SAMUEL	1956	New York, New York		1966
HURWITZ, ALFRED	1964	Portland, Maine		
HUTCHINSON, JAMES A.	1913	Montreal, Canada		1929
HUTCHINSON, JAMES P.	1907	Philadelphia, Pa.		1943
HUTCHISON, JOSEPH C.	1880	Brooklyn, New York	Vice-President-1885	1887
IMPARATO, ANTHONY M.	1977	New York, New York		
INGRAHAM, FRANC DOUGLAS	1948	Boston, Massachusetts		1965
ISHAM, R.N.	1882	Chicago, Illinois	Forfeited Membership 1898	
IVY, ROBERT H.	1937	Philadelphia, Pa.		1974
JACKSON, FRANCIS CHARLES	1969	Pittsburgh, Pa.		
JACKSON, JABEZ NORTH	1913	Kansas City, Missouri		1935
JACOBSON, NATHAN	1901	Syracuse, New York		1913
JAFFE, BERNARD M.	1977	St. Louis, Missouri		
JANES, ROBERT M.	1942	Toronto, Canada		1966
JANNETTA, PETER J.	1979	Pittsburgh, Pa.		
JENKINS, HILGER P.	1942	Chicago, Illinois		1970
JENNINGS, JOHN EDWARD	1930	Brooklyn, New York		1945
JESSEPH, JOHN ERVIN	1967	Columbus, Ohio		
JOHNSON, ALEXANDER B.	1901	New York, New York		1917
JOHNSON, DALE G.	1978	Salt Lake City, Utah		
JOHNSON, GEORGE, Jr.	1976	Chapel Hill, N.C.		
JOHNSON, JULIAN	1947	Philadelphia, Pa.	Vice-President-1956	
JOHNSON, ROBERT W.	1905	Baltimore, Maryland		1930
JOHNSTON, CHARLES G.	1940	Detroit Michigan		1960
JOHNSTON, CHRISTOPHER	1880	Baltimore, Maryland	Vice-President-1886	1891
JOHNSTON, GEORGE BEN	1896	Richmond, Virginia	President-1905	1916
JONAS, AUGUST F.	1901	Omaha, Nebraska	Vice-President-1907	1934
JONASSON, OLGA	1978	Chicago, Illinois		
JONES, DANIEL FISKE	1917	Boston, Massachusetts	Vice-President-1931 President-1934	1937
JONES, JOHN C.	1948	Los Angeles, Calif.		1976
JONES, RAYFORD SCOTT	1977	Durham, N.C.		
JONES, THOMAS E.	1938	Cleveland, Ohio		1949
JOPSON, JOHN H.	1910	Philadelphia, Pa.	Recorder-1920–1930	1954
JORDAN, GEORGE L., Jr.	1965	Houston, Texas	Vice-President-1980	
JORDAN, PAUL HOWARD, Jr.	1970	Houston, Texas		

NAME	YEAR OF ELECTION	LOCATION AT TIME OF ELECTION	OFFICES AND YEAR HELD	YEAR OF DEATH
JOYCE, THOMAS M.	1930	Portland, Oregon	Vice-President-1940	1947
JUDD, EDWARD STARR	1914	Rochester, Minnesota	Vice-President-1926	1935
JUDD, EDWARD STARR, Jr.	1956	Rochester, Minnesota	Vice-President-1971	
JUDE, JAMES RODERICK	1966	Miami, Florida		
JULIAN, ORMAND C.	1953	Chicago, Illinois		
JURKIEWICZ, MAURICE JOHN	1971	Bethesda, Maryland		
KAISER, GERARD	1978	Miami, Florida		
KAISER, GEORGE CHARLES	1973	St. Louis, Missouri		
KAMMERER, FREDERIC	1899	New York, New York		1928
KANAVEL, ALLEN BUCKNER	1913	Chicago, Illinois		1938
KAPLAN, EDWIN L.	1977	Chicago, Illinois		
KARLSON, KARL E.	1962	Brooklyn, New York		
KAUFMAN, JOSEPH J.	1975	Los Angeles, Calif.		
KEELEY, JOHN L.	1960	Chicago, Illinois		
KEEN, WILLIAM WILLIAMS	1880	Philadelphia, Pa.	Vice-President-1893 President-1899	1932
KELLER, JAMES McDONALD	1880	Hot Springs, Kansas	Forfeited Membership	1887
KELLER, WILLIAM L.	1923	Washington, D.C.		1959
KENNEDY, ROBERT HAYWARD	1935	New York, New York		1978
KENT, EDWARD M.	1953	Pittsburgh, Pa.		1970
KERGIN, FREDERICK GORDON	1952	Toronto, Canada	Vice-President-1959	1974
KERR, HARRY H.	1924	Washington, D.C.		1963
KETCHAM, ALFRED SCHUTT	1973	Bethesda, Maryland		
KEY, JOHN ALBERT	1935	St. Louis, Missouri		1955
KIEHN, CLIFFORD L.	1969	Shaker Heights, Ohio		
KIESEWETTER, WILLIAM B.	1965	Pittsburgh, Pa.		
KILGORE, ALSON R.	1937	San Francisco, Calif.		1959
KILIANI, OTTO G.T.	1911	New York, New York	Expelled Membership	1918
KILMAN, JAMES W.	1974	Columbus, Ohio		
KING, ALFRED	1911	Portland, Maine		1916
KING, HAROLD	1968	Indianpolis, Indiana		
KING, THOMAS C.	1978	New York, New York		
KINLOCH, ROBERT A.	1880	Charleston, S.C.		1891
KINNEY, JOHN MARTIN	1967	New York, New York		
KIRBY, CHARLES K.	1958	Philadelphia, Pa.		1964
KIRK, NORMAN T. (Col.)	1942	Washington, D.C.		1960
KIRKLIN, JOHN W.	1959	Rochester, Minnesota	Recorder-1968–1972	
KIRSH, MARVIN M.	1977	Ann Arbor, Michigan		
KIRTLEY, JAMES A., Jr.	1952	Nashville, Tennessee		1968
KITTLE, C. FREDERICK	1961	Kansas City, Kansas		
KLOPP, EDWARD J.	1932	Philadelphia, Pa.		1936
KOCH, SUMNER L.	1930	Chicago, Illinois		1976
KOONTZ, AMOS R.	1941	Baltimore, Maryland		1965
KOOP, CHARLES EVERETT	1959	Philadelphia, Pa.		
KOUCHOUKOS, NICHOLAS T.	1978	Birmingham, Alabama		
KOUNTZ, SAMUEL LEE	1971	Brooklyn, New York		
KREDEL, FREDERICK E.	1944	Charleston, S.C.		1961
KREMEN, ARNOLD J.	1952	Minneapolis, Minnesota		
KREMENTZ, EDWARD THOMAS	1962	New Orleans, Louisiana		
KRIPPAEHNE, WILLIAM W.	1969	Portland, Oregon		
LADD, WILLIAM E.	1931	Boston, Massachusetts		1967
LaGRADE, LOUIS A.	1901	Washington, D.C.	Resigned	1906
LAHEY, FRANK H.	1925	Boston, Massachusetts		1953
LAM, CONRAD R.	1948	Detroit, Michigan		
LANDOR, JOHN H.	1973	Piscataway, New Jersey		
LANE, LEVI COOPER	1889	San Francisco, Calif.	Vice-President-1892	1902
LANGE, FREDERICK E.	1889	New York, New York		Resigned 1904

NAME	YEAR OF ELECTION	LOCATION AT TIME OF ELECTION	OFFICES AND YEAR HELD	YEAR OF DEATH
LANGFITT, THOMAS W.	1976	Philadelphia, Pa.		
LANGSTON, HIRAM THOMAS	1962	Chicago, Illinois		
LANMAN, THOMAS H.	1938	Boston, Massachusetts		1961
LAUFMAN, HAROLD	1958	Chicago, Illinois		
LAW, ARTHUR A.	1916	Minneapolis, Minnesota	Vice-President-1927	1930
LAWRENCE, WALTER, Jr.	1969	Richmond, Virginia		
LEADBETTER, WYLAND F.	1961	Boston, Massachusetts		Resigned?
LECONTE, ROBERT G.	1901	Philadelphia, Pa.	Secretary-1907–1915 President-1916	1924
LEE, BURTON JAMES	1919	New York, New York		1933
LEE, WALTER ESTELL	1923	Philadelphia, Pa.	Recorder-1931–1946	1951
LEFFALL, LaSALLE D., Jr.	1976	Washington, D.C.		
LEHMAN, EDWIN P.	1931	University, Virginia	Vice-President-1947	1954
LELAND, GEORGE A., Jr.	1935	Boston, Massachusetts		1943
LeMESURIER, ARTHUR B.	1939	Toronto, Canada		
LENHART, CARL H.	1933	Cleveland, Ohio		1955
LeVEEN, HARRY H.	1968	Brooklyn, New York		
LEVEN, N. LOGAN	1949	Minneapolis, Minnesota		
LEVENSON, STANLEY M.	1968	Bronx, New York		
LEVIS, RICHARD J.	1880	Philadelphia, Pa.		1890
LEWIS, DEAN D.	1912	Chicago, Illinois	Vice-President-1929	1941
LEWIS, FLOYD JOHN	1955	St. Paul, Minnesota		
LEWIS, FREDERICK I.	1947	Toronto, Canada		1976
LEWIS, STEPHEN R.	1972	Galveston, Texas		
LILIENTHAL, HOWARD	1910	New York, New York		1946
LILLEHEI, CHARLES W.	1956	Minneapolis, Minnesota		
LILLEHEI, RICHARD C.	1967	Minneapolis, Minnesota		
LIND, JAMES F.	1974	Ancaster, Canada		
LINDSKOG, GUSTAF ELMER	1943	New Haven, Connecticut		
LINTON, ROBERT RITCHIE	1950	Brookline, Massachusetts		1979
LISCHER, CARL EDWARD	1955	St. Louis, Missouri		
LITTLE, JAMES LAWRENCE	1882	New York, New York		1885
LITTLEFIELD, JAMES B.	1967	Charlottesville, Virginia		
LITWIN, MARTIN S.	1978	New Orleans, Louisiana		
LIVINGSTON, WILLIAM K.	1948	Portland, Oregon		1966
LOCALIO, S. ARTHUR	1968	New York, New York		
LOCKWOOD, JOHN S.	1942	Philadelphia, Pa.		1950
LONGMIRE, WILLIAM P., Jr.	1948	Baltimore, Maryland	President-1968	
LORD, JERE WILLIAM, Jr.	1955	New York, New York		
LOTHROP, HOWARD AUGUSTUS	1908	Boston, Massachusetts		1928
LOUCKS, HAROLD H.	1947	Peiping, China		
LOWER, RICHARD ROWLAND	1969	Richmond, Virginia		
LOWER, WILLIAM E.	1916	Cleveland, Ohio		1948
LUND, CHARLES CARROLL	1935	Boston, Massachusetts		1972
LUND, FREDERICK BATES	1910	Boston, Massachusetts	President-1930	1950
LUTZ, FRANK J.	1903	St. Louis, Missouri		1916
LYLE, HENRY H.M.	1917	New York, New York		1947
LYNCH, JOHN B.	1978	Nashville, Tennessee		
LYNN, FRANK S.	1934	Baltimore, Maryland		1938
LYONS, CHAMP	1947	New Orleans, Louisiana		1965
McARTHUR, LEWIS L.	1901	Chicago, Illinois	Vice-President-1913 President-1923	1934
McBURNEY, CHARLES	1892	New York, New York		Resigned 1897
McCANN, JAMES	1883	Pittsburgh, Pa.		1893
McCLELLAND, ROBERT N.	1974	Dallas, Texas		
McCLURE, ROY D.	1932	Detroit, Michigan		1951
McCORKLE, HORACE J.	1949	San Francisco, Calif.		

NAME	YEAR OF ELECTION	LOCATION AT TIME OF ELECTION	OFFICES AND YEAR HELD	YEAR OF DEATH
McCORMACK, ROBERT MORRIS	1968	Rochester, New York		
McCOSH, ANDREW J.	1896	New York, New York		1908
McCREERY, JOHN ALEXANDER	1937	New York, New York		1948
McCUNE, WILLIAM S.	1953	Washington, D.C.	Vice-President-1963	
McDERMOTT, WILLIAM V., Jr	1958	Boston, Massachusetts		
McDONALD, JOHN CLIFTON	1979	New Orleans, Louisianna		
McDOWELL, FRANK	1964	St. Louis, Missouri		
McGLANNAN, ALEXIUS	1930	Baltimore, Maryland		1940
McGOON, DWIGHT CHARLES	1966	Rochester, Minnesota		
McGRAW, ARTHUR B.	1941	Grosse Pointe, Michigan		1954
McGRAW, THEODORE A.	1882	Detroit, Michigan	Vice-President-1897	1921
McGUIRE, EDGAR R.	1923	Buffalo, New York		1931
McGUIRE, HUNTER	1880	Richmond, Virginia	President-1887	1900
McGUIRE, STUART	1917	Richmond, Virginia	Vice-President-1928	1948
McINTOSH, CLARENCE A.	1941	Montreal, Canada		
McKEEVER, FRANCIS M.	1948	Los Angeles, Calif.		1973
McKENNA, HUGH	1925	Chicago, Illinois		1957
McKENZIE, KENNETH G.	1944	Toronto, Canada		1964
McKHANN, CHARLES F.	1974	Minneapolis, Minnesota		
McKITTRICK, LELAND S.	1932	Boston, Massachusetts	Treasurer-1944–1950 President-1966	1978
McLAUGHLIN, ANGUS DUNCAN	1952	London, Canada	Vice-President-1967	
McLAUGHLIN, CHARLES W., Jr	1973	Omaha, Nebraska		
McLAUGHLIN, JOSEPH S.	1977	Baltimore, Maryland		
McCLEAN, LEROY	1882	Troy, New York	Forfeited Membership1890	
McMURTRY, LEWIS S.	1903	Louisville, Kentucky		1924
McPHEDRAN, NORMAN TAIT	1975	Calgary, Canada		
McQUARRIE, DONALD GRAY	1979	Minneapolis, Minnesota		
McRAE, FLOYD WILCOX	1915	Atlanta, Georgia		1921
McSHERRY, CHARLES K.	1975	New York, New York		
McSWAIN, BARTON	1962	Nashville, Tennessee		
McVAY, CHESTER BIDWELL	1954	Yankton, S.D.	Vice-President-1973	
McWILLIAMS, CLARENCE A.	1918	New York, New York		1927
MacBETH, ROBERT A.L.	1967	Edmonton, Canada		
MACDONALD, WILLIS G.	1900	Albany, New York	Vice-President-1908	1910
MacFARLANE, JOSEPH A.	1946	Toronto, Canada		1966
MacFEE, WILLIAM FRANK	1935	New York, New York		1974
MacGUIRE, CONSTANTINE J.	1941	New York, New York		1965
MacKENZIE, KENNETH A.J.	1908	Portland, Oregon		1920
MacKENZIE, WALTER C.	1955	Edmonton, Canada		1978
MacLAREN, ARCHIBALD	1904	St. Paul, Minnesota	Recorder-1911–1915 Vice-President-1916	1924
MacLAREN, MURRAY	1914	St. Johns, Canada		1942
MacLEAN, DONALD	1882	Detroit, Michigan	Resigned1890	
MacLEAN, LLOYD DOUGLAS	1965	Montreal, Canada		
MacMILLIAN, BRUCE GREGG	1968	Cincinnati, Ohio		
MacMONAGLE, BEVERLY	1906	San Francisco, Calif.		1912
MACOMBER, WALTER BRANDON	1950	Albany, New York		
MADDEN, JOHN LEO	1957	New York, New York		
MADDOCK, WALTER G.	1940	Ann Arbor, Michigan		1962
MAES, URBAN	1920	New Orleans, Louisiana	Vice-President-1944	1954
MAGNUSON, PAUL B.	1949	Washington, D.C.		1968
MAHONEY, EARLE B.	1947	Rochester, New York		
MAHORNER, HOWARD	1956	New Orleans, Louisiana		1977
MAIER, HERBERT C.	1947	New York, New York		
MALM, JAMES ROYAL	1968	New York, New York		
MALONEY, JAMES V., Jr.	1962	Los Angeles, Calif.	Secretary-1975–1979	

NAME	YEAR OF ELECTION	LOCATION AT TIME OF ELECTION	OFFICES AND YEAR HELD	YEAR OF DEATH
MALT, RONALD A.	1970	Boston, Massachusetts		
MANNICK, JOHN ANTHONY	1967	Boston, Massachusetts		
MANSBERGER, ARLIE R., Jr	1969	Baltimore, Maryland		
MARCHIORO, THOMAS LOUIS	1976	Seattle, Washington		
MARKOE, FRANCIS H.	1899	New York, New York		1907
MARKOE, THOMAS MASTERS	1883	New York, New York	Declined Membership1883–84	
MARKS, SOLON	1880	Milwaukee, Wisconsin	Vice-President-1899	1914
MARSHALL, SAMUEL F.	1947	Boston, Massachusetts		1970
MARSHALL, VICTOR FRAY	1960	New York, New York		
MARTIN, EDWARD	1898	Philadelphia, Pa.	Vice-President-1919	1938
MARTIN, JOHN DANIEL, Jr.	1943	Atlanta, Georgia	Vice-President-1962	
MARTIN, LESTER WARREN	1976	Cincinnati, Ohio		
MARTIN, WALTON	1915	New York, New York		1949
MASON, EDWARD EATON	1973	Iowa City, Iowa		
MASON, GEORGE ROBERT	1974	Baltimore, Maryland		
MASON, JAMES M.	1931	Birmingham, Alabama	Vice-President-1937	1952
MASON, JAMES M., III	1949	Birmingham, Alabama		1975
MASON, JAMES TATE	1930	Seattle, Washington		1936
MASON, MICHAEL L.	1938	Chicago, Illinois		1963
MASSIE, FRANCIS MILTON	1964	Lexington, Kentucky		
MASSON, JAMES CARRUTHERS	1934	Rochester, Minnesota		1975
MASTERS, FRANK	1974	Shawnee, Kansas		
MASTIN, CLAUDIUS HENRY	1880	Mobile, Alabana	Vice-President-1884, 1890 President-1891	1898
MASTIN, WILLIAM McDOWELL	1887	Mobile, Alabama		1933
MATAS, RUDOLPH	1895	New Orleans, Louisiana	Vice-President-1902 President-1910	1957
MATHEWS, FRANCIS S.	1918	New York, New York		1936
MATHEWSON, CARLETON, Jr.	1948	San Francisco, Calif.	Vice-President-1960	
MATSON, DONALD DARROW	1959	Boston, Massachusetts		1969
MAYO, CHARLES H.	1903	Rochester, Minnesota	President-1932	1939
MAYO, CHARLES W. (Lt. Col)	1944	Rochester, Minnesota		1968
MAYO, WILLIAM J.	1899	Rochester, Minnesota	Vice-President-1903 President-1914	1939
MEACHAM, WILLIAM FELAND	1971	Nashville, Tennessee		
MEARS, J. EWING	1880	Philadelphia, Pa	Recorder-1883–1893 President-1894	1919
MEIGS, JOE VINCENT	1934	Chestnut Hill, Mass.		1963
MELENEY, FRANK L.	1938	New York, New York		1963
MENGUY, RENE	1965	Chicago, Illinois		
MERENDINO, K. ALVIN	1950	Seattle, Washington	Vice-President-1973	
MEYER, HERBERT WILLY	1952	New York, New York		1973
MEYER, WILLY	1901	New York, New York		1932
MICHAEL, JACOB EDWIN	1885	Baltimore, Maryland		1897
MIKKELSEN, WILLIAM P.	1964	Los Angeles, Calif.		
MILES, ALBERT BALDWIN	1893	New Orleans, Louisiana		1894
MILLARD, PERRY H.	1893	St. Paul, Minnesota		1897
MILLER, DON R.	1976	Irving, Calif.		
MILLER, EDWIN M.	1932	Chicago, Illinois		1972
MILLER, FLETCHER A.	1966	Omaha, Nebraska		
MILLER, GEORGE GAVIN	1944	Montreal, Canada		1964
MILLER, LEONARD D.	1975	Philadelphia, Pa.		
MILLER, RICHARD H.	1928	Boston, Massachusetts		1952
MILLER, ROBERT T., Jr.	1919	Pittsburgh, Pa.		1960
MILLER, TRUMAN W.	1898	Chicago, Illinois		1900
MITCHELL, CHARLES F.	1917	Philadelphia, Pa		1962
MITCHELL, JAMES F	1912	Washington, D.C.	Vice-President-1921 Vice-President-1952	1961

NAME	YEAR OF ELECTION	LOCATION AT TIME OF ELECTION	OFFICES AND YEAR HELD	YEAR OF DEATH
MIXTER, CHARLES G.	1924	Boston, Massachusetts	Secretary-1937–1942	1965
MIXTER, SAMUEL JASON	1893	Boston, Massachusetts	Vice-President-1911 President-1917	1926
MIXTER, WILLIAM JASON	1920	Boston, Massachusetts		?
MONACO, ANTHONY PETER	1973	Boston, Massachusetts		
MONCRIEF, JOHN ARTHUR	1965	Fort Sam Houston, Texas		1979
MONKS, GEORGE HOWARD	1896	Boston, Massachusetts	Vice-President-1910	1933
MONTGOMERY, ALBERT HORR	1934	Chicago, Illinois		1948
MOODY, FRANK G.	1972	Salt Lake City, Utah		
MOORE, EDWARD CLARENCE	1925	Los Angeles, Calif.	Vice-President-1943	1944
MOORE, FRANCIS D.	1949	Boston, Massachusetts	President-1972	
MOORE, GEORGE EUGENE	1956	Buffalo, New York		
MOORE, JAMES E.	1895	Minneapolis, Minnesotta	Vice-President-1906	1918
MOORE, ROBERT MILO	1940	Galveston, Texas	Vice-President-1955	1977
MOORE, SAMUEL WILSON	1950	New York, New York		1975
MOORE, THOMAS C.	1960	Muncie, Indiana		
MORETZ, WILLIAM H.	1960	Augusta, Georgia		
MORRIS, GEORGE C., Jr.	1967	Houston, Texas		
MORROW, ANDREW GLENN	1960	Bethesda, Maryland		
MORTON, CHARLES B., 2nd	1956	Charlottesville, Virginia		
MORTON, DONALD LEE	1972	Los Angeles, Calif.		
MORTON, JOHN H.	1975	Rochester, New York		
MORTON, JOHN JAMIESON	1927	Rochester, New York	Vice-President-1950	1977
MORTON, THOMAS GEORGE	1880	Philadelphia, Pa.		Resigned1902
MORTON, THOMAS S.K.	1898	Philadelphia, Pa		Resigned1908
MOSCHCOWITZ, ALEXIS V.	1914	New York, New York		1933
MOSS, GERALD S.	1977	Chicago, Illinois		
MOULDER, PETER VINCENT	1965	Chicago, Illinois		
MOYER, CARL A.	1946	Ann Arbor, Michigan		1970
MUDD, HARVEY G.	1904	St. Louis, Missouri	Vice-President-1921	1933
MUDD, HENRY HODGEN	1886	St. Louis, Missouri		1899
MUELLER, CHARLES BARBER	1958	Syracuse, New York		
MULDER, DONALD G.	1970	Los Angeles, Calif.		
MULHOLLAND, JOHN HUGH	1943	New York, New York	President-1958	1974
MÜLLER, GEORGE P.	1919	Philadelphia, Pa.		1947
MÜLLER, WILLIAM HENRY, Jr	1955	Charlottesville, Virginia	Recorder-1962–1967 President-1975	
MUMFORD, JAMES G.	1906	Boston, Massachusetts		1914
MUNDTH, ELDRED DEAN	1975	Boston, Massachusetts		
MUNRO, JOHN C.	1900	Boston, Massachusetts	Vice-President-1906	1910
MURPHY, FRED T.	1913	St. Louis Missouri		1948
MURPHY, GERALD P.	1977	Buffalo, New York		
MURPHY, JOHN B.	1902	Chicago, Illinois		1916
MURPHY, JOHN JOSEPH	1968	Philadelphia, Pa.		
MURRAY, CLAY RAY	1939	New York, New York		1947
MURRAY, DONALD W. GORDON	1946	Toronto, Ontario		1976
MURRAY, FRANCIS W.	1898	New York, New York		1929
MURRAY, JOSEPH EDWARD	1961	Boston, Massachusetts	Vice-President-1979	
MUSSELMAN, MERLE McNEIL	1957	Omaha, Nebraska	Vice-President-1972	
MUSTARD, WILLIAM T.	1970	Toronto, Canada		
MYERS, RICHARD T.	1974	Winston-Salem, N.C.		
NABSETH, DONALD CLARK	1968	Boston, Massachusetts		
NAFFZIGER, HOWARD C.	1928	San Francisco, Calif	Vice-President-1941 President-1954	1961
NAHRWOLD, DAVID L.	1977	Hershey, Pa.		
NAJAFI, HASSAN	1973	Chicago, Illinois		
NAJARIAN, JOHN SARKIS	1968	Minneapolis, Minnesota		
NANCE, FRANCIS C.	1975	New Orleans, Louisiana		

NAME	YEAR OF ELECTION	LOCATION AT TIME OF ELECTION	OFFICES AND YEAR HELD	YEAR OF DEATH
deNANCRÈDE, CHARLES B.	1882	Philadelphia, Pa.	Vice-President-1890, 1900 President-1909	1921
NANSON, ERIC MUSARD	1963	Saskatoon, Canada		
NARDI, GEORGE LIONEL	1962	Boston, Massachusetts		
NEALON, THOMAS F., Jr.	1963	Philadelphia, Pa.		
NEILSON, THOMAS R.	1903	Philadelphia, Pa.		1939
NELSON, NORMAN C.	1978	Jackson, Mississippi		
NELSON, RUSSELL MARION	1968	Salt Lake City, Utah		
NEMIR, PAUL, Jr.	1960	Philadelphia, Pa.		
NESBIT, REED M.	1948	Ann Arbor, Michigan		
NEUHOF, HAROLD	1942	New York, New York		1964
NEVILLE, WILLIAM EVANS	1972	Newark, New Jersey		
NEWTON, FRANCIS CHANDLER	1934	Newton Centre, Massachusetts		1967
NICHOLS, EDWARD HALL	1915	Boston Massachusetts		1922
NOER, RUDOLPH J.	1949	Detroit, Michigan	Vice-President-1964	
NOLAND, STANTON PEELLE	1977	Charlottesville, Virginia		
NORMAN, JOHN C.	1971	Boston, Massachusetts		
NORRIS, BASIL E.	1882	Washington, D.C.		1895
NORTH, JOHN PAUL	1952	McKinney, Texas		1977
NYHUS, LLOYD M.	1962	Seattle, Washington	Recorder-1977–1980	
OBERHELMAN, HARRY A., Jr.	1964	Palo Alto, Calif.		
OCHSNER, ALBERT J.	1900	Chicago, Illinois	Vice-President-1918 President-1925	1925
OCHSNER, ALTON	1931	New Orleans, Louisiana		
OCHSNER, JOHN LOCKWOOD	1969	New Orleans, Louisiana		
ODOM, GUY LEARY	1969	Durham, N. C.		
OLDBERG, ERIC	1940	Chicago, Illinois		
OLDHAM, H. NEWLAND, Jr.	1979	Durham, N.C.		
OLIVER, JOHN C.	1900	Cincinnati, Ohio		1946
OLMSTED, INGERSOLL	1915	Hamilton, Canada		1936
O'NEILL, JAMES A., Jr.	1974	Nashville, Tennesee		
ORLOFF, MARSHALL JEROME	1965	Torrance, Calif.		
ORR, THOMAS G.	1929	Kansas City, Missouri	Vice-President-1947 President-1950	1955
OSBORNE, MELVIN P.	1967	Jamaica Plain, Massachusetts		
OTTINGER, LESLIE W.	1979	Boston, Massachusetts		
OUGHTERSON, ASHLEY W.	1936	New Haven, Connecticut		1956
OVIATT, CHARLES W.	1905	Oshkosh, Wisconsin		1912
OWENS, JAMES CUTHBERT	1974	Denver, Colorado		
OWENS, JOHN E.	1882	Chicago, Illinois	Vice-President-1901	1922
PACE, WILLIAM G., III	1977	Columbus, Ohio		
PACKARD, JOHN H.	1880	Philadelphia, Pa.	Treasurer-1881–1884	Resigned1901
PADGETT, EARL C.	1940	Kansas City, Missouri		1946
PAINE, JOHN RANDOLPH	1942	Minneapolis, Minnesota		1972
PALMER, DUDLEY WHITE	1923	Cincinnati, Ohio		1949
PALOYAN, EDWARD	1975	Hines, Illinois		
PANCOAST, WILLIAM HENRY	1880	Philadelphia, Pa.		1897
PAPPER, EMANUEL M.	1971	Miami, Florida		
PAQUIN, ALBERT J., Jr.	1965	Charlottesville, Va.		1967
PAREIRA, MORTON D.	1968	Philadelphia, Pa.		1978
PARHAM, FREDERICK W.	1899	New Orleans, Louisiana	Vice-President-1917	1927
PARK, ROSWELL	1885	Buffalo, New York	Vice-President-1894 President-1901	1914
PARKER, EDWARD FROST	1959	Charleston, S.C.		
PARKES, CHARLES T.	1882	Chicago, Illinois		1891
PARKHILL, CLAYTON	1896	Denver, Colorado	Vice-President-1901	1902

NAME	YEAR OF ELECTION	LOCATION AT TIME OF ELECTION	OFFICES AND YEAR HELD	YEAR OF DEATH
PARMENTER, JOHN	1893	Buffalo, New York		1932
PARSONS, LANGDON	1950	Boston, Massachusetts		
PARSONS, WILLARD H.	1947	Vicksburg, Mississippi		1969
PARSONS, WILLIAM B., Jr.	1935	New York, New York		1973
PASSARO, EDWARD, Jr.	1977	Los Angeles, Calif.		
PATE, JAMES WYNFORD	1969	Memphis, Tennessee		
PATON, BRUCE CALDER	1969	Denver, Colorado		
PATTERSON, HOWARD A.	1946	New York, New York		
PAULSON, DONALD L.	1975	Dallas, Texas		
PAYNE, J. HOWARD	1975	Los Angeles, Calif.		
PAYNE, ROBERT LEE	1933	Norfolk, Virginia		1967
PAYNE, W. SPENCER	1979	Rochester, Minnesota		
PEACOCK, ERLE EWART, Jr.	1966	Chapel Hill, N.C.		
PEARSE, HERMAN ELWYN, Jr.	1937	Rochester, New York		
PEARSON, FREDERICK G.	1971	Toronto, Canada		
PECK, CHARLES HOWARD	1908	New York, New York	Treasurer-1916–1925	1927
PECK, WASHINGTON, F.	1883	Davenport, Iowa		1891
PEET, MAX MINOR	1937	Ann Arbor, Michigan		1949
PELTIER, LEONARD FRANCIS	1961	Kansas City, Kansas		
PEMBERTON, JOHN deJ.	1929	Rochester, Minnesota	Vice-President-1945, 1946	1967
PENBERTHY, GROVER C.	1934	Detroit, Michigan		1959
PENFIELD, WILDER G.	1936	Montreal, Canada	Vice-President-1949	1976
PENICK, RAWLEY M., Jr.	1950	New Orleans, Louisiana		1963
PENN, ISRAEL	1975	Denver, Colorado		
PERCY, NELSON M.	1919	Chicago, Illinois		1958
PEREY, BERNARD JEAN F.	1977	Sherbrooke, Canada		
PERRY, JOHN FRANCIS, Jr.	1972	Minneapolis, Minnesota		
PESKIN, GERALD WILLIAM	1967	Chicago, Illinois		
PETERS, GEORGE A.	1882	New York, New York	Resigned 1884	
PETERS, RICHARD MORSE	1962	Chapel Hill, N.C.		
PETERSON, FRANK R.	1941	Iowa City, Iowa		
PFEIFFER, DAMON B.	1925	Philadelphia, Pa.	Vice-President-1943	1966
PHEMISTER, DALLAS B.	1917	Chicago, Illinois	Vice-President-1931 President-1939	1951
PICKETT, LAWRENCE K.	1973	New Haven, Connecticut		
PICKHARDT, OTTO C.	1931	New York, New York		1972
PICKRELL, KENNETH LEROY	1963	Durham, N.C.		
PIERCE, WILLIAM S.	1978	Hershey, Pa.		
PILCH, YOSEF H.	1979	San Diego, Calif.		
PILCHER, COBB	1948	Nashville, Tennessee		1949
PILCHER, LEWIS STEPHEN	1889	Brooklyn, New York	Vice-President-1894, 1915 President-1919	1934
PILCHER, PAUL M.	1916	Brooklyn, New York		1917
PLUMMER, SAMUEL C.	1914	Chicago, Illinois		1952
POLK, HIRAM CAREY, Jr.	1973	Louisville, Kentucky		
POLLOCK, ALEX M.	1881	Pittsburgh, Pa.	Forfeited Membership 1890	
PONKA, JOSEPH L.	1972	Detroit, Michigan		
POOL, EUGENE H.	1914	New York, New York	Treasurer-1926–1933 President-1936	1949
POPPEN, JAMES LEONARD	1956	Boston, Massachusetts		
PORIES, WALTER J.	1973	Cleveland, Ohio		
PORTER, CHARLES A.	1904	Boston, Massachusetts		1931
PORTER, CHARLES BURNHAM	1887	Boston, Massachusetts	Vice-President-1893	1909
PORTER, MILES FULLER	1915	Fort Wayne, Indiana		1933
PORTER, WILLIAM GIBBS	1882	Philadelphia, Pa.		1906
POTH, EDGAR JACOB	1951	Galveston, Texas		
POTTS, WILLIS JOHN	1948	Chicago, Illinois		1968

NAME	YEAR OF ELECTION	LOCATION AT TIME OF ELECTION	OFFICES AND YEAR HELD	YEAR OF DEATH
POWERS, CHARLES A.	1896	Denver, Colorado	Vice-President-1904 Treasurer-1907–1912 President-1913	1922
POWERS, SAMUEL R., Jr.	1965	Albany, New York		
PRESTON, FREDERICK W.	1959	Chicago, Illinois		
PREWITT, THEODORE F.	1882	St. Louis, Missouri	Vice-President-1887 President-1898	1904
PRICE, PHILI B.	1947	Salt Lake City, Utah		
PRIESTLEY, JAMES T.	1947	Rochester, Minnesota		1979
PRIMROSE, ALEXANDER	1908	Toronto, Canada	Vice-President-1922, 1927 President-1931	1944
PRINCE, DAVID	1882	Jacksonville, Illinois		1889
PROHASKA, JOHN VAN	1963	Chicago, Illinois		1969
PRUITT, BASIL A., Jr.	1972	Fort Sam Houston, Texas		
PUESTOW, CHARLES B.	1941	Chicago, Illinois		1973
PUGH, HERBERT LAMONT	1952	Arlington, Virginia		
QUIGLEY, THOMAS BARTLETT	1963	Boston, Massachusetts		
RAAF, JOHN	1973	Portland, Oregon		
RAFFUCCI, FRANCISCO L.	1966	San Juan, Puerto Rico		1971
RAKER, JOHN WILLIAM	1956	Philadelphia, Pa.		
RAND, ROBERT WHEELER	1968	Los Angeles, Calif.		
RANDALL, ALEXANDER	1937	Philadelphia, Pa.	Forfeited Membership1943	
RANDALL, HENRY T.	1956	New York, New York		
RANDOLPH, JUDSON D.	1975	Washington, D.C.		
RANKIN, FRED WHARTON	1928	Rochester, Minnesota	President-1949	1954
RANSOHOFF, JOSEPH	1886	Cincinnati, Ohio	Vice-President-1912	1921
RANSOM, HENRY K.	1939	Ann Arbor, Michigan		
RAPAPORT, FELIX T.	1973	New York, New York		
RAVDIN, ISIDOR S.	1939	Philadelphia, Pa.	President-1959	1972
RAVDIN, ROBERT GLENN	1965	Philadelphia, Pa.		1972
RAVITCH, MARK MITCHELL	1950	Baltimore, Maryland	Vice-President-1974	
RAY, BRONSON S.	1947	New York, New York		
READ, RAYMOND CHARLES	1974	Little Rock, Arkansas		
REDO, S. FRANK	1964	New York, New York		
REED, THOMAS BAIRD	1882	Philadelphia, Pa		1891
REEMTSMA, KEITH	1963	New Orleans, Louisiana		
REICHERT, FREDERICK LEET	1935	San Francisco, Calif.		1969
REICHLE, FREDERICK A.	1975	Philadelphia, Pa.		
REID, MONT ROGER	1926	Cincinnati, Ohio	Vice-President-1935	1943
REMINE, WILLIAM HERVEY	1971	Rochester, Minnesota		
REYNOLDS, FRED C.	1969	St. Louis, Missouri		
REYNOLDS, JOHN TODD	1952	Chicago, Illinois		
RHOADS, JONATHAN EVANS	1943	Philadelphia, Pa.	President-1973	
RICHARDS, VICTOR	1952	San Francisco, Calif.		
RICHARDSON, EDWARD P.	1923	Boston, Massachusetts		1944
RICHARDSON, MAURICE HOWE	1887	Boston, Massachusetts	Secretary-1895–1897 Vice-President-1898 President-1903	1912
RICHARDSON, TOBIAS G.	1880	New Orleans, Louisiana	Vice-President-1889	1892
REINHOFF, WILLIAM F., Jr.	1931	Baltimore, Maryland		
RITCHIE, HARRY P.	1924	St. Paul, Minnesota		1942
RIVES, JAMES DAVIDSON	1942	New Orleans, Louisiana		1975
RIXFORD, EMMET	1901	San Francisco, Calif.	Vice-President-1905 President-1928	1938
ROB, CHARLES G.	1961	Rochester, New York	Vice-President-1979	
ROBERTS, BROOKE	1962	Philadelphia, Pa.		

NAME	YEAR OF ELECTION	LOCATION AT TIME OF ELECTION	OFFICES AND YEAR HELD	YEAR OF DEATH
ROBERTS, JOHN B.	1882	Philadelphia, Pa.	Treasurer-1892–1894 Vice-President-1889, 1895 President-1921	1924
ROBERTS, STUART SHERWOOD	1969	Columbus, Ohio		
ROBERTSON, DAVID E.	1929	Toronto, Canada	Vice-President-1937	1944
ROBERTSON, H. ROCKE	1957	Vancouver, Canada		
ROBINSON, DAVID WEAVER	1953	Kansas City, Kansas	Vice-President-1966	
ROBINSON, ROBERT A.	1967	Baltimore, Maryland		
ROCKEY, EUGENE W.	1940	Portland, Oregon		1970
RODMAN, JOHN STEWART	1924	Philadelphia, Pa.	Vice-President-1954	1958
RODMAN, WILLIAM LOUIS	1898	Louisville, Kentucky		1915
ROE, BENSON BERTHEAU	1963	San Francisco, Calif.		
ROSATO, ERNEST F.	1977	Philadelphia, Pa.		
ROSATO, FRANCIS E.	1975	Norfolk, Virginia		
ROSEMOND, GEORGE PARROTT	1962	Philadelphia, Pa.		
ROSOFF, LEONARD	1971	Los Angeles, Calif.		
ROSS, DUDLEY E.	1947	Montreal, Canada		1967
ROSS, GEORGE G.	1914	Philadelphia, Pa.		1922
ROUSSELOT, LOUIS M.	1949	New York, New York	Vice-President-1965	1974
ROWAN, CHARLES J.	1917	Iowa City, Iowa		1948
ROWE, MARC I.	1974	Miami, Florida		
ROYSTER, HENRY PAGE	1954	Philadelphia, Pa.		
ROYSTER, HUBERT A.	1922	Raleigh, N.C.		1959
RUSH, BENJAMIN F., Jr.	1970	Newark, New Jersey		
RUSHMORE, JOHN DIKEMAN	1882	Brooklyn, New York		1929
RUSSELL, PAUL SNOWDEN	1963	Boston, Massachusetts		
RUSSELL, THOMAS PEMBER	1880	Oshkosh, Wisconsin	Vice-President-1886 Forfeited Membership1893	
RYAN, ROBERT F.	1979	New Orleans, Louisiana		
SABINE, THOMAS TAUNTON	1882	New York, New York		1888
SABISTON, DAVID C., Jr.	1960	Baltimore, Maryland	President-1978	
SALZMAN, EDWIN WILLIAMS	1970	Boston, Massachusetts		
SAMSON, PAUL CURKEET	1956	Oakland, Calif.		
SANDUSKY, WILLIAM R.	1952	Charlottesville, Va.		
SANTULLI, THOMAS V.	1966	New York, New York		
SAWYERS, JOHN LAZELLE	1970	Nashville, Tennessee		
SAYRE, LEWIS ALBERT	1880	New York, New York		1900
SCANLON, EDWARD F.	1974	Evanston, Illinois		
SCANNELL, JOHN GORDON	1957	Boston, Massachusetts		
SCHAFER, PAUL WILLIAM	1952	Kansas City, Kansas		Resigned?
SCHENK, WORTHINGTON G., Jr.	1960	Buffalo, New York		
SCHILLING, JOHN A.	1955	Rochester, New York	Treasurer-1971–1975 Vice-President-1978	
SCHLICKE, CARL PAUL	1971	Spokane, Washington	Vice-President-1977	
SCHLOERB, PAUL RICHARD	1968	Kansas City, Kansas		
SCHMIDT, ERWIN R.	1936	Madison, Wisconsin		1961
SCHULLINGER, RUDOLPH N.	1944	New York, New York		1969
SCHWARTZ, HENRY GERARD	1966	St. Louis, Missouri	Vice-President-1976	
SCHWARTZ, SEYMOUR IRA	1965	Rochester, New York		
SCHWEGMAN, CLETUS W.	1961	Philadelphia, Pa.		
SCHWYZER, ARNOLD	1928	St. Paul, Minnesota		1944
SCOTT, HENRY WILLIAM, Jr.	1953	Nashville, Tennessee	Treasurer-1960–1965 President-1974	
SCOTT, W.J. MERLE	1933	Rochester, New York		1973
SCRIMGER, FRANCIS A.C.	1930	Montreal, Canada		1937
SCUDDER, CHARLES L.	1909	Boston, Massachusetts		1949

NAME	YEAR OF ELECTION	LOCATION AT TIME OF ELECTION	OFFICES AND YEAR HELD	YEAR OF DEATH
SEALY, WILL CAMP	1957	Durham, N.C.		
SEARLS, HENRY HUNT	1948	San Francisco, Calif.		1974
SEDGWICK, CORNELIUS E.	1967	Boston, Massachusetts		
SEELIG, M.G.	1919	St. Louis, Missouri		1953
SEIGLER, HILLIARD FOSTER	1978	Durham, N.C.		
SELIGMAN, ARNOLD MAX	1958	Baltimore, Maryland		1976
SENN, NICHOLAS	1882	Milwaukee, Wisconsin	Vice-President-1888 President-1893	1908
SHAW, ROBERT ROEDER	1966	Dallas, Texas		
SHELDON, GEORGE F.	1979	San Francisco, Calif.		
SHENSTONE, NORMAN S.	1934	Toronto, Canada		1970
SHEPHERD, FRANCIS J.	1902	Montreal, Canada		1929
SHERMAN, HARRY M.	1905	San Francisco, Calif.		1921
SHERMAN, ROGER TALBOT	1965	Memphis, Tennessee		
SHERWOOD, WALTER A.	1927	Brooklyn, New York		1931
SHINGLETON, WILLIAM W.	1961	Durham, N.C.		
SHIPLEY, ARTHUR MARRIOTT	1923	Baltimore, Maryland	Vice-President-1944	1955
SHIRES, GEORGE THOMAS	1965	Dallas, Texas	Secretary-1970–1974 President-1980	
SHUCK, JERRY M.	1979	Albuquerque, New Mexico		
SHUMACKER, HARRIS B., Jr.	1947	New Haven, Connecticut	Vice-President-1961 Secretary-1965–1968	
SHUMWAY, NORMAN EDWARD	1967	Palo Alto, Calif.		
SIEGEL, JOHN H.	1978	Buffalo, New York		
SILEN, WILLIAM	1966	Boston, Massachusetts		
SILER, VINTON E.	1954	Cincinnati, Ohio		1971
SILVER, DONALD	1974	Durham, N.C.		
SIMEONE, FIORINDO A.	1952	Cleveland, Ohio		
SIMMONS, CHANNING C.	1926	Boston, Massachusetts		1953
SIMMONS, RICHARD L.	1975	Minneapolis, Minnesota		
SINGLETON, ALBERT OLIN	1935	Galveston, Texas	Vice-President-1945, 1946	1947
SISTRUNK, WALTER E.	1920	Rochester, Minnesota		1933
SKILLMAN, JOHN JOAKIM	1975	Boston, Massachusetts		
SKINNER, DAVID B.	1974	Chicago, Illinois		
SLAUGHTER, DANELY PHILIP	1950	Chicago, Illinois		1970
SLOAN, HERBERT E., Jr.	1958	Ann Arbor, Michigan		
SLOAN, LAWRENCE W.	1947	New York, New York		
SMITH, ALAN PENNIMAN	1882	Baltimore, Maryland	Forfeited Membership1894	
SMITH, GARDNER WATKINS	1974	Baltimore, Maryland		
SMITH, LOUIS LIVINGSTON	1975	Loma Linda, Calif.		
SMITH, MORRIS K.	1931	New York, New York		1950
SMITH, REA	1918	Los Angeles, Calif.		1935
SMITH, ROGER FIELDING	1975	Detroit, Michigan		
SMITH-PETERSEN, MARCUS N.	1948	Boston, Massachusetts		1953
SMITHWICK, REGINALD H.	1939	Boston, Massachusetts		
SMYTH, CALVIN M., Jr.	1940	Philadelphia, Pa.		1967
SNYDER, HOWARD ERROL	1952	Winfield, Kansas		
SNYDER, WILLIAM H., Jr.	1957	Los Angeles, Calif.		1974
SOROFF, HARRY S.	1971	Boston, Massachusetts		
SOUCHON, EDMOND	1895	New Orleans, Louisiana	Vice-President-1900	1924
SOUTHWICK, HARRY WEBB	1963	Chicago, Illinois		
SPARKMAN, ROBERT S.	1959	Dallas, Texas	Vice-President-1978	
SPEED, KELLOGG	1919	Chicago, Illinois		1955
SPEESE, JOHN	1922	Philadelphia, Pa.		1933
SPELLMAN, MITCHELL W.	1972	Los Angeles, Calif.		
SPENCER, FRANK COLE	1960	Baltimore, Maryland		
SPRATT, JOHN S., Jr.	1973	Columbia, Missouri		

NAME	YEAR OF ELECTION	LOCATION AT TIME OF ELECTION	OFFICES AND YEAR HELD	YEAR OF DEATH
SQUIRE, TRUMAN HOFFMAN	1882	Elmira, New York		1889
ST. JOHN, FORDYCE BARKER	1923	New York, New York	Treasurer-1934–1943	1973
STABINS, SAMUEL J.	1954	Rochester, New York		
STAFFORD, EDWARD STEPHEN	1951	Baltimore, Maryland		
STAHL, WILLIAM M., Jr.	1970	New York, New York		
STAMEY, THOMAS ALEXANDER	1974	Stanford, Calif.		
STARK, RICHARD BOIES	1963	New York, New York		
STARR, ALBERT	1964	Portland, Oregon		
STARR, CLARENCE L.	1918	Toronto, Canada	Vice-Pres. elect-1929 (d.12/25/28)	1928
STARR, FREDERIC N.G.	1914	Toronto, Canada	Vice-President-1933	1934
STARZL, THOMAS EARL	1966	Denver, Colorado		
STATE, DAVID	1964	New York, New York		
STEICHEN, FELICIEN M.	1977	Pittsburgh, Pa.		
STEMMER, EDWARD A.	1975	Long Beach, Calif.		
STEPHENS, H. BRODIE	1951	San Francisco, Calif.		
STEPHENSON, GEORGE W.	1969	Chicago, Illinois		
STEPHENSON, SAMUEL E., Jr.	1963	Nashville, Tennessee		
STERN, WALTER EUGENE	1959	Los Angeles, Calif.		
STEWART, FRANCES T.	1911	Philadelphia, Pa.		1920
STEWART, GEORGE DAVID	1915	New York, New York		1933
STEWART, JOHN DUNHAM	1943	Buffalo, New York	Vice-President-1959 President-1961	
STILLMAN, STANLEY	1907	San Francisco, Calif.	Vice-President-1925	1934
STIMSON, LEWIS A.	1889	New York, New York	Resigned1898	
STINCHFIELD, FRANK E.	1959	New York, New York		
STOKES, CHARLES F.	1912	U.S. Navy	Resigned1923	
STONE, CALEB S., Jr.	1967	Seattle, Washington		
STONE, HARRY HARLAN	1975	Atlanta, Georgia		
STONE, HARVEY BRINTON	1926	Baltimore, Maryland	President-1942	1977
STOOKEY, BYRON	1938	New York, New York		1966
STORCK, AMBROSE HOWELL	1949	New Orleans, Louisiana		1975
STORER, EDWARD H.	1972	New Haven, Connecticut		
STRANDNESS, DONALD E., Jr.	1973	Seattle, Washington		
STRODE, JOSEPH E.	1948	Honolulu, Hawaii		1972
STUART, FRANK PAUL, Jr.	1978	Chicago, Illinois		
STUCKEY, JACKSON H.	1969	Brooklyn, New York		
STURGEON, CHARLES T.	1936	Los Angeles, Calif.		1967
STURGIS, SOMERS HAYES	1958	Boston, Massachusetts		
SUMMERS, JOHN EDWARD	1907	Omaha, Nebraska	Vice-President-1917	1935
SWAN, HENRY	1950	Denver, Colorado		
SWAN, KENNETH G.	1979	Newark, New Jersey		
SWEET, RICHARD HARWOOD	1943	Boston, Massachusetts	Vice-President-1960	1962
SWEET, WILLIAM HERBERT	1961	Boston, Massachusetts		
SWENSON, ORVAR	1953	Boston, Massachusetts		
SWINBURNE, JOHN	1880	New York, New York	Forfeited Membership1886	
SYMBAS, PANAGIOTIS N.	1978	Atlanta, Georgia		
SZILAGYI, D. EMERICK	1960	Detroit, Michigan		
TALBERT, JAMES L.	1975	Gainesville, Florida		
TAYLOR, ALFRED S.	1920	New York, New York		1942
TAYLOR, FREDERIC WILLIAM	1955	Indianapolis, Indiana		
TAYLOR, GRANTLEY W.	1940	Boston, Massachusetts		1966
TAYLOR, WILLIAM EDWIN	1883	San Francisco, Calif.	Forfeited Membership1895	
TAYLOR, WILLIAM J.	1900	Philadelphia, Pa.		1936
TEMPLETON, JOHN Y., III	1957	Philadelphia, Pa.		
TERRY, WALLACE, I.	1916	San Francisco, Calif.		1950
THAL, ALAN PHILIP	1963	Detroit, Michigan		

NAME	YEAR OF ELECTION	LOCATION AT TIME OF ELECTION	OFFICES AND YEAR HELD	YEAR OF DEATH
THOMAS, COLIN G., Jr.	1965	Chapel Hill, N.C.		
THOMPSON, ALAN GIBB	1969	Montreal, Canada		
THOMPSON, JAMES CHARLES	1971	Galveston, Texas		
THOMPSON, JAMES E.	1909	Galveston, Texas	Vice-President-1922	1927
THOMPSON, JAMES EDWIN	1950	New York, New York		
THOMPSON, JESSE ELDON	1968	Dallas, Texas		
THOMPSON, JOSEPH FORD	1885	Washington, D.C.		1917
THOMPSON, JOSEPH W.	1882	Paducah, Kentucky		1886
THOMSON, WILLIAM	1882	Philadelphia, Pa		1907
THORBJARNARSON, BJORN	1976	New York, New York		
THORLAKSON, PAUL H.T.	1941	Winnipeg, Canada		
THORNDIKE, AUGUSTUS (Col)	1944	Boston, Massachusetts		
TIDRICK, ROBERT T.	1958	Iowa City, Iowa	Vice-President-1970	
TIFFANY, LOUIS MCLANE	1882	Baltimore, Maryland	Vice-President-1892 President-1896 President-1896	1916
TINKER, MARTIN BUEL	1920	Ithaca, New York		1954
TOLAND, CLARENCE G.	1932	Los Angeles, Calif.		1947
TOMPKINS, RONALD K.	1975	Los Angeles, Calif.		
TOREK, FRANZ	1928	New York, New York		1938
TOUROFF, ARTHUR S.W.	1952	New York, New York		1973
TREMAINE, WILLIAM S.	1880	Buffalo, New York	Forfeited Membrship	1895
TRIMBLE, I. RIDGWAY	1942	Baltimore, Maryland		1979
TROUT, HUGH H.	1925	Roanoke, Virginia		1950
TRUESDALE, PHILEMON E.	1918	Fall River, Massachusetts		1945
TRUSLER, GEORGE A.	1976	Toronto, Canada		
TRUSLER, HAROLD M., Sr.	1946	Indianapolis, Indiana		1972
TURCOT, JACQUES	1974	Quebec, Canada		1977
TURCOTTE, JEREMIAH G.	1973	Ann Arbor, Michigan		
TURNBULL, RUPERT B., Jr.	1957	Cleveland, Ohio		
TUTTLE, WILLIAM M.	1954	Detroit, Michigan		1963
TYSON, RALPH ROBERT	1978	Philadelphia, Pa.		
ULFELDER, HOWARD	1954	Boston, Massachusetts		
URSCHEL, HAROLD C., Jr.	1976	Dallas, Texas		
VALK, WILLIAM LOWELL	1955	Kansas City, Kansas		
VanBEUREN, FREDERICK, Jr.	1928	New York, New York		1943
VANDERVEER, ALBERT	1882	Albany, New York	Vice-President-1899 President-1906	1929
VANDERVEER, EDWARD A.	1910	Albany, New York		1953
VARCO, RICHARD L.	1948	Minneapolis, Minnesota	Vice-President-1968	
VARICK, THEODORE ROMEYN	1885	Jersey City, New Jersey		1887
VAUGHAN, GEORGE T.	1902	Washington, D.C.		1948
VAUGHAN, JOHN WALTER	1921	Detroit, Michigan		1949
VEAL, JAMES ROSS	1951	Washington, D.C.		1964
VEITH, FRANK J.	1972	Bronx, New York		
VERDI, WILLIAM FRANCIS	1920	New Haven, Connecticut	Vice-President-1933	1957
VÈZINA, CHARLES	1949	Quebec, Canada		1955
VINCENT, BETH	1922	Boston, Massachusetts		1962
VOORHEES, ARTHUR B., Jr.	1975	New York, New York		
WADDELL, WILLIAM RHOADS	1960	Boston, Massachusetts		
WADE, PRESTON ALLEN	1961	New York, New York		
WAINWRIGHT, JONATHAN M.	1918	Scranton, Pa.	Vice-President-1932	1934
WALDHAUSEN, JOHN ANTON	1971	Hershey, Pa.		
WALES, PHILIP SKINNER	1880	Washington, D.C.	Resigned	1887
WALKER, EDWARD W.	1891	Cincinnati, Ohio		1925
WALKER, IRVING J.	1933	Boston, Massachusetts		1960
WALKER, JOHN B.	1907	New York, New York		1943

NAME	YEAR OF ELECTION	LOCATION AT TIME OF ELECTION	OFFICES AND YEAR HELD	YEAR OF DEATH
WALKER, MATTHEW	1972	Nashville, Tennessee		1978
WALKLING, ADOLPH A.	1948	Philadelphia, Pa.		1966
WALLACE, ROBERT BRUCE	1974	Rochester, Minnesota		
WALT, ALEXANDER JEFFREY	1972	Detroit, Michigan		
WALTER, CARL W.	1974	Boston, Massachusetts		
WALTERS, WALTMAN	1932	Rochester, Minnesota		
WANGENSTEEN, OWEN H.	1933	Minneapolis, Minnesota	Vice-President-1952 President-1969	
WANGENSTEEN, STEPHEN L.	1972	Charlottesville, Va.		
WARD, SAMUEL B.	1882	Albany, New York		Resigned?
WARDEN, HERBERT EDGAR	1970	Morgantown, West Va.		
WARREN, JOHN COLLINS	1882	Boston, Massachusetts	Vice-President-1891 President-1897	1927
WARREN, KENNETH W.	1962	Boston, Massachusetts		
WARREN, RICHARD	1952	Brookline, Massachusetts	Vice-President-1975	
WARREN, WALTER DEAN	1963	Miami, Florida		
WARTHEN, HARRY J., Jr.	1949	Richmond, Va.		
WATSON, BERIAH ANDREW	1882	Jersey City, New Jersey		1892
WATSON, FRANCIS S.	1896	Boston, Massachusetts		1942
WATTS, STEPHEN HURT	1913	Charlottesville, Va.		1953
WAUGH, JOHN McMASTER	1948	Rochester, Minnesota		1962
WAY, LAWRENCE WELLESLEY	1976	San Francisco, Calif.		
WEBB, WATTS RANKIN	1961	Jackson, Mississippi		
WEBSTER, DONALD R.	1953	Montreal, Canada		
WEBSTER, JEROME P.	1940	New York, New York		1974
WEEKS, STEPHEN H.	1889	Portland, Maine	Vice-President-1904	1909
WEIR, ROBERT F.	1889	New York, New York	President-1900	1927
WEIST, JACOB ROWLAND	1880	Richmond, Indiana	Secretary-1881–1894 Vice-President-1895	1900
WELCH, C. STUART	1947	Boston, Massachusetts		
WELCH, CLAUDE EMERSON	1951	Boston, Massachusetts	President-1977	
WELDON, CLARENCE SCHOCK	1973	St. Louis, Missouri		
WELLS, SAMUEL A., Jr.	1976	Durham, N.C.		
WEST, JOHN PETTIT	1951	New York, New York		1978
WESTMORELAND, W. F.	1880	Atlanta, Georgia	Forfeited Membership	1888
WHARTON, HENRY R.	1892	Philadelphia, Pa.		1925
WHEAT, MYRON W., Jr.	1969	Gainesville, Florida		
WHEELER, HEWITT BROWNELL	1979	Worcester, Massachusetts		
WHELAN, THOMAS J., Jr.	1965	Honolulu, Hawaii		
WHIPPLE, ALLEN O.	1912	New York, New York	President-1940	1963
WHITE, JAMES C.	1939	Boston, Massachusetts		
WHITE, JAMES WILLIAM	1882	Philadelphia, Pa.		1916
WHITE, RALEIGH R., III	1971	Temple, Texas		
WHITE, THOMAS TAYLOR	1976	Seattle, Washington		
WHITE, WILLIAM CRAWFORD	1937	New York, New York		1962
WHITTEMORE, WYMAN	1926	Boston, Massachusetts		1957
WIGHT, JARVIS SHERMAN	1891	Brooklyn, New York		1901
WILCOX, BENSON R.	1975	Chapel Hill, N.C.		
WILKIE, ARCHIBALD	1938	Montreal, Canada		1971
WILKINS, EARLE W., Jr.	1966	Boston, Massachusetts		
WILLARD, DeFOREST	1882	Philadelphia, Pa.	Recorder-1894–1901 President-1902	1910
WILLARD, DeFOREST P.	1934	Philadelphia, Pa.		1957
WILLIAMS, CARRINGTON	1939	Richmond, Virginia		1978
WILLIAMS, GEORGE M.	1972	Baltimore, Maryland		
WILLIAMS, GEORGE RAINEY	1963	Oklahoma City, Oklahoma		
WILLIAMS, HUGH	1912	Boston, Massachusetts		1945

NAME	YEAR OF ELECTION	LOCATION AT TIME OF ELECTION	OFFICES AND YEAR HELD	YEAR OF DEATH
WILLIAMS, LESTER J., Jr.	1975	Boston, Massachusetts		
WILLIAMS, ROGER DAVIS	1962	Columbia, Ohio		
WILLMAN, VALLEE LOUIS	1966	St. Louis, Missouri		
WILSON, BEN J.	1958	Dallas, Texas		Resigned?
WILSON, HARWELL	1950	Memphis, Tennessee	Vice-President-1977	1977
WILSON, PHILIP DUNCAN	1946	New York, New York		1969
WILSON, RICHARD EMANUEL	1969	Boston, Massachusetts		
WINFIELD, JAMES Mac.	1946	Detroit, Michigan		1964
WINSLOW, RANDOLPH	1914	Baltimore, Maryland		1937
WISE, WALTER D.	1935	Baltimore, Maryland		1968
WOLFER, JOHN A.	1931	Chicago, Illinois		1955
WOMACK, NATHAN A.	1939	St. Louis, Missouri	Secretary-1949–1953 Vice-President-1962	1975
WOOD, ALFRED C.	1918	Philadelphia, Pa.		1959
WOOD, JAMES RUSHMORE	1880	New York, New York	Vice-President-1881	1882
WOODHALL, BARNES	1948	Durham, North Carolina		
WOODWARD, EDWARD ROY	1960	Gainesville, Florida		
WOOKEY, HAROLD W.	1941	Toronto, Canada		
WOOLSEY, GEORGE	1901	New York, New York		1950
WRIGHT, ARTHUR M.	1933	New York, New York		1948
WRIGHT, HASTINGS KEMPER	1970	New Haven, Connecticut		
WYLIE, EDWIN J.	1959	San Francisco, Calif.		
WYLIE, ROBERT H.	1949	New York, New York		
YATES, JOHN L.	1916	Milwaukee, Wisconsin	Vice-President-1934	1938
YEAGER, GEORGE H.	1944	Baltimore, Maryland		
YOUNG, WILLIAM GLENN, Jr.	1964	Durham, N.C.		
ZEPPA, ROBERT	1969	Miami, Florida		
ZIEROLD, ARTHUR A.	1937	Minneapolis, Minnesota		1976
ZIFFREN, SIDNEY EDWARD	1969	Iowa City, Iowa		
ZIMMERMAN, BERNARD	1958	Minneapolis, Minnesota		
ZIMMERMAN, HARRY BERNARD	1935	St. Paul, Minnesota		1960
ZINNINGER, MAX M.	1938	Cincinnati, Ohio		1973
ZINTEL, HAROLD ALBERT	1950	Philadelphia, Pa.		
ZOLLINGER, ROBERT M.	1948	Boston, Massachusetts	President-1965	
ZUIDEMA, GEORGE D.	1964	Baltimore, Maryland		
ZUKOSKI, CHARLES F, III	1972	Tucson, Arizona		

HONORARY FELLOWS

NAME	YEAR OF ELECTION	LOCATION AT TIME OF ELECTION	OFFICES AND YEAR HELD	YEAR OF DEATH
ALLGOWER, MARTIN	1978	Basel, Switzerland		
ALLISON, PHILIP ROWLAND	1959	Oxford, England		1974
ANNANDALE, THOMAS	1885	Edinburgh, Scotland		1907
ATKINS, HEDLEY JOHN B.	1966	London, England		
ATLEE, JOHN LIGHT	1882	Lancaster, Pa.		1885
BALLANCE, CHARLES ALFRED (Sir)	1907	London, England		1936
BARRETT-BOYES, BRIAN G. (Sir)	1975	Auckland, New Zealand (Corresponding Member 1972)		
BASTIANELLI, RAFFAELLE	1919	Rome, Italy		1961
vonBERGMANN, PROF. ERNST	1894	Berlin, Germany		1907
BIGELOW, HENRY JACOB	1886	Boston, Massachusetts		1890
BILLINGS, JOHN SHAW	1882	Washington, D.C. (Elected Honorary Member 1905)		1913
BILLROTH, C.A. THEODOR	1885	Vienna, Austria		1894
BJÖRK, VIKING (Prof)	1979	Stockholm, Sweden (Corresponding Member 1974)		
BOWLBY, ANTHONY (Sir)	1919	London, England		1929
BRAND, PAUL WILSON	1967	Carville, Louisianna		
BROCK, RUSSELL CLAUDE (Lord)	1966	London, England		
BROSTER, LENNOX ROSS	1942	London, England		1965
BRUCE, JOHN	1961	Edinburgh, Scotland		1976

NAME	YEAR OF ELECTION	LOCATION AT TIME OF ELECTION	OFFICES AND YEAR HELD	YEAR OF DEATH
BRYANT, THOMAS	1891	London, England		1914–15
CHIENE, JOHN	1891	Edinburgh, Scotland		1923
CHUTRO, PIETRO	1922	Buenos Aires, Argentina		1937
CRAFOORD, CLARENCE	1951	Stockholm, Sweden		
CZERNY, VINCENZ	1885	Heidelberg, Germany		1916
deMARTEL, THIERRY	1927	Paris, France		1940
DENK, WOLFGANG	1948	Vienna, Austria		1970
DÉPAGE, ANTOINE	1916	LePanne, Belgium		1925
DUBOST, CHARLES	1974	Paris, France		
DURHAM, ARTHUR EDWARD	1891	London, England		1895
EDWARDS, HAROLD CLIFFORD	1964	London, England		
EISELSBERG, ANTON F. von	1911	Vienna, Austria		1939
ERICHSEN, JOHN ERIC	1885	London, England		1896
ESMARCH, J. FRIEDRICH	1885	Kiel, Germany		1908
EWING, (Prof.) MAURICE R.	1972	Parkville, Australia		
FONTAINE, RENÉE	1961	Strasbourg, France		
FRASER, JOHN BART (Prof)	1933	Edinburgh, Scotland		1947
FRIEDRICH, P.L. (Prof)	1910	Marburg, Germany		1916
GELIN, LARS-ERIK	1977	Göteborg, Sweden (Corresponding Member 1972)		
GIERTZ, KNUT HAROLD	1937	Stockholm, Sweden		1950
GOLIGHER, JOHN C.	1978	London, England		
GORDON-TAYLOR, GORDON	1956	London, England		1960
GORGAS, WILLIAM C.	1916	Washington, D.C.		1920
GREY-TURNER, GEORGE	1949	Taplow, Bucks, England		1951
GUSSENBAUER, CARL (Prof)	1893	Wengelsplatz, Germany		1903
HARRISON, REGINALD	1891	London, England		1908
HARTMANN, HENRI	1919	Paris, France		1952
HORSLEY, VICTOR ALEX. C.B.	1890	London, England		1916
HORWITZ, PHINEAS J.	1882	Philadelphia, Pa.		1904
HUMPHREY, GEORGE MURRAY (Sir)	1896	Cambridge, England		1896
HUNT, WILLIAM	1882	Philadelphia, Pa.		1897
ILLINGWORTH, CHARLES (Sir)	1966	Glasgow, Scotland		
IRELAND, MERRITTE W.	1934	Washington, D.C.		1952
KAY, ANDREW WATT (Sir)	1977	Glasgow, Scotland (Corresponding Member 1972)		
KEOGH, ALFRED	1918	London, England		1936
KEYNES, GEOFFREY	1938	London, England		
KOCHER, E. THEODOR (Prof.)	1894	Berne, Switzerland		1917
von LANGENBECK, BERNHARD	1886	Weisbaden, Germany		1887
LEGER, LUCIEN (Prof)	1979	Paris, France		
LERICHE, RENÉ	1922	Lyons, France		1955
LINDER, FRITZ	1968	Heidelberg, Germany		
LISTER, JOSEPH	1885	London, England		1912
LOEWENTHAL, JOHN	1973	Melbourne, Australia		
LORTHIOIR, JULES	1927	Brussels, Belgium		1931
LOUW, JOHN	1973	Cape Town, South Africa		
McINTIRE, ROSS T.	1942	Washington, D.C.		1959
MacCORMAC, WILLIAM	1886	London, England		1901
MACEWEN, WILLIAM (Sir)	1894	Glasgow, Scotland		1924
MAGEE, JAMES C. (Maj. Gen)	1942	Washington, D.C.		1976
MAKINS, GEORGE (Sir)	1918	London, England		1933
MAUNOURY, GABRIEL	1920	Chartres, France		1925
MERCADIER, MAURICE P.A.	1976	Paris, Frances (Corresponding Member 1972)		
von MIKULICZ-RADECKI, JOHANN	1904	Breslau, Germany		1905
MOORE, EDWARD MOTT	1880	Rochester, New York	Vice President-1883 President-1884 (Elec. Hon. 1896)	1902
MORGAN, CLIFFORD N. (Sir)	1963	London, England		

NAME	YEAR OF ELECTION	LOCATION AT TIME OF ELECTION	OFFICES AND YEAR HELD	YEAR OF DEATH
MOYNIHAN, BERKELEY G.A.	1908	Leeds, England		1936
MYLES, THOMAS (Sir)	1907	Dublin, Ireland		1937
von NUSSBAUM, J.N.	1885	Munich, Germany		1890
NYSTRÖOM, GUNNAR (Prof)	1930	Uppsala, Sweden		1964
OLLIER, LÉEOPOLD	1885	Lyons, France		1900
ONG, GUAN BEE	1977	Hong Kong, China (Corresponding Member 1974)		
PAGET, JAMES (Sir)	1885	London, England		1899
PARKER, WILLARD	1882	New York, New York		1884
PATEY, DAVID HOWARD	1964	London, England		1977
PÉAN, JULES E.	1894	Paris, France		1898
PETROVSKY, BORIS	1972	Moscow, Russia		
PORRITT, (Lord) ARTHUR	1973	London, England		
POST, ALFRED C.	1882	New York, New York		Resigned 1884
POWER, d'ARCY (Sir)	1925	London, England		1941
POZZI, SAMUEL JEAN (Prof)	1907	Paris, France		1918
ROBSON, A.W. MAYO (Sir)	1902	Leeds, England		1933
ROSS, JAMES PATTERSON (Sir)	1956	London, England		
SANDBLOM, JOHN PHILIP	1960	Lund, Sweden		
SCHEDE, MAX H.E.W.	1894	Hamburg, Germany		1903
SENNING, ÅKE (Prof)	1979	Zurich, Switzerland (Corresponding Member 1974)		
SIMS, J. MARION	1882	New York, New York		1883
SMITH, STEPHEN	1882	New York, New York	Vice President-1891 (Elec. Hon. 1896)	1922
SMITH, THE LORD OF MARLOW	1978	London, England		
STILES, HAROLD J.	1912	Edinburgh, Scotland		1946
TAYLOR, WILLIAM (Sir)	1924	Dublin, Ireland		1933
TERRIER, LOUIS FELIX	1896	Paris, France		1908
THIERSCH, KARL	1894	Leipsig, Germany		1895
THOMSON, ALEXIS	1914	Edinburgh, Scotland		1924
TRENDELENBURG, F. REIDRICH (Prof)	1907	Leipzig, Germany	(dropped 1919-WWI)	1924
TUFFIER, THEODORE	1918	Paris, France		1929
VERNEUIL, ARISTIDE A.S.	1885	Paris, France		1895
von VOLKMANN, RICHARD	1885	Halle, Germany		1889
WALLACE, CUTHBERT (Sir)	1920	London, England		1944
WALTHER, CHARLES	1920	Paris, France		1935
WEBB-JOHNSON, ALFRED	1950	London, England		1958
WELBOURN, RICHARD B.	1976	London, England (Corresponding Member 1974)		
WELLS, THOMAS SPENCER (Sir)	1894	London, England		1897
WOODRUFF, MICHAEL F.A.	1965	Edinburgh, Scotland		
WU, YING-K'AI	1978	Peking, China		
YANDELL, DAVID WENDELL	1880	Louisville, Kentucky	President-1890 (Elec. Hon. 1896)	1898
YOUNG, ARCHIBALD	1930	Glasgow, Scotland		1939
ZENKER, RUDOLPH	1968	Munchen, Germany		

CORRESPONDING FELLOWS

NAME	YEAR OF ELECTION	LOCATION AT TIME OF ELECTION		
CALNE, ROY YORKE	1972	Cambridge, England		
CHARTIKAVNIJ, KASARN	1972	Bangkok, Thailand		
DuPLESSIS, DANIEL JACOB	1972	Johannesburg, South Africa		
FORREST, ANDREW P. McEWEN	1972	Edinburgh, Scotland		
NANSON, ERIC M.	1972	Auckland, New Zealand		
PATINO, JOSE FELIX	1972	Bogota, Columbia		
PAULINO, FERNANDO	1974	Rio de Janeiro, Brazil		
SANO, KEIJL	1972	Tokyo, Japan		
WILLIAMS, DAVID INNES	1974	London, England		
YONG, NEU KHIONG	1972	Kuala Lumpur, Malaya		

SIGNERS OF THE CONSTITUTION OF THE AMERICAN SURGICAL ASSOCIATION

The 44 men in this list are on record as having signed the Constitution on May 5, 1880. In addition, two others were made Fellows in 1880, William H. Pancoast, of Philadelphia, and John Swinburne, of New York. Ever since, there has been some confusion about the Founding or Original members. The Association's records designate these two as Original members. Mears, in 1908, and others took the more exclusive view.

John Ashhurst, Jr.,
Philadelphia, Pennsylvania
S. N. Benham,
Pittsburgh, Pennsylvania
D. D. Bramble,
Cincinnati, Ohio
W. T. Briggs,
Nashville, Tennessee
John H. Brinton,
Philadelphia, Pennsylvania
Hugh W. Brock,
Morgantown, West Virginia
Wm. A. Byrd,
Quincy, Illinois
James L. Cabell,
University of Virginia, Virginia
Henry F. Campbell,
Augusta, Georgia
John S. Coleman,
Augusta, Georgia
P. S. Conner,
Cincinnati, Ohio
Saml. T. Davis,
Lancaster, Pennsylvania
W. W. Dawson,
Cincinnati, Ohio
L. A. Dugas,
Augusta, Georgia
J. W. S. Gouley,
New York, New York

Wm. Warren Greene,
Portland, Maine
Samuel D. Gross,
Philadelphia, Pennsylvania
Samuel W. Gross,
Philadelphia, Pennsylvania
Moses Gunn,
Chicago, Illinois
H. Lenox Hodge,
Philadelphia, Pennsylvania
John T. Hodgen,
St. Louis, Missouri
J. C. Hughes,
Keokuk, Iowa
J. C. Hutchison,
Brooklyn, New York
Christopher Johnston,
Baltimore, Maryland
J. M. Keller,
Hot Springs, Arkansas
W. W. Keen,
Philadelphia, Pennsylvania
R. A. Kinloch,
Charleston, South Carolina
R. J. Levis,
Philadelphia, Pennsylvania
Solon Marks,
Milwaukee, Wisconsin
C. H. Mastin,
Mobile, Alabama

Hunter McGuire,
Richmond, Virginia
J. Ewing Mears,
Philadelphia, Pennsylvania
E. M. Moore,
Rochester, New York
T. G. Morton,
Philadelphia, Pennsylvania
J. H. Packard,
Philadelphia, Pennsylvania
T. G. Richardson,
New Orleans, Louisiana
Thos. P. Russell,
Oshkosh, Wisconsin
L. A. Sayre,
New York, New York
Wm. L. Tremaine,
Buffalo, New York
P. S. Wales,
Washington, D. C.
J. R. Weist,
Richmond, Virginia
W. F. Westmoreland,
Atlanta, Georgia
James R. Wood,
New York, New York
D. W. Yandell,
Louisville, Kentucky

The Presidents of the American Surgical Association and the Offices They Held

Name	President	Age Elected	Vice President	Secretary	Treasurer	Recorder
* Gross, S.D.	1880–1883	75				
* Moore, E.M.	1884	70	1883			
* Briggs, W.T.	1885	56				1880–1882
* Gunn, M.	1886	64	1883			
* McGuire, H.	1887	52				
Agnew, D.H.	1888	70				
Cheever, D.W.	1889	58				
* Yandell, D.W.	1890	64				
* Mastin, C.H.	1891	65	1884;1890			
* Conner, P.S.	1892	53			1887-1891	
Senn, N.	1893	49	1888			
* Mears, J.E.	1894	56				1883–1893
Dennis, F.S.	1895	45	1888			
Tiffany, L. Mc.	1896	52	1892			
Warren, J.C.	1897	55	1891			
Prewitt, T.F.	1898	66	1887			
* Keen, W.W.	1899	62	1893			
Weir, R.F.	1900	63				
Park, R.	1901	49	1894			
Willard, DeF.	1902	56				1894–1901
Richardson, M.H.	1903	52	1898	1895–1897		
Dandridge, N.P.	1904	58			1895–1897	
Johnston, G.B.	1905	52				
VanderVeer, A.	1906	65	1899			
Allen, D.P.	1907	55		1902–1906		
Carmalt, W.H.	1908	72	1896			
Nancrède, C.B.G.de	1909	62	1890;1900			
Matas, R.	1910	50	1902			
Harte, R.H.	1911	56				1902–1910
Gerster, A.G.	1912	64	1909			
Powers, C.A.	1913	55	1904		1907–1912	
Mayo, W.J.	1914	53	1903			
Armstrong, G.E.	1915	60	1911			
LeConte, R.G.	1916	51		1907–1915		
Mixter, S.J.	1917	62	1911			
Huntington, T.W.	1918	69	1907			
Pilcher, L.S.	1919	74	1894;1915			
Brewer, G.E.	1920	59	1914			
Roberts, J.B.	1921	69	1889;1895		1892–1894	
Finney, J.M.T.	1922	59	1910			
McArthur, L.L.	1923	65	1913			
Crile, G.W.	1924	60	1912;1919			
Ochsner, A.J.	1925	67	1918			
Gibbon, J.H., Sr.	1926	55		1916–1922		
Cushing, Harvey	1927	58				
Rixford, E.	1928	63	1905			
Eliot, E., Jr.	1929	65	1923			

1594   * Original Member

The Presidents of the American Surgical Association and the Offices They Held

Name	President	Age Elected	Vice President	Secretary	Treasurer	Recorder
Lund, F.B.	1930	65				
Primrose, A.	1931	70	1922;1927			
Mayo, C.H.	1932	67				
Bevan, A.D.	1933	72				
Jones, D.F.	1934	66	1931			
Archibald, E.W.	1935	63	1926			
Pool, Eugene H.	1936	62			1926–1933	
Graham, E.A.	1937	54				
Elting; A.W.	1938	66	1936			
Phemister, D.B.	1939	57	1931			
Whipple, A.O.	1940	59				
Cheever, David	1941	65	1935			
Stone, Harvey B.	1942	60				
David, V.C.	1943	61	1938	1932–1936		
Coller, F.A.	1944	57				
NO MEETING 1945						
Darrach, W.	1946	70				
Churchill, E.D.	1947	52				
Cutler, E.C.	died 8-16-47	60				
Gallie, W.E.	1948	66	1936;1948			
Rankin, F.W.	1949	63				
Orr, T.G.	1950	66	1947			
Harvey, S.C.	1951	65				
Elkin, D.C.	1952	59	1942			
Dinsmore, R.S.	1953	61				
Naffziger, H.C.	1954	70	1941			
Gibbon, J.H., Jr.	1955	52	1953			1947–1951
Blalock, A.	1956	67				
Davis, Loyal	1957	61	1942			
Mulholland, J.H.	1958	58				
Ravdin, I.S.	1959	65				
Cole, Warren H.	1960	62	1948			
Stewart, John D.	1961	58	1959			
Dunphy, J.E.	1962	54				1957–1961
Cope, O.	1963	61	1957			
Firor, W.M.	1964	68	1951	1943–1948		
Zollinger, R.M.	1965	62				
McKittrick, L.S.	1966	73			1944–1950	
Creech, O., Jr.	1967	51				
Longmire, W.P., Jr.	1968	55				
Wangensteen, O.H.	1969	71	1952			
Altemeier, W.A.	1970	60		1958–1964		
Holden, W.D.	1971	59			1966–1970	
Moore, F.D.	1972	59				
Rhoads, J.E.	1973	66				
Scott, H.W., Jr.	1974	58			1960–1965	
Muller, W.H., Jr.	1975	56				1962–1967
Hardy, J.D.	1976	58				
Welch, C.E.	1977	71				
Sabiston, D.C.	1978	54				
Beahrs, Oliver	1979	65				
Shires, G. Thomas	1980	55		1970–1974		

OFFICERS OF THE
AMERICAN SURGICAL ASSOCIATION

	*Year indicated is the year the President was in the Chair		
Year	Meeting Place	President	Vice-Presidents (1st and 2nd VP's were not so designated until 1933)
June 1 1880	College of Physicians and Surgeons, New York, N.Y.		
May 5 1881	House of Delegates, Richmond, Virginia	SAMUEL D. GROSS	Louis Alexander Dugas James Rushmore Wood
Sept. 1881	Hotel Brighton Coney Island, New York	SAMUEL D. GROSS	Louis Alexander Dugas James Rushmore Wood
1882	Hall of Physicians, Philadelphia, Pennsylvania	SAMUEL D. GROSS	Louis Alexander Dugas James Rushmore Wood
1883	College Hall, University of Cincinnati, Cincinnati, Ohio	SAMUEL D. GROSS	Edward Mott Moore Moses Gunn
1884	Hall of the National Museum Building, Washington, D.C.	EDWARD MOTT MOORE	William Wirt Dawson Claudis Henry Mastin
1885	Reading Room of the Army Medical Museum, Washington, D.C.	WILLIAM THOMPSON BRIGGS	Joseph Chrisman Hutchison Elisha H. Gregory
1886	Army Medical Museum, Washington, D.C.	MOSES GUNN	Christopher Johnston Thomas P. Russell
1887	Army Medical Museum, Washington, D.C.	HUNTER McGUIRE	T.F. Prewitt J.W.S. Gouley
1888	Main Hall, Grand Army Building, Washington, D.C.	D. HAYES AGNEW	N. Senn F.S. Dennis
1889	New Army Medical Museum, Washington, D.C.	DAVID WILLIAMS CHEEVER	T.G. Richardson John B. Roberts
1890	Army Medical Museum, Washington, D.C.	DAVID W. YANDELL	C.H. Mastin C.B. Nancrede
1891	Grand Army Building, Washington, D.C.	CLAUDIUS HENRY MASTIN	John Collins Warren Stephen Smith

	Secretary	Treasurer	Recorder
	Jacob Rowland Weist	John H. Packard	William Thompson Briggs
	Jacob Rowland Weist	John H. Packard	William Thompson Briggs
	Jacob Rowland Weist	John H. Packard	William Thompson Briggs
	Jacob Rowland Weist	John H. Packard	J. Ewing Mears
	Jacob Rowland Weist	John H. Packard	J. Ewing Mears
	Jacob Rowland Weist	John H. Brinton	J. Ewing Mears
	Jacob Rowland Weist	John H. Brinton	J. Ewing Mears
	Jacob Rowland Weist	Phineas S. Conner	J. Ewing Mears
	Jacob Rowland Weist	Phineas S. Conner	J. Ewing Mears
	Jacob Rowland Weist	Phineas S. Conner	J. Ewing Mears
	Jacob Rowland Weist	Phineas S. Conner	J. Ewing Mears
	Jacob Rowland Weist	Phineas S. Conner	J. Ewing Mears

*Year	Meeting Place	President	Vice-Presidents (1st and 2nd VP's were not so designated until 1933)
1892	Hall of Natural History Society, Boston, Massachusetts	PHINEAS SANBORN CONNER	Louis McLane Tiffany Levi Cooper Lane
1893	Alumni Hall, Buffalo, New York	NICHOLAS SENN	Charles B. Porter W.W. Keen
1894	Main Hall, Preparatory Dept. Columbian University, Washington, D.C.	JAMES EWING MEARS	Roswell Park Lewis S. Pilcher
1895	New York Academy of Medicine, New York, New York	FREDERIC SHEPARD DENNIS	Jacob Rowland Weist John B. Roberts
1896	Detroit College of Medicine, Detroit, Michigan	LOUIS MCLANE TIFFANY	Christian Fenger William H. Carmalt
1897	Chemical Laboratory, Columbian University, Washington, D.C.	JOHN COLLINS WARREN	Theodore A. McGraw John Ashhurst, Jr.
1898	Tulane Medical College, New Orleans, Louisiana	THEODORE F. PREWITT	James McFadden Gaston Maurice Howe Richardson
1899	Chicago Medical Society, Chicago, Illinois	WILLIAM W. KEEN	Albert VanderVeer Solon Marks
1900	Columbia University Building, Washington, D.C.	ROBERT F. WEIR	Charles Beylard Nancrede Edmond Souchon
1901	Library Building, Medical & Chirurgical Faculty of Maryland, Baltimore, Maryland	ROSWELL PARK	John E. Owens Clayton Parkhill
1902	Senate Chamber of the Capitol, Albany, New York	DEFOREST WILLARD	Robert Abbe Rudolph Matas
1903	Medical Building of Columbia University, Washington, D.C.	MAURICE H. RICHARDSON	N.B. Carson W.J. Mayo
1904	Assembly Room of the Board of Education, St. Louis, Missouri	NATHANIEL P. DANDRIDGE	S.H. Weeks C.A. Powers

Secretary	Treasurer	Recorder
Jacob Rowland Weist	John B. Roberts	J. Ewing Mears
Jacob Rowland Weist	John B. Roberts	J. Ewing Mears
Jacob Rowland Weist	John B. Roberts	DeForest Willard
Maurice H. Richardson	Nathaniel P. Dandridge	DeForest Willard
Maurice H. Richardson	Nathaniel P. Dandridge	DeForest Willard
Maurice H. Richardson	Nathaniel P. Dandridge	DeForest Willard
Herbert L. Burrell	George Ryerson Fowler	DeForest Willard
Herbert L. Burrell	George Ryerson Fowler	DeForest Willard
Herbert L. Burrell	George Ryerson Fowler	DeForest Willard
Herbert L. Burrell	George Ryerson Fowler	DeForest Willard
Dudley P. Allen	George Ryerson Fowler	Richard H. Harte
Dudley P. Allen	George Ryerson Fowler	Richard H. Harte
Dudley P. Allen	George Ryerson Fowler	Richard H. Harte

*Year	Meeting Place	President	Vice-Presidents (1st and 2nd VP's were not so designated until 1933)
1905	Banquet Hall of the Hotel St. Francis, San Francisco, California	GEORGE BEN JOHNSTON	Emmet Rixford James Bell
1906	Assembly Room of the Hollenden Hotel, Cleveland, Ohio	ALBERT VANDERVEER	James E. Moore John C. Munro
1907	Assembly Room of the Shoreham Hotel, Washington, D.C.	DUDLEY P. ALLEN	Thos. W. Huntington A.F. Jonas
1908	Meeting Hall of the Jefferson Hotel, Richmond, Virginia	WILLIAM H. CARMALT	Willis G. Macdonald John F. Binnie
1909	Clover Room of the Bellevue-Stratford Hotel, Philadelphia, Pennsylvania	C.B.G. DE NANCRÈDE	A.G. Gerster Leonard Freeman
1910	Cabinet Room of the New Willard Hotel, Washington, D.C.	RUDOLPH MATAS	J.M.T. Finney George H. Monks
1911	Ordinary of the Brown Palace Hotel, Denver, Colorado	RICHARD H. HARTE	Samuel J. Mixter George E. Armstrong
1912	Windsor Hotel, Montreal, Canada	ARPAD G. GERSTER	Joseph Ransohoff George W. Crile
1913	Auditorium of the New National Museum, Washington, D.C.	CHARLES A. POWERS	Lewis L. McArthur Francis B. Harrington
1914	Ball Room of the Hotel Astor, New York, New York	WILLIAM J. MAYO	George E. Brewer William S. Halsted
1915	Assembly Room of the Mayo Clinical Building, Rochester, Minnesota	GEORGE E. ARMSTRONG	Lewis S. Pilcher Frank E. Bunts
1916	New National Museum, Washington, D.C.	ROBERT G. LECONTE	Charles L. Gibson Archibald MacLaren
1917	A Lecture Room of the Harvard Medical School, Boston, Massachusetts	SAMUEL J. MIXTER	Frederick W. Parham John E. Summers

Secretary	Treasurer	Recorder
Dudley P. Allen	George Ryerson Fowler	Richard H. Harte
Dudley P. Allen	George Ryerson Fowler	Richard H. Harte
Robert G. LeConte	Charles A. Powers	Richard H. Harte
Robert G. LeConte	Charles A. Powers	Richard H. Harte
Robert G. LeConte	Charles A. Powers	Richard H. Harte
Robert G. LeConte	Charles A. Powers	Richard H. Harte
Robert G. LeConte	Charles A. Powers	Archibald MacLaren
Robert G. LeConte	Charles A. Powers	Archibald MacLaren
Robert G. LeConte	Charles L. Gibson	Archibald MacLaren
Robert G. LeConte	Charles L. Gibson	Archibald MacLaren
Robert G. LeConte	Charles L. Gibson	Archibald MacLaren
John H. Gibbon	Charles H. Peck	John F. Binnie
John H. Gibbon	Charles H. Peck	John F. Binnie

*Year	Meeting Place	President	Vice-Presidents (1st and 2nd VP's were not so designated until 1933)
1918	Auditorium of New Cincinnati Medical College, Cincinnati, Ohio	THOMAS W. HUNTINGTON	A.J. Ochsner John B. Deaver
1919	Belvedere Room of the Hotel Traymore, Atlantic City, New Jersey	LEWIS S. PILCHER	George W. Crile Edward Martin
1920	Meeting Room Floor 17 of the Hotel Statler, St. Louis, Missouri	GEORGE E. BREWER	John F. Binnie Alexis Carrel
1921	Hart House, University of Toronto, Toronto, Canada	JOHN B. ROBERTS	Harvey G. Mudd James F. Mitchell
1922	National Museum, Washington, D.C.	JOHN M.T. FINNEY	Alexander Primrose James E. Thompson
1923	Kahler Hotel, Rochester, Minnesota	L. L. McARTHUR	Ellsworth Eliot, Jr. Donald C. Balfour
1924	Hotel Belvedere, Baltimore, Maryland	GEORGE W. CRILE	E. Wyllys Andrews Homer Gage
1925	National Museum, Washington, D.C.	ALBERT J. OCHSNER	Joseph C. Bloodgood Stanley Stillman
1926	Hotel Statler, Detroit, Michigan	JOHN H. GIBBON	Edward Starr Judd Edward W. Archibald
1927	Jefferson Hotel, Richmond, Virginia	HARVEY CUSHING	Alexander Primrose Arthur Ayer Law
1928	National Museum, Washington, D.C.	EMMET RIXFORD	Robert B. Greenough Stuart McGuire
1929	Auditorium of Allen Memorial Library, Cleveland Medical Library Assn., Cleveland, Ohio	ELLSWORTH ELIOT, JR.	Clarence L. Starr Dean D. Lewis
1930	Mitchell Hall of the College of Physicians, Philadelphia, Pennsylvania	FRED B. LUND	Carl A. Hamann Astley P.C. Ashhurst
1931	Fairmont Hotel, San Francisco, California	ALEXANDER PRIMROSE	Daniel Fiske Jones Dallas B. Phemister

Secretary	Treasurer	Recorder
John H. Gibbon	Charles H. Peck	John F. Binnie
John H. Gibbon	Charles H. Peck	John F. Binnie
John H. Gibbon	Charles H. Peck	John H. Jopson
John H. Gibbon	Charles H. Peck	John H. Jopson
John H. Gibbon	Charles H. Peck	John H. Jopson
Robert B. Greenough	Charles H. Peck	John H. Jopson
Robert B. Greenough	Charles H. Peck	John H. Jopson
Robert B. Greenough	Charles H. Peck	John H. Jopson
Robert B. Greenough	Eugene H. Pool	John H. Jopson
Robert B. Greenough	Eugene H. Pool	John H. Jopson
Lincoln Davis	Eugene H. Pool	John H. Jopson
Lincoln Davis	Eugene H. Pool	John H. Jopson
Lincoln Davis	Eugene H. Pool	John H. Jopson
Lincoln Davis	Eugene H. Pool	Walter Estell Lee

*Year	Meeting Place	President	Vice-Presidents (1st and 2nd VP's were not so designated until 1933)
1932	Sterling Hall of Medicine, Yale University, New Haven, Connecticut	CHARLES H. MAYO	Lincoln Davis Jonathan M. Wainwright
1933	National Museum, Auditorium, Washington, D.C.	ARTHUR DEAN BEVAN	F.N.G. Starr William F. Verdi
1934	Theatre of Hart House, University of Toronto, Toronto, Ontario	DANIEL FISKE JONES	LeGrand Guerry John L. Yates
1935	Harvard Medical School, Building B, Boston, Massachusetts	EDWARD WILLIAM ARCHIBALD	David Cheever Mont R. Reid
1936	Thorne Hall, Northwestern University, Chicago, Illinois	EUGENE H. POOL	Arthur W. Elting William E. Gallie
1937	Sert Room, Waldorf-Astoria Hotel, New York, New York	EVARTS A. GRAHAM	James M. Mason D.E. Robertson
1938	Assembly Room, The Traymore Hotel, Atlantic City, New Jersey	ARTHUR W. ELTING	John Homans Vernon C. David
1939	The Homestead, Hot Springs, Virginia	DALLAS B. PHEMISTER	Barney Brooks Seward Erdman
1940	George Warren Brown Hall, Washington University, St. Louis, Missouri	ALLEN O. WHIPPLE	John Staige Davis Thomas M. Joyce
1941	The Greenbrier, White Sulphur Springs, West Virginia	DAVID CHEEVER	Howard C. Naffziger Roscoe R. Graham
1942	The Cleveland Hotel, Cleveland, Ohio	HARVEY B. STONE	Loyal Davis Daniel C. Elkin
1943	Netherland Plaza Hotel, Cincinnati, Ohio	VERNON C. DAVID	Damon B. Pfeiffer Edward C. Moore
1944	Thorne Hall, Northwestern University, Chicago, Illinois	FREDERICK A. COLLER	Urban Maes Arthur M. Shipley

	Secretary	Treasurer	Recorder
	Vernon C. David	Eugene H. Pool	Walter Estell Lee
	Vernon C. David	Eugene H. Pool	Walter Estell Lee
	Vernon C. David	Fordyce B. St. John	Walter Estell Lee
	Vernon C. David	Fordyce B. St. John	Walter Estell Lee
	Vernon C. David	Fordyce B. St. John	Walter Estell Lee
	Charles G. Mixter	Fordyce B. St. John	Walter Estell Lee
	Charles G. Mixter	Fordyce B. St. John	Walter Estell Lee
	Charles G. Mixter	Fordyce B. St. John	Walter Estell Lee
	Charles G. Mixter	Fordyce B. St. John	Walter Estell Lee
	Charles G. Mixter	Fordyce B. St. John	Walter Estell Lee
	Charles G. Mixter	Fordyce B. St. John	Walter Estell Lee
	Warfield M. Firor	Fordyce B. St. John	Walter Estell Lee
	Warfield M. Firor	Leland S. McKittrick	Walter Estell Lee

*Year	Meeting Place	President	Vice-Presidents (1st and 2nd VP's were not so designated until 1933)
1945*	The meeting of the Association which had been scheduled for Philadelphia in the spring of 1945 had to be postponed because of Government restrictions on travel. By the time these restrictions were lifted, it was too late in the year to prepare for a meeting. In order to maintain the continuity of the Transactions of the Association, the President and the Council decided to publish as many of the papers listed on the Program as it was possible to obtain from the authors. Accordingly, nineteen papers, which were to have been presented at the meeting, were published in the *Annals of Surgery,* and then bound together as the 63rd Volume of the *Transactions of The American Surgical Association.*		
1946	The Homestead, Hot Springs, Virginia	WILLIAM DARRACH	Albert O. Singleton John deJ. Pemberton
1947	The Homestead, Hot Springs, Virginia	EDWARD D. CHURCHILL	Thomas G. Orr Edwin P. Lehman
1948	Chateau Frontenac, Quebec, Canada	ELLIOTT CARR CUTLER (died 8/16/47) WILLIAM E. GALLIE	William E. Gallie Warren H. Cole
1949	Jefferson Hotel, St. Louis, Missouri	FRED WHARTON RANKIN	Wilder Penfield Emile Holman
1950	Broadmoor Hotel, Colorado Springs, Colorado	THOMAS G. ORR	John J. Morton B. Noland Carter
1951	Shoreham Hotel, Washington, D.C.	SAMUEL CLARK HARVEY	Warfield M. Firor John M. Foster
1952	The Greenbrier, White Sulphur Springs, West Virginia	DANIEL C. ELKIN	Owen H. Wangensteen James F. Mitchell
1953	Statler Hotel, Los Angeles, California	ROBERT S. DINSMORE	John H. Gibbon, Jr. R. Kennedy Gilchrist
1954	Hotel Cleveland, Cleveland, Ohio	HOWARD C. NAFFZIGER	J. Stewart Rodman Lawrence Chaffin
1955	Warwick Hotel, Philadelphia, Pennsylvania	JOHN H. GIBBON, Jr.	Robert M. Moore Donald M. Glover
1956	The Greenbrier, White Sulphur Springs, West Virginia	ALFRED BLALOCK	Stuart William Harrington Julian Johnson
1957	Palmer House, Chicago, Illinois	LOYAL DAVIS	Brian Blades Oliver Cope
1958	The Waldorf-Astoria, New York; New York	JOHN H. MULHOLLAND	R.K. Gilchrist Henry Harkins

Secretary	Treasurer	Recorder
Warfield M. Firor	Leland S. McKittrick	Walter Estell Lee
Warfield M. Firor	Leland S. McKittrick	John H. Gibbon, Jr.
Warfield M. Firor	Leland S. McKittrick	John H. Gibbon, Jr.
Nathan A. Womack	Leland S. McKittrick	John H. Gibbon, Jr.
Nathan A. Womack	Leland S. McKittrick	John H. Gibbon, Jr.
Nathan A. Womack	B. Noland Carter	John H. Gibbon, Jr.
Nathan A. Womack	B. Noland Carter	John H. Gibbon, Jr.
Nathan A. Womack	B. Noland Carter	Brian Blades
R. K. Gilchrist	B. Noland Carter	Brian Blades
R. K. Gilchrist	B. Noland Carter	Brian Blades
R. K. Gilchrist	John C. Burch	Brian Blades
R. K. Gilchrist	John C. Burch	J. Englebert Dunphy
William A. Altemeier	John C. Burch	J. Englebert Dunphy

*Year	Meeting Place	President	Vice-Presidents (1st and 2nd VP's were not so designated until 1933)
1959	The Fairmont Hotel, San Francisco, California	I. S. RAVDIN	John D. Stewart Frederick G. Kergin
1960	The Greenbrier, White Sulphur Springs, West Virginia	WARREN H. COLE	Richard H. Sweet Carleton Mattewson, Jr.
1961	The Boca Raton Hotel & Club, Boca Raton, Florida	JOHN D. STEWART	Harris B. Shumacker, Jr. Joel W. Baker
1962	The Sheraton-Park Hotel, Washington, D.C.	J. ENGLEBERT DUNPHY	Nathan Anthony Womack John Daniel Martin, Jr.
1963	The Westward Ho Hotel, Phoenix, Arizona	OLIVER COPE	Frank Leven Albert Gerbode William S. McCune
1964	The Homestead, Hot Springs, Virginia	WARFIELD M. FIROR	Rudolph J. Noer Virgil S. Counseller
1965	Bellevue Stratford Hotel, Philadelphia, Pennsylvania	ROBERT M. ZOLLINGER	Clarence E. Gardner, Jr. Louis M. Rousselot
1966	The Boca Raton Hotel & Club, Boca Raton, Florida	LELAND S. McKITTRICK	Lawrence Chaffin David W. Robinson
1967	The Broadmoor, Colorado Springs, Colorado	OSCAR CREECH, JR.	Eugene M. Bricker Angus D. McLachlin
1968	Sheraton-Boston Hotel, Boston, Massachusetts	WILLIAM P. LONGMIRE, JR.	Truman G. Blocker, Jr. Richard L. Varco
1969	Netherland Hilton Hotel, Cincinnati, Ohio	OWEN H. WANGENSTEEN	Leon Goldman Bentley P. Colcock
1970	The Greenbrier, White Sulphur Springs, West Virginia	WILLIAM A. ALTEMEIER	Leonard D. Heaton Robert T. Tidrick
1971	The Boca Raton Hotel & Club, Boca Raton, Florida	WILLIAM D. HOLDEN	J. Hartwell Harrison Edward S. Judd, Jr.
1972	Fairmont Hotel, San Francisco, California	FRANCIS D. MOORE	Clarence Dennis Merle M. Musselman
1973	Century Plaza Hotel, Los Angeles, California	JONATHAN E. RHOADS	K. Alvin Merendino Chester B. McVay

	Secretary	Treasurer	Recorder
	William A. Altemeier	John C. Burch	J. Englebert Dunphy
	William A. Altemeier	H. William Scott, Jr.	J. Englebert Dunphy
	William A. Altemeier	H. William Scott, Jr.	J. Englebert Dunphy
	William A. Altemeier	H. William Scott, Jr.	William H. Muller, Jr.
	William A. Altemeier	H. William Scott, Jr.	William H. Muller, Jr.
	William A. Altemeier	H. William Scott, Jr.	William H. Muller, Jr.
	Harris B. Shumacker, Jr.	H. William Scott, Jr.	William H. Muller, Jr.
	Harris B. Shumacker, Jr.	William D. Holden	William H. Muller, Jr.
	Harris B. Shumacker, Jr.	William D. Holden	William H. Muller, Jr.
	Harris B. Shumacker, Jr.	William D. Holden	John W. Kirklin
	C. Rollins Hanlon	William D. Holden	John W. Kirklin
	George Thomas Shires	William D. Holden	John W. Kirklin
	George Thomas Shires	John A. Schilling	John W. Kirklin
	George Thomas Shires	John A. Schilling	John W. Kirklin
	George Thomas Shires	John A. Schilling	Jack W. Cole

*Year	Meeting Place	President	Vice-Presidents (1st and 2nd VP's were not so designated until 1933)
1974	The Broadmoor, Colorado Springs, Colorado	H. WILLIAM SCOTT, JR.	Mark M. Ravitch Allen M. Boyden
1975	Le Chateau Frontenac, Quebec City, Quebec, Canada	WILLIAM H. MULLER, JR.	Richard Warren Fraser N. Gurd
1976	Fairmont Hotel, New Orleans, Louisiana	JAMES D. HARDY	Henry G. Schwartz Clarence J. Berne
1977	Boca Raton Hotel and Club, Boca Raton, Florida	CLAUDE E. WELCH	Harwell Wilson Carl P. Schlicke
1978	Sheraton-Dallas Hotel, Dallas, Texas	DAVID C. SABISTON	John A. Schilling Robert S. Sparkman
1979	The Homestead, Hot Springs, Virginia	OLIVER H. BEAHRS	Joseph E. Murray Charles G. Rob
1980	Hyatt Regency, Atlanta, Georgia	G. THOMAS SHIRES	William G. Anlyan George L. Jordan, Jr.

Secretary	Treasurer	Recorder
George Thomas Shires	John A. Schilling	Jack W. Cole
James V. Maloney, Jr.	John A. Schilling	Jack W. Cole
James V. Maloney, Jr.	Walter F. Ballinger, II	Jack W. Cole
James V. Maloney, Jr.	Walter F. Ballinger, II	Lloyd M. Nyhus
James V. Maloney, Jr.	Walter F. Ballinger, II	Lloyd M. Nyhus
James V. Maloney, Jr.	Walter F. Ballinger, II	Lloyd M. Nyhus
W. Gerald Austen	Walter F. Ballinger, II	Lloyd M. Nyhus

INDEXES

INDEX OF SCIENTIFIC MATTERS

SUBJECTS

Page numbers within circles indicate figures.

3

4 Adrenals
adrenogenital syndrome, 754–55
aldosteronism, 1103–04, 1227–28
cortex, effect of stimulation on thyroid
function, 979
cortical function and sodium
retention, 948
Cushing's syndrome, 754–55, 1076–77,
1205
autotransplantation, 1492–94
cortical adenoma, 1205
hirsutism, 754
hyperplasia, 754–55
and Cushing's syndrome, 1205
injury by DDD, 1493
Nelson's syndrome, 1492–94
pheochromocytoma, 711
first in vivo diagnosis, 677
and medullary thyroid carcinoma,
1235, 1432
resection, 676–77, 711
transplantation of cortex, 753
tumors of, with Zollinger-Ellison
tumor, 1157
Agammaglobulinemia, and
homotransplantation, 1019
Air embolism. See Embolism, air
Albumin, macro-aggregated, radioisotope
tagged, in pulmonary embolism,
1193–95
Aldosteronism, primary, 1103–04,
1227–28
Aleuronat, intrapericardial, to develop
myocardial collateral circulation,
839
Alkalosis
hypokalemic in aldosteronism, 1104
in shock, 1248–49
Alloxan, experimental diabetes, 1420
Alpha-fetoprotein, 1411–12
Ambulances, horse, 272
Ambulation, early, 888–89
American Board of Surgery, 997. See
also Appendix C
certification, effect on army rank, 845
impetus to formation of, 758
suggestion for, 763, 775
American College of Surgeons. See also
Index of Organization Matters
qualifications for fellowship, 758–59
rejection of education papers, 759
and young Turks, 759
American Medical Association
disappearance of major figures from,
1216
stand on chiropractic, 582
Amino acids, for intravenous
administration, 821–22, 1354
Ammonemia, in parenteral nutrition,
1354
Ammonia, intoxication, in cirrhosis,
1044–46
Ammonium chloride, "of no value in
plasma repair", 806
Amphotericin, in prevention of
Candidiasis, 1355

Ampulla of Vater, cancer of, 768, 852–55
history of resection, 624
transduodenal resection, 768
Amputations, 534
technique
aperiosteal (Bunge), 467
Gritti-Stokes, 534
kineplastic, objected to in trauma,
467
major, performed in stages, 468
neuroma formation after, 561
prevention of neuroma by alcohol
injection, 562
osteoplastic, Pirogoff, 467, 534
secondary hemorrhage from, 39
tissue by tissue dissection, for
hemostasis, 467
for trauma, 466–68
delayed, 468
time of performance, 467–68
use of spinal anesthesia, 468
for war wounds, guillotine decried, 548
for war wounds, secondary
hemorrhage in, 548
Amputations by level
arm, for cancer of the breast, 126–27
foot
Chopart, 467
Hay, 467
Pirogoff, 467
Syme, 467, 836–37
forequarter
for melanoma, 932
transthoracic, 1085–86
hindquarter, 115
for melanoma, 932
hip, disarticulation (Brashear, Walter,
1806), 108
lower extremity, 836–37
Gritti-Stokes, 836–37
prostheses, 836–37
site of election, through knee-joint,
467
site of election, preserve knee-joint,
468
shoulder, 153–54
shoulder girdle, 153–54, 374
thumb, proscribed, 50
translumbar, 1225–26
transmetatarsal, 944
Amylase
in pancreatic fistula, 218
serum, in pancreatic transplantation,
1270
serum, in pancreatic trauma, 864–65
Anastomosis. See also under Shunt. See
also under organ or structure
adrenal-splenic, venous, 1016
aortocoronary, 424, 1292–94, 1400,
1425–27, 1496–98, 1521–23
arteriovenous
for coronary sclerosis, 473
for epilepsy, 473, 927
failure to provide distal perfusion,
473
for hemiplegia, 474
for threatened gangrene, 473–74

for vascular insufficiency, end-to-
end preferred, 474
biliary-intestinal, compatibility with
long survival, 771
coronary-internal mammary, 1175
ileo-anal, after proctocolectomy,
1055–56
portacaval. See Shunt, portacaval
Anemia
Cooley's, splenectomy for, 661
pernicious
and Balantidium coli, 569
cause, toxic absorption from
intestinal tract, 569
cholecystectomy in, 569
focal infection in, 569
operations to remove foci of
infection in, 566
splenectomy for, 490, 569, 662
transfusions for, 566
sickle cell, splenectomy in, 662
splenic, splenectomy for, 707
Anergy
in sepsis, 1460
in trauma, 1460, 1513–15
Anesthesia
anociassociation. See Anociassociation
changing trends in, 646–47
choice of, 438–44, 501
dangers of, 47, 645
deaths from, 438–39, 441–43
preceded by acapnia and overdosage
of anesthetic, 441
risk of at conclusion of operation,
441
duration of operations, 186–87
effect on temperature and blood
pressure, 186–87
evils of, 94
experimental, study of, 46
explosions, ethylene, 646
history of, 438
hypothermia, prevention, 186–87
increase in numbers of operations, 196
influence upon surgery, 120, 191–96
influence on wound infection, 196
inhalation agents
chloroform, 46, 167, 438–39
cardiac arrest, 84–85
for laryngectomy, 222
in military hospitals, 224, 444
necrosis of guinea pig livers from,
502
ether, 46, 167
controversy, 191–95
drop, standard anesthetic, 501
effect on kidneys, 167
the "first sponge" for, 191, 194
intrapharyngeal for head and
neck cases, 501
parties, 194
red cell counts, 250
Warren, J. C., Oct, 16, 1846, 195
ethyl bromide, 46
ethylene, 646–48
nitrous oxide, 441, 501
polypharmacy in, 438, 997

19

extracorporeal for lymphocyte
        depletion, 1265
of kidney grafts, 1217, 1265
Strontium[90], of blood for rejection
        crises, 1217
total body, 1059, 1150
        and marrow refusion, 1523
        and transplantation, 1111–12
Ischemia, chronic, visceral, 1475–76
Islet cell
        autotransplantation, 1495
        transplantation. *See* Transplantation,
                pancreas, islets
        tumor
                insulimonas, with Z-E tumors, 1157
                non-Beta, 1502–04
                non-Beta cells, 1271–72
Isotope, radioactive, colloidal gold, 1168
Ivalon
        aortic wrapping, 1037
        buttons, for cardiac suturing, 1131

J

Jaundice
        in biliary obstruction, 142
        bleeding in, 634
        congenital, hemolytic, splenectomy for,
                662, 707
        postoperative, cause of, 645
        serum, prevention of by room storage
                of plasma, 1001–03
Jaw
        dental root abscess, abstention from
                curettage, 640
        phosphorus necrosis of, 65
Jejunal interposition
        for dumping, 1378–80
        for esophagitis, 1024
        after total gastrectomy, 1118–20
Jejunostomy
        for gastric cancer, 727
        with gastroenterostomy for bleeding
                duodenal ulcer, 299
Jejunum
        pouch, (Poth) for dumping syndrome,
                1378
        pouch, stasis in, 1379
        ulcer
                anastomotic, 388–89, 618, 631–32,
                        955, 1011
                after posterior gastroenterostomy,
                        573–74
                after total pancreatectomy, 1495
                vagotomy for, 908
                antethoracic, 993
                with islet cell tumors of pancreas,
                        1039–41
Jews, peculiarities of, 591–92
        Mayo, W. J., 542–43
Joints
        cartilage and synovium uninjured by
                Dakin solution, 532
        excision, 88–89
        projectile wounds, 265
        pyarthrosis, Willems treatment of, 534
        resection, antisepsis in, 89

Kanamycin
        in bowel preparation, 1389
        topical in vascular surgery, 1454
Kasai, operation for biliary atresia,
        1448–49, 1500
Keloid
        in Negroes, 83
        after operations for pectus excavatum,
                1038
Kidney
        autotransplantation, 1407
                for study of renal hypertension,
                        798–99
        blunt force injury of, 731
        chronic failure, and
                parathyroidectomy, 1344
        cysts of, puncture at operation, 599
        decapsulation for nephritis, 328
        electrolyte conservation by, 821
        embryoma of, 598, 808, 1252–53
        floating, Dietl's crises, 116–18, 325
        horseshoe, resection of suppurating
                half, 437
        intravenous urography in diseases of,
                695
        movable, and neurasthenia, 428
        nephrolithiasis
                preference for pyelolithotomy over
                        nephrolithotomy, 598
                staghorn calculi, 598–99
        nephrolithotomy, 61
        operations, oblique incision, 328
        pyonephrosis, 109
        renal artery ligation, effect of, 186
        renal failure due to crush injuries, 835
        resection. *See* Nephrectomy
        revascularization, 1289–91
        stone
                difficulty in diagnosis, 391
                inaccuracy of diagnosis, 328
                nephrotomy preferred to pyelotomy,
                        391
                pyelotomy preferred to nephrotomy,
                        390, 598
                X-ray diagnosis, 199–200, 390–91
        surgery of, 325, 598–99
        transplantation. *See* Transplantation
        trauma, 185–86, 328
        tuberculosis of, 178
                nephrectomy for, 328
        unilateral, multicystic, mistaken for
                embryoma, 598
        ureterovesical obstruction from
                aberrant artery, 640
        Wilms' tumor, 598, 808, 1252–53
Knee
        internal derangements, 147–48
Knee joint, fractures involving, 464
Kraske operation, for imperforate anus,
        187
Kwashiorkor, and constrictive fibrous
        endocarditis, 1441
Kyphosis. *See* Spine

Laboratory
        in medical education, 253
        unnecessary recourse to, 730
Laminar air flow, in hip replacement,
        1346
Laminectomy
        for fracture and paraplegia, 331–33
        for intervertebral disc, need for fusion
                after, 797
Laminography, in cholangiography, 1017
Lane's (Arbuthnot) kinks, never
        symptomatic, 570
Laparotomy, exploratory
        ("diagnostitial"), for intestinal
        obstruction and for gunshot
        wounds, 70–72
Laryngectomy
        for cancer, 402, 474
                preceded by bilateral neck
                        dissection, 475
                two-stage operation, 403, 482
        death from "vagitis", 474
        preliminary gastrostomy, 403
        total, technique of, 222
        useful speech after, 402
Larynx
        inflammation, intubation for
                (O'Dwyer), 92–93
        inflammation, tracheotomy for, 92–93
        tuberculosis, laryngotomy for, 118
Laser, surgical applications of, 1198
Lavage, gastric, for acute renal failure,
        889
League of Nations, American Surgical
        Association urged to endorse, 581
Leeches, anticoagulant effect of hirudin,
        804
Leukemia
        and Budd-Chiari syndrome, 1508–09
        extracorporeal blood irradiation for,
                1084
        splenectomy for, 86, 278–79, 662
Leukocyte typing, 1265
Leukocytes, abnormalities of and
        infection, 1356
Leukocytosis, in appendicitis, 250–51
Leukotomy, frontal, 1153–54
Liability. *See* Malpractice liability
Library, of the Surgeon General, and
        Billings, John S., 155
Ligatures, absorbable, 33
Limb, replantation, experimental, 584
Limulus lysate assay, for sepsis, 1422
Lip, cancer, 164
Lipidemia, ileal bypass in, 1339, 1396–97
Lipids, serum, in renal transplant
        patients, 1447
Listerism
        Briggs, W. T., 4
        and elective joint operations, 111
        The Great Debate, 28–29
        and herniorrhaphy, 111
        Mastin, C. H., in 1891, 120
        reception of, 463–64

INDEX OF SCIENTIFIC MATTERS

NAMES

See *also* INDEX OF ORGANIZATION MATTERS — NAMES

Page numbers within circles indicate figures.

A

Abbe, Robert: catgut rings for intestinal anastomosis, 105; anesthesia, ether versus chloroform, 167–68; cases from New York Hospital, 173; operation for tic douloureux, 176; tuberculous peritonitis, 178–79; castration for prostatic hypertrophy, 183; anesthesia, burns from warming mattress, 187; thoracotomy, pneumothorax, use of Fell-O'Dwyer respirator, 188; spinal cord suture, 266; abdominal route for rectal tumors, 287; intracranial trigeminal resection for tic douloureux, 295; tic douloureux, due to nerve root inflammation, 295; string technique for esophageal stricture, 316; radium, effects of, 321–22; Quenu abdominoperineal rectal resection, 348; radium, effect of on malignant tissue, 492

Abbott, Maude: on patent ductus, cited by Gross, 812

Abbott, Osler A.: polyethylene wrapping of aneurysms, cited by Bahnson, 999

Abbott, W. Osler: intestinal tube for fluid and nutritional maintenance, 822–23; indwelling intestinal tube, cited by Ravdin, 900

Abbott, Walter P.: coauthor of DeBakey, 1197

Abbott, William E.: discussion of Glenn on Cushing's syndrome, 1078; postgastrectomy malfunction, 1082; discussion of Beal, total gastrectomy, 1119–20; discussion of Barnes and Cope on magnesium requirements, 1127

Abel, John J.: extracorporeal dialysis, cited by Rhoads, 890

Abernethy, John: skull fracture, 40

Abrams, Berel L.: coauthor of Haller, 1176

Abrams, L. D.: coauthor of Williams and Schenk, 1331

Abrasanhoff: first use of muscle flap for bronchopleural fistula, cited by Wangensteen, 779

Ach, A.: resection of cardia for cancer, 507

Ackerman, Lauren V.: classification of breast cancer, 1135; local excision and irradiation of breast cancer, 1333

Adair, Frank E.: coauthor of Lee, B. J., 563; local excision of breast cancer, cited by Wise and Ackerman, 1334

Adami, George J.: attack on Lane's (Arbuthnot) doctrine, 523

Adams, Donald S.: coauthor of Gage, Homer, 583, 598

Adams, Forrest H.: endocardial elastosis, cited by Maloney, 1441

Adams, Herbert D.: prolonged successful cardiac massage, cited by Lahey, 850; cancer of lung, discussion of Gibbon, 1004

Adams, J. T.: colleague of DeWeese, vena cava clip, 1374

Adams, William E.: caustic occlusion of bronchus, cited by Archibald, 746; first transthoracic esophagogastrectomy, cited by Phemister, 897

Adamsons, Roland J.: gastroepiploic artery-umbilical vein shunt, cited by Dennis, 1350

Adey, W. R.: astronaut's EEG, cited by Maloney, 1274

Adkins, Paul C.: resection of multiple pulmonary metastases, 1381–83

Adler, F. L.: immune RNA transfer, cited by Ramming, 1474

Admirand, William H.: choledocholithiasis, 1359

Adson, Alfred W.: sympathectomy for Raynaud's disease, 638; sympathectomy for angina pectoris, 649; coauthor of Judd, 664; coauthor of Mayo, W. J., 718; sympathectomy for hypertension, cited by Heuer, 780; discussion of Heuer, sympathectomy for hypertension, 781; discussion of Dandy on pseudotumor, 789; discussion on sympathectomy and renal hypertension, 799; cranial osteomyelitis and brain abscess, 801; locating facial nerve, cited by Byars, 980

Agnew, D. Hayes: carotid artery aneurysm, 75; operation for

38 Agnew, D. Hayes (*continued*)
  stone, 79; medico-legal liability in cranial and heart
    wounds, 82; medicolegal liability in laparotomy for
    penetrating wounds, 82; hernia, follow-up in, 101; hernia,
    fecal fistula closure, 105; fracture, shaft of femur, 110;
    contributions, (121;) brain surgery, 121–22; craniotomy
    for microcephaly, 132; liver abscess, 204; flap cleft palate
    operations, 316; operations for epilepsy (1891), 990
Agote, Luis: citrate anticoagulation of blood, 535
Aikins, W. T.: cited by Starr, F. N. G., 713
Albarran y Dominguez, Joaquin: perineal prostatectomy, 409
Albers, Heinrich E.: fractures, lower extremities, early weight
    bearing, 183
Albert, Eduard: hernia, recurrences, 302
Albert, Harold M.: extracorporeal circulation, homologous
    lungs and mechanical heart, 984–85; operation for
    transposition, cited by Senning, 1423
Albright, Fuller: adrenocortical response to major operative
    stress, 948; cited by Cope, 987; protein nutrition with
    intravenous plasma, cited by Allen, 1046
Alden, John: gastric bypass, cited by Mason, 1480
Aldrete, J. S.: coauthor of Hallenbeck, 1451
Aldridge, H. E.: coauthor of Bigelow, 1222
Alexander, Emory G.: early operation for acute cholecystitis,
    736
Alexander, J. Wesley: heptavalent pseudomonas vaccine, cited
    by MacMillan, 1318; leucocyte antibacterial action, 1356
Alexander, John: results of thoracoplasty for tuberculosis, 653;
    technique of thoracoplasty, 777
Alexander, M. K.: coauthor of Priest, 1157
Alexandre, Guy W.: kidney transplantation, 1150
Allbritten, Frank F., Jr.: cancer of the lung, 1003; discussion of
    Koop on esophageal atresia, 1204
Allbutt, Sir Clifford: angina pectoris, seat of in ascending aorta,
    625
Allen, Arthur W.: discussion of symposium on sympathectomy,
    718; sympathectomy for peripheral vascular disease, 719;
    duodenal ulcer, acute massive hemorrhage, 733; discussion
    of Brooks, B., ligation of concomitant vein, 745; gastric
    ulcer, 840; subtotal gastrectomy for duodenal ulcer, 887;
    on bleeding ulcer, cited by Churchill, 921; discussion of
    Lahey and Marshall on total gastrectomy, 952;
    contributions of, (1072;)
Allen, Carroll W.: coauthor of Matas, 469
Allen, Dudley P.: anesthesia, effect upon temperature and
    blood pressure, 186; hysterectomy, 197; Larrey and
    pericardiotomy, 202; appendectomy and fecal fistula, 228;
    gastric cancer, operation after diagnosis, 243; surgical
    physiology and pathology for students, 271; vaginal
    hysterectomy, 288; traction for fracture with spinal cord
    injury, 333; aseptic surgical technique, 339; teaching of
    surgery, 362–64; contributions, (363;) proposal for a
    national examining board in surgery, 364; peritonitis,
    irrigation, 383; tetanus, from toy pistol wounds, 400;
    accreditation of surgeons ignored in 1907, 582
Allen, Duff S.: experimental cardiac valvotomy, 610; coauthor
    of Graham, 934
Allen, J. Garrott: pooled plasma and homologous serum
    jaundice, 1001–02; discussion of Hoxworth, stored liquid
    plasma, 1046; homologous serum jaundice, 1046; protein
    nutrition with intravenous plasma, 1046; total body
    irradiation, 1059; hepatitis from blood transfusion,
    1095–96; discussion of Langston on autotransfusion, 1165;
    discussion of Starzl on hepatitis in homograft recipients,
    1343
Allen, Terry R.: coauthor of Kaiser and Dale, 1490

Alley, Ralph D.: ruptured aorta, cited by Kirsh, 1443
Allingham, Herbert W.: anticipation of Mikulicz colon
    resection, 296
Allis, Oscar H.: pelvis, fractures, 118; fractures, open reduction,
    carpenter's screws, 141; hip, dislocation of, 435
Allison, Philip R.: discussion of Lahey and Marshall on total
    gastrectomy, 953; discussion of Gray on esophageal
    varices, 959; splenectomy and pancreatectomy with
    gastrectomy for cancer, 997; hiatus hernia, 1377–78
Alpert L. I.: thymus in myasthenia, cited by Buckingham, 1455
Altemeier, William A.: infected burns with hemorrhage, 846;
    quality of study of infection, 860; discussion of Cohn,
    antibiotics and colonic anastomoses, 1054; discussion of
    Howe, staphylococcal wound infections, 1061; infection,
    and regression of cancer of rectum, 1097; postoperative
    infection, 1139; infection after thoracotomy for cardiac
    arrest, 1177–78; staphylococcal enterocolitis, 1192; gram-
    negative septicemia, 1246; President 1970, 1314;
    contributions of, (1315;) antibacterial agents in burns,
    1316–17; changing pattern in surgical infections, 1387;
    discussion of Nichols, antibiotic colon preparation, 1389;
    on intestinal antibiotics, cited by Judd, 1410; discussion of
    Stone, prophylactic antibiotics, 1454
Altman, R. Peter: portoenterostomy for biliary atresia, 1500–02
Amad, Kamel H.: coauthor of Cooley, 1100
Amdrup, E.: proximal gastric vagotomy, cited by Sawyers, 1481
Ament, Marvin E.: home parenteral nutrition, 1504
Amerson, J. R.: coauthor of Humphrey, 1333
Amussat, J. Z.: anus, imperforate, 206
Anderson: cited by Crile, on thyrocardiacs, 677
Anderson, Danny: Scott versus Payne operation for morbid
    obesity, 1455
Anderson, Roger: fractures, percutaneous skeletal fixation,
    204–05; external fixation of fractures, cited by Wilson,
    835–36
Andresen, A. F. R.: treatment of gastroduodenal hemorrhage,
    cited by Enquist, 1208
Andrews, Edmund: nitrous oxide oxygen anesthesia, 438;
    cholesterol gallstone formation, 714
Andrews, E. Wyllys: Gasserian ganglionectomy for tic
    douloureux, 146, 175; operation for tic douloureux, 176;
    hernia, overlapping repair, 256; resolution of ulcer mass by
    gastroenterostomy, 311; law of accelerating risk in cancer,
    372; advantages of aseptic anastomosis (Halsted), 425;
    internal hydrocephalus, glass tubes for subdural drainage,
    435–36; contributions, (436;) intravenous ether anesthesia,
    advantages of, 491; unimportance of lung inflation in
    unilateral thoracotomy, 498; focal infection theory, 515
Andrews, Frederick W.: microorganisms of saliva, 308
Andrus, E. Cowles: colleague of Blalock, 973
Andrus, William DeW.: coauthor with Heuer, 613; atelectasis,
    688; adrenal extract for shock from closed loop extracts,
    751; adrenal cortical extract in shock, cited by Blalock,
    837; twin of Andrus, E. C., 973
Ankeney, Jay L.: discussion of Dunphy on disappearance of
    polyps, 1097
Anlyan, William G.: discussion of Goldman on
    hyperparathyroidism, 1062
Annandale, Thomas: lithotomy, perineal, 90; peroral
    intratracheal anesthesia, 93; resuture of bucket handle
    meniscus, 148
Ansell, Jack E.: bleeding varices—vasopressin, 1473
Anthony, Milton: pulmonary resection (1823), 180
Antyllus: operations for aneurysm, 282
Apostoli, Georges: electrical treatment of uterine myomas, 133
Appleby, L. H.: pelvic exenteration, cited by Bricker, 1238

54 Dubost, Charles (*continued*)
and homograft replacement, cited by Bahnson, 999;
constrictive endocarditis, 1441

Duckett, John: primary urethral valvotomy, cited by Murphy, 1407

Dudley, Benjamin W.: epilepsy, trephining for, 49;
Transylvania University, 108

Dudley, Hugh F.: antidiuresis after trauma, 1010–11

Dudrick, Stanley J.: parenteral alimentation, 1354; discussion of Fonkalsrud on home parenteral nutrition, 1504

Duff, John H.: coauthor of MacLean, 1246

Duffell, David: coauthor of Aust and Urdaneta, 1224

Dugas, Louis A.: contributions, ④; sign of dislocated shoulder, 4

Dugger, Gordon: hypophysectomy for breast cancer, cited by Womack, 1048

Duisberg, E. H.: coauthor of Green, 992

Dumont, Allan E.: thoracic duct fistula for immunosuppression, 1185; discussion of Starzl on thoracic duct drainage for immunosuppression, 1526

Dunham, Edward K.: pneumonia and empyema in army camps, 561

Dunham, Theodore: string passing for esophageal stricture, 316

Dunlop, George R.: cancer cells in bloodstream, cited by Lund, 1067

Dunn, James H.: esophagus, stricture, 316

Dunott, Thomas J.: cardiac puncture, 84

Dunphy, J. Englebert: pilonidal sinus, cited by Burch, 865; discussion of Karlson, massive gastrointestinal hemorrhage, 1083; polyposis and carcinoma of colon, 1096; discussion of Lillehei on transplantation, 1099; irradiation and bone marrow regeneration, 1112; President 1962, 1149; contributions, ⑴⑴⑤⑴; comment on Ravdin, 1155; discussion of Altemeier on infection in thoracotomy for cardiac arrest, 1178; treatment of gastroduodenal hemorrhage, cited by Enquist, 1208; discussion of Dennis and of Thal on gastroduodenal hemorrhage, 1209; discussion of Madden on electrocoagulation of rectal cancer, 1236; discussion of Turnbull on no-touch colon resection, 1236; discussion of Farris on bleeding duodenal ulcer, 1251; discussion of Ravitch on intestinal healing, 1253; discussion of Murray on renal transplantation, 1270; discussion of Kirklin and of Maloney on computers, 1276; discussion of DeCosse, irradiation bowel injury, 1288; discussion of Madden on electrocoagulation of rectal cancer, 1336; choledocholithiasis, 1359; discussion of Wolff on colonoscopy, 1383; and abdominal angina, cited by Campbell, 1476

du Plessis, Daniel J.: bile reflux and gastric ulcer, cited by Dragstedt, 1338

Dupuytren, Baron Guillaume: skull fracture, 40; enterotome for division of enterostomy spur, 105; innominate artery ligation, 170; enterotome, for spur crushing in fecal fistula, 346; intestinal ulceration in burn patients, 388; closure of total fecal fistula, 607

Durand: pericardium, incision for access to, cited by Roberts, 210

Durand, Marius: anus, imperforate, 206

Durante, Francesco: nerve xenograft, 317

Durham, Arthur E.: lithotomy, techniques, 90; colostomy, 443

DuShane, James W.: coauthor of Kirklin, 1122, 1210

Duval: operation for procidentia, cited by Ashhurst, A. P. C., 622

DuVal, Merlin K., Jr.: caudal pancreatojejunostomy, 571; caudal pancreatojejunostomy, cited by Dennis, 1039; caudal pancreatojejunostomy, cited by Mulholland, 1053; discussion of Longmire on pancreatitis, 1053

Dworken, H. J.: coauthor of DeCosse, 1286

Dye, Williams S.: coauthor of Julian, 982, 999; ruptured aortic aneurysms, 1035; aortic commissurotomy, 1079–80; balloon occlusion of vena cava, 1477

E

Earlam, Richard J.: coauthor of Ellis, 1251

Eastcott, Sir H. H. G.: carotid resection for arteriosclerosis, 1064; carotid resection and reconstruction, cited by Connolly, 1468; antibiotics in vascular surgery, cited by Barker, 1491

Eastman, J. R.: local anesthesia in thyroidectomy for hyperthyroidism, 592

Eaton, L. M.: thymectomy for myasthenia, cited by Buckingham, 1455

Eccles: inguinal hernia and cryptorchidism, cited by Jopson, 680

Eck, Nicolai V.: experimental portacaval shunt, 882; portacaval shunt, cited by McDermott, 1280

Eckert, Charles: discussion of Clatworthy, bleeding varices in children, 1093; discussion of Howard, pancreaticoduodenectomy, 1277; discussion of Wells on medullary carcinoma of thyroid, 1432

Edebohls, George M.: tubercle bacilli in Fallopian tubes, 178

Edgerton, Milton T., Jr.: ocular hypertelorism, 1322–23

Edkins, John S.: postulate of antral secretory hormone, cited by Herrington, 1097

Edmounds, W.: anticipation of Mikulicz colon resection, cited by Mikulicz, 296

Edmunds, L. Henry, Jr.: gastrointestinal fistulae, 1120–22

Edwards, C.: coauthor of Rob, 1064

Edwards, J. E.: pulmonary hypertension, suggestion of pulmonary constriction, cited by Muller, 985

Edwards, Leonard W.: cited by Scott, postgastrectomy malfunction, 1082; vagotomy and antrectomy for duodenal ulcer, 1097; vagotomy-antrectomy experience, cited by Scott, 1172; antrectomy and vagotomy, 1482

Edwards, M. Lowell: mitral replacement, 1145–47; coauthor of Starr, 1195

Edwards, W. Sterling: discussion of Connolly on carotid endarterectomy, 1469

Edwards, William H.: coauthor of Herrington, 1097; coauthor of Kaiser and Dale, 1490

Effler, Donald B.: cardiac arrest, cited by Lam, 1064; discussion of Bahnson, surgery of aortic valves, 1126; discussion of Bigelow on mitral annuloplasty, 1131; internal mammary myocardial implant, 1173; coronary endarterotomy, 1211–12; and Vineberg internal mammary implant, 1222; aneurysms of left ventricle, 1385–86; discussion of Spencer on coronary bypass, 1401; contributions of, ⑴⑷⑴②

Egan, R. L.: clinical mammography, cited by Barker, 1288

Egdahl, Richard H.: coauthor of Hume, 1111; RNA transfer, 1151; colleague of Mannick, 1475

Eggers, Carl: transpleural esophagectomy, 669; diverticulitis and sigmoiditis, 704; discussion of Burdick and Coley on cryptorchidism, 726; discussion of Graham, on empyema, 727

Ehrenfeld, William K.: visceral revascularization, 1475–76

Ehrenhaft, Johann L.: contributions of, ⑴⓪②⑥⑴; discussion of Kirklin on tetralogy of Fallot, 1211

Ehrlich, Paul: transformation of carcinoma into sarcoma, 477; therapia sterilisans magna, 627

Ehrmann, J.: uranoplasty, improvement of results with age of patients, cited by Brophy, 314

Eichelter, P.: caval filter, cited by DeWeese, 1374

Eichwald, E. J.: islet cell transplantation, 1270

56

Escher, Doris J. W.: coauthor of Furman, 1223

Esmarch, J. Friedrich: Listerism, 30; breast cancer, 126

Esterhazy, Marie Charles Ferdinand: Dreyfus affair, 211

Estes, William L.: spinal cord, transection with recovery, 266; skepticism over radiotherapy, 287; myofibroma of colon, 350; discussion of rectal cancer (Mayo), 452; end results of fracture of shaft of femur, 458; amputations for trauma, 466–67; discussion of Cotton on fractures of femoral neck, 504; tetanus antitoxin, not needed in railroad injuries, 513; discussion of Gibson on tetanus, 514; professors versus practical surgeons, 514; abdominal injury, blunt versus penetrating, 538; Committee on Fractures, final report, 578; clinic use of gallbladder radiographic visualization, 609; implantation of ovary, 629

Estes, William L., Jr.: immediate treatment of open fractures, 671; discussion of Lewis and Trimble, abdominal injuries, 732; survival of patients with aortic aneurysm, 999; discussion of McVay on herniorrhaphy, 1082

Estlander, Jakob A.: operation for empyema, 152; thoracoplasty for empyema, 179; operation for chronic empyema, 406

Evans, C. S.: bladder tumor, 109

Evans, Everett I.: no capillary leak in shock, cited by Blalock, 862; discussion of Coller, renal insufficiency, 916; discussion of Allen, plasma and jaundice, 1003

Evans, H. M.: thyroid and parathyroid drawing for Halstead, 367; drawings of myenteric plexuses for Finney, 396

Evans, John: coauthor of Glenn, 1017

Eve, Duncan: hand disinfection, 231; discussion of Cotton on fracture of neck of femur, 503

Everson, Tilden: discussion of Harkins on Billroth I, 1012

Ewing, James: giant cell tumor, a case of malignancy, 457; histological report on Coley's specimen, 476; discussion of Lee, irradiation in carcinoma of breast, 620

Ewing, Maurice R.: discussion of Starzl on renal transplantation, 1414

Exner: fluoroscopy 1897, cited by White, 198

Exner, A.: Heyrovsky operation for achalasia, 596

F

Fabri, Peter J.: coauthor of Pace, 1519

Fagge, Charles H.: appendicitis, 91

Fahimi, H. D.: coauthor of McGuff and Deterling, 1198

Fairley, H. B.: clinical hypothermia, 1065

Falk, Gerald: coauthor of LeVeen, 1410

Fallis, Laurence F.: total pancreatoduodenectomy, 915; discussion on colectomy, 1056

Farber, Sidney: aminopterin and leukemia, cited by Cole, 1111; Wilms' tumor, cited by Swenson, 1252

Farina, Guido: attempted suture of heart wound, 407

Fariñas: retrograde aortography, cited by Freeman, 923

Farmer, Douglas A.: ulcer operations and gastric acidity, 964–65

Farrand, Robert E.: coauthor of Harken, 973

Farris, Jack M.: discussion of Herrington on vagotomy-antrectomy, 1098; vagotomy and pyloroplasty for bleeding ulcer, 1115–18; discussion of Dennis and of Thal on gastroduodenal hemorrhage, 1209; bleeding duodenal ulcer, 1250–51; discussion of selective vagotomy, 1337; discussion of Hoerr on operations for duodenal ulcer, 1361

Fattah, Farouk: coauthor of Wangensteen, 1090

Fauntleroy, A. M.: surgical lessons of the European War, 508

Favaloro, Rene: coronary endarterotomy, 1211–12; first saphenous coronary bypass at Cleveland Clinic, cited by Effler, 1401

Feinman, Z. R.: no benefit from antietanus serum, 514

Felix, W. Robert: portacaval shunt, 1348

Fell, Egbert H.: aortic commissurotomy, cited by Dye and Julian, 1079; discussion of Kirklin, tetralogy of Fallot, 1123

Felton, Warren J., II: pectus excavatum, 1038

Fenger, Christian: brain abscess, 47–49, 58; contributions, (48;) pancreas carcinoma, 75; on empyema, 152; ureteral surgery, 158–59; cancer of the tongue, intratracheal anesthesia, 165; bladder in groin hernia, 171; on tic douloureux, 177; operation for tuberculosis of the seminal vesicles, 178; tuberculous adenitis, resection, 181; fractures, lower extremities, opposition to ambulant treatment, 184; anesthesia, need to warm patient, 187; appendiceal abscess, 228; tuberculous peritonitis; nonoperative treatment, 278; hyperthyroidism, cardiac degeneration in, 320; teacher of Murphy, J. B., 381; nephrolithiasis, 390

Fenwick: appendicitis, cited by Bull (1888), 91

Fenwick, Samuel and W. S.: stress ulcers with sepsis, 388

Ferebee, N. M.: The Battleship in War, 225

Ferguson, Alexander H.: inguinal hernia, operation, 172; inguinal herniorrhaphy without transplantation, 258; contributions, (302;) inguinal herniorrhaphy without cord transplantation, 302–03; choice of operation for duodenal ulcer, 311; opposition to Brophy, preference for flap palatal operations, 315–16; hemostasis in liver resection, 319; decapsulation of kidney in nephritis, 328; breast cancer, arm amputation, 373; breast cancer, neck dissection, 373; visceral pleurectomy, 406; perineal prostatectomy, 410; Halsted's recognizing sarcoma of mandible as benign, 421; biliary fistula into colon, 425; crushing bowel ends to permit aseptic anastomosis, 425; unimportance of cord transplantation in inguinal herniorrhaphy, 552

Ferguson, Donald J.: hemodynamics of portal hypertension, 1167–69

Ferguson, L. Kraeer: discussion of Aust on ureterosigmoidostomy and colon cancer, 1225

Ferguson, Lewis K.: discussion on colectomy, 1056

Ferguson, Sir Wiliam: flap cleft palate operation, 316

Ferrebee, W.: coauthor of Rapaport, 1523

Fetter, D.: coauthor of Humphrey, 1333

Fierst, Sidney M.: coauthor of Karlson, 1082; coauthor of Enquist, 1207

Fifield, William C. B.: tracheotomy, 57–58

Fine, Jacob: discussion of intestinal obstruction, 765; traumatic shock, 861; peritoneal irrigation for acute renal failure, 889; host resistance to bacteria in traumatic shock (1955), 1461

Fink, F.: subcutaneous gastric esophageal substitute, cited by Ochsner, Alton, 747

Finland, Maxwell: and staphylococcal infections, cited by Sandusky, 1061

Finney, John M. T.: operations for tic douloureux, 176; breast, comedocarcinoma, 214; breast cancer, operations, 216; perforating ulcer, 240; wiring for aneurysm, 259; pyarthrosis, drainage of, 267; prostatectomy, Bottini, transurethral fulguration, 268; prostatectomy, for tuberculosis, 268; pyloroplasty, 275; 389; interest in wire filigree herniorrhaphy, 281; value of large opening in pyloroplasty, 299; rhinoplasty, use of finger graft, 366; diagnosis of renal stone, 391; congenital idiopathic dilatation of colon, 393; enterotomies and saline intestinal flush, 393; aneurysm, wiring, 404; wiring aortic aneurysm, 419; pancreas, resection, 426; deprecation of X-ray therapy and Coley's toxins, 426–27; discussion of Hartmann on gastroenterostomy, 490; splenectomy for Banti's disease and pernicious anemia, 490; breast, cystic disease, choice of operation, mastectomy, 493; cited by Bloodgood, 506;

Gaspar, Max R.: Scott versus Payne operation for morbid obesity, 1455; discussion of Connolly on carotid endarterectomy, 1470; discussion of Ravitch on jejunoileal shunt, 1520

Gaston, J. McFadden: prostatic hypertrophy, secret cure with prostatic extract, 183; thoracotomy, trap-door incision, 187–88; pericarditis, 201; obstruction of common bile duct, 217

Gatch, Willis D.: experimental surgery of lungs, with Halsted, 404; box for animal positive pressure anesthesia, 405; rebreathing anesthesia apparatus, 439, 442; 1911 introduction of rebreathing technique in anesthesia, 647; circulatory disturbances in bowel caused by intestinal obstruction, 764; discussion of Moore, G. E., tumor cells in bloodstream, 1067

Gatewood: peptic ulcer, mortality and late results of operation, 689; discussion of Lahey on biliary fistulae, 692; carcinoma of the stomach, 713; subphrenic abscess, aspiration followed by operation, 790

Gay, George H.: tracheotomy, 58

Gay, George W.: Listerism, 27; ether versus chloroform, 47; tracheotomy, for croup, 56–57; tracheotomy and intubation for croup, 92–93; shock, 94; breast, cancer, 127; anesthesia, ether versus chloroform, 167; tuberculosis, surgical treatment, 180; fractures, lower extremities, ambulant treatment, medico-legal rights, 185; anesthesia, effect upon temperature, 187; on Homans, John, 197

Gaylord, Harvey R.: organisms causing cancer, 248–49

Geary, Joseph E.: coauthor of Linton, 1136

Geelhoed, Glenn W.: coauthor of Morton, 1381

Geheber, Carol E.: coauthor of Stone, 1453

Gelin, Lars-Erik: discussion of Connolly on hypothermia and cardiac arrest, 1212; discussion of Starzl on renal transplantation, 1414; discussion of Lee on arteriosclerosis in kidney recipients, 1447

Generali, Francesco: parathyroid discovery, 97

Genkins, G.: thymus in myasthenia, cited by Buckingham, 1455

Geoghegan, Thomas: air embolism in cardiac surgery, 984

Gerber, I. E.: coauthor of Doubilet, 915

Gerbode, Frank, L. A.: replacement of aorta by venous autograft, 976; control of heart action, 985–87; contrbutions of, (1026;) discussion of Julian, on ruptured aortic aneurysm, 1035; discussion of Bahnson on silk suture infection in cardiac surgery, 1061; discussion of Cooley, aneurysmectomy, 1101; discussion of Kirklin on tetralogy of Fallot, 1211; discussion of Kirklin and of Maloney on computers, 1276; prolonged membrane oxygenation, 1292

Gerota, D.: bladder lymphatics, 211

Gerrish, Edwin W.: primary entero-anastomoses in infants, cited by Gross, R. E., 1172

Gerrish, Frederic H.: prostatism, permanent cystostomy, 145; breast, cancer, 216; Matas on postoperative tetanus, 400

Gerster, Arpad G.: laryngotomy for tuberculosis, 118; contributions, (123;) and Mayo, W. J., 123; asepsis and antisepsis, 123–24; asepsis, skin preparation, 129; sterilization of materials, 130; elbow fractures, position, 133; tongue, cancer, 135; carotid occlusion, for intraoperative control of hemorrhage, 144; vagal section, cardiorespiratory effects, 144; cancer of the rectum, 165, 173; castration for benign prostatic hypertrophy, 166; operation for tic douloureux, 176; aspersions on Coley's cures, 280; aneurysm, preference for Antyllus' operation, 283; pylephlebitis in appendicitis, 291; citation of personal experience, 294; thrombectomy in pylephlebitis, 294; preference for sacral approach for cancer of rectum, 351; Murphy treatment for peritonitis, 382; Matas on

postoperative tetanus, 400; Friedrich thoracoplasty, 408; hepaticojejunostomy, Roux-Y, 425; discussion of Bevan, 427; ureteral transplantation into ileum, danger of uremia, 433; discussion of Martin, fractures, 435; discussion of MacKenzie, 438; chloroform, requires trained anesthetist, 443; nephrectomy, 112 cases, 448; pancreatitis, drainage from behind, 450; cirrhotic ascites, spontaneous resolution, 451; intratracheal insufflation anesthesia, 456; osteomyelitis cavities, skin grafting, 461; open reduction, clostridial infection, 465; two-stage operations rarely necessary, 483; gastroenterostomy for ulcer, development of carcinoma after, 485; advantages of drainage and of open wounds in military surgery, 512; injuries to surgeons in operating rooms, 514; attack on Arbuthnot Lane's intestinal stasis, 523; quoted as favoring cholecystectomy over cholecystostomy, 525; earlier reference to Maunsell, 997

Gersuny, Robert: twisting rectal stump for incontinent sacral anus, 165; operation for vesical exstrophy, 345; twisting rectum for a continent sacral anus, 347; twisting rectal stump for continent sacral anus, 351

Gerwig, Walter H., Jr.: discussion of Sawyers and Herrington on dumping, 1379

Getzen, Lindsay G.: the "Navy stitch", 1253

Gewurz, Henry: coauthor of Najarian, 1302

Gey, George O.: coauthor of Stone, 753; tissue culture laboratory, 753

Gibbon, John H.: anastomotic ulcer after gastroenterostomy, 388; tetany, post-thyroidectomy, recovery in one year, 400; transfusion, Brewer's paraffined glass tubes, 402; high rectal cancer, preliminary colostomy, 452; fistula-in-ano, injection with methylene blue, 453; instruction in fractures, 461; duodenal ulcer, two-stage operation, justification of, 485; fluoroscopy superior to films in gastric diagnosis, 485; typhoid perforation, laparotomy and closure, 504; guillotine amputation, an unfortunate resurrection, 548; importance of Carrel-Dakin treatment, 548; support for Coley, 551; discussion of Jackson, Jabez, on radical mastectomy, 563; postoperative irradiation for carcinoma of breast, 564; discussion of Meyer on cholecystitis, 572; carcinoma of breast, improvement in results due to postoperative irradiation, 583; patient included in report of Klopp, 586; discussion of peptic ulcer papers, 591; discussion of Müller on periarterial sympathectomy, 597; technic of renal and ureteral surgery, 598; endoaneurysmorrhaphy, 615; gratitude to Jackson, Chavalier, 629; President 1926, 631; discussion of plastic surgery, 642; discussion of Lewis and Trimble, abdominal injuries, 732

Gibbon, John H., Jr.: resection and anastomosis of colon for carcinoma, 841; and saddle embolectomy on Lockwood, 842; extracorporeal circulation, cited by Dennis, 951; contributions of, (970;) mechanical heart and lung apparatus, 970–71; discussion of Fischer and Potts, et. al, on extracorporeal oxygenators, 984; mechanical oxygenator, cited by Dennis, 984; cancer of the lung, 1003–04; oxygenator, cited by Blalock, 1023; discussion of Lillehei and Varco on open correction of tetralogy of Fallot, 1024; screen oxygenator, 1025; discussion of DeBakey on thoracoabdominal aneurysms, 1050; discussion of Spencer and Bahnson, postoperative cardiac output 1102; heart lung machine, cited by Shumacker, 1222

Gibbon, John and John, Jr.: father and son Presidents, 835

Gibbon, Mary H.: mechanical heart and lung apparatus, 970–71

60   Gibbons, E. C.: "assistant" to Archibald on experimental pancreatitis, 570

Gibbs, E. L.: psychomotor epilepsy, cited by Penfield, 992

Gibbs, F. A: coauthor of Bailey, 992; psychomotor epilepsy, cited by Penfield, 992

Gibson, Charles L.: is failure of ulcer operation accompanied by continued hyperacidity?, 389; tuberculous pericarditis, 406; end-to-end intestinal anastomosis by the invagination method, 425; special skill needed for open reduction of fractures, 460; methods of treating tetanus, 513; support for Mikulicz procedure, 523; Carrel method of treating wounds, 526; impressed by Carrel-Dakin method in military hospitals abroad, 533; surgical treatment of war wounds, 533; operation for cure of large ventral hernia, 562; acute perforation of stomach and duodenum, 590; hyperparathyroidism, hypercalcemia crises, 675

Gibson, Frank: progressive exopthalmos, cited by Dinsmore, 980

Gibson, J. G.: no capillary leak in shock, cited by Blalock, 862

Gibson, William: iliac artery ligation, 39

Giertz, Knut H.: discussion of Nyström on pulmonary embolectomy, 687

Giffin, H. Z.: clinical notes on splenectomy, 505

Gilchrist, R. Kennedy: pathological factors in carcinoma of colon and rectum, 898; espousal of Miles abdominoperineal resection, 916; discussion of Johnson on ventricular fibrillation, 969; discussion of McGuff and Deterling on lasers, 1198; discussion of Madden on electrocoagulation of rectal cancer, 1336

Gilchrist, Thomas C.: X-rays, effects on bone, 199

Gilder, Helena: coauthor of Beal, 1118

Gill, George P.: report from Kocher, 515

Gill, Sarjit S.: coauthor of Cooley, 1218

Gillison, D. Walford: discussion of Dragstedt on bile reflux and gastric ulcer, 1338

Gilman, A.: nitrogen mustard effect on tumors, cited by Cole, 1111

Ginzburg, Leon: regional ileitis, 767; ileocolostomy with exclusion for regional ileitis, 816

Giraldo, Nelson: islet cell transplantation, 1270

Girard, Charles: esophageal diverticulum, invagination of, 565; use of fascial sutures in herniorrhaphy, 602

Glass, Bert: pulmonary embolectomy, cited by Cohn, 1195

Glassman, Ephraim: coauthor of Spencer, 1466

Glenn, Frank: experimental renal hyertension, 799; pancreatic duct anastomosis in pancreaticoduodenectomy, cited by Dragstedt, 864; acute acalculous cholecystitis, 898; intravenous cholangiography, 1017; Cushing's syndrome, 1076–78; discussion of Scott on adrenal-Cushing's, 1206; discussion of Hardy on Cushing's disease, 1493

Glenn, William W. L.: contributions of, (1026;) radiofrequency stimulation, 1181; discussion of Furman on transvenous pacemakers, 1223; discussion of Senning on transposition, 1424

Gley, Eugène: parathyroid discovery, 97

Gleysteen, J. J.: coauthor of Hallenbeck, 1451

Gliedman, Marvin: mesocaval shunts, cited by Lord, 1280; coauthor of Veith, 1390

Gluck: ivory prosthetic joints, cited by Senn, 140

Gluck, Themistokles: pneumonectomy, experimental, 180; thoracic surgery, experimental, 188; pneumectomy for tuberculosis, 406

Gobbel, Walter: cited by Scott, duodenum after total gastrectomy, 1120

Godlee, Rickman J.: cerebral localization, 61

Goepel, R.: herniorrhapy with silver wire netting, 281

Goetsch, Emil: three-stage right colectomy, cited by Cheever, 705; discussion of Mixter and Cutler, thyroidectomy for angina, 744; coauthor of Lillehei, R. C., 1318

Goff, M.: coauthor of Andrews, Edmund, 714

Goggans, W. H.: control of heart action, 985

Gold, E.: hyperparathyroidism, 675

Gold, H. K.: coauthor of Mundth and Austen, 1384

Gold, Philip: carcinoembryonic antigen, cited by Grace, 1262

Goldberg, H.: creation of pulmonic stenosis for pulmonary hypertension, cited by Muller, 985

Goldblatt, H.: production of hypertension by renal artery constriction, 798; adrenalectomy abolishes renal hypertension, cited by Blalock, 799

Goldenberg, Ira S.: breast cancer, 1134

Goldin, Marshall D.: balloon occlusion of vena cava, 1477

Goldman, Leon: discussion of Glenn on cholangiography, 1017; hyperparathyroidism, 1061; coauthor of Wylie, 1072; discussion of Howard on pancreaticoduodenectomy, 1278

Goldman, Mitchell H.: coauthor of Moore, 1355

Goldschwend, Franz: Roux-Y after total gastrectomy, cited by Wangensteen, 998

Goldthwait, Joel E.: contribution to intervertebral disc problem, cited by Mixter, W. J., 796

Goligher, John C.: one-stage proctocolectomy, cited by Ravitch, 1056; comment on Turnbull's no-touch technic, 1238; discussion of Hoerr on operations for duodenal ulcer, 1360; parietal cell vagotomy cited by Nyhus and by Hallenbeck, 1452; proximal gastric vagotomy, cited by Sawyers, 1481; discussion of Enker on wide resection for colorectal cancer, 1515

Gomez, Cesar: discussion of Griffen on shunting for morbid obesity, 1480

Gompertz, Michael L.: coauthor of Kehne, 1473

Gonzalez, Luis L.: coauthor of Culbertson, 1139

Good, Robert A.: agammaglobulinemia and transplantation, 1019

Goodfellow, George: perineal prostatectomy, 268

Goodman, L. S.: nitrogen mustard effect on tumors, cited by Cole, 1111

Goodpasture, Ernest W.: pathologic study of Blalock's thymus specimen, 814

Goodrich (of St. Paul): gastroenterostomy for congenital pyloric stenosis, cited by MacLaren, 359

Goodwin, Willard E.: discussion of Hume on renal homotransplantation, 1179; discussion of Reemtsma, renal heterograft, 1187; discussion of Scott on adrenal-Cushing's, 1206; discussion of Starzl on renal transplantation, 1214; discussion of Aust on ureterosigmoidostomy, 1225; discussion of Swenson on Wilms' tumor, 1253; contributions of, (1266;) discussion of Belzer and Kountz on cadaver kidney transplantation, 1318; discussion of Kountz and Belzer on renal transplantation, 1368; ureterosigmoidostomy, in discussion of Clatworthy, 1380; discussion of Hendren, urinary tract reconstruction, 1407

Goott, Bernard: coauthor of Lillehei, R. C., 1098

Gorbach, Sherwood L.: antibiotic colon preparation, 1388

Gordon, Esther B.: coauthor of Barnes and Cope, 1127

Gordon, Gilbert S.: coauthor of Goldman, 1062

Gorgas, General William C.: and World War I, cited by Cutler, 838

Goswitz, John T.: coauthor of Zollinger, 1157

Gottlieb, L. S.: coauthor of McGuff and Deterling, 1198

Gould, Alfred H.: coauthor with Harrington, 313

Gouley, John W. S.: Listerism, 26–28; contributions, (28;) suprapublic lithotomy, 50; prostate, hypertrophy, surgery of, 62–63; prostatectomy, transurethral, 62–63, prostate, transurethral punch, 90

Gowans, J. L.: thoracic duct drainage for immunosuppression, cited by Starzl, 1526

Grace, James T., Jr.: discussion of Humphrey on immunologic response in cancer patients, 1261

Graham, A. Stephens: coauthor of Rankin, 714

Graham, Christopher: coauthor with Mayo, C. H., 310

Graham, Evarts A.: assistant to Bevan, A. D., 501; pathogenesis of cholecystitis, 571; cholecystitis, due to "lymphogenous" spread, 573; influence of Crile and Mayo on American College of Surgeons, 606; roentgenologic visualization of the gallbladder, 609; experimental cardiac valvotomy, 610; discussion of Cutler on valvotomy, 611; discussion of Brooks on peripheral vascular disease, 615; physiology of the biliary tract, 635; discussion of plastic surgery, 642; studies on pneumothorax effects, 647; pulmonary suppuration, 649–50; cholecystography, 686; colleague of Elman, 714; acute empyema, 726; Empyema Commission, 726–27; opposition to early operation for acute cholecystitis, 735; first successful one-stage pneumonectomy, cited by Archibald, 746; failure to discuss Archibald on pneumonectomy, 747; young Turks attack on American College of Surgeons, 759; discussion of symposium on surgical education, 763; discussion of Whipple on ampullary carcinoma, 770; discussion of Shenstone on muscle flap closure of bronchial fistulae, 779; President 1937, 785; contributions of, 786; discussion of Beck on cardiac defibrillation, 791; discussion of Morton on etiology of cancer, 792; intrathoracic surgery, cited by Coutard, 792; discussion of Keynes, radium treatment of breast cancer, 795; prophylactic use of sulfanilamide, 807; discussion of Cournand and Berry on pneumonectomy, 847; discussion of Rienhoff on bronchial closure, 848; discussion of Huggins on cancer of prostate, 852; discussion of Meleney, infections in wounds from trauma, 859; principles versus details, cited by Koch, 860; Hogan on gelatin in 1912, 861; discussion of Lindskog, bronchogenic carcinoma, 887; discussion of Doubilet and Mulholland on pancreatitis, 915; mitral valvotomy, cited by Blalock, 934; rectosigmoid myotomy for Hirschsprung's disease, 964; early mitral valvotomy, cited by Dinsmore, 996; discussion of Gibbon on cancer of the lung, 1004; discussion of Glenn on intravenous cholangiography, 1017; and Wu, Ying-k'ai, 1517–18

Graham, Henry F.: acute cholecystitis, cited by Smith, M. K., 737; discussion of Key and Frankel on local sulfonamide therapy, 831

Graham, Roscoe R.: coauthor with Starr, 542; discussion of Maes, gastric cancer, 728; discussion of Whipple and Elliott on wound closure, 805; discussion of Lehman on appendiceal abscess, 808; support of Allen and Welch on gastric ulcer, 841; discussion of Clute on thiouracil, 875; discussion of Allen on gastrectomy for duodenal ulcer, 888; discussion of Ransom, subtotal gastrectomy, 904; cited by Dinsmore, 995

Graham, Ruth M.: coauthor of Ulfelder, 916

Grambort, David E.: coauthor of Orloff, 1419

Grant, Francis C.: report of case of Frazier, reinfusion of venesection blood, 585; discussion of Adson on brain abscess, 802; discussion of Horrax and Poppen on acoustic tumors, 941

Grant, George N.: coauthor of Zollinger, 1157

Grant, General Ulysses S.: tongue, cancer, 134

Grantham, E. G.: frontal leukotomy by electrodesiccation, cited by White, 1153

Graves, Amos M.: coauthor of Ochsner, Alton, 738, 790

Gray: Surgeon General's Museum, cited by Billings, 73

Gray, Howard K.: hemorrhage from esophageal varices, 959

Gray, Laman A., Jr.: coauthor of Kirsh, 1442

Gray, S. J.: treatment of gastroduodenal hemorrhage, cited by Enquist, 1208

Green: work on intralaryngeal pressure anesthesia, reported by Blake, 408

Green, Edward: coauthor of Lam, 1062

Green, George: internal mammary-coronary bypass, cited by Spencer, 1294

Green, J.: temporal lobe resection for epilepsy, 992

Greenberg, Jack: cloth covered valve prosthesis, cited by Beall, 1297

Greenfield, Lazar J.: caval filter, cited by DeWeese, 1374; discussion of DeWeese, caval filters, 1374; extraluminal prosthesis, cited by DeWeese, 1374; transvenous catheter pulmonary embolectomy, 1403–04

Greenough, Robert B.: breast cancer, results at Massachusetts General Hospital, 368; pancreatitis, spontaneous recovery, 450; cystic disease of the breast, conservative operation, 492; treatment of septic gunshot fractures, 510; extension as well as plaster to be used in military fractures, 513; radium treatment of uterine cancer, 516; discussion of Lee, 613; cited by Bloodgood, cancer of the breast, 620; discussion of Moschcowitz, carcinoma of the breast, late results, 637

Greenough, W. B.: diarrhea of cholera, cited by Zollinger, 1271

Gregersen, M. I.: no capillary leak in shock, cited by Blalock, 862

Gregory, Elisha H.: bloodletting, 34; blood vessel ligation, use of silk, 55; tracheotomy, 57; neoplasms, 58; Negro, surgical diseases of, 84; cervix, amputation for cancer, 85

Gregory, R. A.: gastrin in pancreatic tumors, cited by Zollinger, 1157; gastrin from Z-E tumors, cited by Dragstedt, 1158; gastrin radioimmunoassay, cited by Way, 1502

Griepp, Randall B.: heart transplantation, 1366; valve prostheses, 1464

Griffen, Ward O., Jr.: coauthor of Wangensteen, 1090; immunologic response in cancer patients, 1261; discussion of Eisenberg on vagotomy and drainage, 1284; jejunoileal versus gastric bypass for morbid obesity, 1479

Griffin, H. Z.: coauthor with Mayo, W. J., 375–76

Griffith: collaborator of Archibald, 746

Griffith, Charles A.: coauthor of Harkins, 1011; coauthor of Harkins and Nyhus, 1171; selective vagotomy, cited by Sawyers, 1337; proximal gastric vagotomy, cited by Sawyers, 1481

Grillo, Hermes C.: circumferential tracheal resection, 1201–03

Grimson, Keith S.: collaborator of Phemister, 782; total and partial paravertebral sympathectomy for hypertension, 798; discussion of symposium on vagotomy, 906; vagotomy for ulcer, cited by Walters, 906; total sympathectomy, cited by Ray, 941; discussion of Herrington on vagotomy-antrectomy, 1098

Griswold, H. E.: coauthor of Bing and Blalock, 921

Griswold, R. Arnold: vagotomy and gastric function, 905

Gritti (Rocco)-Stokes (William): amputation, cited by Gallie, 836

Grogan, James B.: parenteral alimentation infections, cited by Hardy, 1355

Grosberg, Saul: coauthor of LeVeen, 1410

Grosfeld, Jay L.: rhabdomyosarcoma, 1380

Gross, Frederick S.: alkaline esophagitis, cited by Wangensteen, 1338

Gross, Robert E.: results in biliary atresia, 768; patent ductus arteriosus, 811; coarctation of aorta, 921; atrioventriculostomy for mitral bypass, cited by Blalock, 935; homologous grafts for coarctation of aorta, 974–76; and cardiac surgery, cited by Dinsmore, 996; atrial well,

76 McCann, James: extremity injuries, 50–51; tourniquets, 51; splenectomy for wandering spleen, 86; middle meningeal hemorrhage, wooden plug, 116; mobile kidneys, 118

McClenahan, John: coauthor of Glenn, Frank, 1017

McClure, Roy D.: discussion of symposium on surgical education, 764; colleague of Park, 815; discussion of Lee, adrenal cortical extract in burn shock, 837–38; wound and burn project, 858; discussion of Schullinger on appendicitis, 902

McClure, W. L.: colleague of McKittrick, 707; transverse abdominal incision, cited by Haight, Cameron, 840

McCombs, R. K.: control of heart action, 985

McCord, Colin W.: coauthor of Starr, 1195

McCorkle, Horace J.: serum amylase test in pancreatic trauma, 864

McCormick, John: coauthor of Ravitch, 1253

McCosh, Andrew J.: choledocholithotomy and suture of common duct, 173; thyroidectomy, 173; ventral herniorrhaphy with celluloid prosthesis, 256; operation for paraplegia with spine fracture, 257; myomectomy versus hysterectomy, 287

McCreary, Charles: resection, clavicle, 108

McCune, William S.: malignant melanoma, 931–32; viability of long blood vessel grafts, 976; discussion of Fry and Child of 95% pancreatectomy, 1027; carotid endarterectomy, 1065; discussion of Wanebo on melanoma, 1428

McDermott, William V., Jr.: colonic defunctionalization for hepatic encephalopathy, 522; bleeding esophageal varices, 1044–46; double portacaval shunt, cited by Warren, 1094; double portacaval shunt, 1095; discussion of Moore's liver transplantation, 1113; contributions of, (1241;) discussion of Rousselot on portacaval shunts for ascites, 1280; discussion of Buchwald and Varco on ileal bypass for hyperlipidemia, 1397; discussion of Malt on portasystemic shunts, 1440; discussion of Griffen on jejunoileal shunt, 1480; discussion of Warren on distal splenorenal shunt, 1489; discussion of Orloff on Budd-Chiari syndrome, 1509

McDill, John R.: bloodless surgery of the liver, 448

McDonald, Gerald O.: coauthor of Morales and Cole, 1067

McDonald, Richard T.: coauthor of Szilagyi, 1078

McDonald, V. G.: coauthor of Holder, 1202

McDowell, Ephraim: monument to, 5; ovariotomy, technique of, 33; fee for ovariotomy, 108; ovariotomy, 108, 316

McFarland, John: and gastric freezing, cited by Artz, 1170

McFetridge, Elizabeth M.: coauthor of Maes, Urban, 727

McGill, A. F.: suprapubic prostatectomy, 90

McGoon, Dwight C.: coauthor of Kirklin, 1210; shunts for tetralogy of Fallot, cited by Barratt-Boyes, 1387; contributions of, (1399;) report of first success in repair of truncus, 1399; truncal valvular regurgitation, 1399; discussion of Shumway and of Spencer on valve replacement, 1467

McGrath, Ruth: coauthor of Cole and Roberts, 1133

McGrath, W. B.: coauthor of Green, 992

McGraw, Arthur B.: coauthor of Szilagyi, 978

McGraw, Theodore A.: tracheotomy, 57; gunshot wounds of intestine, 103; cholecystenterostomy, experimental, 143; cancer of the breast, arm amputation, 165; cancer of the breast, axillary dissection, 165; castration for benign prostatic hypertrophy, 166; rubber-band gastroenterostomy, 243; gastroenterostomy, vicious circle, 260; military medical statistics, worthlessness of, 266; war wounds, effect of delay, 267; gastroenterostomy mishaps, 277; splenectomy in leukemia, 278; X-ray effect on sarcoma, 280; preliminary colostomy for carcinoma of rectum, 288

McGrew, Elizabeth A.: coauthor of Cole and Roberts, 1133

McGuff, Paul E.: surgical applications of laser, 1198

McGuire, Edgar R.: choice of operation for biliary lithiasis, 633; prevention of common duct injuries, 635

McGuire, Hunter: skull fracture, 40, 61; publications in surgery, 77; contributions of, (78;) opposed trephining for depressed fractures, 78; suprapubic cystostomy, 78; cystostomy, continent suprapubic, 90; suprapubic cystotomy for tumor, 109; teaching of surgery, 157; cancer of male genitals, 164–65

McGuire, Stuart: opposition to early operation for acute cholecystitis, 735

McIver, Monroe A.: discussion of intestinal obstruction, cited by Fine, 765

McKenna, Hugh: fractures of neck of femur, 696

McKhann, Charles F.: discussion of Ramming on RNA cancer therapy, 1475

McKinley, President William: and imperialism, 236

McKittrick, John B.: coauthor of McKittrick, L. S., 943

McKittrick, Leland S.: pulmonary complications in spinal anesthesia, cited by Müller, 707; idiopathic ulcerative colitis, 766; interstitial radiation of cancer of the breast, 793; discussion of Lund on burns, 861; transmetatarsal amputations, 943–44; ileostomy dysfunction, cited by Crile, 1015; President 1966, 1216

McLachlin, Angus D.: venous stasis in lower extremities, 1127–28, discussion of Haller on iliofemoral thrombectomy, 1177

McLachlin, John A.: coauthor of McLachlin, Angus, 1128

McLanahan, Samuel: coauthor of Stone, H. B., 841

McLean, A. P. H.: coauthor of MacLean, L. D., 1246

McLean, W. S.: coauthor of Archibald, 528

McLeod, Neil: anus, imperforate, combined approach (1880), 206

McLoughlin, Gerald A.: circulating immunosuppressive factor, 1513–15

McMaster, P.: coauthor of Calne, 1462

McMurtry, Lewis S.: silk ligatures in nephrectomy, 329

McNaughton, George: pelvic abscess, drainage through rectum or vagina, 396

McPherson, Harry T.: coauthor of Wells, 1431

McQuiston, William O.: controlled intraoperative hypothermia, 932

McSherry, Charles K.: coauthor of Beal, John, 1118

McVay, Chester B.: inguinal and femoral hernioplasty, 1080–82; discussion of Farris on bleeding duodenal ulcer, 1250

McVey, John L.: coauthor of Ellis, F. H., 1251

McWhirter, R.: simple mastectomy and radiotherapy, 930; axilla sparing mastectomy, cited by Humphrey, 1333

McWilliams, Clarence A.: knee-joint war injuries, 548

MacArthur, General Douglas: recalled by President Truman, 961

MacCallum, William G.: calcium metabolism and parathyroid deficiency, 400; examination of Halsted dog thyroid, 401; experimental cardiac valvotomy, 610–11; atelectasis, 688

MacCormac, Sir William: joints, excision of, 89; cystotomy, 90; breast cancer, 127

MacDonald, I. G.: ineffectiveness of early diagnosis in cancer, cited by Barker, 1288

MacDonald, Willis G.: techniques of hysterectomy, 287; thyroidectomy, anesthesia deaths, 355; anesthesia specialists, 365

Macewen, Sir William: Listerism, 27; cerebral localization, 61; hernia, inguinal, operation for, 100, 171; decalcified chicken bone drains, 102; paraplegia in Pott's disease, 124; pneumonectomy for tuberculosis, 132; aneurysms, needling of, 143; apical thoracoplasty for tuberculosis, 405; two-

78 Martell, Captain Charles: hyperparathyroidism of, 675
Martin: tubercle bacilli in Fallopian tubes, cited by
VanderVeer, 178
Martin, Alfred J., Jr.: liver transplantation, 1262
Martin, E. W.: CEA in colon cancer, cited by Wanebo, 1507
Martin, Edward: fractures, lower extremities, ambulatory
treatment, 183; occlusive dressings for war wounds, 226;
peritoneal toilet in biliary tract operations, 293; treatment
of shock with adrenalin, 304; open treatment of fractures,
352; transverse femoral fractures, open treatment, 433–35;
pancreatitis, accurate diagnosis by physicians, 450; Eck
fistula, desirability of, 451; experimental mesenteric-iliac
shunt for cirrhosis (1912), 451; carotid-cavernous
aneurysm, cure by partial occlusion of common carotid
artery, 505; acacia as a blood substitute, 536; myotomy for
Hirschsprung's disease, 648; surgical significance of
rectosigmoid sphincter, 648
Martin, Edward W., Jr.: coauthor of Pace, 1519
Martin, Franklin H.: and the Australasian College of Surgeons,
758; and control of American College of Surgeons, 759
Martin, John J.: discussion of Palmer on intestinal obstruction,
730
Martin, Lester, W.: total colonic aganglionosis, 1358; colectomy
and endorectal mucosal stripping, 1476
Martin, Walton: discussion of Greenough on septic gunshot
fractures, 512; etiology of chronic empyema, 560;
septicemia, the fate of microbes in the bloodstream, 627;
discussion of Judd and Adson, sympathectomy for
Hirschsprung's disease, 665; maggots and osteomyelitis,
721
Mascagni, Paolo: breast, lymphatics, 216
Mason, Aubrey York: local excision and irradiation of breast
cancer, 1333
Mason, Edward E.: gastric bypass for obesity, 1285–86;
discussion of Williams on ischemic colitis, 1434; discussion
of Griffen on gastric bypass, 1480; discussion of Pace and
Carey on gastric partitioning, 1520
Mason, James C.: discussion of Meigs on ovarian fibroma-
ascites, and hydrothorax, 816
Mason, James M.: discussion of Graham on empyema, 727;
discussion of Lewis and Trimble, nonpenetrating
abdominal injuries, 731
Mason, Morton F.: collaborator of Blalock, 799, 814
Mason, R. L.: parathyroid autotransplantation, cited by Lahey,
676
Massover, Alfred J.: coauthor of Stewart, 920
Mastin, Claudius H.: contributions of, ⟨28;⟩ recants opposition
to Listerism, 28; and Listerism, 28, 32; hernia, inguinal,
operations for, 99–102; antisepsis, 120; Presidential
Address, 1891, 120; surgery, progress of, 131–32
Matas, Rudolph: anesthesia, nerve block, 32; appendicitis, 91;
Negro, surgical peculiarities of, 188; anus, imperforate,
206–07; breast cancer, recurrence, 216; arteriovenous
aneurysm, 255; aortic aneurysm wiring, mishaps, 260;
laryngeal intubation and positive pressure anesthesia, 260;
teaching of medical students, 270–71;
endoaneurysmorrhaphy, 282, 340–42; splint for lower jaw
fractures, 322; contributions of, ⟨341;⟩ breast cancer,
recurrence after 25 years, 372; fecal origin of some forms
of postoperative tetanus, 399; positive pressure anesthesia
apparatus, 409; collected experience with
endoaneurysmorrhaphy, 416; surgery of the vascular
system, testing collateral circulation, 416; suture and
plication of aorta, 446; endoaneurysmorrhaphy, low
incidence of gangrene, 455; plication of wall of aorta to
reduce caliber, 469; positive pressure anesthesia in thoracic
surgery, 473; cited by Kümmell, 494; the continued

intravenous "drip", 602; continuous saline drip into
common duct, 602; discussion, symposium on surgery of
the colon, 608; discussion of Butler on valvotomy, 611;
ligation of the abdominal aorta, 615; intravenous fluids,
cited by Gallie, 682; discussion of Nyström on pulmonary
embolism, 687; discussion of Stone, Harvey, on saphenous
thrombophlebitis, 716; discussion of Dandy, carotid-
cavernous aneurysm, 773; discussion of breast cancer
papers, 795; on Gross, S. D., 795; vascular surgery, 824;
arterial occlusion, discussion of Pearse, 828; discussion of
Bigger and of Elkin on aortic aneurysm, 828; discussion of
Gage and Ochsner on sympathetic blocks, 830; compressor
for development of collaterals, cited by Elkin, 872;
discussion of Blalock, pulmonic stenosis, 893;
contributions to surgery of aneurysms, cited by Freeman,
894; discussion of Elkin, vertebral arteriovenous
aneurysms, 894; discussion of Freeman, on aneurysm, 894;
length of discussions, 894; comment on Murray, D. W. G.,
cardiac infarctectomy, 904; discussion of Blakemore on
endoaneurysmorrhaphy, 909
Matherstock: appendicitis, cited by Bull, 91
Mathews, Francis S.: cited by MacLaren, pelvic abscess at
Roosevelt Hospital, 570; discussion of Whipple on typhoid
carriers, 673; discussion of Miller, tuberculosis of cervical
nodes, 701; cryptorchidism and anterior pituitary extract,
726
Mathewson, Carleton, Jr.: discussion of Emmett, gastrectomy
for perforation, 999; discussion of Nance on penetrating
abdominal wounds, 1300
Matloff, J. M.: discussion of Mundth and Austen on acute
myocardial ischemia, 1385
Matson, Donald D.: coauthor of Dunphy, 865;
hypophysectomy for breast cancer, cited by Moore, 1048;
discussion of Miller on translumbar amputation, 1226
Matthews, Stella S.: nitrous oxide oxygen experience, 440
Maunsell, Henry, W.: rectum, operation for cancer, 165, 288,
348; operation of adapted by Swenson, cited by Dinsmore,
997
Mauro, A.: coauthor of Glenn, W. W. L., 1181
Maury, J. W. Draper: McGraw ligature with twine, 314; cited
by Hartmann, 490
Mautz, Frederick R.: coauthor of Beck, C. S., 790
Maxwell, T. J.: fracture femoral neck, traction method, 460
Maydl, Karl: colostomy technique, 105; gastrectomy mortality,
241; ureterosigmoidostomy for vesical exstrophy, 345;
implantation of vesical trigone in rectum, 432, 478–79
Mayer, Doanld J.: coauthor of Dumont, 1185
Maylard (of Glasgow): early user of transverse incision, cited
by Binnie, 516
Maynard, Anthony T.: coauthor of Dudrick, 1354
Maynes, E. A.: membrane oxygenator, 1175, 1292
Mayo: technique of drainage in choledochotomy, cited by
Ochsner, Albert, 309
Mayo Brothers: tribute by Beahrs, 1513
Mayo, Charles H.: and Fenger, 48; gastroenterostomy, 273;
thyroidectomy for exophthalmic goitre, 319; 50
thyroidectomies for Graves' disease, 335; contributions of,
⟨336;⟩ cancer of sigmoid and rectum, 347; combined
abdominoperineal resection, 349; no mention of
sigmoidoscopy, 349; thyroidectomy experience, 356;
thyroidectomy, avoidance of parathyroid, 366;
thyroidectomy, treatment of posterior capsule, 366–67;
compared to Hunter, John, 381; recognition of
diverticulitis of sigmoid, 381; cases included in ulcer report
of Mayo, W. J., 1908, 385; comment by Halsted, 400; the
parathyroid question, 400; caution in resort to open
reduction of fractures, 411; occlusion carotid artery for

82 Moore, Francis D. (*continued*)
hip replacement, 1347; President 1972; 1353; candidemia in parenteral alimentation, 1355; discussion of Alexander on leukocyte antibacterial action, 1356; discussion of Brant and Krippaehne on visceral angiography, 1362; discussion of Wolff on colonoscopy, 1384; discussion of Burke, skin allografts in burns, 1419; discussion of Mueller on breast cancer, 1429; and liver transplantation, cited by Murray, 1464

Moore, George E.: tumor cells in bloodstream, 1066–67; Chairman of cancer chemotherapy trials, cited by Cole, 1068; cancer cells in bloodstream, cited by Cole, 1133; Surgical Adjuvant Chemotherapy Projects, NIH, 1141; tumor transplants and lymphocyte transfer, 1223; Adjuvant Chemotherapy Breast Cancer Report, 1260; Co-chairman, National Surgical Adjuvant Breast Project, 1260; immunologic response in cancer patients, cited by Grace, 1261; antilymphocyte serum, 1302–03

Moore, James E.: tuberculosis, heredity questioned, 181; patella, operation for fracture, 212; gastric cancer, 243; ventral hernia, 256; prostatectomy, preference for perineal route, 267; reciprocal physical examinations for students, 271; caution in use of X-ray, 287; nature of papillary ovarian tumors, 312; spina bifida, 333; no loop gastroenterostomy, 338; breast cancer, retrograde spread from metastases, 373; peritonitis, usefulness of morphine, 383; perineal prostatectomy, treatment of sequels, 409–10; discussion of Martin, fractures, 435; chloroform anesthesia, 438; surgery of the long bones, 457; fracture, femur, traction method, 460; fractures, opposition to early passive motion in, 465; appendiceal abscesses, two-stage operation favored for, 483; favors two-stage operations "in selected cases", 483; prostatism with urinary tract infection, preliminary cystostomy, 483; radium therapy, failure of, 492; Buck's extension and lateral traction for fracture of femoral neck, 503; unwilling to accept need for impaction of fractures of neck of femur, 503; inadequacy of teaching of wound care, 515; agreement with Bevan on Lane, Arbuthnot, 523

Moore, Richard B.: coauthor of Buchwald and Varco, 1396

Moore, Samuel Wilson: discussion of DeBakey on occlusive disease, branches of aortic arch, 1145

Moore, Thomas C.: discussion of Murray on renal transplantation, 1269; discussion of Belzer and Kountz, cadaver kidney transplantation, 1318; discussion of Starzl on renal homotransplantation, 1321; discussion of Kountz and Belzer on renal transplantation, 1368; discussion of Starzl on renal transplantation, 1414; discussion of Swenson on Hirschsprung's disease, 1422

Morales, Francisco: prophylactic chemotherapy of cancer, 1067–68

Moran, Walter H., Jr.: coauthor of Zimmerman, 1103

Morehead, Donald E.: coauthor of Dye and Julian, 1079

Morelli, Eugenio: three bottle irrigation and siphon system for empyema, 561

Moreno, Augusto H.: coauthor of Rousselot, 1093

Morestin, Hippolyte: tongue, cancer, resection technique, cited by Bloodgood, 489

Moretz, William H.: acidosis after aortic clamping, in discussion of Campbell, 1197; discussion of Ravitch on intestinal healing, 1253; removable vena caval occlusion clip, cited by DeWeese, 1374

Morgan, Hugh J.: coauthor of Blalock, 814

Morgan, John: Surgery in 1776, 1464

Morison, Alexander: chest wall resection for cardiomegaly, 611

Morison, Rutherford: omentopexy, first publication, 450

Moritz, Allen R.: production of collateral cardiac circulation, cited by Beck, C. S., 771

Morris: perineal prostatectomy, cited by Bevan, 409

Morris, George C., Jr.: and DeBakey, 1037; coauthor of DeBakey, 1048, 1071, 1143; coauthor of Cooley and DeBakey, 1064; abdominal aortic aneurysm, 1197; discussion of DeWeese on venous bypass grafts, 1331

Morris, Henry: X-rays of gallstones (1896), 199; nephrolithiasis, low mortality, 390

Morris, Robert T.: endoaneurysmorrhaphy with complete arterioplasty, 342

Morrow, Andrew Glenn: mitral replacement, cited by Starr, 1145

Morse, Plinn F.: coauthor of Ballin, 703

Morson, Basil C.: polyps and cancer, cited by Wolff, 1383; ischemic colitis, cited by Williams, 1432

Morton: fractured spine, cited by Burrell, 331

Morton, Donald L. resection and immunotherapy for pulmonary metastases, 1381; discussion of Parks on alpha fetoprotein, 1412; immunotherapy of malignant melanoma, 1415; discussion of Wanebo on melanoma, 1428; delayed hypersensitivity and tumor resistance, cited by MacLean, 1461; discussion of Wanebo on CEA, 1508; discussion of Mannick on immunosuppressive factors, 1514

Morton, J. C.: external iliac artery ligation, 39

Morton, John J.: studies on activity of lumbar sympathetic nervous system, 696; vasoconstrictor spasm in peripheral arterial disease, 717; etiology of cancer, 791; discussion of Whipple and Elliott on wound closure, 805; radiation burns, 1059

Morton, Thomas G.: amputations and sepsis, Pennsylvania Hospital, 25; club foot, astragalectomy, 111; appendectomy, safety of, 114

Morton, William T. G.: ether inhaling apparatus, 195; ether anesthesia, cited by Bevan, 438

Moschcowitz, Alexis V.: consent for laparotomy to be obtained in all typhoid patients, 504; cholecystostomy abandoned for cholecystectomy, 506; transverse incision in upper abdomen, 516; preference for cholecystectomy over cholecystostomy, 525; converted to Carrel-Dakin method by Carrel, 533; citrate transfusion, 536; costal cartilages, infections of, 541; hernia recurrence, 544; empyema, Carrel treatment and cavity closure, 549; discussion of Eliot, appendicitis, 570; denial of existence of precancerous stage in breast cancer, 583; discussion on exophthalmic goiter, 615; uterine prolapse, operation for, 622; discussion on symposium on gallbladder disease, 635; late results of amputation for carcinoma of the breast, 637; discussion of Brewer on Meleney's ulcer, 641; pleural and pericardial suppuration, 654; discussion of Bevan on cryptorchidism, 680; silence in peptic ulcer symposium, 691; tuberculosis of thyroid versus Riedel's struma, 714; discussion of Graham on empyema, 727; discussion of Miller, intussusception, 733

Moser, K. M.: balloon caval occlusion catheter, cited by DeWeese, 1374

Mosler: condemnation of pneumectomy, cited by Fowler, 180

Moss, William L.: and blood groups, 535

Moszkowicz, Ludwig: hyperemia test, to demarcate level of amputation, 417; arteriovenous fistula and proximal venous ligation, for arterial insufficiency, 473

Mott, Valentine: iliac artery ligation, 39; resection, clavicle, 108; innominate artery ligation, 170

Moulder, Peter V., Jr.: cardiac arrest, cited by Lam, 1064; discussion of Sabiston and Wagner on pulmonary emoblism, 1193

Moullin, Charles W.: prostatectomy, cited by White, 145

84 Murray, Joseph E. (*continued*)
discussion of Rapaport on induced unresponsiveness to organ transplant, 1522; total body irradiation for immunosuppression, cited by Starzle, 1525; discussion of Starzl on thoracic duct drainage for immunosuppression, 1526

Muscatello: operation for vesical exstrophy, cited by Trendelenburg, 345

Musser, J. H.: cholecystotomy for stone, 65

Musser, John H.: pancreatitis, proficiency in diagnosis, 450

Mustard, William T.: extracorporeal circulation, cited by Potts, 984; monkey lungs in clinical extracorporeal circulation, cited by Janes, 984; animal lungs as oxygenators, 1025; clinical use of hypothermia, cited by Bigelow, 1065; operation for transposition, cited by Senning, 1423

Mütter, Thomas D.: middle meningeal hemorrhage, wooden plug for, 116

Myers, Nate A.: extrahepatic portal hypertension in children, 1404–05

Myers, R. T.: gastric freezing and acid secretion, 1170–71

N

Nabseth, Donald C.: discussion of Malt on portasystemic shunts, 1440; bleeding varices—vasopressin, 1473; discussion of Warren on distal splenorenal shunt, 1489

Nadler, Sigmond H.: tumor transplants and lymphocyte transfer, 1223; immunologic response in cancer patients, cited by Grace, 1261

Naef, A. P.: discussion of Paulson, bronchogenic carcinoma, 1445

Naffziger, Howard C.: progressive exophthalmos, pathology and treatment, 702; discussion of Dandy, carotid-cavernous aneurysm, 773; discussion of Mixter, W. J., ruptured intervertebral disc, 798; progressive exophthalmos, operative relief, 802; serum amylase test in pancreatic trauma, 864; discussion of Horrax and Poppen on acoustic tumors, 941; discussion of Craig, on progressive exophthalmos, 980; President 1954, 1006; contributions of, (1007;) discussion of Glenn on Cushing's syndrome, 1077

Nageotte, Jean: fate of homografts, cited by Key, 982

Najafi, Hassan: balloon occlusion of vena cava, 1477

Najarian, John S.: contributions of, (1267;) renal transplantation, cited by Dunphy, 1270; antilymphocyte serum, 1302–03; coauthor of Lillehei, R. C., 1318; renal transplantation in children, 1341–42; discussion of Starzl on hepatitis in homograft recipients, 1343; discussion of Kountz and Belzer on renal transplantation, 1368; discussion of Starzl on renal transplantation, 1414; islet cell autotransplantation, cited by Braasch, 1495

Nance, Francis C.: stab wounds of abdomen, 1299–1300

Nancrede, Charles B. (Nancrède, Charles B. G. de): Listerism, 23, 27, 29, 32; contributions, (29;) bloodletting, 33–34, 45; aneurysm, femoral arteriovenous, 39; brain abscess, 48; blood vessel ligation, use of catgut, 55; value of experiments, 55; air embolism, 64; laparotomy for gunshot wounds, 80–82; medico-legal liability in laparotomy for gunshot wounds, 80–82; hysterectomy for cancer, 85; appendicitis, 91; shock and anesthesia, 94; gunshot wounds of abdomen, 103; posttraumatic epilepsy, 122; breast, cancer, 127; arterial aneurysms, treatment, 143–44; on empyema, 152; teaching of surgery, 157–58; animal operative surgery course, 158; nephrectomy, 159; inguinal hernia, operation, postoperative care, 172; fractures, lower extremities, opposition to ambulant treatment, 185; anesthesia, blood loss and shock, 187; x-ray for

localization of foreign bodies, 199; treatment of gunshot wounds, 224–25; volunteer line officers and Medical Corps, 226; gastroenterostomy versus gastrectomy for cancer, 243; war wounds of large joints, 265; difference between Civil War wounds and "modern" wounds, 266; statistics, value of, 267; operative surgery course in cadavers and animals, 272; principles of asepsis, 310; frozen section for diagnosis of cancer, 351; breast, cancer, multiple sections to classify, 373; diverticulitis of sigmoid, 376; diagnosis of renal stone, 390; tetanus, geographic variation in incidence, 400; chloroform for military use, 444; breast, cystic disease, radical operation for, 493; 1911 plea for chloroform for war surgery, 647; operations for epilepsy (1891), 990

Nanson, Eric M.: I^{131} fibrinogen localization of venous thrombosis, 1193

Nardi, George L.: discussion of portal hypertension papers, 1169

Nash, Ogden: cited by Elkin, 978

Nassetti, Francesco: aorta, occlusion with fascia lata strips, cited by Matas, 470–71

Nassiloff, I.: posterior mediastinal approach to esophagus, 129

Nathanson, Ira: breast cancer, life expectancy, cited by Welch, 1429

National Research Council: Contaminated Wound and Burn Project, 858; Subcommittee on Blood Substitutes, 860; and penicillin, 873

Naunyn, Bernard: cholesterol content of bile, cited by Andrews, 714

Navia, Jose A.: aneurysms of left ventricle, 1385–86

Nealon, Thomas F., Jr.: cancer of the lung, 1003; discussion of Powers on PEEP, 1376

Neibling, Harold A.: coauthor of Walters, 905

Nélaton, Auguste: scapulo-humeral arthroplasty, cited by Murphy, 324

Nelsen: Zollinger-Ellison tumors, cited by Dragstedt, 1158

Nelson, Charles A.: coauthor of Kremen, 1012

Nelson, Russell M.: discussion of extracorporeal circulation, 972; discussion of Williams and Schenk on cardiac output measurements, 1332

Nemir, Paul, Jr.: coauthor of Hawthorne, 1052; discussion of Szilagyi on vein grafts, 1374; The Ritual of Congratulations, (1435;) discussion of Stone, Harlan, on prophylactic antibiotics, 1453; discussion of Connolly on carotid endarterectomy, 1470

Nesiloff: *See* Nassiloff, I.

Neuber, Gustav A.: decalcified bone for drains, cited by Weeks, 102

Neuhof, Harold: assistant to Lilienthal, 575; pulmonary embolism, 874; lamb kidney heterograft, cited by Reemtsma, 1186

Neutze, J. M.: tetralogy of Fallot, 1386–87

Neville, Williams E.: discussion of Maloney on coronary revascularization, 1426

Newburger, B.: early ambulation, cited by Burch, 888

Newlin: spinal cord, severance, cited by Harte, 266

Newman, David: nephrectomy, cited by Keen, 42

Newmark, S.: coauthor of Rowe, 1422

Newton, F. C.: adoption of Miller-Abbott tube, cited by Ranklin, 900

Newton, William A., Jr.: rhabdomyosarcoma, 1380

Newton, William T.: thoracic duct fistula for immunosuppression, cited by Starzl, 1526

Niazi, Suad: coauthor of Lewis and Varco, 1020

Nichols, Ronald L.: antibiotic colon preparation, 1388–90

Nichols, W. Kirt: coauthor of DeWeese, 1374; discussion of Starzl on glycogen storage disease, 1391

Nickel, William F., Jr: coauthor of Cave, 823; ileostomy mortality, cited by Crile, 1015; one-stage proctocolectomy, cited by Ravitch, 1056

Nicoladoni, Carl: gastroenterostomy devised by, 275

Nicolaysen, Johan: Gluzinski's gastric acidity test for differentiation cancer and ulcer, 484

Nicoll, James H.: pyloroplasty for congenital pyloric stenosis, 359

Nietert: attempted cardiorrhaphy in United States, cited by Peck, 407

Nimberg, Richard: circulating immunosuppressive factor, 1513

Nissen, Rudolph: first successful pneumonectomy, cited by Archibald, 745

Nitze, Max: cystoscope (1898), 211

Noer, Rudolph J.: discussion of Butcher on breast cancer, 1135; Breast Adjuvant Chemotherapy, 1141; Adjuvant Chemotherapy Breast Cancer Report, 1260; Surgical Adjuvant Chemotherapy Breast Group, 1260

Nora, James J.: coauthor of Hallman and Cooley, 1301

Norman, John C.: nuclear-fueled artificial heart, 1364; discussion of Weldon on ventricular aortic shunt, 1443; ventricular aortic shunt, cited by Weldon, 1443; discussion of Kaiser and Willman on myocardial revascularization, 1497

Norris, Basil: astragalus dislocation, 36; tracheotomy, 57; gunshot wounds, 58

Northrup, William Perry: Fell-O'Dwyer positive pressure anesthesia, 260

Nothnagel: convulsive center, cited by Briggs, 48

Nugent, F. Warren: coauthor of Braasch, 1495

Nusbaum, Moreye: intestinal angiography in hemorrhage, 1298–99; visceral arteriography, cited by Brant, 1362; visceral angiography, vasoactive drip, cited by Brant, 1362; mesenteric artery vasopressin infusion, cited by Johnson, 1473

Nussbaum, Johann N.: nerve stretching, cited by Dandridge, 93

Nyhus, Lloyd M.: coauthor of Harkins, 1011; discussion of Meredith and Myers on gastric freezing, 1170; selective gastric vagotomy, 1171–72; discussion of Eiseman on heterologous liver perfusion, 1201; discussion of Mason on gastric bypass, 1285; discussion of Sawyers and Scott on selective vagotomy, 1337; antibiotic colon preparation, 1388; discussion of DeMeester on esophageal reflux, 1409; discussion of Judd on antibiotic colon preparation, 1410; discussion of Hallenbeck on parietal cell vagotomy, 1452; discussion of Sawyers on proximal gastric vagotomy, 1481; and Harkins, 1482; contributions of, (1483)

Nyström, Gunnar: pulmonary embolectomy, successes, 472; Trendelenburg operation for pulmonary embolism, 686–88; discussion of peptic ulcer symposium, 691

O

O'Bannon, William: coauthor of Pierce, 1397

Oberhelman, Harry A., Jr.: coauthor of Dragstedt, 953; hyperfunctioning antrum and ulcer, 965–67; Zollinger-Ellison tumors, cited by Dragstedt, 1158

O'Brien, Peter C.: coauthor of Buckingham, 1454

Ochsner, Albert J.: umbilical herniorrhaphy, 256; prostatectomy, perineal route, 268; medical school control of hospitals, 272; gastroenterostomy mishaps, 277; tuberculous peritonitis, 278; X-ray cures of cancer, 287; toilet of peritoneum in tuberculous peritonitis, 291; aseptic requirements in nonuniversity hospitals, 307–09; osteomyelitis, usable bone in sequestrum, 312; papillary ovarian tumors, 312; mechanical aids to anastomosis still superior, 314; thyroid storm, 320; plaster cast for fracture of spine, 333; benefit of iodoform pack in thyroidectomy

wounds, 335; operation for exophthalmic goitre, 335; anastomotic ulcer with anterior gastroenterostomy, 338; manipulation versus operation for congenital hip dislocation, 352; breast, cancer, systematic postoperative X-ray therapy, 371; Theodore Roosevelt-J. B. Murphy episode, 381; Mayo thyroidectomy technique for preserving parathyroids, 400; fistulae and abscesses after operations for empyema, 406; techniques of prostatectomy, 410; sarcoma, Coley's toxin, 476–77; stomach, cancer, diagnosis of, superiority of history and physical examination to X-ray and laboratory, 485; breast, cancer of, preliminary biopsy always fatal, 493; radium treatment of uterine cancer, 516; safe elimination of colon for relief of intestinal stasis, 521; discussion of Primrose on blood transfusion, 535; bismuth paste for chronic empyema, 549; discussion of Percy on transfusion in pernicious anemia, 566; discussion of Summers on intestinal obstruction, 566; bypass of colon and ileosigmoidostomy for Hirschsprung's disease, 568; observation of Sauerbruch's patients in Zurich (1912), 586; discussion of Jopson, 587; discussion of Cheever on gastric cancer, 596; President 1925, 617; proposal for sterilization of imbeciles, perverts and criminals, 617; contributions of, (619;) treatment of peritonitis of appendiceal origin, 636; treatment of appendicitis, cited by Ladd, 856; electrocoagulation of cancer, cited by Ochsner, Alton, 1236

Ochsner, Alton: discussion of Palmer on intestinal obstruction, 730; subphrenic abscess, 738–39; contributions of, (739;) antethoracic esophagoplasty, 747; introduction of staged thoracoplasty, cited by Alexander, 777; subphrenic abscess, extraserous aspiration, 790; subphrenic abscess mortality, cited by Lehman, 790; coauthor with Gage, 830; discussion of Rienhoff on bronchial closure, 850; discussion of Churchill and Sweet on transthoracic esophagogastrectomy, 851; wound and burn project, 858; discussion of Neuhof on pulmonary embolism, 874; discussion of Lindskog, bronchogenic carcinoma, 887; gastric lavage, in discussion of Fine on peritoneal dialysis, 889; sympathectomy with paradoxical contralateral effect, 910; discussion of Doubilet and Mulholland on pancreatitis, 915; Oddi sphincteroplasty, in discussion of Doubilet and Mulholland, 915; and DeBakey, 1037; discussion of Hawthorne on achalasia, 1052; discussion of McLachlin on venous stasis, 1128; discussion of Madden on electrocoagulation of rectal cancer, 1236; on reverse intestinal loops, cited by Schlicke, 1379

Ochsner, John L.: discussion of Spencer on coronary bypass, 1402

O'Connell, J. C.: case of traumatic diaphragmatic hernia, cited by Truesdale, 577

O'Connell, Ruary C.: coauthor of Moore, 1355

O'Dwyer, Joseph P.: intubation for croup, 92–93

Oerum, H. P. T.: intussusception, cited by Miller, 733

Ogilvie, Sir Heneage: antral exclusion, cited by Nyhus, 1285; ulcer operation questionnaire, cited by Hoerr, 1361

Ogston, Sir Alexander: hand disinfection, cited by Senn, 230

Olch, Peter D.: account of Evarts Graham, American College of Surgeons and American Board of Surgery, 759

Olinger, Gordon N.: coronary revascularization, 1425–27

Oliver, G.: vasopressor pituitary extracts, cited by Nabseth, 1473

Oliver, John Chadwick: breast, cancer, end results, 371; Murphy treatment for perforation of abdominal wounds, 383; pyloric stenosis, gastroenterostomy, 390

Ollier, Léopold L. X. E.: pericardium, incision for access to, cited by Roberts, J. B., 201; treatment of compound fractures, cited by Cheever, 834

for thyroidectomy, 355; radical cure of hernia, 359; laryngectomy, first successful in United States, 403; etiology of cancer, 791; operation for epilepsy (1891), 990

Parker, Edward F.: discussion of Langston, pulmonary tuberculosis, 1227

Parker, Willard: appendicitis, abscess, extraperitoneal drainage, 91

Parker, William H.: coauthor of Lehman, 808

Parkes, Charles T.: air embolism, 47; artificial respiration, 47; cholecystotomy for stone, 65; intestinal obstruction, and operation, 70; gunshot wounds of abdomen, 103; talipes, manipulation, 111; herniorrhaphy, sac excision, 113; nephrorrhaphy, doubt over, 117–18; nephrolithiasis, 390; cited by Bevan, abdominal injuries, 732

Parkhill, Clayton: fractures, percutaneous skeletal fixation, 204–05, 354, 432, 434, 458

Parkin, A.: hydrocephalus, drainage of fourth ventricle, cited by Andrews, 436

Parkman, Samuel: first operation under ether, 191, (194)

Parks, Leon C.: alpha fetoprotein, 1411

Parmenter, John: inflammation and infection, 170; brain surgery, technique, 203

Parsons, William Barclay: coauthor of Whipple, 768; discussion of Gibbon on colonic resection and anastomosis, 841

Passavant, P. G.: compression to correct pubic separation in exstrophy, cited by Trendelenburg, 345

Passet: bactericides, for staphylococci, cited by Ernst, 73

Pasteur, Louis: micorcoccus of pus, 72; pneumococcus, 169

Pasteur, William: christened acute massive collapse of lungs, 629

Pate, J. W.: caval filter, cited by DeWeese, 1374

Paterson, James R. S.: coauthor of Wangensteen, 1090; breast cancer, randomized trial, cited by Crile, G., 1260

Patman, R. Don: coauthor of Thompson, 1324; carotid bruit, 1494

Patterson, Howard, A.: discussion of peptic ulcer symposium, 957

Patterson, Russel H., Jr.: hypothermia for intracranial surgery, 1152

Patterson, W. B.: coauthor of Dunphy, 1096

Pauchet, Victor: megacolon, operation for, by intussusception, cited by Summers, 565

Paulson, Donald L.: bronchogenic carcinoma, 1444

Pavlov, Ivan P.: gastric secretion, cited by Dragstedt, 967

Pawlik, Karel J.: ureteral catheterization, 159

Paxton: and pancreatitis, cited by Dinsmore, 996

Payne, J. Howard: and pancreatitis, cited by Dinsmore, 996; discussion of Gaspar on operations for morbid obesity, 1456; jujunoileal shunt, cited by Ravitch, 1518; discussion of Ravitch on jejunoileal shunt, 1519

Payne, W. Spencer: coauthor of Kirklin, 1122; thymectomy for myasthenia gravis, 1454

Payr: *See* Frangenheim

Payr, Erwin: arthroplasty, preference for pedicled fascia and fat, cited by Jurasz, 488

Peacock, Erle E., Jr.: discussion of Humphrey on immunologic response in cancer patients, 1261

Péan, Jules E.: contributions, 222

Pearl, Felix L.: aortic commissurotomy, cited by Dye and Julian, 1079

Pearse, Herman E.: gradual occulsion of large arteries, 828; Vitallium tubes in biliary surgery, 852, 895; discussion of pancreaticoduodenectomy, 854; discussion of Burch on early ambulation, 889; discussion of Cole, common duct strictures, 915; discussion of Yeager on cellophane wrapping, 919; atomic bomb injuries, 1060

Pearson, F. Griffith: Collis-Belsey operation, cited by Ellis, 1498; discussion of Ellis on short esophagus with stricture, 1498

Pearson, Olof H.: coauthor of Ray, 1047

Pease, Herbert D.: coauthor with Jacobson, 357

Peck, Charles H.: facility in languages, 407; operative treatment of heart wounds, 407; observation of Elsberg's intratracheal anesthesia, 440; intratracheal insufflation (Meltzer-Auer), 455; discussion of Jackson, Jabez, on radical mastectomy, 564; late results in gastric and duodenal ulcer, 587, 591; discussion of Miller on colon carcinoma, 597; carcinoma of the colon, 607; support of gastroenterostomy for ulcer, 619

Peet, Max Minor: sympathectomy for hypertension, cited by Adson, A. D., 781; discussion of Smithwick on sympathectomy, 833; sympathectomy, cited by Ray, 941

Pemberton, John de J.: splenectomy, 707; reactions following operation for hyperthyroidism, 775; discussion of Ginzburg on regional ileitis, 816; discussion of Clute on thiouracil, 875; citation of Moersch's sclerotherapy of esophageal varices, 898

Penberthy, Grover C.: empyema in children, 779; appendicitis in infants and children, 855–56; discussion of Schullinger on appendicitis, 902

Pendergrass, E. P.: pulmonary hyperventilation (atelectasis), 688

Penfield, Wilder G.: discussion of Dandy on pseudotumor, 789; discussion of Siler and Reid on burns, 845; temporal lobectomy for seizures, 990

Penn, Israel: liver transplantation, 1262; coauthor of Starzl, 1412

Pennell, R.: coauthor of Willman, 1245

Pennington, M. E.: coauthor with Martin, E., 304

Pensky: experimental liver resection, cited by Freeman, 318–19

Percy, Nelson M.: end-to-side ileosigmoidostomy, 522; blood transfusion and other surgical procedures in the treatment of pernicious anemia, 566; pernicious anemia treated by splenectomy and removal of foci of infection, 569

Perloff, Dorothee L.: coauthor of Wylie, 1160, 1289

Perrett, T. S.: colleague of Murray, D. W. G., 804

Perrin, Edward .: portacaval shunt, 1348

Perry, E. C.: stress ulcers with sepsis, 388

Persijn, J. P.: estrogen receptors, cited by Benfield, 1430

Person, Cooper: pancreatic duct anastomosis in pancreaticoduodenectomy, cited by Dragstedt, 864

Perthes, Georg Clemens: surgeon's gloves, 229; valve-action obstruction in Hirschsprung's disease, cited by Finney, J. M. T., 394; transverse abdominal incisions, superiority of, 516; rectosigmoidoplasty for Hirschsprung's disease, cited by Wangensteen, 964

Peskin, Gerald W.: discussion of Zollinger on diarrheogenic islet cell tumors, 1273

Peter, E. T.: gastric freezing, 1158

Peterman, M. G.: coauthor with Graham, Evarts, 571

Peters, John P.: structure of blood in relation to surgical problems, 820

Peters, Richard M.: pulmonary measurements, cited by Maloney, 1274; discussion of Kirklin and Maloney on computers, 1275

Peters, V. M.: local excision of breast cancer, cited by Wise and Ackerman, 1334

Peterson: regression of cancer nodules due to giant cells, cited by Ransohoff, 372

Petersson, Reuben: nerve grafting, 317

Peyton, Marvin D.: coauthor of Greenfield, 1403

Pezzer: perineal prostatectomy, cited by Bevan, 409

Pfaff, Franz: amylase in pancreatic fistula, 218

88 Pfahler, G. E.: coauthor with Rodman, W. L., 300

Pfeiffer, Damon B.: coauthor with Deaver on pancreatitis, 571; coauthor with Jopson, 586; praise of Whipple resection of ampullary carcinoma, 770; compound fractures, cited by Smyth, 836

Pfiffner, Joseph J.: adrenal extract, provided to Heuer and Andrus, 751; adrenal extract, 756

Phelps, A. M.: "mattress of wire" in herniorrhaphy, 281

Phelps, Charles: patella, fracture, operation, 173

Phemister, Dallas B.: jejunal anastomotic ulcers, 573; calcium carbonate gallstones, 713; discussion of Ballin on hyperparathyroidism, 716; discussion of Mixter and Cutler on thyroidectomy for angina, 744; inability to demonstrate toxic substance in shock, cited by Cannon, W. B., 750; primary shock, 750–52; discussion of Churchill on hyperparathyroidism, 753; discussion of Heuer on sympathectomy for hypertension, 782; total and partial paravertebral sympathectomy for hypertension, 798; President 1939, 811; contributions of, (812;) discussion of Churchill and Sweet on transthoracic esophagogastrectomy, 851; clinic of, and Huggins, 852; nervous system in shock, 861; esophagogastrectomy and total gastrectomy for bleeding varices, 897; first transthoracic esophagogastrectomy, 897; and Dragstedt, 954; and Dragstedt, cited by Wangensteen, 1338; esophagectomy for cancer, cited by Lischer, 1518

Phillagrius: excision for aneurysm, cited by Matas, 282

Phillips, G. W.: fracture femoral neck, priority in traction method, 460

Phillips, J. Roberts: coauthor of Judd, E. Starr, 737

Phillips, Winfred M.: coauthor of Pierce, 1397

Physick, Philip Syng: enterotome for division of enterostomy spur, 105

Piccoli, E.: umbilical herniorrhaphy, 256

Pickering, Sir George W.: carotid resection for arteriosclerosis, 1064–65, 1468; carotid arterosclerosis, 1491

Pierce, James: colleague of Varco, 1151

Pierce, William S.: paracorporeal pump for left ventricular bypass, 1397–99

Pierie, William R.: coauthor of Hodam and Starr, 1294

Pilch, Yosef H.: RNA transfer, cited by Mannick, 1152; colleague of Ramming, cited by Mannick, 1475

Pilcher, Cobb: discussion of Horrax and Poppen on acoustic nerve tumors, 941

Pilcher, Lewis S.: nephrorrhaphy, pride in, 117; breast, cancer, 127; castration for benign prostatic hypertrophy, 166; fractures of leg, walking casts, 173; castration for prostatic hypertrophy, 183; fractures, lower extremities, ambulant treatment of, 183–85; hemorrhoidectomy, 350; breast, cancer, neck operation justified, 370; war not thought of at April 1914 meeting, 481; influence of the war on civil practice, 547

Pincoffs, Maurice: first in vivo diagnosis of pheochromocytoma, 676

Pinto, Douglas: coauthor of Richards, 1166

Pirogoff, Nikolai I.: innominate artery ligation, 170; osteoplastic ankle amputation, 534

Playfair, William S.: drainage of empyema, 359

Ploman, John: distal splenorenal shunt, cited by Warren, 1489

Plummer, Henry S.: dilatation for cardiospasm, 595; coauthor of Mayo, C. H., 615; odor of gas gangrene, 672; iodine for hyperthyroidism, 677; tuberculosis of the thyroid, 714; effect of thyroxin on hyperthyroid patients, 776

Po, Jonathan: coronary revascularization, 1425–27

Poirier, P.: breast, cancer, early supraclavicular metastasis, cited by Rodman, 374

Polk, Hiram C., Jr.: discussion of Wanebo on melanoma, 1428; discussion of Child on pancreatectomy for pancreatitis, 1450; prophylactic antibiotics, cited by Stone, 1453; discussion of MacLean on acquired failure of host defenses, 1461; discussion of Dale on antibiotic prophylaxis, 1491; discussion of Wanebo on CEA, 1508

Polk, President James K.: lithotomy on by McDowell, Ephraim, 108

Polk, W. M.: visceral ptoses, end results of operation, 427

Pollack, Marilyn: alpha fetoprotein, 1411

Polley, Theodore Z., Jr.: coauthor of Block and Jensen, 1430

Pollock, Lee W.: coauthor with Judd, E. Starr, 607

Ponfick, Emil: fatal outcome of temporary occulsion of hepatic artery and portal vein, cited by McDill, 448

Pool, Eugene H.: recent wounds of the knee-joint, 548; late results of gastroenterostomy for gastric and duodenal ulcer, 588, 590–91; gynecologic surgery, 622; pectoralis major flap for bronchial fistula closure, 650; discussion of peptic ulcer symposium, 691; discussion of Shipley on appendicitis, 712; discussionnof symposium on surgical education, 762; pedicled muscle flaps for closure of bronchial fistula, cited by Wangensteen, 779; cancer cells in bloodstream, cited by Lund, C., 1067

Poppen, James L.: acoustic tumors, complete versus incomplete removal, 940–41; sympathectomy, cited by Ray, 941; and acoustic neuromas, 1347

Porell, William J.: coauthor of Farmer, 964

Porritt, Sir Arthur: local excision of breast cancer, cited by Wise and Ackerman, 1334

Porta, Luigi: partial occlusion of an artery, first attempt, cited by Halsted, 471; post-stenotic dilatation of aorta, cited by Halsted, 545

Porter, Charles A.: tetanus, serum therapy, 357; carcinomata from X-ray dermatitis, 378; acute hemorrhagic pancreatitis, 450; intratracheal insufflation anesthesia, 456; discussion of Greenough on septic gunshot fractures, 512; tetanus, advantage of intrathecal administration of antitoxin, 514; end results in thyroid surgery, 591–92; axillary aneurysm, 615; discussion of Kerr, sympathectomy for angina pectoris, 626; discussion of Brewer, Meleney's ulcer, 641; discussion of Bevan on cryptorchidism, 681; radiation injury, 1286

Porter, Charles B.: appendicitis, recurrent, 115; fractures, passive motion, 133; Surgical Constellation at Massachusetts General Hospital, (193;) pericardiotomy for purulent pericarditis, 201; chest wall resection for sarcoma, 261

Porter, Ken A.: liver transplantation, 1262; coauthor of Starzl, 1412

Porter, Miles F.: injection of boiling water into thryoid for hyperthyroidism, 478; no tetanus in railroad injuries, 513; wound treatment in Civil Practice (railroad injuries), 513; cholecystotomy preferred to cholecystectomy, 524; fascia lata in ventral herniorrhaphy, 563; discussion of Jackson, Jabez, on radical mastectomy, 564; technique of common duct drainage, 636; discussion of Moschocowitz on carcinoma of the breast, 638

Portmann, B.: coauthor of Calne, 1462

Post, Alfred: Listerism, 31

Potain: siphon and irrigation for empyema, cited by Bryant, 359

Poth, Edgar J.: sulfanilylguanidine intestinal antisepsis, 842; discussion of Blakemore on arterial prostheses, 1010; discussion of Harkins on Billroth I, 1012; plastic cloth arterial prostheses, 1037; biliary division for pancreatitis, cited by Bowers, 1039; discussion of Bowers on choledocojejunostomy for pancreatitis, 1039; discussion of Zollinger and Ellison on ulcerogenic pancreatic tumors,

102 Wangensteen, Owen H. (*continued*)
fistula, 779; discussion of Lehman on appendiceal abscess, 808; intestinal obstruction, discussion of Peters and of Maddock and Coller, 822; intravenous amino acid administration, 822; discussion of Key and Frankel on local sulfonamide therapy, 831; citation of Ravdin, Whipple and Elman in discussion of Brunschwig and Clark, 855; acid peptic factor in variceal bleeding, 898; discussion of Gilchrist and David, 899; discussion of symposium on vagotomy, 908; discussion of Colp on subtotal gastrectomy and vagotomy, 919; cervical dissection for breast cancer, 931; the second look operation for cancer, 953; discussion of Doubilet and Mulholland on chronic pancreatitis, 959; achalasia of esophagus, 963–64; histamine in beeswax ulcer production, 965–66; physiology of intestinal obstruction, cited by Dinsmore, 996; discussion of Sweet, transthoracic gastrectomy, 998; discussion of Harkins on Billroth I, 1012; discussion of Allen, protein from intravenous plasma, 1046; discussion of Hawthorne on achalasia, 1052; gastric cooling for peptic ulcer, 1090; discussion of Lillehei on transplantation of intestine, 1099; experimental work on peptic ulcer, cited by Coller, 1117; super-radical mastectomy, 1136; gastric freezing, 1158–59, 1169; discussion of Meredith and Myers on gastric freezing, 1170; discussion of Dennis and of Thal on gastroduodenal hemorrhage, 1209; President 1969, 1282; contributions of, (1283;) Medallion for Distinguished Service to Surgery, (1308;) discussion of Dragstedt on bile reflux and gastric ulcer, 1338; second look for colon cancer, cited by Wanebo, 1507; near total colectomy for colorectal cancer, 1516

Wagensteen, Stephen: and gastric freezing, cited by Barker, 1171

Warbasse, James P.: fractures, lower extremities, ambulatory treatment, 183

Ward, John T.: operations for duodenal ulcer, 1360

Warden, Herbert E.: tetralogy of Fallot, open correction, 1022–24

Wareham, Joan: coauthor of McDermott, 1044

Warren, J. Collins (1842–1927): arteries, healing after ligature, 58, 62; air embolism, 63; pyogenic bacteria, 63; bacteria in surgical disease, 72; suprapubic cystotomy, 79; intestine, healing, 80; cancer, early diagnosis, 98; cancer, frozen section diagnosis, 98; cancer, needle aspiration biopsy, 98; local anesthesia, 98; asepsis and antisepsis, 124; asepsis, skin preparation, 129; lingual thyroid, 135; fracture, non-union, thyroid extract, 141; omphalocele, 148; teaching of surgery, 156; Coley's toxin, 160; inguinal hernia, operation, postoperative care, 172; anesthesia, 191-96; contributions, (192;) Surgical Constellation at Massachusetts General Hospital, (193;) Committee on Nomenclature and Study of Tumors, 217; typhoid perforation, 245; inguinal herniorrhaphy, 258; trephining for osteomyelitis, 312; spinal cord tumors, 333; spina bifida closure followed by hydrocephalus, 334; request to Greenough for paper on breast cancer, 368; tetanus, a tropical disease, 400; breast, subcutaneous mastectomy for cystic disease, 492; cystic disease of breast, conservative operation for, 492

Warren J. Mason: perineal lithotomy, 79; first operation under ether, 191–92, (194;) operations, increasing infection rate, 196

Warren, James V.: physiological basis of cardiac surgery, cited by Dinsmore, 996

Warren, John (1753–1815): and Harvard Medical School, 192; Surgery in 1776, 1464

Warren, John C. (1778-1856): first operation under ether, 191,

(194;) permission to Wells to anesthetize, 195; ether anesthesia, 316

Warren, Joseph (erroneously in text as John C.): fell at Bunker Hill, 192

Warren, Joseph H.: hernia, inguinal, injection treatment, 100

Warren, Kenneth W.: colleague of Cattell, 1053; discussion of Howard on pancreaticoduodenectomy, 1277; pancreaticoduodenectomy, cited by Welch, 1324; discussion of Stinchfield on him replacement, 1347; discussion of Child on pancreatectomy for pancreatitis, 1450

Warren, Richard: Vice-President 1975, 192, 194; collaborator of Abbott, W. O., 823; discussion of Crile and Turnbull on ileostomy, 1015; ileostomy dysfunction, cited by Crile, 1015; discussion of Linton on femoral artery replacement, 1033; discussion of Szilagyi on graft failures, 1051; discussion of DeBakey, arteriosclerotic vascular occlusive disease, 1074

Warren, Stafford L.: mammography, cited by Barker, 1288

Warren, W. Dean: hemodynamics in cirrhosis, 1094; barb at Linton, 1095; coauthor of Muller, 1126; hemodynamics of portal hypertension, 1168–69; distal splenorenal shunt, 1239–44, 1486–90; contributions, (1242;) discussion of Jackson on portacaval shunt, 1350; discussion of Drapanas on mesocaval shunt, 1363; central splenorenal shunt, cited by Malt, 1439; discussion of Malt on portasystemic shunts, 1440

Warthin, A. S.: collaborator of Cabot, Hugh, 623

Washington, John A., II: antibiotic colon preparation, 1409

Wassink, W. F.: electrocoagulation of rectal cancer, cited by Madden, 1236

Watkins, David: discussion of Merendino on jejunal interposition, 1031

Watkins, Elton, Jr.: discussion of Parks on alpha fetoprotein, 1412

Watne, Alvin C.: cancer cells in bloodstream, cited by Cole, 1133

Watson, Beriah A.: contributions, (29;) supports Lister, 29, 31; anesthetics, 46; blood vessel ligation and antisepsis, 55; hermorrhage, secondary, 55; cardiac resuscitation by ventricular puncture, 84–85; chloroform death, cardiac arrest in, 84–85; appendicitis, 91; typhoid, intestinal perforation, 92

Watson, Francis S.: hourglass stomach, 242; prostatectomy, perineal route, 268; permanent ureterostomy, 479; simultaneous bilateral operations for renal stone, 598

Watson, Frank R.: coauthor of Turnbill, 1236

Watson, James W.: prefrontal lobotomy, 1153; discussion of White on frontal lobotomy, 1154

Watts, Stephen H.: as house officer, demonstrating to Mikulicz, 296; drainage in pancreatitis, 449; discussion of Moschcowitz on costochondral infections, 541; discussion of Archibald on pancreatitis, 542; achalasia, cardioplasty by Finney technique, 595

Waugh, John M.: rectal cancer survival, cited by Best, 940; discussion of Longmire on pancreatitis, 1053; regional enteritis, 1154–55

Way, Lawrence W.: choledocholithiasis, 1359; Zollinger-Ellison syndrome, 1502

Wayne, Eli: superior mesenteric artery syndrome, 1329–30

Webb, Charles W.: experimental surgery of lungs, with Halsted, 404

Webb, Watts R.: discussion of Wylie on fibromuscular hyperplasia, 1163; coauthor of Hardy, 1189; and cardiac transplantation, 1300; discussion of Maloney on coronary revascularization, 1426; discussion of Warren on distal splenorenal shunt, 1488

rectum through gluteus maximus for a continent sacral anus, cited by Armstrong, 347; intravenous ether anesthesia, introduced by, 491

Wolf, J.: uranoplasty in infancy, cited by Brophy, 314

Wolff, William A.: coauthor of Rhoads, 837

Wolff, William I.: colonoscopy for polyps, 1383–84

Wölfler, Anton: rectum, operation for cancer, cited by Gerster, 165; arterial ligation for hyperthyroidism, 279; Y gastrojejunostomy, 281

Wolfson, Sidney K., Jr.: hypothermia and cardiac arrest, cited by Rhoads, 1212

Wollner, L. B.: medullary carcinoma of thyroid, 1234

Womack, Nathan A.: discussion of Gray on esophageal varices, 959; discussion of Wangensteen on achalasia, 964; discussion of Ray, hypophysectomy for cancer of breast, 1048; discussion of Crile on simple mastectomy for cancer of breast, 1259

Wood, Alfred C.: discussion of Lee, B. J., on carcinoma of breast, 613

Wood, David A.: coauthor of Galante, M., 1016

Wood, Francis C.: coauthor of Ravdin, I. S., 842

Wood, H. C.: epilepsy, clinical trial of mock operations, 122

Wood, James: coauthor of Starr, 1195

Wood, John: hernia, inguinal, operation for, 100

Woodhall, Barnes: nerve repair, cited by Elkin, 872; hypothermia by partial bypass, cited by Ray, 1152; discussion of Ray on hypothermia for intracranial surgery, 1153

Woodruff, James: coauthor of Wanebo, 1427

Woodruff, Michael F. A.: change in graft antigenicity, cited by Sturgis, 1152; thoracic duct diversion and immunosuppression, cited by Dumont, 1185; discussion of Reemtsma, renal heterografts, 1188; early renal transplantation, 1268; discussion of Najarian on antilymphocyte serum, 1302

Woodward, Edward R.: vagotomy for ulcer, 906; coauthor of Dragstedt, 953; and Dragstedt, 954; invitation to Dragstedt, 1284; vagotomy and drainage for duodenal ulcer, 1284–85; bile reflux and gastric ulcer, 1337–38; discussion of Scott on intestinal bypass, 1340; reflux after hiatus hernia repair, cited by Hill, 1378; discussion of Sawyers and Herrington on dumping, 1379; stasis in jejunal pouches, cited by Sawyers, 1379; discussion of DeMeester on esophageal reflux, 1409; parietal cell vagotomy, cited by Herrington, 1452; discussion of Gaspar on operations for morbid obesity, 1456; morbid obesity, cited by Gasper, 1456; contributions of, (1483)

Wookey, Harold W.: discussion of Sweet on carcinoma of esophagus, 886; discussion of symposium on vagotomy, 908; reconstruction of cervical esophagus, 1202

Woolley, Morton M.: coauthor of Holder, 1202

Woolsey, George: surgery of cerebral tumors, 304; pancreatitis, importance of drainage, 450; choice of operation for gastric ulcer, 589, 591

Woolsey, John H.: discussion of Mayo and Truesdale on diaphragmatic hernia, 656

Woolston, W. H.: associate of Kanavel, 602

Wormsley, K. G.: secretin and diarrhea, cited by Zollinger, 1272

Wright, A. E.: formed elements of the blood, 346

Wright, Sir Almroth: opposition to use of antiseptics in war wounds, 509; saline solution for wounds, 527

Wright, Hastings K.: discussion of Ravitch on jejunoileal shunt, 1520

Wright, R.: intraluminal vena cava partitioning prosthesis, cited by DeWeese, 1374

Wu, Andrew V.: circulating immunosuppressive factor, 1513

Wu, Ying-k'ai: carcinoma of esophagus, Chinese experience, 1517

Wylie, Edwin J.: aortic endarterectomy, fascia lata support, cited by Julian, 982; aortic thromboendarterectomy, cited by Julian, 999; endarterectomy for aortic occlusive disease, 1007; aortography in arteriosclerotic disease of lower extremities, 1072–73; contributions of, (1075;) discussion of Spencer on renal hypertension, 1143; fibromuscular hyperplasia of renal arteries, 1160; renal arterial surgery for renal hypertension, 1289–91; discussion of Connolly on carotid endarterectomy, 1470; visceral revascularization, 1475

Wylie, Robert H.: duodenal ulcer mortality, cited by MacGuire, 957

Wyman: gallstone, ileus, cited by Richardson, 142

Y

Yamagiwa, Katsuaburo: experimental tar cancer, cited by Morton, 791

Yandell, David W.: Listerism, 26–27; Western Journal of Medicine and Surgery, 45; cystotomy, 79; hernia, inguinal, radical cure for, 101; hernia, operations and antisepsis, 101; gunshot wounds of abdomen, 103; fracture, shaft of femur, 110

Yankauer, Sidney: esophagoscopy of Lilienthal's esophagectomy patient, 576

Yates, A. J.: lung transplantation, cited by Hardy, 1191

Yates, John L.: nitrous oxide oxygen experience, 440; discussion of Moschcowitz, carcinoma of the breast, 637; untoward effects of narcotics and anesthetics, 644; pressure inhalation anesthesia, 647; factors in the treatment of pulmonary tuberculosis, 653

Yeager, George H.: polythene as a fibrous tissue stimulant, 919

Yeoh, K. S.: teflon portacaval H-graft, cited by Drapanas, 1363

Yore, Richard W.: coauthor of Elman, 943

Young, Hugh Hampton: infections of urinary tract, 211; suprapubic aspiration of bladder, cited by Halsted, 211; ureteral catheterization of the male, 253; transurethral (Bottini) fulguration of prostate, 268; Harrington's solution for hands, 309; perineal prostatectomy, 375, 409; supply of mercurophen to Europe (World War I), 527; partial nephrectomy, 621; mercurochrome in the treatment of septicemia, 627–29; opposition to one-stage cystectomy, 681; transurethral bladder neck resection, cited by Beer, 783; castration for prostatic cancer, cited by Huggins, 852

Young, V. Leroy: coauthor of Griffen, 1479

Young, W. Glenn: coauthor of Sealy and Brown, 1103

Younger, Rachel K.: coauthor of Scott, 1339

Younis, M. T.: vasopressin control of variceal bleeding, cited by Nabseth, 1473

Z

Zaaijer, Johannes H.: resection of cardia for cancer, 507

Zarsky, Leona R. N.: coauthor of Zoll and Frank, 1131

Zech, Ralph K.: coauthor of Harkins, 1011

Zeldis, L. J.: coauthor of Barker, 1288

von Zenker, Friedrich A.: pharyngeal diverticulum, 231, 421, 884; accurate description of achalasia, 295

Zeppa, Robert: distal spenorenal shunt, 1239; contributions, (1242;) discussion of Warren on splenorenal shunt, 1488

von Ziemssen, Hugo W.: pharyngeal diverticulum, 231

Zimmerman, H. Bernard: discussion of Coller, 949; primary aldosteronism, 1103; discussion of Silen on aldosteronism, 1228

Zimmerman, K. A.: and saddle embolectomy on Lockwood, 842

INDEX OF ORGANIZATION MATTERS

SUBJECTS

Page numbers within circles indicate figures.

110

N

National Institutes of Health: diminished support from, 1437
National Research Council: Crile, G. W., representative from American Surgical Association, 553; Division of Medical Sciences, 642
New York: costs of meetings in, 1085
Nixon Administration: impact on medicine, 1394–95
Nomenclature: National Committee on, 741; of disease, standard, endorsed by American Surgical Association, 774
Nurse anesthetists: attack upon, 929
Nurses: shortage of, 667, 896, 1087, 1316; bedside, need for, 911
Nursing: Committee, to grade schools of, 667; deleterious effect of university emphasis, 896; Committee on, 911; trends, 911; problem of, 929; hospital schools of, 1087

O

Officers: Recorder, 8, 10, 19; Corresponding Secretary, 8, 19; flamboyant, controversial surgeons passed over, 227; overlapping terms, 1392, 1417
Operations: unnecessary, report of Committee on, 994, 1004, 1017, 1042, 1057, 1070, 1085, 1104
Osteopaths: in Michigan hospitals, 1085

P

Papers: read by title, 58, 343; discussion of, when not heard, Tiffany, L. McL., Weist, J. R., 64; time limit, 77, 87, 157, 161, 220; discussion, grouping for, 78, 345; bibliography in, 79; junior authors, 109; printed abstracts, 119; selection, 120, 130, 219; delivery of manuscripts, 174; publication in journals, 207; publication, in *Transactions*, 220; motion to dispense with reading, 263; length of, 264, 809, 811; not read, but published in *Transactions*, 343; cost of alterations to be borne by authors, 360; journal publication, 360; publication of, 630; publication, excessive cost of, charged to author, 642, 658; publication, recommendation for an official journal, 658; publication, all in *Annals of Surgery*, 666; publication, satisfaction with, in *Annals of Surgery*, 683; time limit, ten minutes, proposal for, 789; manuscripts of, due date, 843; time limit, ten minutes, 895, 929; from departments of Program Committee members, 1057; instructions concerning invited abstracts, 1057; recommendation to cease printing titles and abstracts not accepted for program, 1057; submission to two programs, 1069; multiple, or in successive years, from same author or department, 1070; cancelled (on two programs), 1517
Pathology: poor performance in on Boards, 817
Pediatric Surgery: Board of, 1256; Certificate of Special Competency, 1256, 1369
Peer review: 1459–60
Philadelphia: as home of American Surgical Association, 1087
Physicians: supply of in wartime, 843; shortage, 1316; and society, 1328; distribution, 1329
Physicians assistants: need for, 1327
Placement: surgical, national service for, 1354, 1369
President: failure to vote on, 1458
President of the United States: appeal to on training of surgeons, 878; appeal to on medical student numbers, 879
Presidential Address: nature, 69; not at annual dinner, 809
President's Dinner, 809
President-Elect: motion to create, 1180
Press: admission to meetings, 231, 233; Secretary to censor all communications to, 567
Program: selection, 10; publication, 13; abstracts, 13, 124; demonstrations in, 14; number of papers, 14–15; papers,

time limit, 15, 38; 1882, ㉑ two papers per day, 59; method of arranging, 150; Business Committee, 208; volunteer papers, 219; printed, format of, 288; basis of selection, 1069; night sessions, 1135; session, last afternoon, 1135; divided sessions to accommodate specialties, 1282–84; multiple sessions opposed, 1325
PSRO: economic base for, 1395
Public issues: Surgeon General's Library, 13; support of cancer laboratory in Buffalo, 220; support of yellow fever quarantine regulations, 220; Society for Advancement of Research, 221; *Transactions* to San Francisco after earthquake, 360; resolution, patients with breast lumps to see surgeons, 374; resolution supporting "National Council of Public Health", 379; condemnation of fee splitting, 480; move to preserve separateness of Surgeon General's Library, 500; resolution to abrogate German patents on salvarsan (1917), 530; history of the war, petition to Surgeon General to make records available for, 554
Publications: of candidates, 1280
Publicity: at meetings, undesirability of, 567; Secretary empowered to censor all communications to the lay press, 567; of Fellows, criticized, 896
Purpose, 5–6

R

Race prejudice, 1316
Recertification, 1459
Recorder: overlapping term of office, 1392
Register: separate for members and guests, 1311
Relicensing, 1459–60
Research: progress under H.E.W., 1393
Research support: federal, decreased, 1315; lobbying effort, 1327; and federal control, 1353
Residency positions: proposed legislation, 1418
Residency training: danger of federal control, 1435
Residency Training Program, 1438
Resident surgeon: status of, 1070
Residents: deferments for during Korean War, 977; matching plan for selection of, 1326; distribution of, 1369
Resolution: to President of United States, protesting bill limiting research, 207

S

Scholarship: recognition of, 1372
Seal, 8– ⑨ vignette of Gross, S. D., 67
Secretary: overlapping term of office, 1392; expenses of, 1434
Selective Service: deferment of medical students, 843
Sex prejudice, 1316
Smithsonian Institution: role in distributing *Transactions*, 630
Society, International of Surgery: American Surgical Association to be host for, 480; joint meeting (1914), 500
Society for Promotion and Protection of Research Work, 246
SOSSUS, 1329, 1350–52, 1436, Appendix D; similarity of problems to those of Nursing Committee in 1928, 667; surgical manpower calculations, 1316; purposes of, 1353–54; on production of surgeons, 1371; interim report at breakfast meeting, 1392; importance of, 1396; completed, 1434; interpreted to legislative committees, 1435; surgical manpower predictions, 1437
Specialists: role of in American Surgical Association, 787; proposal to select as Fellows, 809; as President of American Surgical Association, 884; recommendation to increase number, in American Surgical Association, 895; production of, 1354
Specialization: negative aspects, 960
Specialties: representation in program, 1325
Sputnik: effect on American education, 1215

NAMES

See *also INDEX OF SCIENTIFIC MATTERS—NAMES*

Page numbers within circles indicate figures.

114

221; Society for Advancement of Research, 221; reelected
Secretary 1899 and 1900, 233, 246; composition of
Nominating Committee, 262
Butcher, Harvey R., Jr.: Fellow 1961, 1148
Byrnes, James F.: Economic Stabilization Board, 880

C

Cabell, James L., 7
Cabot, Arthur T.: Fellow 1889, 105; M.D. *sine* "Harvard", 172;
death, 481
Cabot, Hugh: Fellow 1924, 616
Calne, Roy Y.: Corresponding Fellow 1972, 1370
Campbell, Gilbert S.: Fellow 1960, 1128
Campbell, Henry F., 5, 7, 19
Cannon, Walter Bradford: experimental surgery, A.E.F., 546
Carmalt, William H.: proposed 1884, 58; elected Vice-
President, 174; membership increase, proposed 343;
elected President 1907, 378; President 1908, 380, 396;
motion to raise membership limit, 480; on Surgeon-
General's Library, 500; complaint of inaccuracies in
Souchon's historical article, 554
Carrel, Alexis: proposed 1907, 379; Fellow 1909, 412; elected
Vice-President 1919, 553; death, 884
Carson, Norman B.: advertisements of abortionists, 288; elected
Vice-President 1902, 288
Carter, B. Noland: Fellow 1935, 774; on active duty 1943, 866;
elected second Vice-President 1949, 944
Case, James Thomas, Chief X-ray, A.E.F., 546
Cattell, Richard B.: Fellow 1940, 833
Chaffin, Lawrence G.: elected second Vice-President 1953,
1005; elected first Vice-President 1965, 1215
Chartikavanij, Kasarn: Corresponding Fellow 1972, 1370
Chase, Robert A.: SOSSUS, financing and delivery of surgical
services, 1351
Cheever, David: Fellow 1922, 593; reinstatement of German
and Austrian Honorary Fellows, 658; elected first Vice-
President 1934, 757; elected President 1940, 833; President
1941, 843
Cheever, David W., 21; President 1889, 97; M.D. *sine*
"Harvard", 172; death, 508
Chiene, John: Honorary Fellow 1891, 130
Child, Charles G., III: and American Medical Association
meeting, 1215; Michigan curriculum change, cited by
Cope, 1255
Churchill, Edward G.: Fellow 1932, 724; elected President
1946, 896; President 1947, 897; past President, presence
noted by Blalock, 1057; wives at dinner, 1105–06;
Committee to Consider *Transactions*, 1307; death, 1371
Churchill, Mary: cited by Wangensteen, 1105–06
Clark, Dwight E.: Committee on Arrangements 1957, 1070
Cleveland, Grover: reception for Fellows, 95
Clinton, Marshall: Governor of American College of Surgeons,
710
Clowes, George H. A., Jr.: Fellow 1963, 1180
Codman, Ernest A.: Registry of Bone Sarcomas, 579
Colcock, Bentley P.: elected second Vice-President 1968, 1281
Cole, Charles E.: Fellow 1896, 190
Cole, Charles K.: rejected 1894, 161
Cole, Jack W.: SOSSUS, professional interrelationship, 1351
Cole, R. Beverly, 7, 19; resignation, 88
Cole, Warren H.: Fellow 1937, 800; elected second Vice-
President 1947, 912; elected President 1959, 1106;
President 1960, 1128
Coley, Bradley L.: death, 1149
Coley, William B.: name withdrawn 1894, 161; Fellow 1898,
220; death, 775
Coller, Frederick A.: Fellow 1928, 666; elected President 1943,
867; missing at time of election, 867; Committee on
Postwar Surgical Training, 877; President 1944, 877;

examination in surgery for specialties, 878; on membership
limit, 879; report of Committee on Unnecessary
Operations, 994, 1004, 1017, 1042, 1057, 1070, 1085, 1104;
past-President, presence noted by Blalock, 1057; request to
discontinue Committee on Unnecessary Operations, 1058;
terminal illness, 1148; collaboration with Maddock,
Walter, 1165; cited by Dunphy, 1180; death, 1200;
Committee on Unnecessary Operations, 1327
Colp, Ralph: Fellow 1936, 784
Conner, Phineas S., 5, 7; surviving founder, 6; surviving founder
1908, 69; Fellows, election, age of, 105; President 1892,
131; move to suppress names of rejected candidates, 189;
defense of medical care in Cuba, 233; memorial by
Dandridge, N. P., 412
Connolly, John E.: Fellow 1964, 1199
Conway, Herbert: death, 1314
Cooley, Denton A.: Fellow 1955, 1042
Cope, Oliver: proposed 1942, 857; Fellow 1943, 867; Chairman,
Committee on Undergraduate Medical Education, 960,
1199, 1215, 1255; Committee on Graduate Surgical
Education, 1004; elected second Vice-President 1956, 1058;
elected President 1962, 1164; President 1963, 1179;
motion, Vice-Presidents to sit with Council, 1199
Cotton, Frederick J.: Fellow 1914, 500
Counsellor, Virgil S.: elected second Vice-President 1963, 1180
Crafoord, Clarence: Honorary Fellow, 977
Crawford, Ernest Stanley: Fellow 1962, 1164
Creech, Oscar, Jr.: Fellow 1957, 1070; elected President 1966,
1231; lymphoma at time of election as President, 1232;
President, 1232; President 1967, 1255; death, 1257
Crile, George W.: Fellow 1905, 343; elected Vice-President
1911, 447; Chief, Research, A.E.F., 546; elected Vice-
President 1918, 546; first representative of ASA to
National Research Council, 553; Committee on X-rays and
Radium Therapy of Neoplasms, 579; elected President
1923, 604; President 1924, 616; death, 866
Cullen, Thomas S.: proposed 1904 (never elected), 324
Cushing, Harvey W.: Fellow 1906, 361; Committee on Surgeon-
General's Library, 500; Chief, Neurological Surgery,
A.E.F., 546; sponsor of Reid, Mont R., 616; elected
President 1926, 643; President 1927, 658; death, 820;
neurosurgical specialist President of American Surgical
Association, 884
Cushing, Hayward W.: Fellow 1896, 190; operative clinic 1899,
231; Audit Committee, 262; death, 758
Cutler, Elliott C.: Fellow 1925, 630; proposal to limit papers to
ten minutes, 789; on active duty 1943, 866; elected
President 1947, 912; President 1948, death in office, 913,
929; carcinoma of prostate at time of election as President,
1232
Czerny, Vincenz: Honorary Fellow 1885, 67; death, 519

D

DaCosta, John Chalmers, Sr.: Philadelphia Pathological
Society, 1; Gross, Samuel D., Professor at Jefferson, 698;
death, 742
Dandridge, Nathaniel P.: appeal from the Chair on
nominations, 221; elected President 1903, 306; President
1904, 307; death, 432
Dandy, Walter E.: Fellow 1925, 630; death, 897
Darrach, William: Committee on Grading of Nursing Schools,
667; sponsor of Auchincloss 1928, 667; elected President
1944, 879; President 1945, request for meeting denied, 880;
orthopedic specialist President of American Surgical
Association, 884; President 1946, 884, 895
David, Vernon C.: Fellow 1923, 604; elected Secretary 1931,
710; reelected Secretary 1932 through 1935, 724, 741, 757,
774; elected second Vice-President 1937, 800; elected
President 1942, 857; President 1943, 866; proposal for

116 David, Vernon C. (*continued*)
basic surgical examination for all specialties, 877; past-President, absence noted by Blalock, 1057
Davis, John Staige, 21; death, 88
Davis, John Staige, Jr.: Fellow 1917, 530; 1926 discussion of elections, 642; elected first Vice-President 1939, 817; death, 897
Davis, Lincoln L.: elected Secretary 1927, 658; reelected Secretary 1928 through 1930, 666, 683, 698; elected Vice-President 1931, 710
Davis, Loyal: on Murphy's (J.B.) candidacy for American Surgical Association, 209; passed over 1931, 710; passed over 1932, 724; Fellow 1933, 741; elected first Vice-President 1941, 843; neurosurgical specialist President of American Surgical Association, 884; elected President 1956, 1058; President 1957, 1069; letter, wives at dinner, 1105; discussion of *Transactions,* 1307
Dawbarn, Robert H. M.: proposed 1898, never elected, 221
Dawson, William Wirt: founding of American Surgical Association, 3, ④, 5, 7, 22; elected Vice-President 1883, 19
Deaver, Harry Clay: death, 699
Deaver, John B.: Fellow 1892, 136; flamboyance, 227; elected Vice-President 1917, 530; death, 699; frank memorial by Ashhurst, 699; John Rhea Barton Professor, 1087
DeBakey, Michael E.: nominated 1943, 867; Undergraduate Education Committee, 960
Dennis, Clarence W.: elected first Vice-President 1971, 1352; Constitution Revision Committee, 1510
Dennis, Frederic S.: Fellow 1882, 21; Business Committee 1890, 119; President 1895, 162; death, 742
Dépage, Antoine: funds to, from International Society meeting, 507; Honorary Fellow 1916, 518
Dépage, Madame: death on Lusitania, 507
Dinsmore, Robert S.: Fellow 1935, 774; Coller Committee, 994; elected President 1952, 994; President 1953, 1004; Nominating Committee, 1057; death, 1071
Dixon, Claude F.: Fellow 1936, 784; death, 1282
Dornan, William J.: former printer of *Transactions,* 698; excess copies of *Transactions* to Lippincott, 710
Dowd, Charles N.: elected assistant Treasurer 1917, 530
Dragstedt, Lester R.: passed over 1932, 710; passed over 1933, 724; Fellow 1934, 757; Development Committee, 895; anti-research intent of federal laboratory regulations, 1148; Medallion for Distinguished Service to Surgery, 1307, ⑧, 1311, 1327; award of Association's Medallion, 1417; death, 1437
Drake, Daniel, 1, 44
Drapanas, Theodore: Fellow 1964, 1199; death, 1437
Drenen, Earle: sponsor of Auchincloss 1928, 667
Dripps, Robert D.: rejected 1954, 1018; anesthesiologist, 1130
Dubost, Charles: Honorary Fellow 1974, 1417
Dugas, Louis A.: founding of American Surgical Association, 3, ④, 5, 7, 22; elected Vice-President 1880 and 1881, 19; death, 88
Dunn, James H.: proposed for Fellowship 1898, 220; rejected 1898, 220; Fellow 1899, 233
Dunphy, J. Englebert: Recorder, cost of *Transactions,* 1085; wives after Presidential Dinner, cited by Davis and Welch, 1105; elected President 1961, 1148; President 1962, 1163; move to increase membership, 1179; comment against wives at dinner, 1180; host to Eisenhower, 1180; invention of Bill Wilson, 1180; motion to create President-Elect, 1180; increase in membership, 1199; Committee on Pending Legislation, 1369
Dunphy, Nancy: cited by Davis, Loyal, 1105
du Plessis, Daniel J.: Corresponding Fellow 1972, 1370
Durgin, S. H.: trip down the Boston Harbor 1892, 135
Durham, Arthur E.: Honorary Fellow 1891, 130

E

Eberts, Edmond M.: Fellow 1925, 630
Eckert, Charles: Fellow 1958, 1087
Edgerton, Milton Thomas, Jr.: Fellow 1962, 1164
Effler, Donald B.: Fellow 1959, 1106
Egdahl, Richard H.: Fellow 1963, 1180
Eggers, Carl: Fellow 1930, 698; Council on Medical Education, licensure and hospitals, 809; death, 1059
Ehrenhaft, Johann L.: Fellow 1964, 1199
von Eiselsberg, Anton F.: invited European guest, 430; proposed for Honorary Fellow, 430; Honorary Fellow 1911, 447; dropped from Honorary Fellowship, 553; reinstated as Honorary Fellow, 666
Eiseman, Ben: Fellow 1958, 1087
Eisenhower, Dwight D.: speaker at Dunphy Presidential Dinner, 1105; and wives at annual dinner, 1180
Eliason, Eldridge L.: Fellow 1926, 642; John Rhea Barton Professor, 1087
Eliot, Ellsworth, Jr.: Fellow 1901, 263; motion to withdraw nomination of Fellow after three years, permitting renomination, 507; elected Vice-President 1922, 593; 1926 discussion of elections, 642; elected President 1928, 666; President 1929, 683; death, 884
Elkin, Daniel C.: Fellow 1935, 774; elected second Vice-President 1941, 843; Committee on Postwar Surgical Training, 877; Undergraduate Education Committee, 960; elected President 1951, 977; President 1952, 978; Nominating Committee, 1057; death, 1088
Elliott, John Wheelock: "M.D. Harvard", 172; death, 631
Ellis, Franklin H., Jr.: Fellow 1965, 1215; Program Committee, 1351
Ellison, Edwin H.: Fellow 1957, 1070; death, 1328
Elman, Robert: Fellow 1938, 810; death, 1059
Eloesser, Leo: Fellow 1936, 784; with Chinese Communist Army, 895; on overspecialization, 960; publication of *Transactions,* as is, by subscription, 1306; contributions of, ⑦ escorts President-Elect Welch to Chair, ⑧ death, 1459
Elting, Arthur W.: proposed 1909, 412; Fellow 1911, 447; motion to withdraw Governors from American College of Surgeons, 757; elected first Vice-President 1935, 774; member, Graham Committee, 774–75; American Surgical Association representative to American Board of Surgery, 784; elected President 1937, 800; President 1938, 809; report, American Board of Surgery, 877; death, 913
Erdman, John F.: proposed 1903, 306; privilege of discussing, 430
Erdman, Seward: Fellow 1926, 642; elected second Vice-President 1938, 810
Erichsen, Sir John Eric: Honorary Fellow 1885, 67; death, 191
Ernst, Harold C.: invited guest 1885, 67
von Esmarch, J. Friedrich, 88; Honorary Fellow 1885, 67
Estes, William L.: rejected 1894, 161; Fellow 1896, 190; motion to petition Surgeon-General to make records available, 554
Estes, William L., Jr.: Fellow 1927, 658; reinstatement of German and Austrian Honorary Fellows, 658
Evans, Everett I.: death, 1006
Eve, Duncan: Fellow 1898, 220; death 799
Ewing, James: Registry of Bone Sarcoma, 579
Ewing, Maurice R.: Honorary Fellow 1972, 1370

F

Fenger, Christian, 14, 21; suspension for nonpayment of dues, 149; elected Vice-President, 174; operative clinic, 1899, 231; proposal of unlimited membership, 235; death, 264
Ferguson, Alexander H.: Fellow 1901, 263; death, 448
Ferguson, Colin C.: Fellow 1964, 1199
Fifield, William C. B., 6, 21

Fine, Jacob: Fellow 1941, 843

Finney, John M. T.: Fellow 1899, 235; first President of American College of Surgeons, 381; elected Vice-President 1909, 412; Committee on Surgeon-General's Library, 500; Chief, Surgical Consultant, A.E.F., 546; letter of, from France, 546; motion to have Secretary censor communications to the press, 567; Committee on X-ray and Radium Therapy of Neoplasms, 579; elected President 1921, 579; President 1922, 592; move to reinstate von Eiselsberg, 666; proposal to increase membership, 741; 1922 plea for certification, 774; and Surgeon General, 843; death, 866; and specialty certification, cited by Longmire, 1257

Finney, John M. T., Jr.: Fellow 1932, 724

Firor, Warfield M.: Fellow 1937, 800; elected Secretary 1942, 857; Secretary 1943, 866; reelected Secretary 1943 through 1948, 867, 879, 896, 912, 929; on membership limit, 879; on request for bibliography of candidates, 879; papers, all received by deadline to be accepted, 895; elected first Vice-President 1950, 960; unnecessary operations, 977; elected President 1963, 1180; President 1964, 1199; defense of decision on *Transactions*, 1307

Fisher, William A., Jr.: General Finney's "official family", 546; Fellow 1921, 579; sponsor of Reid, Mont R. and Follis, Richard, 616; 1926 discussion of elections, 642

Fite, Ila: Secretary to Shires, 1434

Fitz, Reginald H., 88; invited guest, 378

Flint, Austin, 1, 3

Flint, Joseph Marshall: dropped for nonattendance, 604

Folkman, Judah M.: Fellow 1969, 1311

Follis, Richard H.: proposed 1924, 616

Fontaine, René: Honorary Fellow 1961, 1148

Ford, President Gerald, 1418

Forrest, Andrew P.: Corresponding Fellow 1972, 1370

Foster, John M.: elected second Vice-President 1950, 960

Fowler, George Ryerson: hirsutes of surgeons, 69; Fellow 1891, 130; death, 362

Frazier, Charles H.: death 799

Freeman, Leonard: elected Vice-President 1908, 397; reinstatement of German and Austrian Honorary Fellows, 658; proposal to increase membership, 741; death, 775

Friedrich, Paul Leopold: guest from Europe, 412; proposed Honorary Fellow 1909, 412; Honorary Fellow 1910, 430; death, 508

G

Gage, Homer: elected Vice-President 1923; 604

Gage, Idys Mims: Fellow 1941, 843

Galen, Claudius: S. D. Gross' conference with, 789

Gallie, William E.: Fellow 1922, 593; elected second Vice-President 1935, 774; elected first Vice-President 1947, 912; President 1948, 929; Nominating Committee, 1057; death 1110

Gallinger, Jacob Harold: antivivisection bill 1899, 233

Gardner, Clarence E., Jr.: elected first Vice-President 1964, 1199

Garrison, H. Fielding: source for Souchon, 567

Gatch, Willis D.: Fellow 1934, 757; motion against too numerous boards, 960; death, 1149

Gatewood: no first name, 643; proposed 1926, 643; death, 820

Gay, George W., 19; M.D. *sine* "Harvard", 172

Gelin, Lars-Erik: Corresponding Fellow 1972, 1370; Honorary Fellow 1977, 1484

Gerbode, Frank L. A.: elected first Vice-President 1962, 1164; Trustee, American Surgical Association Foundation, 1457

Gerrish, Frederic H.: Fellow 1892, 136; motion to admit Canadians, 263; memorial of Lister, 463

Gerster, Arpad G.: Fellow 1890, 119; elected Vice-President

1908, 397; elected President 1911, 447; President 1912, 462; motion on attendance at meetings, 480

Gibbon, John H., Jr.: Fellow 1940, 833; on active duty 1943, 866; elected first Vice-President 1952; 994; elected President 1954, 1018; President 1955, 1042; Chairman, Nominating Committee 1956, 1057; past-President, presence noted by Blalock, 1057; death, 1371

Gibbon, John H., Sr.: proposed 1903, 306; Fellow 1906, 361; elected Secretary 1915; 507; reelected Secretary 1916 through 1920, 518, 530, 546, 553, 567; Secretary, in Armed Forces, 530; stock of old *Transactions* to be kept at College of Physicians, 530; Consultant in Surgery, A.E.F., 546; undesirability of newspaper publicity, 567; announcement of Helen LeMaistre's death, 579; elected President 1925, 630; President 1926, 642; motion to withdraw Governors from American College of Surgeons, 757; presence at election of President John H. Gibbon, Jr., 1018; memorial, 1043; past-President, presence at J. H. Gibbon, Jr.'s election cited by Blalock, 1057

Gibson, Charles L.: elected Vice-President 1915, 507

Gilchrist, R. Kennedy: on Gatewood, 643; elected second Vice-President 1952, 994; elected Secretary 1953, 1005; reelected Secretary 1954 through 1956, 1018, 1042, 1058; elected first Vice-President 1957, 1070; discussion on *Transactions*, 1310

Glenn, Frank: Fellow 1942, 857

Glover, Donald M.: elected second Vice-President 1954, 1018; resolution for American Surgical Association to study undergraduate surgical education, 1180

Goetsch, Emil: Fellow 1928, 666

Goldman, Leon: elected first Vice-President 1968, 1281

Goldthwait, Joel Ernest: Chief, Orthopedics, A.E.F., 546

Goldwin, Thomas H.: proposed as Honorary Fellow, 546

Goligher, John C.: Honorary Fellow, 1978, 1510

Goode, John V.: Coller Committee, 994

Goodwin, Thomas H.: proposed as Honorary Fellow, 546

Goodwin, Willard E.: Fellow 1961, 1148

Gordon-Taylor, Sir Gordon: Honorary Fellow 1956, 1058; death, 1129

Gorgas, William C.: Honorary Fellow 1916, 518; death, 568

Gouley, John W. S., 19

Graham, Evarts, A.: membership ages, 69; Fellow 1920, 567; representative to Division of Medical Sciences, National Research Council, 642; motion to study problems of postgraduate surgical education and qualifications, 774; proposal to discuss increase in membership following year, 774; Chairman, Committee on Postgraduate Education and Qualifications of Surgeons, 774–75; American Surgical Association representative on American Board of Surgery, 784; elected President 1936, 784; Samuel Gross looks in on the American Surgical Association, 785–89; President 1937, 799; reorganization of American Surgical Association, 809; report on American Board of Surgery, 817; discussion of Postwar Surgical Training, 878; on membership limit, 879; selection of candidates, 911; Membership Committee, 929; past-President, presence noted by Blalock, 1057; death, 1059; need for younger members, cited by Wangensteen, 1284; Committee to Consider *Transactions*, 1307

Graham, Roscoe R.: Fellow 1932, 724; elected second Vice-President 1940, 833; death, 913

Gray, Howard K.: proposed 1942, 857; Fellow 1943, 867

Gregory, Elisha H., 6

Greenough, Robert B.: Committee on X-ray and Radium Therapy of Neoplasms, 579; elected Secretary 1922, 593; reelected Secretary 1923 through 1926, 604, 616, 630, 643, 1926 discussion of elections, 642; elected Vice-President 1927, 658

Grey-Turner, George: death, 978

S

Sabiston, David C., Jr.: Fellow 1960, 1128; Advisory Membership Committee, 1325; need for increasing active membership, 1325; elected President 1977, 1485; President 1978, 1510

St. John, Fordyce B.: Fellow 1923, 604; unsuccessful sponsor of Auchincloss, 642; Treasurer, funds inadequate, 774

Sandblom, Philip: Honorary Fellow 1960, 1128

Sano, Keiji: Corresponding Fellow 1972, 1370

Sayre, Lewis A.: founding of American Surgical Association, 5, 7, 10, 22; death, 247

Schede, Max H. E. W.: Honorary Fellow 1894, 161; death, 306

Schilling, John A.: Program Committee, 1199; elected first Vice-President 1977, 1485

Schlicke, Carl P.: elected second Vice-President 1976, 1458

Schmieden, Victor: invited guest, 378

Schwartz, Harry: defense of American medicine, 1395

Schwartz, Henry G.: Fellow 1966, 1231; SOSSUS, legal and ethics, 1351; elected first Vice-President 1975, 1436

Schwartz, Seymour I.: Fellow 1965, 1215

Scott, H. William, Jr.: diploma, 8; Fellow 1953, 1005; Program Committee, 1069, 1085; cost of *Transactions*, 1128; Treasurer, cost of *Transactions*, 1215; elected President 1973, 1392; President 1974, 1417; Committee to Select Writer of History, 1435

Scott, W. J. Merle: Fellow 1933, 741

Scudder, Charles L.: proposed 1904, 324; proposed 1908, 397; Fellow 1909, 412

Senn, Emmanuel J.: proposed 1899, 235; rejected 1900, 246

Senn, Nicholas, 21 (138;) papers, time limit, 38; President 1893, 137; elections, negative votes defeating, 149; delegate to International Medical Congress, Moscow, 207; Chairman, Committee on Arrangements 1899, 231; operative clinic 1899, 231; dinner at 1899 meeting, 233; death, 380; length of papers, 666

Senning, Åke: Corresponding Fellow 1974, 1417; Honorary Fellow 1979, 1527

Shenstone, Norman S.: Fellow 1934, 757

Shipley, Arthur M.: Fellow 1923, 604; 1926 discussion of elections, 642; unreliability of catgut, 799; elected second Vice-president 1943, 867

Shires, G. Thomas: Fellow 1965, 1215; elected Secretary 1969, 1311; Secretary, report of Council 1970, 1326; reelected Secretary 1970 through 1973, 1327, 1352, 1370, 1392; completion of applications, 1351; and publication of Minutes, 1369; Secretary, report of Council 1975, 1434; elected President 1979, 1527; ascent to the rostrum, (1528)

Shumacker, Harris B., Jr.: nominated 1943, 867; elected first Vice-President 1960, 1128; Program Committee 1962, 1163; comment *for* wives at meetings, 1180; elected Secretary 1964, 1199; reelected Secretary 1965 through 1967, 1215, 1231, 1256

Shumway, Norman E.: Fellow 1967, 1256

Sideris, George: SOSSUS, statistics, 1351

Silen, William: Fellow 1966, 1231

Sims, J. Marion: Honorary Fellow 1882, 22; death, 44

Singleton, Albert O.: Fellow 1935, 774; elected first Vice-President 1944, 879

Sistrunk, Walter E.: Fellow 1920, 567

Smith, Alan P., 6

Smith, Rodney, Lord: Honorary Fellow 1978, 1510

Smith, Stephen: Honorary Fellow 1896, 190

Smithwick, Reginald H.: Fellow 1939, 817

Smyth, Calvin M., Jr.: Coller Committee, 994

Souchon, Edmond: elected Vice-President 1899, 233; correction of errors in his historical paper, 567

Sparkman, Robert S.: Fellow 1959, 1106; publication of past

minutes, 1326, 1351, 1369; elected second Vice-President 1977, 1485

Speed, Kellogg: Fellow 1919, 553; proposer of Gatewood, 643

Spencer, Frank C.: Fellow 1960, 1128; urgency for SOSSUS data, 1352

Starr, Albert: Fellow 1964, 1199

Starr, Clarence L.: elected Vice-President 1928, 666

Starr, Frederic N. G.: reinstatement of German and Austrian Honorary Fellows, 658; elected first Vice-President 1932, 724

Starzl, Thomas E.: Fellow 1966, 1231

Stephenson, George W.: on Gatewood, 643; on American Surgical Association-American College of Surgeons relations, 757; Constitution Revision Committee, 1510

Sternberg, George M.: Gross Statue, address of acceptance, 191; Honorary Fellowship tabled 1899, 233; privilege of discussing, 430

Stewart, Francis T.: Fellow 1911, 447; elected Assistant Secretary 1917, 530; Secretary 1918, 546; death, 558

Stewart, John D.: elected first Vice-President 1958, 1087; elected President 1960, 1128; President 1961, 1147

Stiles, Harold J.: invited European guest, 447

Stillman, Stanley: elected Vice-President 1924, 616

Stimson, Lewis A.: Fellow 1889, 105; resignation, 220

Stokes, Charles F.: Committee on Surgeon-General's Library, 500; resigned under pressure, 604

Stone, Frederick L.: Academic Surgery Training Program, 1230

Stone, Harvey B.: Fellow 1926, 642; Committee to Assist Surgeon-General in event of war, 833; elected President 1941, 843; President 1942, 857; past-President, absence noted by Blalock, 1057; Committee to Consider *Transactions*, 1307

Summers, John E.: elected Vice-President 1916, 518

Sweet, Richard H.: proposed 1942, 857; Fellow 1943, 867; Chairman of Program Committee 1957, 1069; elected first Vice-President 1959, 1106; death, 1149

Swenson, Orvar: Fellow 1953, 1005

Symington, Stuart: National Security Resources Board, 977

T

Taylor, Grantley W.: Fellow 1940, 833; death, 1232

Terrier, Louis Felix: Honorary Fellow 1896, 190; memorial by Richardson, M. H., 412

Thiersch, Karl: Honorary Fellow 1894, 161; death, 162

Thompson, James C.: no relation to Thompson, James E., both of Galveston, 579

Thompson, James E.: elected Vice-President 1921, 579

Thompson, Joseph Ford: proposed 1884, 58

Thompson, Joseph W.: papers read by title, 58

Tidrick, Robert T.: elected second Vice-President 1969, 1311

Tiffany, Louis McLane, 6, 21; elected President, 174; President 1896, 175; proposal to elect all Fellows nominated by Council, 208; death, 530; memorial 1918, 531

Tillmanns, Hermann: invited guest, 306

Toland, Clarence G.: Fellow 1932, 724

Torek, Franz: Fellow 1928, 666; death, 811

Trendelenburg, Friedrich: guest from abroad, 360; nominated Honorary Fellow 1906, 361; Honorary Fellow 1907, 378; dropped from Honorary Fellowship, 553

Trout, Hugh H.: Fellow 1925, 630; Catgut Committee, 809

Trudeau, E. L.: message of death of Ricketts, Howard T., 430

Truesdale, Philemon E.: Fellow 1918, 546

Tuffier, Theodore: death, 668

V

VanderVeer, Albert: elected Vice-president 1898, 221; motion to admit press 1899, 233; elected President 1905, 343, President 1906, 344, 360; death, 686